Children's Orthopaedics and Fractures

Michael Benson · John Fixsen ·
Malcolm Macnicol · Klaus Parsch
Editors

Children's Orthopaedics and Fractures

Third Edition

Foreword by Eugene E. Bleck

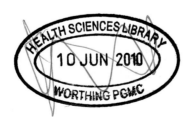

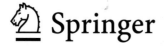

Editors
Michael Benson
University of Oxford
Nuffield Orthopaedic Centre
Windmill Road
Oxford
Headington
United Kingdom OX3 7LD
mbenson-stlukes@btconnect.com

Malcolm Macnicol MBChB BSc(hons) FRCS MCh FRCP
FRCSEd(Orth) Dip Sports Med.
University Orthopaedic Department
Royal Hospital for Sick Children
Sciences Road
Edinburgh
United Kingdom
mmacnicol@aol.com

John Fixsen
Great Ormond Street Hospital
for
Sick Children
Greater Ormond Street
London
United Kingdom WC1N 3JH
jafixsen@btinternet.com

Klaus Parsch
Olgahospital
Orthopädie
Bismarckstr. 8
70176 Stuttgart
Germany
KParsch@t-online.de

ISBN 978-1-84882-610-6   e-ISBN 978-1-84882-611-3
DOI 10.1007/978-1-84882-611-3
Springer London Dordrecht Heidelberg New York

British Library Cataloguing in Publication Data
A catalogue record for this book is available from the British Library

Library of Congress Control Number: 2009940002

Printed on acid-free paper

Springer is part of Springer Science+Business Media (www.springer.com)

Foreword

Confirming the British genetic trait for writing and publishing (as well as acting), two English (Oxford and London) and a Scottish orthopaedic surgeon (Edinburgh) have produced a third edition of their comprehensive text, joined, as in the second edition by an editor from Germany, recognizing its part in the European community. The 62 physician contributors are drawn from pink-colored countries in our childhood geography books—the old British Empire from Australia to Zambia and two from the former colony, the USA.

The original purpose of the book was to give residents or registrars an easily accessible and concise description of diseases and conditions encountered in the practice of paediatric orthopaedic surgery and to prepare for their examinations. But the practicing orthopaedic surgeon will find an update of current practice that can be read for clarity and constraint—enough but not too much. A foreword might be a preview of things to come, but a "back word" of what was thought to be the final say on the subject is needed for a perspective in progress.

A "back word" look reveals the tremendous progress in medical diagnosis and treatment of which paediatric orthopaedics and fracture care is a component. Clubfoot treatment based on the dictums of Hiram Kite has had a revolutionary change by Ponseti. The chapter by Eastwood has the details on cast application and orthotics follow-up to obtain the 95% correction without the extensive surgery many of us thought was needed.

Paediatric fracture care has also changed from traction for fractures of the femoral shaft in the ages of 5–15 years to intramedullary fixation with elastic stable nails originated in Nancy and Metz, France—"Nancy nails." Klaus Parsch's chapter tells us that it is their preferred method of treatment in Stuttgart, Germany.

Robert Dickson's lucid writing on idiopathic scoliosis as primarily a rotation of the lordotic thoracic spine again bears study to deepen the understanding that it is a three-dimensional deformity. As in the past editions, a coat hanger helps to appreciate the distortion of curvatures in a one-dimensional radiograph. Those orthopaedists who need courage to resist pressure to encase children in casts or braces or orthoses will be heartened to know that none of these conservative measures have shown any effect in prevention or curve progression. What to do instead of "treatment"? Read on.

This is not a book to learn the details of surgical technique–other texts and only experience can do that. Even though a seasoned orthopaedic surgeon does not need this knowledge to pass an examination, he or she is expected to know something about the subject. Once identified as an orthopaedic surgeon, your opinion is often sought at social events usually standing with a drink in hand. And commonly it is advice sought by your married children about a grandchild's musculoskeletal problem. Can you answer sensibly? If, "I'll get back to you later" is your response, a quick perusal of the contents of this volume should help maintain your professional standing and as is now the fashion of school teachers, your "self-esteem." And you won't have to log on to the Internet.

Eugene E Bleck

Preface

As in the two previous editions of this textbook, we record here the debt we owe to the children we treat. Ours is a privileged specialty: we watch our patients grow and mature, often developing a close bond with both child and family. When matters go well, there is a very personal sense of fulfillment; when matters go ill, we share a family's distress. We must learn how children develop physically and emotionally, striving to harness their growth potential and minimize progressive deformity.

It is a truism that children are not just small adults. Our approach must recognize this by understanding the natural history of childhood disease and how this may be modified by treatment. Outcome studies are even more important in children than they are in adults, so responsible audit and careful long-term assessment are critical.

This edition further strengthens the chapters dealing with trauma. However, no textbook can hope to be comprehensive and we have tried to be concise and relevant. This is not an operative text, although some procedures at the heart of children's surgery are described in more detail. The reader will recognize that children's orthopaedic practice needs daily experience, initially under careful supervision, coupled with frequent reference to atlases and other sources of information. We hope this book, although not pocket-sized, will prove a valuable companion in times of doubt.

All sections of the book have been rewritten. Recent references have been added but key older ones retained. New authors have joined us and, to both old and new contributors alike, the editors offer their gratitude. It is difficult in a busy life to make time to marshal ideas and present them with clarity and precision. Yet our authors have made the time willingly to share with us their commitment to improve the lot of the injured or disabled child.

As before, the early chapters describe normal child development and growth, offering insight into how the disabled child should resourcefully integrate into society. How to control pain, understand gait, and consider which images to take complete the introduction. Subsequent chapters deal with generalized skeletal problems including metabolic disease, infection, arthritis, and neoplasia. Later chapters cover neurological and regional disorders, while the concluding chapters cover the range of fractures and injuries to which the immature skeleton is prone.

It is a pleasure to record our indebtedness to our publishers; we could not have been better served than by Barbara Lopez-Lucio, who co-ordinated our efforts with wit, charm, and precision, and Grant Weston, who supervised the project with tact and encouragement.

We hope trainees and young surgeons will benefit from the contents of our book; we wish them well both in training and in the fruitful years that follow.

Michael KD Benson, Oxford, UK   John A Fixsen, London, UK
Malcolm F Macnicol, Edinburgh, UK   Klaus Parsch, Stuttgart, Germany

Contents

Part I   Overview **1**

1   **General Principles** **3**
Roderick D. Duncan

2   **Growth and Its Variants** **11**
Roderick D. Duncan

3   **Children and Young People with Disability: Management and Support** **23**
Zoë M. Dunhill

4   **Anesthesia and Analgesia in Children** **37**
Edward Doyle

5   **Paediatric Imaging** **49**
David J. Wilson and Gina M. Allen

Part II   Generalized Disorders **65**

6   **Gait Analysis** **67**
Tim N. Theologis

7   **Bone, Cartilage, and Fibrous Tissue Disorders** **75**
William G. Cole

8   **Metabolic and Endocrine Disorders of the Skeleton** **105**
Roger Smith

9   **Blood Disorders and AIDS** **123**
Christopher A. Ludlam and John E. Jellis

10   **Infections of Bones and Joints** **135**
Klaus Parsch and Sydney Nade

11   **Skeletal Tuberculosis** **161**
Kenneth C. Rankin and Surendar M. Tuli

12   **Children's Orthopaedics in the Tropics** **179**
Sharaf B. Ibrahim and Abdul-Hamid Abdul-Kadir

13   **Juvenile Idiopathic Arthritis** **195**
Günther E. Dannecker and Martin N. Arbogast

    Part 1: Classification, Symptoms, and Medical Treatment **195**
    Günther E. Dannecker

    Part 2: Surgery for Juvenile Idiopathic Arthritis **202**
    Martin N. Arbogast

14 Bone Tumors **213**
Gérard Bollini, Jean-Luc Jouve, Franck Launay, Elke Viehweger,
Yann Glard, and Michel Panuel

Part III   Neuromuscular Disorders **229**

15 Neuromotor Development and Examination **231**
Robert A. Minns

16 Hereditary and Developmental Neuromuscular Disorders **249**
Eugene E. Bleck and James E. Robb

17 Neural Tube Defects, Spina Bifida, and Spinal Dysraphism **265**
H. Kerr Graham and Klaus Parsch

18 Poliomyelitis **287**
Wang Chow, Yun Hoi Li, and Chi Yan John Leong

19 Orthopaedic Management of Cerebral Palsy **307**
James E. Robb and Reinald Brunner

20 Arthrogryposis multiplex congenita **327**
John A. Fixsen

Part IV   Regional Disorders **335**

Section 1 The Upper Limb **337**

21 Developmental Anomalies of the Hand **339**
Peter D. Burge

22 The Shoulder and Elbow **357**
John A. Fixsen

23 Brachial Plexus Injuries Peripheral Nerve Injuries **365**
Alain L. Gilbert and Rolfe Birch

   Part 1: Management of the Injury **365**
   Alain L. Gilbert

   Part 2: Birth lesions of the brachial plexus Peripheral nerve injuries **370**
   Rolfe Birch

Section 2 The Lower Limb **387**

24 Leg Deformity and Length Discrepancy **389**
John A. Fixsen, Robert A. Hill, and Franz Grill

   Part I: Classification and Management of Lower Limb Reduction Anomalies **389**
   John A. Fixsen and Robert A. Hill

   Part II: Leg Length Inequality **406**
   Franz Grill

25 The Limping Child **423**
F. Stig Jacobsen and Göran Hansson

26 Developmental Dysplasia of the Hip **435**
Michael K.D. Benson and Malcolm F. Macnicol

27 Legg–Calvé–Perthes Disease **465**
Andrew M. Wainwright and Anthony Catterall

28 **Slipped Capital Femoral Epiphysis** **481**
Malcolm F. Macnicol and Michael K. D. Benson

29 **The Knee** **495**
David M. Hunt and Malcolm F. Macnicol

Section 3 The Foot and Ankle **521**

30 **The Foot** **523**
John A. Fixsen

31 **The Clubfoot: Congenital Talipes Equinovarus** **541**
Deborah M. Eastwood

32 **Pes Cavus** **559**
John A. Fixsen

33 **Congenital Vertical Talus (Congenital Convex Pes Valgus)** **565**
John A. Fixsen

Section 4 The Spine **569**

34 **Congenital Disorders of the Cervical Spine** **571**
Robert N. Hensinger

35 **Back Pain in Children** **587**
Robert A. Dickson

36 **Spinal Deformities** **599**
Robert A. Dickson

37 **Spondylolisthesis** **639**
Robert A. Dickson

Part V Fractures **647**

Section 1 Overview **649**

38 **Principles of Fracture Care** **651**
Malcolm F. Macnicol and Alastair W. Murray

39 **Fracture Epidemiology** **665**
Lennart A. Landin

40 **Polytrauma in Children** **671**
Peter P. Schmittenbecher and Cathrin S. Parsch

41 **Management of Growth Plate Injuries** **687**
Franck Accadbled and Bruce K. Foster

42 **Birth and Non-accidental Injuries** **701**
Peter J. Witherow†, Michael K.D. Benson, and Jacqueline Y.Q. Mok

Part I: Birth Injuries **701**
Peter J. Witherow and Michael K.D. Benson

Part II: Non-Accidental Injuries **708**
Jacqueline Y.Q. Mok

Section 2 Fractures of the Shoulder, Upper Limb, and Hand **715**

43 **Fractures Around the Shoulder and the Humerus** **717**
J. B. Hunter

44 Fractures of the Elbow and Forearm **731**
James B. Hunter and Klaus Parsch

45 Wrist and Hand Fractures **743**
Malcolm F. Macnicol and Klaus Parsch

Section 3 Fractures of the Pelvis, Femoral Neck, Lower Limb, and Foot **751**

46 Fractures of the Pelvis **753**
Peter W. Engelhardt

47 Femoral Neck Fractures **759**
Peter W. Engelhardt

48 Femoral Shaft Fractures **765**
Klaus Parsch

49 Fractures of the Knee and Tibia **775**
Carol-C. Hasler

50 Ankle Fractures **793**
Klaus Parsch and Francisco Fernandez Fernandez

51 Fractures and Dislocations of the Foot **805**
Francisco Fernandez Fernandez

Section 4 Spinal Fractures **817**

52 Traumatic Disorders of the Cervical Spine **819**
Robert N. Hensinger

53 Fractures of the Thoracic and Lumbar Spine **835**
Robert N. Hensinger and Clifford L. Craig

Index **859**

Contributors

Abdul-Hamid Abdul-Kadir Assunta Hospital, Petaling Jaya, Malaysia

Franck Accadbled Hôpital des Enfants, Toulouse, France

Gina M. Allen University Hospitals Birmingham, Birmingham, UK

Martin N. Arbogast Klinik für Rheuma-Orthopädie, Rheuma-Zentrum Oberammergau, Oberammergau, Deutschland

Michael K. d'A. Benson Nuffield Orthopaedic Centre, Oxford, UK

Rolfe Birch Peripheral Nerve Injury Unit, Royal National Orthopaedic Hospital, Stanmore, UK

Eugene E. Bleck Department of Orthopaedic Surgery, Stanford University School of Medicine, Stanford, CA, USA

Gérard Bollini Department of Paediatric Orthopaedics, Timone Children's Hospital, Marseille, France

Reinald G. Brunner Department of Neuro-Orthopaedics, University Children's Hospital Basel, Basel, Switzerland

Peter D. Burge Hand Surgery Unit, Nuffield Orthopaedic Centre, Oxford, UK

Anthony Catterall Catterall Unit, Royal National Orthopaedic Hospital, Stanmore, UK

Wang Chow Department of Orthopaedics and Traumatology, Hong Kong, China

William G. Cole Stollery Children's Hospital, University of Alberta; Edmonton, Alberta, Canada; Division of Pediatric Surgery, Department of Surgery, University of Alberta; Edmonton, Alberta, Canada

Clifford L. Craig Department of Orthopaedic Surgery, University of Michigan, Ann Arbor, MI, USA

Günther E. Dannecker Department of Pediatrics, Olgahospital, Klinikum Stuttgart, Stuttgart, Germany

Robert A. Dickson Academic Unit of Orthopaedic Surgery, Leeds General Infirmary, Leeds, UK

Edward Doyle Royal Hospital for Sick Children, Edinburgh, UK

Roderick D. D. Duncan Royal Hospital for Sick Children, Glasgow, UK

Zoë M. Dunhill Royal Hospital for Sick Children, NHS Lothian, University of Edinburgh Edinburgh, UK

Deborah M. Eastwood Department of Paediatric Orthopaedics, Great Ormond Street Hospital, London, UK

Peter W. Engelhardt Department of Orthopedic Surgery, Hirslanden Clinic Aarau, Aarau, Switzerland

Francisco Fernandez Fernandez Department of Pediatric Orthopaedic Surgery, Olgahospital, Stuttgart, Germany

John A. Fixsen Orthopaedic Department, Great Ormond Street Hospital for Sick Children, London, UK

Bruce K. Foster Department of Orthopaedic Surgery, Women's and Children's Hospital, Adelaide, SA, Australia

Alain L. Gilbert Clinique Jouvenet, Paris, France

Yann Glard Department of Paediatric Orthopaedics, Timone Children's Hospital, Marseille, France

H. Kerr Graham Department of Orthopaedics, The Royal Children's Hospital, Parkville, Victoria, Australia

Franz Grill Department of Pediatric Orthopaedics, Orthopaedic Hospital Vienna, Vienna, Austria

Göran Hansson Department of Pediatric Surgery, The Queen Silvia Children's Hospital, Goteborg, Sweden

Carol-C. Hasler Department of Orthopaedics, University Children's Hospital Basel, Basel, Switzerland

Robert N. Hensinger Department of Orthopaedic Surgery, University of Michigan, Ann Arbor, MI, USA

Robert A. Hill Orthopaedic Department, Great Ormond Street Hospital NHS Trust, London, UK

David M. Hunt Department of Orthopaedics, St. Mary's Hospital, London, UK

James B. Hunter Departments of Trauma and Orthopaedics, Nottingham University Hospital, Nottingham, UK

Sharaf B. Ibrahim Departments of Orthopaedics and Traumatology, Hospital Universiti Kebangsaan Malaysia, Bandar Tun Razak, Kuala Lumpur, Malaysia

F. Stig Jacobsen Orthopaedics Department, Marshfield Clinic, Marshfield, WI, USA

John E. Jellis University of Zambia, Lusaka, Zambia; Zambian Italian Orthopaedic Hospital, Lusaka, Zambia

Jean-Luc Jouve Department of Paediatric Orthopaedics, Timone Children's Hospital, Marseille, France

Lennart A. Landin Department of Orthopaedics, Malmö University Hospital, Malmö, Sweden

Franck Launay Department of Paediatric Orthopaedics, Timone Children's Hospital, Marseille, France

Chi Yan John Leong The Open University of Hong Kong, Hong Kong, China

Yun Hoi Li Departments of Orthopaedics and Traumatology, Hong Kong Pediatric Orthopaedics Centre, Hong Kong, China

Christopher A. Ludlam University of Edinburgh, Edinburgh, UK; Department of Clinical and Laboratory Haematology, Royal Infirmary Edinburgh, Edinburgh, UK

Malcolm F. Macnicol University of Edinburgh; Royal Hospital for Sick Children; Edinburgh and Murrayfield Hospital; Royal Infirmary; Edinburgh, UK

Robert A. Minns Department of Child Life and Health, University of Edinburgh, Edinburgh, UK; Royal Hospital for Sick Children, Edinburgh, UK

Jacqueline Y. Q. Mok Community Child Health Department, Royal Hospital for Sick Children, Edinburgh, UK

Alastair W. Murray Department of Children's Orthopaedics, Royal Hospital for Sick Children, Edinburgh, UK

Sydney Nade Department of Surgery, The University of Sydney, Sydney, NSW, Australia

Michel Panuel Department of Medical Imaging, North Hospital, Marseille, France

Cathrin S. Parsch Emergency Department Lyell McEwin Health Services and Medstar Emergency Retrieval Services, Adelaide, South Australia, Australia

Klaus Parsch Orthopaedic Department, Pediatric Centre Olgahospital, Stuttgart, Germany

Kenneth C. Rankin Department of Orthopaedic Surgery, Rob Ferreria Provincial Hospital, Nelspruit, Mpumalanga, South Africa

James E. Robb Department of Orthopaedic Surgery, Edinburgh, UK; Royal Hospital for Sick Children, Edinburgh, UK; University of Edinburgh; University of St. Andrews; Edinburgh, UK

Peter P. Schmittenbecher Department of Pediatric Surgery, Municipal Hospital, Karlsruhe, Germany

Roger Smith Department of Orthopaedic Surgery, Nuffield Orthopaedic Centre, Oxford, UK

Tim N. Theologis Nuffield Orthopaedic Centre, Oxford, UK

Surendar M. Tuli Department of Orthopaedics and Rehabilitation, Vidyasagar Institute of Mental Health and Neurosciences, New Delhi, India

Elke Viehweger Department of Paediatric Orthopaedics, Timone Children's Hospital, Marseille, France

Andrew Wainwright Nuffield Orthopaedic Centre, Oxford, UK

David J. Wilson Department of Radiology, Nuffield Orthopaedic Centre, Oxford, UK

Peter J. Witherow[†] Bristol Royal Hospital for Sick Children, Bristol, UK

Part I
Overview

Chapter 1

General Principles

Roderick D. Duncan

Introduction

The correction of deformities in children may be regarded as the purest form of orthopaedics, which translated literally means correct (*ortho-*) child rearing (*paideia*). In the field of adult orthopaedics, the concept of straightening deformed children, as exemplified by the internationally recognized tree of Andry, seems a little remote, but not to the children's orthopaedic surgeon for whom this is part of routine practice. Andry would have been familiar with deformities arising from a number of causes which have become much less common in orthopaedic practice in the developed world, such as pyogenic sepsis and tuberculosis. The problems of deformity resulting from infection, congenital malformations, and trauma remain major causes of disability in the developing world. In Rwanda, for example, it is estimated that 5% of the population has significant musculoskeletal impairment, nearly half of which is the consequence of congenital abnormality, infection, or trauma (CBD Lavy, MD: written communication, 2007). Deformity leads to disability. Disability, particularly in developing countries, is associated with poverty. Correction of the deformity may lift an individual out of poverty. The clubfoot programs running through many parts of the developing world provide good examples: an untreated clubfoot makes it very difficult to walk or stand for long periods because of painful callosities on the lateral border of the foot; this limits the ability to earn a living or even to contribute to the family's everyday life. In the past the families had to travel long distances and raise funds for surgery. Where Ponseti's clubfoot programs [1] are in place, this is no longer required and the prospects have improved greatly over the last 10 years. The children's orthopaedic surgeon can often change lives without relying on complex instrumentation and technology.

The scope of children's orthopaedic practice is immense, ranging from the management of simple normal growth variants to the most complex limb reconstructive surgery and spinal deformity corrections. Challenges are numerous, but so too are the rewards. Simply gaining the trust of a fractious 2-year-old child can be the highlight of an outpatient clinic. The experience of working with a family as their child grows is very rewarding indeed, particularly when the child has overcome the hurdles posed by disability or serious illness. At the present time it is still possible for the children's surgeons to review their patients long term but, sadly, financial restrictions may in future drive follow-up care and supervision to nursing staff or others, a retrograde step.

Many surgeons regard the study of children's orthopaedics as a necessary evil, undertaken simply to pass postgraduate exams. With improved care however, children with major disabilities, such as cerebral palsy and Duchenne muscular dystrophy, survive well into adult life; the surgeon with an adult practice needs to become familiar with the problems they face and how their quality of life can be improved. Close liaison between services for the child and adult is essential.

Children in Hospital

Many governmental and voluntary organizations around the world have produced comprehensive reports relating to children in hospital [2, 3]. Most recommend that children should be treated as individuals in their own right in areas that are physically separate from those where adults are treated. They should be treated by health professionals trained to treat children. The UK General Medical Council [4] recently issued guidance on the duties of any doctor dealing with those younger than 18 years of age. It stresses that all treatment must be given with the *child's* best interest foremost, not the interest of the parents. The document reminds clinicians of the need to communicate at a level appropriate to the child. It covers the difficult area of consent: the emphasis is on deciding whether the child has sufficient understanding to

R.D. Duncan (✉)
Consultant Paediatric Orthopaedic Surgeon, Royal Hospital for Sick Children, Glasgow, UK
e-mail: Roderick.duncan@nhs.net

M. Benson et al. (eds.), *Children's Orthopaedics and Fractures*,
DOI 10.1007/978-1-84882-611-3_1, © Springer-Verlag London Limited 2010

agree, which is not based solely and arbitrarily on age. The laws relating to consent and children are complex and vary considerably from one country to another.

Children do not like coming to hospitals or clinics, particularly if they have been there before. It can be very stressful. It is important to make the atmosphere as welcoming as possible. The child and family should feel relaxed in surroundings which should be appropriate to the child's age or level of social development. Clinic or emergency department waiting areas can be intimidating: educational material, toys, games consoles, and television sets all help to make the environment less threatening. Play specialists are particularly helpful in distracting anxious children with games and activities. They are invaluable also in distracting children of all ages undergoing unpleasant procedures such as cast and wire removal or dressing changes. A crowded waiting area is likely to increase anxiety levels. Children come to hospital with at least one adult and often other siblings and family members: waiting areas should be big enough to accommodate the families and their accompanying buggies or wheelchairs. There must be facilities to change babies and for mothers to feed their children in private. There is merit in holding clinics in the evenings, particularly for older children.

Clinic rooms must be child-friendly and bigger than those for adult consultations: there must be room for a child in a wheelchair, two parents, siblings, medical staff, and other staff. Clinic space should ideally be flexible to accommodate, for example, the increasingly common multidisciplinary clinic. Children unable to transfer independently will need a tracking hoist to allow safe transfer from chair to couch. Ideally, there should be a private corridor where the child can be watched and recorded while walking or running.

It is best to reduce hospital visits to a minimum: a one-stop service is ideal, allowing all necessary investigations to be done on the same day as the clinic visit. It may be hard to organize, but investigations such as routine radiographs, hip ultrasounds, and computed tomography (CT) leg length examinations are suitable. Magnetic resonance imaging (MRI) scans are used more frequently in paediatric orthopaedic practice; while scans in children younger than 6 years usually need sedation or a general anesthetic, older children can be investigated and reviewed on the same day. If intravenous contrast is necessary, the child and family should be appropriately warned.

The children's ward should also be child-friendly and appropriate to the child's age, physical, and emotional development. (It is of course essential that this should not compromise clinical care.) Children should not be admitted to adult wards. The nursing staff must have the skills necessary to look after children and their musculoskeletal problems: it takes special training to recognize orthopaedic complications of treatment. Space for play and leisure is important

and a play specialist is best equipped to supervise the supply of books, board games, electronic toys, and televisions. Traction is still used for some children's conditions and the ward must be able to accommodate traction beds and the hoists needed for transfers. Toileting and bathing facilities should suit both the able-bodied and those with disabilities.

The Paediatric Orthopaedic Service

The team which looks after children includes doctors, nurses, and members of the professions allied to medicine (PAMS) (Table 1.1). Physiotherapists have a key role in managing both inpatients and outpatients; while their input after childhood injury is often less than that needed in the adult, children require prolonged rehabilitation after, for example, multi-level surgery in cerebral palsy, where success or failure of the rehabilitation depends heavily upon the therapist. Extended scope physiotherapists play an increasing role in the diagnosis and treatment of children referred with minor orthopaedic concerns, using clearly defined protocols and working alongside medical staff. Physiotherapists are particularly important in units providing a limb reconstruction service, offering support and advice to families with a child treated by external fixation. There should be a tight link with the occupational therapists to ensure that aids to daily living are available promptly when needed. They can assist in supplying loaned equipment such as car seats, wheel chairs, buggies, or specially adapted seating (Fig. 1.1).

Close working relationships and careful planning with the orthotic services ensure that there are no delays between children coming out of plaster and orthosis fitting. Delays in supply hinder walking and recovery.

Plaster casts, including hip spicas, are more commonly used in paediatric than adult practice. The complications of immobility which are so well recognized in the adult are much less common in children, whose bones heal considerably faster. External cast immobilization is the mainstay of

Table 1.1 Members of the paediatric orthopaedic multidisciplinary team

Surgical team
Secretarial staff
Physiotherapist
Occupational therapist
Orthotist
Plaster team
Theater staff
Ward and outpatient nursing staff
Extended team members
Musculoskeletal radiologist
Paediatric pathologist
Anesthetic and pain service

Fig. 1.1 A girl who had recently undergone hip surgery. She is in a one-and-a-half hip spica. She can sit and eat or play in a specially designed seat (**a**), and with care, a suitable seat can be found to enable her to travel in a car (**b**)

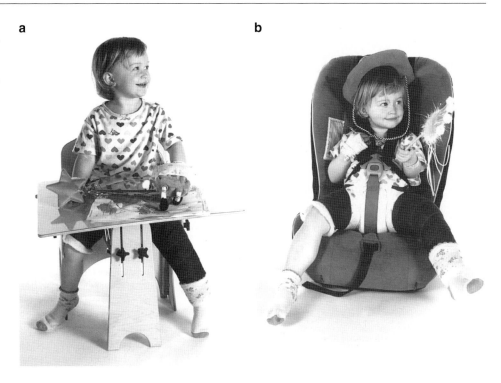

a   b

fracture treatment in children. Hip spicas are commonly used as part of the treatment for hip disorders such as developmental dysplasia of the hip (DDH) and Perthes disease. Most parents find the prospect of their child in a hip spica daunting and a well-trained team of plaster technicians can give indispensable support. They often work in theater alongside the surgical team to ensure excellence in plaster application. They are well placed to deal with carers' concerns and rectify plaster problems.

More and more children are admitted for operation as day cases or on the day of surgery, not only to reduce costs but to disrupt family routine as little as possible. Children and their families often find it helpful to visit the hospital before surgery. An efficient pre-admission program is needed if cancellations are to be minimized and early discharge facilitated. Discharge planning should be an integral part of the pre-admission program, enabling the timely provision of aids and appliances.

Fundamentals of the Paediatric Musculoskeletal Clinical Examination

It is widely recognized that pressures on the medical school curriculum have reduced the time available to teach musculoskeletal medicine and surgery. This has implications: doctors in future may lack competence and skill in diagnosing and managing bone and joint disorders. In one study

[5], 79% of medical students and staff physicians failed a basic musculoskeletal cognitive examination. Those who had undertaken an orthopaedic course during their training scored significantly better than those who had not. The assessment of the musculoskeletal system is every bit as important as any other body system. In the UK, the Gait Arms Legs Spine (GALS) musculoskeletal screening examination has become widely taught: it is a simple, structured method of screening patients for musculoskeletal problems [6]. While more suited to rheumatology, its introduction has been shown to increase competence in musculoskeletal examination. A paediatric version shows promise [7]. The physical examination tends to concentrate on the joints, so it is important that children's orthopaedic surgeons remind students that the "bits between the joints" are also important as children's infections and tumors often develop in the shafts of long bones and the pelvis (Fig. 1.2).

Table 1.2 illustrates the wide differential diagnosis possibilities in children. All clinicians need basic paediatric knowledge if important diagnoses are not to be missed: the child with leukemia may present with a limp.

History

The objective of any consultation is to find out why the parents are seeking medical advice and to reach a diagnosis. There is often a problem in establishing the parents' main concern as it may differ from that outlined in the letter of

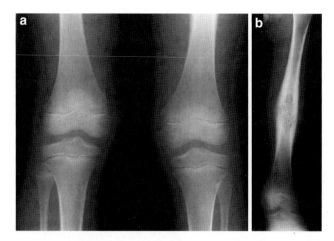

Fig. 1.2 Radiographs of a 12-year-old boy with a Ewing's sarcoma. The image of the knees (**a**) were taken six months before the image of the femur (**b**). Periosteal reaction from the sarcoma is visible at the edge of the film showing both knees on the right leg

Table 1.2 Differential diagnosis in a child with a limp

Congenital—short limb caused by developmental dysplasia of the hip
Limb deformities associated with skeletal dysplasias
Chromosomal abnormalities
Myopathies, muscular dystrophy
Neuropathies
CNS malformations
Acquired—infection—septic arthritis, osteomyelitis   Inflammation—reactive arthritis, juvenile idiopathic arthritis
Tumor—primary bone tumor, leukemia, metastatic neuroblastoma
Trauma—transient synovitis, fracture, accidental and non-accidental injury
Toxin—heavy metal poisoning
Metabolic or nutritional—rickets, vitamin C deficiency
Idiopathic—Perthes disease

Table 1.3 History template

Name
Age
Unit number
Referred by
Presenting complaint
History of presenting complaint
Family history
Past medical history
Gestational history—place of birth, gestation, presentation, weight, complications
Developmental history–gross motor milestones (e.g., walking age), concerns from child health surveillance
Medication
Allergies—drug and non-drug
Social history—siblings, schooling, hobbies, aspirations
Additional information for those with complex needs—include names and addresses of therapists (physiotherapist, orthotist, occupational therapist, school doctor, community paediatrician)
Communication
ADL assessment—feeding, dressing, toileting
Mobility—aids and appliances, seating, ability to transfer
Walking ability
Gross Motor Function Classification System
LEVEL I—Walks without restrictions; limitations in more advanced gross motor skills
LEVEL II—Walks without assistive devices; limitations walking outdoors and in the community
LEVEL III—Walks with assistive mobility devices; limitations walking outdoors and in the community
LEVEL IV—Self-mobility with limitations; children are transported or use power mobility outdoors and in the community
LEVEL V—Self-mobility is severely limited even with the use of assistive technology

referral. In any consultation for a musculoskeletal problem it is vital to exclude tumor, trauma, and infection. In children it is essential also to identify juvenile idiopathic arthritis as 50% will develop chronic anterior uveitis and approximately 10% have it at presentation (J Gardner Medwin, MD: oral communication, 2007).

It is imperative to have enough time to see children and their families in a clinic. The British Orthopaedic Association recommends that 20–30 min appointments be allocated to new orthopaedic patients but that complex cases may need half as much time again [8]. Always speak directly to children in language they understand but avoid being patronizing. Children want to be involved in decisions that affect them.

Taking a history is often challenging: it may be "second hand" history from the carer of a young child who has not learned to talk or who has communication difficulties. An interpreter may be required for those with a different first language. While some older children are exceedingly talkative, some adolescents are exactly the opposite!

Some children see their children's surgeon on and off throughout childhood. Some have conditions which require regular follow-up; others will be re-referred by their family doctor for further reassurance or with a new problem. Find out about the child and family at the first meeting: knowing an older sibling died of a malignancy may explain apparently abnormal concern. It does not help the doctor–patient relationship if a key part of the history is uncovered only on the second or third visit. This applies particularly to children with complex needs. A history template may help trainees who are more used to taking histories from adults. Table 1.3 illustrates a "minimum data set" for the first consultation.

Pain in Children

Pain is a very common reason for referral to a children's orthopaedic clinic. Over a 2-year period, one-third of children seen in our clinic presented with pain: one-quarter of these had knee pain, one-fifth had benign "growing" leg pains, and one-fifth had foot or heel pain. Fourteen percent had groin pain and 8% had back pain. The majority did not have a serious underlying condition, but it can sometimes be difficult to exclude serious pathology.

Benign leg pains or "growing pains" are poorly understood. Their cause is unknown but there are many theories. They are surprisingly common and may occur in over one-third of otherwise normal children [9]. It is important to define their characteristics clearly: the pain is commonly bilateral, but location is vague and may involve the thighs, knees, or calves; symptoms usually occur at night, but may, less frequently, occur during the day as well. The pains are intermittent, with some pain-free days and nights. In benign leg pains the physical examination is always normal. The natural history is favorable but symptoms may persist for several years. One study [10] suggested that range-of-motion exercises performed before bedtime might speed up the resolution of the problem.

A history of a persistent or progressive unilateral pain, systemic symptoms (such as fever), or pain confined to one anatomical site—particularly if associated with swelling—should raise concerns. It is imperative not to miss bone and joint infection, trauma, or tumor. Widhe et al. [11] looked at the initial symptoms of 149 young people diagnosed with either Ewing's tumor or an osteosarcoma to see if there was a distinctive pattern to their pain. They found that 70% had consulted their family doctor purely because of pain but night pain was present only in 20%. Exertional pain was the most common feature and was reported in 84% of those with osteosarcomas and 64% of those with Ewing's tumors.

Neurological symptoms should prompt further investigations. A comprehensive examination is necessary to seek bone tenderness or a mass. In the last 20 years osteomyelitis has become more frequently subacute in presentation: tenderness may be the only clue that infection is present [12].

Children do get chronic regional pain syndromes (reflex sympathetic dystrophy), so the presence of allodynia (pain from a non-painful stimulus) and stiffness should prompt a referral to a paediatric physiotherapist or to the local pain service. Chronic pain syndromes in children are well recognized and a paediatric pain team is indispensable in managing these difficult and often highly complex cases [13].

Examination

The clinical orthopaedic examination of a child should be similar to that of an adult but there are important differences. The differential diagnosis of a limp in a child is much broader than that in the adult and the examination has to take account of this. Often pain in children is poorly localized and not confined to the regions of the major joints. Some children find it difficult to localize the point of maximal tenderness, particularly around the knee. Others will not allow a clinician anywhere near them. Examining the small child on a parent's lap may be much more successful than trying to get the child up on to the examination couch. Very occasionally it is not possible to perform a satisfactory examination and the only alternatives may be a return appointment or a second opinion.

In general paediatric orthopaedic practice, lower limb problems predominate, so this section will concentrate on the examination of the child presenting with a gait variant.

It is important to be able to see a child standing, walking, and running, both in shoes and out of shoes. A private walking corridor where the child can be watched while walking in short trousers is ideal. In some cases, particularly those with neuromuscular conditions, the facilities to record gait in the clinic will enable a more accurate assessment [14]. A quick and simple way to record gait in most children is to observe five easily remembered parameters of gait (Table 1.4). Observe and listen to whether or not the rhythm is normal. Is it antalgic, Trendelenburg, or short-legged? To assess whether the step length is adequate, watch how far the leg during swing passes the limb in stance. Does the limb in swing clear the ground? Is the foot in swing prepared to start loading with a heel strike? During the stance phase, check whether the limb in stance is stable (i.e., supported on a stable foot) or whether there is a valgus or varus thrust at the knee. It is also important to record the foot progression angle (i.e., the angle subtended by the long axis of the foot relative to the line of progression of gait) as part of the rotational profile, which will be discussed in Chapter 2. It is important to observe the arm swing as asymmetry may suggest hemiplegia.

Inspection while standing will allow evaluation of limb deformity, limb length discrepancy, muscle wasting, and the position of the foot. Asking the child to walk on tiptoes will reveal whether or not a flattened medial longitudinal arch is restored in a physiological flat foot. The hindfoot swings from valgus when weight bearing into varus when standing on tiptoes. Watching the act of walking on tiptoes will also give an indication of the child's muscle power balance, co-ordination, and proprioception. Blocks placed under the short limb will enable an assessment of leg length inequality: it is more accurate than using a tape measure where the errors are significant. Forward flexion of the spine may reveal

Table 1.4 The five parameters of gait
Foot preposition
Stability in stance
Clearance in swing
Step length
Rhythm

stiffness or a spinal deformity. Investigations are merited in a child with non-mechanical back pain or stiffness.

Palpation is a key step in the paediatric orthopaedic clinical examination for a number of reasons. As noted above, some children find it very hard to localize pain, and the site of the problem can only be localized by eliciting tenderness. One common pitfall is to assume that all knee pain in adolescents is due to overuse syndromes such as Osgood–Schlatter's condition. Tumors, both benign and malignant, are not uncommonly found around the knee. Unless the child has a point of maximum tenderness precisely on the tibial tuberosity, the diagnosis cannot be Osgood–Schlatter's.

Osteitis of the pelvis can present with hip pain and a limp. Careful palpation may reveal tenderness over the ischium or pubis, areas not routinely included in routine examination. In thin patients the femoral head and neck can be palpated through the buttock. It is also important to palpate the limbs between the joints as infection, tumors, and fractures do occur in the diaphyses of long bones. Palpation of the spine is important in a child who is refusing to walk as tenderness and muscle spasm may suggest discitis.

Hip problems very often present with pain referred to the knee. It is worth stressing that an adolescent with knee pain who has no abnormal physical findings on knee examination must be assumed to have a slipped capital femoral epiphysis until proven otherwise.

Examining the range of joint movement follows the same principles as in adult orthopaedics, but some special tests, such as McMurray's test, are unlikely to be helpful because of the infrequency of meniscal lesions in the younger child. Scenarios, such as the neonatal hip check and the examination of children with neuromuscular conditions, will be covered in the relevant sections of this book.

Investigations

A plethora of special tests cannot take the place of a well-structured history and examination. Radiographs can be difficult to interpret because of the presence (or absence) of secondary centers of ossification. The diagnosis of fractures in children therefore depends upon clinical findings, which are confirmed by radiography. Radiographs are usually normal in early osteitis—tenderness may be the only clue to the diagnosis. Tumors will be missed if the wrong body part is imaged (Fig. 1.2).

An investigation which concentrates on the wrong anatomical site is worse than no investigation at all. Investigations have to be ordered and interpreted with care, remembering that there is no point in ordering a test unless it will affect management. The traction apophysis at the base of the fifth metatarsal and the secondary ossification centers around the elbow are commonly mistaken for fractures by junior doctors. MRI has largely replaced isotope bone scanning and CT as the second-line investigation following inconclusive radiographic findings; however, the large number of normal MRI scans concerns many radiologists. A normal MRI scan can, however, be immensely reassuring to both the clinician and the family.

Certain blood tests are of great value in diagnosing musculoskeletal sepsis and differentiating between a reactive arthritis and a septic arthritis. Kocher et al. [15] found that the probability of septic arthritis in a child with hip pain was 58% if the child refused to weight bear and had a history of pyrexia, but if there was also an erythrocyte sedimentation rate (ESR) over 40 mm/h and a blood white cell count of over 14×10^9/ml, then the probability was greater than 99%. Screening children with joint pain for juvenile idiopathic arthritis (JIA) using tests for antinuclear antibodies and rheumatoid factors is of doubtful value however.

References

1. Tindall AJ, Steinlechner CW, Lavy CB, et al. Results of manipulation of idiopathic clubfoot deformity in Malawi by orthopaedic clinical officers using the Ponseti method: a realistic alternative for the developing world? J Pediatr Orthop 2005; 25(5):627–629.
2. Department of Health. Standards for children in hospital: a guide for parents and carers. 2003. London: Department of Health; available from: http://www.dh.gov.uk/en/Publicationsandstatistics/Publications/PublicationsPolicyAndGuidance/DH_4008383. Accessed 12 August, 2008.
3. Department of Health. Getting the right start: National service framework for children, young people and maternity services: Standards for hospital services. London: Department of Health; 2003. Available from: http://www.dh.gov.uk/en/Consultations/Closedconsultations/DH_4085150. Accessed 23 September 2008.
4. General Medical Council, ed. *0–18 Years: Guidance for all Doctors.* 2007. GMC, Regent's Place, 350 Euston Road, London NW1 3JN.
5. British Orthopaedic Association. Advisory book on consultant trauma and orthopaedic services. British Orthopaedic Association; 2007.
6. Matzkin E, Smith EL, Freccero D, Richardson AB. Adequacy of education in musculoskeletal medicine. J Bone Joint Surg Am 2005; 87(2):310–314.
7. Fox RA, Dacre JE, Clark CL, Scotland AD. Impact on medical students of incorporating GALS screen teaching into the medical school curriculum. Ann Rheum Dis 2000; 59(9):668–671.
8. Foster HE, Kay LJ, Friswell M, et al. Musculoskeletal screening examination (pGALS) for school-age children based on the adult GALS screen. Arthritis Rheum 2006; 55(5):709–716.
9. Evans AM, Scutter SD. Prevalence of "growing pains" in young children. J Pediatr 2004; 145(2):255–258.
10. Baxter M, Dulberg C. "Growing pains" in childhood—a proposal for treatment. J Pediatr Orthop 1988; 8(4):402–406.
11. Widhe B, Widhe T. Initial symptoms and clinical features in osteosarcoma and Ewing's sarcoma. J Bone Joint Surg Am 2000; 82-A(5):667–674.

12. Blyth M, Kincaid R, Craigen M, Bennet G. The changing epidemiology of acute and subacute haematogenous osteomyelitis in children. J Bone and Joint Surg Br 2001; 83 (1): 99–102.

13. Currie J. Management of chronic pain in children. Arch Dis Child 2006; 91:111–114.

14. Read H, Hazlewood M, Hillman S, et al. Edinburgh visual gait score for use in cerebral palsy. J Pediatr Orthop 2003; 23(3):296–301.

15. Kocher M, Zurakowski D, Kasser J. Differentiating between septic arthritis and transient synovitis of the hip in children: An evidence-based clinical prediction algorithm. J Bone Joint Surg Am 1999; 81-A (12):1662–1670.

Chapter 2

Growth and Its Variants

Roderick D. Duncan

Normal Growth

Growth of the body (somatic growth) and of the individual skeletal elements is a phenomenally complex process. Huge advances have been made in recent years in the understanding of how the classical endocrine pathways, neural mechanisms, and local growth factors interrelate, but there are still large gaps in our knowledge. Skeletal growth determines body proportions and height and therefore has been the subject of intense investigation. It must be remembered that the mechanisms influencing overall growth also control the growth of individual organs, nerves, vessels, and muscles, but this discussion will concentrate on somatic growth and skeletal development.

Limb Development

The development of a recognizable limb in the fetus, with separated fingers and toes, takes place over a period of just 25 days [1]. Measurements of fetal limb length using ultrasound illustrate the rapid growth of the limbs in utero. The femur is 10 mm in length at 11 weeks gestation and just over four times longer 10 weeks later [2].

The upper limb buds appear 26–28 days after conception, the lower limb following 2 days later. Limb development proceeds in a proximo-distal pattern under the control of a number of different cytokines and growth factors which work together to produce the perfectly formed limb. Congenital abnormalities of the upper limb occur in between 1 in 600 and 1 in 1000 live births [1, 3], which, considering the complexity of limb formation, is quite incredible.

R.D. Duncan (✉)
Consultant Paediatric Orthopaedic Surgeon, Royal Hospital for Sick Children, Glasgow, UK
e-mail: Roderick.duncan@nhs.net

The bud forms as a flat paddle from the lateral plate of the embryo and consists of somatic mesoderm covered by ectoderm. The structure and the number of skeletal elements within the limb are determined by pre-cartilage condensations of cells within the limb bud and their formation is crucial [4]. The cartilaginous element which forms is initially continuous but joints are formed within it as a result of condensation of tissue and programmed cell death (apoptosis). Distally, apoptosis leads to separation of the digits, a process which is determined by the homeobox (*Hox*) genes. Abnormalities in the Hox pathway can lead to duplication or syndactyly. T-Box (TBX) transcription factors are involved in limb development and are also expressed in other regions, such as the heart. An anomaly of TBX5 is the cause of the Holt–Oram syndrome (cardiac and upper limb malformations) [3]. Further research in this area may explain the frequent links between limb and visceral abnormalities.

Patterning of the limb is described according to three axes: proximo-distal, antero-posterior, and dorso-ventral (see Table 2.1). Proximo-distal development is determined by the apical ectodermal ridge (AER) which lies at the distal end of the limb bud. It overlies a zone of undifferentiated mesoderm, the progress zone. Anomalies in this axis give rise to truncation of the limb. Implantation of a bead containing fibroblast growth factors (FGF) will restore longitudinal growth following ablation of the AER, and it is clear that FGF is important in the formation, maintenance, and signaling within the AER. An FGF-impregnated bead will also

Table 2. 1 The factors controlling limb development

Axis	Signaling center	Responsible substance	Defects
Proximo-distal	Apical ectodermal ridge/progress zone	Fibroblast growth factors	Truncation of limb
Antero-posterior	Zone of polarizing activity	Sonic hedgehog protein/BMPs	Duplications/mirror hand/multiple synostoses
Dorso-ventral	Wnt pathway	–	Double dorsal limb

M. Benson et al. (eds.), *Children's Orthopaedics and Fractures*,
DOI 10.1007/978-1-84882-611-3_2, © Springer-Verlag London Limited 2010

initiate ectopic limb bud development when implanted in animal embryos [3]. However, the AER model of limb development may be incorrect: the limb elements may develop from a population of progenitor cells formed in the limb early in development. Apoptosis of these cells causes limb truncation. These progenitor cells are maintained by FGF [4].

The antero-posterior axis is under the control of the zone of polarizing activity (ZPA) on the posterior aspect of the limb bud. It determines the differentiation of the axial and postaxial aspects of the limb. The main morphogen in this site is the sonic hedgehog protein (Shh). It is closely related to the Indian hedgehog protein (Ihh) which is important in growth of the physis (see below). Shh activity is closely linked with bone morphogenetic proteins (BMP) and the *Hoxd* gene, and a feedback loop exists between the ZPA and the AER such that they depend upon each other for normal function [4]. Transplantation of the ZPA leads to duplication of the digits, as seen in the mirror hand deformity.

The dorso-ventral axis is regulated through the Wnt pathway. Mice which lack the Wnt-7a have double dorsal limbs.

Structure of the Skeleton

There are three types of bone in the skeleton: flat bones (e.g., the flat bones of the pelvis and the skull), cuboid bones (e.g., the vertebrae and the bones of the tarsus/carpus), and the long bones. Their formation and structure are different but they are all made up of cells (osteoblasts, osteoclasts, and chondrocytes) and matrix. The matrix is partly organic (principally type I collagen) and partly mineral (calcium salts). The organic matrix is best at withstanding tension forces and the mineral at resisting compression. This explains the different morphology of bones in different anatomical sites and the variable structure within each bone, depending upon the forces it is required to resist.

Bone in children is structurally and therefore mechanically different from adult bone. It is weaker but less brittle and is able to absorb more energy before fracture. The patterns of crack initiation and propagation are different, hence greenstick fractures occur only in children, and a child's bone can undergo plastic deformation while an adult bone cannot [5]. It is well recognized that bone can respond to the forces applied through it. The mechanism by which this occurs is called mechano-transduction. It remains poorly understood but may involve the osteoblasts responding to shear, bending, and compression forces. A mechanical stimulus is thought to generate a fluid shift within the extracellular fluid in the bone canaliculi. This induces bone modeling through the cyclo-oxygenase-2 pathway and an increase in local nitric oxide production [6].

Long bones are formed in the fetus from a condensation of mesenchymal tissue which appears in the limb bud. Initially a cartilaginous model (or anlage) is formed. Vessels from the limb bud artery invade the cartilage, delivering pluripotent stem cells, which initiate the formation of a primary center of ossification. The process by which this occurs is similar to that seen in the mature growth plate (proliferation, hypertrophy, apoptosis, and mineralization). Secondary ossification centers form at each end of the long bone and between the primary and secondary ossification centers the growth plate, or physis, develops. A number of secondary ossification centers may form within a single epiphysis, most notably in the distal humeral epiphysis. The secondary ossification centers unite with the primary ossification centers in a predictable pattern throughout childhood. The growth plate is the target organ for the majority of the mechanisms which control somatic growth. It is responsible not only for longitudinal growth of the long bone but also for transverse or latitudinal growth. The latter occurs through cell proliferation and matrix deposition in the region of the perichondrial ring.

The process by which long bones grow is termed endochondral or enchondral ossification. The other main way by which bone forms is by intramembranous ossification: mesenchymal cells within the embryonic connective tissue proliferate, producing focal condensations of cells from which osteoblasts differentiate directly. The osteoblasts synthesize woven bone which subsequently matures into lamellar bone [6].

Tissues and organs grow not simply by cell division (mitogenesis) which increases cell numbers (hyperplasia), but also by an increase in cell size (hypertrophy), an increase in the volume of the extracellular matrix, and as a result of regulation by programmed cell death (apoptosis). The mechanisms which determine the final size of an organ, such as a long bone, are not fully understood.

The Growth Plate

The structure of the growth plate or the physis has been recognized for many years, but the complex nature of the interactions that occur within it is only slowly being unraveled. The physis consists of several well-defined zones. Chondrocytes start within the resting zone, then proliferate, hypertrophy, and finally die. Their lacunae become calcified (see Fig. 2.1). The process includes both cartilage differentiation and growth (chondroplasia) and calcification and ossification of the cartilaginous tissue (osteogenesis). The zone nearest to the end of the long bone consists of resting cartilage cells and is termed the reserve zone. The cells within it are stem-like cells which, when activated by factors including growth hormone (GH) or insulin-like growth factor-I (IGF-I), give rise to proliferative chondrocytes. The proliferative zone contains chondrocytes aligned in vertical

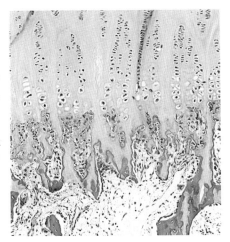

Resting Zone

Proliferating Zone

Hypertrophic Zone
Type X Collagen
Alkaline Phosphatase
Matrix Vesicles
Calcification
Apoptosis

Vascular Ingrowth
and Primary Bone
Formation

Fig. 2.1 Photomicrograph of a human growth plate. From Ballock RT, O'Keefe RJ. The biology of the growth plate. *J Bone Joint Surg* 2003;85:715–726. Reprinted with permission from The Journal of Bone and Joint Surgery, Inc.

columns which become more rounded and secrete matrix rich in type II collagen, type IX collagen, and proteoglycan core proteins. The Indian hedgehog protein (Ihh) is the main mitogen in the proliferative zone. Within the hypertrophic zone, the cells increase in size and accumulate glycogen. Type X collagen predominates within the matrix of the hypertrophic zone. Energy metabolism is repressed in the hypertrophic cells and apoptosis begins. The cells produce angiogenic stimulators which attract metaphyseal blood vessels. In the zone of provisional calcification, apoptosis is complete. The lacunae of the cells calcify and vascular elements from the metaphysis invade, bringing osteoclasts and osteoblasts [6].

The Control of Skeletal Growth

The mechanisms which control skeletal growth are not completely understood, but involve intrinsic (genetic and endocrine) and extrinsic (nutrition and acquired disease) factors [7]. There are interactions between the systems controlling growth and those which regulate energy balance, body weight, and food intake. Malnutrition and chronic diseases retard growth. The control mechanisms act via traditional endocrine pathways [GH, thyroid hormones, or adrenocorticotropic hormone (ACTH), which are secreted into the bloodstream from ductless glands] and also through a variety of local cytokines. The most important cytokines are from the families of insulin-like growth factors (IGF), epidermal growth factors, fibroblast growth factors (FGF), the transforming growth factor-β (TGF-β) superfamily, and the neurotrophic growth factors. The cytokines act locally in several different ways. They can be secreted locally and act on

nearby cells (juxtacrine), can act on the cell which secreted them (autocrine), or can remain attached to the surface of their cell of origin (paracrine). Some also have an endocrine function. The same cytokine receptor, when present on different cells, may result in a different response. In this way cytokines can produce alternative actions depending upon the cell being stimulated [8].

GH, thyroid hormones, and glucocorticoids are the principal hormones acting on the physis, with the sex hormones assuming more importance at the time of puberty. It is largely through IGF-I that GH acts on the physis, but it does act through other cytokines. GH is secreted from the anterior pituitary in response to GH-releasing hormone (GHRH) produced in the hypothalamus. GH and IGF-I promote the clonal proliferation of resting cartilage cells and accelerate chondroplasia. IGF-I is a key cytokine. It is produced in most tissues, including the liver. A protein-bound amount is present in the bloodstream. Circulating levels are reduced in malnutrition. Synthesis in the liver is regulated by insulin. Local production of IGF-I is regulated by GH, parathyroid hormone, glucocorticoids, thyroid hormones, vitamin D, FGF, TGF-β, and platelet-derived growth factor, which serves to illustrate the complex interactions which control growth.

The factors responsible for terminating growth and closing the growth plates are not clear but relate to the increased circulating and local levels of sex hormones at the end of puberty.

Somatic Growth

It is important for the orthopaedic surgeon who treats children to have a basic understanding of the pattern of growth in childhood and the factors which control it. Growth is a process which we take for granted—it is what children do. Healthy, adequately nourished, and emotionally secure children grow normally. Poor growth is the final common pathway for many organic and emotional problems of childhood [9]. The process of growth sometimes works in our favor but on other occasions does not. It is impossible to plan treatment for a child with a limb length discrepancy, a physeal arrest, or scoliosis without having a grasp of normal somatic growth, particularly in later childhood.

It has become clearer over time that many conditions which appear in adult life are related to the fetal environment. Fetal growth is controlled by both genetic and environmental factors. The important environmental processes which can have an effect on growth include maternal factors such as chronic disease and malnutrition, smoking, alcohol, and drug abuse. Low birth weight is related to the subsequent development of hypertension, insulin resistance, type 2 diabetes, and cardiovascular disease [9, 10].

Growth is not continuous throughout childhood. There are two rapid phases of growth, the first in infancy and the second in adolescence. In infancy the rate of growth is by and large nutritionally determined. Poor growth in infancy is very difficult to catch up later. An infant will grow, on average, 25 cm in the first year of life and doubles birth length by the age of 3–4 years. A 3-year-old child has a tibia and a femur which are half their eventual adult length. During infancy and early childhood the body proportions also change. Babies have large heads relative to their bodies. The center of body mass of a toddler is significantly higher than in an older child: it lies at the umbilicus rather than at the adult level just in front of the second sacral vertebral body.

As the child grows its body size becomes proportionately smaller and growth slows. In middle childhood growth is fairly constant at about 4–7 cm per year, although there may be a mini-growth spurt at around 7 years which results from increased adrenal androgen secretion (adrenarche). This pre-adolescent growth spurt may be accompanied by the development of some axillary or pubic hair. The onset of puberty heralds the start of the second period of rapid growth.

The first signs of puberty are an increase in testicular size in boys and an enlargement of breast tissue in girls. Pubertal growth lasts around 6 years and starts, on average, 2 years earlier in girls than in boys. The growth rate in puberty is accelerated, but the rate is not constant: growth velocity increases and then falls. The peak height velocity (PHV) occurs 1 year after the first signs of puberty in girls and 1.7 years in boys. The maximum rate of growth is in the region of 9.8 cm per year in boys and occurs at age 14.1 years, and in girls it is 8.1 cm per year and occurs around the age of 12.1 years. Menarche occurs generally 1 year after the PHV. The ages at which children go through puberty vary significantly, with 80% of boys starting puberty between the ages of 11.2 and 13.2 years, and girls between 10 and 12.3 years. As pubertal growth will last for 6 years, regardless of the age when the first signs appear, estimation of the potential growth remaining should take into account factors other than chronological age. Longitudinal studies of growth in adolescence suggest that pubertal growth prior to the PHV occurs predominantly in the limbs and afterward in the spine [11].

The most reliable signs of the start of puberty are changes in the testes and breasts, which is why most orthopaedic surgeons rely on bone age (*v.i.*). Body weight increases proportionately more than height, but most of the weight gained in puberty is in lean body mass and not fat. As a result the body mass index (weight in kg/height in m^2) rises in normal subjects throughout puberty, making it less reliable than in adults. The other important change in puberty is the increase in bone mass. One-quarter of adult bone is laid down in the 2 years spanning the PHV. While exercise is good for increasing bone mass, extreme forms of exercise have been shown to delay puberty and to reduce height gained during the growth spurt [11].

Implications for Limb Length Equalization

It is useful for the surgeon to be able to calculate the target height for an individual who is contemplating the choice of epiphysiodesis or leg lengthening. This can be calculated from the parental heights. The target height (in centimeters) for a boy is [father's height + mother's height/2] + 7. The target height (in centimeters) for a girl is [father's height + mother's height/2] – 7. In 95% of children, their final height will be within the target height + 10 cm for boys and + 8.5 cm for girls. This is the target range [12].

Several methods are in use to monitor children with limb length discrepancies. They include Moseley's straight line method, which can be used to give a depiction of past growth, a prediction of future growth, and an estimate of the effect of and timing of surgery [13]. Paley's multiplier method can be used to predict the timing of epiphysiodesis but is particularly helpful in providing a quick method of estimating the leg length discrepancy at skeletal maturity for children diagnosed with congenital limb deficiencies. To calculate the likely final discrepancy, the difference in length is simply multiplied by an age-specific constant, calculated from well-established data on limb length [14]. The most straightforward way of predicting the timing of epiphysiodesis is using a method which relies on chronological age and predicted growth around the knee. The authors believe that the assessment of bone age is inaccurate and that chronological age will therefore suffice [15]. The distal femur is assumed to grow 1.0 cm per year after the age of 9 years and the proximal tibia at 0.6 cm per year. Boys are predicted to stop growth at 16 and girls at 14. To equalize a predicted leg length difference of 3 cm in a boy, an epiphysiodesis of the distal femur would need to be performed at the age of 13 years.

Spine Growth and Development

Knowledge of normal growth and development of the spine helps an understanding of its common developmental anomalies and the interpretation of spinal imaging in children.

The adult vertebral column is formed from the spinal cord and nerves (derived from neuroectoderm), the ossified vertebral and costal bones (derived from sclerotomal mesoderm), the spinal muscles and ligaments (derived from myotomal mesoderm), and the intervertebral discs (derived from the notochord). The Wnt pathway and *Hox* genes have roles in determining whether a vertebra develops as a cervical, a thoracic, or a lumbar vertebra [16].

The most important aspects in the postnatal growth of the spine are continuous, symmetrical growth (longitudinal and axial), the development of the normal curves in the sagittal plane (lordosis in the cervical and lumbar spine, and kyphosis in the thoracic and sacral regions), and the development of the bony structures which will provide protection for the neural elements. Variants of growth may lead to scoliosis. Asymmetrical loading of the spine can lead to a "biomechanical modulation of growth," which is retarded on the compression side and accelerated where loading is reduced. The sagittal plane is more stable and resistant to unequal loading than the coronal plane [17].

It is worth remembering that the spinal cord terminates at the bottom of the spinal canal during early fetal life. The bony elements grow more than the neural elements, so that the distal end of the cord appears to migrate proximally. Nerve roots exit the cord at their own level in fetal life, but exit at a higher level as the spinal column grows. The conus medullaris lies at the level of the first or the second lumbar vertebra at birth.

The processes by which the vertebrae form are similar to those seen in the long bones. Each vertebra forms as a cartilaginous model which progressively ossifies. A typical vertebra, however, has three primary ossification centers: one anterior in the vertebral body (the centrum) and one on each side posteriorly. Each ossification center is separated by a synchondrosis (one posterior and one at the junction of the body with the pedicles). These are responsible for the growth of the spinal canal. Premature fusion will cause canal stenosis. The maximum canal diameter is achieved at 5–8 years [18].

The atlas (C1) and the axis (C2) are atypical vertebrae. Their growth is described in detail in Chapter 34. Worth highlighting here is the observation that the child's head is proportionately larger than the rest of the body, so when a child is positioned for a straight lateral radiograph, the neck assumes a position of flexion; this may suggest subluxation of C2 on C3, which is spurious (see Fig. 2.2) [2].

Longitudinal growth of the spine occurs by endochondral ossification at the chondro-osseous vertebral end plate, which functions as a slow-growing epiphysis. The end plate is thicker peripherally than centrally. Ossification of the thickened peripheral end plate at the age of 12–15 years produces the appearance of the *ring apophysis*. Latitudinal growth occurs by a combination of periosteal and perichondrial appositional bone growth [18]. Spinal growth is particularly rapid during the first 2 years of life and also during adolescence. Longitudinal growth of the spine is complete by the age of 16–18 years.

In the assessment and management of spinal deformity, it is important to determine the age during puberty at which the rate of growth is most rapid. This peak growth age is of value in determining the prognosis for scoliosis and

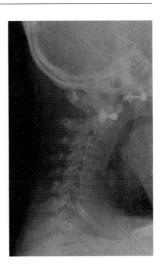

Fig. 2.2 Lateral radiograph in flexion of a normal 2-year-old child showing pseudosubluxation of C2 on C3. The spino-laminar line is intact and there is no increase in the prevertebral soft tissue shadow

has also been used to determine the optimal age for treatment. Prior to the peak growth age a curve is more likely to progress rapidly and the risk of progressive deformity occurring after spinal instrumentation and fusion (crankshaft phenomenon) is higher if surgery is performed before that age. Traditionally, the age at menarche and the Risser stage have been used to assess skeletal maturity in scoliosis, but menarche occurs after the peak growth age and is not reliably associated with the Risser stage [19].

Assessment of Skeletal Maturity

The assessment of skeletal maturity is important not only in the management of scoliosis but also in those with a leg length discrepancy or a growth disturbance as a result of physeal arrest. It must be remembered at the outset that skeletal maturation is nonlinear and that each child is different. It has been said that "maturity advances according to a developmental rather than a chronological clock" [7]. Skeletal age estimation can be used in the calculation of the growth remaining in a limb and in predicting both the limb length difference at the end of growth and the chronological age at which growth is likely to cease. The assessment of skeletal age is based upon the presupposition that bones grow and physes mature in an orderly sequence. Its relation to pubertal status is variable, but less so than chronological age. Because of the nonlinear relationship of skeletal age, it cannot be assumed that a child who has a bone age of 6.5 years will have a bone age of 7 years 6 months later. Serial measurements are therefore essential. There are several methods in widespread use.

The Risser grade is based upon the appearance of the iliac crest apophysis on an AP radiograph of the pelvis. An orderly progression of ossification is seen from the anterior superior iliac spine posteriorly, followed by fusion of the apophysis to the ilium. There are five grades. The first four relate to the extent of ossification (up to 25% grade 1, 25–50% grade 2, and so on), with grade 5 indicating fusion. Risser grade 1 appears around a skeletal age of 13.5 years in girls and 15.5 years in boys, after the peak height velocity in the majority of children [20]. It does not correlate with skeletal age and growth remaining [19]. The Oxford score uses other pelvic landmarks in addition to the iliac crest.

The Greulich and Pyle and Tanner–Whitehouse methods use radiographs of the hand and wrist to estimate skeletal age. A score is calculated based upon the appearances of the bones of the hand and the carpal bones. The Greulich and Pyle system was developed from radiographs of 1,000 white children of "above average economic and educational status" in Cleveland, Ohio, in the 1930s. There is significant inter-observer variation in using this method, and it may be less reliable when used in populations which differ significantly from the original study group. The Tanner–Whitehouse system is similar to the Greulich and Pyle but was developed in the United Kingdom [7].

The Sauvegrain method can be used to assess skeletal maturity and is used during puberty. Fusion of the elbow physes indicates that the accelerated phase of pubertal growth is complete and that the peak height velocity has been attained. The method uses an AP and lateral radiograph of the elbow and examines differences in the appearance of the physes and secondary ossification centers which occur during puberty. These changes are apparent only on radiographs taken between the ages of 9 and 13 years in girls and 11 and 14 years in boys. An advantage of using this system in adolescence is that there are no Greulich and Pyle standards which correspond to skeletal ages of 11.5 and 12.5 years in girls and 14.5 years in boys. It therefore allows a detailed examination of skeletal maturity at this time of rapid growth [21]. A simplified system of assessing bone age using the olecranon apophysis alone has also been described [20]. Each surgeon should be consistent in the techniques used for sequential measurement.

Neuromuscular Development

Knowledge of normal neuromuscular development is required by all clinicians who treat children. Parents concerned about a delay in their child's walking are likely to be referred to an orthopaedic surgeon, despite the fact that the most likely causes are not musculoskeletal. These children require a limited developmental assessment and the key milestones are shown in Table 2.2 [22]. It is more important to be aware of these when dealing with families of children suspected of having cerebral palsy. Children with total body involvement or spastic diplegia are more likely to have a generalized developmental delay than those with hemiplegia.

Table 2.2 Developmental milestones indicating the age by which 90% children would have achieved the particular milestone [22]

	Milestone	Age
Gross motor	Lifts head when prone	0.7 months
	Sits without support	8 months
	Stands alone well	14 months
	Walks well	14.3 months
	Jumps on the spot	3.0 years
Fine motor	Reaches for object	5 months
	Thumb finger grasp	10.6 months
	Tower of two cubes	20 months
	Tower of four cubes	2.2 years
Personal social	Smiles responsively	1.9 months
	Smiles spontaneously	5 months
	Drinks from cup	16.5 months
Speech and language	Laughs	3.3 months
	"Dada" and "Mama" (non-specific)	10 months
	"Dada" and "Mama" (specific)	13.3 months
	Three words other than "Mama," "Dada"	20.5 months

Gait variants are a common cause for referral. A child's gait matures through the early part of childhood, up to the age of about 7. For this reason, surgical treatment of gait problems in children with neuromuscular conditions is usually deferred where possible until after this age. In children with motor delay, it is widely believed that the later they start to walk independently, the less likely they are to maintain independent walking into adult life. It is important to recognize the differences between a child's and an adult's gait and these differences are discussed in Chapter 6. Although the 7-year-old child is generally thought to have an adult pattern of gait, there are still minor differences, most noticeably a higher cadence, a lower walking velocity, and different hip and pelvic rotations [23].

Normal Variants

Children with normal variants of growth or gait are commonly referred to orthopaedic clinics. The reason for this may be concern regarding the diagnosis or simply a wish for reassurance, either on behalf of the family or the referring clinician. Some of these referrals may appear unnecessary but there may often be a good reason for anxiety. Parents may have been treated for these conditions as a child in the belief that treatment will prevent problems in later life. They will expect the same treatment for their child. There may be particular concerns about anomalies seen in firstborn or particularly precious children, for example, those born as a result of in vitro fertilization, or in families where there has been the loss of a previous child. Sometimes children are referred simply to reassure older members of the family that "something is being done" or that "things are being checked out."

The term *normal* is used to describe a precise distribution and pattern of a series of measurements such as height. The profile of the heights of individuals in a given population conforms to a normal or Gaussian distribution. The normal range is, by convention, defined as lying between two standard deviations on either side of the mean, encompassing 95% of individuals. In studies which are designed to examine normal values, the data must be interpreted taking into account the mean and the range which are considered to be normal for that population. In some instances the range of normal is very narrow, but in many situations, such as the age of onset of puberty, it is broad. It must be stressed that simply because a child falls out of the normal range does not necessarily mean that there is a pathological process going on or that treatment is required. There are great rewards, both financial and professional, for those who choose to treat normal variants as their prognosis is rarely anything but good. Ethically, however, such an approach cannot be justified; while some cases may require treatment, most do not.

The diagnosis of a normal variant is based upon the pattern recognition and the exclusion of other pathologies. A useful system to help identify normal variants has been described (DHA Jones, FRCS: oral communication, 1997). It is particularly useful in educating general practitioners and medical students. Normal variants are generally symmetrical (see Fig. 2.3). Children with a normal variant rarely have symptoms or stiffness of the joints. They do not have a systemic illnesses or symptoms and do not have an underlying skeletal dysplasia. Therefore if a child presents with a *S*ymmetrical deformity, with no *S*ymptoms, underlying *S*ystemic illness, or *S*keletal dysplasia and there is no *S*tiffness on examination, then it is likely that they have a normal variant. This is easily remembered as the *five Ss*. Examples are given in the following sections.

Rotational Anomalies

The commonest rotational problems are in-toeing and out-toeing. Children can present at any age with these, although the commonest presentation is within the first few years of starting to walk. The children are usually either in-toe or out-toe on each side (symmetry), though it is not uncommon for there to be slight differences between the two sides. They rarely have symptoms, although some parents say that their children with in-toeing tend to trip over their feet. There are usually no signs of skeletal dysplasia or systemic illness and on examination there is no joint stiffness. To identify the source of the problem one has to be familiar

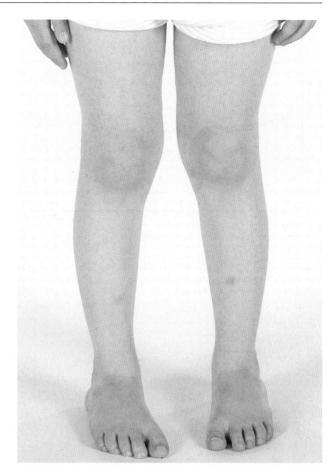

Fig. 2.3 Photograph of a 4-year-old boy with symmetrical in-toeing and flat feet

with the rotational profile, popularized by Dr. Lyn Staheli [24]. Examination of the rotational profile is performed with the child walking and then examined prone with the hips extended and the knees flexed to 90° (see Fig. 2.4). The

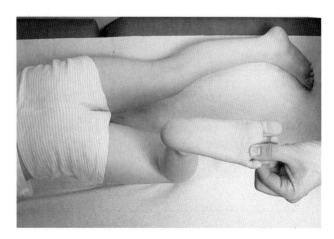

Fig. 2.4 Photograph of a 4-year-old boy being examined for rotational anomalies. He is lying prone with his knees flexed at 90°. The angle subtended between the longitudinal axis of the thigh and the foot is the thigh–foot angle

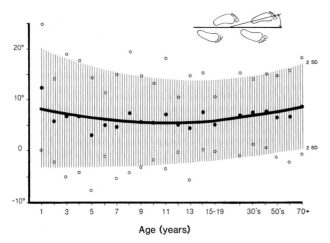

Fig. 2.5 Graph showing the foot progression angle at different ages. The *circles* represent the extremes, the *solid circles* indicate the mean values, and the *shaded areas* represent two standard deviations from the mean. From Staheli et al. [24]. Reprinted with permission from The Journal of Bone and Joint Surgery, Inc.

examination consists of several clinical measurements which were validated in a cross-sectional study of 1,000 limbs in children and adults from Seattle, WA, USA. The foot progression angle is the end result of the rotational limb anomaly and describes the axis of the foot relative to the line of progression of gait (see Fig. 2.5). Positive values indicate out-toeing and negative values indicate in-toeing. The normal range is wide, in excess of 15°, and as indicated above, there is a tendency for the externally rotated gait of infancy to reduce throughout childhood. Assessment of the angle subtended by the long axis of the foot relative to the thigh—the thigh–foot angle (see Fig. 2.6)—will determine whether the torsion is the result of a foot or a tibial anomaly. There is a

tendency for infants to in-toe because of internal tibial torsion; this occurs partly because of the internal rotation of the fetal limb and partly because of in utero molding. It tends to persist longer in infants who sleep prone with their legs flexed under the abdomen and their tibiae internally rotated. The change in the transmalleolar axis (the angle between the long axis of the thigh and a line perpendicular to the axis of the malleoli) mirrors the change in thigh–foot angle (see Fig. 2.7). In-toeing may be due to metatarsus adductus, which is assessed by comparing the axis of the hind foot and the line of the second metatarsal. Increased internal rotation of the hip relative to external rotation will favor an in-toeing gait, and increased external rotation favor an out-toeing gait. Increased femoral anteversion will result in an increase in internal rotation at the hip and is the commonest cause for in-toeing in the older child, usually girls. As can be seen in Fig. 2.8 the range of normal internal rotation in girls is large and tends to increase throughout early childhood, but then reduces during puberty. Increased femoral neck anteversion is associated with increased joint laxity. In older children with dominant internal rotation of the hip, it is not uncommon to find compensatory external rotation of the tibia. As a result of examining the foot progression angle, the hip rotations, the transmalleolar axis, and the thigh–foot angle, the extent and site of the problem will become clear. Examination of the rotational profile can be challenging in the younger child as it is done prone, but with practice, it can be carried out efficiently on the mother's lap. The natural history of the commoner rotational anomalies is illustrated in the accompanying figures. It is recognized that femoral neck retroversion is associated with slipped capital femoral epiphysis, but there is controversy about the long-term prognosis for those with increased femoral neck anteversion. There is no good evidence from longitudinal studies that it predisposes to hip osteoarthrosis [25, 26].

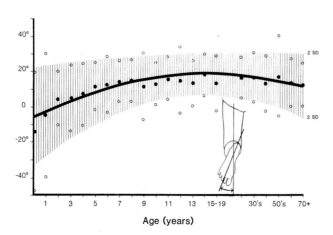

Fig. 2.6 Graph showing the change in the thigh–foot angle at different ages. From Staheli et al. [24]. Reprinted with permission from The Journal of Bone and Joint Surgery, Inc.

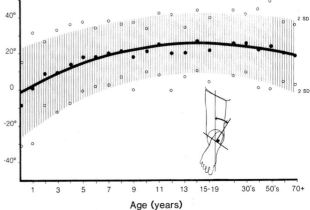

Fig. 2.7 Graph showing the change in the transmalleolar axis at different ages. Staheli et al. [24]. Reprinted with permission from The Journal of Bone and Joint Surgery, Inc.

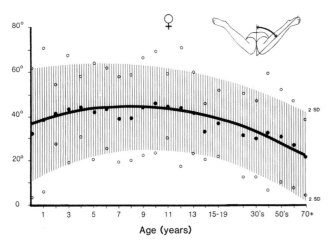

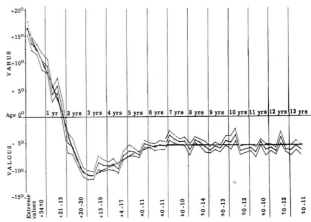

Fig. 2.8 Graph showing internal rotation of the hip in girls and women of different ages. Staheli et al. [24]. Reprinted with permission from The Journal of Bone and Joint Surgery, Inc.

Fig. 2.9 Graph showing the tibiofemoral angle, measured from radiographs in individuals of different ages. The smooth *solid line* represents a line of best fit. The other three lines represent the mean values and the standard error of the mean. Note that the standard deviation across the whole series was 8°. From Salenius and Vankka [27]. Reprinted with permission from The Journal of Bone and Joint Surgery, Inc.

Angular Anomalies

Children frequently present with angular anomalies in the lower limbs. The clinician has to be careful not to miss treatable conditions such as one of the many causes of rickets or progressive conditions such as infantile tibia vara (Blount's disease). Fortunately most children have no underlying medical diagnosis and the angulation of the limb is usually a result of a normal variant in growth. Almost all concerns about angulation relate either to the knee joint or to valgus of the hind foot associated with a flat foot. Children with knock knees or bow legs, occurring as a normal variant, present with a symmetrical deformity, no symptoms, no sign of skeletal dysplasia (such as achondroplasia), no systemic illness, and examination reveals no joint stiffness. The femoro-tibial angle in children is different depending upon the age of the child. Salenius and Vankka examined 1,480 radiographs of children up to the age of 13 years [27]. They found that neonates and children under the age of 2 years tended to be bowlegged. The legs became straighter and angulated into valgus with a mean angle of 10° (valgus) at the age of 3 years. Thereafter, there is a gradual reduction in valgus toward a final mean of 7° (see Fig. 2.9). The standard deviation of the entire series was 8°, indicating the wide normal range. The authors found differences between boys and girls: boys tended to have a greater valgus at 3 years. It is generally accepted that a child with bow legs after the age of 3 years should be investigated.

It is worth pointing out that bow legs in toddlers can appear quite impressive because they tend to walk with their hips externally rotated. As a result, the plane of knee flexion is externally rotated, so that when they flex their knees during walking, the knees separate. Associated medial tibial torsion results in the feet pointing forward, so it is important to assess the rotational profile in these children.

The differentiation between physiological bow legs and Blount's disease can be challenging, but the only completely reliable way to tell them apart is that physiological bowing improves with age, whereas the latter does not. Various radiographic criteria have been used to predict if a child with tibia vara and features suggesting Blount's disease will develop a progressive deformity or not [28–31]. Most techniques measure the metaphyseal–diaphyseal angle (MDA), either of the tibia alone or in comparison with the same measurement on the distal femur. The angle is measured by drawing a line up the lateral cortex of the tibia and another between the most prominent medial and lateral beaks of the metaphysis of the tibia. The MDA is the angle subtended by the metaphyseal line and a perpendicular to the line along the lateral tibial cortex. A value of greater than 11° was found to be a predictor of Blount's disease [32], but other studies have not found it reliable; one group found that 87% of infants with an MDA over 11° resolved without treatment [33]. Physiological bowing will resolve with time. The only reliable way to distinguish between them is to follow the child in the clinic if there is doubt.

Foot Problems

One of the most common reasons for referral of a child with a foot problem to an orthopaedic clinic is a flat foot. A cross-sectional observational study of 441 normal subjects by Staheli et al. showed that the arch is usually completely flat in infants but is present in older children (see Fig. 2.10) [34].

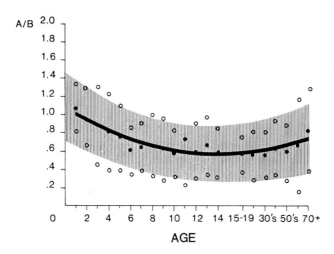

Fig. 2.10 Graph showing the change in the ratio between the width of the midfoot and the width of the heel from footprints of subjects of different ages. A ratio of 1 implies that the widths are equal and that the foot is flat. Values less than 1.0 imply that an arch is present. From Staheli et al. [34]. Reprinted with permission from The Journal of Bone and Joint Surgery, Inc.

A wide range of normal was encountered in this study population. Flattening of the medial longitudinal arch in young children is, therefore, a normal variant and is termed a physiological or flexible flat foot. A child with a physiological flat foot has a symmetrical deformity, with no symptoms, no systemic illness or skeletal dysplasia, and no stiffness. For the deformity to be physiological they must have no restriction of ankle dorsiflexion: a tight Achilles tendon predisposes to a planovalgus foot. In the physiological flat foot, the arch restores with extension of the great toe and on tiptoe standing (see Fig. 2.11)

Occasionally, adolescents with physiological flat feet do have pain related to the excessive pressure over the medial aspect of the midfoot; however, these feet remain mobile. Pain accompanied by stiffness in the foot suggests other causes, such as inflammatory arthritis or tarsal coalition. There are no studies which relate physiological flat foot to the development of degenerative joint disease in the foot. Some have found that lower limb and back pain are no more common in children with flat feet than in those with normal arches [35]. Others have found that some children with flat feet do have diffuse activity-related pain in the leg or in the foot. This may represent an overuse syndrome and these

children may benefit from shoe inserts [36]. It has been suggested that flat feet may be protective against stress fractures of the tibia and the femur in military recruits because of the capacity for the flat foot to act as a better shock absorber. However, these authors also found that they may predispose to metatarsal stress fractures in their selected group [37]. There is no evidence that flat feet predispose to anterior knee pain [38].

It is clear that orthotic treatment of a physiological flat foot does not alter the eventual shape of the arch. A prospective randomized clinical trial was performed by Wenger et al. [39]. They studied four groups of children aged 1–6 years with flexible flat feet over 3 years. Besides a control group, the children were managed with either heel cups, corrective shoes, or shoe inserts. Researchers found that arch development was completely independent of any footwear modification. These findings were confirmed by Gould et al. [40]. Shoe inserts may be useful in prolonging the life of shoes in children with severe flat foot and may help those with exertional leg pains [36], but the claim that they will alter the final profile of the foot has not been substantiated. Although the use of corrective shoe wear in children may seem harmless, one group of investigators found that in a group of adults their use was perceived as a negative experience in childhood and was associated with a lower self-esteem in adult life [41].

Hypermobility Syndromes

Recently there has been a lot of interest in joint hypermobility both in adults and children. A recent review of the topic draws attention to links between joint hypermobility in adults and mitral valve prolapse, osteoarthritis, pelvic floor insufficiency, chronic pain, proprioceptive dysfunction, and osteoporosis, but these links have been established only through cross-sectional studies which are not population based [42]. Hypermobility is, however, normal in children. It is more marked when they are younger and less evident when they become older [43]. It is essential to differentiate symptomatic from asymptomatic children with joint hypermobility. Those with symptoms are described as having the benign joint hypermobility syndrome (BJHS). Symptoms include exercise-related limb pain, back pain, and so-called

Fig. 2.11 Photograph of a child with flexible flat feet. On standing, the medial longitudinal arch is flat (**a**) but is restored both on dorsiflexion of the great toe (**b**) and when standing on tiptoe (**c**)

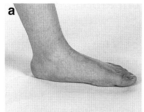 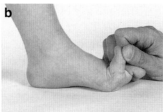 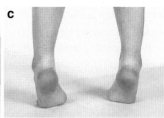

Table 2.3 Beighton's modification of the Carter-Wilkinson criteria of hypermobility

Palms flat on the floor with knees extended 1
Opposition of thumb to flexor aspect of forearm 2
Hyperextension of fingers parallel to extensor aspect of forearm 2
Hyperextension of elbows by more than 10° 2
Hyperextension of knees by more than 10° 2
Score (1 mark for each, including left and right, hypermobile if >6) 9

benign leg pains (see Chapter 1.). Those with no symptoms should be considered normal.

The Beighton score is used to diagnose hypermobility (see Table 2.3) [44]. BJHS is diagnosed on the basis of this Beighton score, which includes major and minor diagnostic criteria similar to those used in the diagnosis of Marfan's or Ehlers–Danlos syndrome. Hypermobile children may appear awkward while running and complain of difficulty with fine motor tasks such as writing. A link with developmental co-ordination disorder (formerly known as dyspraxia) has been postulated [42]. The treatment for symptomatic hypermobility may include the use of insoles, but their efficacy is unproven.

Acknowledgments We acknowledge with grateful thanks to the staff of the Medical Illustration Department, Yorkhill; and to the Rowland family.

References

1. Zguricas J, Bakker WF, Heus H, et al. Genetics of limb development and congenital hand malformations. Plast Reconst Surg 1998;101(4):1126–1135.
2. Hensinger R. Standards in Pediatric Orthopedics. Tables, Charts and Graphs Illustrating Growth. New York: Raven Press; 1986.
3. Manouvrier-Hanu S, Holder-Espinasse M, Lyonnet S. Genetics of limb anomalies in humans. Trends Genetics 1999;15(10):409–417.
4. Tuan RS. Biology of developmental and regenerative skeletogenesis. Clin Orthop Rel Res 2004;(427 Suppl):S105–S117.
5. Currey J, Butler G. The mechanical properties of bone tissue in children. J Bone Joint Surg Am 1975;57-A(6):810–814.
6. Tiosano D, Hochberg Z. Bone and cartilage growth and metabolism. In: Kelnar C, Savage M, Saenger P, Cowell C, eds. Growth Disorders, 2nd ed. London: Hodder Arnold; 2007:25–47.
7. Preece M, Cameron N. Historical background and worldwide perspectives. In: Kelnar C, Savage M, Saenger P, Cowell C, eds. Growth Disorders, 2nd ed. London: Hodder Arnold; 2007:1–12.
8. Holly J. Peripheral hormone action. In: Kelnar C, Savage M, Saenger P, Cowell C, eds. Growth Disorders, 2nd ed. London: Hodder Arnold; 2007:114–126.
9. Drake A, Kelnar C. Growth in infancy and childhood. In: Kelnar C, Savage M, Saenger P, Cowell C, eds. Growth Disorders, 2nd ed. London: Hodder Arnold; 2007:132–149.
10. Johnston L. Normal fetal growth. In: Kelnar C, Savage M, Saenger P, Cowell C, eds. Growth Disorders, 2nd ed. London: Hodder Arnold; 2007:127–131.
11. Buckler J. Growth at adolescence. In: Kelnar C, Savage M, Saenger P, Cowell C, eds. Growth Disorders, 2nd ed. London: Hodder Arnold; 2007:150–164.
12. Wales J. Practical auxology and skeletal maturation. In: Kelnar C, Savage M, Saenger P, Cowell C, eds. Growth Disorders, 2nd ed. Hodder Arnold; 2007:208–218.
13. Moseley C. A straight line graph for leg length discrepancies. Clin Orthop Rel Res 1977;136:33–40.
14. Paley D, Bhave A, Herzenberg J, Bowen J. Multiplier method for predicting limb-length discrepancy. J Bone Joint Surg Am 2000;82-A(10):1432–1446.
15. Eastwood D, Cole W. A graphic method for timing the correction of leg-length discrepancy. J Bone Joint Surg Br 1995;77-B: 743–747.
16. Kusumi K, Turnpenny PD. Formation errors of the vertebral column. J Bone Joint Surg Am 2007;89(Suppl 1):64–71.
17. Sarwark J, Aubin CE. Growth considerations of the immature spine. J Bone Joint Surg Am 2007;89(Suppl 1):8–13.
18. Labrom RD. Growth and maturation of the spine from birth to adolescence. J Bone Joint Surg Am 2007;89-A(Suppl 1):3–7.
19. Sanders JO. Maturity indicators in spinal deformity. J Bone Joint Surg Am 2007;89-A(Suppl 1):14–20.
20. Charles YP, Dimeglio A, Canavese F, Daures J. Skeletal age assessment from the olecranon for idiopathic scoliosis at Risser grade 0. J Bone Joint Surg Am 2007;89(12):2737–2744.
21. Dimeglio A, Charles YP, Daures J, et al. Accuracy of the Sauvegrain method in determining skeletal age during puberty. J Bone Joint Surg Am 2005;87(8):1689–1696.
22. Frankenburg W, Dodds J. The Denver developmental screening test. J Pediatr 1967;71:181–191.
23. Sutherland DH, Olshen R, Cooper L, Woo SL. The development of mature gait. J Bone Joint Surg Am 1980;62(3):336–353.
24. Staheli L, Corbett M, Wyss C, King H. Lower-extremity rotational problems in childhood. J Bone and Joint Surg Am 1985;67-A(1): 39–47.
25. Lievense A, Bierma-Zeinstra S, Verhagen A, et al. Influence of hip dysplasia on the development of osteoarthritis of the hip. Ann Rheum Dis 2004;63(6):621–626.
26. Terjesen T, Benum P, Anda S, Svenningsen S. Increased femoral anteversion and osteoarthritis of the hip joint. Acta Orthop Scand 1982;53(4):571–575.
27. Salenius P, Vankka E. The development of the tibiofemoral angle in children. J Bone Joint Surg Am 1975;57-A(2):259–261.
28. Bowen RE, Dorey FJ, Moseley CF. Relative tibial and femoral varus as a predictor of progression of varus deformities of the lower limbs in young children. J Pediatr Orthop 2002;22(1): 105–111.
29. Davids JR, Blackhurst DW, Allen BL Jr. Radiographic evaluation of bowed legs in children. J Pediatr Orthop 2001;21(2): 257–263.
30. Levine AM, Drennan JC. Physiological bowing and tibia vara. the metaphyseal–diaphyseal angle in the measurement of bowleg deformities. J Bone Joint Surg Am 1982;64(8):1158–1163.
31. McCarthy JJ, Betz RR, Kim A, et al. Early radiographic differentiation of infantile tibia vara from physiologic bowing using the femoral–tibial ratio. J Pediatr Orthop 2001;21(4):545–548.
32. Feldman M, Schoenecker P. Use of the metaphyseal-diaphyseal angle in the evaluation of bowed legs. J Bone and Joint Surg Am 1993;75-A(11):1602–1609.
33. Shinohara Y, Kamegaya M, Kuniyoshi K, Moriya H. Natural history of infantile tibia vara. J Bone Joint Surg Br 2002;84(2): 263–268.
34. Staheli L, Chew D, Corbett M. The longitudinal arch. J Bone Joint Surg Am 1987;69-A(3):426–428.
35. Widhe T. Foot deformities at birth: A longitudinal prospective study over a 16 year period. J Pediatr Orthop 1997;17: 20–24.
36. Mosca V. Flexible flatfoot and skewfoot. J Bone Joint Surg Am 1995;77-A(12):1937–1945.

37. Simkin A, Leichter I, Giladi M, et al. Combined effect of foot arch structure and an orthotic device on stress fractures. Foot Ankle 1989;10(1):25–29.

38. Hetsroni I, Finestone A, Milgrom C, et al. A prospective biomechanical study of the association between foot pronation and the incidence of anterior knee pain among military recruits. J Bone Joint Surg Br 2006;88-B(7):905–908.

39. Wenger D, Maudlin D, Speck G, et al. Corrective shoes and inserts as treatment for flexible flatfoot in infants and children. J Bone Joint Surg Am 1989; 71-A(6):800–810.

40. Gould N, Moreland M, Alvarez R, et al. Development of the child's arch. Foot Ankle 1989;9(5):241–245.

41. Driano A, Staheli L, Staheli L. Psychosocial development and corrective shoewear use in children. J Pediatr Orthop 1998;18(3): 346–349.

42. Grahame R, Hakim AJ. Hypermobility. Curr Opin Rheumatol 2008;20(1):106–110.

43. Grahame R. Joint hypermobility and genetic collagen disorders: Are they related? Arch Dis Child 1999;80(2):188–191.

44. Gardner-Medwin J, Galea P, Duncan R. Musculoskeletal and connective tissue disorders. In: Beattie J, Carachi R, eds. Practical Paediatric Problems—a Textbook for MRCPCH. London: Hodder Arnold; 2005:485–517.

Chapter 3

Children and Young People with Disability: Management and Support

Zoë M. Dunhill

Introduction

Support for children and young people with disabling conditions and their families is a hallmark of a civilized society. A host of conditions can present to the orthopaedic surgeon, both known complications of the disorder and as conditions seen in the general population (see Table 3.1). Through early diagnosis, new therapeutic interventions, and better social and health care, children are surviving longer [1], in many cases into adult life, with multiple and complex needs. Innovations, especially in the realms of supportive equipment and biomechanics, surgical techniques such as minimal access surgery, information technology, and advances in educational theory and pharmacology, have significantly improved the day-to-day life of disabled children and their parents. Much still remains to be done to achieve optimal participation of the disabled child in society and to enable them to attain their potential.

The multi-disciplinary team approach to supporting and managing these children and young people has been recognized as offering the best outcome [2] but requires intensive long-term effort from diagnosis to adult life, with good communication between the team and the family. Sometimes 20 professionals or more may be involved with a family and the orthopaedic surgeon may be only one of many clinicians and practitioners interacting with the family. The concept of *care coordination* [3] has been developed in the United Kingdom (UK) to overcome some of the inherent difficulties of a large team, with the identification of a *key worker* to facilitate overall management of the child and the family. Generally, it is best if the family nominate their preferred key worker from amongst the team members.

Z.M. Dunhill (✉)
Community Child Health Service, Royal Hospital for Sick Children,
NHS Lothian, University of Edinburgh, Edinburgh, UK
e-mail: Zoe.dunhill@euht.scot.nhs.uk

Table 3.1 Common disabling conditions in childhood

Genetic conditions	Down syndrome
	Fragile X syndrome
	Osteogenesis imperfecta
	Achondroplasia
	Duchenne/Becker muscular dystrophy
	Spinal muscular atrophy
	Neurofibromatosis
Congenital anomalies	Neural tube defects
	Arthrogryposis multiplex
	Limb reduction deformities
Acquired conditions	Traumatic brain injury (accidental/non-accidental)
	Cerebral palsy (hypoxic/ischemic encephalopathy)
	Spinal injury
Inflammatory conditions	Juvenile arthropathies
Neurodevelopmental disorders	Autistic spectrum disorders
	Attention-deficit/hyperactivity disorders
	Learning disability syndromes
	Developmental coordination disorder

In the United Kingdom [4], 18% of those aged 0–19 years have a long-standing disability or illness, while 8 per 10,000 of the population aged 0–16 years live with severe disability:

- 25% autism and behavioral disorders
- 15% severe learning difficulties
- 8% cerebral palsy
- 4% global developmental delay
- 3% epilepsy
- 2% asthma

With improved survival of very low birth weight infants, Bracewell et al. found that by the age of 6 years, 25% of survivors had moderate to severe disability [5].

Therefore, it is important to ensure there is a comprehensive system in place to support and care for this important minority of children and young people with disabling conditions.

M. Benson et al. (eds.), *Children's Orthopaedics and Fractures*,
DOI 10.1007/978-1-84882-611-3_3, © Springer-Verlag London Limited 2010

The Multi-disciplinary Team

Throughout the child's management from diagnosis onward, practitioners need to be aware of those involved in the team, to make referrals as appropriate, and to ensure that colleagues are informed of the management plan (see Fig. 3.1). Problems may become apparent before conception (i.e., pre-diagnosed genetic conditions), during pregnancy, at birth, or during childhood. Clearly, conditions with disabling sequelae may develop at any time (i.e., meningitis or head injury).

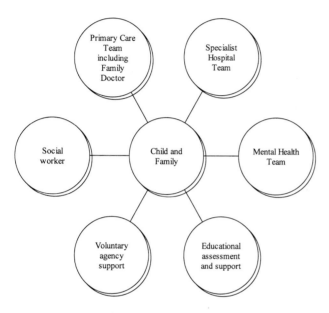

Fig. 3.1 The child and the family at the center of the multi-disciplinary team

Therapeutic abortion, selection of embryos, or chorionic villous sampling may be chosen by parents following appropriate, skilled genetic counseling. Identification of gene loci is possible for many conditions, with more being added regularly. However, cures may not be available even if the gene has been located.

Breaking Bad News

The implications of breaking the news to parents have been scrutinized [6] and best practice guidelines have been formulated by the Scope charitable organization [7]. It is essential that both parents are present, that adequate time is allocated by an experienced senior clinician, and that written and/or recorded information is provided. The parents should be free to come back with further questions on a later occasion. Voluntary organizations, such as Contact a Family [8], provide excellent information and support to families on the

Internet or directly and will put them in touch with other bodies who may specialize in support for a particular condition. The provision of psychological counseling may be needed for some families. If there are already social or emotional difficulties within the family, the stress of caring for a disabled child greatly increases the likelihood of marital breakdown and financial difficulties.

The Impact of Having a Disabled Child in the Family

Researchers commissioned by the Joseph Rowntree Foundation [9] have noted how parents of disabled children can be marginalized and how family, friends, and professionals alike may ignore their role as expert carers. Financial hardship can also ensue with child disability, adversely affecting employment for both lone parents and mothers with partners [10]. Poor housing and a lack of access to aids and adaptations for the home compound these problems. Siblings are reported to suffer increased psychological morbidity [11] but may also assume a very positive role in supporting their brother or sister.

Legislation

In the United Kingdom, there has been a raft of legislation relating to human rights for disabled people, specifically for children. The United Kingdom is a signatory to the UN Convention on the Rights of the Child (see Table 3.2) [12]. Laws differ slightly in Northern Ireland and Scotland.

Families are often unaware of their rights and may need support to obtain financial and social services and appropriate education for their child.

Multi-disciplinary Assessment

The United Kingdom has a comprehensive system of child health surveillance and immunization with universal access to screening by family doctors and health visitors (known in some areas as public health nurses). A recent report recommended changes in the system to ensure the most vulnerable children and their families receive enhanced support [13]. Neonatal hearing screening is now in place for all children and vision screening by an orthoptist is recommended at the age of 4 years.

Table 3.2 Legislation in England and Wales affecting disabled children and their families, 1970–2006

Name	Year	Focus	Results
Chronically Sick and Disabled Persons Act	1970	Access to services	Local authorities must ensure that a range of support services are available
The Children Act (s17)	1989	Assessing need	Social services departments in England and Wales have a duty to assess the needs of a child with a disability
The Disability Discrimination Act (DDA)	1995	Disability discrimination	This Act gives disabled people rights in the areas of employment, education, access to goods, facilities, services, and transport
Health and Social Care Act	2001	Direct payments	Direct cash payments in lieu of social services
Special Educational Needs and Disability Act	2001	Education	This amended the 1995 DDA to make it unlawful for education providers to discriminate against disabled pupils and adult learners
The Carers (Equal Opportunities) Act	2004	Carers assessments	This seeks to give those with caring responsibilities the opportunities that those without caring opportunities take for granted
The Childcare Act	2006	Childcare	This places a duty on local authorities to provide childcare up to age 18 for parents with disabled children

If developmental concerns arise, a child may be referred to a community paediatrician based in a local Child Development Center or to a hospital-based paediatrician with an interest in neurodisability who will undertake a structured assessment and make referrals to therapists and others as appropriate. They may use a variety of test instruments (see Table 3.3) to comprehensively assess a child's development against nationally established norms. The Griffiths Scales are the most commonly used in the United Kingdom.

These findings will aid in referral decisions as well as in diagnosis and should be shared with parents and other members of the team. Parental consent for the sharing of information should be sought, especially with professionals outside the health setting.

Further investigations may be needed to rule out chromosomal or metabolic disorders and antenatal infection. If magnetic resonance imaging (MRI) scans of the head have not been performed already, further diagnostic information can be gleaned, especially in the presence of microcephaly or focal neurological deficit.

If a child is diagnosed at, before, or after birth with a significant or complex disorder, a neonatologist or other specialist should involve the local community paediatrician in order to ensure that support in the community is in place. Community paediatricians should receive copies of relevant correspondence. They are often the interface with professionals from the local authority, supporting access to social and financial benefits, modifications to housing, and so on.

Table 3.3 Test instruments to assess development

Griffiths Mental Development Scales
Bayley Scales of Infant Development
Denver Developmental Screening Test

Early and Continuing Intervention

Paediatric Physiotherapist

The paediatric physiotherapist (PPT) is best involved at an early stage if any form of motor disorder is suspected. The PPT assesses the child's motor function and needs in terms of head control, lying, sitting, standing, and walking, and recommends appropriate aids including orthoses and wheelchairs. Children with high or low tone are vulnerable to deformity through muscle imbalance, abnormal persistence of reflexes, and gravitational forces. Therefore, positioning and stretching exercises need to be taught to parents.

In the beginning, very frequent visits may be needed to build rapport with the family and to consolidate skills in helping the child. If splinting is required (i.e., an ankle/foot orthosis to maintain position at the ankle), parents may need encouragement to use the splints regularly. If the child is placed outside the family, in an *early years* center or with a carer or other family member, staff in these settings will need to be trained and supported. For children with multiple and complex needs who may be in multiple placements (respite or social care, early years nursery, frequent hospital admissions), maintaining effective therapy and communication across the different sites can be difficult. A handheld record which travels with the child can be helpful.

After orthopaedic procedures, due allowance must be made for post-operative rehabilitation, which will be more intensive than the usual day-to-day regimen. If the child lives some distance from the orthopaedic center, liaison with the local district team is essential.

Occupational Therapist

The occupational therapist (OT) provides help and advice relating to the child's activities of daily living (ADL) including play, learning, continence, washing, dressing, eating, and drinking. The OT can supply equipment, including seating and materials to facilitate play and learning, including sophisticated electronic switches to operate toys or computers. Very young children now access computers as part of play, so they can be of immense use to this group of disabled children. The OT can work with *early-years staff* in modifying and using toys for learning and cooperate with speech and language therapists in introducing appropriate communications equipment which is known collectively as augmented and alternative communication (AAC). Such equipment can be mounted on a wheelchair for non-ambulant children.

The family home often requires modifications such as stair rails, stair lifts, ramps, and bathroom changes including the provision of a wet room area. Funding for these may be available from the local authority. Clinicians are often asked to write letters of support to confirm that a specific need exists.

Speech and Language Therapist

The speech and language therapist (SALT) works on all aspects of communication, both diagnostically and therapeutically. He or she is an expert in the assessment of oro-motor function and advises about feeding difficulties, including those caused by poor bulbar function associated with gastro-esophageal reflux.

The SALT can use a variety of standardized tests to assess the child's understanding and expressive language, leading to a specific program for the child in conjunction with teachers, parents, and the other therapists treating the child. Additionally the SALT can be involved with the OT in tailoring an AAC system for the child, comprising picture boards, signing, and information technology (IT).

Community or Specialist Children's Nurse

Most areas now have specialist children's nurses who will visit in the community and provide support for the family, such as medication and dressings, portacath management, continence and stoma care, and parenteral or enteral feeding. They can teach techniques to parents and carers, thus minimizing hospital admissions and enabling early discharge. Some nurses may have specialist expertise in the care of children with cancer or other serious conditions, while others may be skilled in behavior management and learning disability. Nurses can often act as the key worker and be the link for families with other members of the multi-disciplinary team.

Educational Psychologist

The educational psychologist is qualified in both educational theory and child development and can assess and advise how to meet a child's special educational needs. The psychologist works for the local education authority and helps parents to choose what kind of school would best suit their child's needs. Since the publication of the Warnock Report in 1978 [14], many more children have attended their local school with appropriate support instead of attending special schools or classes. This is generally thought to be beneficial for both disabled children and their peers but requires teamwork between teachers, parents, and therapists; good communication; and facilities.

Social Worker and Voluntary Organizations

For families with a disabled child, a social worker can make a huge difference in the provision of state benefits, respite and other forms of care, and housing. Parents may suffer from poor mental health or with alcohol or drug dependence. Sometimes there may be more than one disabled child in the family.

There are a large number of voluntary bodies which provide support and information to families on a generic or condition-specific basis. The Contact a Family directory and web site acts as a useful source of information for professionals and families [8].

Disability Registers

There have been a number of attempts over the past 50 years to create disability registers in parts of the United Kingdom [15]. The Children Act (England) 1995 proposed that local authorities keep a database of disabled children in their area, but no specific resources were allocated and these registers were not kept up to date in many localities.

In Scotland, a national special needs register was set up in 1997 by the National Health Service and remains in operation in 11 of the 14 health board areas [16]. There are cerebral palsy registers in north-west England, north-east England, and the Oxford region [17].

Such registers improve audit and research, keep families informed, and facilitate the regular follow-up of children who may otherwise become lost.

Nature of Disabling Conditions

Disabling disorders encountered by the orthopaedic surgeon include the following:

- Short-term and treatable conditions such as major limb fractures.
- Long-term conditions, such as infections, paraplegia, or acquired brain injury.
- Congenital and lifelong abnormalities, including neural tube defects and osteogenesis imperfecta.
- Degenerative or progressive conditions, such as mucopolysaccharidosis and muscular dystrophy.

Care of these children and young people extends for many years, so the orthopaedic surgeon will develop a close relationship with the child and the family. This makes the formulation of a long-term treatment plan and decision making much easier. Surgical outcome should not be described overoptimistically, lest disappointment ensues, souring the relationship the surgeon may have with the child and the family in the future.

Exemplar Conditions

Neural Tube Defects

Spina bifida and associated hydrocephalus is the most common of all central nervous system malformations, although selective termination and pre-conception folate supplementation have greatly reduced prevalence [18]. Ultrasound scanning is now routinely offered at about 20 weeks of pregnancy and some parents may opt to terminate a severely affected pregnancy. The lesion may occur at any point along the spinal cord and may present as anencephaly or as an encephalocoele. The former condition is not compatible with life. More typically a child may have a lumbar, lumbosacral, or sacral lesion. The lesion may be skin covered or have only a thin covering of meninges which often rupture during delivery. The spinal lesion may be associated with an Arnold–Chiari malformation, with herniation of the cerebellar tonsils through the foramen magnum. Hydrocephalus may also be caused by aqueduct stenosis or blockage of the fourth ventricle.

The condition affects many systems of the body and has lifelong consequences for bowel and urinary tract function, mobility, skin care, and cognitive function. Asymmetrical involvement of the lower limbs is often seen. Vision may be affected if raised intracranial pressure has damaged the optic nerves. Central nervous system complications include epilepsy.

The role of the orthopaedic surgeon in the management of spina bifida is described in Chapter 17.

Management from Birth

Repair of the lesion is undertaken immediately after birth in a specialist center following detailed assessment by a neurosurgeon, an orthopaedic surgeon, and a paediatric neurologist (see Fig. 3.2). Hydrocephalus often requires to be treated by a ventriculo-peritoneal shunt with insertion of an access device to monitor pressure (see Fig. 3.3). Careful surveillance of the child is required in case of shunt malfunction so that parents

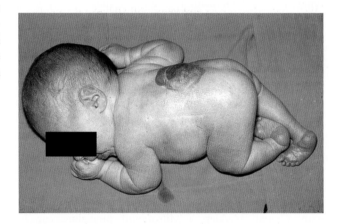

Fig. 3.2 Neural tube defect before repair

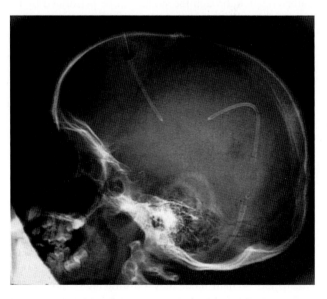

Fig. 3.3 Radiograph showing hydrocephalus controlled by ventriculo-peritoneal shunt device

should be informed about the common symptoms and seek advice when necessary.

The child should attend a combined clinic including a physiotherapist, an orthopaedic surgeon, a paediatric neurologist, a paediatric urologist, and a specialist incontinence nurse. After birth and a comprehensive assessment by the specialist team, parents should be given advice about the prognosis for their child, depending upon the motor and sensory level of the lesion. Rarely, a child may succumb in the early weeks from complications of surgery.

Management of the Renal Tract

Renal investigations at birth and over subsequent years are needed to make sure that the child has a *safe bladder*, with low vesical pressure that does not jeopardize the upper renal tract. Catheterization in infancy may be necessary if there is reflux and evidence of damage to the kidneys. Decisions about continence management rely upon regular isotope-labeled dimercaptosuccinic acid (DMSA) and Mag3 isotope renal scans, renal tract ultrasound examination, and cystometrograms. Preservation of the upper renal tract is important and so symptomatic urinary tract infections need to be treated vigorously. A lower dose of a suitable prophylactic antibiotic may be needed if infections are recurrent.

If there is adequate bladder capacity and sphincter tone, intermittent self-catheterization is recommended for both boys and girls as soon as they can participate. For children with poor sphincter tone and dribbling incontinence with a small bladder, a Mitrofanoff procedure can be undertaken to achieve continence by creating a cystostomy with the appendix, following an augmentation cystoplasty. Catheterization through the stoma can be performed by the child or the carer.

In the case of a child with severe cognitive impairment who is unable to self-catheterize, if there is a tight sphincter, a sphincterotomy can create a safe bladder or a vesicostomy can be performed. Management with incontinence pads may be the only option in the longer term, although in boys a sheath urinal may be effective.

Bowel Incontinence and Constipation

Fecal continence correlates directly with anal sphincter tone (external sphincter nerve supply from the internal rectal nerve and the internal sphincter from parasympathetic branches from S4). There may also be reduced peristalsis in the lower bowel and impaired or absent sensation. Evacuation of hard stool may be difficult or impossible, so the use of stool bulking agents and softeners or bowel stimulants may be necessary. Mini-enemas may also assist.

Manual evacuation of stool from the rectum is found to be effective by many parents. The avoidance of constipation and related megacolon is essential. Occasionally, phosphate enemas are required for fecal impaction.

Toilet training before the child attends school may be possible if the child has some sensation and can push, but recently the use of retrograde bowel washouts, either gravitational or via a pump, has been found to be very effective. Children can have a washout over the toilet in the evening and are then free of incontinence for 24 h or more. In some cases the formation of a stoma (ACE procedure) [19] for antegrade washouts of the large bowel can be performed with good results and a high level of patient satisfaction.

Skin Care in the Paraplegic Child

From the earliest days of the child's life, the parents and carers (and later on the child) need to be taught about the hazards relating to anesthetic skin. Areas at risk need to be inspected daily, especially over bony prominences such as a kyphos, the ischial tuberosities, greater trochanters, the sacrum, the feet, and the toes. Thermal injury (including sunburn) and friction or shearing forces are also damaging. Shoes, wheelchair straps or foot rests, orthoses, or poorly fitting jackets may produce pressure areas. At the first sign of reddening, pressure needs to be relieved until the skin appears healthy.

Prevention is far better than cure since established lesions take many weeks to heal. A preventative regimen includes inspection, avoidance of dampness, positional changes on a regular basis (with press-ups every half hour for wheelchair users), suitable padding in a wheelchair, and a weight-distributing cushion. Great care needs to be exercised when fitting rigid jackets or splints to avoid pressure points. At home the child needs to be aware not to sit near radiators and to avoid hot meal plates on the lap. If sores do occur, a tissue viability nurse needs to be involved and referral to a plastic surgeon may be necessary.

Posture, Seating, and Mobility

A child needs to be able to achieve a stable sitting position to access play materials, to draw and write, and to use a computer keyboard. For thoracic lesions the child will need supportive seating, which may be in the form of a molded seat or foam blocks. Trunk stability may be affected when there is low tone and ataxia related to hydrocephalus. The upper limbs may be involved if there are abnormalities in the cervical cord such as a syrinx, and fine motor function can be compromised. Typically, children may have poor writing and visual/spatial skills.

There are a variety of mobility aids available to suit the toddler such as small-wheeled vehicles. Parents will need a buggy-type pushchair with the capacity to accommodate a seating insert if necessary. For social mobility a child can be prescribed a self-propelling wheelchair if cognitive and upper limb function permits this. Modern wheelchairs are very light and easy to maneuver.

Orthoses

Orthoses may be needed to prevent deformity, to maintain position, to enhance gait, and to enable walking. Depending upon the level of the lesion, appropriate support can be given (see Table 3.4).

The use of standing frames at the right developmental stage promotes awareness of the upright posture in young children and allows weight bearing through the lower limbs, thus promoting skeletal mineralization and renal tract drainage. Prior to prescribing an ambulatory device, a swivel walker is used from around the age of 2 years, provided the child and the parent are motivated and the child can achieve the swivel movement of the trunk and arms required to move the device forward. Once the child is confident in the swivel walker, they may progress to using a hip guidance orthosis (HGO) which works in a similar way, utilizing contraction of latissimus dorsi of the contralateral arm on a crutch or a rollator to transfer weight to the leg in front. The hinges on the HGO are free between a prescribed range of flexion and extension, so the other leg will then swing forward. The process is continued with the opposite arm pressing down and back (see Fig. 3.4).

Some centers use the reciprocating gait orthosis (RGO), which works in a different way and requires normal triceps and latissimus dorsi function. The device is lighter than the HGO and is designed to be worn under clothes. The RGO hip hinges are linked by a cable so that flexion on one side causes flexion in the other. The child moves by pushing down with both arms and pulling the pelvis forward and upward on one side. The weight-bearing leg is left behind and the cable advances the other leg. Children learn to use this device first with parallel bars and then progress to a rollator and possibly to crutches (see Fig. 3.5).

These devices are effective but tend to be used in a complementary fashion with wheelchair mobility, enabling the

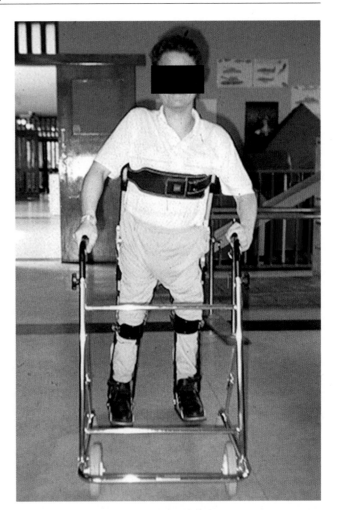

Fig. 3.4 Hip guidance orthosis in use

child to keep up with their peers and to be less dependent upon adult supervision. Most children will need assistance to apply and remove both the HGO and the RGO until they go to secondary school. Young people frequently reject the devices and opt for wheelchair transport as they mature.

Children with lower level lesions may need only above or below knee orthoses for walking. In general the guiding principle is to offer the least splintage consistent with the most functional gait.

Cognitive Issues and Education

Children with hydrocephalus may exhibit learning difficulties, either global or specific, and require careful assessment so that they can be offered a suitable curriculum with adequate support tailored to their needs. They may have problems with concentration and require one-to-one help. Most schools are now wheelchair accessible but the child may still need escorted transport to and from school. In England

Table 3.4 Ambulatory orthoses according to segmental level

Level	Under 4 years	Over 4 years
Thoracic	Swivel walker	HGO with spinal brace
L1-L3	Swivel walker	ARGO, RGO, or HGO
L4-L5	KAFO	KAFO
Below L5	AFO	AFO

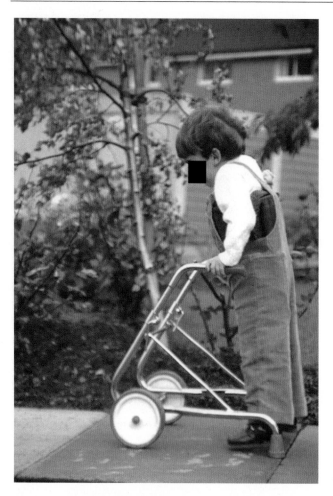

Fig. 3.5 Reciprocating gait orthosis in use

who will be living away from home, at college or university, contact should be made with the local specialist team. Some specialists may have a mixed child and adult practice in which case they may be able to continue caring for the young adult in an adult clinic. Major treatment decisions should not be made at the time of handover, unless absolutely necessary.

Cerebral Palsy

The classification and orthopaedic treatment of cerebral palsy is covered in Chapter 19. Although it is a non-progressive condition neurologically, disability may increase as the child grows because of growth factors, muscle imbalance, and resultant deformity.

Like spina bifida, the role of parents and carers is vital in enabling the child to achieve maximum function and participation in society. The disorder will frequently come to light during the first year of life with a failure to meet developmental and motor milestones and persistence of abnormal reflexes. Frequently other sequelae of hypoxic ischemic encephalopathy are present such as epilepsy, visual and hearing impairment, and cognitive impairment. Once the problem has come to light, the multi-disciplinary team of therapists should be involved to advise on positioning, a program of stretching, and to make sure that feeding and nutrition are satisfactory. Medical problems such as epilepsy will require treatment with anticonvulsants.

Feeding and Nutrition

Difficulties with biting, chewing, and swallowing are common, with persistence of primitive rooting and gag reflexes and hypersensitivity around the mouth and palate causing tongue thrust. A poor cough reflex may result in silent aspiration. A specialized speech and language therapist can advise on feeding methods and can help parents to position the child correctly, thus minimizing adverse motor patterns during mealtimes. Liquids may need to be thickened to reduce the likelihood of aspiration.

Some children with poor sucking may require tube feeding initially and conversion to gastrostomy feeding if there is a risk of aspiration or inadequate intake. A barium swallow may be needed to exclude aspiration. A gastrostomy can be performed by minimal access surgery, avoiding a major abdominal procedure, thus reducing morbidity. Fundoplication, which can be performed laparoscopically, may be necessary if pharmacological management of reflux is ineffective.

The improvement in nutrition of children with cerebral palsy has been one of the major factors in improved survival [22], reflecting the involvement of a gastrointestinal

and Wales, a Statement of Special Educational Needs may be drawn up following consideration of detailed reports. In Scotland, an Individual Education Plan or a Coordinated Support Plan for children with more complex needs may be agreed with parents. Excellent information for teachers has been developed by the Association for Spina Bifida and Hydrocephalus (ASBAH) [20].

Transition to Adult Services

Young people with disabling conditions require special measures when transferring to adult services. It is a time of concern for them and their parents as they are leaving school for a stage in their lives which usually entails an educational or training placement. They are also leaving behind a familiar team of clinicians. Viner [21] has written of the pitfalls and difficulties in the process and how they may be avoided. Paediatric clinicians can ease the handover by holding joint clinics with their adult counterparts and by introducing the new team gradually over a period of time. For young people

team comprising a nutrition support nurse, a paediatric gastroenterologist, and a dietician. Regular measurements of the child's height, weight, and skinfold thickness are required to make sure that intake is sufficient for satisfactory growth. Parents may feel that gastrostomy feeding removes much of the enjoyment at mealtimes, so compromises can be made, with the child receiving tiny tastes of food by mouth.

Management of Drooling

Children with poor lip closure may drool saliva which soaks their clothes and can result in significant fluid loss. If training the child to swallow and to keep the lips closed is unsuccessful, transdermal scopolamine patches can be applied behind the ears. They must to be titrated to the child's particular need to avoid side effects such as blurred vision. Oral anticholinergics, such as glycopyrrolate, can also be effective [23]. Surgical diversion of the submandibular salivary ducts to the pharynx offers a radical solution.

Communication and Speech

Impairment of oro-motor function may greatly impair speech in cerebral palsy. A child may be so dystharthric that no intelligible sounds are possible. Co-existing impairment of cognitive function may also affect both language expression and comprehension. Assessment of intellectual function in children with severe motor impairment affecting speech is extremely difficult as most standardized methods rely upon an intact motor system. Parents and the team interacting with the child on a daily basis will usually be in the best position to assess the child's level of function.

Alternative communication methods should be introduced at an early stage. These can begin with a simple cause-and-effect switch and then progress to low-technology picture or photograph boards with one or two choices, which the child can indicate by eye pointing or gesture. With sufficient hand function a sign language can be taught. Also available are more complex systems with symbol boards and computer-generated synthetic speech production. An integrated therapy and teaching team accustomed to working with these systems is essential, as is funding to purchase the equipment, which is evolving rapidly but is increasingly expensive.

The choice and positioning of access switches may require much trial and error as the child may need to use a head-mounted switch, a chin switch, one which is attached to a finger, or another variation. Access to skilled bioengineering expertise to program and design switches is therefore essential.

It is important to take into account the position in the wheelchair and seating as changes in tone may radically alter the child's ability to work the switch. Digital speech recognition systems may be suitable for a very few children but are not very effective if speech quality and volume fluctuate. When the child starts schooling the communication system needs to go into the classroom, with implications for the training of teachers and support workers.

Control of Tone and Positioning

In cerebral palsy, the imbalance of muscle power across joints results in progressive deformity unless a rigorous program of positioning, stretching, and exercise is instituted. Particularly challenging is the child with dystonia, where tone can vary with position, level of arousal, and emotional state. Head and trunk positions are very important and the child may benefit from the use of a Lycra suit including arm gaiters. Pharmacological management of tone has improved recently with the use of local measures such as botulinum toxin injections and of baclofen pumps which administer the drug directly into the subarachnoid space.

Putting the child in a standing frame will improve posture, bone mineralization, and bladder drainage. Knee orthoses may be needed to prevent flexion at the knee. Serial casting is useful if deformity develops.

Surgical intervention may be needed if secondary deformities develop. Subluxation of the hips can cause pain and requires surgical intervention. If a windswept deformity develops (see Fig. 3.6), surgical treatment is necessary, followed by measures to prevent recurrence, such as a molded seat and sleep positioning system.

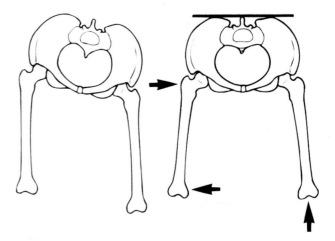

Fig. 3.6 Windsweeping deformity in cerebral palsy

Seating

Supported seating allows the child to see the world around, to interact, and to feed. At first, a foam-molded seat such as

Fig. 3.7 Wheelchair seating

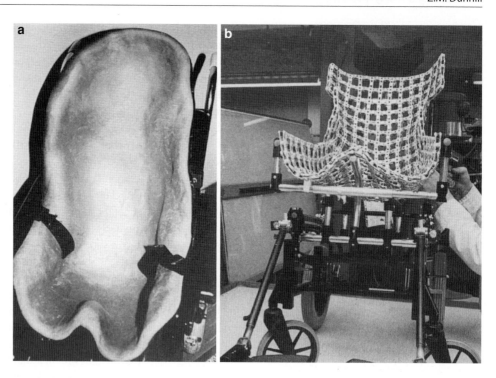

that made by Tumble form is helpful. As they grow, children can move on to a proprietary adjustable seat such as a Saturn chair, which can be wheeled around and customized for each child, varying trunk and head supports, foot rests, and the pommel. A tray in front of the child is useful for feeding, playing, and learning.

A molded seat for the child is made by casting (see Fig. 3.7). The child sits on a casting bag of polystyrene beads which moulds to the body in the optimum position. The beads are then consolidated and a plaster mold is created, allowing a rigid shell to be fashioned. The seat can be used in a variety of ways: as an insert for a pushchair or buggy, in a wheelchair, or as a car seat with appropriate and approved anchorages. Seating needs to be kept under constant review as the child grows and seats for the different settings, particularly school and home, should be provided.

Mobility Aids

The child needs to be supplied with a range of mobility aids tailored to each stage of motor development. Once used to an upright posture, a rollator can be supplied, progressing to elbow crutches, and then to walking unaided, especially if ataxia is the sole manifestation.

Modern wheelchairs have greatly improved in design and maneuverability. Social mobility for the child is paramount, so an electrical chair should be prescribed for those who cannot self-propel. Initially the vehicle moves along magnetic tracks and may then be substituted by a *smart* or a

programmable wheelchair [24] which recognizes obstacles, progresses at chosen speeds, and provides verbal feedback to the child. If these devices are not available, standard wheelchair training can be provided.

In the United Kingdom, wheelchairs are provided by the National Health Service through a network of wheelchair centers, where specialist teams, including a rehabilitation consultant and a physiotherapist or an OT, can assess individual needs. These centers also supply buggies and push chairs for families, including double buggies when necessary.

Inability to self-propel, but with adequate vision and cognitive function, is necessary for the supply of an electric chair. Detailed reports from the team who know the child are helpful in ensuring that the right chair is supplied. An individual chair may need to be modified with a molded seat, restraining straps, head and trunk supports, and mounts for communication devices. A suitable cushion to ensure equal distribution of weight to avoid pressure sores is essential. These can be made from a variety of materials, trial and error determining which is the most suitable.

If the child exhibits extensor spasms/dystonia, the pelvis will tend to shift forward, so the seat should be inclined, being higher at the front, or a wedge cushion used. A lap strap can also be used to prevent the pelvis shifting forward. If there is adductor spasm, an adjustable pommel can be supplied. The child should be safe to travel in the wheelchair in a tail-lift vehicle and there are international standards for the anchor points. Families sometimes wish to purchase a chair privately and it is important to make sure that insurance and maintenance of the chair are funded.

Modifications can be advised for the family car, to assist in carrying a wheelchair, and to install a swivel seat for ingress and egress. Young people who wish to drive can be assessed using test rigs, and adapted cars can be provided. If awarded the mobility component of the Disabled Living Allowance benefit, a suitable car can be leased to the family or the young person when they pass their driving test. The ability to drive is very important for a young disabled person in terms of independence and in being able to move away from home. The clinician may be asked to make a referral specifically for a driving assessment. This should be done before the young person's 16th birthday.

Cognitive Issues and Education

The child with cerebral palsy may suffer complex patterns of cognitive deficit which require skilled assessment. As stated earlier, with profound motor impairment it may be very difficult to assess the cognitive level with any degree of certainty. Assessment is best viewed as an ongoing process, not a one-off event, and those familiar with the child will build up a picture of the relevant strengths and weaknesses. As the child learns to use communication aids, it may be possible to undertake formal testing.

Ascertainment of vision and hearing should to be carried out as early as possible. In very young children indirect methods may need to be used. For children born with low birth weight and extreme prematurity, the finding of periventricular leukomalacia on brain MRI is associated with damage to the visual pathways and presents as cognitive visual impairment [25]. Children with cognitive visual impairment may have fluctuating visual function and difficulty in distinguishing objects against a background. Advice should be sought from a paediatric ophthalmologist, an orthoptist, and a teacher of the visually impaired. The educational environment and teaching materials need to be adapted to make vision easier. Acquiring safe wheelchair mobility may be more difficult for these children.

Neonatal hearing assessment is universal in the United Kingdom but conductive hearing loss may develop later in childhood. If sensorineural deafness is diagnosed, then early fitting of hearing aids should be arranged. For some children with profound deafness, a cochlear implant can be considered. The management of all these developmental difficulties requires constant review to obtain the maximum benefit for the child.

Duchenne Muscular Dystrophy

Duchenne muscular dystrophy is a sex-linked autosomal recessive disorder. It occurs only in boys. About 50% of cases arise de novo and the rest result from a mother carrying an affected X chromosome (see Chapter 16. for further details).

Management and Support

The aim of treatment is to maximize participation, to maintain mobility, and to avoid contractures and excessive weight gain. Parents may need a great deal of support and the voluntary Muscular Dystrophy Campaign group has local support workers in most areas. Genetic counseling is advised if further offspring is desired. With a carrier mother, 50% of daughters will also be carriers. They should receive counseling when appropriate.

About 30% of boys have significant learning difficulty and some develop marked behavioral problems. Developmental assessment and involvement of the local paediatric liaison mental health team may be necessary. Between the ages of around 8 and 11 years the ability to walk is lost and the child becomes wheelchair dependent. Frustration may build up if the child and family are not supported at this difficult time.

Regular stretching and exercise combat contractures in the lower limbs. Night splints to counteract plantar flexion deformity are helpful if tolerated. Swimming and hydrotherapy allow exercise with less gravitational force until quite late in the course of the disease. If contractures develop, Achilles tenotomies may be needed but must be followed by splintage to avoid recurrence. The use of a standing frame can help to maintain the feet in a plantigrade position and improve bone mineralization in the lower limbs. Nevertheless, osteopenia can lead to pathological fractures of long bones during transfers and lifting. These should be treated by minimal splintage and activity resumed as early as possible.

Maintenance of Ambulation

Evidence shows that boys who walk for longer have less need for spinal surgery [26]. Knee–ankle–foot orthoses (KAFO) can assist walking when quadriceps weakness causes sagging at the knees. Carefully monitored steroid therapy with 0.75 mg/kg/day of prednisolone orally has been shown to improve muscle strength and function in the short term (6 months to 2 years) before walking ability is lost, but adverse short-term steroid effects were identified in a recent review [27].

Management of Spinal Deformity

Refer to Chapter 16.

Respiratory Care

Weakness of the thoracic muscles and spinal deformity eventually cause a restrictive type of ventilatory defect. Coughing also becomes weaker. Regular monitoring of respiratory function will show a fall in vital capacity and since chest infections can cause serious respiratory compromise, antibiotics should be prescribed early.

Reduced oxygen saturation and retention of carbon dioxide during sleep can result in restless sleep, morning headaches, and poor concentration. After sleep studies by the respiratory team, intermittent positive pressure ventilation via a mask can be instituted, which usually results in an immediate cessation of symptoms and an increase in well-being. Eagle et al. [26] have shown that the combination of respiratory support and spinal fusion increases survival by many years and improves the quality of life (see Figs. 3.8 and 3.9).

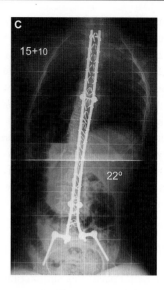

Fig. 3.9 Treated spinal deformity in Duchenne muscular dystrophy

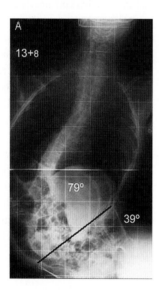

Fig. 3.8 Pre-fusion spinal deformity in Duchenne muscular dystrophy

pressure-reducing mattress can improve the quality of sleep. Eventually a night-time carer may be requested to give the parents a rest. Referral for respite stays in a children's hospice offers welcome relief to the family. The consultant responsible for the child usually has to make this referral as the service is available only for children and young people with life-limiting conditions.

Educational Support

Attendance at the local school is encouraged by recent education policies. If the school has stairs, the provision of a stair-climber chair, or moving classrooms around to avoid stairs, is usually possible. There is an increasing need for support in the classroom and for personal care. Educational legislation provides for this kind of support following comprehensive assessment. Transport to and from school is also necessary.

If there are learning difficulties, a modified curriculum and additional input for reading and number skills can be made available. A laptop computer and a scribe are provided as writing becomes more difficult. A reassessment of the support package is needed at the secondary school transfer stage to ensure a smooth transition. Teacher training and ongoing advice can be given via regular educational review meetings. If absence from school for surgery or other reasons occurs, hospital or home teaching can be instituted.

Activities of Daily Living

During the course of the disorder, the multi-disciplinary team and especially the OT must reassess the child's abilities and provide aids and adaptations to maintain independence as far as possible. Gradually the young person will become dependent for all daily activities including eating. A powered swing arm fixed to the chair should be provided as it supports the forearm and allows movement at the shoulder when eating and drinking or when touching the face and head. For toileting, a pedestal with support may be needed. A shower chair for use in a wet room makes bathing much simpler.

At night the young person may wake with discomfort and require to be turned frequently. An adjustable bed with a

Leaving School and Adult Services

When leaving school, specialist carers' advice should be sought and transition to adult services organized. Different social benefits are available to the family including funds to support the direct employment of carers in the home or at the university'. Each university or further education college has staff dedicated to helping students with additional needs. Residences now have wheelchair-friendly accommodation.

Independent living facilities for young disabled people have been developed by many voluntary housing organizations and local authorities. However, moving away from home is still a huge step for these young people and necessitates a great deal of support. Employment is often possible and successful with the help of an understanding employer.

Summary

The management of the child and young person with disability is best achieved in a team setting with the parents and the child at the center of assessment and planning. Early intervention and coordination of care are necessary to maximize the child's potential, which will be enhanced if the child is encouraged to participate in decision making. Particular attention should be paid to times of transition: from nursery to primary school, to secondary school, and to adult services.

The orthopaedic surgeon is an important member of the team and can make a significant difference to the child's quality of life and prognosis by timely and appropriate intervention.

References

1. Plioplys AV. Survival rates of children with severe neurologic disabilities: a review Sem Pediatr Neurol 2003; 10(2): 120–9.
2. Greco V, Sloper P. Care co-ordination and key worker schemes for disabled children: results of a UK-wide survey. Child Care Health Dev 2004; 30(1):13–20.
3. Greco V, Sloper P, Webb R, Beecham J. An exploration of different models of multi-agency partnerships in key worker services for disabled children: effectiveness and costs. Department for Education and Skills Research Brief, RB656. Nottingham: Department for Education and Skills Publications; 2005.
4. UK Statistics Authority. At: http://www.statistics.gov.uk/. Accessed 23 August 2008.
5. Bracewell MA, Hennessy EM, Wolke D, Marlow N. The EPICure study: growth and blood pressure at 6 years of age following extremely preterm birth. 2008; 93(2):F108–14.
6. Jan M, Girvin JP. The communication of neurological bad news to parents. Can J Neurol Sci 2002; 29(1):78–82.
7. Scope. Right from the Start template 2003. Produced with the support of the Department.
8. Contact a Family: for families of disabled children. At: http://www.cafamily.org.uk/. Accessed 23 August 2008.
9. Dobson B, Middleton S, Beardsworth A. The impact of childhood disability on family life. York, UK: Joseph Rowntree Foundation. 2001. Published for the Foundation by YPS.
10. McKay S, Atkinson A. Disability and caring among families with children, DWP Research Report No. 460. Leeds, UK: Corporate Document Services; 2007.
11. Connors C. The views and experience of disabled children and their siblings: a positive outlook. London: Jessica Kingsley Publishers; 2003.
12. Office of the High Commission for Human Rights. Convention on the Rights of the Child. Adopted and opened for signature, ratification and accession by General Assembly resolution 44/25 of 20 November 1989. At: http://www.unhchr.ch/html/menu3/b/k2crc.htm Accessed 23 August 2008.
13. Hall D, Elliman D, Joint Working Party on Child Health Surveillance (Great Britain), Health for All Children, 4th ed. Oxford, NY: Oxford University Press, 2003.
14. Warnock HM. Special Educational Needs: Report of the Committee of Enquiry into the Education of Handicapped Children and Young People. London: HMSO; 1978.
15. Dunhill Z, Zealley H, Donaghy M. Evaluation of a revised systematic approach to the assessment, registration and monitoring of children with special needs. Chief Scientists Office (CSO); 1991.
16. Johnson A. Prevalence and characteristics of children with cerebral palsy in Europe. Developmental Med Child Neurol 2002; 44(9):633–40.
17. Rankin J, Glinianaia S, Brown R, Renwick M. The changing prevalence of neural tube defects: a population-based study in the north of England, 1984–96. Northern Congenital Abnormality Survey Steering Group. Pediatr Perinat Epidemiol 2000; 14(2): 104–10.
18. Lorber J, Salfield SA. Results of selective treatment of spina bifida cystica. Arch Dis Child 1981; 56(11):822–30.
19. Zickler CF, Richardson V. Achieving continence in children with neurogenic bowel and bladder. J Pediatr Health Care 2004; 18(6):276–83.
20. Association for Spina Bifida & Hydrocephalus. At: http://www.asbah.org/ Accessed 23 August 2008.
21. Viner RM. Transition of care from pediatric to adult services: one part of improved health services for adolescents. Arch Dis Child; 2008; 93(2):160–3.
22. Strauss D, Shavelle R, Reynolds R, et al. Survival in cerebral palsy in the last 20 years: signs of improvement? Dev Med Child Neurol 2007; 49(2):86–92.
23. Jongerius PH, van Tiel P, van Limbeek J, et al. A systematic review for evidence of efficacy of anticholinergic drugs to treat drooling. Arch Dis Child 2003; 88(10):911–4.
24. Simpson RC. Smart wheelchairs: A literature review. J Rehabil Res Dev 2005; 42(4):423–36.
25. Dutton GN, Jacobson LK. Cerebral visual impairment in children. Sem Neonatol 2001; 6(6):477–85.
26. Eagle M, Bourke J, Bullock R, et al. Managing Duchenne muscular dystrophy—the additive effect of spinal surgery and home nocturnal ventilation in improving survival. Neuromuscular Disord 2007; 17(6):470–5.
27. Manzur AY, Kuntzer T, Pike M, Swan A. Glucocorticoid corticosteroids for Duchenne muscular dystrophy. Cochrane Database Syst Rev 2008;(1):CD003725.28.

Chapter 4

Anesthesia and Analgesia in Children

Edward Doyle

Anesthesia

Most children undergoing orthopaedic surgery are healthy with no intercurrent disease to complicate anesthesia. A few have significant cardiac, respiratory, or neuromuscular diseases. Local anesthetic techniques alone, without general anesthesia, are used much less often than in adult orthopaedic patients and are usually most suitable for those patients whose intercurrent disease makes general anesthesia particularly dangerous. A light general anesthetic is often supplemented by local anesthesia. This reduces the requirement for anesthetic agents and opioids during surgery and allows children to experience a rapid, pain-free recovery from operation. For most children and their families, particularly those who need multiple procedures, the main problems associated with anesthesia are pre-operative anxiety and poorly treated post-operative pain. Attention to these and, of course, the anesthetic itself is essential for the well-being of children with orthopaedic problems.

Pre-operative Preparation

A combination of psychological and pharmacological methods helps to alleviate anxiety and fear. The opportunity to visit the hospital, ward, and reception area of the operating theaters before admission may familiarize the patient and parents with what will later happen. This gives children an opportunity to watch an explanatory film of the admission and anesthetic procedures and to be given an age-appropriate explanation of what to expect. Children's hospitals have dedicated play specialists to spend time with children and to discover and reassure their apprehension and

anxiety. They also help to distract the child during induction of anesthesia. Parents are encouraged to accompany their children to the anesthetic room and to remain until their child is anesthetized. Should children remain anxious despite pre-operative preparation, then pharmacological sedation or pre-medication shortly before induction helps to create calm and cooperation. Benzodiazepines usually produce amnesia for the events immediately preceding surgery and may be particularly helpful for children who need a series of procedures, preventing unpleasant memories leading to future difficulties.

Intercurrent Conditions

Some children with orthopaedic problems have either corrected or uncorrected congenital heart disease and its pathophysiological effects may require modification of anesthetic technique. Respiratory function may be sub-optimal, particularly in children undergoing correction of severe scoliosis. Pre-operative physiotherapy may help but only a little. As respiratory function may be further impaired by major surgery, some patients will require post-operative ventilation in an intensive care unit until their respiratory function improves sufficiently to allow extubation. A variety of conditions requiring orthopaedic surgery are associated with neuromuscular diseases that increase sensitivity to opioids and increase the risk of post-operative respiratory depression. These include the muscular dystrophies, myotonia dystrophica, and arthrogryposis. Miscellaneous conditions that may complicate anesthesia are osteogenesis imperfecta, syndactyly, juvenile rheumatoid arthritis, and cervical spine anomalies, such as the Klippel–Feil syndrome, which may make airway management and endotracheal intubation difficult.

In patients undergoing anesthesia for emergency surgery after trauma, there is a risk of pulmonary aspiration of gastric contents. Whenever possible operation should be delayed until the following day to allow gastric emptying. Immediate

E. Doyle (✉)
Royal Hospital for Sick Children, Edinburgh, UK
e-mail: edoyle2@nhs.net

M. Benson et al. (eds.), *Children's Orthopaedics and Fractures*,
DOI 10.1007/978-1-84882-611-3_4, © Springer-Verlag London Limited 2010

surgery should be undertaken only if delay will compromise the outcome. Whenever possible and feasible children at risk of aspiration should undergo a rapid sequence induction of anesthesia to synchronize the onset of muscle relaxation and endotracheal intubation and to minimize the chances of aspiration.

Airway Management

As many orthopaedic operations are on the limbs, most are amenable to local anesthetic/analgesic techniques. Neuromuscular blockade, intermittent positive pressure ventilation, and large doses of opioids are relatively unusual. This means that many elective cases need no endotracheal intubation and the airway may be maintained during anesthesia with a laryngeal mask. This soft, flexible form of airway sits in the pharynx and allows the patient to breathe, unlike an endotracheal tube which is passed through the larynx and vocal cords to lie in the trachea. Endotracheal intubation requires a deep level of anesthesia or neuromuscular blockade, unlike a laryngeal mask airway. The use of a laryngeal mask airway avoids some of the complications which may be caused by endotracheal intubation, particularly laryngeal irritation and its resulting post-operative laryngeal spasm, hypoxia, and croup. It is particularly important to avoid these complications in patients undergoing day-case surgery (see Fig. 4.1).

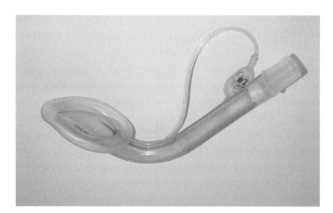

Fig. 4.1 Laryngeal mask airway

Pharmacokinetics

For those infants who need an operation in their first 6 months, drug elimination is very variable owing to diminished clearances and prolonged half-lives. The volume of distribution of opioids and local anesthetics is greater than in older children and there are reduced plasma protein concentrations (especially α-1-acid glycoprotein) with consequently high levels of free drug. Clinically, there is an increased sensitivity to the depressant effects of anesthetic agents and opioids in the first 6 months. The rate of metabolism and elimination of local anesthetic agents is slower. These factors make it necessary to reduce dosages, have longer intervals between doses, or reduce infusion rates for anesthetic and analgesic drugs in the young. Modern volatile agents such as desflurane and opioids such as remifentanil are very rapidly eliminated or metabolized even in neonates and infants. Their use, along with appropriate monitoring techniques, has reduced the risks traditionally associated with anesthetizing very young children.

Venous Access

In many children, gaining adequate venous access for the intra- and post-operative periods may be a major challenge. In well-nourished infants, especially those who will be put into a hip spica or bilateral leg plasters, there are limited options for venous access. When cannulation fails in the upper limbs, the external jugular or scalp veins may be used. Unfortunately, these may not prove long-lasting post-operatively and central venous access via an internal jugular vein may be needed.

Cannulation of the internal jugular vein is difficult in infants because of their relatively short necks. The technique of insertion is similar to the adult except that shorter needles and catheters are used. The right side is preferred when possible. The internal jugular vein lies deep to the sternocleidomastoid muscle and passes from just anterior to the mastoid process to behind the sternoclavicular joint. The internal jugular vein, superior vena cava, and right atrium are in line on the right and correct placement of the tip is almost guaranteed. On the left side the catheter tip frequently ends up in a sub-optimal position and the thoracic duct is at risk. The child is positioned head down with the head turned to the contra-lateral side with a roll or a bolster under the shoulders. The carotid artery is identified and the needle is inserted just lateral to it at an angle of 30° to the skin surface and directed toward the ipsilateral nipple while aspirating gently. The end point is aspiration of venous blood into the syringe. A standard Seldinger technique is then used to place the definitive catheter.

Ultrasound is now very commonly used to guide the insertion of central lines and in most institutions is preferred to the landmark-guided technique. The ultrasound probe identifies the vein before or provides real-time imaging during needle insertion. Its advantages include defining the anatomy, confirming that a patent vein is present, checking the position of the artery, and guiding the needle into the vein.

The complications which may follow attempted internal jugular cannulation include the generic complications of central venous access (air embolus, hematoma, thrombosis, sepsis) and those peculiar to the site of insertion (carotid artery puncture, pneumothorax, hemothorax, damage to the brachial plexus, phrenic nerve, and, on the left, the thoracic duct).

For children in whom the groins are accessible, the femoral veins are usually easier to cannulate and offer central venous access with fewer potential complications.

In emergencies, intraosseous access may be used in place of intravenous access: a short, wide-bore cannula is inserted through the cortex into the medulla of a long bone. The commonest site is the anterior surface of the tibia 1 cm below the tuberosity to avoid the growth plate. This allows immediate fluid resuscitation and drug administration until adequate venous access is secured at a more leisurely pace. Unlike venous access and particularly central venous access, intraosseous access requires no special expertise and may be performed by anyone appropriately trained. This technique is widely used in paediatric emergency departments.

Tourniquets

The pH and the oxygen tension fall steadily and the lactate and the carbon dioxide tension increase in the exsanguinated limb. After tourniquet deflation the products of anaerobic metabolism are released into the circulation and can cause a transient, mixed respiratory and metabolic acidosis. Acid metabolites are buffered by bicarbonate with the production of carbon dioxide and there may be a temporary increase in arterial and end-tidal carbon dioxide tension in the region of 0.5–1.5 kPa. These effects are greater if two limbs rather than one are exsanguinated, if the legs rather than arms are involved, and if the tourniquet has been applied for a long time. Tourniquets reduce the effective body surface area available to dissipate heat and may occasionally cause the body temperature to rise. There may be local adverse pressure effects and blistering, especially if alcohol preparation lies beneath the tourniquet. Recommendations for safe tourniquet use emphasize its use for less than 90 min and an increase in pulmonary ventilation just before and after release to enhance the elimination of excess carbon dioxide.

Depth of Anesthesia

Monitoring the depth of anesthesia to reduce the risk of awareness and aid the titration of anesthetic drugs against

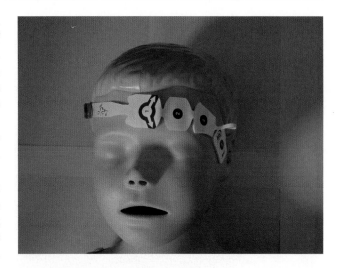

Fig. 4.2 Positioning of the BIS electrode

need is now common in children over 1 year. This is referred to as Bispectral Index^{TM} Monitoring (BIS); a processed electroencephalogram (EEG) parameter that measures the hypnotic effects of anesthetic and sedative agents on the brain. The BIS value is derived from the EEG by a computer algorithm that produces a single numerical value, scaled from 0 to 100, which reflects a patient's state of hypnosis and unresponsiveness.

Practically, BIS involves placing an adhesive electrode strip on the forehead and connecting this by a cable to a compact monitor. The monitor screen displays a value for the BIS and a trend line over time. A value of 100 is seen in the normal awake state; 0 reflects absence of any EEG activity; 80 corresponds to sedation (response to command); and 45–60 corresponds to general anesthesia. Adjusting anesthetic delivery to maintain BIS values within the target range of 45–60 reduces the consumption of anesthetic agents and speeds emergence from anesthesia. The technique is particularly useful in scoliosis surgery, where the need for evoked potential monitoring limits the range of possible anesthetic agents. It is also valuable when using total intravenous anesthesia to minimize the risk of awareness (see Figs. 4.2 and 4.3).

Fluid Balance and Intravenous Fluids

Water turnover in infants is more than double that of adults and approximately 40% of extracellular water is lost every day as urine, stool, sweat, and insensible losses via the skin, airways, and lungs. Dehydration can easily follow a reduction in intake or an increased fluid loss in the peri-operative period (see Table 4.1).

The clinical assessment of fluid balance in children is aided by recognizing those situations where deficits are

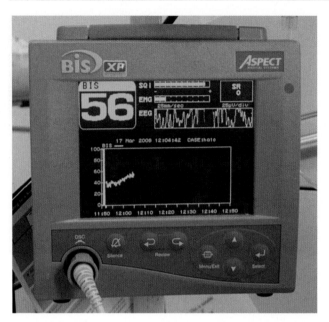

Fig. 4.3 BIS monitor display showing numeric value for BIS, signal quality indicator, and BIS trend over time

Table 4.1 Extracellular volume and blood volume with age

	Extracellular volume (% body weight)	Blood volume (ml/kg)
Premature neonate	60	100
Term neonate	40–45	90
One year	25–30	80
Adult	18	70

likely, such as trauma, intra-, and post-operative bleeding. Hypovolemia and dehydration are diagnosed clinically by

- tachycardia (can also be caused by pain, fever, and anxiety)
- cool peripheries
- capillary refill time of over 2 s
- sunken fontanelle
- thready pulse
- increased core–peripheral temperature gradient
- oliguria
- reduced level of consciousness

Children compensate very well for hypovolemia and hypotension is a late sign that often occurs only after over 30% of the blood volume is lost. Shock is the clinical state when demand is higher than the delivery of oxygen and nutrition to the cells.

Pre-operative Fluids and Fluid Resuscitation

During the pre-operative period, extracellular fluid losses are replaced with isotonic crystalloid solutions such as 0.9% saline or Hartmann's solution. Blood volume is estimated at 90 ml/kg in neonates, 85 ml/kg in infants, and 80 ml/kg in children. Circulating volume is replaced with crystalloids or colloids (plasma protein solution, Gelfusine, or a starch solution). Blood products are given for major or ongoing losses. For shock, the child is given fluid boluses of 20 ml/kg of crystalloid or colloid and then reassessed. Blood is usually given after 15–20% of the circulating volume is lost and fresh frozen plasma and platelets in addition after the loss of 50% of the circulating volume.

Intra-operative Fluid Administration

Intra-operative fluids are required to replace any fluid deficit, to provide maintenance requirements, and to replace intra-operative losses. Fluid deficits are rarely a problem for elective cases. Current fasting times are relatively brief and intravenous fluids are given to children unable to drink. Some non-elective cases may come to theater with a fluid deficit but in most cases this should be dealt with during pre-operative resuscitation and preparation.

Maintenance fluids during surgery can be given as a dextrose-containing solution or as a dextrose-free crystalloid (e.g., Hartmann's solution or 0.9% saline). Dextrose-free solutions are currently preferred. Glucose-containing fluids are usually unnecessary other than in neonates and some at-risk children such as those receiving parenteral nutrition. Hypoglycemia is rare in healthy children during anesthesia and surgery. Most children show an increase in plasma glucose concentration during the peri-operative period as part of the response to fasting and surgery. Fluids containing 4% or 5% dextrose usually cause hyperglycemia during surgery. Glucose-containing solutions are isotonic when administered but once the glucose is metabolized they become hypotonic and effectively result in the administration of free water. There is a risk of hyponatremia if hypotonic solutions are given. Antidiuretic hormone is secreted during the peri-operative period and further reduces plasma sodium concentration and osmolarity. Children develop hyponatremia more readily than adults and are more susceptible to its effects on the central nervous system. This is now considered to be a major risk in the peri-operative care of children. Most fluid losses during surgery are isotonic. Losses are replaced with crystalloid, colloid, or blood products depending upon the clinical situation.

Post-operative or Maintenance Fluid Regimens

Neonates

Fluid and electrolyte requirements during the first 5 days of life are the following:

- Day 1, 60 ml/kg/day
- Day 2, 90 ml/kg/day
- Day 3, 120 ml/kg/day
- Day 4, 150 ml/kg/day
- Day 5, 150 ml/kg/day
- Sodium, 2–4 mmol/kg/day
- Potassium, 2–3 mmol/kg/day

Dextrose requirements are usually provided using a 10% solution for maintenance.

Infants and Children

A common formula is the 4–2–1 regimen:

- 4 ml/kg for the first 10 kg
- plus 2 ml/kg for next 10 kg
- plus 1 ml/kg thereafter

When this formula is used, a child of 17 kg requires 54 ml/h (40 + 14) and a child of 24 kg requires 64 ml/h (40 + 20 + 4).

Electrolyte requirements are the following:

- Sodium, 2–4 mmol/kg/day
- Potassium, 2–3 mmol/kg/day

Common solutions for intravenous maintenance are the following:

- 0.45% saline/5% dextrose
- 0.45% saline/2.5% dextrose
- 0.225% sodium/5% glucose
- 0.18% sodium/4% glucose
- 10% dextrose is commonly used in premature children and neonates

Fluids should be administered through a volumetric pump with a pressure limit set. Monitoring of electrolyte concentrations is required if intravenous maintenance fluids are given for more than 24–48 h. The formulae described are only a guide and generally overestimate fluid requirements. Under these circumstances, electrolyte derangements can occur. Hyponatremia is a particular risk and may be devastating. Some anesthetists restrict maintenance fluids to 50–75% of the calculated requirement during the post-operative period to reduce the risk of these problems. Fortunately, most children undergoing orthopaedic surgery are able to resume oral intake early after operation and thus avoid the potential risks associated with prolonged intravenous fluid administration.

Post-operative Analgesia

Giving children adequate post-operative analgesia is very rewarding. Most operations are peripheral and the absence of prolonged post-operative ileus allows oral drugs and a multi-modal approach to be used for most. Dense intra-operative analgesia provided by a local anesthetic technique means that a light general anesthetic is possible. This reduces the requirement for anesthetic agents and opioids during surgery and allows children to experience a rapid, pain-free recovery with little or no post-operative vomiting. Children can quickly resume oral intake and, as long as adequate oral analgesia is both prescribed and administered before the local anesthetic block wears off, the post-operative course is usually smooth. In general, it is preferable to prescribe oral analgesic drugs on a regular as opposed to an "as required" basis for at least 24 h. This ensures timely administration of analgesia and avoids unnecessary delays in its administration. If parents have to ask for medication and then nurses verify that the child is sore before analgesia is given, the beneficial effect is sub-optimal.

Children's pain may be treated physically, psychologically, and pharmacologically. Simple measures such as warmth and early feeding help. The presence of parents, reassurance, and distraction are important. Older children should be given a simple explanation of what is to happen and an assurance that any pain will be treated quickly. The main groups of drugs used for analgesia after surgery or trauma are the same as in adults: local anesthetics, opioids, and non-steroidal anti-inflammatory drugs (NSAID) including paracetamol.

While mild pain of brief duration can be treated with a single analgesic, it is usually impossible to provide adequate pain relief with one type of analgesic after major surgery or trauma, when analgesia has traditionally been provided by systemic opioid administration. It is difficult to provide complete analgesia using opioids alone without a significant risk of side effects including respiratory depression, nausea, and oversedation. Multi-modal or combined analgesic regimens are better. It is preferable to use two or more analgesic drugs such as a local anesthetic block plus an opioid or a combination of opioid, local anesthesia technique, and an NSAID.

Table 4.2 Post-operative analgesia

Severe pain
- Epidural infusion of local anesthetic solution and opioid started in theater and continued post-operatively
- Single injection local anesthetic technique given in theater and followed post-operatively by a combination of intravenous opioid, NSAID, and paracetamol
- Intravenous opioid given in theater and followed post-operatively by a combination of intravenous opioid, NSAID, and paracetamol
Whenever possible opioid, NSAID, and paracetamol should be used together if there are no contraindications

Moderate pain
- Single injection local anesthetic technique given in theater and followed post-operatively by a combination of oral opioid (morphine sulfate or codeine phosphate), NSAID, and paracetamol
- Intravenous opioid given in theater and followed post-operatively by a combination of oral opioid, NSAID, and paracetamol
This combination of oral opioid, NSAID, and paracetamol should be used after major surgery when intravenous opioids are no longer required

Mild pain
- Paracetamol may be given with oral opioid and an NSAID

These combinations tend to have synergistic effects and provide equivalent or superior analgesia to that obtained with opioids alone but with smaller doses and fewer side effects (see Table 4.2).

Local Anesthetic Techniques

Several local anesthetic techniques combined with general anesthesia play a major role in providing good analgesia for children. Dense analgesia will last into the post-operative period and reduce the requirements for anesthetic agents and opioids. Local anesthetic techniques include infiltration of the surgical field, single nerve blockade, plexus blockade, and central neuraxial blockade (epidural and spinal analgesia). Local anesthetics produce a lack of sensation, which may distress children if this has not been explained beforehand, and present a potential risk of injuries from incorrect positioning of a limb, plaster cast pressure sores, or a compartment syndrome.

The drug of choice for a local anesthetic technique is usually a long-acting amide-type local anesthetic such as ropivacaine (*Naropin*®) or levobupivacaine (*Chirocaine*®), the pure levo- or S-enantiomer of bupivacaine. These have a longer duration of action than lidocaine and are marginally safer in the event of intravenous injection or overdose than racemic bupivacaine (*Marcain*®). The main exceptions are topical cutaneous anesthesia (*EMLA*® cream or amethocaine gel) and Bier's block where prilocaine is the local anesthetic of choice.

Topical Cutaneous Anesthesia

The use of topical cutaneous anesthesia prior to venepuncture is an essential part of anesthesia for elective surgery. This is particularly important for children who will undergo a series of surgical procedures. *EMLA* cream (a eutectic mixture of lidocaine and prilocaine) is an effective topical anesthetic preparation with a very low incidence of side effects. It should be applied 2 h before venepuncture to ensure efficacy. There is also a preparation of amethocaine (*Ametop*®) that has a shorter onset time of 40 min and a longer duration of action than *EMLA* cream. One of these preparations should be used in every child undergoing venepuncture or blood sampling.

Infiltration Analgesia

Infiltration techniques are widely used in paediatric surgery, particularly those limited to the body surface. Local infiltration under direct vision is a technique which can be carried out simply, without the identification of landmarks or knowledge of the anatomy of nerves. However, analgesia is limited to the skin and superficial tissues and for anything other than superficial procedures it is insufficient as the sole analgesic technique.

Bier's Block

Intravenous regional anesthesia (IVRA or Bier's block) is an effective anesthetic technique in older children. The limb is exsanguinated and a tourniquet is inflated to 50 mmHg above systolic blood pressure. Prilocaine (7 mg/kg) is the local anesthetic of choice for this technique and is injected via an intravenous cannula placed distal to the operative site. The tourniquet should be left inflated for a minimum of 20 min even if the surgical procedure is shorter than this. The main limitation to this technique is the tolerance of the patient for the tourniquet, which limits its use to procedures of 30–60-min duration.

Peripheral Nerve Blockade

Digital Nerve Block

This is a simple and effective technique for procedures limited to single digits. In the hand, 0.5–1 ml of 0.25 or 0.5%

levobupivacaine is injected on either side of the base of the digit keeping the needle at right angles to the plane of the hand. This allows both palmar and dorsal branches to be blocked. A similar technique is employed for blockade of the toes although metatarsal block may be more effective. For this the needle is introduced on the dorsal surface of the foot and directed toward the sole passing the side of the metatarsal bone in the space to be blocked. Prior to the sole being punctured, the needle is aspirated and local anesthetic is deposited as the needle is slowly withdrawn. The process is repeated on the other side of the metatarsal. Similar volumes of local anesthetic are used. Adrenaline should not be used because of the risk of vasoconstriction and ischemic damage.

Lower Limb Blocks

Two of the most common indications are fractured shaft of the femur and surgery below the knee. Femoral nerve blockade is used for the former, while both sciatic and femoral nerve blockade are usually required for adequate analgesia after surgery below the knee.

Femoral Nerve Block

This may be performed as a single injection technique (with or without a nerve stimulator) below the inguinal ligament lateral to the femoral artery. The technique has the benefit of simplicity. Continuous femoral nerve blockade by means of an indwelling catheter may be used as an analgesic technique for fractures of the femur to avoid the use of opioids in patients with head injuries.

Sciatic Nerve Block

Blocking the sciatic nerve provides anesthesia of the anterolateral leg and the foot. If used in combination with a saphenous or femoral nerve block, full anesthesia of the leg below the knee is obtained. There are three principal approaches to the proximal sciatic nerve: posterior, anterior, and lateral. The posterior approach is the most commonly used: the patient lies supine with the thigh and the knee flexed to 90°; the sciatic nerve lies midway between a line drawn between the greater trochanter and the ischial tuberosity.

As the leg is flexed, the nerve tends to be fixed in a groove against the pelvis as it emerges from the greater sciatic foramen. The use of a nerve stimulator elicits dorsiflexion of the foot and allows safe identification of the nerve. A short-beveled stimulating needle is introduced and is advanced while a stimulus of 1 mA is produced each second. Once

dorsiflexion is obtained the needle should be localized to the nerve by reducing the stimulating current to approximately 0.5 mA. If the sciatic nerve is blocked at the buttock, the back of the thigh will be anesthetized due to the proximity of the posterior cutaneous nerve of the thigh.

The sciatic nerve or its terminal branches may also be blocked more distally in the popliteal fossa. This approach is most suitable for operations on the ankle or the foot when it is usually combined with a saphenous or a femoral nerve block. The patient is positioned prone or lateral (operative side uppermost). A line between the midpoint of the popliteal crease and the apex of the popliteal fossa is identified and the popliteal artery palpated. The needle of the peripheral nerve stimulator is inserted perpendicular to the skin just lateral to the arterial pulsation. Plantar flexion and inversion indicate tibial nerve stimulation; dorsiflexion and eversion indicate stimulation of the common peroneal nerve. The most reliable method of identifying the sciatic division is by using ultrasound as this improves the success rate of the block to virtually 100%. About 0.3–0.5 ml/kg of 0.25 or 0.5% levobupivacaine is appropriate.

Fascia Iliaca Compartment Block

The fascia iliaca compartment block has been described as an alternative to femoral nerve block and the *3-in-1* block for unilateral analgesia in the thigh. The technique involves passing a needle from an insertion point 1 cm below the lateral inguinal ligament through the fascia lata and fascia iliaca and injecting local anesthetic into the potential space between the iliacus muscle and the fascia iliaca. This solution moves cephalad and blocks the femoral, lateral cutaneous, and obturator nerves as they emerge from psoas. This block has been shown to have a significantly higher success rate (95%) than the 3-in-1 block (20%) in children [1], although blockade of the obturator nerve is less consistent than that of the femoral and lateral cutaneous nerves. It is an excellent block for children undergoing femoral osteotomy or removal of a femoral blade plate. The fascia iliaca compartment block does not require a nerve stimulator or the production of paraesthesia. The injection site is distant from blood vessels and nerves so that the chances of inadvertent nerve injury or intravascular injection of local anesthetic are remote.

Ankle Block

An ankle block requires injection of local anesthetic solution around the saphenous, posterior tibial, sural, deep peroneal, and superficial peroneal nerves. The technique provides analgesia to the foot and is suitable for procedures such as osteotomy of the first metatarsal and distal tendon transfers.

All the injections are superficial, side effects are rare, and special equipment is not required. It is, therefore, quick and simple. The injection to the sural nerve may be omitted for medial surgery and that to the saphenous nerve for lateral procedures.

Plexus Blockade

Brachial Plexus Blockade

Upper limb blockade is usually carried out by the axillary route since this is free of the risks of pneumothorax, phrenic, and recurrent laryngeal nerve block that are associated with the supraclavicular and parascalene techniques. The axillary approach to the brachial plexus is particularly valuable in hand and forearm procedures. More proximal brachial plexus blocks will provide analgesia of the shoulder and may include areas innervated by the cervical plexus. Analgesia of the ulnar nerve distribution may, however, be less predictable. Unsupplemented brachial plexus blocks will be tolerated by few children and are most useful as an adjunct to general anesthesia. The technique is usually contraindicated if there is a risk of a post-operative compartment syndrome.

Lumbar (Psoas) Plexus Blockade

This uses a posterior approach to the lumbar plexus. The anterior rami of the lumbar nerve roots (and T12) enter psoas and merge within it to form the lumbar (psoas) plexus and thence the ilioinguinal, hypogastric, obturator, femoral, and lateral cutaneous nerve of thigh. This plexus can be approached through the quadratus lumborum and the posterior part of the psoas muscle. The aim is to anesthetize the lumbar plexus and some of the sacral plexus by injecting local anesthetic solution between the quadratus lumborum and the psoas major muscles. It produces analgesia in the distributions of the obturator and femoral nerves and the lateral cutaneous nerve of thigh, with some upper branches of the sciatic plexus also being affected. The distribution of this block is similar to that of a 3-in-1 block or a fascia iliaca compartment block. Indications are unilateral procedures on the hip, femur, thigh, or knee. It may be a good choice following previous hip surgery as adhesions can limit the spread of local anesthetic through the tissue planes required for a 3-in-1 block or a fascia iliaca compartment block.

The patient is positioned laterally with the hips and knees flexed to 90° and the operative side uppermost. The insertion point is at the intersection of the intercristal line (superior borders of both iliac crests) and a paraspinous line passing through the ipsilateral posterior superior iliac spine. The

insulated needle of a peripheral nerve stimulator is inserted perpendicular to the skin and then advanced with a slight medial direction. The needle is advanced until it makes contact with the transverse process of L5, then "walked off" the cranial border until either contractions of the quadriceps are visible or a loss of resistance is felt as the needle exits the anterior edge of quadratus lumborum. Either of these end points should be reached within 20 mm of contacting the transverse process.

Central Neuraxial Blocks

Epidural Analgesia

The availability of small gauge epidural needles and fine epidural catheters makes epidural analgesia feasible in the smallest of children. Single injection and infusion epidural analgesia are popular, often permitting light anesthesia, minimal opioid use, and early extubation of the trachea. Physiological differences between adults and children, namely a reduced sympathetic tone and a reduced blood volume in the splanchnic circulation and lower limbs in children, result in remarkable cardiovascular stability in infants undergoing high central neuraxial blockade which in adults would cause hypotension because of sympathetic blockade.

The epidural space in children may be approached at thoracic, lumbar, sacral, or caudal levels. Up to the age of 6–12 months it is usually possible to cannulate the epidural space via the caudal hiatus, which avoids the potential complications of higher approaches.

The main concern during epidural infusions is to keep the total dose of local anesthetic low to minimize the possibility of systemic toxicity. In general, an opioid is required in addition to local anesthetic after major surgery. This acts synergistically with the local anesthetic to improve analgesia and to reduce the requirement for local anesthetics. It also treats discomfort not blocked by the epidural and provides mild sedation.

Side Effects

Epidural analgesia requires close nursing supervision. Potential side effects include urinary retention, leg weakness, and intravenous or subarachnoid injection. Hypotension is rarely a problem, especially in children below 8 years, but the lack of sensation may cause problems if not anticipated. Pressure sores may occur in analgesic skin unless patients are repositioned regularly. Following trauma, the technique is generally contraindicated because of the possibility of a compartment syndrome. Urinary retention occurs with an incidence of 11% in patients receiving epidural infusions of 0.125% bupivacaine and diamorphine [2], and this often needs urinary catheterization which itself has a low but definite risk of complications.

Caudal Epidural Analgesia

A single injection of local anesthetic into the epidural space via the caudal approach combines the advantages of simplicity with a high success rate. It is one of the commonest local anesthetic techniques used in children's anesthesia. The technique has a wide range of indications including lower limb and pelvic orthopaedic surgery. Several large series describe its high success rate and low incidence of complications. Injection is made through the sacral hiatus (formed by a deficiency in the neural arch of the fifth sacral vertebra and covered by the sacrococcygeal membrane). The landmarks for this hiatus are the sacral cornua superiorly and the coccyx inferiorly. Under aseptic conditions, a needle is advanced through the sacrococcygeal membrane until a pop or loss of resistance is felt. After a negative aspiration test, the selected dose of local anesthetic solution is injected slowly (see Fig. 4.4).

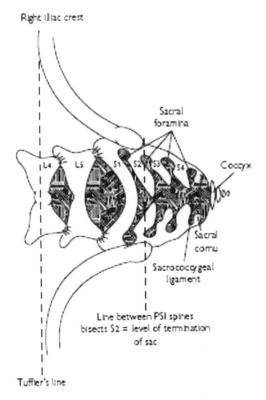

Fig. 4.4 Sacral anatomy at 8 years. From: Bell G. Regional anaesthetic techniques: central blocks. In. Doyle E. Paediatric Anaesthesia. Oxford: Oxford University Press; 2007:201. By permission of Oxford University Press

Side Effects

Failure of the technique is usually caused by failure to inject the local anesthetic into the correct space. The primary determinant of this is the experience of the anesthetist: the "failed caudal" may be due to an inappropriate indication with the use of an inadequate volume to block the required nerve roots. In older children the technique may fail due to the development of fibrous septa within the epidural space. These may result in unilateral or limited blocks despite appropriate volume injections. Weakness of the legs is common and may be found in over 30% of subjects given 0.5% bupivacaine. Motor block is less frequent when more dilute solutions of local anesthetic are used. It is often unnecessary for the child to walk in the first few post-operative hours.

Spinal (Subarachnoid) Anesthesia

Subarachnoid anesthesia may be used in high-risk patients including those with congenital abnormalities and muscular and neuromuscular disease as these conditions increase operative and anesthetic risk.

Ultrasound-Guided Nerve Blocks

The use of ultrasound (10–15 MHz) to help perform some peripheral nerve and nerve plexus blocks is now common and is likely soon to become the norm. Recent advances in ultrasound technology enable imaging of neural structures with good resolution and image quality. When imaged in the transverse view, nerves appear round or oval with a characteristic honeycomb appearance. Longitudinal imaging shows parallel longitudinal fibers. Ultrasound allows accurate identification of nerves or plexuses, helps to guide the blocking needle to the target structure while avoiding adjacent structures such as blood vessels, and assesses the spread of local anesthetic solution around the nerve or the plexus. It will also identify intra-neural injection at an early stage and allow the injection to be terminated quickly. Outcome data suggest that ultrasound guidance improves the success rate for many nerve and plexus blocks and reduces the time of onset and the volume of local anesthetic required [3, 4].

Brachial plexus blockade is well suited to an ultrasound-guided approach. The plexus is relatively superficial and therefore easy to image. The technique is also useful when blocking the femoral nerve in the groin and the sciatic nerve proximally or in the popliteal fossa (see Fig. 4.5).

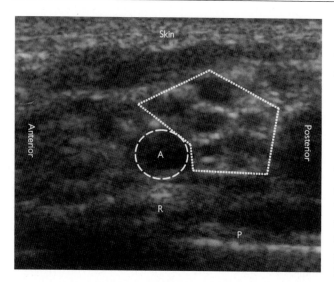

Fig. 4.5 Ultrasonographic appearance of the brachial plexus (*dotted area*) showing the proximity of the pleura (P), the rib (R), and the subclavian artery (A). From: Roberts S. Regional anaesthetic techniques: peripheral blocks. In: Doyle E. Paediatric Anaesthesia. Oxford: Oxford University Press; 2007:185. By permission of Oxford University Press

Opioids

The most commonly used opioid is morphine and there is more experience with this than with any other opioid. As well as producing analgesia, all opioids cause a similar spectrum of side effects. They have the disadvantage of a relatively narrow therapeutic range and marked variability in response between patients because of differing pharmacokinetics and pharmacodynamics. This is particularly marked in children under 6 months as drug elimination is very variable owing to diminished clearance and prolonged half-life. There is also an increased sensitivity to their depressant effects. Nevertheless, it is still possible to provide excellent analgesia with safety in these infants if sensible dosage regimens and appropriate monitoring procedures are used. There are, of course, some older children who, because of specific conditions or sensitivities, are particularly susceptible to the depressant effects of opioids. These include those with severe respiratory disease, upper airway obstruction, and renal or hepatic impairment. The concurrent administration of other centrally acting sedative drugs, such as benzodiazepines, puts any child at considerable risk of oversedation and respiratory depression. These drugs should rarely be administered concurrently.

The intermittent intramuscular administration of opioids is no longer used in children. It produces fluctuating plasma concentrations and periods of analgesia and excessive sedation alternating with periods of inadequate pain relief. The intermittent administration of intravenous bolus doses of

an opioid on an as-required basis provides extremely good analgesia with a high degree of safety and is particularly useful in the post-operative recovery area and the emergency department.

Opioids by Infusion

The technique of continuous intravenous infusion of an opioid solution is popular because of its efficacy, simplicity, and wide range of indications. Continuous infusion will maintain a steady blood concentration of opioids once equilibration is reached. A loading dose is required to avoid the prolonged period of 4–5 half-lives required to reach a steady state. Dosages in the range 10–40 µg/kg/h of morphine are adequate in most patients and infusions are usually started in the middle of this range for children over 6 months and at 5–10 µg/kg/h for the younger child. The effective use of intravenous infusions requires close nursing supervision so that the infusion rate is adequate and titrated against changing requirements during mobilization and physiotherapy.

An alternative way to deliver a continuous infusion of an opioid is the subcutaneous route. This technique has been shown to be effective in adults and children. It is subject to the same potential dangers as the intravenous route.

Patient-Controlled Analgesia

Patient-controlled analgesia (PCA) allows the patient to self-administer bolus doses of opioid with a degree of flexibility within the prescription: this sets the bolus dose administered, the obligatory delay between boluses (lockout interval), and the presence or absence of a background infusion. Most machines have an infusion pump with software which allows a trigger device to deliver bolus doses with or without a variable background infusion.

When used appropriately, PCA has the potential to provide good flexible analgesia which takes into account the changing needs of patients: uncomfortable events, such as physiotherapy and mobilization, are managed with a prophylactic bolus. The technique adjusts for the great variability between patients of pain perception and their pharmacokinetic and pharmacodynamic sensitivity. Children are able to self-administer safely within the prescription limits without reference to medical or nursing staff.

Selection for PCA depends on a number of features including the age of the child, developmental stage, and intelligence. The absolute requirements are the ability to understand the concepts of demand analgesia and a lockout interval, and to be physically able to operate the trigger

Table 4.3 Common dilutions and dosages for the use of morphine sulfate

Technique	Dilution	Dose
Bolus dose IV	–	100–200 μg/kg
Intravenous infusion	1 mg/kg in 50 ml 0.9% saline (20 μg/kg/ml)	10–40 μg/kg/h (0.5–2 ml/h); 5–20 μg/kg/h under 6 months
Subcutaneous infusion	1 mg/kg in 20 ml 0.9% saline (50 μg/kg/ml)	10–40 μg/kg/h (0.2–0.8 ml/h)
PCA	1 mg/kg in 50 ml 0.9% saline (20 μg/kg/ml)	Bolus dose 20 μg/kg (1 ml); lockout interval 5 min
NCA	1 mg/kg in 50 ml saline (20 μg/kg/ml)	Infusion 10 μg/kg/h (0.5 ml/h); bolus dose 20–40 μg/kg (1–2 ml); lockout 20 min
Oral	–	300 μg/kg 4 hourly

of the PCA machine. With adequate explanation and post-operative supervision, many children aged 8 years and above can use PCA appropriately. Sensible use of a PCA machine requires pre-operative tuition of the parent(s) and child and post-operative reinforcement of this tuition, particularly of the lockout interval concept.

A successful variation of PCA has been nurse-controlled analgesia. With this technique a modest infusion of morphine (10–20 μg/kg/h) is supplemented by boluses (10–20 μg/kg) given at the discretion of the nurse caring for the child with a lockout interval. This offers the advantages of a basal level of analgesia which can be supplemented as required and titrated to the needs of the child. It has the further advantage of requiring an obligatory assessment by the nurse before opioid boluses are administered. When used appropriately, nurse-controlled analgesia is very effective and safe, combining some of the better features of both fixed infusions and PCA (see Table 4.3).

Monitoring

The potential problems with opioid infusions or PCA may be divided into those due to medical and nursing errors, misuse by the patient or others, and faults in the equipment. These make it necessary to have a monitoring protocol to detect potential problems early and to provide warnings which can be acted upon to prevent the situation from deteriorating. We need to measure respiratory depression or hypoventilation, to assess the level of sedation or consciousness, the amount of opioid consumed, and the machine performance. The intermittent recording of respiratory rate has been shown to be a late and insensitive monitor of hypoventilation and this cannot be relied upon to give early warning. Pulse oximetry

while breathing air is a more sensitive monitor of hypoventilation [5] and in the absence of other causes of hypoxia, such as impaired gas exchange, mild hypoxia [arterial oxygen saturation $(S_pO_2) < 94\%$] indicates mild hypoventilation.

Somnolence caused by opioids tends to occur early and is a valuable early warning of excessive opioid administration. When used in conjunction with pulse oximetry it helps to discriminate between the possible causes of hypoxia. The components of the Glasgow Coma Scale which relate to eye opening are used to score sedation.

It is essential to regularly check the performance of the infusion pump or the PCA machine to ensure that appropriate doses of opioid are being administered.

Nonsteroidal Anti-inflammatory Drugs

There are several groups of NSAIDs which exert their analgesic effect by means of an anti-inflammatory action, specifically the inhibition of the enzyme cyclo-oxygenase, to reduce the synthesis of the inflammatory mediators: prostaglandins, thromboxane, and prostacyclin. Their efficacy has been well described in minor surgery when used alone or in combination with local anesthesia where they prolong the effective duration of regional blocks [6] and in combination with opioids after major orthopaedic surgery when they exert a useful opioid-sparing effect (a 30% reduction in requirements) [7]. The limitations of NSAIDs are their relative lack of potency, with a ceiling effect on the analgesia provided. This makes them inadequate as the single analgesic technique after intermediate and major surgery.

Adverse effects of NSAIDs include impaired platelet function, bronchospasm, and renal impairment. Prostaglandins inhibit gastric acid secretion and stimulate the production of mucus. Blood flow to the gastric mucosa is reduced by inhibitors of prostaglandin synthesis and this may play a part in the spectrum of gastric effects which NSAIDs produce including erosions, petechiae, and ulcers. In paediatric practice the potential side effects of these drugs rarely cause problems. Most anesthetists and orthopaedic surgeons are prepared to use these drugs for most types of orthopaedic surgery, provided there are no specific contraindications. Commonly used and effective NSAIDs are diclofenac sodium and ibuprofen.

Paracetamol in a dose of 15 mg/kg 4 hourly is a useful analgesic in many forms of minor surgery or non-specific pain. Its anti-pyretic effect is of great value and will not prevent the recognition of post-operative infective complications. It is effective and safe in neonates. The drug has a wide therapeutic ratio and few contraindications. It does not cause gastritis or renal impairment. Paracetamol may also be given intravenously (15 mg/kg 6 hourly) or rectally. The

Table 4.4 Non-steroidal analgesic drugs

Diclofenac sodium	1 mg/kg 8 hourly oral or rectal
	Maximum 3 mg/kg/day
	Maximum adult dose 150 mg/day
Ibuprofen	10 mg/kg 6 hourly oral
	5 mg/kg 6 hourly oral if age less than 6 months
	Maximum dose 400 mg/6 hourly
Paracetamol	Oral 15 mg/kg 4 hourly
	Intravenous 15 mg/kg 6 hourly
	Rectal 40 mg/kg loading dose (20 mg/kg in neonates) followed by 20 mg/kg 6 hourly
	Maximum dose by oral and rectal routes 90 mg/kg/day above 3 months of age (4 g/day in adolescents); 60 mg/kg/day in neonates and infants up to 3 months of age. Maximum IV dose 60 mg/kg/day at all ages

rectal route has a lower bioavailability than the oral and intravenous routes and higher doses in the region of 20–30 mg/kg are required (see Table 4.4).

References

1. Dalens B, Vanneuville G, Tanguy A. Comparison of the fascia iliaca compartment block with the 3-in-1 block in children. Anesth Analg 1989; 69:705–713.
2. Wilson PTJ, Lloyd-Thomas AR. An audit of extradural infusion analgesia in children using bupivacaine and diamorphine. Anesthesia 1993; 48:718–723.
3. Casati A, Baciarello M, Di Cianni S, et al. Effects of ultrasound guidance on the minimum effective anesthetic volume required to block the femoral nerve. Br J Anesth 2007; 98:823–827.
4. Oberndorfer U, Marhofer P, Bösenberg A, et al. Ultrasonographic guidance for sciatic and femoral nerve blocks in children. Br J Anesth 2007; 98:797–801.
5. Hutton P, Clutton-Brock T. The benefits and pitfalls of pulse oximetry. Br Med J 1993; 307:457–458.
6. Gadiyar V, Gallacher TM, Crean PM, Taylor RH. The effect of a combination of rectal diclofenac and caudal bupivacaine on postoperative analgesia in children. Anesthesia 1995; 50:820–822.
7. Teiria H, Meretoja OA. PCA in pediatric orthopedic patients: influence of a NSAID on morphine requirement. Pediatr Anesth 1994; 4:87–91.

Chapter 5

Paediatric Imaging

David J. Wilson and Gina M. Allen

General Principles

Diagnostic and therapeutic imaging of children poses particular challenges. First it is vital to limit the radiation dose. The younger the child, the more radiosensitive the bone marrow and the greater the potential harm. In addition children have to be persuaded to cooperate to obtain adequate imaging studies and particular radiographic skills are essential [1].

When performing conventional radiography the image acquisition must be adjusted to maximize contrast and to provide adequate coverage of the area of interest while minimizing radiation dose. Using conventional film, a fast screen/film system will reduce radiation exposure. The more widespread modern image acquisition systems, computed radiography (CR) and digital radiography (DR), especially direct capture devices, allow greater reduction in exposure. With all systems of image acquisition, short exposure times and good collimation will reduce radiation dose. Adequate gonad protection should be used unless it is essential to examine the central or lower pelvis (see Fig. 5.1). Protection for the thyroid and breast tissue should be provided where necessary, as they are particularly radiosensitive [2]. Ultrasound (US) and magnetic resonance imaging (MRI) should be considered as alternatives to conventional radiography whenever possible although sedation or anesthesia may be needed for MRI, making it less practical in children [3].

The environment in which imaging is performed should be child friendly with pictures and soft toys. Children's waiting areas should be separate from those used by adult patients. Parents should be made welcome in the examination room but care should be taken to protect them if necessary, for example, when a mother is pregnant and her child is being examined by conventional radiography. Fluoroscopy and computed tomography (CT) should be performed only

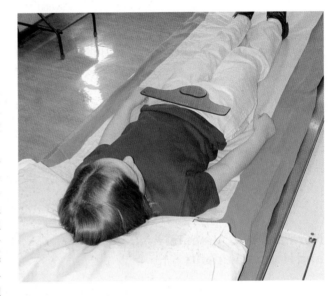

Fig. 5.1 A child with gonad protection in place

for specific indications when the potential benefit outweighs the risk.

The referring clinician should be aware of the risks of ionizing radiation and should be prepared to discuss the issues involved with the child's parents or guardian. On occasion it may be necessary to refer to a radiologist for additional advice.

In the UK, Europe, and many other countries, a doctor with sufficient training and experience to understand the risks, radiation-limiting techniques, and alternative nonionizing methods must clinically direct examinations involving ionizing radiation. Statutes and directives ensure that the necessary specialized training takes several years and in practice in most countries this person will be a qualified radiologist. The individual clinically directing the exposure has a personal responsibility to the patient and should not accept referrals that contravene safety principles. In general the referrer should request an examination for a specified clinical indication and take advice when alternative techniques are safer or more effective.

D.J. Wilson (✉)
Department of Radiology, Nuffield Orthopaedic Centre, Oxford, UK

M. Benson et al. (eds.), *Children's Orthopaedics and Fractures*,
DOI 10.1007/978-1-84882-611-3_5, © Springer-Verlag London Limited 2010

Table 5.1 Dose of common radiographs with risks (Courtesy of Dr A Woodward, Swansea)

Examination	Age group	Effective dose (mSv)	Risk of harm (detriment)*
AP/PA chest	1 to <12 month	0.011	1 in 71,000
	1 to <5 years	0.010	1 in 78,000
	5 to <10 years	0.009	1 in 84,000
	10 to <16 years	0.008	1 in 92,000
AP hip	1 to <12 months	0.024	1 in 32,000
	1 to <5 years	0.032	1 in 24,000
	5 to <10 years	0.021	1 in 37,000
	10 to <16 years	0.087	1 in 89,000
AP skull	1 to <12 months	0.009	1 in 890,000
	1 to <5 years	0.011	1 in 730,000
	5 to <10 years	0.012	1 in 660,000
	10 to <16 years	0.015	1 in 530,000

*Calculated from original paper. To give some idea of these risks, 0.25 mSv of radiation is equivalent to smoking 10 cigarettes, 15 min of rock climbing, or traveling 4000 miles by air. For comparison, traveling 600 miles by air has a 1:100,000 risk of fatality.

Table 5.1 illustrates the radiation dose and the risks of harm which are incurred with a single radiograph of the chest, pelvis, or skull.

Normal Developmental Anatomy and Normal Variants

One of the most challenging aspects of interpreting the child's X-ray is recognizing normal developmental anatomy and normal variants (see Fig. 5.2). It is unlikely that even the dedicated paediatric musculoskeletal radiologist will memories all the epiphyseal centers and their age of appearance with the many variants that occur in bone. Help is at hand with excellent bench books [4, 5].

In assessing bone age in an overdeveloped or underdeveloped child, the left-hand radiograph (see Fig. 5.3) has been well documented by Greulich and Pyle [6] and Tanner et al. [7]. The former uses standard male and female images for direct comparison, indicating the time of appearance of the ossification center in the epiphysis of each bone of the digits and carpus with the timing of their fusion. The latter is a more complex and arguably a more accurate method. Each bone of the carpus and digits is individually scored. This is a time-consuming process but it may be worthwhile when management choices are dependent on precise bone age. When either method is used we recommend that the standard deviation from normal is recorded.

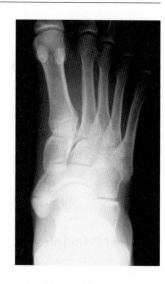

Fig. 5.2 Os tibiale externum, an accessory ossification center on the navicular which is a normal variant

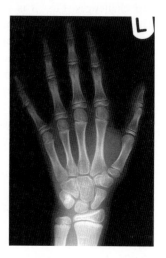

Fig. 5.3 Left hand for bone age—according to the standards of Greulich and Pyle 12 years, standard deviation 10.24 months

The elbow poses a particular challenge to the clinician because of its multitude of epiphyses. A good aide-memoir is CRITOL, as shown in Table 5.2.

Fusion of the epiphyses starts with the radial head and ends with the lateral epicondyle, with the others fusing at approximately the same age.

Table 5.2 Critol aide-memoir

Letter	Ossification centers of the elbow	Time of appearance
C	Capitellum	2 months–2 years
R	Radial head (bipartite)	3–6 years
I	Internal (medial) epicondyle	4–7 years
T	Trochlea (two centers)	1–2 years
	1. Lateral condyle	8–10 years
	2. Medial (bipartite)	
O	Olecranon (bipartite)	8–10 years
L	Lateral epicondyle	10–13 years

Techniques Available

Conventional Radiographs

Radiographs remain the workhorse of imaging. They are mandatory in cases where trauma is suspected and when there is implanted metal in a joint or bone. There are now over a hundred years of accumulated experience in interpreting conventional radiographs and radiologists and clinicians are more familiar at interpreting their abnormalities than more modern imaging techniques. They do have significant limitations which the clinician and imager should understand. They use radiation and give only very limited information about muscles, ligaments, tendons, and soft tissues. A 2D representation will lead to overlap of normal on abnormal bone masking some diseases that would be apparent when using cross-sectional imaging. Bones may appear normal using conventional radiographs in cases of significant abnormality, for example, early osteonecrosis, osteomyelitis, or minimally displaced fractures.

A number of techniques may reduce radiation dose. For film-based systems the newest film screen combinations using rare earth screens should always be used in paediatric practice. Digital capture devices should be employed whenever possible and consideration should be given to replacing older film-based imaging and computed radiographic devices with the latest technology.

CR (computed radiography) uses a phosphor plate to replace the photographic film and a separate piece of apparatus reads the image from this plate directly into a computer archive. The images may be viewed on a monitor via PACS (Patient Archive and Communications System) or printed on photographic film. These computer-based image acquisition systems have much wider latitude to faulty exposure. Over- and underexposures are less likely to obscure or over-penetrate the image. This leads to fewer repeated exposures and the radiation load to patients is reduced. Computer-based images have the advantage that they may be viewed on different "window levels" to allow for a more penetrated examination of bone or a softer view of the muscles and subcutaneous tissues.

The latest digital capture systems allow the image to be virtually instantly transferred to the computer archive for viewing in storage in the same way as computed radiography. These latest systems have advantages similar to computed radiography but also considerably shorten the time they take to perform an examination and have an even greater saving in radiation dose. They have a particular advantage in children as the instant image tells the radiographer that the examination is adequate allowing repeats when necessary to be performed at once. This aids cooperation in the anxious child.

When thicker or wider areas of the body such as the chest or abdomen are being examined, scattering artifact may degrade the quality of the image. A Bucky or grid placed between the film and the patient reduces the scatter but increases the radiation dose required to achieve the same exposure. In general Bucky techniques are not required in the peripheral skeleton and should probably be avoided in small children.

Ultrasound

Musculoskeletal US techniques have improved considerably over the last few years. More sophisticated equipment with high frequency probes and a better understanding of anatomy and disease have lead to its widespread use in orthopaedic, rheumatologic, and other musculoskeletal practice. It does not use ionizing radiation and is easy to perform for the experienced examiner. Children generally tolerate US examinations very well. It helps to warm the contact jelly either in hot water or on a nearby radiator. If you do not use a purpose-built warmer, always test the temperature before use. A careful explanation, including demonstration on the examiner's own arm or limb, usually proves effective in reducing anxiety.

The principle disadvantage of the technique is that it is very observer dependent and there is a considerable learning curve. US is the examination of choice in the assessment of developmental dysplasia of the hip in the infant, irritable hip, tendon disease, and soft tissue lumps. It is also useful in guiding biopsies and aspirations [3].

Computed Tomography

Most hospitals have been re-equipped with helical CT machines. These are less precisely known as spiral CT and differ from conventional CT in their speed of examination and the ability to produce much better quality reconstructions in orthogonal planes. Their principle disadvantage is that it is very tempting to use CT over extensive areas and significantly increases the radiation dose. Care must be taken in planning and judging the area of interest.

CT is still the main workhorse in the general hospitals for cross-sectional imaging. Its use in children should be limited due to its radiation dose. It is used to detect metastasis in the lung in bone sarcomas and to examine the abdomen when looking for the primary tumor in cases where metastases are present, e.g., in neuroblastoma and nephroblastoma.

CT is the best technique for examining bone disease of in detail and for defining the nature and extent of complex fractures. CT is extremely useful for detecting the nidus in osteoid osteoma, as this may not be visible on MRI. For this condition, MRI is useful to detect an area of bone edema and CT is then a second line test to confirm its nature by using very thin sections at the site of MRI abnormality.

CT is now rarely used to assess bone and soft tissue tumors, having been replaced by MRI.

CT is of particular value in bony coalitions and abnormalities of the skeleton. These include complex spinal malformations and hindfoot coalitions.

Magnetic Resonance Imaging

MRI imaging is particularly valuable in children because it does not use ionizing radiation. Children vary considerably in their tolerance of the technique, particularly when using a solenoid (conventional bore-type magnet). Claustrophobia can be a problem. Open MRI systems are better tolerated and also have the advantage that children's parents can sit next to them, but if the field (Tesla) of the magnet is low this can lead to long examination times and the resolution of the images may be poor. More recently high-field open MRI systems achieve good quality images in less time while preserving the advantage of the open architecture.

Radiographers experienced in examining children can normally perform good quality studies on any child able to understand the preliminary explanation of the study. In general, children under the age of four are very difficult to examine without sedation or anesthesia. If a small infant is in a plaster cast it may be practical to perform the examination despite lack of cooperation. It helps if the examination is performed when the child is drowsy after a milk feed. It is always wise to attempt MRI without sedation when there is even an outside chance of achieving a diagnostic study. If sedation or anesthesia is necessary for children in a MRI unit, it should be performed by an experienced paediatric anesthetist with full monitoring equipment. MRI safe monitoring and anesthetic devices are available but they are very expensive and are usually installed only in systems with a particular requirement for anesthesia. An MRI room is a difficult place to observe response to sedation and monitoring is complex. The anesthetist must be used to the environment and familiar with the relatively restricted equipment.

MRI is the investigation of choice in patients suspected of an internal disruption of a joint, bone infection, bone tumor, soft tissue tumor, spinal anomaly, and congenital malformation.

Nuclear Medicine

Nuclear medicine examinations are now used less often since the wider application of US and MRI.

The radiation burden is significant and most examinations require intravenous injection of a radiopharmaceutical. The images can, however, be easily repeated if the child moves.

Nuclear medicine studies are expensive because of radiopharmaceutical costs and in many institutions cost as much if not more than MRI.

Bone scintigraphy is, however, particularly useful both in searching for metastases and assessing their extent. It is useful in the detection or exclusion of osteomyelitis, especially multifocal osteomyelitis. MRI, however, now rivals this technique and is the preferred imaging method.

In children the interpretation of bone scintigrams may be confused by high activity at the growth plates that may obscure significant disease such as tumors and infections.

White cell-labeled indium chloride studies and gallium citrate scintigraphy may be used with or without emission CT (ECAT) in suspected osteomyelitis. However, MRI is the preferred technique and scintigraphy is now used less frequently in bone infection.

Other Imaging

Angiography is of use in treating children with complex vascular malformations, for whom embolization is being considered. This is an area of special expertise available only in specialist centers. Fortunately MRI can be used diagnostically to judge the extent of congenital vascular lesions prior to deciding the need for invasive angiographic intervention. US can also be useful in peripheral lesions to compare the amount of venous with arterial flow.

DEXA (dual X-ray absorptiometry) examinations are sometimes useful in children for the diagnosis of osteoporosis and osteogenesis imperfecta. They may also be used to monitor the treatment of osteoporosis. Sedation is often necessary in the very young as data acquisition is time consuming. There are relatively small numbers of normal examinations in the database for reference and this may cast doubt on the significance of abnormal findings.

Protocols

Antenatal Diagnosis

One of imaging's most significant contributions is the antenatal diagnosis of skeletal disorders [8]. The routine use of

US in pregnancy at 20 weeks gestation to detect fetal anomalies can help the clinician and parent-to-be plan ahead for the newborn if the pregnancy is allowed to continue.

US may detect serious abnormalities such as arthrogryposis, neural tube defects, and reduction defects [9] but it is also useful in the diagnosis of subtle problems such as clubfoot and polydactyly [10–12].

In hereditary disorders US-guided amniocentesis may be used to obtain material for DNA analysis.

Spinal Anomalies

In the newborn with a sacral dimple or hair tuft the spinal canal can be visualized with US. This allows the diagnosis of an occult spina bifida or a tethered cord. In the newborn when other skeletal abnormalities are found, an US examination of the cord is an accepted screening test to exclude associated spinal anomalies. Spinal cord tethering (see Fig. 5.4), myelomeningocele, syringomyelia, and diastematomyelia can be diagnosed. The only alternative would be MRI (see Figs. 5.5, 5.6, 5.7, and 5.8). Infants are difficult to examine and the images provided by even the best MRI systems on anaesthetized infants lack the resolution of good quality US. US is the screening technique of choice in infants suspected of spine anomalies [13].

DDH (Developmental Dysplasia of the Hip)

There is a window of opportunity to treat children with hip dysplasia. Splint therapy for instability and dysplasia is most useful in the first 6–8 weeks of life. US examination is proven

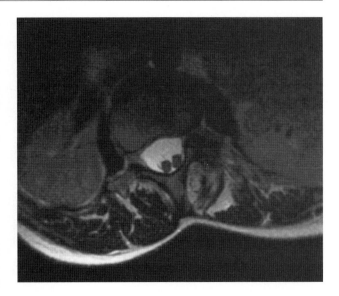

Fig. 5.5 MRI of diastematomyelia

to enhance the accuracy of clinical assessment and is now established as routine practice in many centers. Frank dislocation is usually detected clinically; US is principally of use in showing milder forms of acetabular dysplasia that might lead to late subluxation or even dislocation [14] (see Figs. 5.9 and 5.10). In the newborn the hips are commonly subluxatable, but within 4 weeks many stabilize. It is wise to delay the initial examination for 3–4 weeks to reduce the number of positive examinations while keeping within the treatment window of 6–8 weeks [15]. There are a variety of methods employed for the examination of infants' hips by US [16, 17]. Each has its advocates, but all that have been reported are similar in their efficacy. Rather than argue the merits of a particular technique it is more useful to advise

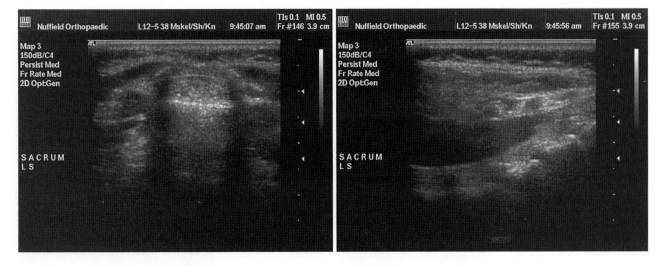

Fig. 5.4 Ultrasound of an infant with a tethered cord, the canal should only contain the cauda equina on the axial view, while the tip of the conus can be seen too low down on the longitudinal image

Fig. 5.6 MRI of tethered cord

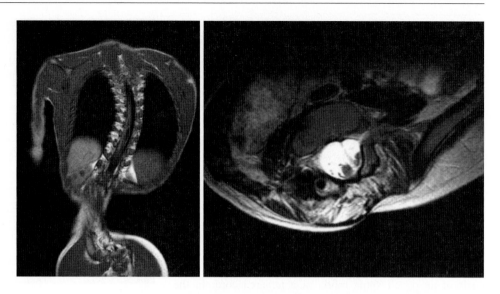

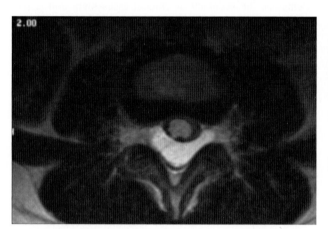

Fig. 5.7 MRI of lipoma of the cord

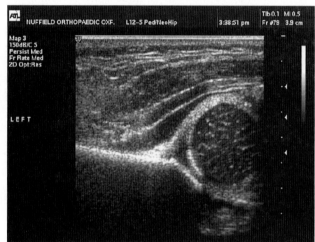

Fig. 5.9 Ultrasound of a shallow (dysplastic) hip

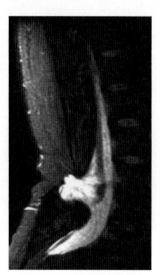

Fig. 5.8 MRI of myelomeningocoele

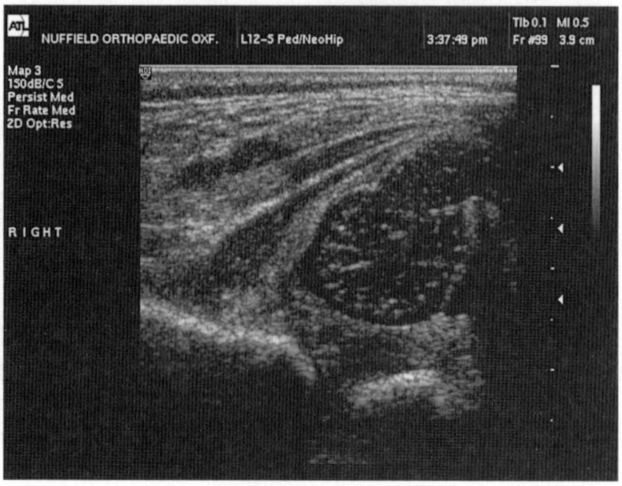

Fig. 5.10 Ultrasound of a dislocated hip

that a standard technique is employed by each hospital so that there is a method of quantifiable measurement of acetabular shape, which can be reproduced. It is recommended that dynamic studies be used as an adjunct. For all methods a precise coronal or axial plane should be recorded. The choice of method will depend on the institution, but those described by Graf, Morin, and Harke are all effective [18]. It is important to arrange regular audit and clinical outcome review as this allows the maintenance of high standards and enhances the continued training of sonographers.

Radiographs are of limited value before the age of 3 months; thereafter they are the preferred method of judging hip morphology.

Irritable Hip

This common condition has a variety of causes—Chapter 26. Investigation and management focus on excluding those conditions that require urgent treatment, in particular septic arthritis [19]. US is a sensitive and powerful method of detecting a hip joint effusion [16, 20–22]. Less than 1 ml of excess fluid can be detected by a careful technique. The hip is examined with the patient supine. The anterior part of the hip capsule is relatively slack. An oblique US plane along the axis of the femoral neck provides an image that will demonstrate fluid as a dark (echo-free) collection. Comparison is made with the opposite side and a difference of 2 mm or more in depth of the synovial space indicates an effusion (see Fig. 5.11) Unfortunately the characteristics of the fluid or synovial hypertrophy do not differentiate a clear effusion from blood or pus. Indeed some septic joints in children occur without any clinical or serological markers and they may produce only a small effusion [23]. We, with others,

feel that emergency US-guided aspiration has great merit. Any tamponade is reduced and the patient becomes pain-free rapidly. Sepsis may be excluded by Gram stain and culture. If the initial gram stain is negative it is safe to discharge the patient providing that if the cultures grow organisms immediate recall is possible. This reduces the duration of symptoms for all and saves many overnight admissions [24]. The techniques are easy to learn and have proved to be safe. By applying a local anesthetic skin cream 90 min prior to the patient being imaged by US, the hip aspiration can be performed at the same time as the diagnostic study [25]. With careful technique the procedure should be less traumatic than venepuncture. To make this process effective a system must be in place for the rapid receipt and feedback of the microbiology results.

US examination may also detect a slipped upper femoral epiphyses [26] or fragmentation of the epiphysis in Perthes disease [27–29] (see Fig. 5.12). However, it is not proven to be sufficiently sensitive to be used to exclude these diagnoses. Unexplained and persistent joint effusions should be investigated further to rule out osteomyelitis, Perthes disease, and other subarticular diseases. While a plain film can be helpful the most useful test is MRI, as most abnormalities are excluded by a normal study [30].

Slipped Upper Femoral Epiphysis

Those children who present with hip pain over the age of 8 years should always be suspected of suffering from a slipped upper femoral epiphysis (see Fig. 5.13). A frog or lateral conventional radiographic view of both hips is mandatory in all cases. It may be argued that the conventional AP view may be omitted, as 14% of AP films may be normal in the presence of a SUFE. Some authors, however, claim that the frog lateral view can provoke the slip! Remember that 75% of children with SUFE show a joint effusion on US and may be confused with those suffering from transient synovitis [31, 32]. The inclusion of a plain film with an appropriate projection should remove the risk of oversight in this age group. If there is doubt about minor degrees of slip, especially on the "normal" side when SUFE is apparent in one hip, then MRI using an oblique plane of axial imaging along the femoral neck is very useful [33]. It could be argued that all patients with a unilateral SUFE should be examined by MRI because in some studies the incidence of bilateral slip is 60%. Furthermore pre-slippage signs such as posterior widening of the growth plate and juxta-epiphyseal osteopenia may be seen. Imaging after treatment will assist in detecting complications of surgery and the disorder itself, a combination of conventional radiographs and MR will be important in many cases [34].

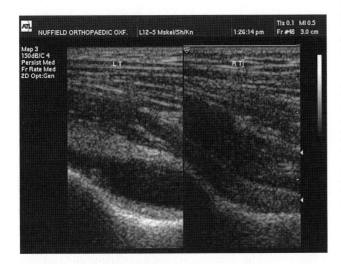

Fig. 5.11 Ultrasound of an irritable hip showing an effusion on one side due to transient synovitis

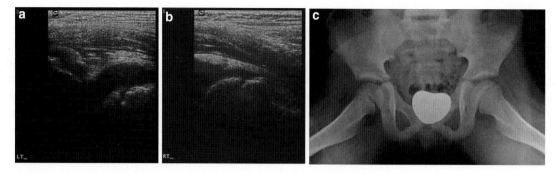

Fig. 5.12 (**a**) Perthes disease detected using ultrasound, (**b**) normal side, and (**c**) confirmed with a radiograph

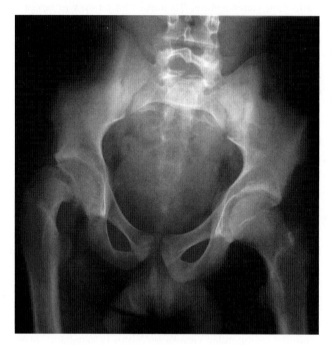

Fig. 5.13 A child with a slipped upper femoral epiphysis

Limb Lengthening

Operations to correct leg length discrepancies or fracture deformity may be monitored by a combination of US and conventional radiographs (see Fig. 5.14). The gap at the osteotomy will contain developing callus [35, 36]. Too slow a distraction may allow premature bridging. Too fast a distraction can cause hemorrhagic cysts to form in the gap preventing healing. Weekly or fortnightly review with the combination of a radiograph that includes a measurement marker plus US measurement of the width of the gap allows effective and safe management. If the gap is filling too fast more speedy distraction is indicated. If there is delayed filling on US with or without cysts then it is wise to slow down. Cysts that do not resolve rapidly may be aspirated with US guidance [37].

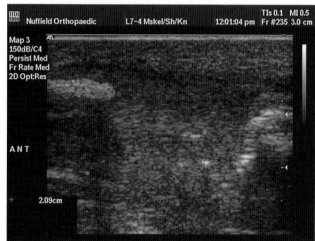

Fig. 5.14 Ultrasound of the gap during a leg lengthening procedure; there are no cysts

Scoliosis

Children present with scoliosis because of deformity, pain, or a rib hump. Imaging is useful in assessing the degree of scoliosis, underlying congenital bony abnormalities and underlying neurological tissue abnormalities [38].

Imaging is particularly important prior to operation. Defects of neural tissues including tethering, myelomeningocele, and diastematomyelia are especially dangerous if they are not diagnosed prior to corrective surgery [39]. The routine follow-up for patients with spinal deformity is a concern because of the substantial radiation load for organs and tissues that are sensitive in young people.

The initial diagnosis should include assessment of curve severity and bony abnormalities on plain films taken standing. This should include an AP and lateral radiograph to include the whole spinal column. The angle of curvature (scoliosis or kyphosis) may be measured from these films. A line should be drawn along the end plate of the vertebral body at the point of which the curve reverses, effectively measuring the maximum angle within each element of the curve (Cobb's angle). Curvature is described by the direction in which it produces the convexity. Marks made on the film should be made in erasable crayon so as to avoid obscuring details that may be clinically important at a later stage. Angle measurements are particularly easy using PACS monitors with in-built measurement software.

The report should include a description of hemivertebrae, fused vertebrae, butterfly vertebrae, and other segmentation anomalies.

In cases of simple scoliosis without congenital vertebral anomalies, further imaging for the neurological structures is not normally indicated until such time as surgery is considered or planned. If there were significant bony abnormalities, it would be reasonable to perform an MRI series early (see Fig. 5.15). Most surgeons would now consider MRI to be a requirement prior to elective surgery for scoliosis [40]. The sequences employed should include images of the foramen magnum for Chiari and other hindbrain abnormalities. Sagittal images are required to assess spinal cord tethering and lipoma of the cord. Coronal images are particularly useful to look for vertebral anomalies and to examine the adjacent organs. Renal abnormalities are commonly associated with the spinal region. A series of axial images should be taken throughout the spinal cord, as diastematomyelia and syringomyelia may be very difficult to identify on sagittal and coronal images alone. The MRI protocol is lengthy but to exclude any of these images' risks missing a significant abnormality.

MRI protocol for scoliosis imaging:

- Sagittal TSE T2 (thoraco-lumbar)
- Coronal CSE T1 (thoraco-lumbar)
- Axials through the apex of the curve (TSE T2 or GE T2*)
- Axial TSE T2 from conus to filum terminale
- Sagittal TSE T2 (cervical spine)

The assessment of curvature should include plain film lateral-bending views. Reactive and secondary curves will be obliterated by motion, while the primary structural curve remains.

Follow-up studies may use photographic methods of back shape assessment, for example, the ISIS scanner marketed by Oxford Metrics or Moiré Fringe technique [41] (see Fig. 5.16). These methods have the advantage of not using ionizing radiation and being recorded in a repeatable electronic form. They are also probably a better assessment of the physical deformity of the patient giving a measure of the rib hump as well as the rotational abnormalities in the spine. They are particularly useful for serial follow-up under conservative or surgical treatment.

After operations plain films are mandatory to assess the placement and integrity of the instrumentation. When there is doubt over the positioning, especially of pedicle screws, CT is the best means of assessing their location. Metal artifact reduction software is improving and it is usually possible to define the position of the implants with considerable accuracy. If there is a question of impingement on nerve roots or spinal cord, CT may not be sufficient to make this diagnosis. An attempt should be made to use MRI. Fast spin echo techniques with the minimum of additional RF pulses (pre-saturation, fat saturation, etc.) produce the least artifacts. Low-field systems similarly produce fewer artifacts than high-field systems. If MRI fails it may be necessary to resort to conventional myelography with or without CT. These are difficult examinations and need to be performed by a radiologist with expertise in myelography.

Osteomyelitis

Isotope scintigraphy is useful when searching for multifocal areas of infection [42]. Children are restless and therefore after one injection of isotope they can be repeatedly examined as necessary. Whole-body MRI may be the technique of the future to look for multiple site infection as unlike scintigraphy it locates precisely the anatomical site of abnormality without the use of radiation [43, 44].

US examination helps detect early infection as it demonstrates sub-periosteal abscesses long before conventional radiographs show an abnormality [45, 46]. This technique works well in the extremities, but for spinal infection MRI is mandatory to examine not only the skeleton but also possible epidural and disc involvement.

Conventional radiographs may strongly suggest infection, for example, the well-defined metaphyseal lesion of a Brodie's abscess, and therefore the initial investigations for possible infection should be by US and conventional radiography [47, 48].

The organism that has caused the infection may rarely give a characteristic appearance on imaging, but specimens should always be obtained after adequate imaging to guide the appropriate antibiotic therapy (see Figs. 5.17 and 5.18).

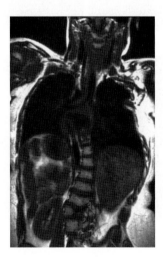

Fig. 5.15 MRI of scoliosis with a butterfly vertebra

Fig. 5.16 Printout and "ISIS" study of a child with scoliosis and rib hump

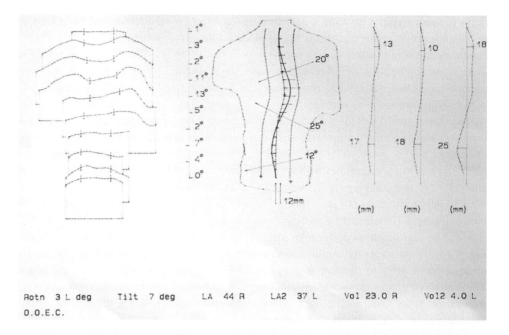

Fig. 5.17 (**a**) Periosteal reaction in the tibia due to osteomyelitis, (**b, c**) MRI shows the soft tissue extension, (**d**) ultrasound shows the periosteal reaction, and (**e**) the sinus track through the muscle

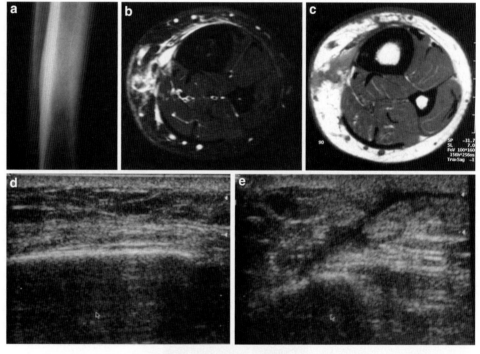

Fig. 5.18 Distal tibia acute osteomyelitis. Normal radiograph and focal lesion on MR imaging (age 10)

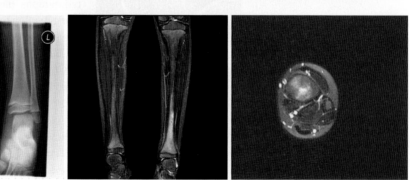

Juvenile Arthritis

Conventional radiographs have long been used to look for erosive changes in the skeleton. MRI and US have been shown to detect erosions and other soft tissue abnormalities much earlier in the disease enabling earlier and perhaps more effective treatment [49]. MRI is the most sensitive imaging in these patients, but US is an excellent screening test. US is easier to use in children than MRI and it is also more sensitive than conventional radiographs as it detects the synovitis and shows erosions in profile. The benefit of intravenous contrast agents for US is still being investigated. The use of gadolinium-enhanced MRI is accepted practice in the detection of synovitis (see Fig. 5.19). Both MRI and US will also detect any associated teno-synovitis [49, 50].

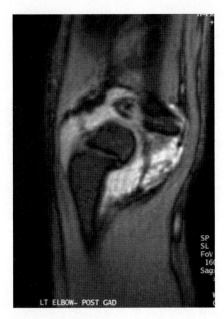

Fig. 5.19 MR arthrogram of a child with juvenile rheumatoid arthritis and profound synovitis of the right hip

Tumors—Soft Tissue and Bone; Diagnosis, Staging, and Follow-Up

In any child who presents with bone pain, malignancy must be excluded. A conventional radiograph will show most lesions, but should it appear normal and doubt persists about diagnosis then an MRI examination should be performed [51].

For soft tissue lesions, US examination is the best initial screening test. It may provide the definitive diagnosis, such as a popliteal cyst or ganglion, but it will also detect those lesions that require further imaging. In general, echogenic or mixed echo pattern lesions require further investigation by MRI (see Fig. 5.20) and probably biopsy [3].

All lesions should be investigated by a staged approach, with assessment of local and distant spread only after a definitive diagnosis of malignancy is made [52].

MRI should be performed to assess the extent of local involvement of bone or soft tissue before a biopsy is performed. Any biopsy should be undertaken by a route that may be excised at operation in case the lesion is found to be malignant, taking into account the compartmental anatomy in the limbs. Preliminary discussion with the involved tumor surgeon is mandatory.

Biopsies of soft tissue and bone lesions with soft tissue extension (e.g., sarcomas) may be performed with US guidance [53].

Doppler US examination and MRI angiography can also be used to assess the vascularity and vascular involvement of a lesion allowing the surgeon to plan excision of the lesion or to assess the need for selective embolization before operation (see Fig. 5.21).

Fractures

Exclusion of fractures is the most common reason for imaging a child's skeleton. Radiographic examination is routine following trauma or suspected trauma. The necessity for good quality images cannot be overemphasized [54]. When a radiograph is not clinically indicated but the parents expect it, the risks and benefits of radiation should be discussed. When a radiographic examination is negative but a fracture is strongly suspected other imaging techniques should be considered.

CT is very useful in this situation and details not easily seen on radiographs will be revealed and it is invaluable in delineating the extent and nature of complex fractures prior to reconstruction. This is especially true for injuries to the pelvis and face. The radiation dose is high and it is tempting to use modern helical CT systems to excess. Even with very thin slices there is a risk that fractures in the plane of the section may be obscured by volume-averaging artifact. The use of 3D reformatting to reduce errors of interpretation is now an accepted practice (see Fig. 5.22). Radiologists will insist on seeing conventional radiographs prior to CT and the examination will be easier and safer if they are available in the CT room. The use of lead shielding to the radiosensitive areas of the patient should also be considered, as these are nearer to the radiation beam in a child [55].

US examination can help in trauma. It may show subperiosteal hematoma at the fracture site, a break in the cortex or periosteal reaction, when the fracture is a few days old [3].

A posterior effusion of the elbow is often difficult to detect using conventional radiographs, especially as a true lateral view may be impossible to obtain when the elbow

Fig. 5.20 Aneurysmal bone cyst of the proximal humerus with fluid levels seen on MRI (age 5)

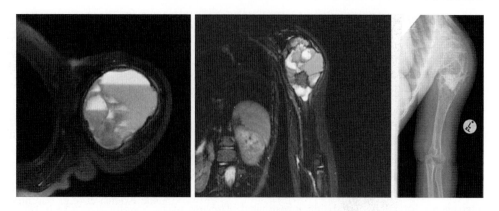

Fig. 5.21 (**a**) Plain films of a destructive lesion in the femur, (**b**, **c**) MRI shows a more extensive lesion. The diagnosis on biopsy was Ewing's sarcoma

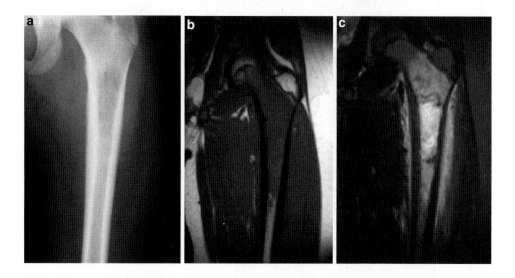

Fig. 5.22 A child who suffered C1/2 subluxation in a road traffic accident. (**a**) Plain films and (**b**) CT 3D surface reconstruction

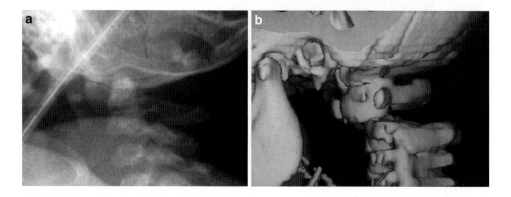

is particularly painful. US examination will sensitively and easily detect elbow joint effusion in such cases; this finding may support the diagnosis of a fracture that is being considered. US examination may show synovitis suggesting infection or arthropathy.

It could be argued that US examination should be a first line test in the very young infant, but the current availability of machines and more importantly those with expertise limit its application. MRI can also be used as an adjunct to conventional radiography as it may show subtle fractures invisible on radiographs (see Fig. 5.23). If there is doubt about the extent of an epiphyseal lesion, MRI may help the surgeon to decide whether to operate. For example, if Salter Harris IV fracture fragments involve the articular surface they should be fixed operatively but if the fracture is seen on MRI to stop in the epiphyses, it will be stable.

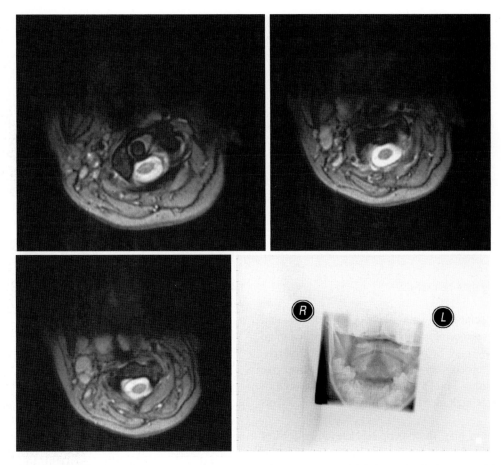

Fig. 5.23 Rotatory subluxation of the C1/2 junction. Note the change in alignment on the axial MR and the displacement of the peg on the AP radiograph

MRI can also determine the displacement of a fracture fragment although the signal from bone is poor and edema may make interpretation difficult. MRI is a tomographic technique and may reveal detail inside bone not seen on plain films. Hematoma and soft tissue injury are readily apparent using MRI. Currently, MRI is not routinely used for trauma but this may change in the future.

Nonaccidental Injury

A skeletal survey for nonaccidental injury should be performed only if there is clinical suspicion of abuse. Signs that raise this suspicion include retinal hemorrhage, a torn frenulum, and skin lesions (Chapter 42). Nonaccidental injuries may be suspected after inexplicable fractures, for example, those not corresponding to the history of injury, fractures of differing ages, metaphyseal fractures, anterior and posterior rib fractures, or long bone fractures in the infant younger than 1 year [56–58].

It is important that all the administration and image labeling for these radiographs are exemplary, because they may be needed in future legal proceedings. A parent, nurse, doctor, or social worker must accompany the child to the examination.

Routine X-radiographic views for nonaccidental injury include:

- Skull AP and lateral (plus Towne's view if there is an occipital fracture)
- Spine (thoracic and lumbar) lateral
- AP chest (supine)
- AP both arms
- Both hands (oblique) if clinically suspicious
- Abdomen and pelvis (supine)
- AP both legs
- Both feet AP if clinically suspicious

Coned down views, centered on the joints, are required to see metaphyseal fractures. Therefore, an overview image known as a *babygram* is not acceptable as it centers over the body and the extremities are therefore blurred.

If a fracture is suspected or demonstrated, lateral views of the affected limb must be obtained.

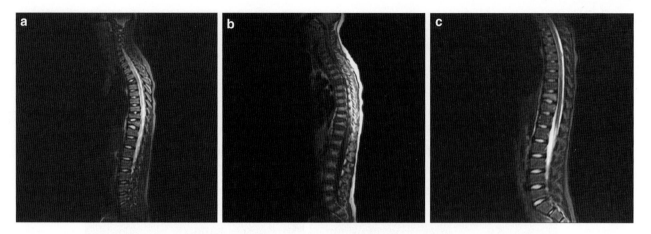

Fig. 5.24 (**a, b**) Infantile osteoporosis with fractures of different ages and (**c**) 18 months later (age 10)

Other imaging may be useful:

- Isotope bone scintigraphy may show occult fractures and confirm the presence of metaphyseal fractures when there is doubt. They may help resolve the issue of ambiguous fractures on conventional radiographs. Studies may be positive within 7 h of injury, but if negative and clinical suspicion is high then they should be repeated 3 days later.
- US examination may show periosteal elevation at sites of suspected fracture. It can be also be used to look for intracranial hemorrhage while abdominal US examination may detect small amounts of fluid in the abdomen should intra-abdominal injuries be suspected.
- Repeating radiographic examinations when there are findings is sometimes helpful as callus will start to form 10 days after injury.
- CT may be useful in detecting intracranial hemorrhage and significant abdominal trauma.
- MRI can be used to judge the age of subdural collections of blood. It is the best means of examining the brain stem and posterior fossa and of detecting subtle structural or ischemic/anoxic changes, for which CT is poor. Whole-body MRI may become important in detecting fractures but this indication is not yet established.

Table 5.3 gives a guide to the age of a fracture from its conventional radiograph appearances.

Rare conditions, such as infantile osteoporosis, may lead to fracture with minimal trauma (see Fig. 5.24).

Sports Injuries

In children there may be a poor or equivocal history of trauma. The mechanical demands on the developing skeleton

Table 5.3 A guide to fracture age assessment on plain radiograph

Benchmark	Fracture age
Resolution of soft tissue swelling	4–10 days
Fracture without periosteal reaction	<7 days
Slight periosteal reaction	4–7 days
Peak periosteal reaction	10–14 days
Blurring of fracture line	2–3 weeks (earliest 10 days)
Well-defined florid callus	>3–6 weeks (earliest 2 weeks)
Bony union/remodeling	3 months–1 year (earliest 1 month)

can be great in many sports. Injuries may occur due to excessive or repetitive load. Apophyseal injuries are not seen in the adult population and may be overlooked by those with less experience of paediatric imaging. They may present as a mass that mimics a bone tumor. They occur at the site of tendinous attachment and lead to overgrowth or detachment of the epiphysis [59]. The commonly encountered injuries occur at

- the anterior superior iliac spine—where sartorius inserts
- the anterior inferior iliac spine—where rectus femoris originates
- the pubic tubercle—the adductor origin
- the medial epicondyle of the elbow—the common flexor origin in throwing athletes

However, any tendon origin may be traumatically avulsed.

An initial conventional radiograph may give the diagnosis but if there is doubt then an MRI should confirm the diagnosis.

Soft tissue injuries are much less common in the young and should always alert the doctor to the possibility of an underlying tumor unless there has been a history of a significant relevant injury. They are best detected with US or MRI; the latter will also exclude more sinister disease.

References

1. Cook J, et al. Guidelines on Best Practice in the X-Ray Imaging of Children. 1999: RPC. London

2. Kyriou J, et al. Comparison of Doses and Techniques Between Specialist and Non-Specialist Centres in the Diagnostic X-Ray Imaging of Children. Br J Radiol 1996 69; 437–50

3. Wilson D. Paediatric Musculoskeletal Disease with an Emphasis on Ultrasound. 2005: Springer Verlag, Dordrecht.

4. Kohler A, Zimmer E. Borderlands of the Normal and Early Pathology in Skeletal Roentgenology. 1961: Grune and Stratton, New York.

5. Keats T, Anderson M. Atlas of Normal Roentgen Variants That May Simulate Disease, 8th ed. 2006: Mosby.

6. Greulich W, Pyle S. Radiographic Atlas of Skeletal Development of the Hand and Wrist, 2nd ed. 1959: Stanford University Press. Palo Alto

7. Tanner J, et al. Assessment of Skeletal Maturity and Prediction of Adult Height (TW2 Method), 2nd ed. 1983: Academic Press, London.

8. Petrikovsky B, Boris M. Fetal Disorders: Diagnosis and Management. 1998: John Wiley and Sons Ltd., New York

9. Hadi HA, Wade A. Prenatal diagnosis of unilateral proximal femoral focal deficiency in diabetic pregnancy: a case report. Am J Perinatol 1993; 10(4): 285—7.

10. Treadwell MC, Stanitski CL, King M. Prenatal sonographic diagnosis of clubfoot: implications for patient counseling. J Pediatr Orthop 1999; 19(1):8–10.

11. Pagnotta G, et al. Antenatal sonographic diagnosis of clubfoot: a six-year experience. J Foot Ankle Surg 1996; 35(1):67–71.

12. Burgan HE, Furness ME, Foster BK. Prenatal ultrasound diagnosis of clubfoot. J Pediatr Orthop 1999; 19(1):11–13.

13. Korsvik HE, Keller MS. Sonography of occult dysraphism in neonates and infants with MR imaging correlation. Radiographics 1992; 12(2):297–306; discussion 307–308.

14. Castelein RM, et al. Natural history of ultrasound hip abnormalities in clinically normal newborns. J Pediatr Orthop 1992; 12(4):423–427.

15. Berman L, Klenerman L. Ultrasound screening for hip abnormalities: preliminary findings in 1001 neonates. Br Med J (Clin Res Ed) 1986; 293(6549):719–722.

16. Harcke HT, Grissom LE. Pediatric hip sonography. Diagnosis and differential diagnosis. Radiol Clin North Am 1999; 37(4):787–796.

17. Harcke HT. Imaging methods used for children with hip dysplasia. Clin Orthop Relat Res 2005(434):71–77.

18. Marks DS, Clegg J, al-Chalabi AN. Routine ultrasound screening for neonatal hip instability. Can it abolish late-presenting congenital dislocation of the hip? J Bone Joint Surg Br 1994; 76(4):534–538.

19. Shah SS. Abnormal gait in a child with fever: diagnosing septic arthritis of the hip. Pediatr Emerg Care 2005; 21(5):336–341.

20. Wilson DJ, Green DJ, MacLarnon JC. Arthrosonography of the painful hip. Clin Radiol 1984; 35(1):17–19.

21. Adam R, et al. Arthrosonography of the irritable hip in childhood: a review of 1 year's experience. Br J Radiol 1986; 59(699): 205–208.

22. Alexander JE, et al. High-resolution hip ultrasound in the limping child. J Clin Ultrasound 1989; 17(1):19–24.

23. Del Beccaro MA, et al. Septic arthritis versus transient synovitis of the hip: the value of screening laboratory tests. Ann Emerg Med 1992; 21(12):1418–1422.

24. Fink AM, et al. The irritable hip: immediate ultrasound guided aspiration and prevention of hospital admission. Arch Dis Child 1995; 72(2):110–113; discussion 113–114.

25. Berman L, et al. Technical note: identifying and aspirating hip effusions. Br J Radiol 1995; 68(807):306–310.

26. Terjesen T. Ultrasonography for diagnosis of slipped capital femoral epiphysis. Comparison with radiography in 9 cases. Acta Orthop Scand 1992; 63(6):653–657.

27. Wirth T, LeQuesne GW, Paterson DC. Ultrasonography in Legg-Calve-Perthes disease. Pediatr Radiol 1992; 22(7):498–504.

28. Terjesen T. Ultrasonography in the primary evaluation of patients with Perthes disease. J Pediatr Orthop 1993; 13(4):437–443.

29. Eggl H, et al. Ultrasonography in the diagnosis of transient synovitis of the hip and Legg-Calve-Perthes disease. J Pediatr Orthop B 1999; 8(3):177–180.

30. Ranner G, et al. Magnetic resonance imaging in children with acute hip pain. Pediatr Radiol 1989; 20(1–2):67–71.

31. Castriota-Scanderbeg A, Orsi E. Slipped capital femoral epiphysis: ultrasonographic findings. Skeletal Radiol 1993; 22(3): 191–193.

32. Kallio PE, et al. Ultrasonography in slipped capital femoral epiphysis. Diagnosis and assessment of severity. J Bone Joint Surg Br 1991; 73(6):884–889.

33. Umans H, et al. Slipped capital femoral epiphysis: a physeal lesion diagnosed by MRI, with radiographic and CT correlation. Skeletal Radiol 1998; 27(3):139–144.

34. Tins B, Cassar-Pullicino V, McCall I. Slipped upper femoral epiphysis: imaging of complications after treatment. Clin Radiol 2008; 63(1):27–40.

35. Terjesen T, et al. Leg-length discrepancy measured by ultrasonography. Acta Orthop Scand 1991; 62(2):121–124.

36. Young JW, et al. Sonographic evaluation of bone production at the distraction site in Ilizarov limb-lengthening procedures. AJR Am J Roentgenol 1990; 154(1):125–128.

37. Derbyshire ND, Simpson AH. A role for ultrasound in limb lengthening. Br J Radiol 1992; 65(775):576–580.

38. Hedequist D, Emans J. Congenital scoliosis: a review and update. J Pediatr Orthop 2007; 27(1):106–116.

39. Oestreich AE, Young LW, Young Poussaint T. Scoliosis circa 2000: radiologic imaging perspective. I. Diagnosis and pretreatment evaluation. Skeletal Radiol 1998; 27(11):591–605.

40. Gupta P, Lenke LG, Bridwell KH. Incidence of neural axis abnormalities in infantile and juvenile patients with spinal deformity. Is a magnetic resonance image screening necessary? Spine 1998; 23(2):206–210.

41. Weiss I, et al. ISIS scanning: a useful assessment technique in the management of scoliosis. Spine 1988; 13(4):405–408.

42. Sundaram M, et al. Chronic recurrent multifocal osteomyelitis: an evolving clinical and radiological spectrum. Skeletal Radiol 1996; 25(4):333–336.

43. Dormans JP, Moroz L. Infection and tumors of the spine in children. J Bone Joint Surg Am 2007; 89 Suppl 1:79–97.

44. Pineda C, Vargas A, Rodriguez AV. Imaging of osteomyelitis: current concepts. Infect Dis Clin North Am 2006; 20(4):789–825.

45. Nath AK, Sethu AU. Use of ultrasound in osteomyelitis. Br J Radiol 1992; 65(776):649–652.

46. Larcos G, et al. How useful is ultrasonography in suspected acute osteomyelitis? J Ultrasound Med 1994; 13(9):707–709.

47. Jaramillo D, et al. Osteomyelitis and septic arthritis in children: appropriate use of imaging to guide treatment. AJR Am J Roentgenol 1995; 165(2):399–403.

48. Kaiser S, Jorulf H, Hirsch G. Clinical value of imaging techniques in childhood osteomyelitis. Acta Radiol 1998; 39(5):523–531.

49. Wakefield RJ, et al. The value of sonography in the detection of bone erosions in patients with rheumatoid arthritis: a comparison with conventional radiography. Arthritis Rheum 2000; 43(12):2762–2770.

50. Johnson K. Imaging of juvenile idiopathic arthritis. Pediatr Radiol 2006; 36(8):743–758.

51. Lang P, et al. Advances in MR imaging of pediatric musculoskeletal neoplasms. Magn Reson Imaging Clin N Am 1998; 6(3):579–604.

52. Stacy GS, Dixon LB. Pitfalls in MR image interpretation prompting referrals to an orthopedic oncology clinic. Radiographics 2007; 27(3):805–826; discussion 827–828.

53. Saifuddin A, Burnett SJ, Mitchell R. Pictorial review: ultrasonography of primary bone tumours. Clin Radiol 1998; 53(4):239–246.

54. Thornton A, Gyll C.Childrens fractures: A Radiological Guide to Safe Practice. 1999: Bailliere Tindall.

55. Beaty J, Kasser J. Rockwood and Wilkins Fractures in children, 6th ed. 2005: Lippincott Williams and Wilkins.

56. Rao P, Carty H. Non-accidental injury: review of the radiology. Clin Radiol 1999; 54(1):11–24.

57. Carroll DM, Doria AS, Paul BS. Clinical-radiological features of fractures in premature infants – a review. J Perinat Med 2007; 35(5):366–375.

58. Kleinman P. Diagnostic Imaging in Child Abuse, 2nd ed. 1998: Mosby-Elsevier Science Health Sciences.

59. Auringer ST, Anthony EY. Common Pediatric Sports Injuries. Semin Musculoskelet Radiol 1999; 3(3):247–256.

Part II
Generalized Disorders

Chapter 6

Gait Analysis

Tim N. Theologis

Normal Gait

Definitions

The term *gait* describes the characteristics of body motion during walking or running. The study of bipedal gait in humans is called *gait analysis* and refers to the objective and systematic study of human locomotion, including both visual observation and measurement using instrumentation.

Normal gait is a complex activity that relies on control by the central nervous system and the integrity of the spinal cord, peripheral nerves, and the musculoskeletal system. Its purpose is to propel the body forward while maintaining an upright posture and conserving energy. The neurological control of gait is based on an automated central nervous system mechanism, which may be modified by visual, sensory (including somatosensory), and acoustic stimuli while it remains under voluntary control.

From the biomechanical viewpoint, the prerequisites of normal gait include stability of the weight-bearing limb, appropriate pre-positioning of the limb for initial contact, adequate clearance of the non-weight-bearing limb, efficient step length, and energy conservation [1]. In order to achieve these, normal neurological control and an intact musculoskeletal system are necessary.

The description of gait is based on the definition of its unit, the *gait cycle*. The gait cycle is the period of time between the initial contact of one foot with the ground and its next contact with the ground. The timing of events occurring during a gait cycle is usually described as a percentage of this cycle, considering the initial contact as 0% and the second contact of the same foot as 100%. The gait cycle is divided into *stance phase* when the limb under consideration is in contact with the ground and *swing phase* when the limb is off the ground

and moving forward. Stance occupies approximately 60% of the cycle and swing the remaining 40%.

Another important subdivision of the gait cycle is into single and double limb support time. At initial contact both feet are on the ground, the first double support phase. At about 10% through the cycle the contralateral limb lifts off the ground. At this point double support time finishes and single support time commences. Fifty percent through the cycle, the contralateral limb contacts the ground again, which marks the beginning of the second double support time of the cycle; this finishes at the end of stance phase of the first limb 60% through the cycle. Therefore, there are two periods of double limb support time at the beginning and the end of the stance phase, each lasting 10% of the cycle.

Walking speed, usually expressed in meters per second, depends on cadence (steps per minute) and stride length (the sum of left and right step lengths). Stride time and step time are often measured in the temporal and spatial assessment of gait.

Description of Normal Gait

Systematic description of gait should always consider all three anatomical planes: sagittal, coronal, and transverse. Consideration should also be given to all moving body segments, including the head, upper limbs, trunk, pelvis, and lower limbs (see Fig. 6.1). A detailed description of motion in the lower limb segments and joints will follow later in this section.

Human gait characteristics depend on age, anatomical/structural characteristics, and walking speed. Each individual has a preferred or self-selected speed, which is optimal for energy conservation. Deviations from this optimal speed alter gait characteristics. Despite these individual variations, human gait characteristics are largely universal and the inter- and intra-subject variations are relatively small. When considering pathological gait, however, the variability of normal gait patterns should be taken into account. Some perceived

T.N. Theologis (✉)
Nuffield Orthopaedic Centre, Oxford, UK

M. Benson et al. (eds.), *Children's Orthopaedics and Fractures*,
DOI 10.1007/978-1-84882-611-3_6, © Springer-Verlag London Limited 2010

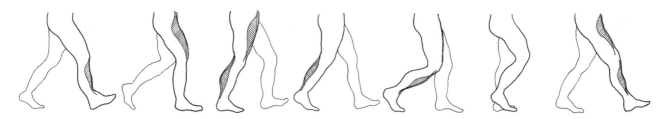

Fig. 6.1 The gait cycle subdivided into stance including initial contact, loading response, mid-stance, and late stance; and swing including initial, mid, and terminal swing. The predominant muscle activation during each phase is also shown

gait abnormalities may be normal variants or compensations for other underlying problems.

The gait cycle begins with the initial contact of the heel with the ground, often described as *heelstrike*. To achieve heel contact the foot is in neutral plantar/dorsiflexion and this requires activation of the dorsiflexors. The knee is slightly flexed at 5–10° and the hip is flexed at 30°. Following initial contact, the foot plantarflexes in relation to the tibia to allow forefoot ground contact. This is known as the *first ankle rocker* and is controlled by eccentric contraction of the dorsiflexors (see Fig. 6.2). In this early part of stance, knee flexion increases to 15–20° to allow smooth acceptance of body weight onto the weight-bearing limb. This increase in flexion is known as the *loading response* and is controlled by eccentric quadriceps activity. It coincides with the first double support time and is also characterized by progressive extension of the hip, driven by the gluteal muscles and the hamstrings. Mid-stance commences at the point of the opposite foot toe-off. During mid-stance the knee and hip progressively extend fully. At the hip, extension occurs passively through inertia. Some quadriceps activity is necessary at the knee to control the speed of flexion. While the weight-bearing foot remains in contact with the ground, the tibia progresses forward over it and the whole body is propelled forward. This is described as the *second ankle rocker* and is controlled by an eccentric contraction of the triceps surae.

In late stance, the foot plantarflexes on the tibia as the concentric contraction of the triceps surae propels the body forward. This phase is known as push-off or the *third ankle rocker*. The knee begins to flex at this stage in order to reach the flexion required in swing phase. The hip remains extended until the end of stance.

During initial swing the ankle dorsiflexes rapidly toward neutral through concentric contraction of the dorsiflexors. At the same time the knee and hip flex rapidly to allow clearance of the foot from the ground. Proximally, the iliopsoas actively flexes the hip. Knee flexion is a passive pendulum effect of the hip flexion. The knee reaches over 60° of flexion within the initial third of swing. Any pathology preventing this flexion results in foot clearance problems (e.g., spasticity of the rectus femoris muscle).

In mid-swing, the foot passes the opposite weight-bearing side and actively dorsiflexes further. The knee extends while the hip remains flexed. There is little muscle activity at hip and knee during this stage.

In terminal swing, the foot lowers toward the ground and dorsiflexion reduces. This is controlled by the dorsiflexors. At the knee, concentric activity of the quadriceps and eccentric activity of the hamstrings drive the knee toward extension. The hip remains flexed at 30°.

In the coronal plane there is a limited range of pelvic motion. The weight-bearing side is higher than the opposite one and the hip on the swing side is slightly abducted. In the transverse plane there is also a small range of pelvic rotation, which remains normally within 5–10° and aids forward propulsion. The hips rotate slightly around the neutral position and maximum internal rotation occurs in terminal stance. Foot progression (the angle between the axis of the

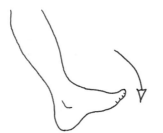
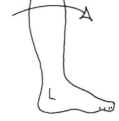
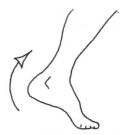

Fig. 6.2 The three ankle rockers. During the first rocker, the heel contacts the ground and the foot plantarflexes to allow the sole and forefoot to reach the ground. During the second rocker, the foot remains in contact with the ground, while the tibia progresses forward over it, producing dorsiflexion at ankle level. During the third rocker, the foot plantarflexes again to lift the heel off the ground and push forward

foot and the line of gait progression) is normally between 0° and 30° external rotation.

The upper body moves forward during walking but its speed is variable, accelerating during double support and decelerating during single support. The trunk also moves up and down twice during the gait cycle. The highest points coincide with mid-stance and mid-swing. In the coronal plane there is lateral leaning of the trunk toward the weight-bearing limb. In the transverse plane, the shoulders and trunk rotate toward the opposite direction in relation to the pelvis. The arms swing out of phase with the lower limbs. The leg swings forward simultaneously with the arm and shoulder of the opposite side.

The *ground reaction force* is important as it influences the stability of gait in general and the lower limb joints in particular. The fore-aft or antero-posterior component of the force vector is directed posteriorly in early and mid-stance, as a braking mechanism tending to decelerate the forward movement of the body. During transition from mid- to late stance the direction of the ground reaction force becomes anterior to contribute toward the forward acceleration of the body (see Fig. 6.3). The lateral component of the ground reaction force is relatively small and the direction of acceleration is toward the non-weight-bearing limb during most of stance.

The acceleration and deceleration of body speed coincide with energy conversion between potential and kinetic. During the first double support time, the body is at its lowest position and at its highest speed. Following this, kinetic energy is converted to potential energy and the body reaches its highest position and slowest speed during single support. Later in stance, the body lowers again and its speed increases. The rotation of the shoulders and pelvis in opposite directions is another example of an exchange between kinetic and potential energy.

Development of Gait

Gait Maturation

Most infants achieve independent bipedal walking at 12–18 months. Infant gait, characterized by its broad base of support, persists for 2–3 years. The arms are usually held up and out for balance and reciprocal swinging is not achieved until the age of 4–5 years. Infants make initial contact with the foot flat on the ground and the hip externally rotated while there is no knee flexion for loading response. Heel strike, normal hip rotation, and loading response are achieved around the age of 2 years. Although most infants walk with external hip rotation, some with persistent foetal alignment have an in-toe gait. Increased femoral anteversion, internal tibial torsion, metatarsus adductus, or a combination of these rotational variations may lead to internal foot progression.

Stride length depends on leg length and is, therefore, height and age dependent. Infants compensate for their reduced stride length by increasing their cadence. By the age of 7–8 years, their speed and cadence, normalized for height, are similar to that of an adult. In absolute terms, children achieve normal adult walking speed around the age of 12–15 years. It should be noted here that speed affects gait parameters, including kinematics and kinetics. Therefore, when assessing gait parameters, walking speed as well as the subject's anthropometric parameters (height or leg length) should be taken into account [2].

Electromyographic studies have shown that infants activate their lower limb muscles for longer periods during the walking cycle but reach adult patterns by the age of 2 years [3].

Variations of Gait

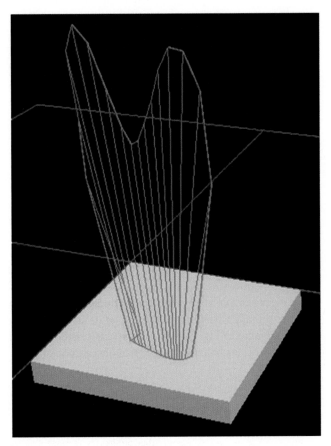

Fig. 6.3 The butterfly-shaped diagram of the ground reaction force throughout stance

Most children achieve independent ambulation by the age of 18 months. Children who are late in achieving their motor milestones may achieve independent walking later. After 18 months children who are not walking require assessment to rule out an underlying neurological or orthopaedic condition that could be responsible for the delay.

It is not uncommon for toddlers to walk weight bearing on the forefoot only when they start to walk. Such "toe-walking" is common up to the age of 2 years but prolonged or acquired toe-walking should be investigated for an underlying neurological condition or the plantarflexor tightness often seen in idiopathic toe-walking.

Children may use a variety of compensatory mechanisms for leg length discrepancy. Small discrepancies are compensated in the coronal plane by tilting the pelvis down on the short side. This is accompanied by hip adduction on the higher side of the pelvis and hip abduction on the shorter side. A compensatory postural scoliosis may develop. In larger discrepancies, increased plantarflexion on the short side or *vaulting* may be observed. Increased flexion of the hip and knee and dorsiflexion of the foot on the long side are additional compensatory mechanisms for leg length inequality. In order to aid clearance of the longer limb in swing phase, increased hip and knee flexion or hip circumduction in swing may be employed. When these variations of gait are seen, careful clinical assessment is needed to identify the primary problem. If there is no true leg length discrepancy, structural spinal deformity, joint, or muscle contracture may be responsible. It should also be noted that late-diagnosed hip dysplasia often presents as gait asymmetry and leg length inequality.

Gait asymmetry due to lower limb pain is associated with a variety of musculoskeletal conditions, including trauma. This type of gait is often described as antalgic. Its main characteristic is the short stance phase on the affected side. Other secondary characteristics depend on the pain site and the nature of the underlying condition.

Compensations around the pelvis are often observed in response to hip pathology. The Trendelenburg gait is characterized by hip adduction on the affected weight-bearing side and coronal plane pelvic obliquity, with the affected side being higher than the opposite side. The trunk leans toward the weight-bearing side. This type of gait is caused by hip instability and/or weakness or insufficiency of the hip abductors. In Duchenne gait, the pelvis rotates toward the affected weight-bearing hip in the coronal plane. The hip is therefore abducted during weight bearing. The trunk leans toward the affected weight-bearing side.

Analysis of Gait

Gait assessment is an integral part of the clinical evaluation of the patient. A multitude of musculoskeletal and

neurological conditions can affect it. Important information that may influence diagnosis and treatment is revealed by observation and analysis of gait. This information should be evaluated together with the patient's history, clinical examination, and other diagnostic investigations.

The particular parameters of walking that need analysis and the complexity of the necessary assessment should be determined on an individual patient basis. Instrumented three-dimensional gait analysis using sophisticated equipment is well established for patients with cerebral palsy. Gait analysis for less difficult conditions, such as an isolated leg length discrepancy or drop foot, requires less sophisticated techniques.

An understanding of the capabilities and limitations of the various techniques will avoid over- or under-interpretation of results. Gait analysis is also an important measure of the outcome of treatment. When the aim of treatment is to improve walking, it is essential that gait is objectively evaluated before and after treatment.

Observational Analysis

Systematic observation of gait should form part of the orthopaedic clinical examination. The three anatomical planes should be considered and observation should involve all the mobile segments of the body. The patient's gait should be compared with normal patterns. Deviations of gait that compromise the prerequisites of gait should be given particular attention. Slow-motion video or digital imaging can assist with the detailed assessment of walking. Systematic observation can be enhanced by using validated scores, such as the Edinburgh visual gait score [4].

A significant limitation of observational gait analysis is the difficulty in discriminating between movements that occur in more than one of the three anatomical planes. The degree of knee flexion in the sagittal plane, for example, may be significantly underestimated if the hip is internally rotated at the time of observation. Another typical example of this limitation of visual gait analysis relates to the scissoring of the legs at hip level in diplegic patients: discrimination between hip adduction and internal rotation in this context is challenging (see Fig. 6.4). Quantitative assessment of gait deviations is also challenging by visual observation alone.

Kinematics

The study of kinematics, as part of gait analysis, describes the motion of body segments. It includes their position and

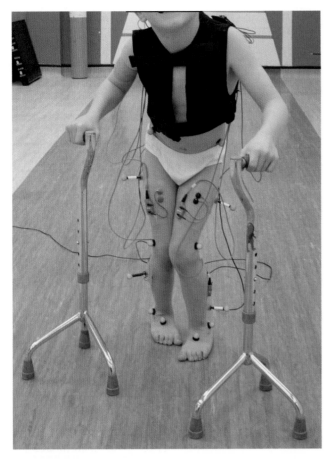

Fig. 6.4 Limitations of observational gait analysis. Discriminating between hip adduction and internal rotation in this patient would be challenging. Quantifying the degree of adduction and/or internal rotation would not be possible through simple observation

orientation, the angles of the joints, and the corresponding linear and angular velocities and accelerations.

Typically, three-dimensional kinematic analysis involves optico-electronic cameras tracking markers placed on anatomical landmarks of the body. The information on the position of the markers is digitized through an appropriate interface. A computerized biomechanical model of the musculoskeletal system is then used to convert the information on the position and movement of the markers to a description of body movements. The output usually involves the graphic representation of individual joint movements during the gait cycle (see Fig. 6.5). Comparison of those graphs with a normal database offers a quantification of the gait deviations observed in the individual patient. State-of-the-art equipment can acquire images at 100 Hz with accuracy of under 1 mm.

Instrumented kinematic analysis can provide accurate, detailed, and quantifiable information on the motion of body segments in the three anatomical planes. It is an objective assessment method which offers invaluable information for managing patients and in evaluating the outcome of treatment. Its main limitation is that it relies on a sophisticated and expensive laboratory setup, which assesses walking on level ground and does not necessarily reproduce real-life conditions. Furthermore, interpretation of gait data is complex and requires specific training.

Kinematic data can also be expressed in terms of muscle length variation (as opposed to angular joint changes). This offers potentially useful information, particularly in neuromuscular conditions. The current biomechanical muscle models, however, are susceptible to error, particularly when anatomical variations and deformities coexist.

Electrogoniometers can be attached to the limbs to measure the dynamic range of joint motion during gait. They are portable but less precise than conventional kinematic equipment. Accelerometers and gyroscopes have also been introduced: they measure, respectively, the acceleration and orientation of body segments. While they can record data for long periods of time and can be used during activities of daily living, they lack precision by comparison with conventional gait analysis.

Kinetics

The information obtained from kinematic analysis can be combined with information obtained from a force platform set into the floor, which measures the ground reaction force of a single step. This combination of data helps to calculate the *inverse dynamics*, a close estimate of the forces and moments acting on individual segments and joints, together with the power generation or absorption in these areas. These data help our understanding of gait deviations and the discrimination between true gait problems and compensations. The output is similar to the kinematic data: Individual joint kinetic variations are shown graphically against time during the gait cycle.

Dynamic Electromyography

Dynamic electromyography (EMG) records the electrical signals from muscles during walking. Multiple muscles can be recorded simultaneously and the signals compared with published or lab-based data of normal phasic activity. Muscles produce EMG signals with any type of contraction, whether concentric, isometric, or eccentric. Furthermore, the intensity of the EMG signal is not indicative of the force generated by the muscle.

For the purposes of gait analysis, most EMGs are obtained using surface electrodes attached to the skin. Fine wires inserted through a needle can be used for deep muscles, such as the tibialis posterior and gluteus medius. In combination with kinematic and kinetic data, EMGs can contribute toward the understanding of gait deviations.

Fig. 6.5 Example of normal kinematic graphs. The left column of graphs represents the sagittal plane, the middle one the coronal, and the right one the transverse. Lower limb joints and segments as shown from proximal (*top*) to distal (*bottom*). The *x*-axis of each graph represents the percentage of the gait cycle. The *y*-axis represents the joint angle. Each curve, therefore, shows the variation of the relevant joint angle during the gait cycle. Right and left leg angles are superimposed in each graph. The vertical line in each graph represents the separation between stance and swing phase at approximately 60% of the gait cycle

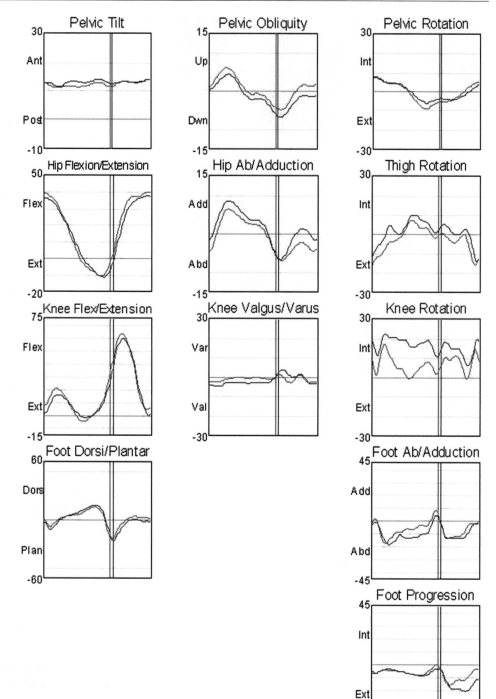

Energy Consumption

Energy consumption during walking indicates the efficiency of gait. Increased consumption suggests an inefficient gait and may contribute to the indications for treatment. Changes in energy consumption which follow treatment are clearly clinically relevant.

Energy consumption is judged indirectly by measuring oxygen consumption. This requires portable equipment to record the exhaled oxygen concentration. In addition, the carbon dioxide produced can be measured. In the absence of sophisticated equipment, the physiological cost index (PCI) of gait can be measured:

$$PCI = (\text{heart rate during walking} - \text{resting heart rate})/\text{speed}.$$

This has been shown to be a reliable indicator of gait energy efficiency.

Plantar Pressure and Foot Kinematics

Information about foot function while walking often helps in planning treatment. State-of-the-art pedobarographs describe the distribution of pressure over the plantar surface of the foot throughout the gait cycle. In recent years the increasing accuracy and resolution of equipment have allowed the development of kinematic foot models. These allow assessment of the motion between different moving segments of the foot during walking. Validation of these models in children is necessary before their clinical use is implemented [5]. Moreover, this information can be synchronized with the kinematic data to allow gait events to be married to changes in plantar pressure [6].

Clinical Application of Gait Analysis

The clinical use of gait analysis was first established in managing children with cerebral palsy [1, 3]. The complex patterns of walking in these children, the interaction between problems in different joints and muscles, and the unpredictability of results following orthopaedic surgery led to the development of motion analysis laboratories. With the support of gait analysis, the concept of single-stage, multi-level orthopaedic surgery replaced the multiple isolated procedures performed year by year and described as the "birthday syndrome" by Mercer Rang [7]. New procedures were developed or refined with the improved understanding of gait abnormalities [8–10]. Currently, most centers managing children with cerebral palsy use gait analysis as part of their preoperative planning of single-stage, multi-level surgery in diplegia as well as in the more complex forms of hemiplegia. Despite some continuing controversy on the repeatability of gait data interpretation, there is evidence that the proper use of gait analysis has led to better results [11].

Gait analysis has also been used extensively in myelodysplasia [12]. Detection of excessive valgus knee strain (valgus thrust) and discrimination between coronal and transverse plane deviations, particularly around the hip, are often the indications for analysis. For example, the combination of dynamic internal hip rotation and external tibial torsion seen in patients with lumbar myelomeningocoele may be mistaken for valgus knee. Transverse plane kinematic data reveal any dynamic rotation while walking, while coronal plane data reveal any valgus knee strain. The differentiation between these two problems is important in management.

Kinematic and kinetic analyses often guide the indications for various orthotics and their modifications to optimize the effects of the ground reaction force. Dynamic spasticity of the plantarflexors persisting throughout the gait cycle may need a rigid ankle foot orthosis (AFO), while equinus in swing may be treated with a flexible AFO which allows dorsiflexion. A ground reaction AFO may help when spasticity of the plantarflexors prevents full knee extension in stance.

Furthermore, after fitting orthoses, gait analysis may be used to tune them. For example, a tendency to knee hyperextension may be managed by pitching an AFO forward by raising the heel. Incomplete knee extension can be treated by pitching the AFO posteriorly and transferring the ground reaction force forward. The video vector technique (video with the ground reaction force superimposed) can be used for this purpose.

Gait analysis, particularly kinetics, may help to resolve treatment dilemmas for common anatomical variants. Genu valgum or varum, in-toeing due to persistent femoral anteversion, internal tibial torsion, or metatarsus adductus, as well as out-toeing due to external hip rotation or tibial torsion are common problems in paediatric orthopaedic clinics. When these normal variants persist beyond the expected remodeling age, a decision has to be made as to whether surgical correction is necessary. In mild cases gait analysis can offer reassurance by demonstrating the absence of any abnormal forces and moments in the proximal joints. With significant anatomical deviation, kinetic abnormalities will be present. This may provide a relative indication for treatment, as abnormal moments may pre-dispose to premature joint degeneration in adult life.

Conclusion

In recent years, several clinical studies on children with orthopaedic problems have used gait analysis as an outcome measure (e.g., congenital club foot, Perthes disease, and end-stage hip arthropathy requiring arthrodesis) [13–15]. These studies underline the importance of assessing gait before and after treatment, particularly when walking ability is the main indication for treatment. By assessing objectively the results of treatment better outcomes should follow. The possibilities for using gait analysis in children with orthopaedic conditions are enormous.

There are promising improvements in gait analysis technology on the horizon. Improved accuracy, speedier acquisition, and strict clinical protocols will improve repeatability. Better biomechanical models and custom-specific models will allow us to combine gait analysis with imaging techniques such as MRI. Forward simulation techniques will permit the creation of biomechanical models where surgery and its outcomes may be simulated before definitive treatment.

References

1. Gage JR. The treatment of gait problems in cerebral palsy series: clinics in developmental medicine, No. 164. London: Mac Keith Press, 2004.

2. Hof AL. Scaling gait data to body size. Gait Posture 1996; 4: 222–3.

3. Sutherland D. The development of mature gait. Gait Posture 1997; 6: 163–70.

4. Read HS, Hazlewood ME, Hillman SJ, et al. Edinburgh visual gait score for use in cerebral palsy. 2003; 23(3):296–301.

5. Stebbins J, Harrington M, Thompson N, et al. Repeatability of a model for measuring foot kinematics in children. Gait Posture 2006; 23(4):401–10.

6. Stebbins J, Harrington M, Giacomozzi C, et al. Assessment of sub-division of plantar pressure measurement in children. Gait Posture 2005; 22(4):372–6.

7. Wenger DR, Rang M. The art and practice of children's orthopaedics. New York: Raven Press; 1993.

8. Ounpuu S, Muik E, Davis RB 3rd, et al. Rectus femoris surgery in children with cerebral palsy. Part II: A comparison between the effect of transfer and release of the distal rectus femoris on knee motion. J Pediatr Orthop 1993; 13(3):331–5.

9. Seniorou M, Thompson N, Harrington M, Theologis T. Recovery of muscle strength following multi-level orthopaedic surgery in diplegic cerebral palsy. Gait Posture 2007; 26(4):475–81.

10. Lee CL, Bleck EE. Surgical correction of equinus deformity in cerebral palsy. Dev Med Child Neurol 1980; 22(3):287–92.

11. Graham HK, Harvey A. Assessment of mobility after multi-level surgery for cerebral palsy. J Bone Joint Surg Br 2007; 89(8):993–4.

12. Duffy CM, Hill AE, Cosgrove AP, et al. Three-dimensional gait analysis in spina bifida. J Pediatr Orthop 1996; 16(6):786–91.

13. Westhoff B, Petermann A, Hirsch MA, et al. Computerized gait analysis in Legg Calvé Perthes disease—analysis of the frontal plane. Gait Posture 2006; 24(2):196–202.

14. Karol LA, Halliday SE, Gourineni P. Gait and function after intra-articular arthrodesis of the hip in adolescents. J Bone Joint Surg Am 2000; 82(4):561–9.

15. Theologis TN, Harrington ME, Thompson N, Benson MK. Dynamic foot movement in children treated for congenital talipes equinovarus. J Bone Joint Surg Br 2003; 85(4):572–7.

Chapter 7

Bone, Cartilage, and Fibrous Tissue Disorders

William G. Cole

Introduction

The disorders to be considered in this chapter are mostly inherited conditions of the musculoskeletal system. There are many hundreds of them, but only the major ones will be considered because the purpose of this chapter is to provide an approach to diagnosis and treatment rather than an encyclopedic account of every known inherited disorder of bone, cartilage, and fibrous tissue.

General Principles

Etiology

The connective tissues contain a wide range of cell types and extracellular matrix components. It is to be expected that mutations of each of the matrix proteins and of the enzymes involved in their synthesis, modification, and degradation will produce diseases with major skeletal involvement. Various examples will illustrate this point. First, mutations of type I collagen, the major collagen of bone, ligaments, tendons, dentin, and sclera, produce osteogenesis imperfecta and one form of the Ehlers–Danlos syndrome. Secondly, mutations of type II collagen, the main collagen of cartilage and intervertebral discs, produce a range of dysplasias with major anomalies of the growth plates, epiphyses, articular surfaces, and intervertebral discs.

The composition of the connective tissues alters during development, aging, and repair. During skeletal development of the limbs, there is a complex series of tightly regulated events that produce mesenchymal and cartilage models of the skeleton. Primary and secondary ossification centers subsequently develop, with definition of the growth plates and articular cartilage. Some of the genes that regulate the embryological events have been identified. They include genes that encode growth factors, growth factor receptors, and transcription factors that switch other genes on and off. For example, a family of genes—the hox genes—encodes transcription factors that regulate segmental development of the axial and peripheral skeleton. Many embryological skeletal events are reproduced during fracture healing, and remodeling of the skeleton and articular surfaces occurs throughout adulthood.

The pathogenesis of the skeletal dysplasias characterized to date can be attributed to a deficiency of a normal component of the tissue, to the addition of mutant components that do not function normally, to the accumulation of normal metabolic intermediates, or to abnormal regulation of development. The tissue distribution of the changes conforms to the normal tissue expression patterns of the relevant genes.

It is to be expected that the genetic causes of an increasing number of the dysplasias will be determined, with consequent improvements in the diagnosis, classification, prediction of prognosis, counseling, and treatment. There are two general approaches to defining the genetic defects. The first approach involves linkage studies in which coinheritance of genetic markers and the clinical phenotype are sought in large families. Such studies can be undertaken quickly because of the ready availability of genetic markers. Linkage analysis was used to identify the fibrillin-1 gene (FBN1) as the Marfan syndromegene and the fibroblast growth factor receptor 3 gene (FGFR3) as the achondroplasia gene. The second approach is to produce a short list of likely candidate genes in which the known distribution of the gene product matches the distribution of the phenotypic features of the disease. The candidate genes are then studied in detail. The candidate gene approach has been successfully used to characterize type I collagen mutations in osteogenesis imperfecta and type II collagen mutations in some of the cartilage dysplasias such as spondyloepiphyseal dysplasia.

W.G. Cole (✉)
Stollery Children's Hospital, University of Alberta, Edmonton, Alberta
Canada; Division of Pediatric Surgery, Department of Surgery,
University of Alberta Edmonton, Alberta, Canada

M. Benson et al. (eds.), *Children's Orthopaedics and Fractures*,
DOI 10.1007/978-1-84882-611-3_7, © Springer-Verlag London Limited 2010

The DNA sequence of the human genome has been completed from DNA fragments obtained from different individuals. Recently, the DNA sequence of an individual has been completed. In addition to these major advances, considerable progress has been made in defining the similarities and differences in DNA sequences between normal individuals as well as between those with various common and rare clinical disorders. It is to be expected that further rapid progress will be made in identifying the disease genes as well as interacting genes and environmental factors that determine a person's susceptibility to a disease. Such studies should also provide new insights into the factors that determine the severity of a given genetic disease within and between families. It has long been recognized that the clinical severity of a given genetic disease, such as osteogenesis imperfecta, can vary significantly amongst affected family members who bear the same collagen mutation. These various molecular advances should result in improved methods and accuracy of diagnosis and are likely to yield new treatment options. The Online Mendelian Inheritance of Man web site provides a portal to new information concerning genetic disorders [1].

Clinical Diagnosis

A child may first be suspected of having an inherited disorder of the skeleton because of obstetric and birth abnormalities, abnormal growth, specific musculoskeletal complaints, family history, or radiographic findings. A detailed history is required and should include information about the family history, pregnancy, birth, growth, development, and the presenting complaints.

A careful clinical examination is also required. If there have been progressive changes in the appearance of the child, families should be asked to provide photographs at various ages for review. It is also useful to examine other affected members of the family in order to assess the variability of the disease and the likely prognosis.

Most children with inherited disorders of the skeleton are either abnormally short or tall, and their bodies are often disproportionate. The limbs may be short relative to the spine, as in short-limbed forms of dwarfism, or long relative to the spine, as in short-trunk forms of dwarfism. The limb segments may also be disproportionate, with more shortening in one segment than in another. For example, children with achondroplasia have more proximal or rhizomelic shortening, those with mesomelic dysplasias have more shortening of the forearms and shins, and those with acromelic dysplasias have greater involvement of the hands and feet. Many children also have anomalies of the head and face.

The height and weight of the child should be recorded on growth charts. Previous measurements and birth measurements are also plotted. Arm span and upper-to-lower segment ratios are recorded, particularly in patients with Marfanoid features. Normally, the upper segment measured from the crown to the pubis is equal to the lower segment measured from the pubis to the heel.

The alignment of the limbs and spine, ranges of movement and stability of joints, limb length discrepancies, and gait anomalies are also recorded.

In many instances, a provisional clinical diagnosis can be rapidly made from the general appearance of the child. This diagnostic process involves pattern matching, in which the clinician compares the general appearance of the child with the features of other children that have previously been seen with known diseases. Syndrome atlases and computer-based diagnostic systems are commonly used to supplement the clinician's memory.

Radiographic Diagnosis

Some disorders, such as achondroplasia, produce characteristic clinical appearances that are unlikely to be confused with other disorders. However, despite confidence in a clinical diagnosis, it is wise to confirm it with radiographs. Furthermore, in many instances a firm clinical diagnosis cannot be made and the definitive diagnosis relies on the radiographic appearances of the skeleton.

A skeletal survey, using standard plain radiographs, is essential and should include the skull, spine, pelvis, and all bones of one arm and leg. Computed tomography (CT) or magnetic resonance imaging (MRI) may be needed to investigate specific lesions such as anomalies of the spinal canal with cord compression. Other imaging methods such as isotope bone scans and ultrasonography are rarely needed for diagnosis.

As the skeletal features of many bone dysplasias change with growth, it is essential that previous radiographs, including birth radiographs, are obtained and kept. All available radiographs are displayed in chronological order. A quick scan will reveal which bones are most affected and these can be examined in detail before re-examining the whole skeleton.

The radiographic pathology is assessed in a manner similar to that applied to a pathology specimen, taking note of the size, shape, and texture of the bone, and the details of localized anomalies. Abnormalities will usually be more marked in one region of the bone, although not necessarily confined to it. The abnormal features are systematically identified and categorized. For example, a dysplasia that has its major effects on epiphyseal development is classified as an epiphyseal dysplasia (e.g. multiple epiphyseal dysplasia). If there is also major spinal involvement, it is classified as a spondyloepiphyseal dysplasia. If the changes are mostly in the metaphyses, the disorder is classified as a metaphyseal dysplasia, such as metaphyseal chondrodysplasia. Similarly, changes that are greatest in the diaphysis are classified as diaphyseal dysplasia.

The distribution of changes between the proximal, middle, and distal segments of the limb is also noted, as is that in the skull and spine. If a child has metaphyseal dysplasia and frontal bone anomalies, the disorder is descriptively named craniometaphyseal dysplasia. Some limb disorders preferentially affect one segment more than another. If the radius, ulna, tibia, and fibula are mainly affected, the disorder is classified as a mesomelic dysplasia.

Various classifications of inherited disorders of the skeleton are available, but all are complex. The most widely used is the International Nomenclature of Constitutional Diseases of Bone [2], which is revised periodically.

Biochemical and Pathological Diagnosis

Routine biochemical diagnosis is available for only a few of the bone dysplasias. Urinary screening tests and enzyme assays are used in children with suspected storage disorders, such as the mucopolysaccharidoses. Metabolic screening is also used to investigate children with various types of rickets.

Characteristic histopathological changes are present in many skeletal dysplasias but they are infrequently used for diagnosis. However, specimens should always be obtained for biochemical and histological examination when a child is having an operation on affected tissues.

General Management

Although there are many inherited disorders of the skeleton, each one is rare and, as a result, most children should be reviewed by staff experienced in the field. Many children's hospitals have multidisciplinary bone dysplasia clinics that involve an orthopaedic surgeon, medical geneticist, social worker, and associated specialists as required. Children should be referred for assessment once an inherited abnormality of the skeleton is suspected.

An accurate diagnosis is essential in order to be able to provide families with appropriate information. It is needed for the prediction of mature height, associated anomalies, prognosis, treatment, and genetic counseling. A diagnosis should not be made if there is any uncertainty about it; it

is preferable to follow the child's progress until the diagnosis becomes obvious when other features appear. Syndrome atlases and computer systems with clinical and radiographic illustrations stored on a laser disc can also be used as aids in diagnosing an unknown syndrome.

The child's height and weight are recorded at each clinic visit. Specific areas, which will vary with the different disorders, are also reviewed. For example, regular ophthalmological examinations are required in children with spondyloepiphyseal dysplasia, Marfan's syndrome, homocystinuria, Stickler syndrome, and Ehlers–Danlos syndrome. Infants with achondroplasia need regular assessment by ear, nose, and throat specialists. Regular cardiovascular assessments are also required in patients with Marfan's syndrome.

Apart from some of the metabolic disorders, considered in the next chapter, no specific treatment is available for any of the inherited disorders of the skeleton. Treatment is, therefore, symptomatic. Initially, the focus is on providing appropriate verbal and written information for the parents about their child's disorder and the risk of recurrence in future pregnancies. This information must be reinforced by regular visits to a bone dysplasia clinic. Medical social workers and various self-help organizations such as the Little People's associations and Brittle Bone societies can also provide valuable support.

Specific assistance will often need to be given when the child starts kindergarten and primary school, in the transition from secondary to tertiary education, and when entering the workforce. Obtaining a driving license, for example, is a challenge that requires expert assistance. Additional information is often sought by affected individuals when marriage and children are contemplated.

Genetic Counseling

Genetic counseling is requested by most families but should be undertaken only by those experienced in the specialty. It involves a discussion of the clinical disorder, the risk of recurrence in another child, and consideration of the burden of the disorder. An unequivocal diagnosis is clearly essential before such discussions commence.

Intrauterine diagnosis by biochemical means is available for a few bone dysplasias, such as the mucopolysaccharidoses and osteogenesis imperfecta. Many bone dysplasias are diagnosed in utero by ultrasonography. The lengths and shapes of individual long bones can be determined with remarkable accuracy, as can anomalies of vertebral development and deformities of the spine and limbs. Fractures can be detected, and osteoporosis is likely if there is a poor echogenic signal from the skeleton.

Orthopaedic Management

Many children need very little orthopaedic treatment, whereas others have major orthopaedic anomalies that almost defy treatment. In general, orthopaedic management is directed toward preventing and correcting deformities, stabilizing lax and dislocated joints, supporting fragile bones, and correcting limb length discrepancies. The treatment is usually more complex than for similar problems in otherwise normal children. It is undertaken with the help of paramedical staff who assist the children to be independent in their activities of daily living.

Some deformities, such as talipes equinovarus, are present at birth, but many develop later. Deformities such as tibia vara and valga may progress rapidly when the mechanical axis of the limb is disturbed to such an extent that abnormal growth from asymmetrical loading of the growth plates is added to the pre-existing growth disturbance. Such deformities should be corrected before they deteriorate rapidly; they may need to be corrected several times during growth. Hemiphyseal tension band plating appears useful for correcting angular deformities in young children. The technique appears safer than alternative procedures such as hemiphyseal stapling.

Malalignment of the limb is corrected surgically because orthoses, particularly in dwarfed children, are poorly tolerated and largely ineffective. The correction of limb alignment often requires osteotomies at multiple levels. The deformities are usually complex, with both angulatory and rotational anomalies, and the adjoining joints may be unstable or stiff. Careful preoperative planning is required. Both limbs should be corrected at the same operation or within a short time of each other. Plaster fixation cannot be relied upon in children with short limbs, so that internal fixation or external unilateral or ring fixation is preferable. Hemiphyseal stapling or tension plating can be used near the end of growth to correct some angular deformities.

Spinal deformities often develop at an early age and are severe and rigid. Orthoses are of limited value in children of short stature because they restrict mobility and are ineffective in children with soft bone and lax tissues. Localized spinal fusion or non-fusion rodding may be needed before the vertebrae are big enough for definitive internal fixation and arthrodesis. Rib distraction can also be used to correct some spinal deformities in young children. Atlanto-axial instability is common in dysplasias with major spinal involvement: Atlanto-axial fusion may be required for gross instability and to relieve cervical myelopathy. Decompression of the lumbar spinal canal and its nerve root canals is frequently required in adults with achondroplasia and cauda equina syndrome.

Premature osteoarthritis is a common outcome of many bone dysplasias. Replacement arthroplasties may be required. These may need to be tailor-made but often improve function greatly.

Specific Bone Disorders

This section will be confined to osteogenesis imperfecta; metabolic and endocrine disorders affecting bone are presented in Chapter 8.

Osteogenesis Imperfecta

Osteogenesis imperfecta (OI) is one of the most common and best known of the skeletal dysplasias. It is a form of genetically determined osteoporosis for which orthopaedic treatment is frequently required.

Etiology

The birth incidence is approximately 1:20,000. About 80% of cases of OI are caused by mutations of the type I collagen genes. Type I collagen is the principal collagen of bone, ligament, dentin, and sclera, the tissues most affected in OI. Most cases result from autosomal dominant mutations that are either inherited from a parent or develop spontaneously as a new mutation. A number of affected children may occur in families with apparently normal parents as a result of autosomal recessive inheritance or gonadal mosaicism. Autosomal recessive inheritance, in which an abnormal allele is inherited from both parents, has a recurrence risk of 25% with each pregnancy. In contrast, gonadal mosaicism, in which one parent carries an autosomal dominant mutation in the sperm or ova, has an unpredictable risk of recurrence. Overall, the recurrence risk of apparently normal parents having a second child with OI is about 7%.

The autosomal dominant mutations of the genes for type I collagen produce two general categories of protein defects. In the first group, the mutations inactivate one copy or allele of the gene and result in a 50% reduction in the amount of normal type I collagen in bone. These patients usually have a mild form of the disease (Type I OI). The bone is osteoporotic, with osteoid seams that are about half the normal thickness. Lamellar bone is found in the trabeculae and with Haversian systems in the diaphysis. In the second group, the tissues contain a reduced amount of normal collagen in addition to type I collagen molecules that contain one or two mutant collagen chains. The patients are usually severely affected and may have a perinatal lethal disease. The bone morphology is grossly abnormal, with defects of bone modeling and lack of normal cortical bone formation. The bone is of a woven type, with minimal amounts of osteoid and without lamellar bone and Haversian systems.

In general, the severity of the clinical disease is greater in those with mutant collagen in the tissues than it is in those with only a reduced amount of normal type I collagen.

Several additional disease genes that are involved in the enzymatic modification of type I collagen have been identified in some patients with autosomal recessive forms of OI. The protein products of two disease genes, cartilage-associated protein (CRTAP) and leprecan (LEPRE1), normally form an enzyme complex that hydroxylates the 3-position of a single proline residue within type I collagen molecules [3]. The severity of the clinical phenotype is determined by the amount of residual enzymatic activity, being absent in lethal cases and reduced in moderately severe cases.

Clinical and Radiographic Features

OI is a heterogeneous disorder. In 1979, Sillence et al. [4] classified the condition into four broad categories which have since expanded into eight (see Table 7.1). The main clinical and radiographic features in the absence of treatment and the inheritance patterns are outlined below.

Table 7.1 Classification of osteogenesis imperfecta

Type	Features	Inheritance
I	IA: Bone fragility, blue sclerae, and normal teeth	Autosomal dominant
	IB: Same as IA but with dentinogenesis imperfecta	
II	IIA: Lethal perinatal form due to mutations of the type I collagen genes	Autosomal dominant
	IIB: Lethal perinatal form due to mutations of cartilage-associated protein	Autosomal recessive
III	Progressive deforming form. Multiple fractures at birth with progressive deformities, normal sclerae, and dentinogenesis imperfecta	Autosomal dominant and recessive
IV	IVA: Moderately severe bone fragility, white sclerae, and normal teeth	Autosomal dominant
	IVB: Similar to IVA but with dentinogenesis imperfecta	
V	Similar to IVA but with interosseous ossification and susceptibility to hyperplastic fracture callus healing	Autosomal dominant
VI	Similar to but more severe than IV and has distinct bone histopathology	Uncertain
VII	Similar but more severe than IV. Rhizomelic shortening with minimally blue sclerae	Autosomal recessive
VIII	Resembles II and III. Severe growth retardation and undermineralization of skeleton	Autosomal recessive

Type I OI (Blue Sclerae and Autosomal Dominant Inheritance)

This is the most common and mildest clinical form. It is the classical type, with blue sclerae, bone fragility, minimal deformities, premature deafness, and autosomal dominant inheritance. Birth weight and length are normal, but one or more bones may be fractured. A family history of OI will prompt careful assessment of the scleral color, as it is the most consistent feature of OI in large families. Although most neonates have light blue sclerae, those with type I OI have dark blue sclerae with a gray tinge.

The osteoporotic skeleton is well formed and modeling of the metaphyses is also normal. The skull usually contains Wormian bones. Fractures commonly occur for the first time when the child starts to walk. The blue sclerae may then be observed for the first time in children with sporadic new mutations. The severity of osteoporosis and the frequency of fractures may differ considerably between affected members of large pedigrees.

The types of fractures that occur in type I OI are similar to those seen in normal children, except that they occur more easily. The fractures heal well. Fractures are less common after puberty but may increase later in life as the effects of age- and sex-related osteoporosis are superimposed upon the effects of the underlying OI.

Dentinogenesis imperfecta also occurs in some patients with type I OI and premature deafness from otosclerosis is common.

Type II OI (Lethal Perinatal)

This is the most severe type of OI and is usually fatal within hours of birth, although some babies survive for several months. The babies are dwarfed and have gray-blue sclerae and short, bowed limbs. The skull is soft and the face is small.

Radiographs show severe osteoporosis, with multiple fractures of limbs and ribs. The long bones are frequently short and crumpled, and the calvarium contains minimal bone. Most cases are the result of new autosomal dominant mutations of the type I collagen genes, referred to as IIA, while some result from autosomal recessive mutations of CRTAP or LEPRE1, referred to as IIB.

Type III OI (Progressively Deforming Type)

Babies with type III OI have severe bone fragility, with multiple fractures at birth. In contrast to babies with type II OI, the chest is usually well formed, with few or no fractures of the ribs. The inheritance is autosomal recessive or autosomal dominant. The autosomal dominant forms are usually the result of mutations of the type I collagen genes. The autosomal recessive forms overlap with types II and VIII OI which result from mutations of genes involved in prolyl 3-hydroxylation of type I collagen.

The birth weight and length of these babies are nearly normal. The sclerae are pale blue and fade over the following years to become white. The limbs are bowed and the calvarium is large relative to the small triangular face (see Fig. 7.1). The long bones progressively bow with growth and multiple fractures are common. The shafts of the long bones may be wide at birth but narrow later. The epiphyses appear large in proportion to the narrow shafts and the growth plates may fracture into many pieces, which round up to form islands of endochondral ossification. These islands produce a "popcorn" appearance on radiographs (see Fig. 7.2), but eventually they disappear, leaving an enlarged lucent epiphysis. Progressive bowing, multiple fractures, and disruption of the growth plates account for the very short skeleton. Progressive flattening of the vertebral bodies and kyphoscoliosis are common. The chest becomes barrel shaped, with a pectus carinatum. As the lumbar spine shortens, the wide

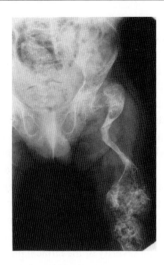

Fig. 7.2 Osteogenesis imperfecta type III. Radiograph showing "popcorn" femur and tibia, with a shepherd's crook (severe coxa vara) femoral deformity and multiple fractures. Courtesy of Dr. R. Smith

rib cage overlaps the narrow pelvis. The iliac wings flare outward as the hip joints migrate toward each other. Severe shortening of the trunk and limbs results in very short stature and reduced sitting height. Children with type III OI may walk for a period, particularly if treated with bisphosphonates, but most cease to walk as they become older.

Dentinogenesis imperfecta is frequent.

Type IV OI (White Sclerae with Autosomal Dominant Inheritance)

This is a form of OI in which there are autosomal dominant inheritance, white sclerae, a moderate number of fractures, and variable severity of bone deformity. It resembles type I OI, except that the sclerae are normal in color. Dentinogenesis imperfecta is common. It is in this group that confusion with child abuse is most common.

Type V OI

Patients in this category resemble patients with type IV OI. However, there are several distinct features. Radiographs of their forearms and lower legs show ossification extending into the interosseous membranes and radiodense metaphyseal bands immediately adjacent to the growth plates. These radiographic features appear to be unique. Another important feature is their susceptibility to hyperplastic fracture callus. It has long been recognized that some patients with OI can produce massive amounts of callus, resembling an osteosarcoma, following a fracture. However, this aberrant response to a fracture appears to be limited to this group of patients who have interosseous membrane ossification. Type V OI is

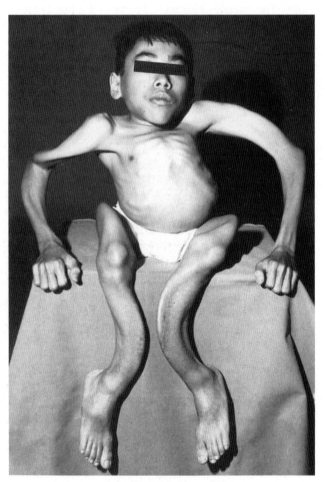

Fig. 7.1 Osteogenesis imperfecta type III. This child presented with multiple deformities and minimal previous treatment

inherited as an autosomal dominant trait but the disease gene has not been identified.

Type VI OI

This form of OI is similar to but more severe than type IV OI. The main distinguishing features from type IV OI are differences in the histopathology of the bone and in the absence of demonstrable type I collagen mutations. The inheritance pattern is uncertain and no disease gene has been identified.

Type VII OI

This type of OI was added as the result of pedigree analysis of a moderately severe form of OI that showed autosomal recessive inheritance. Affected individuals had multiple fractures at birth. Fractures recurred during childhood but diminished in adolescence. The skeleton showed progressive deformities during childhood and produced rhizomelic shortening of the limbs and severe coxa vara. The sclerae were minimally blue. Molecular analyses showed mutations of the CRTAP, which encodes a protein that is involved in the prolyl 3-hydroxylation of a single proline residue of type I collagen.

Type VIII OI

This is a severe autosomal recessive form of OI that overlaps with types II and III OI. The babies have white sclerae, severe growth deficiency, extreme undermineralization of the skeleton, and bulbous metaphyses. Mutational analyses have shown that they bear mutations of the LEPRE1 gene that encodes the prolyl 3-hydroxylase enzyme that forms a complex with cartilage-associated protein. Together they are involved in prolyl 3-hydroxylation of a single proline residue in type I collagen.

Investigations

In most instances, the diagnosis of OI can be made from the clinical appearance of the individual, the family history, and plain radiographs. Diagnostic difficulty is frequent in patients with sporadic forms of type IV OI because such individuals may have normal sclerae and teeth and no bone malformations. In infancy, this form of OI is frequently misdiagnosed as child abuse (see Chapter 42). Careful assessment of the radiographs may reveal osteoporosis, slender bones with fine cortices, and Wormian bones. Dental assessment may also demonstrate subclinical evidence of dentinogenesis imperfecta.

The diagnosis of type IV OI should be suspected in a school-aged child who has repeated fractures and none of the usual clinical features of OI. In this situation, measurement of the bone mineral density is helpful in determining whether osteopenia is present; normal bone density standards for children are available, and help to exclude the condition. Type I collagen analyses provide the definitive evidence of OI but are time consuming and expensive and not routinely indicated.

Management

As with other bone dysplasias, families should be referred to an orthopaedic surgeon and geneticist who specialize in this field, once the diagnosis is suspected.

There is currently no specific treatment that will correct the underlying type I collagen mutations. Specific treatment using somatic gene therapy is likely to be difficult to achieve, as each child with OI has its own particular mutation. In addition, major improvements in somatic gene therapy methods will be needed before the technique can be considered seriously. However, non-specific bisphosphonate treatment of severe and moderately severe types of OI appears to be successful in relieving bone pain, improving strength, reducing the number of fractures, and improving the density of the bones; the effects appear to be greatest when it is commenced within a few months of birth [5]. Current evidence indicates that the natural history of types III and IV OI is significantly improved after bisphosphonate treatment, which reduces bone resorption: Histological studies of iliac crest biopsies show that it increases the thickness and density of the iliac crest. Further trials are in progress to determine the effectiveness of bisphosphonates in the mild type I form of OI.

Treatment of Fractures and Deformities

Severely affected babies usually have multiple fractures, in varying stages of healing, at birth. Unstable fractures require simple splintage to reduce pain and to aid nursing. Analgesics may also be needed. The pain usually decreases after several weeks as the fractures heal. These babies are difficult to nurse and parents need assistance in learning to care for their child. Home visits and regular clinic assessments are essential in the first few months of life. Bisphosphonate treatment may be commenced in the neonatal period.

Thermoplastic splints for upper and lower limbs are provided for home treatment of fractures. The splints are easy to apply and provide good first-aid support for the fractured limb. Radiographs may be obtained, but in many instances it is appropriate to rely on the clinical diagnosis of a fracture.

The methods of treating fractures in OI are the same as in normal children, except that the period of immobilization is kept to a minimum. Home gallows traction kits are useful in the treatment of femoral shaft fractures in young children with OI. Standing and walking with lower limb plasters are encouraged in previously mobile children.

The role of external and internal splintage of the skeleton requires evaluation in children receiving bisphosphonate treatment. External supports such as inflatable suits or polypropylene orthoses can be used to support the limb; they are most effective after deformities have been corrected by osteotomies or osteoclasis. As an alternative, the support can be provided internally, using intramedullary rods (see Fig. 7.3). Fragmentation and rodding were popularized by Sofield et al. in 1952 [6]. It dramatically reduces the number of fractures in the involved bone but has the disadvantage that, with growth, the bone bows beyond the rod and re-fractures. Stress shielding from the rod also leads to further thinning of the diaphysis. These rods may need to be changed several times during growth. To avoid these problems, the telescoping rod was developed. However, this must be inserted correctly; otherwise there is a high technical failure rate. Also, the bone needs to be sufficiently strong to provide an anchor for the ends of the rod or it will not extend. Multiple osteotomies are frequently required to correct deformities and are best made as closing wedge osteotomies with minimal periosteal stripping. If too large a rod is used the bone is stress-shielded and wastes; if too slender it will bend and break.

In adolescents and adults with OI it is usually appropriate to use the internal fixation systems that are commonly used in the management of trauma. Modern intramedullary rods with cross-bolt fixation can provide excellent internal splintage of long bones. The cross bolts are removed once the fracture is healed, but the rod is best left in place.

Scoliosis and kyphoscoliosis are common in untreated, severe forms of OI. In some, arthrodesis with spinal instrumentation is appropriate. In many children with severe OI, however, the vertebral bodies flatten within the first few years of life and scoliosis develops rapidly. Orthotic or plaster management is not practical in most, because the chest wall deforms without any change in spinal shape. The small and severely osteoporotic vertebrae are also unsuitable for most forms of internal fixation. However, the prevalence of spinal deformities requires evaluation in children receiving bisphosphonates. Restoration of vertebral height may follow bisphosphonate treatment.

Mobility

All parents are keen for their child with OI to walk. Bisphosphonates appear to improve significantly the walking ability of children with severe forms of OI. In the absence of bisphosphonates, community walking is rarely achieved in children with type III OI and is not achieved in some patients with severe type I or IV OI. The children who are unable to walk have severe osteoporosis, severe deformities, and muscle weakness. In such children, it is important to set achievable goals in therapy. If the child shows no signs of wishing to walk, it is unlikely that the correction of deformities with external or internal splintage will transform the child into an effective walker. Under these circumstances, it is more desirable to focus on other methods of achieving mobility; children as young as 2 years can use electric mobility devices. Provision of such devices gives the child more independence and stimulates motivation. The provision of an electric mobility device at an early age does not prevent later attempts to stand and walk.

Specific Cartilage Disorders

Achondroplasia

Achondroplasia is the most common and best known form of dwarfism. The clinical and radiographic appearances are remarkably constant.

Etiology

Achondroplasia is inherited as an autosomal dominant but 80–90% of cases result from new mutations of the FGFR3

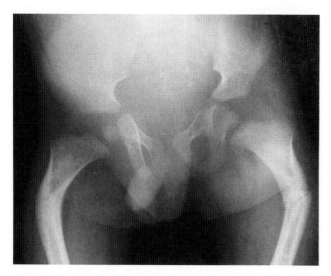

Fig. 7.3 Osteogenesis imperfecta type IV. Radiograph showing subtrochanteric deformities and a pathological fracture of the femur. This child is able to walk, but correction of the femoral deformities and insertion of intramedullary rods were required to prevent recurrent fractures

gene. Histological assessment of growth plates has shown relatively normal architecture, except that the cartilage columns are short and lack the usual linear array of cells.

Clinical Features

At Birth

The most obvious features at birth are the abnormal facies and disproportionate shortness. The skull is large, with a prominent forehead, biparietal bossing, and flattening of the occiput. The nasal bridge is depressed, with midface hypoplasia and prominence of the lower jaw.

Achondroplasia is a rhizomelic, short-limbed form of dwarfism. The limbs are relatively short compared with the trunk and the proximal segments of the limbs are relatively shorter still (rhizomelic) compared with the middle and distal segments. The fingertips usually reach to the iliac crests or greater trochanters. The amount of skin, subcutaneous fat, and muscle appears excessive. The hands are short, and the stubby fingers produce a trident appearance when extended.

The limbs are well aligned at birth. The elbows have fixed flexion deformities of about 30°, whereas most other joints are lax.

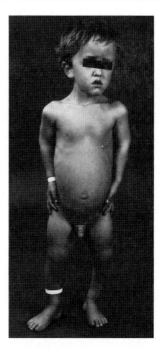

Fig. 7.4 Achondroplasia. Note the frontal bossing, flat nasal bridge, and long torso relative to the short limbs. This child has rhizomelic shortening of the limbs; he developed progressive bowing of the left tibia

During Childhood

The disproportionate short stature becomes more obvious during childhood (see Figs. 7.4 and 7.5). Gross motor development is delayed by about 6 months because of hypotonia and joint laxity. Delay beyond this time may be due to stenosis of the foramen magnum, with compression of the medulla oblongata and cervical spinal cord.

Rapid calvarial development occurs during the first 12–18 months of life. True hydrocephalus can develop, although shunting of cerebrospinal fluid is rarely required. Recurrent middle ear infections are common in the preschool and early school-age child. They are due to facial hypoplasia with constriction and hypoplasia of the Eustachian tubes. Deafness is a frequent sequel unless treated early. Dental crowding may also result from hypoplasia of the jaw.

The children are slow to develop head control, because the skull is relatively large and the spinal muscles are hypotonic. The large head, muscle hypotonia, and ligament laxity also contribute to the rounded thoraco-lumbar kyphosis that develops when the child first starts to sit. The kyphosis is postural in most children. Once the child starts to walk, the kyphosis changes to a marked lumbar lordosis, and the abdomen and buttocks become prominent. A few children develop an angular thoraco-lumbar kyphosis as a result of

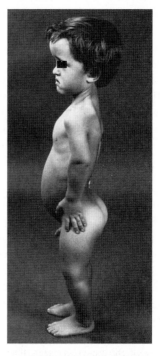

Fig. 7.5 Achondroplasia. Side view of patient shown in Fig. 7.4. Note the prominent calvarium, midface hypoplasia, excessive lumbar lordosis, and rhizomelic shortening of the limbs

wedging of the vertebral bodies at this level. Progressive thoraco-lumbar kyphosis is likely to follow.

The knee is hypermobile because of ligament laxity. Mediolateral stability is present when the knee is hyperextended. The walking child usually has mild genu varum and internal tibial torsion. These deformities give little trouble in early childhood but later may cause aching over the lateral side of the knee as a result of stretching of the lateral collateral ligament. In addition, the overlong fibula may abut against the calcaneus and prevent valgus at the subtalar joint.

The restricted elbow joint motion usually persists. Fixed flexion deformities of the hips are also common in later childhood but are rarely troublesome.

During Adolescence and Adulthood

The average adult height is 131 cm for men and 124 cm for women with achondroplasia. The principal musculoskeletal problem arising in the mid to late teens and early adulthood is neurological deterioration resulting from spinal stenosis. Short pedicles make the spinal canal much smaller than normal, but several additional factors add to the stenosis; these include excessive lumbar lordosis secondary to an angular thoraco-lumbar kyphosis, osteophytes and herniation of degenerative intervertebral discs.

The earliest clinical indication of stenosis is decreased exercise tolerance. Aches and paraesthesia in the limbs may be incorrectly attributed to osteoarthritis of peripheral joints. However, osteoarthritis of peripheral joints is infrequent, and such symptoms are usually due to spinal stenosis. In the early stages, these symptoms are relieved by flexion of the spine and hips or by sitting. Later, progressive neurological impairment occurs, with persistent backache and overt neurological signs caused by compression of the cauda equina. An abrupt deterioration in neurological status may follow an injury.

Radiographic Features

The radiographic features of achondroplasia are present at birth and are diagnostic. Radiographs of the skull, lumbar spine, and pelvis are the minimum required to make a diagnosis. The calvarium is large, with prominence of the frontal, parietal, and occipital bones. The base of the skull and foramen magnum are hypoplastic and occipitalization of the atlas is frequent. The characteristic feature of the achondroplastic spine is the progressive narrowing of the interpedicular distances from the thoracic to the sacral spine, in contrast to the normal widening of the interpedicular distances. The pedicles and the anteroposterior diameters of the vertebral bodies are also short, and posterior scalloping of the vertebrae is usual (see Fig. 7.6).

A rounded thoraco-lumbar kyphosis is common in infancy, but lumbar lordosis develops after walking commences. The sacrum becomes more horizontal as a result of

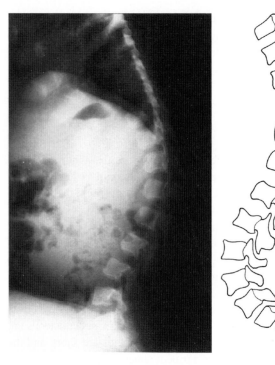

Fig. 7.6 Achondroplasia. Lateral radiograph of the spine of a 1-year-old child, showing short pedicles and posterior scalloping of the vertebral bodies

increasing angulation at the lumbo-sacral junction. In contrast to these normal changes with growth, a few infants develop wedging of the T12/L1 vertebral bodies. It is commonly associated with a progressive gibbus and, later, cauda equina compression.

The pelvis also has a characteristic shape. The ilia are wide, the greater sciatic notches are deep, and the superior margins of the acetabulum are horizontal. The femoral necks are short, but the neck-shaft angles are usually normal. The shafts of the femora and other long bones are broad, with flared metaphyses.

An oval-shaped lucency is common at birth in the proximal humeri and femora but disappears over several years. In infancy, the distal femoral growth plate also has a characteristic inverted-V shape, with a correspondingly shaped ossific center of the distal femoral epiphysis (see Fig. 7.7). The growth plate becomes more horizontal with growth. The fibula is longer than the tibia and may be associated with tibia vara. The distal fibula may also abut against the calcaneus.

Progressive deformity of the radial head and posterior bowing of the radius is frequent and lead to posterior subluxation and dislocation of the radial head in later childhood.

Management

A clinical and radiographic diagnosis of achondroplasia can usually be confidently made at birth. The features are

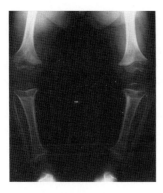

Fig. 7.7 Achondroplasia. Same child as in Fig. 7.6. Radiograph of legs, slowing the short broad bones with inverted, V-shaped distal femoral growth plates

characteristic and there is little clinical and radiographic variability. Achondroplasia needs to be distinguished from other dwarfing conditions evident at this time, including diastrophic dysplasia, lethal short-limbed dwarfing syndromes, and spondyloepiphyseal dysplasia congenita. In the past, many of these conditions were misdiagnosed as achondroplasia.

In school-age children, achondroplasia can resemble hypochondroplasia. This latter dysplasia shares many of the features of achondroplasia, but is less severe; both are caused by mutations of the FGFR3 gene.

Treatment is symptomatic. Initial treatment focuses on providing parents with verbal and written information about achondroplasia. Additional information and continuing support are also available from the Little People's or related associations.

Infants and young children are reviewed regularly in order to provide general support and to follow their development and growth. The height and weight can be plotted on normal growth charts and on normal achondroplastic growth charts. The particular medical problems that may require investigation and treatment are recurrent middle ear infections, possible hydrocephalus, possible cervical cord compression, thoraco-lumbar kyphosis, and tibia vara.

It may be necessary to insert grommets into the middle ears to provide drainage. CT and MRI of the brain and cervical cord are undertaken in infants with possible hydrocephalus or spinal cord compression: A general anesthetic is usually required for these investigations. A cerebrospinal fluid shunt may occasionally be needed to correct hydrocephalus, and occasionally a posterior fossa decompression is needed to release the contents of the posterior fossa and the upper cervical spinal canal.

Infants with wedging of the bodies of the vertebrae at the thoraco-lumbar junction need orthotic treatment in an attempt to prevent progressive kyphosis. Anterior release and grafting may be required in the few children with progressive wedging of the vertebral bodies and an increasing

gibbus. Orthoses are unnecessary and expensive for normal achondroplastic infants who have a rounded thoraco-lumbar kyphosis without anterior wedging of the vertebral bodies.

The treatment of spinal stenosis in early adulthood is difficult. Neurological investigation has been aided considerably by MRI of the cauda equina and spinal cord. Lumbar myelography is often difficult and dangerous because of the narrow spinal canal arid partial or complete blockage of the subarachnoid space. Cisternal puncture is also difficult because of the overhanging occiput and basilar impression. Posterior decompression of the stenotic spinal canal and nerve root canals is usually required to relieve spinal stenosis. The surgery is difficult because of the thick bone and the cramped space and the results are unpredictable.

Progressive unilateral or bilateral tibia vara and internal tibial torsion may develop in early childhood and require correction. Careful preoperative planning is required to ensure full correction of each component of the deformity. Standing radiographs and photographs are essential because the knee is lax. Both legs are draped and sterile tourniquets are used, so that the alignment of both limbs can be observed. Often two osteotomies of the tibia and an osteotomy of the fibula are required in order to restore the mechanical axis of the limb. External fixators are often used to maintain the alignment. Tension band plating of the proximal tibial physis may be used as an alternative to osteotomies in milder deformities. Lengthening of the femora, tibiae, and humeri as a means of increasing height and arm length can be undertaken, but its place in the management of achondroplasia remains controversial.

Pseudoachondroplasia

This dysplasia is distinct from achondroplasia. It is also known as the pseudoachondroplastic form of spondyloepiphyseal dysplasia, in order to highlight the widespread changes in the skeleton.

Etiology

Pseudoachondroplasia is an autosomal dominant trait. The cartilages are disorganized and the chondrocytes contain intracellular inclusions. Mutations of the cartilage oligomeric matrix protein gene, COMP, have been identified in patients with this condition [7–9].

Clinical Features

The child appears normal at birth. By the second to third year, growth retardation, a waddling gait, and angular deformities of the legs are observed (see Figs. 7.8 and 7.9). This

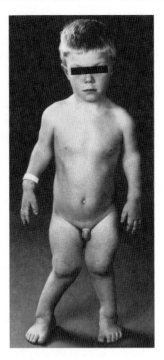

Fig. 7.8 Pseudoachondroplasia. Note the short stature, normal facies, and severe deformities of lower limbs

is a short-limbed form of dwarfism, with body proportions resembling those of achondroplasia. However, the head and face are normal. The lumbar lordosis is exaggerated, and scoliosis may develop.

Ligament laxity and progressive lower limb deformities are common in young children. Typically, the lower limbs have a windswept appearance, with genu valgum and an adducted hip on one side and genu varum and an abducted hip on the other. Occasionally, symmetric bow legs or knock knees develop.

The windswept deformities are progressive. The adducted hip subluxates and is associated with pelvic obliquity and scoliosis. The valgus knee also subluxates. The adducted hip drives the femoral condyles anteromedially, whereas the tibial plateau translates posterolaterally and rotates externally. In late childhood, the patella is chronically dislocated and there is minimal contact between the tibial and femoral condyles. At this stage, the patient may have great difficulty standing, and mobility is severely restricted. The ankles may also subluxate. Premature osteoarthritis is usual.

The adult height is between 82 and 130 cm.

Radiographic Features

The long bones are short, broad, and misshapen, and the metaphyses are cupped and flared. The epiphyses are delayed in their appearance and are small and irregular (see Fig. 7.10). The pubis and ischium are hypoplastic, and the acetabular roof is horizontal. The vertebral bodies are irregular and biconvex, with central projections (see Fig. 7.11). Odontoid hypoplasia is frequent, but atlanto-axial instability is uncommon (see Fig. 7.12). The ribs are spatulate.

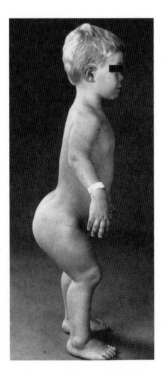

Fig. 7.9 Pseudoachondroplasia. Side view of patient shown in Fig. 7.8. Note the normal skull and face, the short limbs, and flexion contractures of elbows, hips, and knees. The spine is flat

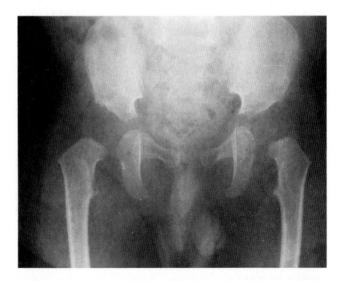

Fig. 7.10 Pseudoachondroplasia. Radiograph of the pelvis in a child aged 2 years. Note the delayed ossification of the femoral epiphyses, the abnormal contour of the acetabulum, and the abnormal ossification of the pubis and ischium

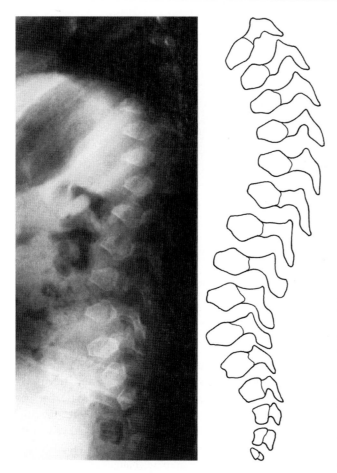

Fig. 7.11 Pseudoachondroplasia. Lateral radiograph of the spine in the same patient as in Fig. 7.10, showing biconvex vertebral bodies with central projections

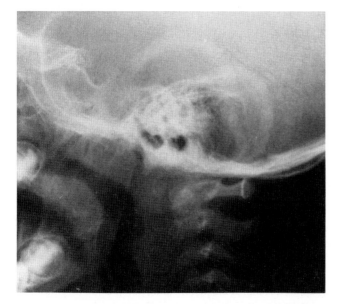

Fig. 7.12 Pseudoachondroplasia. Lateral radiograph of the cervical spine in the same patient as in Figs. 7.10 and 7.11, showing odontoid hypoplasia

Management

Pseudoachondroplasia may be confused with achondroplasia. However, babies with pseudoachondroplasia are normal at birth. Later, when some of the disproportionate features of achondroplasia develop, the pseudoachondroplastic child is noted to have a normal head and face, and there are major differences in the radiographic features of the spine and peripheral skeleton compared with those of the achondroplastic child.

The major orthopaedic problems during childhood involve the alignment of the lower limbs. Progressive deformity usually merits surgical correction. Multiple osteotomies may be required to restore the weight-bearing line and the plane of the various joints. However, epiphyseal development is grossly delayed, so that the shape of the joints is impossible to determine from standard radiographs. MRI, ultrasonography, or arthrograms can be used to determine the plane and shape of the cartilaginous epiphyses. In addition, it is necessary to assess with care the laxity of the knee joints and to determine the alignment with the knee fully extended and when weight-bearing. Rotatory malalignment is also noted. Weight-bearing radiographs and photographs are essential for record keeping and surgical planning.

Corrective lower limb surgery is undertaken with both legs and the pelvis prepared and draped. Multiple osteotomies are often required, and it is best to commence proximally. Three-dimensional corrections are required at most sites. The proximal femoral osteotomies are fixed with a blade plate or screw plate, but distal osteotomies are fixed with crossed Kirschner wires and the limb supported in a hip spica. The second side is corrected 3 weeks later, when the osteotomies are stable on the first side. In older children, monolateral or circular frames can be used to maintain the alignment of the limbs. Lengthening the limbs in pseudoachondroplasia may increase the likelihood of premature osteoarthritis. Many of the older children are obese, and it is desirable to reduce their weight before corrective surgery is undertaken.

Despite the enthusiasm for corrective surgery that exists in some centers, recurrence of deformities is common. Nonetheless, if no procedures are undertaken in young children, many will not be able to walk later in childhood. Hemiphyseal tension band plating of the greater trochanter, distal femur, and proximal tibial is currently being evaluated as a simple method of early restoration and maintenance of mechanical alignment of the lower limb. Total joint arthroplasty, particularly of the hip, may be required in the young adult.

Atlanto-axial instability is not as common as in other forms of spondyloepiphyseal dysplasia. Scoliosis of moderate degree is usually seen in patients with pelvic obliquity. Treatment is directed toward restoring pelvic symmetry. Arthrodesis and instrumentation of the spine are rarely required.

Mobility becomes an increasing problem for older children and adolescents with pseudoachondroplasia. Pain, stiffness and instability of joints, short limbs, and obesity contribute to their inability to keep up with their peers. A mobility device such as a wheelchair or skateboard is often required for school excursions and other group activities, but walking is usually possible within the schoolroom, home, and workplace.

Epiphyseal Dysplasias

Many skeletal dysplasias affect the epiphyses. However, two main groups will be considered here, multiple epiphyseal dysplasia, which has minimal spinal involvement, and the spondyloepiphyseal dysplasias in which the spine is involved.

Multiple Epiphyseal Dysplasia

Etiology

Multiple epiphyseal dysplasia is an autosomal dominant disorder with wide variability in expression. Families tend to have either the mild Ribbing type or the more severe Fairbank type of dysplasia. The radiographic and pathological features suggest that the patients have an anomaly of the matrix of the hyaline cartilage of the growth plates, epiphyses, and articular cartilages. Mutations have been identified in the cartilage oligomeric matrix protein, type IX collagen, and matrilin-3 genes [7–9].

Clinical Features

Multiple epiphyseal dysplasia is not evident at birth. It first becomes apparent because of joint pain and stiffness in childhood. The hips, knees, and ankles are usually involved. The hands and fingers are often short, and the fingers may lack full movement.

Some children have progressive physical difficulties during childhood. They may not be able to keep up with their peers, and attempts to do so increase their pain and limp and accentuate nocturnal limb pain. Hand fatigue is also common during writing. Growth is slower than normal, although dwarfism is rare. Adult heights range from 145 to 170 cm. The face is usually normal.

Radiographic Features

Radiographs of the pelvis, spine, knees, ankles, and wrists are required to make the diagnosis. The epiphyseal changes

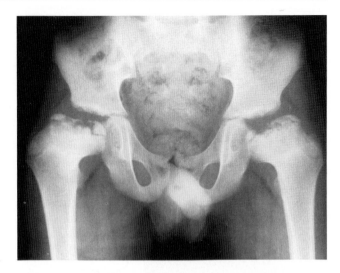

Fig. 7.13 Multiple epiphyseal dysplasia. Radiograph of the pelvis of a child aged 6 years, showing abnormal ossification of the femoral heads and short, broad femoral necks. He developed incongruous hips, with premature osteoarthritis

are usually most evident in the proximal femora (see Fig. 7.13), where the ossific nuclei are small and irregular or fragmented. The features resemble Perthes' disease, but they lack the progressive changes seen in that condition. Any child believed to have bilateral Perthes' disease should be considered to have an epiphyseal dysplasia until proven otherwise, particularly when the radiographic changes are symmetrical.

The severity of the epiphyseal dysplasia varies between families. In some families, the ossific nucleus of the femoral head is fragmented, with multiple centers of ossification, and the femoral neck is short and broad. The fragmented areas coalesce to produce a flattened and often incongruous femoral head. Premature osteoarthritis is common in adolescence and early adult life. In other families, the ossific nucleus of the femoral head is small and irregular but well contained within a relatively normal acetabulum. A congruous hip usually results, which is also prone to premature osteoarthritis, but usually several decades later than those with a fragmented epiphysis [10].

The epiphyses of other bones are often less affected, but ossification is delayed and the ossific nuclei are small and misshapen. The spine is minimally affected. There may be a minor amount of platyspondyly, and the vertebral bodies may be slightly ovoid. If there is more marked spinal involvement, the patient is likely to have spondyloepiphyseal dysplasia.

Management

The diagnosis is currently based on the clinical and radiographic features of the patient and family. DNA diagnoses are available in specialized centers. Treatment is symptomatic. Mildly short stature is usual but is rarely a clinical problem.

Severe hip pain and limp are treated by rest and crutches. Paracetamol taken before going to bed is useful in children with increasing nocturnal limb pain. At other times, the children are encouraged to participate in activities within their limits of comfort. Pain in the hand when writing is eased by using a pen with a wide grip.

It is uncertain whether containment procedures, such as the Salter osteotomy or femoral osteotomy, alter the prognosis of the hips. Premature osteoarthritis of the hip is difficult to treat, because the patients are often young and the disease is bilateral. Femoral osteotomy may be used to delay the need for total hip arthroplasty.

Spondyloepiphyseal Dysplasias

Spondyloepiphyseal dysplasia is the term used to describe a diverse range of conditions involving delayed and abnormal ossification of the epiphyses and the spine. Some of the conditions have known causes and are classified separately, e.g., several patterns of spondyloepiphyseal dysplasia are features of congenital hypothyroidism and mucopolysaccharidoses. These conditions will not be considered here.

Spondyloepiphyseal dysplasia varies in its severity. It includes achondrogenesis, which is lethal; spondyloepiphyseal dysplasia congenita, which produces severe dwarfism; and spondyloepiphyseal dysplasia tarda, which produces mild short stature and premature osteoarthritis. The Stickler syndrome (hereditary arthro-ophthalmopathy) and Kniest dysplasia are also included in this family of dysplasias [11]. The features of spondyloepiphyseal dysplasia congenita and tarda and of the Stickler syndrome will be described.

Spondyloepiphyseal Dysplasia Congenita

Etiology

Spondyloepiphyseal dysplasia congenita is an autosomal dominant disorder in most families. Mutations involving the type II collagen gene have been characterized in some families. This collagen gene was considered to be the likely candidate gene, as it is expressed in growth plate and articular cartilage, intervertebral disc, and vitreous humor.

Clinical Features

At Birth

Fetal growth is delayed, and short-trunk dwarfism is evident at birth. The face is flat with malar hypoplasia and wide-set eyes. Club feet and a cleft palate may be present.

During Childhood

Hypotonia is usual and motor development is delayed, although most children walk by 2 years of age. Excessive delay in walking may be due to cervical myelopathy with atlanto-axial instability and odontoid hypoplasia.

After weight-bearing commences, the lumbar lordosis worsens, causing further shortening of the trunk (see Fig. 7.14). A waddling gait is usual and is due to coxa vara. The coxa vara is progressive and is often associated with a triangular metaphyseal fragment. The hips are also flexed and externally rotated. A moderate degree of bow leg and internal tibial torsion are common.

Children with spondyloepiphyseal dysplasia congenita are prone to develop cervical myelopathy at any age, because of atlanto-axial instability. Progressive kyphoscoliosis may also develop in early childhood.

During Adolescence and Adulthood

Shortness of stature is severe, with an adult height of between 81 and 120 cm. Retinal detachments, with or without myopia, are common (they occur in up to 50% of children) and preventable.

Decreasing endurance and increasing limb pain are common and may be due to premature osteoarthritis or cervical myelopathy.

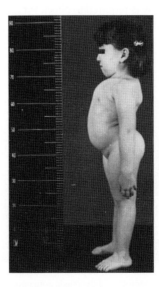

Fig. 7.14 Spondyloepiphyseal dysplasia congenita. Clinical appearance in a child aged 3 years, showing short stature, short trunk, and relatively long limbs. This girl has excessive lumbar lordosis and prominence of the sternum

Radiographic Features

Radiographic abnormalities are present at birth. The ossification centers of the pubis, lower femur, and proximal tibia are severely retarded and the vertebrae are ovoid and flattened.

Ossification of the femoral head is absent through most of childhood (see Fig. 7.15). Progressive coxa vara is accompanied by a high greater trochanter, short femoral neck, and a triangular metaphyseal fragment. The development of other epiphyses is also delayed. Premature osteoarthritis in the hips and knees is common.

The spinal anomalies worsen with growth. The lumbar lordosis becomes severe and is associated with decreased vertical height of the posterior margins of the vertebral bodies and elongation of the pedicles (see Fig. 7.16). A thoracic kyphoscoliosis may also develop. The odontoid is hypoplastic and is often associated with atlanto-axial instability.

The feet and hands are relatively normal at all ages.

Management

The clinical and radiographic features of spondyloepiphyseal dysplasia congenita are usually characteristic. When there is any doubt, mucopolysaccharidosis screening tests are required, and the results of neonatal screening tests for hypothyroidism should be checked and may need to be repeated.

As with other forms of dwarfism, the initial treatment focuses on providing families with appropriate information about the disorder. A full radiographic skeletal survey is required for diagnostic purposes and for comparison with later radiographs.

Regular review is required to check for atlanto-axial instability and cervical myelopathy. If cervical myelopathy is

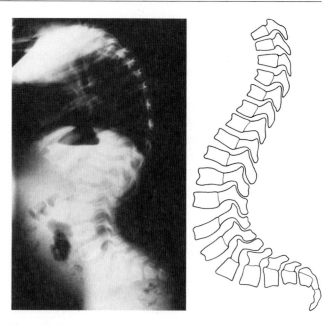

Fig. 7.16 Spondyloepiphyseal dysplasia congenita. Radiograph of the spine from the same child shown in Figs. 7.14 and 7.15. Note the excessive lumbar lordosis and thoracic kyphosis, the decreased height of the posterior margins of the vertebral bodies, and the elongation of the pedicles

suspected, flexion and extension radiographs of the cervical spine and MRI of the spinal cord and brain stem are indicated. Atlanto-axial fusion may be necessary to restore stability.

Coxa vara is usually progressive and may be associated with a triangular metaphyseal fragment, as seen in infantile coxa vara. Coxa vara can be corrected by Pauwel's Y-shaped intertrochanteric osteotomy that corrects the plane of the growth plate and provides support for the triangular metaphyseal fragment [12]. The valgus osteotomy may need to be repeated. Progressive tibia vara and internal tibial torsion infrequently require correction by osteotomy. Progressive tibia valga may occasionally occur and requires correction by osteotomy or hemiepiphyseal stapling. Osteoarthritis of multiple joints is common in adulthood and total joint arthroplasties, particularly of the hips, may be required.

Regular ophthalmological examinations are recommended during childhood to recognize and treat retinal detachments.

Spondyloepiphyseal Dysplasia Tarda

Etiology

Spondyloepiphyseal dysplasia tarda is an X-linked disorder caused by mutations of the SEDL gene. This gene produces a protein involved in the transport of proteins from the chondrocyte.

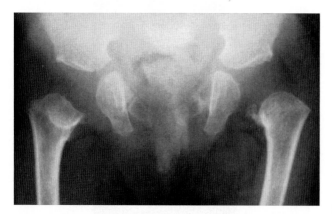

Fig. 7.15 Spondyloepiphyseal dysplasia congenita. Radiograph of the pelvis from the same patient shown in Fig. 7.14. Note the absence of ossification in the femoral heads, the short broad femoral necks, and the triangular metaphyseal fragment of the left proximal femur. The child developed progressive coxa vara that was treated by a Pauwel's Y-shaped intertrochanteric osteotomy of the femur

Clinical Features

The clinical manifestations appear in late childhood. The patients have a short trunk and the adult height ranges from 125 to 157 cm. The chest is broad and there is moderate pectus carinatum. Spine and joint pains are common. Premature osteoarthritis, particularly of the hips and shoulders, develops in the second and third decades of life.

Radiographic Features

There is generalized platyspondyly, with central humps of bone on the upper and lower plates of the lumbar vertebrae. The ring epiphyses are poorly developed. There may also be a thoracic kyphosis or mild scoliosis.

The pelvis is small and the femoral necks are short and broad. The hip joints may also be misshapen and premature osteoarthritis is common.

Management

The clinical and radiographic features are usually sufficient to allow the diagnosis of spondyloepiphyseal dysplasia tarda. The extensive involvement of the spine distinguishes this condition from multiple epiphyseal dysplasia, and the widespread changes within the spine distinguish it from Scheuermann's disease.

The major orthopaedic abnormalities are short stature and premature osteoarthritis. Total joint replacements may be required to relieve progressive osteoarthritis.

Stickler Syndrome (Hereditary Arthro-Ophthalmopathy)

Etiology

Stickler syndrome is transmitted as a dominant trait with highly variable expression. In some families, the phenotype has been linked to the type II and XI collagen genes.

Clinical Features

Children have a Marfanoid habitus, with hypotonia and joint hypermobility. The facies is flat, with midface and mandibular hypoplasia, a depressed nasal bridge, and epicanthal folds. Other cranio-facial features include cleft palate, deafness, and ocular anomalies. Progressive myopia, beginning in childhood, is common and may give rise to retinal detachments in later childhood and young adulthood. The joints are large, and progressive joint degeneration occurs in the second and third decades of life.

Radiographic Features

In childhood, there is a mild epiphyseal dysplasia of the proximal femora and distal tibiae. The tubular bones have long narrow shafts and wide metaphyses. The vertebral bodies show mild flattening and anterior wedging.

Management

The treatment required will vary according to the phenotypic features. A cleft palate may need repair. The joints wear prematurely, and arthroscopic lavage may be required in adolescence, to ameliorate symptoms. Some patients show symptomatic improvement with anti-inflammatory agents. However, arthroplasties are the only means of treating a severely arthritic joint in adult life.

Mucopolysaccharidoses

Etiology

The mucopolysaccharidoses represent a class of storage disorder in which intermediate metabolites from the partial degradation of proteoglycans are stored in various tissues, including the bone marrow and connective tissues. They are caused by autosomal recessive and X-linked recessive genetic deficiencies of various enzymes involved in the degradation of proteoglycans and glycosaminoglycans. The clinical and chemical anomalies are summarized in Table 7.2.

Clinical and Radiographic Features

The mucopolysaccharidoses are heterogeneous, with various types and sub-types attributable to different enzyme deficiencies in the cascade of enzymatic steps in the degradation of the glycosaminoglycan components of proteoglycans. The major clinical features are mental retardation, dwarfism, corneal clouding, and dysostosis.

The typical progressive features of the mucopolysaccharidoses are well illustrated by Hurler's syndrome. The babies appear normal up to about 6–8 months of age; they subsequently become large babies with rhinorrhea, stiff joints, and thoraco-lumbar kyphosis. Over the following year, the

Table 7.2 Main features of the mucopolysaccharidoses

Classification	Enzyme deficiency	Excreted gly-cosaminoglycan	Main organs affected	Appearance	Mental state
IH Hurler	α[alpha]-L-Iduronidase	Dermatan sulfate Heparan sulfate	CNS, skeleton, viscera	Hurler (gargoylism)	Rapid deterioration
IS Scheie	α[alpha]-L-Iduronidase	Dermatan sulfate Heparan sulfate	Skeleton, viscera	Coarse features	Normal
IS/H Hurler/Scheie	α[alpha]-L-Iduronidase	Dermatan sulfate Heparan sulfate	Intermediate phenotype	Coarse features	Variable
II Hunter	Iduronate sulfate sulfatase	Dermatan sulfate Heparan sulfate	CNS, skeleton, viscera	Like Hurler	Variable deterioration
III Sanfilippo—III D	Four distinct biochemical types. Identical phenotype	Heparan sulfate	CNS	Not characteristic	Severe mental deterioration
IV Morquio	Galactosamine 6-sulfatase	Keratan sulfate	Skeleton. Severe deformities. Flat, beaked vertebrae. Thoraco-lumbar gibbus. Odontoid hypoplasia	Not diagnostic	Normal
VI Maroteaux–Lamy	N-Acetylgalactosamine 4-sulfatase	Dermatan sulfate	Skeleton	Like Hurler	Variable
VII—	β[beta]-Glucuronidase	Dermatan sulfate Heparan sulfate	CNS, skeleton, viscera	Like Hurler	Variable

Note that all these disorders are inherited as autosomal recessive disorders, with the exception of MPS II (Hunter), in which the enzyme deficiency is inherited as an X-linked recessive.

There are common skeletal abnormalities in this group of disorders (referred to as dysostosis multiplex): these are seen typically in Hurler's syndrome (MPS I). Specific features occur in MPS IV (Morquio syndrome).

In MPS I there is a large skull, with a J (shoe)-shaped pituitary fossa. In the spine, persistence of infantile biconcave vertebra gives way to a thoraco-lumbar kyphosis. In the thorax, the ribs are paddle shaped; in the hands, the phalanges are pointed distally (bullet shaped) and the metacarpals proximally.

In MPS IV, excessive joint mobility combines with typical skeletal deformity. The spine initially resembles MPS I. Later, platyspondyly with an anterior projecting central tongue is typical. The odontoid is small or absent. There is gross deformity of the chest, shortening of the spine, and genu valgum. The small bones of the hand are well modeled.

accumulation of metabolic intermediates in the tissues produces increasing coarseness of the face, stiffness of joints, hepatosplenomegaly, corneal clouding, severe growth retardation, and developmental delay. These changes progress, with death between 6 and 10 years of age.

The radiographic features in Hurler's syndrome are often referred to as *dysostosis multiplex*. The principal changes are enlargement of the calvarium, with lack of the normal digital markings. The long bones have expanded diaphyses as a result of the storage of metabolic intermediates in the bone marrow. The hands show characteristic features with proximal pointing of the metacarpals; the metacarpals and phalanges are wider than normal. There is generalized platyspondyly, with anterior beaking of the vertebral bodies and a thoraco-lumbar gibbus with wedging of the apical vertebra.

Orthopaedic surgeons may be referred children with the milder forms, such as Morquio, Scheie, Hunter (see Fig. 7.17), or Maroteaux–Lamy syndromes. The orthopaedic problems are likely to consist of progressive kyphoscoliosis, flexion deformities of joints, foot deformities, and atlanto-axial instability.

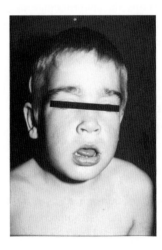

Fig. 7.17 A 9-year-old child with Hunter's syndrome. Note the coarse features: thick eyebrows and lips and wide nostrils. Unlike Hurler's syndrome, there is no corneal clouding

Management

The key to management is to have a biochemical diagnosis so that the likely progress of the disease can be predicted.

There is little point in undertaking orthopaedic procedures in a child with rapid general deterioration. However, progressive deformities may need to be corrected in a child with slow progression and a good life expectancy. For example, soft tissue releases of flexion contractures and correction of foot and spinal deformities may need to be undertaken. Enzyme replacement therapy is effective in some patients. It is to be hoped that somatic gene therapy in the future will provide a lasting supply of the deficient enzyme.

Metaphyseal Chondrodysplasias

This group of dysplasias is characterized by defective endochondral ossification. In metaphyseal chondrodysplasia, the metaphyses and growth plates are abnormal, whereas in spondylometaphyseal dysplasia the spine is also abnormal. The spondylometaphyseal dysplasias are extremely rare and will not be described.

Metaphyseal chondrodysplasia is heterogeneous, with a typical mild-to-moderate Schmid type, a very rare severe Jansen type, a cartilage-hair form also referred to as the McKusick type, a Shwachman–Bodian type associated with pancreatic insufficiency and cyclical neutropenia, and the Davis type associated with thymolymphopenia. The features of the Schmid type are outlined below.

Schmid Type Etiology

It is inherited as an autosomal dominant trait with variable expression. Histologically, there is disorganized growth and ossification of the growth plate. Mutations of the type X collagen gene, COL10A1, which is specifically produced by hypertrophic chondrocytes, have been identified in patients with this dysplasia [13].

Clinical Features

Affected children appear normal at birth. Short stature, bow legs, a waddling gait, and increased lumbar lordosis are noted at about 2 years of age. The facies is normal. Exercise-related and nocturnal leg pain is common.

The adult height is between 130 and 160 cm. Premature osteoarthritis is unusual.

Radiographic Features

The abnormalities are noted principally at the ends of the fastest growing bones. All long bones are short and curved; the growth plates are wide and the metaphyses are irregular and wide (see Fig. 7.18). The appearances are like those of rickets, particularly X-linked hypophosphatemic rickets, except that the bones are normally mineralized and have a normal texture in metaphyseal chondrodysplasia. The epiphyses are normal. There is bilateral coxa vara, with short broad femoral necks.

Management

The clinical and radiographic features of metaphyseal chondrodysplasia are very similar to those of X-linked hypophosphatemic rickets. They can be distinguished by the osteopenia and by the abnormal serum calcium, inorganic phosphate, and alkaline phosphatase concentrations in those with rickets.

Osteotomies may be required to correct tibia vara should the bow legs be progressive (see Figs. 7.18 and 7.19). The osteotomies are planned and undertaken in the same manner as described for achondroplasia. If femoral osteotomies are also required, each limb is corrected in turn. Monolateral or ring fixators can be used to provide three-dimensional control of multiple osteotomies in older children.

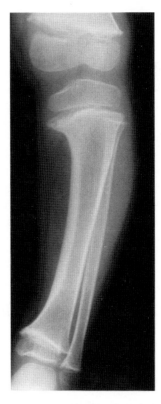

Fig. 7.18 Metaphyseal chondrodysplasia. Radiograph of the tibia of a 3-year-old child, showing tibia vara and widening and irregularity of the growth plates

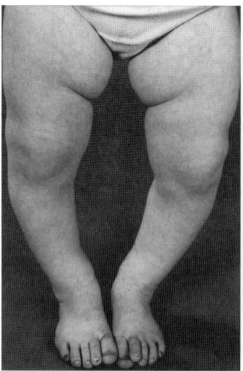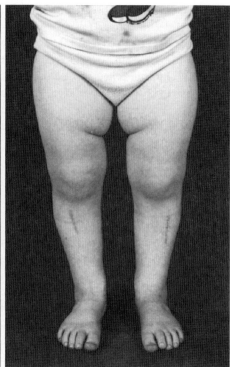

Fig. 7.19 Metaphyseal chondrodysplasia. (**A**) Clinical appearance of the same child shown in Fig. 7.18 at age 4. Note the bilateral bowing and internal tibial torsion. (**B**) Clinical appearance of the same child after correction of the bow legs and internal tibial torsion by tibial osteotomies at age 4

Exostosis Syndromes

Exostoses in childhood are usually osteochondromata rather than true exostoses. They develop from the margins of the growth plates and protrude from the surface of the metaphysis. Rarely, they develop from epiphyses giving rise to dysplasia epiphysealis hemimelica.

Solitary osteochondromas are common and sporadic; they will not be considered further. Multiple osteochondromata typically occur in diaphyseal aclasis, but they also occur as part of other syndromes. The features and management of diaphyseal aclasis and dysplasia epiphysealis hemimelica are described below.

Diaphyseal Aclasis (Hereditary Multiple Exostoses)

Etiology

Diaphyseal aclasis is an autosomal dominant trait. About 30% of cases are new mutations, involving the EXT1 and EXT2 genes.

The growth plates of the osteochondromata grow in a manner similar to the normal growth plates and close at similar times.

Clinical Features

Osteochondromata first become apparent in infancy and increase in both number and size with growth. They stop growing when the growth plates close, unless there is malignant transformation, which occurs in less than 2% of cases. The common sites for osteochondromata are the ends of the long bones, pelvis, shoulder girdle, and fingers; the spine and skull are rarely affected. They may be unsightly and give rise to pressure effects on tendons and neurovascular structures. Joint stiffness is common and some children may complain of aching.

Osteochondromata can also produce major skeletal distortions because of pressure and growth effects. At the deep surface of the scapula, they produce winging of the scapula; at the distal radius and ulna they may produce a Madelung deformity; at the distal tibia or fibula they may distort the ankle mortice, producing a deformed and unstable ankle; and at the femoral neck they may subluxate the hip. Osteochondromata of the phalanges may produce angular deformities of the fingers and joint stiffness.

The average final height of affected individuals is 169 cm for males and 159 cm for females.

Radiographic Features

The trabecular and cortical bone of the osteochondromata is continuous with the equivalent components of the metaphysis (see Fig. 7.20). The attachment to the metaphysis may be broad (*sessile*) or slender (*pedunculated*). The metaphysis is poorly modeled. CT is a useful means of defining the circumferential extent of osteochondromata, particularly around the distal femur and proximal tibia. The lumps may be felt to be discrete, whereas the scan may show them to be continuous, rather like a mountain range with a common base and a series of peaks. Each osteochondroma is much larger than the radiographic appearance because of its radiolucent cartilage cap.

The bone of the osteochondromata has a well-ordered trabecular pattern that is continuous with the underlying metaphyseal bone. Some lesions may have a smooth external surface, whereas others are more lobulated, with a cauliflower appearance. The appearance of bone destruction or patchy calcification after maturity is likely to indicate malignant transformation.

Madelung's deformity frequently develops as a result of disproportionate shortening of the ulna with bowing of the radius. The growth of the distal radius and ulna is often grossly abnormal. Shortening and bowing of the distal fibula and widening of the ankle mortice with progressive valgus deformity are also common.

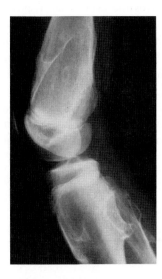

Fig. 7.20 Diaphyseal aclasis. Radiograph of the knee in a 13-year-old adolescent, showing sessile and pedunculated osteochondromata

Management

The diagnosis is usually obvious. Osteochondromata occur in other syndromes such as the Langer–Giedon form of acrodysplasia, which is also called trichorhinophalangeal dysplasia, type II. However, such children have a characteristic facies, with a bulbous pear-shaped nose, sparse hair, and cone-shaped phalangeal epiphyses.

The clinical diagnosis may also be confused with multiple enchondromatosis, which presents with metaphyseal lumps. Madelung deformity is also a feature of dyschondrosteosis, but children with that condition lack the widespread osteochondromata that are characteristic of diaphyseal aclasis.

Excision of selected osteochondromata may be required because of pain, dysfunction, or deformity. If the base of the lesion abuts the growth plate, it is wise to delay removal until the growth plate has grown away from it, otherwise cautious removal of the lesion may lead to recurrence and complete removal a partial growth plate arrest. A surgical approach is selected that provides direct access to the base of the lesion rather than to the cap. The cap is often large and obstructs access to the base. Vital structures may also be closely applied to the base of the lesion. For example, the femoral or popliteal artery may wind around the base of osteochondromata of the distal femur. In such situations, the surgical approach should not only provide direct access to the base of the lesion but also allow the vessels to be isolated above and below the lesion, so they can be retracted from the base before excision.

It is essential that the cartilage cap, with its growth plate, is completely removed, or the lesion may recur. This is easily achieved with small osteochondromata, but considerable care is required when removing large, cauliflower lesions. After removal of the lesion, the metaphysis should have the normal concave shape of a well-modelled metaphysis.

Removal of sessile lesions from the distal femur and proximal tibia is often difficult because the lesions are circumferential. Computed tomographic angiograms will confirm the clinical extent of the lesions and their proximity to the main vessels. The radiographic and clinical findings are used together in planning which osteochondromata to remove. Care should be taken to ensure there is sufficient cortical bone remaining to minimize the risk of post-operative fracture.

Madelung's deformity is difficult to treat. Removal of exostoses, epiphysiolysis and realignment osteotomy of the radius, and lengthening of the ulna have been recommended, but the results are unpredictable.

Osteochondromata of the distal tibia or fibula may widen the ankle mortice. Regular radiographs of the ankles are advisable and if this complication appears likely, the osteochondromata should be excised and medial distal tibial growth arrest considered. It is difficult to restore the ankle mortice to normal once the inferior tibio-fibular joint has been separated.

All excised osteochondromata should be sent for pathological examination, although malignant transformation is rare in childhood. In adults, it is wise to regard any lesion that starts to enlarge or to become painful as being a chondrosarcoma. The radiograph may show some new areas of calcification and bone destruction. Such lesions, even without radiographic evidence of a sarcomatous degeneration, should be removed immediately. The clinical behavior of the lesion is the best indication of whether it is malignant. Biopsy is not helpful in the early stages, and if a suspicious lesion is left alone it may become very large and difficult, or even impossible, to remove later. In general, malignant transformation is more likely in proximal and flat bone lesions. A recent study has related the site of gene mutation both to the severity of the disease and to the risk of sarcomatous change. Patients carrying the EXT1 mutation tend to have a more severe form of the condition and a higher risk of malignant change than those with the EXT2 mutation [14].

Dysplasia Epiphysealis Hemimelica

This disorder is also known as Trevor's disease [15] or epiphyseal osteochondroma.

Etiology

The etiology of this condition is unknown, because most cases are sporadic. The lesions are similar to those of metaphyseal osteochondromata, except that they develop from the epiphysis and protrude into the joint.

Clinical and Radiographic Features

Affected children present with pain, swelling, and deformity; the wrist, ankle, and foot are the most frequent sites of complaint. A lump is palpable on the epiphysis and is often associated with angular deformity of the joint. Radiographs reveal multiple sites of ossification over one-half of the epiphysis, at the ends of the long bones of one or more segments of a limb, or of the tarsal bones (see Fig. 7.21). The multiple centers of ossification gradually coalesce and, by the end of growth, the trabecular pattern is continuous with that of the underlying epiphysis. The end result is enlargement of one side of the epiphysis of one or more long bones or of the tarsal bones.

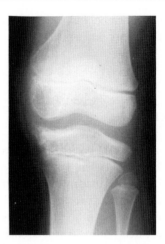

Fig. 7.21 Dysplasia epiphysealis hemimelica. Radiograph of the knee in a 7-year-old child showing abnormal ossification of the medial margin of the proximal tibial epiphysis. A similar lesion of the distal femur was shaved off when the child was 3 years old

Management

The diagnosis is usually obvious from the clinical and radiographic appearances. Chondrodysplasia punctata also produces stippling of epiphyses. However, in chondrodysplasia punctata, the stippling has usually disappeared by the age of 2 years, whereas dysplasia epiphysealis hemimelica becomes apparent at or after this age.

Growth of the epiphyseal osteochondroma frequently leads to angular deformities of the knee or to distortion of the ankle mortise. In both situations, paring down of the osteochondroma may be indicated. This can be undertaken using curved scalpel blades. It is best done when the centers of ossification are deep in the lesion, otherwise more superficial ossific centers are exposed as the lesion is pared. In later childhood, it is preferable to leave epiphyseal osteochondroma of the distal tibia and femur alone and to correct limb alignment by osteotomy or hemiphyseal tension band plating. However, progressive stiffness or subluxation of the hip, knee, or ankle may require decancellation of the affected epiphyses as a means of reducing the intra-articular size of the osteochondromas. At the hip there is often marked valgus deformity, which, in association with a heavy osteochondromatous load, may contribute to subluxation.

Enchondromatosis

Enchondromatosis, also called Ollier's disease, is a skeletal dysplasia that may involve one or more bones. When it is associated with hemangiomata, it is called Maffucci's syndrome. There are also rarer variants in which enchondromata are associated with osteochondromata.

Etiology

The etiology is unknown: almost all cases are sporadic.

Clinical and Radiographic Features

There are two main presentations. The first is with multiple lumps on the fingers or toes. The second is with deformity and limb length discrepancy (see Fig. 7.22). Pathological fractures may also occur.

The radiographs show multiple metaphyseal lesions. Lesions in the metacarpals or phalanges usually have the typical features of benign enchondromata. They expand the bone and the enlarging surface is covered by a thin layer of subperiosteal new bone. The lesion may contain some speckled calcification, characteristic of a cartilage lesion. The number and size of the lesions in the digits often increase during childhood, but they stop growing after skeletal maturity.

The masses of hyaline cartilage in the metaphyses of long bones give rise to long metaphyseal lucencies in the radiographs. The lesions are usually present bilaterally, but the severity of involvement is asymmetric (see Fig. 7.23). The more severely affected limb, commonly the leg, is short

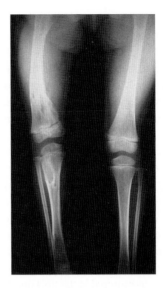

Fig. 7.23 Ollier's disease. Radiograph of legs of same girl as shown in Fig. 7.22. Note the normal long bones of the left leg. The right femur and tibia are short and the distal femur is bowed. The metaphyses of the right leg are abnormal because of the persistence of cartilage columns

and bowed and the metaphyses are enlarged. Mild shortening of one leg may be evident at birth, without evidence of enchondromata.

The lesions stop growing at puberty and remodeling occurs, with replacement of the cartilaginous masses by bone, although some cartilage islands usually remain. Malignant degeneration occurs rarely.

The diagnosis is usually obvious from the clinical and radiographic features. It should be distinguished from diaphyseal aclasis, metaphyseal chondrodysplasia, and fibrous dysplasia.

Management

Surgical treatment of finger lumps may be required to improve finger function and to correct deformities. Selected lesions of the phalanges and metacarpals are treated by curettage, with care to avoid damage to the growth plate if the lesion adjoins it. Asymmetric lesions rarely need bone grafting, because the normal bone acts as a stable buttress and the subperiosteal bone can be invaginated into the defect. An osteotomy may be undertaken at the same time if asymmetric growth of the bone has produced a significant angular deformity. For symmetric lesions, a corticocancellous bone graft may be needed to maintain alignment and length of the bone after subperiosteal excision of the lesion.

No attempt is made to excise enchondromata from the long bones of the leg, as the masses of cartilage are continuous with the growth plates. However, severe and progressive

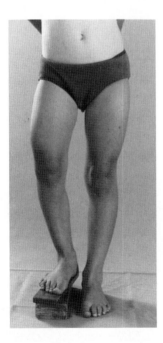

Fig. 7.22 Ollier's disease. Clinical appearance in a girl aged 4 years, showing shortening of the right leg, with bowing and internal torsion of the femur

angular deformities often need to be corrected in early childhood by osteotomy; for example, varus of the distal femur is corrected by metaphyseal osteotomy. Both limbs are prepared and draped free and a sterile tourniquet is applied high on the affected thigh. An osteotomy is made perpendicular to the bone and the deformity is overcorrected. The osteotomy is fixed with crossed Kirschner wires, and the limb is immobilized in a well-molded hip spica.

The osteotomy through the abnormal metaphysis heals in the normal time; however, the deformities in the lower limb recur, and the leg length discrepancy worsens progressively. Correction of the angular and rotary deformities and leg length discrepancy are undertaken together in later childhood. Monolateral or ring fixator methods of limb lengthening and deformity correction provide the three-dimensional control required to achieve satisfactory correction. Multiple osteotomies may be required in the tibia and femur to achieve correct alignment.

Malignant transformation in Ollier's disease is rare. It is, however, common in Maffucci's syndrome. Reactivation of growth of any lesion in adult life should be considered the result of sarcomatous transformation.

Specific Fibrous Disorders

Marfan's Syndrome

This is a relatively common and well-known connective tissue disease.

Etiology

Marfan's syndrome is an autosomal dominant disorder with variable expression. About 15% of patients have new mutations. The abnormal FBN1 encodes a microfibrillar protein that is found in the various tissues affected by the syndrome.

Clinical and Radiographic Features

Patients with Marfan's syndrome are tall, with disproportionately long slim limbs, arachnodactyly, and a decreased upper-to-lower segment ratio. Pectus carinatum or excavatum is common. The face is long and narrow, with a high arched palate. Ocular problems are common and include lens subluxation (usually upward), myopia, and retinal detachment. Mitral valve prolapse and aneurysms of various types are also common.

There are three patterns of spinal deformity: thoraco-lumbar kyphosis, *flat back*, and scoliosis. Thoraco-lumbar kyphosis is noted in late infancy. It is flexible and is caused by hypotonia and ligament laxity. It usually improves as muscle power increases. The flat back consists of flattened lumbar and thoracic spines. Scoliosis is common and may commence in infancy (see Fig. 7.24). The curves are usually progressive, and more than half are double structural curves.

Congenital hip dislocation and dysplasia may occur, as may protrusio acetabuli. The foot is long and narrow with an abnormally long big toe and rolls into planovalgus (see Fig. 7.25). Hallux valgus is common.

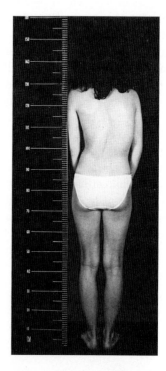

Fig. 7.24 Marfan syndrome. Note the right thoracic scoliosis

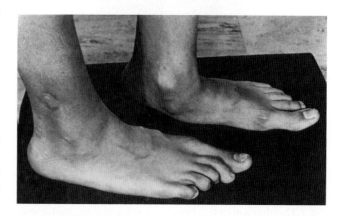

Fig. 7.25 Marfan syndrome. Severe planovalgus feet that were treated with inlay triple fusions because of persistent pain

The diagnosis of Marfan's syndrome is a clinical one at present. It is straightforward in the typical case, but many children lack some of the usual features and either have another syndrome or are classified as having a Marfanoid habitus.

There are many syndromes with a Marfanoid habitus. Homocystinuria, which is very similar to Marfan's syndrome, is an autosomal recessive disease that can be diagnosed by urine analysis. It is important to distinguish it from Marfan's syndrome, because patients with homocystinuria are prone to major thromboses during or after surgery unless precautions are taken. Patients with congenital contractural arachnodactyly (Beal's syndrome) have the Marfanoid habitus and contractures of the knees, elbows, and hands at birth. The face is oval, with micrognathia, and the pinnae are crumpled and flattened. The feet are often held in calcaneus with hindfoot valgus and forefoot adductus and supination; the contractures tend to improve with growth. Patients with Stickler's syndrome (hereditary arthro-ophthalmopathy), Klinefelter's syndrome, diaphyseal dysplasia, and frontometaphyseal dysplasia may all show some Marfanoid features.

Management

Orthopaedic care is best provided in conjunction with a paediatrician or geneticist because of the general and life-threatening complications that may occur. Ankle–foot orthoses may be required in infancy to provide a stable base for the child during stance. Progressive scoliosis may require fusion and instrumentation in late childhood or adolescence. Non-fusion rods may be used in early childhood if the scoliosis is severe and progressive. Progressive genu valgum may occur in late childhood and can be corrected by hemiepiphyseal stapling or tension band plating. Pes plano abductovalgus foot deformities may produce pain or excessive shoe wear. An inlay triple fusion improves the shape, stability, and comfort of the foot. To ensure a solid arthrodesis, it is usually necessary to inlay bone graft along the medial joints of the foot and to use staples or heavy Kirschner wire fixation.

Cardiovascular assessment, including ultrasonography of the heart valves and aorta, should be undertaken regularly in childhood and is essential before undertaking any major orthopaedic surgery in older children and teenagers. Aortic replacement, with or without aortic valve replacement, is frequently required and is best undertaken early because vascular complications are the usual cause of premature death. It is usually wise to keep the blood pressure below normal.

Ehlers–Danlos Syndrome

The Ehlers–Danlos syndrome (EDS) is a heterogeneous disease producing laxity in soft connective tissues (see Fig. 7.26).

Etiology

The Ehlers–Danlos syndrome is divided into several types (see Table 7.3): They are genetically determined and involve autosomal dominant, autosomal recessive, and X-linked inheritance patterns. Abnormalities of various connective tissue macromolecules have been identified in most forms of the syndrome. In the types of EDS that involve collagen abnormalities, the connective tissue laxity and fragility appear to be due to the presence of mutant and poorly cross-linked collagen in the tissues [16].

Clinical Features

There are at least ten main types of Ehlers–Danlos syndrome. Their features and etiology, when known, are outlined below.

Type I EDS (Gravis or Classic Type)

Type I EDS is an autosomal dominant disease caused by mutations of type V collagen [17–19]. This type of collagen is involved in regulating the size and shape of the thick, type I collagen-containing fibrils of dermis, tendon, ligaments, bone, and blood vessels. The principal features include soft, velvety, hyperextensible, and fragile skin that is

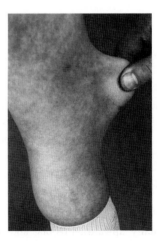

Fig. 7.26 Ehlers–Danlos syndrome. Child with type I EDS, showing marked laxity of the skin of the thigh

Table 7.3 Classification of the Ehlers–Danlos syndrome

Type	Features	Inheritance
I (gravis or classic type)	Lax, fragile skin; lax joints	Autosomal dominant
II (mitis or mild type)	Mild type I features	Autosomal dominant
III (benign hypermobility syndrome)	Severe hypermobility with multiple dislocations	Autosomal dominant
IV (ecchymotic type)	Vascular fragility; mild distal joint hypermobility; thin skin	Autosomal dominant and recessive forms
V (X-linked type)	Type II features	X-linked
VI (ocular-scoliotic type)	Skin laxity and fragility; ocular fragility; scoliosis	Autosomal recessive
VII (arthrochalasis multiplex congenita)	Multiple joint dislocations; mild skin laxity	Autosomal dominant and recessive forms
VIII (periodontitis type)	Skin and joint laxity with periodontitis	Autosomal dominant
IX (occipital horn syndrome)	Cutis laxa	X-linked
X	Skin laxity and fragility and easy bruising	Autosomal recessive

prone to forming paper-thin scars, easy bruising, hypermobility of joints, flat feet, and valvular incompetence. There are also a wide diversity of visceral complaints.

Type II EDS (Mitis or Mild Type)

Type II EDS is also an autosomal dominant disease caused by mutations of type V collagen. The clinical features are similar to those of EDS-I but are much milder.

Type III EDS (Benign Hypermobility Syndrome)

Type III EDS is inherited as an autosomal dominant disorder. In a few cases, mutations have been identified in the type V collagen or tenascin X genes. It is a heterogeneous type of EDS so that additional disease genes are likely to be identified. Joint hypermobility is severe and dislocations are common. The skin is soft, but otherwise normal.

Type IV EDS (Ecchymotic Type)

The ecchymotic type is caused by mutations, usually autosomal dominant, of type III collagen [18], which is the major collagen in vessels and viscera. The skin is thin, and bruising is common. The finger joints are hypermobile, but otherwise there are few skeletal anomalies. Most of the abnormalities involve the vessels and viscera. Premature death may result from vascular ruptures.

Type V EDS (X-linked Type)

Type V EDS is similar in appearance to EDS-II. The molecular defect remains uncertain.

Type VI EDS (Ocular-Scoliotic Type)

Type VI EDS is an autosomal recessive disease caused by a deficiency of the enzyme lysyl hydroxylase, an important collagen-modifying enzyme. The skin is soft and is prone to scarring and bruising. Ocular fragility, keratoconus, and progressive scoliosis are common.

Type VII EDS (Arthrochalasis Multiplex Congenita)

Type VII EDS is characterized by marked joint hypermobility and multiple dislocations at birth. The skin is soft but not excessively lax. It includes autosomal dominant forms with deletions involving the amino-terminal proteinase cleavage sites of the pro-α[alpha]1(I) and pro-α[alpha]2(I) chains of type I procollagen. There is a rarer autosomal recessive form in which there is a deficiency of the amino-proteinase enzyme. These mutations prevent the removal of the amino-terminal propeptide that normally occurs in the processing of procollagen to collagen. The persistent attachment of the propeptide interferes with fibril formation and collagen function.

Type VIII EDS (Periodontitis Type)

Type VIII EDS is an autosomal dominant trait of unknown cause. In addition to the usual features of skin and joint laxity, affected patients have periodontitis.

Type IX EDS (Occipital Horn Syndrome or X-linked Cutis laxa)

Type IX EDS is an X-linked recessive disease involving copper metabolism. Lysyl oxidase (a copper-dependent enzyme) activity, which is important for collagen cross-linking, may be reduced as a result of abnormal copper metabolism. This form of EDS has been reclassified as X-linked cutis laxa.

Type X EDS (Fibronectin Abnormality)

Type X EDS is an autosomal recessive form caused by defects in fibronectin, a widespread glycoprotein of the connective tissues. The skin is moderately hyperextensible and is prone to scarring and bruising. Platelet function is abnormal.

Management

It is important to decide first whether a patient has the Ehlers–Danlos syndrome and then to determine which type it is. It may be difficult to be sure whether a patient has the disease; if the diagnosis is not certain it should not be made. Difficulty is often encountered in children who have hypermobile joints or hypermobility, particularly in selected joints such as the shoulders and knees.

The general aspects of management include referral to a genetics clinic for diagnosis and assessment for ocular, cardiovascular, and visceral involvement. Correct typing of the EDS will assist in genetic counseling.

Skin fragility is a major problem in many young children because they fall so frequently. A protective head orthosis may be temporarily required to protect the forehead which can otherwise become extensively scarred from simple falls.

The orthopaedic problems associated with EDS include congenital dislocation of the hips, congenital laxity of multiple joints, flat feet, and scoliosis. Congenital dislocations of the hips are difficult to treat because the hip joint capsule remains lax and voluminous, despite prolonged use of harnesses and other abduction devices (see Fig. 7.27). The hips may dislocate easily for many months. If the hips remain unstable, it may prove necessary to splint the joints for several months in a hip spica or to carry out an open reduction and capsular reefing. Femoral or acetabular osteotomy is required to ensure that a stable reduction is achieved and maintained. Soft tissue procedures alone are rarely adequate, owing to the torsional abnormality.

Laxity of multiple joints can produce pain, frequent injuries, and impaired function. Limited motion orthoses are often helpful in protecting a joint. For example, pain in the elbow, as a result of hyperextension, is a common complaint in many sporting activities. An orthosis with an extension stop will often allow a child to continue comfortably with sports. Knee orthoses may also be required. Patellar instability is common and is best managed conservatively because soft tissue procedures usually fail.

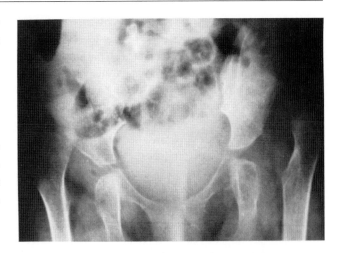

Fig. 7.27 Ehlers–Danlos syndrome. Radiograph of the pelvis of a child with type VII EDS. The dislocations were very unstable. Stability was achieved by open reductions and innominate osteotomies

Severe planovalgus deformity is common and is a source of discomfort and excessive shoe wear. In young children, ankle–foot orthoses prevent excessive valgus. Although the laxity does diminish with growth, a soft or plastic foot orthosis is usually needed long term. In some adolescents a triple arthrodesis of the foot, commonly of the inlay type, will be required as in Marfan's syndrome.

Scoliosis is also common. The deformity is often quite flexible. Arthrodesis with spinal instrumentation may be required in later childhood or adolescence.

Patients with EDS are prone to excessive bleeding during and after surgery. Wound dehiscence and spreading of healed wounds are common. Meticulous hemostasis should be obtained. Subcuticular dermal sutures must be carefully inserted, as the dermis is often thin. The wound should be supported for several months, with adhesive plastic strips or wound dressings.

Fibrous Dysplasia

Etiology

In fibrous dysplasia, the bone and bone marrow are replaced by fibrous connective tissue containing some fragments of bone. There are two forms of the disease: the monostotic and polyostotic. In the latter, skin pigmentation may be present, and some children have endocrine anomalies known as the McCune–Albright syndrome. Protein mutations have been identified in both forms of the disease.

Clinical Features

The monostotic form is more common than the polyostotic. It may produce pain, fracture, or swelling, usually in teenagers, and is occasionally an incidental finding on a radiograph taken for another purpose. The most common sites are the proximal femur and tibia. The lesion may enlarge during growth but usually ceases to grow after puberty.

The polyostotic form produces symptoms in the first decade of life. Although many bones may be affected, it is often most severe in one leg, producing deformity, fractures, and severe shortening. Cranio-facial involvement is common. The McCune–Albright syndrome occurs in girls and causes precocious sexual development, premature closure of epiphyses, and short stature. The skin lesions consist of multiple, well-demarcated melanotic patches that stop at the midline and have irregular margins.

Radiographic Features

The typical appearance is of a lytic area in the medullary cavity of a long bone, producing a "ground glass" appearance. As the lesion expands it erodes and scallops the cortex but is covered by the remaining cortex or by subperiosteal new bone. Additional bone may form on the concave side of the lesion—an appearance that is common in the tibia, where it produces a saber appearance. Progressive coxa vara is common, and in polyostotic forms the proximal femur may produce the characteristic "shepherd's crook" deformity (see Fig. 7.28).

Management

Many monostotic lesions have a typical radiographic appearance and biopsy is not required to confirm the diagnosis. Similarly, polyostotic fibrous dysplasia also produces a typical clinical and radiographic appearance and biopsy is not required for diagnosis. In spite of early enthusiasm bisphosphonate treatment does not appear to improve bone density and strength in children with polyostotic fibrous dysplasia.

Fractures are usually treated by standard methods but the lesion usually persists. Repeated fracture of a deformed bone, such as the proximal femur, requires correction of the deformity and internal fixation, preferably with an intramedullary rod.

Malignant transformation has been reported but is rare.

Summary

The variety of disorders of bone, cartilage, and fibrous tissue is wide, and most are genetically determined. It is essential to make the correct diagnosis, so that families can be given appropriate information regarding the future, associated anomalies, and the risks of recurrence in future pregnancies. Orthopaedic anomalies are frequent, often severe, and progressive. Treatment needs to be carefully planned. It should take into account the specific requirements of children with short limbs and trunks and those with lax and fragile or stiff tissues.

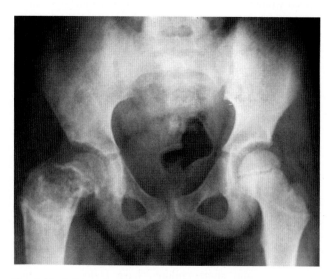

Fig. 7.28 Polyostotic fibrous dysplasia. Radiograph of the pelvis, showing the abnormal bone of the proximal right femur and pelvis. Progressive coxa vara was treated with a Pauwel's Y-shaped intertrochanteric osteotomy of the femur

References

1. Johns Hopkins University. OMIM—Online Mendelian Inheritance in Man. At: www3.ncbi.nlm.nih.gov/Omim. Accessed 31 August 2008.
2. McKusick VA. Mendelian inheritance in man. Catalogs of autosomal dominant, autosomal recessive, and X-linked phenotypes. Baltimore: The Johns Hopkins University Press; 1990.
3. Cole WG. The molecular pathology of osteogenesis imperfecta. Clin Orthop 1997; 343:235–46.
4. Sillence DO, Senn A, Danks DM. Genetic heterogeneity in osteogenesis imperfecta. J Med Gen 1979; 16:101–16.
5. Glorieux FH, Bishop NJ, Plotkin H, et al. Cyclic administration of pamidronate in children with severe osteogenesis imperfecta. New Eng J Med 1998; 339:947–52.
6. Sofield HA, Page MA, Mead NC. Multiple osteotomies and metal-rod fixation for osteogenesis imperfecta. J Bone Joint Surg 1952; 34A:500–2.
7. Briggs MD, Mortier OGR, Cole WG, et al. Diverse mutations in the gene for cartilage oligomeric matrix protein in the pseudoachondroplasia—multiple epiphyseal dysplasia disease spectrum. Am J Hum Gen 1998; 62:311–9.

8. Hecht JT, Deere M, Putnam E, et al. Characterization of cartilage oligomeric matrix protein (COMP) in human normal and pseudoachondroplasia musculoskeletal tissues. Matrix Biol 1998; 17:269–78.

9. Susic S, McGrory J, Ahier J, Cole WG. Multiple epiphyseal dysplasia and pseudoachondroplasia due to novel mutations in the calmodulin—like repeats of cartilage oligomeric matrix protein. Clin Gen 1987; 5:219–24.

10. Treble NJ, Jensen F0, Banhier A, et al. Development of the hip in multiple epiphyseal dysplasia. Natural history and susceptibility to premature osteoarthritis. J Bone Joint Surg 1990; 72B; 1061–4.

11. Cole WG. Abnormal skeletal growth in Kniest dysplasia caused by type I collagen mutations. Clin Orthop 1997; 341:162–9.

12. Cordes S, Dickens DR, Cole WG. Correction of coxa vara in childhood. The use of Pauwel's Y-shaped osteotomy. J Bone Joint Surg 1991; 73B:3–6.

13. Chan D, Cole WG, Rogers JG, Bateman JF. Type X collagen multimer assembly in vitro is prevented by a Gly618 to Val Mutation in the alpha 1 (X)NC1 domain resulting in Schmid metaphyseal chondrodysplasia. J Biol Chem 1995; 270:45558–62.

14. Porter DE, Lonie L, Fraser M, et al. Severity of disease and risk of malignant change in hereditary multiple exostoses. J Bone Joint Surg 2004; 86B:1041–6.

15. Trevor D. Tarso-epiphyseal aclasis. J Bone Joint Surg 1950; 32B:204–13.

16. Wenstrup RJ, Langland UT, Willing MC, et al. A splice-junction mutation in the region of COL5a that codes for the carboxyl propeptide of pro alpha 1(V) chains results in the gravis form of the Ehlers—Danlos syndrome (type I). Hum Mol Genetics 1996; 5:1733–6.

17. Michalickova K, Susic M, Willing MC, et al. Mutations of f alpha2(V) chain of type V collagen impair matrix assembly and produce Ehlers—Danlos syndrome type I. Hum Mol Genetics 1998; 7:249–5.

18. McOromy J, Wieksberg P, Thorner P, Cole WG. Abnormal extracellular matrix in Ehlers—Danlos syndrome type IV due to the Substitution of Glycine 934 by glutamic acid in the triple helical domain of type Ill collagen. Clin Genetics 1996; 50:442–5.

19. Giunta C, Superti-Furga A, Spranger S, et al. Ehlers-Danlos syndrome type VII: clinical features and molecular defects. J Bone Joint Surg 1999; 81A:225–38.

Chapter 8

Metabolic and Endocrine Disorders of the Skeleton

Roger Smith

Introduction

This chapter deals with the metabolic and endocrine disorders that affect the skeleton in childhood. It also considers the results of excess and deficiency of vitamins and the toxic effects of metals on bone. These disorders deal with inherited conditions, such as osteopetrosis, that result from abnormal bone cell biology; with polyostotic fibrous dysplasia, in which endocrine disturbances may also occur; and with ossification in the soft tissues, particularly when this is inherited. Osteogenesis imperfecta—an important metabolic disorder that has become a subject of its own [1]—and the skeletal dysplasias are dealt with in Chapter 7. The prevalence of individual metabolic bone diseases varies with age; in particular osteoporosis, so frequent in adult life, is rare in childhood.

Within the past three decades, the scope of metabolic bone disease has widened. There is increasing recognition of the importance of the organic matrix of bone, particularly collagen and many other non-collagen proteins which contribute to the function of the skeleton. There is also greater understanding of how hormones and cytokines interact through complex signaling pathways to control bone cell activity [2]. This does not mean that classic metabolic bone diseases such as rickets are of less importance, but it emphasizes that the term "metabolic bone disease" now covers a wider range of skeletal disorders than previously envisaged [3, 4].

Rapid advances in gene technology have led to the identification of the causes of numerous bone disorders which are included in our knowledge of the human genome [5]. Those relevant to the skeleton (Table 8.1) are dealt with in detail by Smith and Wordsworth [4]. Some of these disorders, which include the skeletal dysplasias (Chapter 7), are very rare. Many have wide implications in bone biology; for instance pseudoglioma osteoporosis and Wnt signaling, [6] and rare forms of rickets caused by abnormal metabolism of fibroblast growth factor 23.

Physiology

An outline of the physiology of bone, presented here, is necessary to understand the cause, diagnosis, and management of metabolic bone disorders; the subject has been reviewed extensively by Bilezikian et al. [7]. The important components of the skeleton are cells, organic matrix, and mineral. There are two widespread misconceptions about the skeleton: first that it is inert and second that it is composed entirely of chalk. Both conclusions are superficially logical, the first because of the mechanical properties of the skeleton and its persistence after death, the second from the fact that the skeleton contains 99% of the body's calcium. However, neither is correct.

Bone Cells

Bone cells comprise osteoblasts, osteocytes, and osteoclasts. Bone cells (and bone) are constantly being destroyed and replaced. The balance between the activities of the osteoblasts (formation) and osteoclasts (resorption) determines the size and shape of bone. Osteoblasts, which come from preosteoblasts of the mesenchymal stromal system, become transformed to osteocytes that occupy lacunae in mineralized bone, but osteoclasts are derived from the hemopoietic system.

Osteoblasts have many functions and may be regarded as the most important bone cells (Fig. 8.1). They produce all the components of the organic matrix including collagen and important non-collagen proteins such as osteocalcin. They also control the mineralization of this matrix. They influence the activity of other bone cells, particularly osteoclasts, by the use of short-acting messengers (cytokines), only some

R. Smith (✉)
Department of Orthopaedic Surgery, Nuffield Orthopaedic Centre, Oxford, UK

M. Benson et al. (eds.), *Children's Orthopaedics and Fractures*,
DOI 10.1007/978-1-84882-611-3_8, © Springer-Verlag London Limited 2010

Table 8.1 Molecular basis of some metabolic disorders which affect the skeleton

Disorder	Affected gene/protein
X-linked hypophosphatemia	*PHEX*
Autosomal dominant hypophosphatemic osteomalacia	*FGF23*/fibroblast growth factor 23
X-linked nephrolithiasis (Dent disease)	*CLC5*/chloride channel 5
Vitamin D-dependent rickets (type I)	25(OH)D 1α hydroxylase
Vitamin D-dependent rickets (type II)	1,25(OH)$_2$D receptor
Oncogenic rickets/OM	*FGF23*
Paget's disease	SQSTM1/sequestosome
Familial expansile osteolysis	*RANK/TNFRSF 11A*
Expansile skeletal hyperphosphatasia	*RANK/TNFRSF 11A*
Juvenile Paget's disease	*OPG/TNFRSF 11B*
Neonatal hyperparathyroidism	*CASR*
Pseudohypoparathyroidism	*GNAS1*
Jansen metaphyseal dysplasia	PTH/PTHrP receptor
Blomstrand chondrodysplasia	PTH/PTHrP receptor
Osteogenesis imperfecta	COL1A1, COL1A2
Osteoporosis pseudoglioma syndrome	*LRP5*
Familial high bone density	*LRP5*/lipoprotein receptor related protein 5
Marfan syndrome	*FBN1*/fibrillin 1
Congenital contractural arachnodactyly	*FBN2*/fibrillin 2
Loeys–Dietz syndrome	*ITGFBR1/2*
Ehlers–Danlos syndrome (EDS)	
EDS I	*COL5A1*
EDS IV	*COL3A1*
EDS VI	*PLOD1*/Lysyl hydroxylase
EDSVIIa, b	*COL1A1, COL1A2*
Other	Tenascin XB
Homocystinuria	Cystathionine β synthase
Hypophosphatasia	*TNAP*/alkaline phosphatase
Alkaptonuria	*HGD*/homogentisate 1,2-dioxygenase
Gaucher disease	β glucosidase
Mucopolysaccharidoses	Multiple lysosomal enzymes
Achondroplasia	*FGFR3*/fibroblast growth factor receptor 3
Thanatophoric dysplasia	*FGFR3*
Hypochondroplasia	*FGFR3"*
Spondyloepiphyseal dysplasia (SED)	*COL2A1*
Spondyloepiphyseal dysplasia tarda (X-linked)	*SEDLIN*
Stickler syndrome	*COL2A1, COL11A1*
Kniest dysplasia	*COL2A1*
Achondrogenesis	*COL2A1*
Multiple epiphyseal dysplasia	*COL9A1, 2, 3, COMP, SLC26A2 (DTDST), MATN3 (matrilin 3)*
Pseudoachondroplasia	*COMP*
Metaphyseal chondrodysplasia (Schmid)	*COL10A1*
Diastrophic dysplasia	*SLC26A2(DTDST)*
Campomelic dysplasia	*SOX 9*
Apert syndrome	*FGFR2*
Osteopetrosis (marble bone disease)	*TCIRG1, CLCN7, CA2*
Pycnodysostosis	*CTSK*/cathepsin K
Camurati-Engelmann's disease	*TGFB1*
Sclerosteosis	*SOST*/sclerostin
Fibrous dysplasia	*GNAS1*/G$_s$α protein subunit
Familial hyperphosphatemic tumoral calcinosis	*FGF23 and GALNT3*
Fibrodysplasia ossificans progressiva	*ACVR1*/activin receptor 1
Familial chondrocalcinosis	*ANKH*
Progressive osseous heteroplasia	*GNAS1*

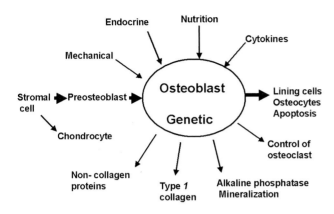

Fig. 8.1 The central position of the osteoblast. *Fine arrows* indicate factors that influence the osteoblast and some functions of the osteoblast. *Broad arrows* indicate the origin of the osteoblast and osteocyte

of which have been identified. Among the most important is receptor activator of nuclear factor κB ligand (RANKL). Details of the RANK/RANKL and osteoprotegerin pathways are discussed by Smith and Wordsworth [4]. Osteoblasts respond to a number of systemic hormones (such as parathyroid hormone, estrogens, and growth hormone) by virtue of their surface receptors.

The functions of the osteocytes are not so well defined but current research emphasizes their importance. They appear to be responsible for the integrity of bone and communicate with each other via their extensions in the canaliculi. They also modulate the response of the skeleton and its cells to mechanical stimuli by mechanisms which are not yet fully understood.

Whereas osteoblasts are synthetic cells, osteoclasts are concerned particularly with bone resorption. Contrary to previous belief, osteoclasts do not have receptors for hormones such as parathormone and dihydroxycholecalciferol ($1,25(OH)_2D$), and their development and activity are controlled largely by the osteoblasts. However, they do respond directly to calcitonin, which temporarily suppresses their activity. The osteoclast has polarity, and resorption begins when the cell seals off an area on the bone surface adjacent to its ruffled border. Within this sealed area the production of lysosomal enzymes and a very acid environment via a proton pump utilizing the enzyme carbonic anhydrase II leads to the digestion of bone. Studies in man and animals have now identified many mutations in the proton pathway which may lead to osteopetrosis [8].

Bone Matrix

The major component of the organic bone matrix is collagen, interspersed with a complex mixture of non-collagen proteins and proteoglycans. Defects in the synthesis of collagen lead to the inherited disorders of connective tissue, notably osteogenesis imperfecta (see Chapter 7). Further mutations in the synthetic pathways of many non-collagen proteins lead to numerous skeletal dysplasias (see Table 8.1). Abnormal breakdown of the complex proteoglycan (mucopolysaccharide) molecules produces a large variety of disorders known as the mucopolysaccharidoses. The enzyme defects responsible produce a variety of skeletal defects.

The skeleton contains more than 50% of the body's collagen, which is essential for its strength and for correct mineralization. Many collagens exist, each with different functions and different polypeptide α[alpha]-chains controlled by their own specific genes, localized to different chromosomes. In normal adult bone, the only collagen molecule is type I, a heteropolymer with two α[alpha]-1 chains and one α[alpha]-2 chain, each represented as $(Gly\ X\ Y)_{338}$. An absolutely accurate triple helix with glycine in every third position in the α[alpha]-chains is essential for the structural integrity of collagen. The chains are formed as precursors within the osteoblast and fibroblast and then exported as triple helical procollagens. These are converted to collagen and self-assemble in the form of fibrils and fibers that overlap by 25% of their length and subsequently cross-link. This cross-linking provides both the strength of collagen and an organized matrix with hole zones upon which early mineralization occurs. Although the non-collagen proteins are less abundant than collagen, their number and functions are considerable and continue to be elucidated. Among them are the bone morphogenetic proteins, which belong to the transforming growth factor beta family, named after their ability to induce bone formation in soft tissues.

Mineralization

Mineralization appears to be an active phenomenon controlled by osteoblasts or components derived from them (matrix vesicles), both of which contain alkaline phosphatase. This enzyme acts also as a pyrophosphatase, and it has been proposed that the local removal of pyrophosphate, itself an inhibitor of mineralization, initiates mineralization at selected sites. The importance of alkaline phosphatase is well demonstrated by the defective mineralization in hypophosphatasia. Mineralization normally occurs in the region of matrix vesicles found in most, if not all, mineralizing tissues, particularly bone and cartilage. It also occurs, apparently without vesicles, on the organized matrix of bone collagen.

Mineral Homeostasis

Little is known about matrix homeostasis. However, there are many factors known to affect the absorption and excretion of calcium and its intracellular and extracellular concentrations. Phosphorus remains a neglected but important ion, for instance, in inherited hypophosphatemia [9]. Calcium is essential for life, regulating neuromuscular transmission, reproduction, endocrine function, blood clotting, and many widespread processes. It circulates in the plasma at a concentration of 2.25–2.60 mmol/1 in ionized (47%), protein-bound (46%), and complexed forms. Its concentration is maintained by a sensitive balance between intestinal absorption, renal reabsorption, and bone resorption, controlled by the classic calciotropic hormones parathyroid hormone, vitamin D (as its $1,25(OH)_2$ derivative) and calcitonin, also by the relatively newly discovered parathyroid-related protein (PTHrP), and a host of locally acting factors in addition to hormones with other important functions, such as growth hormone and estrogens. The actions of these are illustrated in Fig. 8.2; their clinical effects are listed in Table 8.2. Strangely neither deficiency nor excess of calcitonin has any clinical affect on the skeleton. PTHrP, produced by cancer

Table 8.2 The main clinical actions of hormones on the skeleton

	Excess	Deficiency
Parathyroid hormone	Increased bone resorption Osteitis fibrosa cystica	Skeletal changes in pseudohypoparathyroidism (PHP)
Vitamin D (via $1,25(OH)_2D$)	Increased metaphyseal density	Defective mineralization
Thyroxine	Osteoporosis (resorption increased more than formation)	Delayed bone age: fragmented epiphyses
Cortisol	Osteoporosis: short stature	None
Sex hormones	Early epiphyseal closure	Osteoporosis
Growth hormones	Acromegaly and giantism (before growth ceases)	Osteoporosis associated with hypogonadism
PTHrP	Increased bone resorption	

cells, is an important cytokine with a central role in skeletal development.

Parathyroid Hormone

Parathyroid hormone (PTH) is synthesized as a precursor (pre-proPTH), in the manner of proteins packaged for export. It is secreted in response to hypocalcemia and is produced in excess in primary hyperparathyroidism. PTH increases plasma calcium by stimulating intestinal absorption (via its effect on the synthesis of $1,25(OH)_2D$), by increasing renal reabsorption of calcium, and by increasing osteoclastic bone resorption (via the osteoblasts). Its effects on receptor cells are mediated through two separate systems that involve adenyl cyclase and phospholipase. Recent work by Brown [10] has demonstrated important calcium-sensing receptors in the parathyroid and other tissues. Mutations in the genes for these receptors can cause inherited alterations in plasma calcium.

Vitamin D

Vitamin D produces its effects via its active metabolite, $1,25(OH)_2D$. The main physiological source of vitamin D is the skin, where cholecalciferol (vitamin D_3) is synthesized from its precursor, 7-dihydrocholesterol, in the presence of ultraviolet light. Vitamin D also comes from the diet, mainly in the form of ergocalciferol (vitamin D_2). Both vitamins D_3 and D_2 (collectively referred to as vitamin D) undergo hepatic conversion to 25(OH) D and subsequent renal conversion to $1,25(OH)_2D$, the active vitamin D metabolite. As 25(OH)D is the major circulating vitamin D metabolite, it provides an accurate measure of vitamin D status. It is reduced in nutritional rickets, in Asian immigrants, and in geriatric patients.

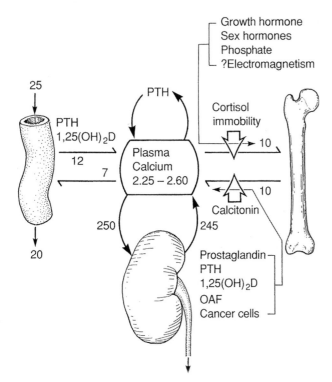

Fig. 8.2 Calcium homeostasis. The numbers represent the daily exchange in adults (in mmol) and the concentration in the plasma (in mmol/1). To convert values to mg, multiply by 40. PTH, parathyroid hormone; OAF, osteoclast activating factor(s). The complex interplay of cytokines is not shown

The effects of 1,25(OH)$_2$D are mediated through its widely distributed receptor. The gene for this receptor has been cloned, and mutations within it cause very rare forms of type II vitamin D-dependent rickets (see below). The main effects of vitamin D on mineral metabolism are to increase intestinal calcium absorption and osteoclastic bone resorption. However, the effects of vitamin D (via 1,25(OH)$_2$D) are not limited to mineral metabolism, as 1,25(OH)$_2$D is known to have important effects on growth, on the differentiation of cells, and on immunological processes [11, 12].

Calcitonin

Calcitonin directly suppresses the osteoclast, thereby reducing bone resorption. It is secreted in response to hypercalcemia, but its physiological role remains undefined. It has been proposed that it prevents bone resorption in times of physiological stress, such as growth and pregnancy.

Parathyroid Hormone-Related Peptide

Investigations of hypercalcemia in non-metastatic solid tumors have identified a hormone with considerable amino-terminal homology with PTH, now known as PTHrP. It has actions very similar to those of PTH and appears to use the same receptor mechanisms. Apart from its secretion by some tumors, there is evidence that it is a naturally occurring fetal hormone that may control calcium flux across the placenta. It is also important in the early development of bone and cartilage. Activating mutations in the PTHrP receptor can cause the very rare Jansen metaphyseal dysplasia.

Clinical Aspects of Metabolic Bone Disease in Children

Metabolic and endocrine bone disease in children differs from that in adults in the relative frequency of its causes, its relationship to growth, and the physiological variations in its biochemistry. The importance of growth is emphasized in Chapter 2. Accurate and consecutive measurements of height against percentile charts for a normal population will detect abnormality and the effects of treatment such as thyroxine in hypothyroidism or phosphate in inherited hypophosphatemia. Short stature (dwarfism) is the most frequent abnormality of height. It is proportional in some genetic conditions and in coeliac disease, hypopituitarism, or malnutrition. Disproportionate short stature is most commonly caused by a skeletal dysplasia, which may lead to relative shortness of the limbs as in achondroplasia, or relative shortness of the spine as in some spondyloepiphyseal dysplasias.

The normal biochemical reference ranges differ with age. Thus plasma phosphate concentration in children is about twice the adult normal level and declines rapidly after puberty. Alkaline phosphatase, urinary total hydroxyproline, and related collagen-derived indices of bone resorption are related to growth velocity and increase temporarily during adolescent growth. The interpretation of new bone markers based on collagen-derived fragments is difficult in children. The radiographic changes, which will be described in the appropriate sections, occur mainly in the growing regions of the bones. The clinical and biochemical features of the main disorders discussed in this chapter are summarized in Table 8.3.

Rickets

Rickets (and osteomalacia in the adolescent and adult) is, with rare exceptions, caused by a deficiency in vitamin D or a disturbance in its metabolism. The bone matrix fails to mineralize and, histologically, there is an excess of osteoid. The causes, some of which are very rare, can be understood in relation to vitamin D metabolism (Table 8.4). The features of nutritional rickets will be described, and the specific differences in other types outlined.

Vitamin D-Deficiency Rickets

This occurs in underprivileged populations throughout the world, particularly in the northern hemisphere. In the UK, it is most common in the Asian immigrant population of northern cities. Affected children lack the exposure to ultraviolet light necessary for the dermal synthesis of vitamin D and have a diet poor in vitamin D in which the components (high fiber and high cereal) probably contribute to the excessive breakdown of vitamin D [4, 13].

Clinical Features

The child with nutritional rickets has delayed growth, bony deformity, proximal myopathy, and tenderness and pain in the bones. The child is typically miserable and apathetic. Classic changes (see Fig. 8.3) are enlarged epiphyses in the long bones, enlarged costochondral junctions (rickety rosary), bossing of the vault of the skull, and deformities of the long bones that depend upon the age at which rickets occurs. Bow legs are common, and knock knees and

Table 8.3 Metabolic and endocrine disorders of the skeleton in children: main features

Disorder	Clinical	Biochemical	Comments
Rickets	Bone pain Deformity Proximal myopathy Many causes Nutritional rickets becoming more common in the UK	Ca↓, P↑ Phosphatase↑	For variations see Table 8.4
Osteoporosis (see Table 8.5)	Uncommon in childhood Bone pain and fractures	Normal (N) unless immobilized	Idiopathic juvenile osteoporosis, rare
Hyperparathyroidsim	Some have osteitis fibrosa cystica		Phosphatase sometimes increased if bone disease present
Hypoparathyroidism	Features of hypocalcemia	Ca↓, P↑, Phosphatase N	Those with PHP have short metacarpals, mental retardation, soft tissue ossification
Hypothyroidism	Lack of development Dull, slow, cold	Low T4, high TSH	Skeletal features resemble mucopolysaccharidoses
Hypophosphatasia	Severe: lethal Juvenile: with cranial synostosis Adult: with long bone fractures	Phosphoethanolamine in urine	Different forms (see text)
Idiopathic hyperphosphatasia, juvenile Paget's disease	Bowing of long bones; large head	Ca N, P N, Phosphatase↑	Very rare. Similar to severe Paget's disease in adults. Deficiency of OPG
Osteopetrosis	Dense bones, fracture, blindness etc	In some acid phosphatase↑	Several different types
Idiopathic hypercalcemia	Mental retardation, aortic stenosis	Plasma Ca↑	Associated with elfin face syndrome
Fibrodysplasia ossificans progressiva (FOP)	Extensive ectopic ossification	Alkaline phosphatase increased in acute phase	
Fibrous dysplasia	Deformity, fracture, pigmentation	Normal (N)	Polyostotic form maybe associated with endocrine abnormalities (McCune–Albright syndrome)

asymmetric deformity can also occur. Proximal myopathy is a striking feature of rickets (and also of osteomalacia). Its cause is unknown, but it can produce delay in standing and walking and, at a later age, difficulty in rising from a low chair or climbing stairs. Hypocalcemia may produce tetany, carpopedal spasm, and occasionally stridor.

Table 8.4 The causes of rickets

Cause	Biochemistry		Comments
	Plasma	Urine	
Vitamin D deficiency	Ca↓, P↓, Phosphatase↑	Ca↓	Particularly Asian immigrants
Malabsorption	Ca↓, P↓, Phosphatase↑	Ca↓	Main cause coeliac disease
Inherited hypophosphatemia	Ca N, P↓, Phosphatase↑	Ca N	X-linked inheritance. Dominant forms exist
Fanconi syndrome	Ca↓, P↓, Phosphatase↑	Ca↓ N Aminoaciduria	Many causes Often systemic acidosis Generalized aminoaciduria
Renal glomerular failure	Ca↓, P↑, Phosphatase↑	Ca↓	Biochemistry of uremia
Vitamin D-dependent rickets	Ca↓, P↓, Phosphatase↑	Ca↓	Two forms, both autosomal recessive: type I 1,25(OH)$_2$D ↓ type II 1,25(OH)$_2$D ↑
Tumor (oncogenic) rickets	Ca N, P↓, Phosphatase↑		Associated with hemangiomatous tumors 1,25(OH)$_2$D ↓

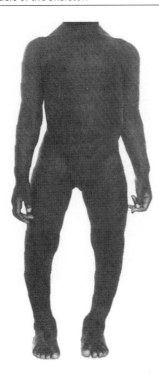

Fig. 8.3 Nutritional rickets. The thickened epiphyses at wrist and ankle and the genu varum are evident

Radiographic Features

In rickets there is failure of the orderly replacement of mineralized cartilage with bone. Radiographs show widening of the growth plate with a ragged, cupped, and widened metaphysis. Additional radiographic changes are due to secondary hyperparathyroidism with bone resorption induced by hypocalcemia. This can occur in relation to the periosteum at the end of the long bones, the phalanges, the medial ends of the clavicles, and elsewhere. Finally, in the adolescent, Looser's zones are diagnostic of osteomalacia. These are ribbon-like areas of failed mineralization that typically occur symmetrically on the medial borders of the long bones, pubic rami, borders of the scapulae, and ribs.

Biochemistry

Plasma calcium concentration is low or normal, phosphate low, and alkaline phosphatase increased. The typical findings vary with the stage of rickets and its cause (see Table 8.4). Secondary hyperparathyroidism will tend to correct hypocalcemia, but increase hypophosphatemia. The increase in plasma alkaline phosphatase is related to the degree of osteoblastic activity. (Despite the fact that mineralization is defective, osteoblastic activity is increased.) In vitamin D deficiency, the plasma 25(OH)D concentration is low. The urine calcium excretion is also very low. Aminoaciduria (which is reversible) may occur in vitamin D deficiency, as in the inherited renal tubular syndromes.

Histology

It is rarely essential to examine bone histologically in order to diagnose rickets, but bone will show an excess of unmineralized bone matrix (osteoid), with both increased thickness and coverage of the mineralized surfaces.

Prevention and Treatment

Nutritional rickets is prevented by exposing the skin to summer sunlight. Where this is not possible or unacceptable, physiological amounts of oral vitamin D (up to 25 μg or 1000 U) daily are effective. Successful preventive programs have been used in Asian rickets.

Differential Diagnosis

In its classic form, nutritional rickets is unlikely to be misdiagnosed. It is not, however, uncommon in premature infants. Furthermore, the diagnosis may be delayed since rickets is, erroneously, now thought to be infrequent. Rare causes may present difficulties. These include some skeletal dysplasias, particularly the metaphyseal dysplasia type Schmid.

Other Forms of Rickets

They are outlined in Table 8.4 and will be summarized here.

Rickets Due to Malabsorption

This will have the added features of the underlying disease—such as coeliac disease.

Rickets Due to Renal Disease

The term "renal rickets" is an over-simplification. Rickets occurs in renal tubular disorders and renal glomerular failure. The causes, clinical features, management, and treatment are different.

Renal Tubular Rickets

Inherited hypophosphatemia (vitamin D-resistant rickets; XLH) is inherited as an X-linked dominant and, excluding

Fig. 8.4 Vitamin D-resistant rickets. Bowing of the femora and tibiae with metaphyseal flaring, especially at the distal femora

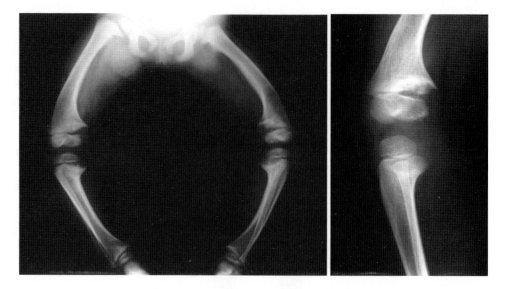

Vitamin D deficiency rickets, is probably the most frequent cause of rickets in orthopaedic practice [14]. The incidence is about 1 in 20,000 births, and the mutant gene has been localized to the X chromosome. Boys carrying the mutant gene may be more severely affected than girls, who have an additional normal X chromosome. Particular features are short stature, lower limb deformity (see Fig. 8.4), absence of proximal myopathy, and persistent hypophosphatemia. The children are normally bright, cheerful, and active. In later years there is a widespread enthesopathy, sometimes with ligamentous calcification leading to paraplegia. The exact cause of the renal loss of phosphate is not known, but the mutant protein is similar to an endopeptidase and may control phosphate metabolism. Quarles emphasized the importance of fibroblast growth factor 23 (FGF23) in XLH

and oncogenic rickets [9]. The main differential diagnosis is from other forms of rickets and from metaphyseal dysplasias (especially the Schmid type). Treatment combines oral phosphate (up to 2 g daily in divided doses) and 1-α-hydroxycholecalciferol (up to 1 μg daily). Corrective surgery requires considerable planning, because the deformities are complex. Surgery should only be undertaken when adequate, sustained medication has failed to prevent deformity (see Fig. 8.5).

Rickets and the Fanconi Syndrome

The term "Fanconi syndrome" refers to multiple renal tubular abnormalities, with generalized aminoaciduria. In children

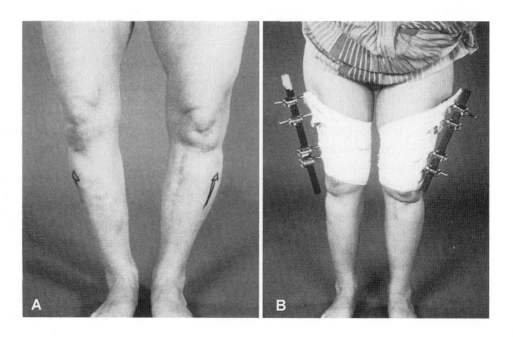

Fig. 8.5 (**a**) Hypophosphatemic rickets in a 15-year-old girl. Despite lifelong medication with phosphate and active vitamin D, she has residual excessive knee valgus. (**b**) After distal femoral osteotomy with external fixation

Fig. 8.6 Cystine crystals in the eye in a child with cystinosis. Reproduced with permission from Smith R [16]

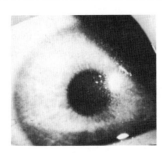

Fig. 8.8 Renal glomerular osteodystrophy. Shows excessive bone resorption and gross deformity in a child with chronic renal failure

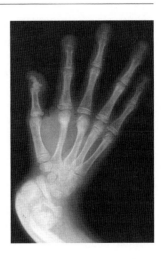

the most frequent cause is cystinosis or cystine storage disease [15]. Cystinosis is due to mutations in the *CTN5* gene on chromosome 17p13 which eliminate expression of the cystine transport protein, cystinosin. In this condition, inherited as a recessive trait, cystine crystals progressively accumulate in the tissues. This leads to multiple renal tubular defects, with rapid dehydration as a result of failure of reabsorption of water, severe acidosis, hypophosphatemia, and a form of renal tubular rickets. Cystinosis can be rapidly confirmed by the finding of cystine crystals in the eyes often associated with photophobia (see Fig. 8.6) [16].

The renal aspects of the disorder can be dealt with by renal transplantation. The rickets is alleviated by correction of the severe acidosis with oral bicarbonate and by giving 1-α-hydroxycholecalciferol.

Other rare renal tubular disorders leading to rickets, which include Dent disease and autosomal dominant hypophosphatemic rickets, are reviewed by Smith and Wordsworth [4].

Renal Glomerular Rickets (Renal Glomerular Osteodystrophy)

When renal failure predominantly involves the glomeruli (as in chronic renal failure, for instance, secondary to undiagnosed renal obstruction) the sequence of events differs from that in tubular disease (see Fig. 8.7). Hyperphosphatemia

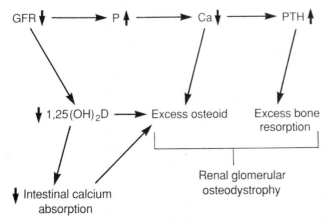

Fig. 8.7 The biochemistry of renal glomerular osteodystrophy. GFR, glomerular filtration rate. P, Ca, PTH, and 1,25(0H),D refer to circulating concentrations

leads to hypocalcemia, secondary hyperparathyroidism, and bone resorption. This is superimposed on failure of bone mineralization and rickets as a result of a lack of $1,25(OH)_2D$ and produces a rapidly deforming bone disease that particularly affects the growing ends of the long bones, giving a "rotting stump" appearance (see Fig. 8.8). Other skeletal changes include osteosclerosis (producing the "rugger-jersey" spine), osteoporosis, osteonecrosis, and deposits of amyloid in the bone. In addition, severe renal glomerular failure delays growth and bone age. Extensive ectopic mineralization (in the blood vessels and soft tissues) may eventually occur.

Diagnosis is based on the association of severe rickets and deformity with renal glomerular failure. Medical treatment of renal glomerular osteodystrophy is based on replacing the deficiency of $1,25(OH)_2D$ and, where necessary, reducing plasma phosphate.

Prolonged dialysis may produce problems of its own. In the past these included aluminum-induced bone disease. Successful renal transplantation is clearly the most effective treatment. The development of autonomous hyperparathyroidism may necessitate parathyroidectomy.

Vitamin D-Dependent Rickets

This is a very rare type of severe rickets that occurs without vitamin D deficiency. Two types exist, both inherited as recessive traits. In the first type (type I), the 1-α[alpha]-hydroxylase enzyme is defective; in the second type (type II), there is apparent end-organ resistance to $1,25(OH)_2D$. This resistance appears to be caused by single base mutations in the gene for the vitamin D ($1,25(OH)_2D$) receptor, affecting either the DNA or steroid binding sites. Interestingly, this form of rickets, also known as 1,25-vitamin D-dependent rickets, has additional features of abnormal teeth and alopecia. Treatment is difficult, but there is a good response to prolonged intravenous calcium, and spontaneous improvement occurs with age.

Oncogenic Rickets

Certain tumors, such as non-ossifying fibromas, fibrosing hemangiomata, and hemangiopericytomas, are associated with rickets, which is cured by their removal. It is likely that the tumor interferes with the hydroxylation of 25(OH)D. There is an excess of fibroblast growth factor (FGF) 23. Similar abnormalities may cause hypophosphatemic rickets in association with osteopetrosis, neurofibromatosis, and polyostotic fibrous dysplasia.

Osteoporosis

In osteoporosis there is a reduction in the amount of bone per given volume, without a change in its composition. Microarchitectural failure leads to fragility predisposing to fracture. The increasing use of dual radiograph absorptiometry has led to another definition of osteoporosis, namely a bone mass, measured as bone mineral density (BMD) or bone mineral content (BMC), which is 2.5 SD or more below the mean peak bone mass. This is useful in adults, but normal ranges for children have not been widely established. However osteoporosis is uncommon in children. Known causes of osteoporosis, such as Cushing's syndrome, have

their own features in addition to the bone disease they produce. Visual impairment is associated with osteoporosis in the rare, recessively inherited, osteoporosis-pseudoglioma syndrome [6]. Rarely, osteoporosis occurs without an identifiable cause, sometimes associated with pre-adolescent growth [17].

Idiopathic Juvenile Osteoporosis

The underlying change in this condition appears to be temporary formation of abnormal osteoporotic bone at the growing ends of the long bones and in the vertebrae, associated with a reduction in osteoblastic activity. Fractures occur in the metaphyses and shafts of the long bones, and in the vertebrae, and growth velocity decreases. Backache, a kyphosis, and characteristic pain around the lower ends of the tibiae develop with weight bearing. The child walks slowly and with difficulty. Radiographically, the compression fractures may simulate Looser's zones; widespread wedging of the vertebrae may produce a fish-like spine with excessive biconcave vertebral collapse (see Fig. 8.9). Routine plasma hematology and biochemistry are normal. Because pain in the bones with fracture is uncommon in children, the differential diagnosis is important (see Table 8.5). It is particularly important to exclude leukemia by bone marrow examination, which can be done at the same time as bone biopsy. In a significant proportion of affected individuals, the bone disorder begins to improve with the onset of puberty, so that the vertebrae may resume an almost normal shape (sometimes leaving a shadow of the osteoporotic bone within them). In

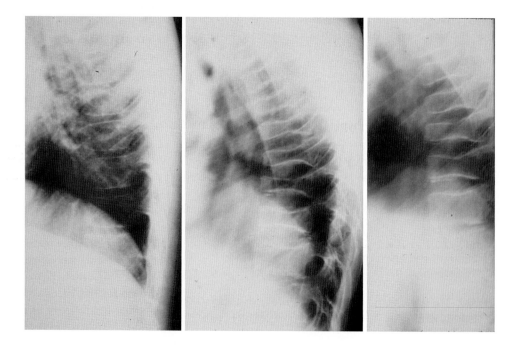

Fig. 8.9 Radiological appearance of the spine in a 14-year-old boy with idiopathic juvenile osteoporosis. There is progressive vertebral collapse, with subsequent spontaneous improvement

Table 8.5 Differential diagnosis of idiopathic juvenile osteoporosis

Other causes of juvenile osteoporosis
Cushings's syndrome
Homocystinuria
Turner's syndrome
Osteogenesis imperfecta (type I)
Osteoporosis pseudoglioma syndrome
Other diseases
Rickets
Acute leukemia

others, the bones continue to be fragile and to fracture, so that it is important to be as certain as possible that mild forms of osteogenesis imperfecta (types I and IV) have been excluded (see Chapter 7), although this can be difficult if a family history is absent.

Provided the diagnosis of idiopathic juvenile osteoporosis is correct, treatment is for symptoms only. Some reports suggest a lack of $1,25(OH)_2D$ and an improvement when this is administered. More recently bisphosphonates, particularly those with an amino substitution, have been used [18].

Parathyroid Disorders

Primary hyperparathyroidism and its associated bone disease are uncommon in childhood, but secondary hyperparathyroidism may be associated with the hypocalcaemia of rickets. The skeleton also alters in pseudohypoparathyroidism (PHP).

Hyperparathyroidism

Skeletal changes are the same as in the adult, with excessive osteoclastic activity, fibrosis, and the formation of cyst-like areas within the bones combining to produce osteitis fibrosa cystica. Bone resorption occurs at the growing ends of the long bones and subperiostially, especially on the medial border of the phalanges. In those children with bone disease, the diagnosis of primary hyperparathyroidism is confirmed by the characteristic biochemistry: an increase in the plasma calcium, reduced plasma phosphate, and increased alkaline phosphatase. Treatment is surgical removal of the primary tumor. The differential diagnosis is from other causes of hypercalcemia in childhood (see Table 8.6).

Table 8.6 Causes of hypercalcemia in childhood

Hyperparathyroidism
Vitamin D overdose
Idiopathic hypercalcemia
Neoplastic disease
Immobilization
Hypophosphatasia

Hypoparathyroidism

Secretion of parathyroid hormone may be defective, or the hormone itself may be ineffective. Hypoparathyroidism may present in the neonatal period as a transient or persistent disorder.

It may be associated with maternal hyperparathyroidism, magnesium deficiency, or as part of the Di George syndrome. In childhood, hypoparathyroidism may be one aspect of an autoimmune disorder or the result of thyroidectomy.

The skeletal abnormalities are restricted to PHP, in which there is end-organ resistance to the action of parathyroid hormone as a result of a loss of function mutation in a component of the G protein signaling system. The circulating PTH concentration is high, yet there is hypocalcemia and hyperphosphatemia. The typical phenotypic changes of PHP are delayed growth, mental retardation, cataracts, and subcutaneous ossification, together with characteristic skeletal changes that mainly affect the hands and feet, with short fourth and fifth metacarpals and/or metatarsals. This last feature can be demonstrated by asking the patient to clench their fist and noting that the knuckles are not in line.

PHP may be familial, and the expression of the dominant gene among family members is variable. Patients within such families may have the PHP phenotype without any biochemical changes. The diagnosis of PHP is important since lifelong treatment with 1-α[alpha]-hydroxycholecalciferol and calcium may be necessary to prevent complications.

Hypothyroidism and Other Hormonal Disorders

The skeleton is affected by altered secretion of other systemic hormones. Probably the most striking effects in infancy occur in hypothyroidism. This is rarely recognized at birth, but by the time the child is about 6 months of age defective thyroid function leads to the clinical features of cretinism. The child becomes sluggish and sleepy, with noisy ventilation and a large tongue. Nasal obstruction and a large abdomen gradually became apparent. The temperature is subnormal, the skin is dry and cold, and there is difficulty in feeding. There is also a marked delay in growth and skeletal age.

The diagnosis is made biochemically: circulating thyroid-stimulating hormone (TSH) is high, thyroxine is low, and the plasma cholesterol is increased. Radiographs show delayed bone age and stippling of the upper femoral epiphyses, which ossify late. The first lumbar vertebra may be hypoplastic, with anterior beaking. The diagnosis of skeletal hypothyroidism in an infant is not difficult, but should be differentiated from multiple epiphyseal dysplasia, spondyloepiphyseal dysplasia, or one of the mucopolysaccharidoses. Prolonged thyrotoxicosis causes bone disease in the adult, but apart from the epiphyseal abnormalities, this does not occur in childhood.

The growing skeleton may also be affected by an excess of corticosteroids—most often administered therapeutically and less frequently in Cushing's syndrome—and by hypogonadism, hypopituitarism, or hyperpituitarism. The effects of these and other hormone disturbances on the skeleton are summarized in Table 8.2.

Hypophosphatasia

Hypophosphatasia is a rare condition associated with a reduction in the tissue non-specific plasma alkaline phosphatase (TNAP) [19]. The incidence is about 1 in 100,000 live births. The inheritance of the severe form is recessive, and in some cases there is consanguinity. For reasons that are not fully understood, there is wide phenotypic variation, from a lethal perinatal disease to a virtually asymptomatic condition in childhood. Numerous missense mutations have now been described in the *TNAP* gene in hypophosphatasia.

The main effect of the absence or reduction of alkaline phosphatase is to produce a disorder of mineralization that histologically resembles rickets, with excessively thick osteoid seams. This is associated with an increase in the urinary excretion of phosphoethanolamine and an increase in plasma pyrophosphate.

Perinatal Lethal Hypophosphatasia

This recessive condition is one of the causes of perinatal lethal short-limbed dwarfism, which includes type II osteogenesis imperfecta, thanatophoric dwarfism, and achondrogenesis. The differential diagnosis depends on the radiological appearances. The skeleton shows grossly defective mineralization, with large Y-shaped defects in the long bones as a result of patchy failure to mineralize (see Fig. 8.10). The cranial bones are ossified only in their central portion. Prenatal diagnosis is possible by ultrasound and radiography, by measurement of alkaline phosphatase in amniotic fluid cells, and by genetic linkage studies.

Infantile Hypophosphatasia

This condition occurs before the age of 6 months and is characterized by poor feeding, inadequate weight gain, and the

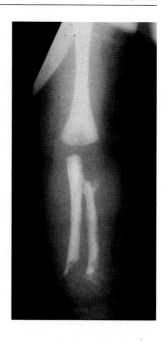

Fig. 8.10 Lethal perinatal hypophosphatasia. There are large mineralization defects in the metaphyses of the long bones

development of rachitic-type deformities. Hypercalcemia, hypercalciuria with nephrocalcinosis, and renal failure are also features. The sclerae may be blue. Premature fusion of the cranial sutures may produce papilledema and proptosis; radiographs show irregular translucencies within the metaphyses.

Childhood Hypophosphatasia

This is characterized by early loss of deciduous teeth (before 5 years of age), the incisors being shed first. Where the teeth, but not the skeleton, are affected the term "odontohypophosphatasia" may be used.

There is short stature, delayed walking, and a waddling gait, with rachitic deformities. Cranial synostosis may lead to proptosis and brain damage if cranial osteotomy/cranioplasty is not undertaken. As in infantile hypophosphatasia, radiographs may show tongues of radiotranslucency extending from the growth plate into the metaphyses.

Adult Hypophosphatasia

In the mild form of the disease, the adult develops pathological fractures across the shafts of the long bones. Chondrocalcinosis (possibly related to an excess of pyrophosphate) may occur. Such adults may represent the heterozygous form of the alkaline phosphatase gene mutation.

Management

Treatment depends on the severity of the disease. In the infantile form, hypercalcemia may be reduced by dietary restriction of calcium and glucocorticoid therapy. The transfusion of alkaline–phosphatase-enriched plasma from patients with Paget's disease has proved unsuccessful. Long bone fractures are probably best treated with intramedullary rods. For the severe infantile form, transplantation of bone marrow-derived stromal cells may be possible in the future.

Hyperphosphatasia

In a very rare condition called idiopathic hyperphosphatasia or juvenile Paget's disease, there is bowing of the long bones, progressive deformity, and increased bone turnover. Cundy et al. have shown that the autosomal recessive inheritance is caused by loss of function mutations in the gene for osteoprotegerin (OPG) [20].

The Osteopetrosis (and Osteosclerosis)

In a number of conditions, there is an excessive amount of mineralized bone within the skeleton. This can be due to defective resorption or increased formation (see Fig. 8.11) [4]. The best recognized is osteopetrosis (marble bone disease) (see Table 8.7).

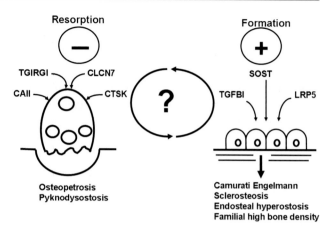

Fig. 8.11 The inherited causes of dense bones. The *curved arrows* between formation (osteoblasts) and resorption (osteoclasts) indicate that the linkage between formation and resorption may still be maintained, but the details are unknown (hence the question mark). Capital letters refer to the genes in which mutations have been identified (see text). Reproduced with permission from Smith R, Wordsworth P. [4]

Marble Bone Disease (Osteopetrosis; Albers–Schönberg Disease)

Marble bone disease has a variable phenotype, from a severe, recessive infantile form to dominantly inherited, mild adult forms [8]. It has recently been further subdivided according to biochemistry and radiology. Rickets is occasionally associated with the disorder. Most advances in understanding

Table 8.7 Different types and features of the osteopetrosis

Type	Clinical features	Radiology	Plasma biochemistry	Chromosome locus	Gene
Mild dominantly inherited type I	Fractures Cranial nerve compression Variable anemia Osteomyelitis of the jaw In both mild types	Bones uniformly dense Sclerosis of the skull Enlarged thick cranial vault	Acid phosphatase normal	11	LRP5 mutations in some
Mild dominantly inherited type II		Variable bone density "Endobones" Sandwich vertebrae Lack of modeling	Acid phosphatase increased Calcium and PTH may be increased	16	CLCN7 mutations most frequent
Severe infantile recessively inherited	Short stature Severe anemia Cranial nerve palsies Fractures Deformity Hepatosplenomegaly	Uniform increased bone density Lack of modeling	Increased acid phosphatase Calcium may be low	11	TCIRG1
Carbonic anhydrase II deficiency, recessive	Cerebral calcification Growth retardation	As in other forms	Systemic acidosis	8	CAII
Pycnodysostosis Cathepsin K deficiency, recessive	Disproportionate short stature Blue sclerae Open anterior fontanelle Kyphoscoliosis	Uniform osteosclerosis Wormian bones Acroosteolysis	Normal	1	CTSK

and treatment have been made in the severe form. There are variable abnormalities in the osteoclasts and some may lack their ruffled border, whereas others have defects in their carbonic anhydrase II enzyme and proton pathway. The multiple causes of infantile recessive osteopetrosis help to explain why some infants are cured by bone marrow transplantation containing compatible normal osteoclasts, whereas others are not.

Severe Infantile Osteopetrosis

The failure of resorption of calcified cartilage and bone leads to excessive amounts of bone because its formation probably continues unabated. This produces two main effects: a lack of bone marrow with a progressive pancytopenia and cranial nerve compression, with deafness, blindness, and eventual death. Diagnosis is based on these clinical features, together with various deformities, including those of the face and skull, and typical radiographic appearances. A number of radiographic changes are described: the two most important are an increase in bone density affecting the skull and long bones and a lack of bone remodeling.

Mild Osteopetrosis

The mild form of osteopetrosis is dominantly inherited and does not have the severe complications of the infantile form. It may be asymptomatic and diagnosed only by radiographs. Characteristically, there is a variation between dense unmodeled bones and less dense bone with normal modeling. This leads to striation, which is transverse in the long bones and circumferential in the pelvis, and to the appearance of a "bone within a bone" in the vertebrae and the small bones of the hands and feet (see Fig. 8.12). The complications of mild osteopetrosis include an increased tendency to fracture, which affects the long bones and also the phalanges (the fractures are typically transverse, as are most pathological fractures), anemia (especially at time of increased physiological requirement), and a tendency to develop mandibular osteomyelitis. Deafness, loss of vision, psychomotor delay, osteoarthritis, and carpal tunnel syndrome have all been recorded. In some patients there is an isolated increase in plasma acid phosphatase.

Management

This differs according to the severity of the disease. Bone marrow transplantation is a complex and dangerous procedure that should be reserved for life-threatening disease in infancy. Successful grafting of allogeneic bone marrow has produced excellent improvement in a few patients, but not all respond. The response depends upon the specific mutation causing the disease.

Other forms of treatment have included restriction of dietary calcium, high-dose calcitriol to encourage bone resorption, and high-dose glucocorticoids for malignant osteopetrosis with pancytopenia. Deterioration of vision and other signs of cranial nerve compression may benefit from surgery. In the rare form of osteopetrosis that is caused by carbonic anhydrase II deficiency, there is no evidence that correction of the systemic acidosis decreases bone density.

Orthopaedic surgery for fractures in osteopetrosis can be very difficult because the bone is very hard and very brittle. Both bone and drills may shatter and diamond-tipped drills are useful.

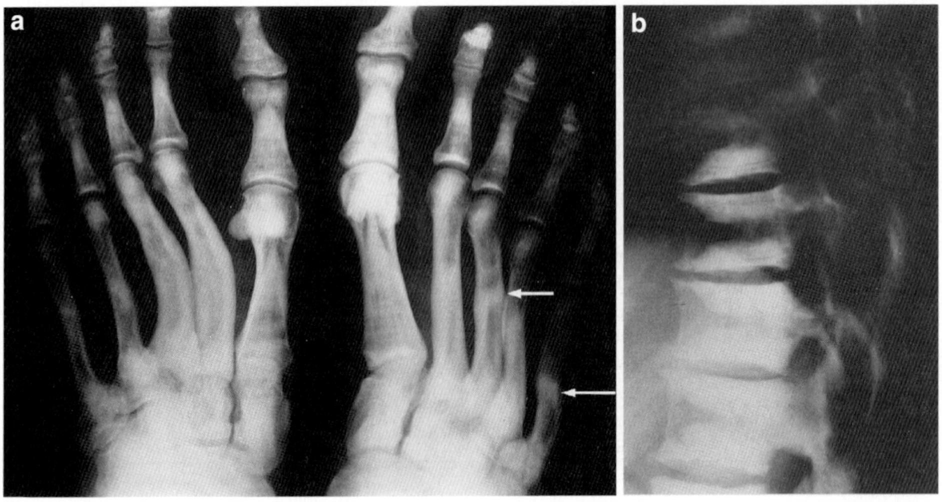

Fig. 8.12 The skeleton in dominantly inherited mild osteopetrosis demonstrates variable bone density. (**A**) AP view of the feet, which shows evidence of previous fractures. (**B**) Lateral view of the lower thoracic and lumbar spine. This form would now be classified as ADOII

Table 8.8 Some causes of ectopic ossification

1. Acquired	Local injury	
	Hip replacement	
	Traumatic paraplegia	
	Tumors	
	Others	DISH
		OPLL
		Ankylosing spondylitis
		Etretinate therapy
		Some metabolic enthesopathies
2. Inherited	Albright's hereditary osteodystrophy (AHO)	
	Fibrodysplasia (myositis) ossificans progressiva (FOP)	
	Progressive osseous heteroplasia (POH)	

Ectopic Mineralization

Mineral may be deposited outside the skeleton, with or without the formation of ectopic bone matrix. Ectopic calcification (without bone formation) can be due to biochemical abnormalities such as vascular calcification in hyperparathyroidism, basal ganglia calcification in hypoparathyroidism, and tumoral calcinosis in inherited hyperphosphatemia. Alternatively, it may occur with normal biochemistry in damaged tissues, as in the dystrophic calcification in systemic sclerosis. In contrast, all the components of bone may be laid down in the soft tissues (see Table 8.8). This often occurs after head and spinal injury, after some forms of surgery, and in the ligaments of adults with inherited hypophosphatemia. Progressive ossification in muscles occurs in the rare, dominantly inherited condition of myositis (or fibrodysplasia) ossificans progressiva. Despite its extreme rarity (fewer than one per million), this is an important disease to recognize. Recently Shore et al. have described an apparently activating mutation in a bone morphogenetic protein (BMP) type I receptor (ACVRI) [21].

Fibrodysplasia (Myositis) Ossificans Progressiva

Ossification in the skeletal muscles progresses from infancy, leading to fixation of major joints and gross disability. This is combined with typical skeletal abnormalities, particularly monophalangic big toes and fusion of the cervical spine [22].

Ossification usually begins in the paraspinal muscles, and at least 50% of patients have had episodes of myositis by the age of 3 years. Typically, there is swelling, redness, and pain in the affected muscle, which feels very hard. At this acute stage, various diagnoses are considered, particularly infection and soft tissue sarcoma. Biopsy shows \hbox{edematous} muscle with many inflammatory cells and fragmented myofibrils. Later, true bone forms, often in cartilage, and this subsequently mineralizes. Clinically, the swelling subsides but is replaced by palpable masses of solid bone that prevent movement of the larger joints. The paraspinal muscles are involved early and the major muscles around the hip late, but all major striated muscles can become involved. Small muscles such as those of the hands and feet, smooth muscle, and cardiac muscle escape ossification. At birth and in infancy, the big toes show abnormal centers of ossification and are short and deviated laterally, so that a diagnosis of congenital hallux valgus may be made. Attempted surgical correction leads to ossification, and subsequent fusion of the epiphyses leads to a short and rigid big toe (see Fig. 8.13).

In the cervical spine the vertebral bodies are small in comparison with the pedicles and spinous processes. There is progressive fusion of all these elements. At this stage, erroneous diagnoses such as Still's disease and Klippel–Feil syndrome may be made.

Because episodes of myositis are quite unpredictable, it is difficult to give a prognosis. However, myositis is less frequent with increasing age, although it may follow injury at any time. There is no evidence that any current form of treatment influences the progress of the condition. Surgical removal of ectopic bone is followed by rapid recurrence and increasing disability. It should be avoided. Prolonged corticosteroids have been used in an attempt to reduce the frequency and effects of myositis, and also in high-dose short courses during acute episodes of myositis.

Progressive Osseous Heteroplasia

This is a very rare disorder with progressive ossification in the soft tissues. The clinical expression is wide. Inheritance is dominant and the identified mutation is in *GNAS1* coding for the $G_s\alpha$ protein.

Fibrous Dysplasia (Monostotic and Polyostotic)

Fibrous dysplasia is a relatively common disorder of bone. Typically, isolated or monostotic lesions are found in the long bones, ribs, or skull. They may be discovered incidentally, or as the result of a pathological fracture, for instance, in the femoral neck. The rarer polyostotic form may be associated with ipsilateral pigmentation and endocrine abnormalities—particularly sexual precocity in girls (McCune Albright syndrome). Cushing's syndrome, thyrotoxicosis, and hypertension are also described.

Fig. 8.13 Fibrodysplasia
ossificans progressiva. (**A**) Neck:
abnormal vertebrae with fusion.
(**B**) Ectopic ossification:
radiograph with bars of ectopic
bone (*arrows*). (**C**) Hands:
radiograph of short abnormal
thumbs (**D**) Toes: the typical
clinical appearance of shortened
(valgus) big toes

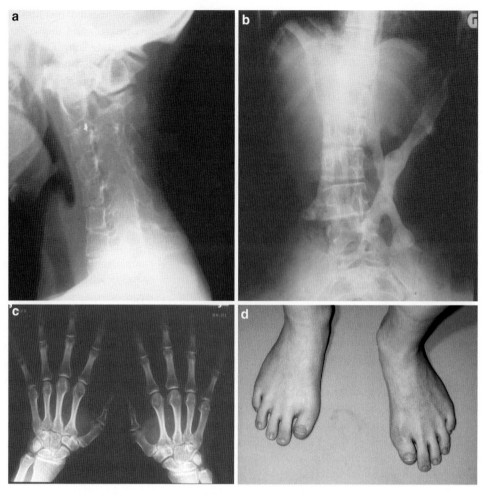

The skeletal lesions are often unilateral and widespread. Cranio-facial fibrous dysplasia causes severe deformity, which can sometimes be corrected surgically. Advanced fibrous dysplasia involving the proximal femur may lead to a "shepherd's crook" deformity, which may be bilateral. Rarely, polyostotic fibrous dysplasia is associated with hypophosphatemic osteomalacia. It is now known that the cause of fibrous dysplasia (both monostotic and polyostotic) is an activating mutation in the G protein involved in cell signaling. The severity of the condition depends on the proportion of cells affected (mosaicism). Weinstein has shown that the skeletal lesions may respond to an amino-bisphosphonate [23].

Vitamins and Minerals

Vitamin C Deficiency

Scurvy occurs typically between the age of 6 and 7 months in infants fed exclusively on vitamin C-deficient food. Vitamin C, ascorbic acid, is necessary for the hydroxylation of proline to hydroxyproline, a vital post-translational step in the synthesis of collagen. In its absence, the underhydroxylated collagen is not correctly exported from the cell.

The onset of scurvy may be precipitated by an acute infection. Perifollicular petechial hemorrhage in the skin may be the earliest sign, and periodontal hemorrhage also occurs. The scorbutic infant is irritable, anorexic, and fails to gain weight. The main skeletal problems are sub-periosteal hemorrhage, with characteristic epiphyseal and metaphyseal changes. The limbs are tender and painful and the infant lies in the frog position. The sub-periosteal lesions produce painful swellings along the shafts of the long bones, radiological changes being most marked where growth is rapid, e.g., at the knees, wrists, and costochondral junctions. There is a loss of bone density, with a thin cortex and a ground-glass appearance of the cancellous bone. The outline of the epiphyses is accentuated to give a ringed appearance, and there is a dense line with spurs at the ends of the metaphyses. Sub-periosteal hemorrhages become radiologically more obvious after treatment is commenced. It is possible to confuse the changes with infection. The changes in the metaphyses resemble those of non-accidental injury (see Chapter 42) but scurvy is far less common. Treatment is with vitamin C.

Vitamin A Excess

Retinoic acid and its derivatives have profound effects on osteoblastic function. Two main skeletal abnormalities result from an excess of vitamin A: cortical hyperostosis and ectopic ossification of the ligaments. In children, prolonged overdose with vitamin A causes pain and tenderness in the long bones and localized swelling. The cortical density of the long bones is increased, but the bones are abnormally fragile and liable to fracture. In adults, the prolonged use of retinoic acid derivatives for skin disease such as psoriasis and ichthyosis can lead to calcification of the ligaments, especially around the spine, with new bone formation, stiffness, and reduced mobility.

Vitamin D Toxicity

This may occur from therapeutic overdosage in inherited hypophosphatemia. In addition to the features of hypercalcemia (nocturia, polyuria, thirst, constipation, anorexia, and vomiting), nephrocalcinosis and renal failure can develop. As in idiopathic hypercalcemia (below), there are deposits of dense bone at the metaphyses of the long bones and increased density of the spine, ribs, and pelvis.

Idiopathic Hypercalcemia

Idiopathic hypercalcemia of infancy (the elfin face syndrome; Williams' syndrome) has been attributed to an excess of vitamin D, although doubt exists as to its true cause. Mild and severe types are described. In the severe type, symptomatic hypercalcemia is associated with supravalvular aortic stenosis, a characteristic pyknic face with low-set ears, and mental impairment. Further study of this disorder suggests abnormal regulation of 25(OH)D, concentrations of which may be increased when the patient is hypercalcemic. Radiographs of the long bones show increased metaphyseal density. There may be calcification of the basal ganglia. There is a mutation in the elastin gene [24] but this does not explain the hypercalcemia.

Lead Poisoning

Increased radiographic density of the metaphyses in children may be produced by an excess of lead, phosphorus, mercury, or bismuth. The extent of environmental lead poisoning is not clear, but established causes include the ingestion of lead-containing paint or of water stored in lead pipes, and exposure to exhaust fumes. Lead has effects upon the gastrointestinal, neuromuscular, and hematological systems,

causing constipation, myopathy, and anemia. There may be discoloration of the gum margins. There is a characteristic punctuate basophilia. Radiographs may demonstrate deposits in the gastrointestinal tract and widening of the sutures of the skull as a result of increased intracranial pressure. However, the most characteristic feature is the lead line—a dense metaphyseal band of varying thickness seen after about 1 month of chronic lead poisoning. Repeated lead lines may form with variations in lead exposure and during the treatment of lead poisoning with chelating agents. The amount of lead in the body increases with chronic renal failure [25]. The diagnosis of lead poisoning is confirmed by an increase in plasma and urinary lead.

Fluorosis

The skeletal effects of fluoride are most often seen in adults treated for osteoporosis with sodium fluoride. The fluoride ion stimulates the osteoblasts to produce new bone, although this is woven rather than lamellar and, unless additional calcium is given, is poorly mineralized. Fluoride is not given therapeutically to increase bone density in children but low concentrations are recommended to prevent dental caries.

Fluoride poisoning is uncommon in western societies, but may be produced by inhalation of fluoride vapor in the cryolith industry, by ingestion of vegetables contaminated with fluorine-containing dust, and from a high concentration in drinking water. Endemic fluorosis is well described in India. In Asia, Whyte et al. have shown that excessive consumption of inferior quality "brick tea" may cause skeletal fluorosis [26].

The changes in the teeth affect the permanent dentition, mainly the incisors, and are seen only if the high fluoride intake begins before the age of 8 years. The teeth are arranged irregularly and the enamel is translucent with patchy opaque areas. The bones are dense but more fragile than normal, the cortex is thick, and the metaphyses are widened, with an irregular edge. The skull is thick and dense, as are the vertebral bodies. Calcium is deposited in the spinal ligaments and at the insertions of tendons into the long bones. The skeletal signs of fluorosis increase with age, and calcification in the spine can lead to spinal and nerve root compression.

Aluminum Excess

An excess of aluminum can lead to a form of osteodystrophy in patients maintained on hemodialysis. The aluminum, derived from the dialysis fluid itself or from tap water, accumulates in the skeleton, where it is deposited at the calcification front. Histologically, there is a failure of normal osteoblast function and of mineralization, producing an aplastic bone disease that is resistant to treatment with vitamin D. Aluminum osteodystrophy, or "dialysis bone disease," also causes bone pain and fracture. Furthermore, amyloid may be deposited in the skeleton of patients on prolonged dialysis.

Copper Deficiency

Copper is essential for the function of many enzymes, particularly amino acid oxidases, and for the hydroxylation of proline and lysine residues. The main skeletal effect of copper deficiency probably arises from its effect on collagen synthesis. Acquired deficiency of copper occurs in premature or low birth weight babies maintained on parenteral nutrition, although it may occur as a transient phenomenon in otherwise normal infants or in protein-energy malnutrition. The effects of copper deficiency on the skeleton are similar to those of scurvy; in the differential diagnosis, non-accidental injury and osteogenesis imperfecta should be excluded.

Menkes' syndrome is an inherited disorder of copper metabolism that is closely related to the occipital horn syndrome (now called Ehlers–Danlos syndrome IX). In both, the inheritance is X-linked. In Menkes' syndrome, the face and hair ("steely" hair) are abnormal. Progressive cerebral degeneration, hypopigmentation, arterial rupture, and thrombosis occur. In the skeleton, there is osteoporosis and widening of the flared metaphyses with spiky protrusions. Rib fractures and Wormian bones occur. Again, non-accidental injury and osteogenesis imperfecta must be excluded.

The occipital horn syndrome is so named because of the palpable protrusions of bone from the occiput. Other features include inguinal herniae, skin and joint laxity, and widespread arterial tortuosity.

Summary

The number of metabolic and endocrine disorders known to affect the skeleton has rapidly increased now that disorders previously thought to be skeletal oddities have been found to have a metabolic basis. With the definition of new syndromes and the increased understanding of rarities, the management of metabolic bone disease in children is more than ever a team effort, and should involve a physician and geneticist in addition to the orthopaedic surgeon.

References

1. Rauch F, Glorieux FH. Osteogenesis imperfecta. Lancet 2004; 363:1377–85.

2. Miyazono K, Maeda S, Imamura T. BMP receptor signaling: transcriptional targets, Regulation of signals, and signaling cross-talk. Cytokine Growth Factor Rev 2005; 16:3251–63.

3. Cohen MM. The new bone biology: pathologic, molecular and clinical correlates. Am J Med Genetics 2006; 140A:2646–706.

4. Smith R, Wordsworth P. Clinical and biochemical disorders of the skeleton. Oxford: Oxford University Press; 2006.

5. McKusick VA, Amberger JS. Morbid anatomy of the human genome. In: Rimoin DL, Connor JM, Pyeritz RE, Korf BR, eds. Principles and Practice of Medical Genetics, 4th ed. London: Churchill Livingstone; 2002:175–298.

6. Johnson ML, Harnish K, Nusse R, Van Hul W. LRP5 and Wnt signaling; a union made for bone. J Bone Miner Res 2004; 19:1749–57.

7. Bilezikian J, Raisz L, Rodan G. Principles of Bone Biology, 2nd ed. San Diego CA: Academic Press; 2002.

8. Tolar J, Teitelbaum SL, Orchard PJ. Osteopetrosis. New Engl J Med 2004; 351:2839–49.

9. Quarles LD. Evidence for a bone-kidney axis regulating phosphate homeostasis. J Clin Invest 2003; 112:642–6.

10. Brown EM. Clinical lessons from the calcium-sensing receptor. Nat Clin Pract Endocrinol Metabol 2007; 3:122–33.

11. Adams JS, Hewison M. Unexpected actions of Vitamin D: new perspectives on the regulation of innate and adaptive immunity. Nat Clin Pract Endocrinol Metabol 2008; 4:80–90.

12. Holick MF. Vitamin D deficiency. New Engl J Med 2007; 357:266–81.

13. Wharton B, Bishop N. Rickets. Lancet 2003; 362:1389–400.

14. Whyte MP. Rickets and osteomalacia (acquired and heritable forms). In: Wass JAH, Shalet SM, eds. Oxford Textbook of Endocrinology and Diabetes. Oxford: Oxford University Press; 2002:697–715.

15. Gahl WA, Thoere J, Scheider JA. Cystinosis. New Engl J Med 2002; 347:111–21.

16. Smith R. Biochemical Disorders of the Skeleton. London: Butterworths; 1979.

17. Smith R. Idiopathic juvenile osteoporosis; experience of twenty-one patients. Br J Rheumatol 1995; 34:68–77.

18. Brumsen C, Hamdy NAT, Papapoulos SE. Long-term effects of bisphosphonates on the growing skeleton. Medicine 1997; 76: 266–83.

19. Whyte MP. Heritable forms of rickets and osteomalacia. In: Royce PM, Steinmann B, eds. Connective Tissue and its Heritable Disorders, 2nd ed. New York: Wiley-Liss; 2002:849–99.

20. Cundy T, Davidson J, Rutland MD, et al. Recombinant osteoprotegerin for juvenile Paget's disease. New Engl J Med 2005; 353:918–23.

21. Shore EM, Xu M, Feldman GJ, et al. A recurrent mutation in the BMP type I receptor ACVR1 causes inherited and sporadic fibrodysplasia ossificans progressiva. Nat Genetics 2006; 38:525–7.

22. Smith R. Fibrodysplasia (myositis) ossificans progressiva. Clinical lessons from a rare disease. Clin Orthop Rel Res 1998; 346:7–14.

23. Weinstein RS. Long-term aminobisphosphonate treatment of fibrous dysplasia: spectacular increase in bone density. J Bone Miner Res 1997; 12:1314–15.

24. Langman CB. Hypercalcemic syndromes in infants and children. In: Favus MJ, ed. Primer on the Metabolic Bone Diseases and Disorders of Nineral Metabolism, 3rd ed. Philadelphia PA: Lippincott-Raven; 1996:209–12.

25. Marsden PA. Increased body lead burden—cause or consequence of chronic renal insufficiency. New Engl J Med 2003; 348:345–7.

26. Whyte MP, Essinger K, Gannon FH, et al. Skeletal fluorosis and instant tea. Am J Med 2005; 118:78–82.

Chapter 9

Blood Disorders and AIDS

Christopher A. Ludlam and John E. Jellis

Disorders of either the hemostatic system or the bone marrow may lead to impaired musculoskeletal development.

Bleeding disorders are of two main types:

1. Those affecting the plasma coagulation factors (e.g., hemophilia), leading predominantly to joint and muscle hemorrhage.
2. Disorders of platelets and von Willebrand factor, in which the bleeding is usually from mucosal surfaces (e.g., epistaxis, gastrointestinal hemorrhage, and menorrhagia).

Permanent damage may follow joint and muscle bleeds, particularly if these are recurrent at the same site or if treatment is delayed. In contrast, musculoskeletal changes are rare in those with platelet disorders and von Willebrand disease.

In many congenital disorders of hematopoiesis, bone marrow hypertrophy occurs; it is particularly marked in the thalassemias and to a lesser extent it accompanies hemoglobinopathies such as sickle cell disease. Increased erythropoiesis leads to hypertrophy and deformity of the surrounding bone; in sickle cell disease bone infarction occurs.

Acute lymphatic leukemia in childhood infiltrates the marrow, but it is uncommon for this to lead to orthopaedic complications. However, back pain from vertebral involvement, a swollen joint, or a limp should alert the orthopaedic surgeon to this possibility, particularly if the child is systemically ill. Occasionally, localized malignant deposits of other tumors cause osteolytic lesions that may cause pathological fracture.

Hemophilia

Congenital deficiencies of the plasma coagulation factors VIII and IX result in hemophilia A and B, respectively. As genes for both these proteins lie on the X chromosome, the diseases are inherited as sex-linked disorders; consequently, in the majority of cases, only males are clinically affected. Female carriers of hemophilia, however, may have reduced levels of factors VIII and XI and thus suffer a bleeding disorder which predisposes to post-operative hemorrhage. Hemophilia A and B are clinically indistinguishable. Approximately one-third of cases of hemophilia arise "sporadically," without a family history. A variety of gene defects, including inversions, point mutations, or deletions, result in the synthesis of a coagulant protein with decreased activity. As the same genetic defect is present in all individuals within a family, all affected individuals have hemophilia with the same degree of severity. Diagnostic and therapeutic guidelines for hemophilia are available from the United Kingdom Hemophilia Doctors Organisation (www.ukhcdo.org).

The propensity to hemorrhage depends upon the level of coagulant protein in the plasma (Table 9.1). Individuals with severe hemophilia (less than 1% factor VIII activity) usually have frequent, apparently spontaneous joint bleeds, whereas those with levels of 1–5% have moderate disease and only bleed significantly following minor trauma; those with more than 5% factor VIII/IX only hemorrhage excessively after trauma or surgery.

Factor VIII is synthesized principally in the liver and endothelial cells. In the plasma it is bound to the carrier protein von Willebrand factor. Its plasma half-life is approximately 12 h. The basal concentration can be increased in

Table 9.1 Classification of severity of hemophilia

Factor VIII/IX level	Clinical manifestation
Severe (<2%)	Frequent, "spontaneous" bleeds
Moderate (2–10%)	Bleeds following minor trauma
Mild (>10%)	Only bleeds after surgery or trauma

For surgery in all patients it is necessary to increase the factor VIII/IX level to greater than 50% of normal.

C.A. Ludlam (✉)
University of Edinburgh, Edinburgh, UK; Department of Clinical and Laboratory Haematology, Royal Infirmary Edinburgh, Edinburgh, UK

M. Benson et al. (eds.), *Children's Orthopaedics and Fractures*,
DOI 10.1007/978-1-84882-611-3_9, © Springer-Verlag London Limited 2010

response to a variety of stimuli, such as stress and exercise. Hemophilia B is caused by a deficiency of factor IX. This protein is also synthesized in the liver but has a longer half-life of approximately 18 h.

In children with severe hemophilia, bleeding is uncommon until the age of approximately 6 months, when excessive bruising may begin to be seen as the baby becomes more active. These infants may initially be assumed to be victims of non-accidental injury or child abuse (see Chapter 42) and it is important that, whenever this diagnosis is suspected, appropriate tests of the hemostatic system are performed at an early stage of investigation [1]. An earlier diagnosis may be made if the baby is circumcised, as prolonged hemorrhage almost inevitably occurs. Diagnosis can be made at birth by measuring the plasma factor VIII or IX concentration, and it is appropriate to do so if the mother is known to have a high probability of being a carrier.

Hemarthrosis results in a distressed infant resistant to all attempts at comforting. An arm or leg is held rigidly and the elbow or knee may be swollen. As children become older, they realize that a bleed is starting as they experience the characteristic discomfort that precedes joint swelling. If treatment is not given at this early stage, stiffness and severe pain ensue and the joint becomes markedly warm, swollen, and very painful. It is held in partial flexion by surrounding muscle spasm since this ensures the maximum volume of the joint capsule; any attempt at movement greatly exacerbates the pain. After relatively few hemarthroses, joint changes become established. The synovium hypertrophies and forms a pannus over the articular cartilage; its increased vascularity and bulk predispose to further hemorrhage. Cartilage is eroded both by the hypertrophied synovium and by the leukocyte enzymes liberated from blood within the joint cavity (Fig. 9.1). During resolution of an acute hemarthrosis, iron accumulates in synovial macrophages, which become laden with hemosiderin. Subchondral hemorrhage and bleeds into the matrix further weaken the bone. Hyperemia of the joint ensues, causing bone overgrowth. Osteoporosis and disuse atrophy of the surrounding muscles develop, and joint instability and deformity progress [2].

Recurrent hemarthroses result in fibrosis within the joint capsule and surrounding muscles. This, together with the bony changes, leads to permanent loss of joint movement. Fixed flexion deformities of the knee and hip result in apparent shortening of the leg and the resultant compensatory pelvic tilt may later induce spinal symptoms. Thus hemophilic arthropathy of the lower limbs may produce skeletal deformities remote from the sites of hemarthrosis.

The incidence and sites of hemarthroses vary with age. Children bleed more often than adults, probably because of greater physical activity and joint laxity early in life. An individual joint particularly prone to recurrent hemarthroses is termed a "target" joint; it is imperative that effective therapeutic measures are initiated to prevent a rapid decline in its function [3].

The knee is the most common site of hemarthrosis (Fig. 9.2). Ridging of the condyles and posterior tibial subluxation may prevent full extension. Wasting of the quadriceps, particularly vastus medialis, becomes obvious. If knee bleeds are not treated early and promptly in childhood, by mid-adult life ankylosis of the knee in partial flexion is frequently observed. Therefore it is essential for long-term protection to minimize the development of fixed flexion deformity by prompt treatment of bleeds: rest, splinting, and later physiotherapy all help. Once fixed flexion is greater than 20°, walking becomes extremely difficult and the joint quickly flexes further. This, along with osteoarthritis of the hips and ankles, inevitably causes severe physical disability.

The elbow is the next most commonly affected joint, particularly on the non-dominant side [4, 5]. Recurrent bleeds lead to loss of both flexion and extension; supination is particularly impaired as a result of enlargement of the radial head. Typical features of ulnar neuritis may develop if the nerve is entrapped or stretched as it passes behind the medial humeral epicondyle.

Acute bleeds into the hip joint cause pain and spasm of the surrounding muscles, limiting all movement. Such bleeds must be distinguished from an iliopsoas hematoma, joint infection, or acute appendicitis. Relatively few acute recurrent hemarthroses may be sufficient to initiate chronic

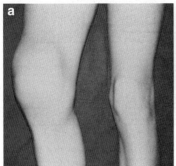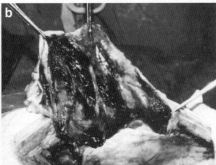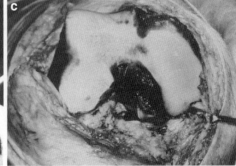

Fig. 9.1 Recurrent hemarthrosis (**a**) Clinical appearance (**b**) Synovial hypertrophy and pannus (**c**) Articular cartilage erosions

Fig. 9.2 Progressive changes of left knee hemophilic arthropathy in a young person aged 11 years (**a**), 14 years (**b**), and 17 years (**c**)

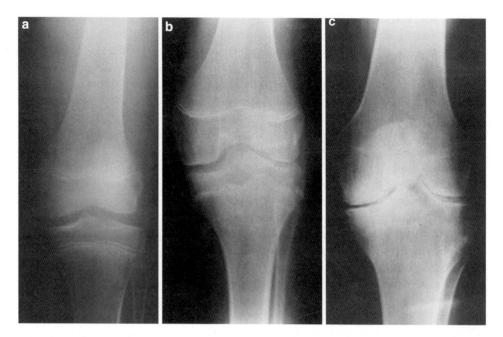

progressive degenerative arthropathy, possibly because the femoral head readily undergoes ischemic necrosis. It is therefore particularly important to treat promptly and effectively all acute bleeds into the hip joint.

As in other joints, acute hemarthrosis of the shoulder leads to loss of articular cartilage and "squaring" of the proximal humeral epiphysis [6]. Marked loss of abduction and rotation can be compensated for by scapular movement, provided that the gleno-humeral joint adopts a position of function.

Recurrent ankle bleeds are a characteristic problem in young children. These result in ankle and subtalar arthropathy. The talus has a particularly vulnerable blood supply because of its extensive articular surfaces. Regular hemarthroses lead to avascular necrosis and progressive collapse of the talar dome [7]. Early joint pathological changes

may be discernible by magnetic resonance imaging (MRI) before any changes become visible on plain radiograph (Fig. 9.3). In later life, loss of ankle joint movement is rarely a handicap, but the pain of the chronic arthropathy can be very disabling. Equinus should be controlled by splintage. An ankle arthrodesis is occasionally indicated to relieve pain.

Muscle hematomas are less common than hemarthroses but are potentially very serious and require early, vigorous treatment with factor VIII or IX concentrate. Hemorrhage dissects between the muscle planes, producing ischemia, which may lead to necrosis and subsequent fibrosis. If the muscle is contained within an inflexible, tough sheath, such as the gastrocnemius and soleus, and hemorrhage continues unabated, compartment pressure increases to the point when the arterial supply is occluded, leading to further

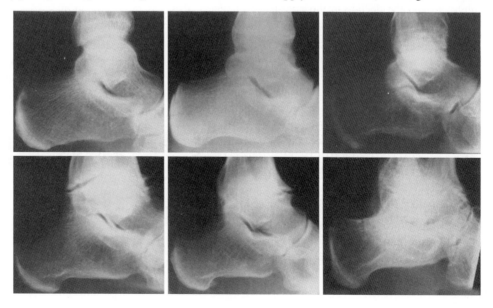

Fig. 9.3 The stages of talar body collapse in late adolescence are shown from *top left* to *bottom right*. Once the talar dome has flattened and anterior ankle impingement developed the ankle becomes irreversibly stiff

muscle ischemia and subsequent necrosis. The resultant fibrosis causes shortening and, in the case of the calf muscle, equinus deformity. In the forearm, a similar process may produce a Volkmann's ischemic contracture.

A bleed into the iliopsoas muscle may present with pain in the lower abdomen, groin, thigh, or knee. The hip is flexed in an attempt to relieve muscle tension. Compression of the femoral nerve from the enlarging hematoma as it passes under the inguinal ligament causes paresthesia over the thigh and inner calf and gross weakness of the quadriceps. The ipsilateral knee jerk may be depressed.

Pseudotumors are rarely seen nowadays in patients who are able to receive prompt treatment with a reasonable supply of factor VIII or IX concentrate. Previously, these tumors arose particularly in the thigh and pelvis as a result of inadequately treated hematomas into which chronic oozing continued unabated. The hematoma, surrounded by a fibrous capsule, gradually expands and then may erode adjacent structures, including bone, causing pathological fractures. Infection may supervene and the ensuing septicemia can be fatal. Treatment with long-term regular factor VIII/IX replacement therapy and antibiotics prevents the progression of these cysts, although later surgical excision may be indicated in some instances.

Hemorrhage may also occur at other sites. Excessive bleeding following dental extraction is common, and all such procedures must be undertaken with appropriate hemostatic cover.

Hemorrhage into the central nervous system, if not promptly treated, is often fatal. Hematuria was previously a common symptom but is now rarely seen. Bleeding is believed to arise from the renal parenchyma but can be from bladder lesions. When peptic ulcers were more common, upper gastrointestinal bleeding was a major source of morbidity and mortality. With the use of proton pump inhibitors and the decline in the prevalence of ulcers, this is now much less of a problem. However, increasing numbers of patients are developing hepatic cirrhosis as a result of hepatitis-C-induced progressive liver disease, and the prevalence of associated esophageal varices is increasing. Hemorrhage from these is liable to be catastrophic. Bleeding from hemorrhoids and fissures should be treated by surgery and prophylactic factor VIII/IX therapy.

For children with severe hemophilia optimal therapy relies upon injections of factor VIII/IX concentrate to prevent bleeds. This prophylactic treatment prevents most hemorrhages and allows the child to lead a nearly normal life, without the worry and disruption that bleeds cause. Furthermore, by preventing most hemarthroses, this strategy enables the child to grow into adulthood with the prospect of normal joints and a life unaffected by severe arthritis. As the half-life of factor VIII is only 12 h, injections need to be given on alternate days, whereas factor IX, because of its longer half-life of 18 h, need be given only twice weekly [8, 9].

If a hemophiliac patient who is not receiving regular prophylaxis suffers recurrent bleeds into a single target joint, a short period of prophylaxis for several weeks or months, along with physiotherapy, reduces the propensity to bleed. Prophylaxis breaks the vicious circle of bleeds and subsequent muscle atrophy which otherwise leads to further joint deformity and recurrent hemarthroses.

Treatment of Acute Hemorrhage

Early treatment of acute hemarthroses with intravenous factor VIII/IX concentrate delays the onset of chronic, crippling hemophilic arthropathy. The child should be taught to report when he considers a bleed has started and his parents should ensure he receives treatment quickly. With children under 3 years, parents usually find it difficult to give intravenous therapy. Once a child reaches school age it is often possible for the parents to give treatment at home (Fig. 9.4). This is the best arrangement, because there is less delay than when the child is brought to hospital for treatment.

The amount of factor VIII/IX required to be infused depends upon the size of the child and the severity of the bleed. Spontaneous hemarthroses require less treatment than those after trauma. If there is delay before treatment is given, larger doses may be necessary over a prolonged period. If a small spontaneous hemarthrosis is treated promptly, a single infusion of concentrate is sufficient to stop bleeding and allow restitution of normal joint function. For more significant bleeds, injections may need to be given twice daily for several days. Provided there is no doubt about the diagnosis of a hemarthrosis, aspiration of the joint is not advisable unless a human immunodeficiency virus (HIV)-positive hemophiliac patient has a fever, with an "atypical" joint swelling suggestive of septic arthritis.

If the hemarthrosis is other than minor, the joint should be rested. With a severe hemarthrosis, resolution of the bleed with rest can be aided by means of a lightweight polypropylene splint (Fig. 9.5). The application of icepacks helps many patients.

Minor bleeds treated early in children usually do not require rest or subsequent physiotherapy. However, if a child has a major hemarthrosis, gentle physiotherapy should be initiated once the bleeding has stopped. It may be necessary to continue factor VIII/IX therapy at a prophylactic dose for several weeks to prevent further bleeding during the phases of mobilization and more intense physiotherapy.

In patients with mild hemophilia, it may be appropriate to offer treatment with desmopressin. This vasopressin analogue increases factor VIII concentrations three- to fourfold

Fig. 9.4 Home therapy with factor VIII/IX by mother

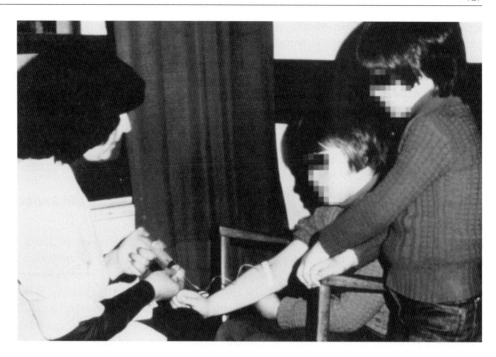

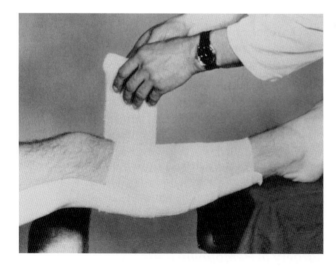

Fig. 9.5 Polypropylene splintage of the knee during a bleed

above the basal level when administered intravenously or subcutaneously. Desmopressin is, therefore, useful for patients with relatively minor bleeds or to cover surgical procedures, such as dental extraction or lymph node biopsy. The advantage of using desmopressin, as opposed to factor VIII concentrate, is that it avoids exposing the patient to exogenous factor VIII or a pooled plasma product, and

Table 9.2 Major complications of hemophilia treatment

- Anti-factor VIII antibodies
- Virus transmission: HIV, hepatitis viruses B, C, and D
- Parvovirus
- HIV infection and AIDS
- Hepatitis, cirrhosis, liver failure, and hepatocellular carcinoma

the potentially serious adverse effects described below and summarized in Table 9.2.

Complications of Therapy with Factor VIII/IX Concentrates

Transmission of Viral Infections

From the early days of treatment in the 1960s it became apparent that the use of blood products could lead to hepatitis in those with hemophilia. During the 1970s widespread infection with hepatitis B was identified and plasma products continued to be infectious, despite screening donors for hepatitis B antigen (because of the insensitivity of the assays).

In addition it was noted in the 1980s that plasma products also appeared to contain a virus that caused non-A non-B hepatitis (NANBH), later identified as hepatitis C in 1989 [10]. By 1985 it became evident that, because of the relatively high carrier rate for hepatitis C viremia among blood donors (approximately 0.5%), virtually all patients became infected who received treatment, either with several infusions of cryoprecipitate (each made from plasma derived from approximately 20 donors) or with factor VIII/IX concentrate (made from a plasma pool contributed by many thousands of donors). Although NANB was initially considered a benign form of mild liver disease, by the mid-1980s it was clear that it was progressive. Recent studies estimate that approximately 30% of those infected will develop cirrhosis over 20 years, with its attendant complications of varices, liver failure, and hepatocellular carcinoma. While 10% of patients spontaneously clear the hepatitis C virus, the majority remain viremic; treatment with pegylated interferon and ribavirin (for up to a year) cures the infection in about 50% of individuals, although those who are also infected with HIV do less well [11].

The other tragedy is the transmission of HIV by blood and blood products [12]. Although the clinical syndrome of AIDS was first described in 1981, when sensitive and specific blood tests were subsequently developed and stored serum samples were examined, it became clear that infection was probably first transmitted by clotting factor concentrates in 1977, although the clinical syndrome of AIDS was not reported in individuals with hemophilia until 1982. Many patients became infected silently during the early 1980s, and by the time specific HIV tests became available it was evident that up to 90% of patients with severe hemophilia had been infected in some countries. In the UK approximately two-thirds of those infected have sadly died. Initially there was no specific antiviral therapy and the only treatment was to prevent the development of pneumocystis carinii pneumonia with nebulized pentamidine and subsequently co-trimoxazole. With the development of a range of anti-HIV drugs the outlook after treatment with four or five drugs simultaneously (highly active antiretroviral treatment [HAART]) has greatly improved.

Initial attempts in the early 1980s to destroy the hepatitis C virus in clotting factor concentrates by heat treatment were unsuccessful because the virus was relatively heat-resistant. By the autumn of 1984 some preliminary data indicated that HIV would be sensitive to heat, resulting in viral inactivation. This led to the introduction of heat treatment of concentrates, which rendered them safe from HIV. An additional, different technique of solvent/detergent treatment during the manufacture of clotting factor concentrates inactivated lipid-coated viruses (including HIV along with hepatitis B and C viruses). Donors at increased risk of HIV and hepatitis now refrain from donating blood and all donations are screened for viral markers. In addition, those with hemophilia are offered protection by hepatitis A and B vaccines; unfortunately, at present there is no vaccine against hepatitis C or HIV. As a result of the introduction of these measures, clotting factor concentrates manufactured after the late 1980s have not transmitted lipid-coated viruses to recipients.

While plasma-derived, virally inactivated clotting factor concentrates now do not transmit HIV or hepatitis viruses, there is still the risk of transmission of non-lipid-coated viruses which are resistant to solvent/detergent and also tend to be heat-resistant. An example is the parvovirus which causes severe anemia, protracted generalized arthropathy, and hydrops fetalis if pregnant women become infected.

With the identification of factor VIII and IX genes in 1984 it became possible to develop processes to synthesize in vitro recombinant concentrates. These have been available for clinical use since the mid-1990s, proving safe from viral infection and effective for treating individuals with hemophilia. Within some countries they have completely replaced the use of plasma-derived concentrates, although at a considerable financial cost.

Anti-factor VIII Antibodies

The transfusion of factor VIII concentrates leads to the development of antibodies to factor VIII. Thirty percent of children with severe hemophilia develop these after approximately 10 injections. When this occurs, infused factor VIII is rapidly neutralized and fails to stop hemorrhage so readily. The antibody can be quantified and, if low, it is often possible to stop bleeding by transfusing larger doses of factor VIII concentrate. If the antibody titer is high, alternative therapy with other blood products (activated prothrombin complex concentrates, porcine factor VIII, or recombinant VIIa) may be effective. In many children with these anti-factor VIII antibodies it is possible to abolish the inhibitor by immune tolerance induction by giving daily injections of factor VIII for up to 3 years. Although it is difficult to ensure frequent intravenous injections in small children over a prolonged period, it is then possible to suppress the antibody. Infused factor VIII becomes hemostatically effective again so that bleeding can again be effectively treated or prevented with factor VIII concentrate. In hemophilia B, antibodies to factor IX are fortunately very rare.

Surgery in Hemophilia Patients

Provided a patient does not have an anti-factor VIII/IX inhibitor, surgery can be safely undertaken, provided that the level of the deficient clotting factor can be increased to an appropriate level with specific therapy.

Immediately before operation, concentrate is infused to bring the level to 100% and repeated infusions are given postoperatively. Alternatively, in those with severe hemophilia, the plasma factor VIII can be maintained by a continuous infusion of concentrate. Initially, it is necessary to keep the factor VIII level about 50%, but this can be gradually reduced during the second and third weeks after surgery. After major orthopaedic surgery, gentle mobilization can begin the day after operation, but treatment with factor VIII/IX should continue for approximately 2–3 weeks until the patient is fully mobile.

Synovectomy is useful in young patients with a target joint when there is significant synovitis. The aim is to reduce the frequency of bleeding, but this is often achieved at the expense of a reduction in joint movement.

If malalignment of the knee causes recurrent bleeds or painful arthritis, a proximal tibial osteotomy is occasionally indicated. This may improve gait and reduce the pain and frequency of hemarthroses. In the adult, total joint replacement or arthrodesis may be indicated when arthropathic pain, recurrent bleeds, and stiffening are severe. Arthrodesis is rarely indicated except for painful ankle arthropathy.

Hemophilia Centers

Within the UK, all individuals with hemophilia are registered at hemophilia centers which offer comprehensive care from hematologists, orthopaedic and dental surgeons, hepatologists, infectious disease specialists, specialist physiotherapists, nurses, and social workers. In addition to treating the acute and chronic hemorrhagic problems, the hemophilia team is able to offer parental support and advise nurseries, schools, and prospective employers. Genetic counseling of potential carriers is important, particularly now that molecular genetic techniques can be used to identify carriers accurately and to provide antenatal diagnosis.

Thalassemias

In the thalassemias, overactivity of the marrow as a result of ineffective erythropoiesis and hemolysis leads to widening of the medullary cavity and thinning of cortical bone. The skull radiograph shows widening of the diploic space, giving the typical "hair-on-end" appearance. Overgrowth of the maxillary and temporal bones reduces the volume of the sinuses. The thickened cranium and prominent cheek bones, depressed nasal bridge, and overgrowth of the maxillae produce a distinctive appearance. Cortical thinning may predispose to pathological fractures of long bones. The skeletal deformities come from many causes of low bone mass including endocrine disturbance and delayed puberty [13].

Management consists of regular red cell transfusions to ensure that the hemoglobin concentration remains relatively normal. This reduces erythropoietic activity and prevents the characteristic skeletal deformities. Furthermore, because these children then have nearly normal hemoglobin values, their growth approaches that of their peers, in marked contrast to the stunted appearance seen in those only occasionally transfused. To reduce the risk of iron overload these patients require regular iron chelation therapy with desferrioxamine.

Hemoglobinopathies

In some sub-Saharan African countries, up to 25% of the population carry the sickle cell gene. From unions of these individuals, some children, about 1% of the indigenous paediatric population, are born with sickle cell disease (HbSS). HbSS is also common in Central India. Increasing migration and ease of travel have raised the incidence of hemoglobinopathies in other countries. Affected children develop chronic hemolytic anemia with hemoglobin concentrations of 5 g/dl in their "normal" state. They may suffer episodes of acute hemolysis: sickle cell crises in which they become jaundiced and the hemoglobin concentration decreases further. In West Africa, hemoglobin C disease (HbSC) and thalassemia complicate the situation, but the effects are generally milder than in the homozygous HbSS state. Sickling tests may be positive in both homozygous and heterozygous individuals, but the homozygous state can be distinguished by hemoglobin electrophoresis. Furthermore, heterozygous children do not suffer the clinical manifestations of HbSS.

Children with sickle cell disease (SCD) are usually thin and small for their age (Fig 9.6). In infancy and early childhood, they may first present to an orthopaedic surgeon with sickle cell dactylitis—the hand–foot syndrome [14]: during a sickling crisis or respiratory infection the child develops a high fever and tender swelling of the hands and feet. The characteristic radiological changes of cortical thinning, periosteal new bone formation, and a moth-eaten bone appearance only appear after 10 days or so. Treatment should be directed to the concomitant crisis or infection plus elevation, splintage, and analgesia for affected limbs.

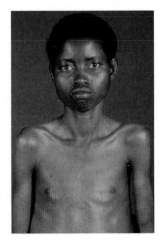

Fig. 9.6 Patient with sickle cell disease showing frontal bossing of the skull

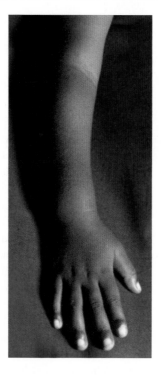

Fig. 9.7 The short stubby fingers of a patient with sickle cell disease. There is also osteomyelitis of the radius

This syndrome may explain why many children with SCD have short stubby fingers (Fig. 9.7). The syndrome may be mistaken for osteomyelitis, which may indeed coexist.

Clinical anemia and slight jaundice are usually obvious and increase during crises. The abdomen is typically protuberant with hepatosplenomegaly.

Children with SCD are prone to bacterial infections, the clinical appearance being very similar to those with advanced HIV infection. They are prone to bone and joint infections and commonly have chronic otitis media. Acute, subacute, and chronic osteomyelitis; septic arthritis; aseptic bone infarction; and Perthes' disease are the usual presentations to the orthopaedic surgeon and it may be difficult to distinguish between them. During a sickling (hemolytic) crisis, the child will have fever, tachypnea, bone pains and tenderness, joint pains, and possible abdominal pain and peritonism. An attack of malaria gives a similar picture and may, indeed, precipitate a crisis. Bone pain and tenderness or joint pain and effusion may be either aseptic as a result of infarction or septic from septicemia. If possible, blood samples or joint or bone aspirates should be obtained for culture and sensitivity before antibiotic treatment is commenced. Gram staining may give a rapid indication of the presence and type of bacteria.

If a joint is found to contain pus, arthrotomy and copious lavage are indicated. Similarly, collections of sub-periosteal pus and soft tissue abscesses should be drained. Every precaution should be taken to ensure that anesthesia will be safe, and if this is not assured repeated aspirations may have to suffice.

Hypoxia and acidosis cause the abnormal hemoglobin in SCD to form liquid crystals that distort the erythrocytes, rendering them fragile and encouraging clumping. Hemolysis, blockage of small vessels, and infarction are the result. Pre-operative determination of hemoglobin concentration and the further investigation of anemic patients are essential to avoid the disasters of rapid circulatory collapse and death, which may occur within a few hours of surgery. The presence of malarial parasites in a blood film of a supposedly well child similarly contraindicates surgery until treated.

Before surgery, the hemoglobin concentration should be increased to as near 8 g/dl as possible. In an emergency, or immediately before major surgery, exchange transfusion or the transfusion of packed red cells should be considered. Pre-operative dehydration should be prevented by giving intravenous fluids, and hypoxia must be avoided during the induction and maintenance of anesthesia.

The use of tourniquets in patients with SCD remains controversial. A bloodless field may shorten an operation, make it safer, and minimize blood loss; these are important considerations, especially if safe blood is not readily available for transfusion. Conversely, and theoretically, any blood that remains in a limb distal to a tourniquet will sickle and the hypoxia and acidosis present in a limb by the time of tourniquet deflation could have deleterious effects. We have carefully monitored the systemic pO_2 by pulse oximetry and have not found any decrease in value after tourniquet release in such patients. If the limb is thoroughly exsanguinated, using an Esmarch bandage before tourniquet inflation, very little blood remains in the vessels. The benefits afforded by the use of a tourniquet should be balanced against the dangers and a decision made for each operation.

After surgery, oxygen should be given by mask for 24 h and the arterial pO_2 monitored by pulse oximetry. Drugs that reduce respiratory drive (such as narcotic analgesics) should be given with great caution or avoided. Aspirin should not be used. Regional analgesia should be employed, if practicable. Attention should be paid to the bandaging and elevation of an operated limb to prevent venous stasis and minimize swelling.

Osteomyelitis in children with SCD tends to have a subacute onset and is often polyostotic. In contrast to the pattern in other children (see Chapter 10), it affects the upper limbs (Fig. 9.7) almost as commonly as the legs and both the diaphyses (Fig. 9.8) and the metaphyses. Osteomyelitis in more unusual sites, such as skull (Fig. 9.9) and pelvis, are relatively common. The usual infecting organisms are *Staphylococcus aureus* and *Salmonella* species; antimicrobial treatment that will cover both possibilities should be used pending culture results. Antibiotics should be given intravenously in high dosage and the limb immobilized and elevated while the child is further investigated or prepared for surgery. In general, bone infection is more diffuse and

Fig. 9.8 Sickle cell osteomyelitis. Note that most of the swelling is diaphyseal

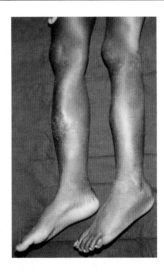

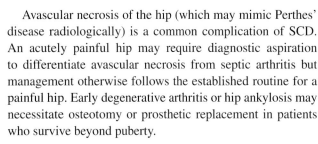

Avascular necrosis of the hip (which may mimic Perthes' disease radiologically) is a common complication of SCD. An acutely painful hip may require diagnostic aspiration to differentiate avascular necrosis from septic arthritis but management otherwise follows the established routine for a painful hip. Early degenerative arthritis or hip ankylosis may necessitate osteotomy or prosthetic replacement in patients who survive beyond puberty.

Acquired Immune Deficiency Syndrome

Children can be infected by HIV by maternal transmission, by infusion of infected blood, or by sexual assault. With the current rigorous screening of blood donors, HIV antibody testing of each donation, and the safe manufacture of factor VIII/IX concentrates, the risk of HIV transmission by transfusion is remote. However, the infection is commonly transmitted heterosexually, and women so infected are liable to infect their children with HIV by prenatal or neonatal transmission of the virus. Such women are often unaware of their infection and therefore the child is not perceived as being at risk. Where the mother's status is known, antenatal treatment with antiretroviral therapy reduces transmission rates considerably.

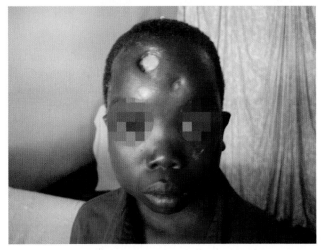

Fig. 9.9 Patient with sickle cell disease and chronic osteomyelitis of skull

surgery to remove large sequestra is less often needed than in the *staphylococcal* osteomyelitis commonly seen in children without SCD. Conversely, involucrum formation is often poor (Fig. 9.10) and the weakened bone needs protection by splinting. Non-unions need to be stabilized and bone grafted. During the periods of often prolonged bed rest, it is essential to keep painful joints from stiffening in flexion by the use of traction or splintage.

HIV primarily infects CD4 lymphocytes (T-helper cells) and leads, over time, to a steady decline in their numbers. The CD4 cells play a pivotal role in the control of the immune system and their loss inevitably impairs immune mechanisms. After infection of an individual cell by the RNA virus, a DNA copy is made by the enzyme reverse transcriptase; this copy is then incorporated as a provirus into the nuclear DNA, where it is immortalized. If the cell undergoes mitosis, each daughter cell will contain HIV in its nucleus. Expression of the proviral DNA leads to the assembly of many virus particles, which then infect other cells. In addition to T cells, glial cells within the central nervous system and epithelial cells within the gut can also become infected. Infected monocytes and macrophages harbor the virus in so-called sanctuary sites, where it evades some antiviral drugs.

Fig. 9.10 (a) Patient with sickle cell disease and chronic osteomyelitis of the right femur. The left leg had previously been amputated for overwhelming infection. (b) Radiograph of the right femur of the same patient. Incomplete involucrum 9 months after onset of sepsis

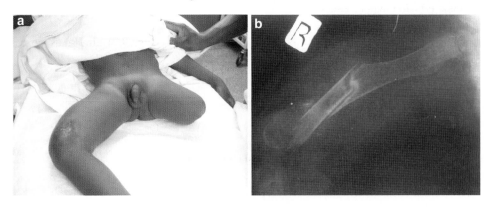

The clinical manifestations of HIV depend upon the route of infection[15]. Children infected at or before birth initially appear healthy but later fail to gain weight and thrive. Recurrent bacterial infection is a prominent feature initially but later there are classical opportunistic infections, such as pneumocystis pneumonia. The common opportunistic infections vary according to the particular organisms most prevalent in the environment. Whereas in Western Europe and in the USA, *Pneumocystis jiroveci* is the most common infective agent; in sub-Saharan Africa, tuberculosis and cryptococcal infection are much more common. As the immune system involutes, high-grade non-Hodgkin lymphomas can occur. The lymphomas appear, not infrequently, at extranodal sites—for example, the central nervous system. Kaposi's sarcoma, caused by human herpes virus 8 (HHV8), is not seen in those infected by transfusion because the virus is sexually transmitted. The classification of HIV disease is different in children than adults, and is summarized in Table 9.3. Various classifications are necessary because the clinical manifestations are so diverse.

Management of HIV is less well defined for infected children than for adults. Any child with HIV infection, or whose mother is known to have HIV infection, should be regularly reviewed. Many infants at birth have passively acquired maternal anti-HIV antibody and therefore all children of infected mothers should be investigated. HIV infection can be established by culturing the virus, identifying it by polymerize chain reaction (PCR), or by detecting the presence of antibody after the child has reached 18 months of age.

Any existing infections should be treated promptly, and there is evidence from the African experience that co-trimoxazole prophylaxis will improve survival in the absence of available antiretroviral therapy. However, the mainstay of managing symptomatic children with HIV is the use of highly active antiretroviral therapy. Prompt initiation of HIV therapy improves the child's immune system and helps to prevent neurodevelopmental problems.

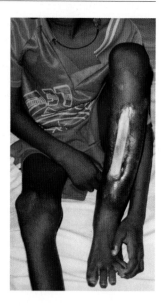

Fig. 9.11 Florid osteomyelitis of the tibia in an HIV +ve child. The breakdown of tissue covering the sequestrated tibia had been spontaneous

The common presentations to the orthopaedic surgeon are of children with septic arthritis, osteomyelitis, or pyomyositis or with paraparesis from spinal tuberculosis or transverse myelitis. Although osteomyelitis may start subacutely, it may not respond to treatment. Florid presentations also occur (Fig. 9.11). That the child is HIV positive may be known or suspected from the history of slow development and recurrent infections, from diffuse symmetrical lymphadenopathy, and from the appearance of the skin. Children with HIV infection require the same spectrum of management and surgical procedures as uninfected children, but with the addition of antiviral therapy. Some HIV-infected individuals are thrombocytopenic. This must be corrected by either platelet infusion or intravenous immunoglobulin before surgery. The best treatment for such thrombocytopenia, however, is antiretroviral therapy.

The prospects for HIV-infected children are progressively improving as greater experience is gained in the management of the clinical difficulties experienced. Antiviral drugs and the prompt treatment of infections, fortunately, seem to improve the prognosis for this unfortunate group of children. The British HIV Association web site offers up-to-date advice on management (www.bhiva.org.uk).

Table 9.3 Classification of HIV disease in children

P-0	Indeterminate infection
P-1	Asymptomatic infection
P-2	Symptomatic infection
	A: Non-specific findings
	B: Progressive neurological disease
	C: Lymphoid interstitial pneumonitis
	D: Secondary infectious diseases (e.g., pneumocystis carinii pneumonia)
	Toxoplasmosis
	Recurrent bacterial infections
	E: Cancers
	Lymphomas
	Kaposi's sarcoma

References

1. Thomas AE. The bleeding child; is it NAI? Arch Dis Child 2004; 89(12):1163–67.
2. Hoots WK. Pathogenesis of hemophilic arthropathy. Semin Hematol 2006; 43(1 Suppl 1):S18–S22.
3. Mulder K, Llinas A. The target joint. Haemophilia 2004; 10 Suppl 4:152–56.
4. Hogh J, Ludlam CA, Macnicol MF. Hemophilic arthropathy of the upper limb. Clin Orthop Relat Res 1987; 218:225–31.

5. Utukuri MM, Goddard NJ. Haemophilic arthropathy of the elbow. Haemophilia 2005; 11(6):565–70.

6. Cahlon O, Klepps S, Cleeman E, et al. A retrospective radiographic review of hemophilic shoulder arthropathy. Clin Orthop Relat Res 2004; 423:106–11.

7. Macnicol MF, Ludlam CA. Does avascular necrosis cause collapse of the dome of the talus in severe haemophilia? Haemophilia 1999; 5(2):139–42.

8. Berntorp E, Astermark J, Bjorkman S, et al. Consensus perspectives on prophylactic therapy for haemophilia: summary statement. Haemophilia 2003; 9 Suppl 1:1–4.

9. Hay CR. Prophylaxis in adults with haemophilia. Haemophilia 2007; 13 Suppl 2:10–5.

10. Kessler CM. Update on liver disease in hemophilia patients. Semin Hematol 2006; 43(1 Suppl 1):S13-7.

11. Posthouwer D, Mauser-Bunschoten EP, Fischer K, Makris M. Treatment of chronic hepatitis C in patients with haemophilia: a review of the literature. Haemophilia 2006; 12(5):473–8.

12. Goedert JJ, Brown DL, Hoots K, Sherman KE. Human immunodeficiency and hepatitis virus infections and their associated conditions and treatments among people with haemophilia. Haemophilia 2004; 10 Suppl 4:205–10.

13. Singer ST, Vichinsky EP. Bone disease in beta-thalassaemia. Lancet 1999; 354(9182):881–2.

14. Babhulkar SS, Pande K, Babhulkar S. The hand-foot syndrome in sickle-cell haemoglobinopathy. J Bone Joint Surg Br 1995; 77(2):310–2.

15. Lindegren ML, Steinberg S, Byers RH Jr. Epidemiology of HIV/AIDS in children. Pediatr Clin North Am 2000; 47(1): 1–20, v.

Chapter 10

Infections of Bones and Joints

Klaus Parsch and Sydney Nade

Infection must be considered as a struggle between two organisms ... the parasite and its host. This brings about adaptations on both sides.

(Elie Metschnikoff, 1891)

Etiology and Biological Cause

In order to produce disease organisms must be able to invade host tissues, multiply, spread and produce toxic substances. The ability to produce disease is known as *pathogenicity* and the comparative pathogenicity of different organisms is expressed as *virulence*. Very small numbers of virulent organisms are able to produce disease, whereas larger numbers of less virulent organisms are required. The *invasiveness* of microorganisms is not clearly related to their toxic properties, but enzymes produced by them allow both spread by tissue dissolution and protection from host phagocytes.

Portals of Entry

There are several ways in which organisms gain access to bones and joints:

- Hematogenous spread from the primary site of colonization (skin, mouth, and gut) if the barriers to spread have been breached. In children this is the most common form.
- Direct access by puncture of the skin and deeper tissues after injury.
- Direct access at the time of elective surgery or after surgery for open injury.
- Local spread from infected adjacent tissues (for example, from a subcutaneous abscess into the adjacent bone or joint).

The Pathology of Bone Infection

In acute hematogenous osteomyelitis in infants and children, bacteria lodge adjacent to the physis, probably in relation to terminal metaphyseal vessels. These vessels are open-ended as they tunnel between the columns of dividing and decaying physeal cartilage cells. It is likely that chondrotropic pathogenic bacteria adhere to cartilage cells at the junction between physis and metaphysis (Fig. 10.1) [1]. They divide and stimulate an acute inflammation that results in vascular engorgement, edema, polymorphonuclear cellular responses, and tissue death secondary to ischemia from either venous or arterial obstruction. The growing bacterial colonies provoke acute suppuration and liquefactive necrosis of medullary tissues. The trabecula of cancellous bone become fragmented, lose their vascular relationship, and die. They lie in the pus

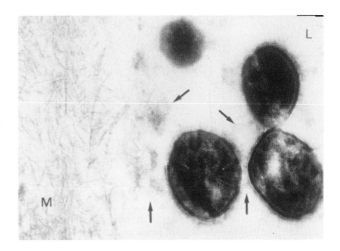

Fig. 10.1 An electron micrograph of *S. aureus* bacteria adhering to physeal cartilage at the metaphyseal junction. Note the strands of adhesive glycocalyx joining bacterial capsule to the cartilage matrix

K. Parsch (✉)
Orthopaedic Department, Pediatric Centre Olgahospital, Stuttgart, Germany

M. Benson et al. (eds.), *Children's Orthopaedics and Fractures*,
DOI 10.1007/978-1-84882-611-3_10, © Springer-Verlag London Limited 2010

Fig. 10.2 Photomicrograph of an abscess forming in physeal cartilage 1 day after inoculation of *S. aureus* into a vein. This is the earliest example of formation of an abscess in hematogenous osteomyelitis

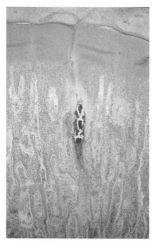

as small *sequestra* (Fig. 10.2). Why hematogenous infections select bone, and even certain bones more than others, remains an enigma.

The inflammatory process extends from the marrow and contained trabecular bone to the adjacent cortex. The inflammatory process spreads within the cortex, probably following the natural pathways of Haversian and Volkmann canals (Fig. 10.3). Both osteoclastic and non-osteoclastic bone resorption occurs. Periosteal tissues may be lifted, thereby disrupting the periosteal blood supply entering the cortex. Further spread through the periosteum and soft tissues may lead to spontaneous discharge of pus to the exterior. The lifting of periosteum from bone ruptures the intra- to extra-medullary vascular connections, thereby increasing the volume of bone made ischemic. The displaced periosteum is stimulated to produce bone which may be seen, on radiographic examination, initially (about 7–10 days after the onset of infection), as fine layers, and later perhaps as a thick *involucrum*.

In the absence of treatment, some of the physeal and metaphyseal bone dies and this dead bone, seeded as it is with bacteria, may act as a permanent reservoir for recurrent infection. The spontaneous or surgical drainage of pus is followed by repair, in favorable cases through the apposition of new bone. The cortex may become thickened by the newly formed bone of the repair process. Where the blood supply is inadequate, necrotic bone persists, as osteoclastic resorption can only take place under conditions of viability. The features found on imaging studies are easily explained if the pathology is understood.

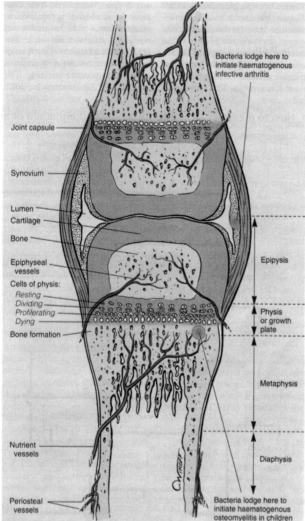

Fig. 10.3 Diagram to show the anatomy of bone and joint in a child. The terms used to describe the parts of the bone are shown. Note the relationship of the site of initiation of a metaphyseal abscess to the blood supply. Note also that the most likely site of sequestration of bacteria causing septic arthritis is within synovial capillaries, causing an abscess. Bacteria that have escaped from the synovial capillaries can then reach the joint cavity

Why Is the Course Different in Infants?

The basic process in the infant is similar to that in the child. However because of the presence of transphyseal vessels that become obliterated in the first year of life, the infection may spread across the physis and epiphysis into the joint (Fig. 10.4). Whereas in childhood infection does not usually involve the germinal cells of the physis and hence does not interfere directly with growth, in infants these cells may be inhibited or die.

The Pathology of Subacute and Chronic Osteomyelitis

In subacute and chronic osteomyelitis the balance between microbe and host is such that the destructive and repair processes do not take place as rapidly as in acute infection.

Fig. 10.4 Spread of bacteria initially deposited at the growing tip of a metaphyseal vessel present in the first year of life through a transphyseal vessel to the epiphysis, producing an abscess in the epiphysis. More commonly, the spread is in the opposite direction entering other metaphyseal vessels to produce an abscess

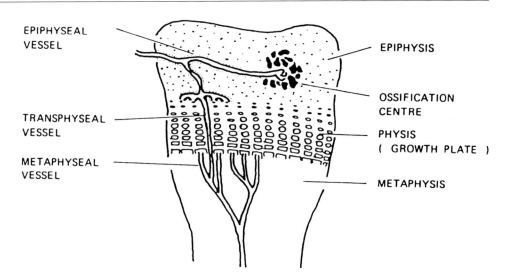

The result is a *bone abscess*, most often in the metaphysis of a long bone. The proximal tibia, distal femur, proximal and distal humerus, or distal radius are most often affected. The calcaneum and metatarsals are also common locations.

The clinical appearance is usually of a mild, sometimes intermittent, limb pain, present for days or weeks, with loss of function and local tenderness, but minor or no systemic signs.

The Pathology of Septic Arthritis

Bacteria may enter a joint from synovial micro-abscesses that communicate directly with the joint lumen Fig. 10.3. An intra-articular infective dose of bacteria produces edema, hyperemia, and acute inflammation of the synovium. Polymorphonuclear neutrophils can be seen within synovial vessels, outside those vessels in the synovium, and within the joint cavity. Synovial fluid dynamics are altered, leading to an effusion.

Bacterial infection may destroy synovial joints because of erosion of articular cartilage. It is usually irreversible and progressive. Articular cartilage has few blood vessels, and it is improbable that hematogenous spread of bacteria leads to their deposition in subchondral bone. Metaphyseal osteomyelitis can spread directly to the epiphysis through the growth plate via transphyseal vessels and may penetrate through articular cartilage into the joint lumen. Usually, however, bacteria reach the joint through synovial capillaries. In infants, in particular, it is a common finding that septic arthritis is present several days before osteomyelitis

of the metaphysis and the epiphysis becomes apparent (Fig. 10.5).

If treatment is commenced early and is successful, resolution of the inflammatory process may take place. When the disease process is not controlled, there may be complete loss of articular cartilage, leading eventually to ankylosis of the joint. Although modern antimicrobial agents are efficient they do not remove the pus sufficiently, or do not do so rapidly enough, to avoid permanent damage to the cartilage. The majority of paediatric orthopaedic surgeons agree that it is important to remove purulent fluid from a joint as soon as its presence is suspected: "ubi pus, ibi evacua" (lat.: Where there is pus, evacuate!).

In infants in particular, but sometimes also in children, intra-capsular inflammation, with synovial proliferation and an exudate of fluid, may distend the joint capsule, causing laxity, subluxation, or dislocation (Fig. 10.6). Pus contained in the joint, by virtue of the thick anatomical barriers around it, increases intra-articular pressure and favors the destruction of articular cartilage. Later, when cartilage has been destroyed, there may be focal or patchy bone loss in the subchondral region. Osteopenia resulting from disuse and hyperemia appears quickly.

As an alternative to blood-borne spread, bacteria may also gain entry by direct, penetrating injury, by diagnostic or therapeutic puncture, as a complication of venipuncture, or by arthrotomy. The virulence of the infecting organism and the resistance of the host determine whether suppuration ensues. Infancy, trauma, or prior arthropathy appears to reduce the resistance to spread of infection. In any acute and painful joint disease without preceding trauma infection must be suspected.

Fig. 10.5 Spread of pus from a metaphyseal focus into (**a**) the joint, (**b**) the subperiosteal tissue, and (**c**) the medullary canal

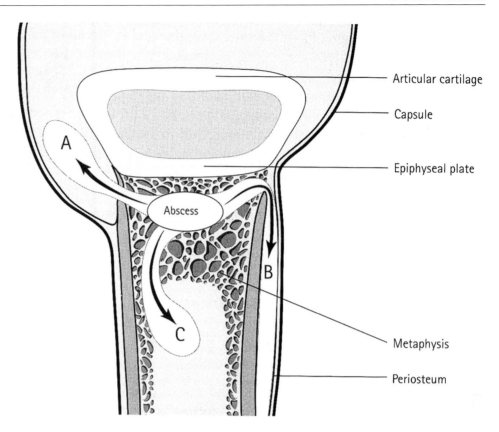

Articular cartilage

Capsule

Epiphyseal plate

Abscess

Metaphysis

Periosteum

How to Determine Which Bacteria Are the Cause?

Blood

When blood is cultured in suspected bacteremia, the number of viable organisms that may be circulating is usually small. A large volume of blood is cultured under conditions that favor the growth of pathogens. The blood sampled should not clot, because the bacteria, if present, may colonize within the clot and not grow in the culture medium. If a patient has febrile rigors, samples should be taken at those times, thus increasing the yield of bacteria.

Aspirate

In suspected bacterial infection, the key to appropriate treatment is the identification of the causative organism. The sample for culture should be taken before antibiotic drugs are given. The manner in which specimens are obtained and the speed with which they are taken to the laboratory may affect the success of culture. Laboratory tests include observation of the specimen, examination of the stained films (with Gram's stain), and culture on laboratory media. Any

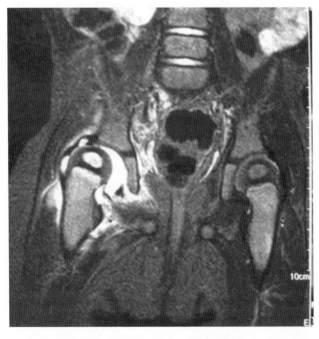

Fig. 10.6 MRI of a boy of 13 months with septic arthritis of his right hip and subluxation of the femoral head. Intra-articular pressure from *S. aureus* infection had pushed the femoral head out of the joint

bacterium isolated from a body fluid that is normally sterile should be regarded as a potential pathogen. In acute osteomyelitis an organism can be identified in about 60% of cases. A higher yield may be found if aspirates are also inoculated into blood culture media. A single needle puncture can be inserted into a bone, a joint, or a subperiosteal fluid collection.

Pus

Although pus is usually sampled with a swab it is more satisfactory, whenever possible, to take a liquid sample with a syringe from an anechoic collection next to bone, demonstrated by ultrasound. Swabs should be placed in Stuart's transport medium for the preservation of anaerobes and microbes sensitive to drying. Note the color, consistency, and odor of the pus. Gram staining of pus smears is undertaken in all cases and, if tuberculosis is considered a possibility, another smear should be stained by the Ziehl–Neelsen method. The use of DNA polymerase chain reaction (PCR) may reveal positive findings in cases of culture-negative samples [2].

Synovial Fluid

If infection is suspected, the following investigations of synovial fluid are of value:

1. Description of fluid appearance: the color and nature of blood staining (if any) should be noted.
2. Smears on slides and stains for bacteria: smears can be made of the joint aspirate directly or after centrifugation. After air-drying, the smear is subjected to Gram staining and direct microscopic examination made for bacteria.
3. Culture followed by antibiotic sensitivity tests: as soon as the arthrocentesis has been performed, the fluid should be cultured, or a centrifuged deposit used to increase the yield. Inoculation in blood culture media will help when *Kingella kingae* is suspected. Antibiotic sensitivity tests (antibiograms) are essential.

Tissue

Culture of tissues removed at surgery may sometimes reveal pathogens that have escaped isolation.

Which Are the Pathogens That Cause Osteomyelitis and Septic Arthritis?

Since the introduction of antibiotics, positive identification of a causative bacterium has become less frequent. The yield of microorganisms from patients with a clinical diagnosis of bone or joint infection is usually between 50 and 75%.

Staphylococci

These Gram-positive cocci are responsible for the majority of acute osteomyelitis, septic arthritis, and post-traumatic osteomyelitis. *Staphylococcus aureus* includes many potentially pathogenic strains, and antibiotic resistance is common in isolates from hospital.

Staphylococcus epidermidis is a common commensal of skin and an opportunistic pathogen cultured occasionally in children with arthritis or osteomyelitis.

Methicillin-Resistant S. aureus (MRSA)

For the last few years infections caused by *methicillin-resistant S. aureus* (MSRA) in patients with established risk factors have been reported increasingly in the United States [3]. While *methicillin-sensitive S. aureus* (MSSA) did not change in incidence, MRSA rose from 4 to 40% in the years 2000–2004. Fulminant *methicillin*-sensitive *S. aureus* infection in healthy adolescents has been observed in young populations globally, highlighting the Panton–Valentine leukocidin syndrome (PVL syndrome) [4].

Streptococci

Streptococci are Gram-positive cocci, quite frequently cultured in cases of septic arthritis in the neonate and older child, but also in osteomyelitis. ß[beta]-Hemolytic *streptococci* account for most human infections. *Streptococcus pyogenes* is sensitive to penicillin and cephalosporins, to which it does not develop resistance. *Streptococcus pneumoniae* infrequently causes septic arthritis; when it does, the patient usually has an underlying disease. *S. agalactiae* has assumed importance as a "nursery pathogen."

Haemophilus Influenzae

In communities where *Haemophilus influenzae* vaccination is routine in infancy it is rarely seen as a pathogen [5].

Escherichia coli

Escherichia coli are Gram-negative and normally found in the gut. They are often cultured in decubitus ulcers. Initially they are sensitive to ampicillin, cephalosporins, and gentamicin but develop resistance quite rapidly.

Pseudomonas aeruginosa

It is common in penetrating injuries, especially of the foot.

Kingella kingae

This microorganism has emerged from obscurity in recent years to become known as an important cause of invasive infections like septic arthritis and osteomyelitis [6]. *Kingella kingae* is a part of the bacterial flora of the pharynx. To identify this germ one should insist that fluid aspirates are inoculated into blood culture media, and not simply plated out on blood agar [7, 8]. These bacteria are highly sensitive to β[beta]-lactam antibiotics and infection resolves quickly with antibiotic treatment. If *K. kingae* is identified surgical intervention will rarely be indicated.

Mycobacteria

Mycobacteria, when infecting man or animals, usually form tubercles. They require special methods for staining, the most common being the acid-fast stain of Ziehl–Neelsen. They are strict aerobes that grow slowly (see Chapter 11).

Mycobacterium bovis infection from bacille Calmette–Guérin (BCG) vaccination is occasionally observed. In some countries, vaccination against tuberculosis using BCG vaccine is used for children in the first weeks of life, which increases the risk of osteomyelitis or septic arthritis.

Others

Unusual or uncommon bacteria may be isolated from some patients, particularly if their natural immunity is compromised or if they are or have been recreational drug abusers.

In all cases of suspected bone and joint infection make every effort to identify the causative microorganisms.

How to Locate the Site of Infection?

Clinical Appearance

The site of pain and the identification of tenderness are the usual clues to the focus of infection. Location of the site of infection can be helped greatly by ultrasonography, radiology, radioisotope imaging and, increasingly, by magnetic resonance imaging (MRI). Confirmation that changes seen on the images obtained are due to infection is achieved by the identification of organisms.

Ultrasound Imaging

Ultrasonography is currently the main imaging method for the detection of septic arthritis and osteomyelitis but cannot detect cavities within bone. In the assessment of soft tissue swelling, however, fluid-filled cysts or abscesses are readily detectable and their size measured accurately by this method, which is free from the hazards of ionizing radiation. Extra-osseous abscesses in osteomyelitis can be identified by ultrasound [9].

In suspected *septic arthritis* in infants a thickened synovium and intra-articular effusion are seen within hours of onset. False-negative ultrasound scans have been reported [10], although not in our experience.

Effusions in the hip, knee, shoulder, or any other joint are visualized by ultrasound. Septic arthritis of the knee or ankle joints is more superficial and obvious from the clinical appearance. There are special features of infantile joint infection, which will be described later.

Ultrasound is the diagnostic tool of choice for the detection of septic arthritis in any joint.

Conventional Radiography

Both the bones and the soft tissues must be examined. In acute hematogenous osteomyelitis the earliest stages of infection produce no radiological signs. Small intramedullary abscesses cannot be detected. Once there is a spread of pus or edema outside the bone, swelling in the soft tissues may be seen.

The changes that occur in bones are those of *destruction*, or failure of formation of metaphyseal bone, and *repair*, which may be seen easily as a result of periosteal osteogenic activity or, less easily, within the medulla.

In typical *long bone osteomyelitis*, the earliest radiographic change is a faint hazy shadow around the shaft of the bone, caused by pus and edema. The first reliable radiographic sign consists of several small lytic areas and a periosteal reaction, 10–14 days after onset of symptoms. The periosteal new bone is a thin linear shadow, parallel to the cortex but separated from it by a translucent zone 2–10 mm wide. If the infection is not controlled, the lytic lesions enlarge and the periosteal response extends to produce an onion skin appearance, with bone deposits separated by narrow translucent zones. As healing takes place, the living bone regains its normal density (Fig. 10.7).

The radiological features of *septic arthritis* also parallel the pathological changes. Edema and hypertrophy of the synovium with effusion can be seen as a swollen joint, limited by capsular attachments. Disuse osteopenia adjacent to the infected joint appears quickly. Bone destruction, initially in the form of erosion next to the cartilaginous articular margin, can be detected long before similar changes in the cartilage are evident radiographically. The evidence of cartilage loss is confirmed by a "loss of joint space" and subchondral bone erosions may be seen. Capsular distension by fluid results in eventual subluxation or dislocation of an infected joint.

Infants pose a special problem in the radiological location of joint infection, because their epiphyses are either radiolucent or partially ossified. Furthermore, in childhood epiphyseal ossification may be irregular while developing normally.

Computed Tomography (CT)

This technique clarifies bone destruction and bone production and the extent of soft tissue swelling or loss. There seems little indication for CT in acute osteomyelitis, but it is of some value in spinal infections and soft tissue sepsis, if MRI is not available [11].

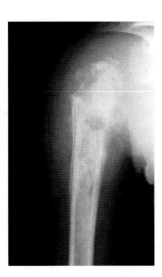

Fig. 10.7 Radiograph of the right proximal humerus of a 4-year-old girl with *S. aureus* osteomyelitis. Lytic zones from bone resorption of the proximal humerus and partial regeneration

Radioisotope Imaging

Radioisotopes can be attached to non-radioactive molecules of which the metabolism is understood and act as markers of the sites in the body to which they are distributed. The radiation source technetium-99m (99mTc) is usually linked to a phosphorus compound: The commonly used radiopharmaceutical is 99mTc-methylene diphosphonate (99mTc-MDP) (Fig. 10.8). In most patients with osteomyelitis, bone scans show evidence of bone formation within 48–72 h of the onset of clinical symptoms and, taken together with the clinical status, may be useful, particularly in multifocal disease and in the detection and localization of infections by unusual organisms or at unusual sites.

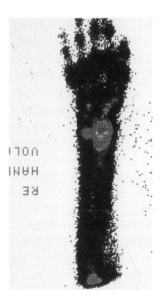

Fig. 10.8 Technetium-99m MDP bone scan of the right distal radius of a boy aged 13 years with multifocal osteomyelitis showing signs of acute osteomyelitis

Magnetic Resonance Imaging

The absence of ionizing radiation makes this an attractive tool for sequential imaging. Subtle changes of soft tissue and bone are detectable within 24 h of infection. Osteomyelitis shows decreased signal intensity in T1-weighted images and an increased signal intensity in T2-weighted images. Short time inversion recovery (STIR) sequences allow visualization of changes in the bone marrow. The contrast medium gadolinium is used to help in the differentiation of tissue changes and to distinguish tumor from infection. MRI enables exact anatomical localization at the adjacent growth plates and joints. If available, MRI images using STIR sequences are best for identifying acute hematogenous osteomyelitis in the early phase. MRI will also identify a medullary abscess as well as the perforation of pus into the subperiosteal space (Fig. 10.9) [11, 12].

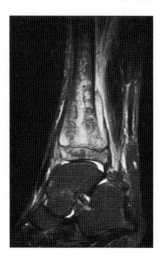

Fig. 10.9 MRI of 12-year-old girl with acute osteomyelitis of the distal tibia showing an abscess in the distal tibial medullary canal, subperiosteal abscesses, and effusion of the ankle joint

made CRP concentrations very useful in the differential diagnosis of suspected bone and joint infection [16]. Values less than 10 mg/L are regarded as insignificant whereas bacterial infections are a common, but not unique, cause of concentrations greater than 100 mg/L, possibly increasing in acute osteomyelitis to values greater then 200 mg/L.

White Cell Count

An increased white blood cell count in peripheral blood in excess of 12,000 cells/mm^3 may help to confirm the diagnosis of infection but has limitations as a measure of disease activity. The white blood cell count may be normal in up to 80% of cases and is not a reliable indicator [16]. A persistent increase should raise concern, but the rate of decline of a leukocytosis to normal has a very variable course.

Antibody Tests

Antibody tests are based on assays of antibodies produced by the host in response to exposure to bacterial antigens. They are not, in themselves, indicators of infection. If an increasing titer can be shown after exposure to potential infection that is presumptive evidence of infection. In staphylococcal infection, serological studies have not proved useful.

MRI should not be necessary in most cases of acute osteomyelitis or septic arthritis. Its great importance lies in the localization of special sites of osteomyelitis such as the spine [13] (spondylitis) or the pelvis, including acute infection of the sacroiliac joint [14]. In these atypical locations MRI is superior to radioisotope scans that would have been performed in the past. Whole body MRI, if available, is used in the localization and monitoring of treatment in chronic recurrent multifocal osteomyelitis (see below). MRI and radioisotope scans have the significant disadvantage of requiring a child to remain calm for up to an hour. Full anesthesia rather than sedation is necessary in the majority of children with painful bone and joint infection.

Several months may elapse before MRI images demonstrate that the tissues have returned to normal after infection.

DNA-Based Assays, PCR

Species-specific and ubiquitous DNA-based assays (polymerase chain reaction, PCR) allow identification of microorganisms in many specimens that do not yield growth on conventional microbiological investigations [2, 17, 18].

Which Laboratory Tests Are Useful?

Sedimentation Rate

An increase in the erythrocyte sedimentation rate (ESR) is the traditional indicator of infection. The ESR is not specific but is useful in the differentiation between trauma and transient synovitis [15]. In osteomyelitis it usually reaches quite high levels.

C-Reactive Protein

C-reactive protein (CRP) has been recognized for many years as a marker of the acute-phase response to inflammation. It lacks specificity and can be demonstrated in a number of infectious diseases. Precise, quantitative assessment has

How to Monitor Progress?

Clinical assessment of improvement or deterioration is the most important observation. Resolving pain and improving movement in a pseudo-paralyzed limb can be taken as the best sign of successful treatment. The child will also improve generally, with increased appetite and involvement in ward activities. The most useful blood test in monitoring progress in treatment of osteomyelitis and septic arthritis is the quantitative measurement of CRP. The values have a high sensitivity. A quick response to antibiotic or surgical treatment can be expected; conversely, if the CRP remains increased, the infection is still active.

Less reliable is the ESR. If it is increased at the time when treatment commences, one expects to see, after a transient increase, a regular, gradual decrease that parallels clinical improvement. Although, in the long term, the ESR generally returns to normal, this may occur quite slowly. The ESR, by itself, should not be used as a guide to duration of treatment or as an indication for primary or secondary intervention.

What Are the Differential Diagnoses of Bone and Joint Infection?

To the experienced clinician, the history given by the patient is the most important part of the diagnostic exercise. After a complete history has been taken, the list of possible causes of the symptoms is usually small. The clinician less familiar with the natural history of the disease may place more reliance upon physical examination, laboratory aids, and imaging methods.

The age of the patient is also relevant: childhood osteomyelitis may be present with symptoms similar to osteosarcoma, Ewing's tumor, neuroblastoma, leukemia, and eosinophilic granuloma.

A child with osteomyelitis may have a fever and vomit, causing malnutrition and dehydration, with metabolic dysfunction. There may be a history of trauma to explain bone pain and lost function. Pseudo-paralysis is an important sign in infancy: the baby who holds a limb still may have septic arthritis and not a fracture or palsy.

Because the hip and shoulder joints are less accessible to clinical examination and also a frequent source of pain in older children the following alternative diagnoses must be considered:

- Irritable hip or Perthes' disease (Kocher's algorithm based upon clinical, radiological, and ESR criteria can be used [15]).
- Juvenile idiopathic arthritis
- Acute rheumatic fever
- Post-traumatic joint effusion
- Acute osteomyelitis
- Cellulitis
- Hemophilia
- Leukemia

How Should Bone and Joint Infection Be Managed?

Because cure is possible in those cases in which treatment is commenced early the principle that should apply is

- If you suspect acute osteomyelitis or septic arthritis treat with antibiotics as soon as a bacteriology specimen is taken and before final diagnosis is confirmed.
- If the infection you suspect is subacute or chronic confirm the diagnosis before treatment.

Acute is defined as a syndrome with rapid onset of symptoms in which pain and dysfunction prevent most normal activities. *Subacute* is defined as a more gradual onset of symptoms, over 7–10 days, with less marked interference of function. *Chronic* is defined as slow onset of symptoms, usually without systemic features and less severe pain (unless there is fracture of the bone with structural failure).

An algorithm for the management of skeletal infection is presented in Fig. 10.10. The three lines of approach to management are aspiration and biopsy, antibiotics, and surgery.

Aspiration and Biopsy

Most joints can be accessed using anatomical landmarks, and tender areas in bone are identified without difficulty or special skills. Modern techniques of imaging allow access to the whole body by an exploratory needle. Sophisticated equipment is not usually required. If necessary, accurate needle positioning in deeper tissues can be aided by ultrasonography. If the clinical picture, ultrasonography, and elevated CRP suggest a septic joint, it is sensible and kind to the child to use the same general anesthesia to aspirate the joint and also perform the arthrotomy or arthroscopy necessary to treat the infection. Although infrequently practiced, aspiration in acute osteomyelitis may also be useful.

Biopsy specimens of bone should be sent for both histopathological examination and direct culture for isolation of bacteria or other organisms. When aspirating, it is important to avoid carrying infection from the exterior to non-infected bone by using a careful aseptic technique and to avoid needle passage through potentially septic sites in skin or soft tissues. If this is done the risk of iatrogenic infection is minimal.

The Choice of Antibiotics

Antibiotic management requires consideration of the choice of drug administered, the dose to be used, the route of administration, and the duration of treatment. The choice of antibiotics is determined by

- The microorganism(s) to be eradicated
- Patient allergy to particular antibiotics

Fig. 10.10 Algorithm for diagnosis and treatment in suspected bone and joint infection

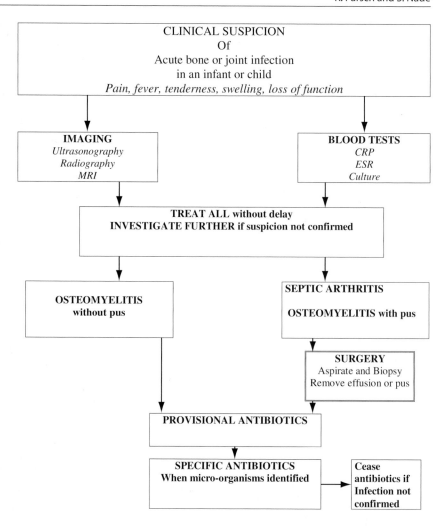

- Associated diseases
- Characteristics of the antibiotics (toxicity, activity and specificity, expense, and potential hypersensitivity)
- Availability of antibiotics

The chosen antibiotic must be effective against the bacteria causing the infection. Before an organism has been identified, or while antibiotic sensitivity of known organisms is being determined, the selection of antibiotic is provisional, based on a best guess and local policy. Once identification and sensitivity are known, the definitive or specific treatment can be used.

In infants and children, the dose is determined in relation to body weight. The efficiency of elimination of an antibiotic should be considered when the frequency of administration is being decided. The concentration of antibiotic in the blood should be greatest soon after administration of a dose and still therapeutic just before a subsequent dose. The aim of treatment is to maintain effective serum (and tissue) concentrations.

If antibiotics are administered intravenously, the physician can be assured of serum concentrations in the therapeutic range, given correct dosage. If they are given orally, absorption from the gut must also be taken into consideration.

If manufacturers' instructions are followed with regard to dosage schedules and timing of administration, regular monitoring of serum concentrations is not usually necessary. However, when using toxic antibiotics, such as aminoglycosides, it is important to measure serum concentrations and renal function frequently and to adjust the drug dose accordingly. Table 10.1 lists the average doses for various antibiotics when used to treat musculoskeletal infections in children.

The Route of Administration

Possible routes of administration are intravenous, intramuscular, oral, rectal, and locally into the infected area by irrigation or slow release. In acute infections, when the patient is unwell, nauseated, or dehydrated, oral treatment is not advised.

Table 10.1 Average doses of antibiotics used for musculoskeletal infections in children older than 4 weeks

Drug	Dose (mg/kg)	Doses per day
Benzyl penicillin G	60–120	4
Cloxacillin	50–100	4
Flucloxacillin	50–100	4
Cefuroxime	50–100	4
Gentamicin	4.5	3
Vancomycin	30–50	3
Clindamycin	8–16	3
Fusidic acid	20–40	3
Erythromycin	30–40	3

Table 10.2 Antibiotic therapy in osteomyelitis and septic arthritis

- 4–7 days parenteral
- 21–28 days oral

Monitoring

- Clinical progress
- CRP and ESR

The most effective route is intravenous. Entry to the blood stream is ensured and the exact dose calculated can be given. Because of antibiotic protein binding and excretion patterns, it is preferable to give a bolus of antibiotic at regular intervals (4–6 h), rather than a continuous, low-concentration infusion [19].

Oral preparations are available for most classes of antimicrobials except aminoglycosides (gentamicin), which are not absorbed from the gut. The major problems with oral use are the breakdown of the drug by gastric secretions or poor absorption across the gastrointestinal mucosa [19].

The criteria for a change to oral administration are as follows:

- Satisfactory clinical response to initial parenteral therapy
- Isolation of a bacterial pathogen that is susceptible to orally administered drugs
- Patient tolerance of an oral agent
- Adequate serum bactericidal activity with oral therapy
- Compliance by the patient

Subacute and chronic infections may respond to oral treatment from the outset. However, if surgical intervention is indicated the intravenous route is used initially.

In chronic osteomyelitis, irrigation with antibiotic solutions can achieve high local concentrations. Antibiotic-impregnated methyl methacrylate cement as a stent or as wire-threaded beads (PMMA beads) placed into the septic bone cavity is used in severe cases of acute or chronic osteomyelitis.

Duration of Therapy

There are very few studies that compare the duration of therapy in musculoskeletal infections. The specter of chronic osteomyelitis from the pre-antibiotic era still looms large, and many clinicians believe that prolonged treatment should be used for all bone and joint infections. What needs to be

determined is the minimum period of treatment necessary to prevent chronicity and relapse of infection. This should be balanced against the cost, exposure to toxicity, and duration of parenteral treatment. There is now sound evidence that intravenous antibiotics are only needed for a limited time. A short-course parenteral antibiotic therapy of 4–7 days followed by oral administration for 4 weeks is probably adequate (see Table 10.2) [19–21]. The same is true if surgical drainage of an acute osteomyelitis or chronic abscess has been performed.

It is essential to follow the clinical progress, loss of pain, and restoration of activity in the involved extremity. In addition CRP and ESR values are monitored.

In septic arthritis, clinical resolution may sometimes take only 2–3 days. Nevertheless oral medication should be continued after initial parenteral therapy for at least 3 weeks, monitored by the CRP.

Whether the child needs to remain in hospital is debatable and is more a matter of domestic circumstance than medical need. After surgical intervention and for the safety of intravenous antibiotic treatment, the acute phase is better taken care of with the patient in hospital. At home oral medication should be supervised by a paediatrician or family practitioner.

What Is the Place of Surgery?

In some centers, surgery is advised only if previous aspiration or MRI images have demonstrated an abscess and pus. Paediatricians and family practitioners are sometimes reluctant to advise surgery in the early stages, but this may jeopardize the chance of cure.

Contraindications to surgery include dehydration, a bleeding disorder (unless hemostasis can be ensured), and parental refusal.

When an operation is indicated, it should be performed as follows:

In acute osteomyelitis a direct approach should be made to the extra-osseous pus. The incision should be centered over the point of maximum tenderness to allow release of pus in the soft tissues and beneath the periosteum. Swabs and specimens must be taken. Pus should be evacuated, followed by copious lavage with isotonic saline solution but not a disinfectant irrigation fluid. If clinical signs or imaging suggest an intra-medullary abscess the cavity must be opened followed by copious lavage. Necrotic soft tissue should be removed, although not so radically as to endanger long bone integrity. Adequate drainage must be provided by one or two suction drains, depending upon the extent of the infected cavities. In case of large cavities application of gentamicin-impregnated bone cement has been of help, either by implanting a surgeon-formed stent, prefabricated PMMA beads, or foam [22–24].

In acute septic arthritis all pus must be evacuated from the joint. This can be done by open arthrotomy or by arthroscopic evacuation and lavage at certain sites if the surgeon is experienced. We advise the insertion of a suction drain. The joint capsule should be left unsutured while subcutaneous tissue and skin are closed.

Post-operatively the limb should initially be immobilized (for short-term relief of pain) in such a way that the wound can be inspected. Prolonged immobilization is advised only if there is a risk of pathological fracture or dislocation of a joint.

Specific Syndromes

Acute Hematogenous Osteomyelitis

Acute hematogenous osteomyelitis is an acute illness characterized by fever, bone tenderness, and reduced function secondary to the establishment of a bacterial colony in bone. Pain and inflammation develop quickly and progress rapidly. Clinical suspicion is the most valuable clue to diagnosis (Fig. 10.11).

Incidence

Osteomyelitis severe enough to require hospital admission is predominantly a disease of children, affecting boys more often than girls. The incidence appears to be greater in countries at lower latitudes, and multifocal disease is more frequently seen there [25]. Seasonal variations, with a peak in autumn and spring, suggest an environmental effect. Although there is an association with lower socioeconomic status, acute osteomyelitis occurs also in children who are perfectly healthy and who live in a good environment. The incidence of acute and subacute hematogenous osteomyelitis has declined during the past 20 years [26].

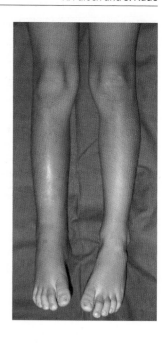

Fig. 10.11 Clinical photograph of both legs of a 6½-year-old boy with acute osteomyelitis of the right tibial shaft and distal metaphysis (patient of Fig. 10.13)

Diagnosis

The diagnosis of acute hematogenous osteomyelitis in the early phase relies upon five features:

1. Clinical examination—the cardinal sign is finger point tenderness localized to the metaphysis of a long bone associated with limb pain and inability to move or to bear weight
2. Ultrasound imaging identifying an epi- or subperiosteal abscess, appearing as an anechoic zone
3. Increased CRP (>10 mg/L) and ESR (>20 mm/first h)
4. Plain radiographs in which there is no evidence of any other diagnosis (e.g., trauma)
5. MRI images in STIR sequences with additional gadolinium contrast demonstrating infection in bone marrow and possible invasion into the periosteum and adjacent tissue

Antibiotics: Which Should Be Used?

In hospitals where several paediatric orthopaedic surgeons and paediatricians are practicing a protocol of management should be agreed upon [27, 28]. It is not always possible to identify the infective microorganism or to determine antibiotic sensitivity since organisms are grown from clinically diagnosed cases of hematogenous osteomyelitis in only 50–66% of patients. The majority of infections are caused by *S. aureus* and β[beta]-hemolytic *Streptococcus*. With the help of PCR *K. kingae* has been identified as a frequent cause of osteo-articular infection in specimens formerly classified as sterile [8].

Bactericidal anti-staphylococcal and anti-streptococcal antibiotics should be administered parenterally in adequate doses. Cefuroxime (100 mg/kg) in four doses per day has been an effective drug for more than 20 years, with very rare exceptions to its sensitivity. The antibiotic is administered parenterally for 4–7 days.

Oral therapy is introduced when the child is clinically well, has no fever, and the local signs have decreased. Flucloxacillin or cefaclor is administered between meals, because of the effect of gastric contents on drug absorption. The dose to be given by mouth is controlled initially on a body weight basis (50–100 mg/kg per day, in divided doses).

For streptococcal osteomyelitis, benzyl penicillin should be given intravenously ($0.25–1.0 \times 10^6$ units, every 6 h) for as long as the intravenous route is necessary (4–7 days if clinical response is obvious). When intravenous is replaced by oral administration, phenoxymethyl penicillin is given in a dose of 100 mg/kg per day every 6 hours. If the child is intolerant of penicillins, a cephalosporin such as cephradine or cephalexin can be given in a dose of 100 mg/kg per day, either intravenously or orally.

When investigation indicates a probable infection, the selection of antibiotics may also be based on the age of the child:

- neonates: gentamicin + flucloxacillin or a cephalosporin
- age 6 weeks–2 years: flucloxacillin or a cephalosporin + ampicillin
- age over 3 years: flucloxacillin or a cephalosporin

Surgery

Surgery gives quick relief from pain and offers the chance of rapid recovery. After decompression, a swab is taken for bacteriology and a tissue specimen to the pathologist.

Surgical cleansing of bone marrow and periosteum of pus and debris is followed by thorough and copious lavage of the infected region. The wound is closed with a drain left in place.

In severely infected bone, gentamicin-impregnated PMMA as stents or beads aligned in a chain can be inserted to fill the gap. The PMMA stent or chain is removed after 10 days or perhaps less depending upon the clinical parameters, which provides the opportunity of a "second look" operation and another curettage. With gentamicin-impregnated collagen carriers (sponges) the second intervention can be avoided (Fig. 10.12a–c).

Some centers prefer the use of an irrigation suction system for several days. However, there can be compliance problems, especially in small children, and its value compared with other methods has not been ascertained. We do not advocate such treatment.

Immobilization

Immobilization of the involved limb is for as short a time as possible; as soon as the patient is able to move the extremity without pain, he or she may do so. Full weight bearing is permitted after 4–6 weeks or even earlier if there is no pain, no tenderness, if the child is generally well, and if laboratory tests have returned to normal.

Re-intervention

In very aggressive infections with virulent organisms, occasionally a second or even a third operation is necessary. As soon as there are signs of the infection spreading, one should not hesitate to look again. This offers a better chance for a complete recovery than a "wait and see" strategy [20]. Additional precautions have to be taken if community-associated MRSA or MSSA is involved. The bacteria carry genes encoding PVL, leading to venous thrombosis and a high complication rate [3, 29].

Complications are more likely in infants, especially if surgical drainage is delayed.

Outcome of Acute Osteomyelitis

Death rarely complicates acute hematogenous osteomyelitis today. When it does, it is from overwhelming septicemia with involvement of multiple organs. The emergence of community-associated MRSA infection in North America, Australia, and also Europe since the year 2000 has produced cases of multifocal infection with septicemia not seen in the previous period [3].

The risk of chronic osteomyelitis remains a major reason for seeking to improve early management in acute hematogenous osteomyelitis. If the child presents early enough and the principles of treatment are followed meticulously, chronic osteomyelitis should become a disease of the past. Unfortunately children living in war zones and in underprivileged countries are still at risk of developing chronic infection and subsequent amputation.

Aberrant growth from metaphyseal infection is of concern if it is marked, affects only a portion of the growth plate, producing an angular deformity, or affects one of a pair of bones (in the forearm or leg) (Fig. 10.13a, b). Anatomical deformity of the contour of a bone does not necessarily produce significant clinical, functional, or cosmetic deformity.

Fig. 10.12 (**a**) Radiograph of the distal radius of a boy aged 12 years. Acute *S. aureus* osteomyelitis was proven by culture. (**b**) After 3 weeks of antibiotic treatment and surgical revision followed by implantation of gentamicin PMMA beads. (**c**) Radiograph of distal forearm after 6 years. Residual sclerosis near the distal growth plate is indicative of the previous infection. Note asymmetric distal radial growth

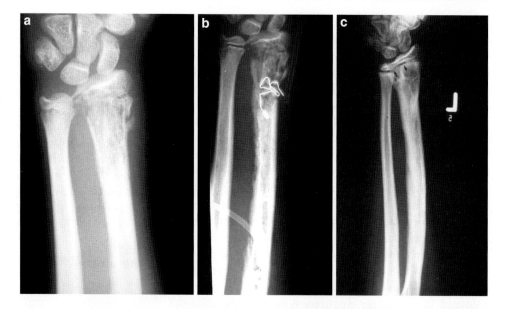

Fig. 10.13 (**a**) Right tibia in two planes: acute osteomyelitis with signs of bone resorption and new periosteal bone formation in a boy of $6\frac{1}{2}$ years. Pus aspiration was followed by parenteral antibiotic treatment (patient of Fig. 10.11). (**b**) Both legs of 20-year-old patient with shortening and valgus deformity of the right ankle joint from post-infectious lateral growth arrest

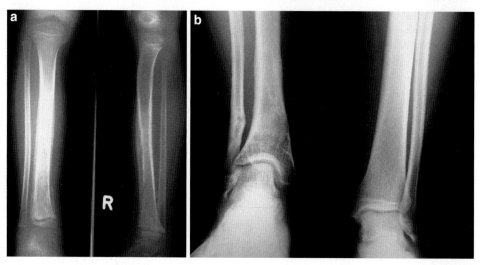

Sequelae are more frequent in the infant group following metaphyseal osteomyelitis after an initial septic arthritis. Major growth disturbances are seen if surgery is delayed.

The process of resorption of bone, either in the acute phase or more often in the chronic phase, may lead to pathological fracture. Provided that the infection is controlled, such fractures usually unite when treated by conventional, non-operative methods.

A very difficult complication to treat is diaphyseal bone loss, often extensive. It usually implies that the ability of the surrounding periosteum to produce reparative involucrum has been lost and that the spontaneous restoration of bone, even when infection is eradicated, cannot occur.

The risk of recurrence of acute osteomyelitis decreases rapidly as time passes after the acute illness. Recurrence seems to be lower in children who have undergone prompt

abscess drainage, an important consideration when counseling the patient and parents.

Chronic Osteomyelitis Following Acute Osteomyelitis

Chronic osteomyelitis subsequent to inadequate treatment of the acute disease carries a substantial morbidity. The fundamental problem in chronic bone infection is the persistence of organisms despite treatment.

The pathological anatomy reflects the consequences of continuing necrosis (sequestrum, abscess, and sinus) and repair (reactive new bone and scar). The balance achieved between these processes determines the outcome; the aim of management is to tip the balance in favor of the host.

Staphylococcus aureus remains the most common isolate, but other organisms are increasingly reported, particularly Gram-negative bacilli and anaerobes. Tissue perfusion in chronic osteomyelitis may be impaired after previous vascular injury, extensive scarring, or small-vessel disease. This in turn reduces the host immune response including phagocytosis and the repair process of fibroblast aggregation, proliferation of collagen matrix, and neo-vascularization.

There is no standard prescription for the treatment of chronic osteomyelitis because the reasons for chronicity are varied. However, the objectives of management are to reduce the number of bacteria in the tissue and to improve repair by the host. The principles are

1. Adequate microbiological diagnosis
2. Assessment and modification of the host response
3. Anatomical definition of the local disease, both in bone and soft tissue
4. Antibiotic therapy after identification of causative microorganisms
5. Surgical removal of necrotic and poorly vascularized tissue
6. Obliteration of dead space left by surgical excision
7. Restoration of functional skeletal stability using the Ilizarov method of bone transport [30, 31]

8. Vascularized free tissue grafts of fibula or iliac crest to fill the space left after surgical excision of infected tissue [32, 33]

Subacute Osteomyelitis

Frequency

The estimated incidence of subacute osteomyelitis is 0.4–0.9 per 100,000 population per year. While the incidence of acute hematogenous osteomyelitis has declined during the last 20 years, the incidence of the subacute form has not changed [26].

Clinical Picture

Subacute osteomyelitis presents as a mild, sometimes intermittent, local limb pain of a few days or weeks duration, with mild systemic signs. A characteristic of subacute presentation is the long history of symptoms dominated by pain and swelling (Fig. 10.14a). Fever is slight or absent and constitutional symptoms are rare. Loss of function is obvious in most cases but may be dramatic in spinal infection.

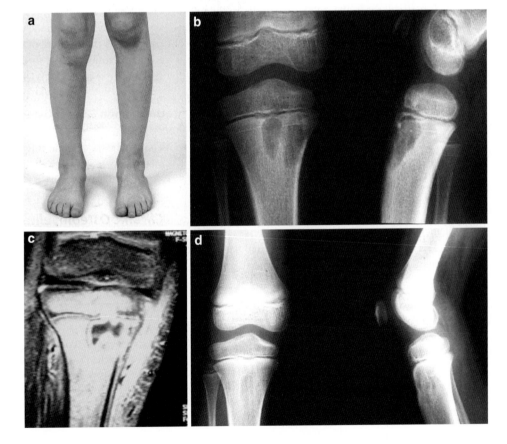

Fig. 10.14 (a) Painful swelling below the right knee. (b) Right knee in two planes showing a lytic lesion of the metaphysis with connection into epiphysis. (c) MRI of proximal tibia shows meta-epiphyseal abscess as well as subperiosteal fluid (pus). (d) Three months after surgical drainage and 3 weeks of antibiotic treatment. Complete recovery and no sign of premature physeal closure

Unlike the acute osteo-articular infections, the diagnosis of subacute infection depends upon imaging techniques. It is often difficult to differentiate subacute osteomyelitis from neoplastic conditions (osteosarcoma, Ewing sarcoma, and eosinophilic granuloma).

Imaging

Most lesions occur in the metaphysis of the tibia, femur, and humerus but the tarsal bones, particularly the os calcis, may be affected [1]. Epiphyseal abscesses are rare, representing an extension of the metaphyseal bone abscess.

Radiological signs are normally established at the time of presentation and include absorption, sclerotic margination, and sequestration. Classically, a "punched-out" lesion of the metaphysis or diaphysis develops, often surrounded by sclerosis (Brodie's abscess) and rarely by cortical destruction [20]. Very occasionally these lesions cross the growth plate (Fig. 10.14b).

The classification derives from the radiological appearances [34, 35]. It has been suggested that a distinction can be made between aggressive lesions which need surgery and non-aggressive metaphyseal or epiphyseal lesions without clinical signs of pus [36].

Radioisotope imaging is a valuable investigation in the early stages when radiological changes are obscure or poorly developed, particularly in the pelvis. Once the radiological changes are established, there is no benefit to be gained from radioisotope scanning.

MRI has greatly advanced our knowledge about bone abscesses. It shows the exact extent of the lesion, periosteal involvement, and the soft tissue response to bone infection. MRI helps to differentiate a bone abscess from histiocytosis X (eosinophilic granuloma) (see Fig. 10.14c and Table 10.3) [37].

Laboratory Signs

A slight increase in the ESR is present in fewer than 50% of cases. The white cell count is usually normal but the CRP can be moderately increased.

Pathology and Microbiology

About 40% of cases of subacute osteomyelitis, although showing histological features of chronic inflammation and plasma cells (plasma cell osteomyelitis), yield no growth on cultures obtained either by aspiration or by surgical biopsy. Blood cultures are rarely positive, whereas cultures obtained from aspiration, biopsy, or at definitive surgery are positive in about 60% of reported cases.

Treatment of Subacute Osteomyelitis

Surgical drainage and curettage used to be advocated for all cases of subacute osteomyelitis [34]. Since infections may mimic bone tumors such as eosinophilic granuloma or even Ewing's sarcoma or osteosarcoma, surgical intervention was advised, if only to assist in the establishment of a correct diagnosis [38, 39].

It is likely that antibiotic treatment alone has an equal chance of curing subacute osteomyelitis, with 87% success rate after a 6-week course [35]. Typical radiological appearances, particularly in the metaphysis, may render diagnostic biopsy unnecessary [40–42].

Antibiotic therapy against *S. aureus* (using cefuroxime or flucloxacillin) is initiated by intravenous therapy for 4–7 days, followed by 3–4 weeks of oral therapy. For other microorganisms the appropriate antibiotic should be selected according to sensitivity.

The outcome in primary subacute osteomyelitis is generally good, with relief of symptoms over days to perhaps a month, followed by slower improvement in radiological appearance (Fig. 10.14d) [38].

Uncommon Sites of Osteomyelitis

The diagnosis of bone infection is often delayed at uncommon sites such as the pelvis or the spine.

Pelvic Osteomyelitis

In acute, subacute, or chronic pelvic osteomyelitis, the child may present with fever and pain in the lower abdomen,

Table 10.3 A classification of subacute osteomyelitis [35]

Type Description
1. Metaphyseal abscess (either of these may involve or cross the physis)
i. Punched-out lucency without significant marginal reaction
ii. Punched-out lucency with sclerotic margin (Brodie's abscess)
2. Eccentrically placed metaphyseal lucency eroding the cortex
3. Diaphyseal cortical abscess with or without sequestrum
4. Diaphyseal medullary abscess (periosteal new bone is common)
5. Epiphyseal abscess (usually eccentric in epiphyseal nucleus) vertebral osteomyelitis

the buttock, or the back, depending upon which direction the pus tracks. In one-third of children the sacroiliac joint is primarily affected. MRI has replaced radioisotope scanning as the preferred method for identifying the site and extent of the lesion [43, 44]. MRI with STIR sequences helps in distinguishing the differential diagnosis of pelvic neoplasm. *Staphylococcus aureus* or *P. aeruginosa* are the most common bacteria involved, although other infections, including tuberculosis and brucellosis, or *K. kingae* (identified by PCR), may present in an identical way. Therapy consists of parenteral antibiotic treatment followed by oral antibiotics. Surgery is indicated if MRI identifies a large abscess (Fig. 10.15).

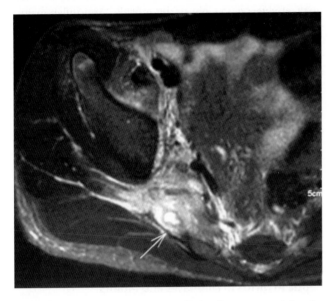

Fig. 10.15 MRI of 12-year-old boy suffering from severe pelvic pain. MRI reveals large abscess in the sacroiliac joint and neighboring soft tissues

Discitis

Subacute vertebral osteomyelitis with adjacent disc space infection is called discitis. Toddlers are most commonly affected. They refuse to walk but do not suffer obvious pain affecting the back or the hip. Older children complain of back pain with reduced mobility. Typically, they are unable to pick up a coin or other object from the ground. Plain radiographs show disc space narrowing, erosion, and sclerosis of the vertebral end plate. A positive blood culture or biopsy is identified in only one half of children from whom a specimen is obtained. The majority reveal Gram-positive *S. aureus.* technetium-99m bone scanning was the method of establishing the diagnosis in the past [45] but MRI is now the diagnostic investigation of choice. Pathological gadolinium enhancement within the disc and adjacent vertebral body

is demonstrated and a paraspinal inflammatory mass may be seen. MRI reduces diagnostic delay and reduces the need for biopsy [46]. If needle biopsy is performed, even with PCR only 61% are positive. *Staphylococcus aureus* and *K. kingae* are the most common organisms found [47].

Simple bed rest encourages gradual resolution, although antibiotics may speed recovery. A multi-center study showed a significant decrease in the duration of symptoms when children were treated with intravenous antibiotics followed by oral therapy compared to only oral or no antibiotics [45]. Patients may be improved by spinal immobilization in a back brace, together with oral antibiotics. Even after full clinical resolution the disc space narrows, sometimes leading to local intervertebral fusion.

Puncture Wound Osteomyelitis

Localized infection in the head of the first metatarsal or heel with progressive pain, tenderness, and swelling has been observed in older boys after penetrating puncture wounds of the foot. The usual pathogen in this "tennis shoe osteomyelitis" is *P. aeruginosa*, which resides in tennis shoe insoles. Surgical exploration helps to identify the causative organisms and allows any coexistent septic arthritis to be drained. At least 7 days of anti-pseudomonal antibiotic therapy should control infection [48, 49].

Chronic Recurrent Multifocal Osteomyelitis

Chronic recurrent multifocal osteomyelitis (CRMO) is seen in children aged 4–15 years and was first described in Switzerland and Scandinavia [50–52]. CRMO affects predominantly the tubular bones of the limbs, followed by the clavicle and the spine. There is localized pain and minimal swelling in the involved limb. Recurrent clinical episodes involve different bones at different times. The ESR and CRP are moderately increased and fever may develop. Radiography shows bone enlargement, periostitis with bone apposition, and zones of osteolysis. 99mTechnetium bone scans help to identify "hot spots" in different locations. Nowadays MRI has taken the place of bone scanning and is the best method for confirming the diagnosis (Fig. 10.16) [53].

To the experienced practitioner CRMO is usually characteristic and a biopsy is not always required to confirm the diagnosis. Cultures do not grow bacteria. Histopathological examination shows inflammation. However, the purpose of biopsy is the differentiation from neoplasia [54]. As soon as the diagnosis is established repeated biopsies are redundant. Antibiotics, steroids, or chemotherapeutic agents should then

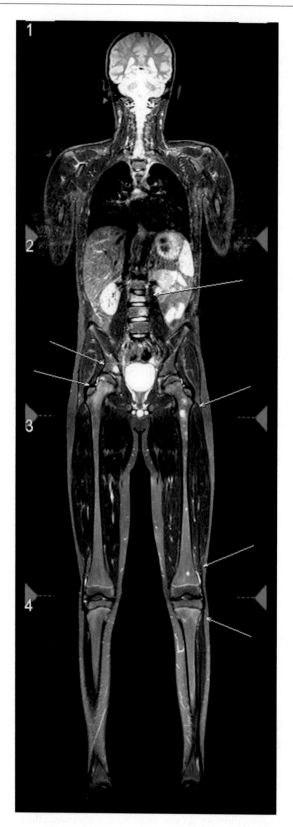

Fig. 10.16 Whole body MRI in a boy with CRMO (spine, long bones, and other sites)

be avoided. Several observations suggest the contribution of genetic factors to the etiology of CRMO [55].

The SAPHO (synovitis, acne, pustulosis, hyperostosis, and osteitis) syndrome belongs to the same group of non-bacterial inflammation. With negative cultures as a constant feature another name has been coined for non-suppurative inflammation: chronic non-bacterial osteomyelitis (CNO) [56].

Treatment of CRMO

CRMO is a benign, self-limiting disease with very few negative effects on the physis or growth. Anti-inflammatory treatment (NSAID) is given until symptoms subside [52–57]. Antibiotic treatment is not advised as it has no rational basis.

Chronic Sclerosing Osteomyelitis

This is a rare sclerosing bone disease also known as Garré's osteomyelitis. In biopsy material bacteria are never cultured. The response to surgical and antibiotic treatment is variable, recurrences may occur. It may be a variant form of CRMO.

Septic Arthritis

Septic Arthritis in Neonates and Infants

In the young infant, the history should include a search for possible maternal sources of infection in pregnancy or during delivery like maternal breast abscess, streptococcal infection, or candidiasis, syphilis, or gonorrhea. Of importance is the obstetric and nursing history. Particular sources of infection include omphalitis, pustular dermatitis and paronychia, purulent rhinitis, infected operative sites (such as circumcision), intramuscular injections, scalp-vein needles, umbilical catheterization, heel puncture, or accidental injury during caesarian section.

Diagnostic delay often characterizes septic arthritis of the hip and shoulder. The very young child with fever and a serious illness may not manifest classic, local signs of acute arthritis. The infective process in a joint, particularly the hip joint, is frequently not obvious, so changes in posture are important. The traditional clinical signs of inflammation, such as swelling and reddish color, may be lacking, especially in the early phase of the disease. In any infant with a septicemia, involvement of the hip or shoulder joint must be suspected. This is manifest by one or more of the following:

Table 10.4 Ultrasonography in neonatal hip joint sepsis	• Day 1—synovial swelling (seen on Graf's lateral view) (Fig. 10.17a, b)
	• Day 3—halo of fluid inside joint, synovial swelling
	• Day >5—distension, subluxation, and metaphyseal bone changes (Fig. 10.17c)

- abnormal posture of the leg or arm
- pain on palpation or passive movement of the leg or arm
- lack of active movement of the limb—pseudo-paralysis
- asymmetrical skin creases
- palpable bulge over the buttock, perineum, or shoulder

Arthritis in the knee and elbow joint of an infant is more obvious on clinical examination. These joints have less muscle and soft tissue to cover them.

The main differential diagnosis is perinatal injury with epiphyseal slip at the hip, knee, shoulder, or elbow. A brachial plexus lesion should be ruled out.

Imaging

Diagnostic ultrasonography is a reliable examination to visualize joint infection in the neonate and small infant. Graf's lateral approach for detecting hip dysplasia is used in addition to the ventral approach commonly done for older children. In neonates, swelling of the synovium is the earliest sign of an infected joint. As the femoral or humeral head is entirely cartilaginous the thickened capsule can be visualized by ultrasound in contrast to the transparent head [58, 59].

After 1 or 2 days fluid inside a hip or shoulder joint can be identified by sonography. Furthermore, ultrasound imaging can detect metaphyseal osteomyelitis with cortical defects in the femoral neck or proximal humerus in cases of aggressive infection. Bony changes are seen in delayed diagnosis (>3 days). The enlarging effusion in a septic hip can lead to lateral displacement and even dislocation of the femoral head (Table 10.4).

Plain radiographs of an infant's hip or shoulder with suspected infection might demonstrate soft tissue swelling. After a few days the infection of the joint may cause the head of the bone to be de-centered, misinterpreted as hip dysplasia or subluxation.

After a minimum of 5–7 days bone changes from osteomyelitis become visible. The earliest sign of osteomyelitis of the femoral neck is a metaphyseal lip. Within a few days cavities develop and new cortical bone formation can be seen (Fig. 10.18).

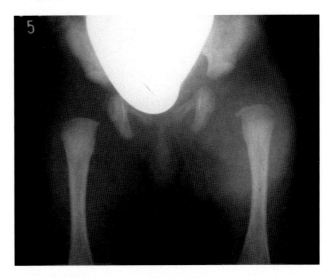

Fig. 10.18 Pelvic radiograph of a 3-week-old girl with septic arthritis of the left hip showing a Metaphyseal lip and lateral displacement caused by metaphyseal osteomyelitis (ultrasound shown in Fig. 10.17b)

The radiographic changes in a septic shoulder are similar to those of a septic hip. Initially only soft tissue swelling is seen, while at a later stage metaphyseal infection can cause cavities or cortical defects and new bone formation.

MRI can be useful to detect and differentiate a septic joint and metaphyseal osteomyelitis. STIR sequences and gadolinium enhancement provide a clear picture of the joint infection.

Fig. 10.17 (**a**) Ultrasonography of normal right hip. (**b**) Ultrasonography of a 3-week-old girl with a 5-day history of septic arthritis of the left hip. Note the thickened synovium and lateralization of the femoral head. (**c**) Ultrasonography of a 5-week-old boy with a 7-day history of septic hip. The femoral head is displaced and there is an effusion

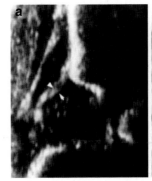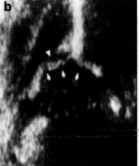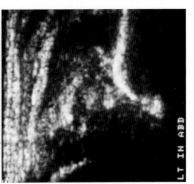

An infant with suspected septic arthritis must be kept under close observation by repeated clinical, laboratory, and ultrasonographic methods.

If ultrasonography is not available, the joint is aspirated under general anesthesia, with image intensifier radiography if available. At an early stage of the infection the aspirate can be transparent, sometimes rose-colored, from blood staining and only in delayed cases is it obviously purulent. Immediately after the aspiration the joint is drained under the same general anesthetic.

The diagnosis of septic arthritis of the infant is made from clinical appearance, CRP elevation, and synovial changes with effusion on ultrasonography.

Treatment

There are two essentials for the effective treatment of septic arthritis: first the joint must be adequately cleansed (evacuate bacterial products and debris) and second antibiotics must be given to diminish the systemic effects of sepsis. If unstable, a septic joint must be reduced and splinted. If there is metaphyseal infection, pus and debris should be evacuated at the same operation.

Surgery

For the neonatal and small infant hip joint, we prefer arthrotomy by an anterior approach. It offers optimum care of the wound post-operatively. The capsule is incised. A swab and small tissue sample of synovium are taken for culture of causative organisms. After adequate irrigation and insertion of a suction drain subcutaneous tissues and skin are loosely closed.

For the infant with septic arthritis of the shoulder, aspiration is followed by anterior arthrotomy with sufficient exposure of the proximal humeral metaphysis to enable thorough evacuation of pus and debris.

Antibiotic Treatment

Staphylococcus aureus and *β[beta]-hemolytic streptococci* are the most common organisms causing septic arthritis in infants and children, but many other organisms have been isolated.

Other causative organisms reported include *Haemophilus influenzae*, *Strep. pneumoniae*, *E. coli*, *Proteus* spp., *Salmonella* spp., *Serratia marcescens*, *Clostridium welchii*, *Neisseria* spp., *Staph. albus*, *Aerobacter* spp., *Bacteroides* spp., *Paracolon bacillus*, and *K. kingae*.

Intravenous antibiotic treatment with a flucloxacillin or with ß[beta]-lactamase-resistant antibiotic (for example, cefuroxime 50–100 mg/kg in four doses) is effective in most cases of *S. aureus* and *Strep. pyogenes* infection. Recovery is prompt and often seen within 3 days. Parenteral treatment is continued for 7 days. Clinical status and CRP levels determine when to institute oral antibiotic treatment.

As septic arthritis of the infant hip is quite often associated with lateralization, subluxation, or even dislocation of the femoral head, a harness for 6 weeks post-operatively or a cast in the human position for a shorter period is recommended (Fig. 10.19).

Recurrence

Scanning may identify a recurrent effusion or another focus in the metaphysis. A second arthrotomy may be necessary. More specimens will be required for laboratory studies and it is sometimes necessary to give two antibiotics simultaneously.

If septic arthritis is recognized too late (after 5 days) osteomyelitis of the epiphysis and metaphysis may develop. Head and neck osteomyelitis in the hip or in the proximal humerus has major impact on the final outcome and post-arthritic sequelae.

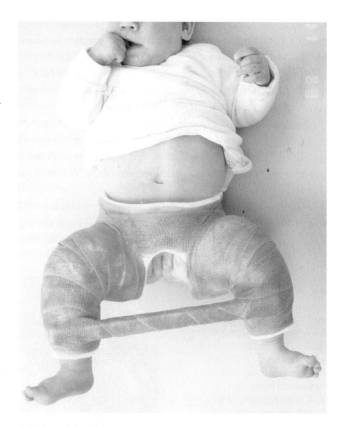

Fig. 10.19 Baby child in spica cast in human position after surgical treatment of a septic hip with dislocation

Outcome

If surgical and antibiotic treatment is started immediately or with a delay of less than 3 days after the beginning of the illness, small infants with septic arthritis of the hip, knee, or shoulder will recover completely.

The potential sequelae of hip sepsis [60] (Fig. 10.20) are

I. Recovery: with no deformity or with coxa magna (Fig. 10.21).
II. Coxa brevis with deformed head causing progressive coxa vara or coxa valga as a result of premature physeal closure, leg length discrepancy (Fig. 10.21).
III. Slipping of femoral epiphysis: with coxa vara or coxa valga or with pseudarthrosis. The femoral head remains in the acetabulum.
IV. Destruction of femoral head and neck: with a small remnant of head or with complete loss of head and neck and no articulation of the hip.

In severe coxa vara with non-union of the femoral neck valgus osteotomy can restore the shaft–neck angle and will consolidate the pseudarthrosis [61]. The leg length discrepancy that follows can be dealt with by contralateral distal femoral epiphysiodesis.

The worst outcome is encountered when adequate treatment is delayed for several weeks, either from antibiotic treatment alone without surgery or by inadequate surgery that fails to eradicate all infection in the metaphysis, with continued destruction of the femoral head and neck in spite of antibiotic treatment [60].

Reconstruction of femoral head and neck pathology has been attempted by greater trochanteric arthroplasty [60].

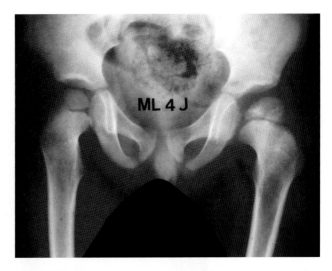

Fig. 10.21 Pelvic radiograph of a 4-year-old boy who had delayed arthrotomy for septic arthritis of the left hip caused by *S. aureus* at the age of 6 months. Coxa magna and coxa brevis have produced shortening of left leg which will eventually necessitate contralateral epiphysiodesis

Reasonable results have been reported, although function is always disappointing (Fig. 10.22a–e) [61–63].

Ilizarov hip reconstruction with subtrochanteric valgus osteotomy has been described as an alternative for type IV sequelae after infantile hip infection [64]. If done at an early age the procedure may need to be repeated.

In the septic knee of infancy, arthrotomy allows good access to the joint space and metaphyseal septic abscess. Arthroscopic lavage is not advised in the infant and delay may result in partial or complete destruction of the growth plate leading to axial deformity and joint instability [65].

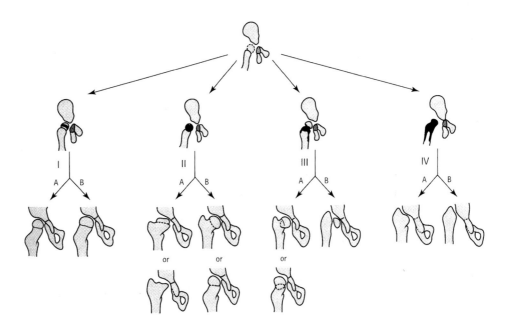

Fig. 10.20 Potential sequelae of hip sepsis. Modified after Choi et al. [60]

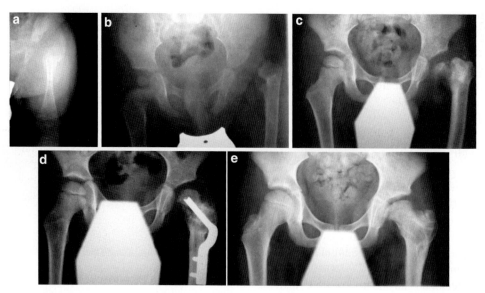

Fig. 10.22 (**a**) Radiograph of left hip of a boy aged 2 months. He had parenteral antibiotic treatment for a septic left hip at the age of 4 weeks, no surgical drainage. The hip dislocated and the femoral neck shows a ring of new bone. (**b**) Pelvic radiograph at 11 months with post-sepsis dislocation of left hip. (**c**) After open reduction and valgus osteotomy of the left hip performed at the age of 13 months the pelvic radiograph taken at age 3 years shows the left hip centered, coxa vara, and coxa brevis. (**d**) Radiograph after valgus osteotomy had been performed at the age of 4. (**e**) Radiograph of the pelvis at age 9 years with satisfactory left hip and signs of premature closure of the proximal femoral growth plate

For septic shoulders in infants, arthrotomy is preferred as metaphyseal involvement is common. After delayed diagnosis, deformation of the humeral head and shortening of the humerus cause marked cosmetic but negligible functional loss [66, 67].

Septic Arthritis of the Older Child

In contrast to the infant, the older child with septic arthritis usually presents with an acute illness. Severe pain, muscle spasm, and reluctance to move the joint or even the whole limb are important criteria. Fever and tachycardia are common, together with evidence of joint effusion. Avoidance of weight bearing and the presence of fever help to differentiate between septic arthritis and transient synovitis of the hip in children [68, 69].

Diagnostic ultrasound is a very reliable imaging technique to visualize joint effusion. Septic arthritis of the hip, the knee, the shoulder, the elbow, or any other joint can be assessed [70]. Ultrasonographic differentiation of purulent from aseptic fluid or blood inside the joint is not yet possible (Fig. 10.23).

Plain radiographs may demonstrate soft tissue swelling but the osseous changes occur later as already discussed.

MRI, if available, can be useful to visualize a joint effusion and also metaphyseal changes.

Features favoring a diagnosis of septic arthritis of the hip and not transient synovitis are clinical appearance including severe pain, elevated CRP, and ultrasound effusion.

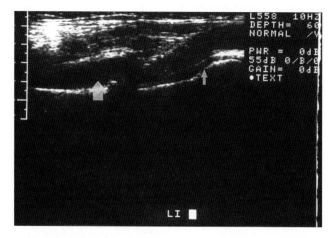

Fig. 10.23 Ultrasonography of both hips in a 13-year-old girl with severe right hip pain and inability to stand or walk. Large effusion on the right side (Bold arrow). No effusion on the left side (arrow)

Management of Septic Arthritis of the Hip

We prefer an anterolateral approach according to Smith Peterson (Fig. 10.24). In the vast majority of cases with septic arthritis, lavage of the joint and antibiotic treatment leads to recovery within 3 days. CRP levels measured after 3 and 6 days post-operatively will show the expected decline. After 4–7 days antibiotic treatment is continued orally with a cephalosporin for another 3–4 weeks. The clinical course is monitored carefully in hospital and then at home if facilities allow.

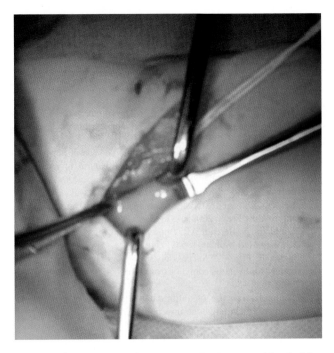

Fig. 10.24 Clinical photograph at time of arthrotomy. After incision of the capsule pus was released under pressure. *Staphylococcus aureus* was cultured

Arthroscopic lavage of the septic hip joint now offers a less traumatic means of decompression [71, 72].

Outcome After Septic Arthritis of the Hip

Early arthrotomy or arthroscopy and parenteral antibiotic treatment offer the chance of full recovery from an infected hip joint [73]. However, if clinical recovery does not promptly follow the initial treatment, the treating surgeon must rethink the strategy (Fig. 10.25a, b).

Delay in diagnosis, inadequate treatment, and virulent microorganisms like *S. aureus* produce chondrolysis (joint cartilage destruction) with reduced motion and possible ankylosis (Fig. 10.26a, b).

Septic Arthritis of the Knee

The majority of centers now use arthroscopic lavage of septic arthritis of the knee. This will achieve joint cleansing by an expert arthroscopist, but the less experienced should consider arthrotomy. Early mobilization is encouraged, but weight bearing is delayed for 3–4 weeks.

Fig. 10.25 (a) Radiograph of a 13-year-old girl with a 3-day history of severe right hip pain caused by septic arthritis (*S. aureus*). (b) Radiograph of the same patient 6 months after arthrotomy, lavage of the joint, and parenteral antibiotic treatment. She has normal function of both hips

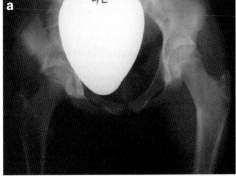
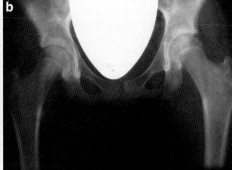

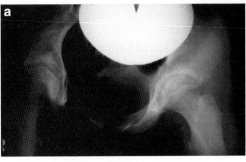
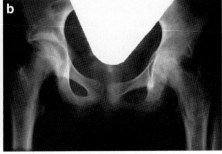

Fig. 10.26 (a) Pelvic radiograph of a 12-year-old girl suffering from unbearable left hip pain for 8 days. *Staphylococcus aureus* was cultured from the joint. At surgery the cartilage was largely destroyed. Antibiotic treatment had controlled the infection but could not prevent articular degeneration. (b) Pelvis at the age of 15 years showing complete destruction of the left hip joint. The hip is stiff in a functional position enabling the girl to walk with a limp and to sit with difficulty. Function is similar to an arthrodesis of the hip

Septic Arthritis of the Shoulder

If there is an expert shoulder arthroscopist arthroscopic lavage of a septic shoulder joints is the treatment of choice. Others will consider arthrotomy for a thorough joint cleansing. If there is metaphyseal abscess this should be surgically evacuated at the same intervention.

Multifocal Septic Arthritis

Septic arthritis in several joints may coexist with multifocal osteomyelitis. Prompt surgical evacuation of pus from the affected joints and metaphyseal sites should be combined with appropriate parenteral antibiotics, offering a reasonably satisfactory outcome.

References

1. Gillespie WJ, Nade S. Musculoskeletal Infections. Melbourne: Blackwell; 1987.
2. Chometon S, Benito Y, Chaker M, et al. Specific real-time polymerase chain reaction places *Kingella kingae* as the most common cause of osteoarticular infections in young children. Pediatr Infect Dis J 2007; 26:377–81.
3. Arnold SR, Elias D, Buckingham SC, et al. Changing patterns of acute hematogenous osteomyelitis and septic arthritis. Emergence of community-associated methicillin-resistant *Staphylococcus aureus*. J Pediatr Orthop 2006; 26:703–8.
4. Swaminathan A, Massasso D, Gotis-Graham I, et al. Fulminant methicillin-sensitive *Staphylococcus aureus* infection in a healthy adolescent, highlighting "Panton-Valentine leucocidin" syndrome. Intern Med J 2005; 36:744–7.
5. Howard AW, Viskontas D, Sabbagh C. Reduction in osteomyelitis and septic arthritis related to *Haemophilus influenzae* Type B vaccination. J Pediatr Orthop 1999; 19:705–9.
6. Morrissy RT. Bone and joint sepsis. In: Morrissy RT, Weinstein SL, eds. Lovell & Winter's Pediatric Orthopaedics. Vol 1. Philadelphia, PA: Lippincott Williams & Wilkins; 2005:579–624.
7. Moumille K, Merckx J, Glorion C, et al. Bacterial aetiology of acute osteoarticular infections in children. cta Paediatr 2005; 94:419–22.
8. Lebel E, Rudensky B, Karasik M, et al. *Kingella kingae* infections in children. J Pediatr Orthop (part B) 2006; 15:289–92.
9. Chau CL, Griffith JF. Musculoskeletal infections: ultrasound appearances. Clin Radiol 2005; 60:149–59.
10. Gordon JE, Huang M, Dobbs M, et al. Causes of false-negative ultrasound scans in the diagnosis of septic arthritis of the hip in children. J Pediatr Orthop 2002; 22:312–6.
11. Mazur JM, Ross G, Cummings RJ, et al. Usefulness of magnetic resonance imaging for the diagnosis of acute musculoskeletal infections in children. J Pediatr Orthop 1995; 15:144–7.
12. Mandell GA. Imaging in the diagnosis of musculoskeletal infections in children. Curr Probl Pediatr 1996; 26:218–37.
13. Wenger DR, Davids JR, Ring D. Discitis and osteomyelitis. In: Weinstein SL, ed. The Pediatric Spine: Principles and Practice. New York, NY: Raven Press; 1994:813–35.
14. Karmazyn B, Loder RT, Kleiman MB, et al. The role of pelvic magnetic resonance in evaluating non-hip sources of infection in children with acute non-traumatic hip pain. J Pediatr Orthop 2007; 27:158–64.
15. Kocher MS, Mandiga R, Zurakowski D, et al. Validation of a clinical prediction rule for the differentiation between septic arthritis and transient synovitis of the hip in children. J Bone Joint Surg 2004; 86 A:1629–35.
16. Lorrot M, Fitoussi F, Faye A, et al. Laboratory studies in pediatric bone and joint infections. Arch Pediatr 2007; 14 Suppl 2:86–90.
17. Martineau F, Picard FJ, Ke D, et al. Development of PCR assay for identification of *Staphylococci* at genus and species levels. J Clin Microbiol 2001; 39:2541–47.
18. Kobayashi N, Bauer TW, Sakai H, et al. The use of newly developed real-time PCR for the rapid identification of bacteria in culture-negative osteomyelitis. Joint Bone Spine 2006; 73:745–7.
19. Nade S. Septic arthritis. In: Bulstrode C, Buckwalter J, Carr A, et al. eds. Oxford Textbook of Orthopaedics and Trauma. Oxford: Oxford Univ Press; 2002:1437–42
20. Hambleton S, Berendt AR. Bone and joint infections in children. Adv Exp Med Biol 2004; 549:47–62.
21. Bachur R, Pagon Z. Success of short-course parenteral antibiotic therapy for acute osteomyelitis of childhood. Clin Pediatr (Phila) 2007; 46:30–5.
22. Klemm K. The use of antibiotic-containing bead chains in the treatment of chronic bone infections. Clin Microbiol Infect 2001; 7:28–31.
23. Mehta S, Humphrey JS, Schenkman DI, et al. Gentamicin distribution from a collagen carrier. J Orthop Res 1996; 14:749–54.
24. Mendel V, Simanowski HJ, Scholz HC, et al. Therapy with gentamicin-PMMA beads, gentamicin-collage sponge and cefazolin for experimental osteomyelitis due to *Staphylococcus aureus* in rats. Arch Orthop Trauma Surg 2005; 125:363–8.
25. Lavy CB. Septic arthritis in Western and sub-Saharian African children-a review. Int Orthop 2007; 31:137–44.
26. Blyth MJG, Kincaid R, Craigen MAC, et al. The changing epidemiology of acute and subacute hematogenous osteomyelitis in children. J Bone Joint Surg 2001; 83B:99–102.
27. Abuarama S, Louis JS, Guyard MF, et al. Osteoarticular infection in children: evaluation of diagnostic and management protocol. Rev Chir Orthop Reparatr App Mot 2004; 90:703–13.
28. Afghani B, Kong V, Wu FL. What would pediatric infectious disease consultants recommend for management of culture-negative hematogenous osteomyelitis? J Pediatr Orthop 2007; 27:805–9.
29. Bocchini CE, Hulten KG, Mason EO, et al. Panton-Valentine leukocidin genes are associated with enhanced inflammatory response and local disease in acute hematogenous *Staphylococcus aureus* osteomyelitis in children. Pediatrics 2006; 117:433–40.
30. Yeargan SA, Nakasone CK, Shaleb MD, et al. Treatment of chronic osteomyelitis in children resistant to previous therapy. J Pediatr Orthop 2004; 24:109–22.
31. Eralp L, Kocaoglu M, Rashid H. Reconstruction of segmental bone defects due to chronic osteomyelitis with use of external fixator and an intramedullary nail. Surgical technique. J Bone Joint Surg 2006; 88A:2137–45.
32. Legré R, Samson P, Tomel F, et al. Treatment of substance loss of the bones of the leg in traumatology by transfer of free vascularized iliac crest. Apropos of 13 cases. Rev Chir Orthop Reparatr App Mot 1998; 84:264–71.
33. Theos C, Koulourvaris P, Kottakis S, et al. Reconstruction of tibia defects by ipsilateral vascularized fibula transposition. Arch Orthop Trauma Surg 2008; 128:179–84.
34. Gledhill RB. Subacute osteomyelitis in children. Clin Orthop Rel Res 1973; 96:57–69.
35. Roberts JM, Drummond DS, Breed AL, et al. Subacute hematogenous osteomyelitis in children. A retrospective study. J Pediatr Orthop1982; 2:249–54.
36. Ross ER, Cole WG. Treatment of subacute osteomyelitis in childhood. J Bone Joint Surg 1985; 67B:443–8.

37. Hoover KB, Rosenthal DI, Mankin H. Langerhans cell histiocytosis. Skelet Radiol 2007; 36:95–104.
38. Lindenbaum S, Alexander H. Infections simulating bone tumors. Clin Orthop Rel Res 1984; 184:193–203.
39. Rasool MN. Primary subacute hematogenous osteomyelitis in children. J Bone Joint Surg 2001; 83B:93–8.
40. Gonzalez-Lopez JL, Soleto-Martin FJ, Cubillo-Martin A, et al. Subacute osteomyelitis in children. J Pediatr Orthop (part B) 2001; 10:101–4.
41. Ezra E, Cohen N, Segev E, et al. Primary subacute epiphyseal osteomyelitis: role of conservative treatment. J Pediatr Orthop 2002; 22:333–7.
42. Hamdy R C, Lawton L, Carey T, et al. Subacute hematogenous osteomyelitis: are biopsy and surgery always indicated? J Pediatr Orthop 1996; 16:220–3.
43. Hammond P, Macnicol MF. Osteomyelitis of the pelvis and proximal femur; diagnostic difficulties. J Pediatr Orthop (part B) 2001; 10:113–9.
44. McPhee E, Eskander JP, Skander MS, et al. Imaging in pelvic osteomyelitis. Support for early magnetic resonance imaging. J Pediatr Orthop 2007; 27:903–9.
45. Wenger DR, Bobechko WP, Gilday DL. The spectrum of intervertebral disc-space infection in children. J Bone Joint Surg 1978; 60A:100–8.
46. Brown R, Hussain M, McHugh K, et al. Discitis in young children: J Bone Joint Surg 2001; 83B:106–11.
47. Garron E, Viehweger E, Launay F, et al. Nontuberculous spondylodiscitis in children. J Pediatr Orthop 2002; 22:321–8.
48. Jacobs RF, McCarthy RE, Elser JM. Pseudomonas osteochondritis complicating puncture wounds of the foot in children: a 10-year evaluation. Infect Dis 1989; 160:657–61.
49. Jarvis JG, Skipper J. Pseudomonas osteochondritis complicating puncture wounds in children. J Pediatr Orthop 1994; 14:755–9.
50. Gideon A, Holtusen W, Masel LF, et al. Subacute and chronic "symmetrical" osteomyelitis. Ann Radiol (Paris) 1972; 15:329–42.
51. Solheim LF, Paus B, Liverud R, et al. Chronic recurrent multifocal osteomyelitis. A new clinical-radiological syndrome. Acta Orthop Scand 1980; 51:37–41.
52. Norden C, Gillespie WJ, Nade S. Conditions that mimic osteomyelitis. In: Infections in Bones and Joints. Malden, MA: Blackwell Science; 1994:274–81.
53. Jurik AG, Egund N. MRI in chronic recurrent multifocal osteomyelitis. Skel Radiol 1997; 26:230–8.
54. Gamble JG, Rinsky LA. Chronic recurrent multifocal osteomyelitis: a distinct clinical entity. J Pediatr Orthop 1986; 6:579–84.
55. El Shanti HI, Ferguson PJ. Chronic recurrent multifocal osteomyelitis. Clin Orthop Rel Res 2007; 462:11–9.
56. Gierschick HJ, Raab P, Surbaum S, et al. Chronic non-bacterial osteomyelitis in children. Ann Rheum Dis 2005; 64:279–85.
57. Abril JC, Ramirez A. Successful treatment of chronic recurrent multifocal osteomyelitis with indomethacin. J Pediatr Orthop 2007; 27:587–91.
58. Couture A, Baud C, Ferran JL. Echographie de la hanche chez l'enfant. Montpellier: Axone; 1988:145–60.
59. Parsch, K, Savvidis E. Die Koxitis beim Neugeborenen und Säugling. Orthopäde 1997; 26:838–47.
60. Choi IH, Pizzutillo PD, Bowen JR, et al. Sequelae and reconstruction after septic arthritis of the hip in infants. J Bone Joint Surg 1990; 72A:1150–65.
61. Choi IH, Shin YW, Chung CY, et al. Surgical treatment of the severe sequelae of infantile septic arthritis of the hip. Clin Orthop Rel Res 2005; 434:102–9.
62. Dobbs MB, Sheridan JJ, Gordon JE, et al. Septic arthritis of the hip in infancy: long-term follow-up. J Pediatr Orthop 2003; 23:162–8.
63. Wang EB, Ji SJ, Zhao Q, et al. Treatment of severe sequelae of infantile hip sepsis with trochanteric arthroplasty. J Pediatr Orthop 2007; 27:165–70.
64. Rozbruch SR, Paley D, Bhave A, et al. Ilizarov hip reconstruction for the late sequelae of infantile hip infection. J Bone Joint Surg 2005; 87A:1007–18.
65. Strong M, Lejman T, Michno P. Sequelae from septic arthritis of the knee during the first two years of life. J Pediatr Orthop 1994; 14:745–51.
66. Bos CF, Mol LJ, Obermann WR, et al. Late sequelae of neonatal septic arthritis of the shoulder. J Bone Joint Surg 1998; 80B: 645–50.
67. Saisu T, Kawashima A, Kamegaya M. Humeral shortening and inferior subluxation as sequelae of septic arthritis of the shoulder in neonates and infants. J Bone Joint Surg 2007; 89A:1784–93.
68. Kocher MS, Zurakowski D, Kasser JR. Differentiation between septic arthritis and transient synovitis of the hip in children: an evidence-based clinical prediction algorithm. J Bone Joint Surg 1999; 81A:1662–70.
69. Kocher MS, Mandiga R, Murphy JM, et al. A clinical practice guideline for treatment of septic arthritis in children. J Bone Joint Surg 2003; 85A:994–9.
70. Zieger M, Doerr U, Schulz R. Ultrasonography of hip joint effusions. Skeletal Radiol 1987; 6:607–11.
71. Chung WK, Slater GL, Bates EH. Treatment of septic arthritis of the hip by arthroscopic lavage. J Pediatr Orthop 1993; 13:444–6.
72. Kim SJ, Choi NH, Ko SH, et al. Arthroscopic treatment of septic arthritis of the hip. Clin Orthop Rel Res 2003; 407:211–4.
73. Nunn TR, Cheung WY, Rollinson PD. A prospective study of pyogenic sepsis of the hip in childhood. J Bone Joint Surg 2007; 89B:100–6.

Chapter 11

Skeletal Tuberculosis

Kenneth C. Rankin and Surendar M. Tuli

Osteoarticular Tuberculosis

Epidemiology and Prevalence

Tuberculous bacilli have lived in symbiosis with mankind since time immemorial. At present there are nearly 30 million people suffering from tuberculosis worldwide, and of these 1–3% have involvement of the skeletal system. Tuberculosis will exist for as long as there are pockets of malnutrition, poor sanitation, and overcrowding.

The advent of the HIV/AIDS pandemic has greatly increased the incidence of tuberculosis, therefore many more cases of skeletal tuberculosis can also be expected.

Tuberculosis is easily spread in conditions of malnutrition, overcrowding, and poor sanitation. Worldwide, the incidence of people living in informal settlements has increased, with an inevitable increase in tuberculosis. The source of spread is the infected person with open pulmonary tuberculosis who is sputum positive. One cough can produce 3000 droplet nuclei, which can stay in the air for a long time, especially in indoor conditions with poor ventilation. Three factors determine a child's risk of contracting the infection: the concentration of droplet nuclei in the air, the duration of his breathing the air, and his immunity status.

Regional Distribution

Vertebral tuberculosis is the most common form of skeletal tuberculosis, accounting for 50% of all cases in reported series [1]. Studies in addition to clinical experience have confirmed these figures. The major areas of predilection are the spine (50%), hip (25%), and knee (10%). Other areas of predilection include the elbow, hand, shoulder, ankle, bursal sheaths, and other sites.

Prophylaxis Against Tuberculosis

Vaccination programs using the Bacillus Calmette-Guerin (BCG) have been established where the disease is prevalent. At the present time vaccination at birth is carried out in Africa and Asia. The practice of universal vaccination has now been discontinued in Europe, North America, and Australia. A policy of selective vaccination using BCG is employed in many countries as follows:

- neonates and children who are likely to travel to or live in countries where tuberculosis is common;
- newborn babies if either parent has leprosy and
- children and adults who have been in contact with tuberculosis and remain Mantoux-negative 3 months after last contact.

In Australia:

- newborn Aboriginal and Torres Strait Islander babies in areas where tuberculosis is prevalent.

Situations in which BCG vaccination may be considered:

- healthcare workers in frequent contact with patients with tuberculosis, especially multidrug-resistant tuberculosis;
- adults who will spend prolonged periods in countries where tuberculosis is common;
- newborn babies living in households where they may be exposed to migrants or visitors from overseas countries with high tuberculosis rates; and
- children under 16 years who are in contact with a patient suffering from tuberculosis where the infection is resistant to treatment or where the child cannot take prophylactic antituberculous treatment.

There is an added difficulty: countries with a high incidence of social deprivation, overcrowding, and malnutrition

K.C. Rankin (✉)
Department of Orthopaedic Surgery, Rob Ferreria Provincial Hospital, Nelspruit, Mpumalanga, South Africa

M. Benson et al. (eds.), *Children's Orthopaedics and Fractures*,
DOI 10.1007/978-1-84882-611-3_11, © Springer-Verlag London Limited 2010

are those in which high rates of vaccination are difficult to achieve. Social unrest, wars, and refugee situations disrupt prevention programs and also lead to a high percentage of unvaccinated children and young people, thus adding to the possibility of infection.

Complications of Vaccination

There is an incidence of 1–2% of complications [2]. This is usually inflammation at the vaccination site with a possible rash and low-grade fever. A number of these children will develop tuberculous osteitis [3]. Fortunately, these patients respond favorably to modern anti-tubercular drugs.

Chemoprophylaxis (using isoniazid with ethambutol) in addition to vaccination is appropriate for infants and children in contact with an infected mother or attendants.

Pathology and Pathogenesis

An osteoarticular tubercular lesion results from hematogenous dissemination from a primarily infected focus that may be active or quiescent, apparently latent, and in the lungs, lymph glands, or other viscera. Prior to the present era of human immunodeficiency virus (HIV) and acquired immunodeficiency syndrome (AIDS), most patients did not have a concomitant active focus in the lung; however, it is now common for this to occur in the HIV-positive patient or in children (Fig.11.1).

The infection reaches the skeleton through vascular channels, generally the arteries, as a result of bacteremia or, rarely, in the axial skeleton through Batson's plexus of veins. Simultaneous involvement of the paradiscal parts of contiguous vertebrae in a typical spinal tuberculous lesion

lends support to the concept that the bacilli are blood-borne. 20% of patients at routine investigation reveal tuberculous involvement of the viscera, lymph nodes, or parts of the skeletal system, suggesting spread of infection through the arterial blood supply. Development of clinical tuberculosis of the skeletal system is a reflection of weakened immune status.

Immunopathogenesis as a Result of HIV Infection

The helper subset of T lymphocytes is central to cell-mediated immunity against tuberculous infection. These cells carry the CD4 antigen on their surface (CD4$^+$ lymphocytes). HIV enters and infects CD4$^+$ lymphocytes, kills these cells, and progressively leads to a decline in the immunity of the host (see Chap. 9).

Experimental Tuberculosis

Hodgson et al. [4] tried to produce spinal tuberculosis in animals by a variety of methods. The only technique that was successful was injection of bacilli into the kidney, prostate, and other abdominal and pelvic organs. This observation suggests that infection may spread directly from visceral foci to the vertebral column through the paravertebral veins.

Chronic osseous lesions were induced consistently in 8 to 10-week-old unvaccinated guinea pigs by the insertion of Gelfoam impregnated with *Mycobacterium tuberculosis* into the metaphyseal region through a drill hole in the distal part of the femur [5]. Localized tissue necrosis and prolonged contact between the bacilli and the damaged bone markedly increased the likelihood of osteomyelitis.

Osteoarticular Disease

Tubercular bacilli reach the joint space via the blood stream through subsynovial vessels, or indirectly from epiphyseal lesions that erode into the joint space. Destruction of the articular cartilage begins peripherally. Since the weight-bearing surfaces are preserved for a few months, there is potential for good functional recovery with effective treatment.

The disease may start in bone or in the synovial membrane, but the one rapidly infects the other. The initial focus starts in the metaphysis in childhood or at the end of the bone in adults. The typical osseous areas of predilection for hip disease are shown in Fig. 11.2.

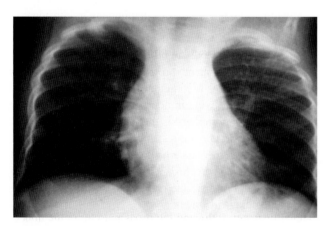

Fig. 11.1 Chest radiograph in a child showing active tuberculosis. This child also developed newly diagnosed spinal tuberculosis

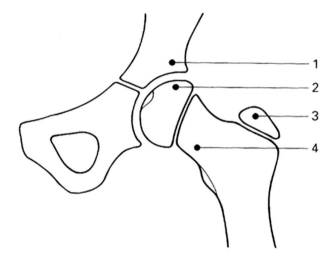

Fig. 11.2 Tuberculous foci that may involve the hip joint. (1) Acetabulum, (2) femoral head/epiphysis, (3) greater trochanter, (4) femoral neck/metaphysis

Radiologically, there is local destruction and marked demineralization. In bones with superficial cortical surfaces (such as metacarpals, metatarsals, phalanges, tibia, and ulna), the lesions may produce reactive subperiosteal new bone formation surrounding lytic areas.

Cartilaginous tissue is resistant to tuberculous destruction. However, penetration of the epiphyseal cartilage plate occurs predominantly in tuberculous disease, rather than in pyogenic infection. Metaphyseal tuberculous lesions may infect the neighboring joint through the subperiosteal space, through the capsule, or through destruction of the epiphyseal plate. Once the tuberculous process has reached the subchondral region, the articular cartilage loses its nutrition and attachment to the bone and may lie free in the joint cavity. Damage to the physis in childhood may result in shortening or angulation of the limb.

When infection starts as tuberculous synovitis, the course is usually slow. The synovial membrane becomes swollen and congested, and an effusion develops. The granulation tissue from the synovium extends over the bone at the synovial reflections, producing erosions. At the periphery of the articular cartilage, granulation tissue forms a pannus that erodes the margins and surface of the joint. Flakes or loose sheets of necrotic articular cartilage and accumulations of fibrinous material in the synovial fluid may produce the *rice bodies* found in synovial joints, tendon sheaths, and bursae. Where articular surfaces are in contact, the cartilage is preserved for a long time because the spread of the pannus is retarded. Necrosis of subchondral bone by the ingrowth of tuberculous granulation tissue produces *kissing lesions* or sequestra on either side of the joint.

The Tubercle

The initial response to infection is in the reticulo-endothelial system. Polymorphonuclear cells accumulate and are rapidly replaced by macrophages and mononuclear cells, both highly phagocytic. The tubercle bacilli are phagocytosed and broken down. Their lipid is dispersed throughout the cytoplasm of the mononuclear cells, thus transforming them into epithelioid cells, characteristic of the tuberculous reaction. These are large, pale cells with a vesicular nucleus, abundant cytoplasm, and indistinct margins and processes, which form an epithelioid reticulum. Langhan's giant cells are probably formed by fusion of a number of epithelioid cells. These are produced only if caseation necrosis has occurred in the lesion and usually contain tubercle bacilli. Their main function is to digest and remove necrosed tissue.

After about 1 week, lymphocytes appear and form a ring around the peripheral part of the lesion. This mass, formed by the reactive cells of the reticulo-endothelial tissues, constitutes a (1–2 mm) nodule popularly known as the tubercle. Tubercles grow by expansion and coalescence. During the second week, in untreated cases, caseation occurs in the center of the tubercle. This coagulation necrosis is caused by the protein fraction of tubercle bacilli. The caseous material may soften and liquefy, and this caseation necrosis (*soft tubercle*) is almost diagnostic of tuberculous pathology or tuberculoid leprosy.

Cold Abscess

A marked, exudative reaction is common in tuberculous infection of the skeletal system. A cold abscess is formed by the products of liquefaction and the reactive exudation. It is composed of serum, leukocytes, caseous material, bone debris, and tubercle bacilli. The abscess penetrates the periosteum and ligaments, and migrates or gravitates in various directions, following fascial planes and the sheaths of vessels and nerves. The cold abscess feels warm, although the temperature is not increased to the same extent as in acute pyogenic infections. A superficial abscess may burst to form a sinus or an ulcer lined with tuberculous granulation tissue. On aspiration, the contents of the cold abscess range from serous fluid to thick pus.

The commonest sites of cold abscesses are those that arise from tuberculosis of the spine in which the cold abscess may present at sites far from the vertebral column. From the lumbar spine they can form in the groin, under and below the inguinal ligament, following the psoas muscle. In the upper lumbar and lower thoracic spine they can track laterally to present in the loin.

Osseous Changes and Tubercular Sequestra

Following the infection, marked hyperemia and severe osteoporosis take place. The softened bone easily yields under the effect of gravity and muscle action, leading to compression, collapse, or deformation. Necrosis may also be caused by ischemic infarction of segments of bone.

Sequestration gives the appearance of coarse sand and rarely produces a radiologically visible sequestrum. Because of loss of nutrition, the adjacent articular cartilage or the intervening disc degenerates and may also become separated as sequestra. Some of the radiologically visible sequestra in tuberculous cavities may result from calcification of the caseous matter.

The Future Course of The Tubercle

Before the availability of anti-tubercular drugs, the 5-year follow-up mortality of patients with osteoarticular tuberculosis was about 30%. Presently available anti-tubercular drugs have changed the outlook. The 5-year mortality depends upon whether the patient is HIV positive or negative. If negative, the mortality is very low. In HIV-positive patients the mortality correlates with the immune status of the patient and whether anti-retroviral drugs are available. Depending upon the sensitivity pattern, the host resistance, and the stage of the lesion at the inception of treatment, the tuberculous lesion may

- resolve completely
- heal with residual deformity and loss of function
- be completely walled off and the caseous tissue may calcify
- persist as a low-grade, chronic, fibromatous, granulating, and caseating lesion
- spread locally by contiguity and systemically by the blood stream

The Organism

Before pasteurization, the bovine-type of bacillus was responsible for a great deal of osteoarticular tuberculosis. Most skeletal tuberculosis is now caused by bacilli of the human type. Because skeletal tuberculosis is a paucibacillary disease, positive cultures for acid-fast bacilli in osteoarticular tuberculous lesions are obtained in fewer than 50% of patients.

The best microbiological specimens appear to be those obtained from centrifuged material from an abscess, curettings from the walls of a cold abscess, or curettings from the lining of sinus tracts as close to the base (source) as possible.

Sensitivity of the Organism

There are only a few reports regarding the culture and sensitivity of tubercle bacilli isolated from osteoarticular lesions. Resistance to various drugs is as follows:

- Streptomycin 7–10%
- *para*-Amino salicylic acid 4–10%
- Isoniazid 8–20%
- Thiacetazone 5–15%
- Ethambutol 2–5%
- Rifampicin 2–3%

The development of resistant strains is minimized by multidrug therapy.

Disease Caused by Atypical Mycobacteria

The term *atypical mycobacteria* refers to mycobacteria other than *Mycobacterium tuberculosis* and *M. bovis*. Rarely, these organisms may be responsible for infective lesions in the skeletal system.

Synovial sheath infections are more common with atypical mycobacteria than infection of osseous tissues. With atypical mycobacterial infections, human-to-human transmission is uncommon. Often a history of trauma such as a puncture wound, steroid injections, surgery, or exposure to contaminated marine life is found. Many patients may have concomitant diabetes or immunodeficiency.

Diagnosis and Investigations

Skeletal tuberculosis mostly occurs during the first three decades of life. The characteristics are insidious onset, monoarticular, or single bone involvement, and the constitutional symptoms of low-grade fever, lassitude (especially in the afternoon), anorexia, loss of weight, night sweats, tachycardia, and anemia. Local symptoms and signs are pain, night cries, painful limitation of movements, muscle wasting, and regional lymph node enlargement. In the acute stage, protective muscle spasm is severe. During sleep, the muscle spasm relaxes and permits movement between the inflamed surfaces, resulting in pain and the characteristic night cries.

This pattern was typical in the era prior to the HIV/AIDS epidemic. Now it is possible for tuberculosis of bone and joint to occur at any age group, including into the fourth and fifth decades.

Patients can present with acute pain as the only major symptom of spinal tuberculosis. This may pose a difficult problem in differential diagnosis, particularly in the spine.

Despite the list of symptoms and signs it is quite common for the patient to present only with local joint symptomatology. The presenting symptoms and signs are low grade and can appear unimportant at first examination. Children can look physically well except for the involved joint.

Diagnosis

In developing countries the diagnosis of tuberculosis of bones and joints can be made reliably on clinical and radiological examination. However in affluent countries, tuberculosis, which formerly was a very rare disease, is now much more common, particularly in areas of high immigrant population. It is ideal to have positive proof of the disease by semi-invasive or invasive investigations. Skeletal tuberculosis must be included in the differential diagnosis of chronic or subacute mono-articular arthritis, chronic abscess, a draining sinus, or chronic osteomyelitis.

Confirming the Diagnosis

Biopsy is the only certain method which can be used to confirm the diagnosis. Due to the delay in obtaining results, since culture and guinea pig inoculation take a long time, histology is the quickest way to obtain the diagnosis. Even here the changes may be non-specific: in some studies the results of biopsy reveal chronic, non-specific inflammation in 50% of cases.

In continental countries with the highest incidence of tuberculosis, namely Africa and Asia, the concept of *trial of treatment* is extremely valuable.

Clinical Trial of Treatment

In countries with limited resources and poor access to histology and bacteriology, one of the best ways to confirm the diagnosis of tuberculosis is to use this empirical method.

If the clinical and radiological evidence point to tuberculosis, anti-tubercular therapy is started, combined with local measures to relieve pain, such as skin traction for hip disease or a back slab for the knee.

If tuberculosis is the cause there will be a dramatic reduction in joint pain and an increase in well-being. This can

be particularly marked in tuberculosis of the spine and may often be the only evidence available on which to base continuation of drug therapy.

In spinal cases it is particularly important since continued destruction of the vertebrae will lead to progressive deformity and paraplegia.

Radiography and Imaging

Localized osteoporosis is the first radiological sign of active disease. The articular margins and bony cortices become hazy and there may be areas of trabecular destruction and osteolysis. The synovial fluid, thickened synovium, capsule, and pericapsular tissues produce soft tissue swelling, and the joint space narrows. As the destructive process advances, bone architecture collapses and joints deform or displace. The epiphyseal growth plate may be destroyed, producing altered growth, angulation, or premature fusion. With healing of the disease process there is remineralization, reappearance of bone trabecula, and sharpening of cortical and articular margins.

In the center of a tuberculous cavity there may be a sequestrum of cancellous bone or calcification of the caseous tissue giving the appearance of an irregular, feathery nidus in a cavity.

If secondary infection supervenes, subperiosteal new bone formation can be seen along the involved bones. The subperiosteal reaction occurs much earlier in pyogenic osteomyelitis. Plaques of irregular (dystrophic) calcification in the wall of a chronic abscess or sinus are almost diagnostic of long-standing tuberculous infection.

Isotope bone scanning and magnetic resonance imaging (MRI) demonstrate the localization and extent of bone and soft tissue lesions (Fig. 11.3), and improve diagnosis of the disease at a very early stage (3–6 weeks).

MRI scanning in the earliest stages reveals inflammation and not infection, just as radioisotope scintigraphy may show a hot area during the active stage of the disease. However, it is neither specific nor does it differentiate between the osseous and soft tissue pathology. The feathery tubercular sequestra and dystrophic calcification are discernible on CT scans, but cannot be seen by MRI.

Blood

A relative lymphocytosis, low hemoglobin, and increased erythrocyte sedimentation rate (ESR) are typically found in the active stage of the disease. A raised ESR, however, is not necessarily proof of activity of the infection. Its repeated estimation at monthly intervals gives a valuable index of the activity of the disease.

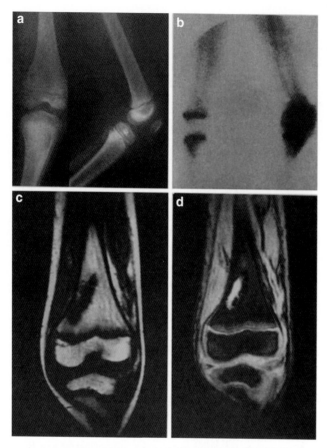

by lymphocytes, even without central necrosis or peripheral foreign body giant cells, is adequate histological evidence of tuberculous pathology in a patient who is suspected to be suffering from the disease. At the time of open biopsy of a joint or bone, the orthopaedic surgeon should perform therapeutic synovectomy or curettage.

The infections of bone and joint that present as granulomatous lesions are, in order of frequency, as follows: tuberculosis, mycotic infection, brucellosis, sarcoidosis, and tuberculoid leprosy.

Guinea Pig Inoculation

The tuberculous pus, joint aspirate, or diseased material obtained at biopsy is injected intraperitoneally into a guinea pig. Examination in positive cases discloses tubercles on the peritoneum 5–8 weeks later. Although no longer considered a cost-effective test, this is perhaps the most reliable proof of tuberculous pathology.

Smear and Culture

The material prepared for guinea pig inoculation may also be submitted for smear and culture examination for acid-fast bacilli.

Fig. 11.3 (**a**) Anteroposterior and lateral radiographs of the distal end of the femur, showing a lytic lesion in the metaphysis. (**b**) An isotope bone scan reveals a hot area in the distal part of the thigh and knee, attributable to localized hyperemia associated with active disease. (**c**) MRI T1-weighted and (**d**) T2-weighted images show that the extent of the disease is greater than suggested radiographically. Histology confirmed the diagnosis of tuberculosis and the disease responded to multidrug treatment

Management of Osteoarticular Tuberculosis

General Principles

Modern drugs (see Table 11.1) promote the healing of sinuses, ulcers, and abscesses previously resistant to extensive surgery. They also eliminate the danger of postoperative miliary and meningeal disease caused by dissemination of the tuberculous infection.

Death as a result of uncontrolled disease, meningitis, miliary tuberculosis, amyloidosis, paralysis, and crippling is now rare in the HIV-negative patient. In those treated early and vigorously joint deformity and ankylosis can be avoided.

In the current HIV epidemic the outlook of patients with tuberculosis who are HIV positive has changed the previous results. Clinical experience has shown that the antitubercular drugs will control the disease for a certain period. If the patient then receives anti-retroviral drugs they may recover from the tuberculosis and enjoy a longer survival. However in many cases the inexorable advance of the HIV infection will not allow long-term survival.

Mantoux Test

As a rule, a positive result on Mantoux testing is present in a patient infected with tuberculosis for more than 1 month. A negative test, in general, excludes the disease. Rarely, the tuberculin test may be negative although active tuberculosis is present, such as in immune deficiency states.

Biopsy

Whenever there is doubt (particularly in the early stages), it is mandatory to prove the diagnosis of tuberculosis by biopsy of the diseased tissue (granulations, synovium, bone, lymph nodes, or the margins of tuberculous ulcers or sinuses). Microscopic examination of an aspiration, core biopsy, needle biopsy, or open biopsy will reveal typical tubercles in untreated cases. The presence of epithelioid cells surrounded

Table 11.1 Commonly prescribed anti-tubercular drugs and their toxicity

Drug	Daily dose and administration	Minimum inhibitory concentration (μg/ml for human mycobacteria)	Main drug toxicity
Streptomycin[a]	20 mg/kg twice/thrice a week (maximum 750 mg)	1–2	Vestibular damage, deafness, fever, rashes, contact dermatitis, nephrotoxicity
Isoniazid[b]	10–20 mg/kg in single/two divided doses	0.1–0.2	Peripheral neuropathy, behavior disorders, convulsions, hepatitis, hypersensitivity
Ethambutol[c]	15–25 mg/kg in single/two divided doses	1–3	Retrobulbar neuritis with loss of vision, preceded by diminution of visual field and acuity, and color blindness
Rifampicin	10–20 mg/kg in single/two divided doses	0.25–1.0	Pinkish staining of urine, sweat and saliva, liver damage, bowel upset, rashes, flu-like symptoms (purpura rarely)
para-Amino salicylic acid	200–400 mg/kg in single/two divided doses	1	Gastrointestinal disturbances, rashes, fever, lymphadenopathy, hepatotoxicity
Thioacetazone[a,d]	3–5 mg/kg single dose	1	Anorexia, nausea, vomiting, liver damage, marrow depression
Ethionamide/ prothionamide	10–20 mg/kg in single/two divided doses	10–20	Gastrointestinal upsets, abnormal liver tests, peripheral neuritis, convulsions, drowsiness
Pyrazinamide	25–30 mg/kg single dose	10–20	Hepatotoxicity, gouty arthritis (hyperuricemic arthralgia)
Cycloserine	15–20 mg/kg in single/two divided doses	5–10	Brain damage, mental disturbances, epilepsy
Capreomycin[a]	15 mg/kg single dose (maximum 750 mg)	2	Nephrotoxicity, others like streptomycin, eighth nerve damage
Kanamycin[a]	15 mg/kg single dose	8–16	Auditory toxicity, nephrotoxicity

[a]To be injected intramuscularly.

[b]Isoniazid must form part of any multidrug therapy. In skeletal tuberculosis there is no osseous barrier or gradient to the penetration of drugs. Avoid more than one hepatotoxic drug in patients in whom surgical intervention is anticipated.

[c]Avoid the use of ethambutol in children younger than 6 years because of possible visual disturbance, which is difficult to assess in the younger child.

[d]Thioacetazone is contraindicated in HIV-positive patients because of the risk of severe skin reactions.

With the use of modern drugs, the indications for surgery have become universally more selective and directed toward the prevention and correction of deformities and the improvement in function of the diseased joints [5, 6]. There is a limited role for excision arthroplasty at the hip and elbow. At the stage of tuberculous arthritis, if the disease remains closed, the natural outcome is generally a fibrous ankylosis. If an abscess discharges and sinuses develop, the outcome may be a bony ankylosis. The prognosis in articular tuberculosis depends upon the stage of the disease when the specific treatment is started (see Table 11.2).

Concomitant disease must be treated. Associated pulmonary involvement is important to recognize (Fig. 11.1). Admission to hospital is necessary only for complications or for those requiring traction under supervision to correct deformities.

Rest, Mobilization, and Bracing

In the treatment of cranio-vertebral, cervical, and cervicothoracic lesions, traction is used in the early stages to rest the diseased part, particularly for those with a neurological deficit and pathological dislocation. In the active stage of the disease, the joints are rested in the position of function by means of removable splints. Prolonged immobilization may lead to spontaneous ankylosis, especially when large joints are destroyed. Patients with early disease are allowed 1-hourly intermittent, guarded active, and assisted exercises under anti-tubercular drug cover, with the aim of retaining a useful range of movement in the functional arc of the involved joint. Traction helps to correct deformity and to rest the diseased part. Gradual mobilization is encouraged, with the help of suitable braces, approximately 3 months after the

Table 11.2 Staging of articular tuberculosis, its suggested management, and the outcome in children

Stages	Clinical	Radiology	Usual effective treatment	Expectation
I Synovitis	Movement present (>75%)	Soft tissue swelling, osteoporosis	Chemotherapy and movement. Rarely synovectomy	Retention of near full mobility
II Early arthritis	Movement present (50–75%)	In addition to I, moderate diminution of joint space and marginal erosion	Chemotherapy and movement. Rarely synovectomy or debridement	Restoration of 50–75% of mobility. Ankylosis
III Advanced arthritis	Loss of movement (<75%) in all directions	In addition to II, marked diminution of joint space and destruction of joint surfaces	Chemotherapy, rarely joint debridement	Ankylosis[a]
IV Advanced arthritis with pathological dislocation/subluxation	Loss of movement (>75%) in all directions	In addition to III, joint is disorganized with dislocation/subluxation	Chemotherapy, rarely joint debridement	Ankylosis[a]

[a]After completion of skeletal growth, elbow and hip arthritis may be treated by excision arthroplasty.

start of treatment, while the healing is progressing. As the disease heals and pain subsides, weight bearing and activity are permitted. If symptoms or signs increase, the patient goes back a stage. If there is steady progress, activity is increased within the limits of discomfort. Bracing is gradually discarded after about 2 years although in most cases this period is much shorter.

Treatment of Abscess, Effusion, and Sinus

Aspiration is the method of choice for large collections. Removal of liquid pus by this method avoids the risk of sinus formation although in the present era of anti-tubercular therapy this risk is much less.

Aspiration is particularly useful in draining large collections in inaccessible areas, such as a psoas abscesses. This can be carried out under ultrasound guidance. Avoiding open operation is even more important in the HIV-positive patient.

Open drainage of an abscess is indicated if aspiration fails. Radiologically visible paravertebral abscess shadows do not require drainage unless decompression is performed for paraplegia or when diseased vertebrae are debrided. A prevertebral abscess in the cervical region is drained if it causes difficulty in swallowing or breathing. Drainage of a large paravertebral abscess may also be considered when its radiological size increases markedly inspite of treatment.

The large majority of ulcers and sinuses heal within 6–12 weeks under the influence of systemic antituberculous drugs. The full course of treatment is still necessary. Fewer than 1% of sinuses require longer treatment and excision of the tract, with or without debridement. Sinus ramification is always greater than can be appreciated, and complete surgical excision is therefore impracticable.

Final End Result

For many patients with advanced disease on diagnosis the ultimate outcome will be poor, the best result in a destroyed joint being an ankylosis in the position of function.

When only one joint is involved the disability may not be great. With more than one joint involved the impact may be significant (Fig. 11.4). This girl of 12 suffered from tuberculosis of both hips many years previously. The resulting bony ankylosis in both hips, although in neutral position, is a grave handicap especially if joint replacement is not available (as in much of the developing world).

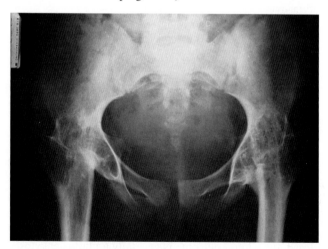

Fig. 11.4 A 12-year-old girl who contracted tuberculosis of the hips many years previously. The end result is bony ankylosis of both hips in extension

Anti-Tubercular Drugs

The commonly used drugs and dosages have been summarized in Table 11.1. Drug regimens conform to World Heath

Organization guidelines. Anti-tubercular drugs now fall into two groups.

First-Line Drugs

First-line drugs are isoniazid, rifampicin, pyrazinamide, and ethambutol. In some countries streptomycin is added but this is generally not used as a first-line drug.

In the intensive phase, which lasts for 2 months, all four drugs are given in a combination tablet. The dose must be worked out according to the age and weight. In the maintenance phase, which lasts for 4 months, two are given. These are usually rifampicin and isoniazid.

These are used in new cases of tuberculosis, in pulmonary cases which are sputum positive or negative, and in tuberculous meningitis.

New cases of bone and joint tuberculosis follow the same drug routine as that for pulmonary cases. It is common practice to extend the length of treatment for up to 9 months on the basis that disease in bone and joint takes longer to heal [7].

In all cases in which first-line drugs are used there is an intensive phase of 2 months followed by a maintenance phase of 4 months.

There are slight differences in the drug regimens for those children who are sputum-negative or for whom the drugs are given because of close contact with known cases of pulmonary disease, usually in the same family. These aspects obviously do not apply to bone and joint cases.

Second-Line Drugs

Cases of recurrent or incompletely treated tuberculosis, failure to complete courses, or gaps in treatment are treated with second-line drugs. These regimens fall into the category of the treatment of multidrug-resistant tuberculosis.

There is a further category of patients who are classed as extreme drug-resistant cases. This group of patients has already undergone several courses of treatment, often with gaps or inconstant therapy. The management of these patients now involves very complex drug regimens. These are almost entirely pulmonary cases and these drug therapies will not be dealt with here.

The combination is of five drugs, which include two of the first-line group, i.e., pyrazinamide and ethambutol. The further three are kanamycin, ethionamide, and ofloxacin. There is again an intensive and a maintenance phase. The maintenance phase consists of ethambutol, ethionamide, and ofloxacin.

However, the treatment regimes for multidrug-resistant disease include a large range of drugs which are used in various combinations which vary between different countries.

In addition to those above, the present list of drugs used as second line in multidrug-resistant disease includes fluoroquinolones (ofloxacin, levofloxacin, moxifloxacin, and gatifloxacin) and aminoglycosides (kanamycin, amikacin, and capreomycin). Isolated drugs include cycloserine and *para*-amino salicylic acid.

Toxicity

All drugs for first and second-line treatment have toxicity and side effects. These are more marked and serious in the second-line drugs, many of which have to be given daily or thrice weekly. It therefore becomes more difficult for patients to continue the full treatment course. Detaining patients in hospital for these regimens is now impossible so the majority have to be treated in the community.

Anti-tubercular drugs are the most important therapeutic measure in skeletal tuberculosis, speeding recovery and minimizing the incidence of complications, recrudescence, and death. Patients with early disease, sensitive organisms, and a favorable pathological lesion (absence of large cavitations, ischemic tissue, and infarcted bone) achieve full clinical healing without recourse to surgery. Osseous tubercular lesions are slower to heal than synovial lesions. After prolonged anti-tubercular therapy the histological appearance ceases to be characteristic. The epithelioid cells become less compact and the tubercle is unrecognizable, because both the epithelioid cells and lymphocytes are widely scattered. Central caseation may disappear, but fibrosis remains a significant feature in advanced tuberculous disease.

Multidrug-Resistant Cases

Six months after receiving multidrug treatment, some patients (5–10%) do not show a healing response. The destructive process increases, and sinuses and ulcers continue to discharge. Some patients develop additional, active tuberculous lesions and operative wounds do not heal despite therapy. These patients then fall into the category of multidrug-resistant cases. Their drug management follows the guidelines described.

Surgery in Tuberculosis of Bones and Joints

No surgery is a substitute for a correct course of anti-tubercular drugs. A trial of conservative treatment is usually adequate in pure synovial tuberculosis, low-grade or early arthritis of any joint, and even advanced (Table 11.2 stage III or IV) arthritis, especially in the upper extremity.

Surgery should be considered only when the general condition of the patient has been stabilized by drug treatment, before the development of drug resistance. In general, a minimum of 1–4 weeks of drug therapy is advisable before any major surgical intervention.

Extent and Type of Surgery

Fusion of a major joint (except in the spine) is seldom indicated as primary treatment during childhood. Juxta-articular osteotomy, soft tissue release, synovectomy, and debridement should produce mobile, stable joints. If a juxta-articular osseous focus is threatening the joint despite adequate antitubercular drugs, excisional surgery of the focus should be performed. Non-responsive cases of tubercular synovitis and early arthritis respond to subtotal synovectomy and synovectomy combined with joint debridement, respectively. At any stage of the disease, if a lesion is proving resistant or the diagnosis is in doubt, operation is mandatory. Debridement should be limited to infected synovium, sequestra, cavities of pus, and sinuses. Repetitive active and assisted movements of the joint should preserve a functional arc of movement after the operation.

In advanced arthritis of the knee, ankle, wrist, hip, and elbow, the *position of function* is achieved by operative debridement followed by splintage for 3–6 months. If the disease has healed leaving a painless range of movement (20° or more) in an unacceptable position, a juxta-articular osteotomy may be performed to yield the best functional arc. Osteotomy may also be indicated to correct varus or valgus deformity particularly in the hip. If the growth plates of the involved joint are open, surgical arthrodesis should be deferred until the child is older than 12 years.

Relapse or Recurrence of Complications

The incidence of relapse or recurrence is unknown, because these complications may occur at any period during the lifetime of a patient, whether the initial treatment included excisional surgery or not. Reactivation may occur as late as 20 years or more after apparent healing, perhaps in 2–5% of patients.

The causes of reactivation include prolonged use of systemic cortisone therapy, malnutrition, the development of diabetes or an immune deficiency state, and any surgical procedure or injury to the previously infected area. Dormant bacilli, persisting in the tissues for years, may start to multiply under such circumstances. The reduction in immunity with advancing age also predisposes those with an old tubercular lesion to reactivation.

Final Result of Untreated Disease

In the past, without the use of antituberculous drugs the final result would be a bony ankylosis. This was considered a satisfactory result if it occurred at one joint in a functional position. Occasionally two joints would be affected in this way (see Fig. 11.4). In this case the young girl had both hips involved at the age of 12, as the radiograph showed, and was seriously disabled, in the era prior to total joint replacement.

Tuberculosis of the Spine

The intervertebral disc is not involved in spinal tuberculosis primarily because it is a relatively avascular structure. However, involvement of the paradiscal regions of vertebrae by the tuberculous process jeopardizes disc nutrition, allowing it to be invaded by the adjacent infectious process. The cartilaginous endplate is a partial barrier but, once it has been transgressed, destruction of the disc progresses rapidly. Radiological narrowing of the disc space may also be a result of the disc breaking through the paradiscal margins of the diseased and softened vertebral endplates.

The tuberculous abscess may be compressed between the sound vertebrae above and below, resulting in lateral extension, propulsion, and retropulsion into the extradural space. The tuberculous process may also spread by osteoperiosteal infiltration, thus destroying distant parts of the vertebral column. Pressure on neural structures is more likely in the thoracic spine, where the caliber of the vertebral canal is relatively small.

Clinical Features

Vertebral tuberculosis accounts for 50% of all cases of skeletal tuberculosis. In developing countries, the disease starts before the age of 16 years in nearly 40% of cases. Fully developed disease is not unusual in infancy.

Symptoms and Signs

The usual clinical symptoms are malaise, loss of weight, anorexia, night sweats, night pain, and an evening increase in temperature. The spine is stiff, painful on movement, and may develop a localized, tender kyphotic deformity. A small kyphosis is the earliest clinical sign of vertebral disease (Fig. 11.5).

Vertebral muscle spasm and a cold abscess may be present clinically. Modern imaging techniques and radiological monitoring after 6–12 weeks of the onset of symptoms assist in

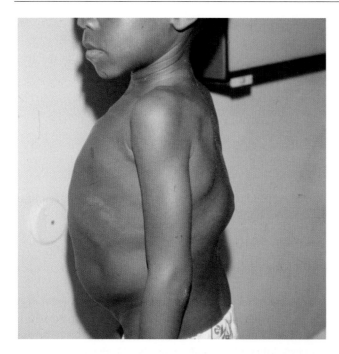

Fig. 11.5 Small kyphosis in a child with spinal tuberculosis. This is often the earliest indication of disease and may be even less obvious

and loss of the disc space (Fig. 11.6 and Table 11.3). In (Fig. 11.7) the earliest signs of tuberculosis can be seen. Such presentation is uncommon in developing countries as few children are brought in the initial stages of the disease, but early treatment with anti-tubercular drugs can result in a normal spine.

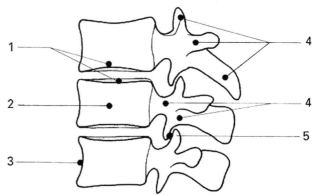

Fig. 11.6 Sites of vertebral tuberculosis. (1) Paradiscal; (2) central; (3) anterior; (4) appendiceal; (5) facet joint. Spondylodiscitis is the most common and facet joint involvement the most rare

Table 11.3 Clinical features of spinal tuberculosis (1965–1974)

Feature	Frequency (%)
Clinical kyphosis	95
Radiological perivertebral abscesses	21
Palpable cold abscesses	20
Neurological involvement	20
Tuberculous sinuses (active/healed)	13
Associated extraspinal skeletal tubercular foci	12
Associated visceral or glandular foci	12
Skip lesions in the spine	7
Lateral shift (radiological)	5

the diagnosis. Biopsy of the diseased vertebrae is not invariably informative. In most series the positive rate of detection of *M. tuberculosis* in biopsy specimens is not greater than 50% and in many instances the histological result only shows chronic fibrosis. This may be a reflection of the few tubercle bacilli in any spinal focus.

Pain referred from the spine may mimic appendicitis, cholecystitis, or renal disease. Sometimes a case of vertebral tuberculosis may present as a spinal tumor syndrome, with neural deficit. Likewise certain conditions in the spine present with clinical and radiological appearances similar to tuberculosis. These cases can progress to paraplegia and it is only from biopsy of the material removed that the true diagnosis is found.

Epidural pus formation can present with long tract signs without there being the normal stigmata of spinal tuberculosis such as a gibbus. These patients, with no bone destruction on plain radiograph, mimic the clinical pattern of various diagnoses including, in the thoracic region, thoracic disc protrusion.

With the use of MRI these cases can be detected early and can be given the opportunity of responding to drug therapy alone.

The Vertebral Lesion

In the majority of patients, typical paradiscal lesions are characterized by destruction of the adjacent vertebral endplates

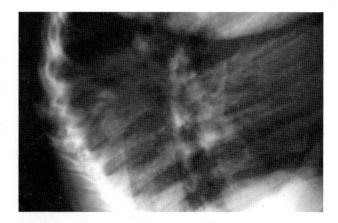

Fig. 11.7 An early radiograph of an 8-year-old child with spinal tuberculosis. The features of contiguous involvement of vertebral bodies and narrowing of the disc between is well seen

In fewer than 2% of all spinal lesions, in which the disc spaces appear to remain intact for a long time, the disease is localized elsewhere (see Fig. 11.6):

1. The anterior type (involvement of anterior surface only)
2. The posterior type (involvement of pedicles, laminae, or spinous processes)
3. The central, cystic type (a lytic lesion in the center or concentric collapse).

Rarely, the tuberculous process involves the atlanto-occipital or atlanto-axial joints or the facet joints.

Abscesses and Sinuses

Abscesses or sinuses from the cervical or thoracic regions may travel along fascial planes or neurovascular bundles to the paraspinal regions, the posterior or anterior cervical triangles, and the intercostal spaces. Abscesses from the thoracolumbar spine track down the psoas sheath to the iliac fossa, the lumbar triangle, the upper part of the thigh below the inguinal ligament, or even the knee.

Psoas abscesses can lead to pitfalls in diagnosis by producing the so-called pseudo hip flexion deformity in which there is no disease in the hip itself and there is no limitation of external or internal rotation.

Spondylodiscitis is the most common variety while facet joint involvement is the most rare (Fig. 11.6).

Psoas abscess is usually associated with tuberculosis of the vertebral column, from the tenth thoracic vertebra to the sacrum, or of the sacroiliac joint, pelvis, or hip joint. The clinical features of spinal tuberculosis have been summarized in Table 11.3.

Radiograph and MRI Appearances

Commonly two or three vertebrae are involved at the sites depicted in Fig. 11.6:

- paradiscal
- central
- anterior
- appendiceal

The appendiceal sites comprise the pedicles, laminae, facet joints, and spinous or transverse processes.

Paradiscal Type of Lesion

Narrowing of the disc is often the earliest radiological finding. Any reduction in disc space, if it is associated with a loss of definition of the paradiscal margins of the vertebrae, suggests tuberculosis and occurs before the appearance of frank osseous destruction. These changes are usually evident only after infection has been present for 3–6 months, although MRI and CAT scanning may detect changes at 6 weeks (Fig. 11.8).

Paravertebral Shadows

A paravertebral shadow is produced by extension of tuberculous granulation tissue leading to an abscess in the paravertebral region. In the cervical region it usually presents as a soft tissue shadow between the vertebral bodies posteriorly and the pharynx and trachea. An upper thoracic abscess casts a V-shaped shadow, striping the lung apices laterally and downward; when it is small, the superior mediastinum shows only squaring of its borders. Abscesses below the level of

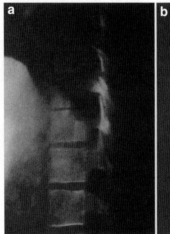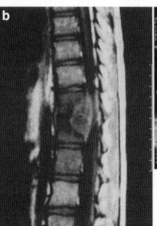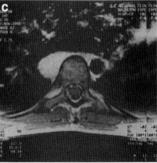

Fig. 11.8 (**a**) A 14-year-old girl was investigated for low-grade spinal pain of 3 months' duration. The radiograph revealed a diminished disc space between the 11th and 12th thoracic vertebrae. (**b**) MRI confirmed an inflammatory lesion extending into the 11th and 12th vertebral bodies. A fluid abscess can be detected in the posterior half of the vertebral bodies and in the peridural space. (**c**) An MRI T2-weighted axial view revealed an abscess connection in the paravertebral gutter

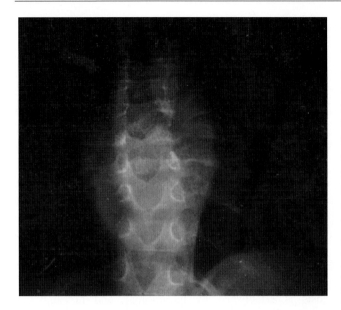

Fig. 11.9 Paravertebral fusiform shadow in mid-thoracic spinal tuberculosis

the fourth thoracic vertebra produce a typical fusiform shape (Fig. 11.9).

However, when the abscess is large, it may take the shape of a generalized broadening of the mediastinum and, if under tension, it may assume a globular shape. Collections of pus above the vertebral attachment of the diaphragm tend to remain within the thorax, whereas those arising below the diaphragm extend along the course of the psoas muscle, causing widening of its radiographic shadow.

The radiographic diagnosis of an abscess is inaccurate because much of the density may represent residual fibrous tissue or calcified and inspissated debris of granulation tissue. Tense paravertebral abscesses may show a scalloping effect (aneurysmal phenomenon) along the anterior margins of the vertebral bodies if they become chronic. Rarely, a small, thin paravertebral abscess casts no radiographic shadow.

A good lateral view of the upper thoracic spine may show anterior convexity of the tracheal shadow caused by a prevertebral abscess in the superior mediastinum. MRI usually allows the distinction to be made between paravertebral shadows cast by liquid abscess, granulations, fibrous tissue, or a combination of these.

Lateral Shift, Scoliosis, and Pathological Subluxation

These are the rare deformities of Pott's disease. Such displacements occur when the posterior spinal articulations are destroyed, in addition to the usual paradiscal lesions (panvertebral disease).

Natural Course of the Disease

When a paradiscal lesion is diagnosed early (pre-destructive stage) and treated adequately, healing may take place, leaving behind no radiological deformity or defect except a moderately diminished disc space. The disease focus may be surrounded by sclerotic bone and a normal trabecular pattern may eventually be restored (see Fig. 11.7). Sharpening of the fuzzy paradiscal margins and the reappearance and mineralization of trabecula that had earlier been absorbed are the radiological signs of healing. With the involvement of only two to three segments and associated discs there will be a noticeable kyphosis clinically (Fig. 11.5). This is a most important clinical sign which should be presumed to indicate tuberculosis and demands the start of treatment. Radiographs can be difficult to interpret but as 95% of children with a clinical kyphosis have spinal tuberculosis (see Table 11.3) it is an indication to start treatment without delay.

If several vertebral bodies are destroyed and a large gap is produced during the process of healing, repair takes place by fibrous tissue. When the disc space is completely destroyed, the gap is obliterated by telescoping of the vertebrae, leading to segmental interbody fusion. If there is delay in effective treatment, the vertebral bodies are collapsed, growth plates are destroyed, and healing takes place with varying degrees of deformity. There can be extensive deformity involving many levels, without the development of paraplegia (see Fig. 11.10).

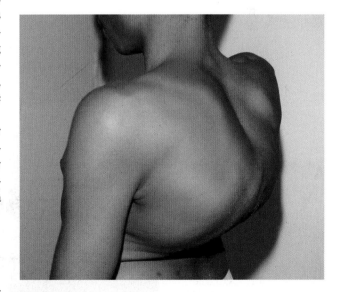

Fig. 11.10 Very large kyphosis in an adult male. The patient was not paraplegic and had involvement of many vertebral segments. Correction of the deformity is possible but only with very great risk to the spinal cord

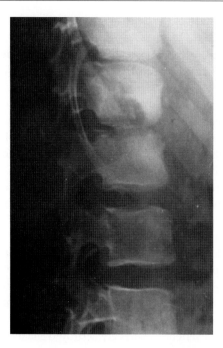

Fig. 11.11 Lateral radiograph showing destruction of at least three vertebral bodies and the development of a kyphosis. This child (the same as Figs. 11.1 and 11.7) had no neurological involvement

Untreated disease invariably leads to more destruction and carries the risk of paraplegia (Fig. 11.11). This may recover on anti-tubercular drugs alone but, in countries with poor resources and late detection, can lead to the tragedy of paraplegia which is irreversible if drugs are unavailable or surgery unlikely (Fig. 11.12).

Differential Diagnosis

In young children, congenital defects of the spine, which generally produce kyphoscoliosis, should be considered. In adolescence, Scheuermann's disease produces no constitutional symptoms but causes an increase in the thoracic kyphosis. The lateral radiograph will show signs of anterior vertebral wedging with irregularities of vertebral end plates.

In acute spinal pyogenic osteomyelitis (spondylitis), the onset is sudden, with severe localized pain, spasm, and a swinging pyrexia. In the early stages there is destruction of bone, rapidly superseded by bony sclerosis and new bone formation. Low-grade pyogenic infection and spondylitis caused by typhoid fever, brucellosis, fungal infection, and syphilis produce an insidious clinical course and radiological features resembling tuberculosis. The diagnosis is established by bacteriology and histology of the diseased tissues, agglutination tests, and therapeutic trials.

Neoplasms are unusual; hemangioma, aneurysmal bone cyst, and histiocytosis X should be considered. Ewing's sarcoma and osteosarcoma occasionally occur, resulting in paraplegia and destruction of vertebrae. Giant cell tumor, 25% of which occur in the spine, can present with an appearance very similar to tuberculosis. It also grows slowly and may produce paraplegia which will recover if the tumor is removed in reasonable time. In our observations and analysis of a large number of giant cell tumors, the location in the vertebral column is around 1–2% only. The incidence would be far less in immature skeletons [8].

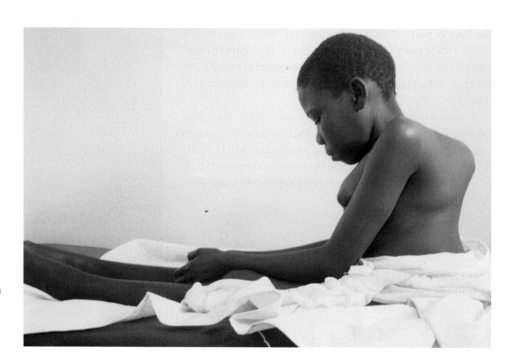

Fig. 11.12 Large kyphosis in an adolescent girl who was paraplegic for many years. Decompression will not assist recovery in this case

Treatment

The basic treatment for spinal tuberculosis is the same as for skeletal tuberculosis. Most individuals can be treated as outpatients. Admission to hospital is indicated if neurological complications develop or when pain and spasm are severe. Inpatient treatment is also required for the drainage of abscesses, debridement of vertebral lesions, and for spinal fusion of an unstable deformity. In the absence of neurological deficit, patients are encouraged to walk as soon as comfort permits.

The Medical Research Council trials [9] showed that spinal braces do not prevent deformity and have no place in the management of spinal tuberculosis.

Most uncomplicated cases of tuberculosis of the spine in childhood heal without surgical intervention. However, progressive bone destruction in spite of chemotherapy and uncertainty about the diagnosis are definite indications for operation in the active stage of the disease (see Table 11.4).

A large percentage of cases with neurological complications recover with drugs and bed rest. Surgical decompression of the cord is indicated if

- neurological complications do not respond to conservative measures after 3–6 weeks
- patients develop neurological complications while on anti-tubercular drugs
- patients with neurological complications become worse (flaccid paralysis, severe flexor spasm, sphincter disturbance)
- patients suffer a recurrence of neurological complications
- patients with prevertebral cervical abscess develop neurological signs or difficulty in swallowing and breathing

Because of the efficacy of modern anti-tubercular drugs, the absolute indications for surgical decompression have been reduced to approximately 5% of uncomplicated cases

Table 11.4 Main indications for various operations in vertebral tuberculosis

- Decompression (± fusion) for neurological complications that fail to respond to 3–6 weeks of conservative treatment or are too advanced
- Debridement ± fusion for failure to respond after 3–6 months of non-operative treatment
- Doubtful diagnosis
- Fusion for mechanical stability after healing
- Debridement ± decompression ± fusion in recurrence of disease or neural complication
- Prevention of severe kyphosis by debridement anteriorly + posterior fusion by panvertebral operation in young children with extensive thoracic lesions

Laminectomy has no place in the treatment of tuberculosis of the spine except for extradural granuloma/tuberculoma presenting as "spinal tumor syndrome" or for the case of old healed disease (without much deformity) presenting with "vertebral canal stenosis" or refractory posterior spinal disease

and to about 60% of those with neurological deficit. An approach to the management of children with vertebral tuberculosis and neural complications is presented in Fig. 11.13.

Radiological Healing of Vertebral Tuberculosis Without Operation

In patients with early disease in whom the intervertebral spaces are preserved, long-term follow-up reveals that the radiological appearance of the disc space remains static. At 5 years following the start of disease, patients with classical paradiscal or metaphyseal tubercular spondylitis show the following radiographic appearances: 19% have fibrous, 12% have fibro-osseous, and 69% have osseous replacement of the intervertebral space. Complete destruction of the disc usually results in bony ankylosis.

Neurological Complications

The overall incidence of neurological complications has been reported to be between 10 and 30% in various studies. Disease below the level of the first lumbar vertebra rarely causes paraplegia which is commonest in tuberculous disease of the lower thoracic region. Tetraplegia from cervical involvement is less common. The youngest child reported to have tuberculous paraplegia was 1 year old [5].

Tuberculous paraplegia has been classified into two main groups [10]:

- *Early onset paraplegia* occurs within the first 2 years of the disease. The underlying pathology includes inflammatory edema, granulation tissue, caseating abscess, or the (rare) ischemic cord lesion.
- *Late onset paraplegia* develops more than 2 years after the vertebral infection. Neurological complications may result from recrudescence of the disease or mechanical pressure on the cord. Compression results from tuberculous caseous tissue, tubercular debris, sequestra from vertebral body and disc, internal gibbus, stenosis of the vertebral canal, or severe deformity.

A more rational classification is paraplegia associated with active disease or with healed disease. In most early onset paraplegia associated with active disease, inflammation causes compression and the prognosis for recovery is favorable. The basic pathology in most cases of late onset paraplegia associated with healed disease is mechanical. Surgical removal of mechanical compression is mandatory, but the prognosis is less favorable. The usual pathology responsible for neurological complications is shown in order of frequency in (Table 11.5).

Fig. 11.13 Suggested algorithm
for the management of children
with vertebral tuberculosis and
neurological complications

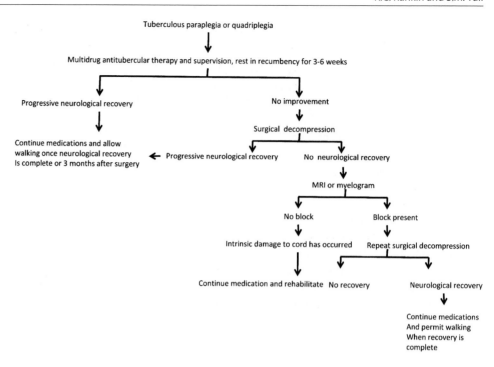

Table 11.5 Usual causes of neurological complications in tuberculosis of the spine

Inflammatory	
Inflammatory edema	Recovers with rest and drug therapy
Tuberculous granulation tissue	Mostly recovers with rest and drug therapy
Tuberculous abscess	Recovers with conservative therapy; rarely requires evacuation and decompression
Tuberculous caseous tissue	May subside with conservative therapy; sometimes requires evacuation and decompression
Mechanical	
Tubercular debris	Solid debris requires operative removal and decompression
Sequestra from vertebral body and disc	Requires operative removal and decompression
Constriction of cord due to stenosis of vertebral canal	Requires operative decompression
Localized pressure due to angulation (internal gibbus) along anterior wall of vertebral canal	Requires operative decompression
Intrinsic	
Prolonged stretching of the cord over a severe deformity	(i) Stretched cord may be more vulnerable to other causes; then decompression, release of cord, and anterior transposition may lead to recovery (ii) Rarely, stretching leads to interstitial gliosis, syrinx formation, or atrophy of cord (difficult to prove/disprove); does not recover, probably seen as myelomalacia on MRI
Infective thrombosis/endarteritis of spinal vessels	Difficult to prove/disprove; does not recover, probably seen as myelomalacia on MRI
Pathological dislocation of spine	Rare complication, usually results from rough manipulation by masseur or panvertebral lesion or indiscriminate laminectomy for crisis spine; irreparable severance of cord
Tuberculous meningomyelitis	Difficult to prove/disprove; myelitis seen on MRI does not recover completely
Syringomyelic changes	Seen on MRI; poor recovery
Spinal tumor syndrome	
Diffuse extradural granuloma or tuberculoma or peridural fibrosis	Present as spinal tumor syndrome; surgical approach is by laminectomy

As a rule more than one cause may be acting in the same case. MRI, whenever available, can demonstrate atrophy of cord, myelomalacia,
syringomyelia, infarction, and arachnoiditis in cases that fail to recover despite adequate surgical decompression.

In children with paraparesis, since they retain some movement and sensation, recovery can be expected after decompression even after 1½–2 years. However, in those who have developed a spastic paraparesis and have remained without operation for up to 2 years the possibility of recovery is much less. After 2 years there is very little chance of recovery since instrinsic cord changes have taken place (Fig. 11.12).

Myelography and Imaging

When there is little difficulty in determining the level of cord compression from clinical, neurological, and radiological examination, myelography is considered unnecessary. However, in cases of paraplegia without radiological evidence of the disease, as in spinal tumor syndrome or in cases with multiple vertebral lesions, myelography is helpful in determining the level of obstruction. Another situation in which myelography is indicated arises when a patient has not recovered after surgical decompression. A myelographic block indicates inadequate mechanical decompression and warrants a second decompression. If a block is not present, failure to recover may be due to intrinsic damage to the cord. Myelography is now being replaced by MRI scanning: T2-weighted images give a myelographic effect, although a block to the flow of contrast medium obviously cannot be portrayed.

Prognosis for Recovery of Cord Function

Recovery depends on many factors (see Table 11.6). However, treatment should never be withheld, as there are many patients with advanced disease who partially recover after a satisfactory mechanical decompression.

Although recovery can take place over many months, in general, with a recent onset paraplegia (i.e., within 6–8

Table 11.6 Clinical factors influencing prognosis in cord involvement

Cord involvement	Better prognosis	Relatively poor prognosis
Degree	Partial	Complete
Duration	Shorter	Longer (>12 months)
Type	Early onset	Late onset
Speed of onset	Slow	Rapid
Age	Younger	Older
General condition	Good	Poor
Vertebral disease	Active	Healed
Kyphotic deformity	<60°	>60°
MRI	Healthy cord	Myelomalacia ± syringomyelia
Operative findings	Wet lesion	Dry lesion

weeks), the time to recovery after decompression is approximately the same time as the paraplegia has been present. Recovery time is extremely variable but in lesions with pus and granulation tissue at operation, neurological function can return to entirely normal within 1 week.

Treatment of Potts Paraplegia

The prevention of paraplegia in tuberculous disease of the spine is of paramount importance. In the usual paradiscal lesion the anterior cord is compressed. Decompression is achieved through an anterior approach. In the cervical region this is through a plane between the pharynx and larynx and carotid sheath. In the thoracic region a thoracotomy is used. Problems arise in the lower thoracic and upper lumbar regions. Disease is frequently in the thoracolumbar junction and may involve T11/T12 and L1 or L2. The deformity can be such that an approach must be made through the lower chest, by removing the crura of the diaphragm on one side. Although an anterior operation, it is made initially from a left lateral approach. At this level the aorta is close and the dissection proceeds deep to it.

In the lumbar region a lateral approach, using that for the kidney, is made. This is a retro-peritoneal dissection. The psoas muscle must be displaced and roots of the lumbar plexus avoided. The ureter usually lies safely anterior. At the lumbo-sacral junction an anterior trans-peritoneal approach is made with care to avoid the pre-sacral plexus.

In all these approaches, particularly from the thoracic region down, the control of bleeding from segmental arteries and veins forms a major part of the operation. Many of these vessels need to be doubly ligated and divided to give clear access to the vertebral lesion. Unless this stage is carried out first, sudden and serious bleeding may occur unexpectedly later in the operation.

Laminectomy is contraindicated as it provides inadequate decompression and renders the vertebral column unstable. Costotransversectomy now has no place; it allows abscess fluid to be drained, but does not give sufficient exposure for the excision of infected tissue.

Anterolateral decompression was most useful in the past in cases of extreme kyphosis in which approach through the thorax is very difficult. It also does not allow complete access. The danger is that in removing sufficient bone to decompress the cord the spine may become unstable.

Kyphosis in Tuberculosis of the Spine

The development of a severe kyphotic deformity is a serious complication, next only to neurological loss (Fig. 11.10). The spine deforms during the phase of active vertebral growth and adults who report with complications related to severe kyphotic deformity (cardiorespiratory compromise, costopelvic impingement, delayed neural deficit) were, as a rule, infected in childhood.

Kyphosis is more common in the thoracic spine, and this region develops the greatest degree of angulation. All patients in whom there is an increase in kyphosis of more than 30% had three or more vertebrae involved in the thoracic region, and all were younger than 10 years at the onset of disease. The normal thoracic kyphosis is accentuated by the effects of gravity. Once the deformity is more than 45°, the posterior spinal muscles work at a mechanical disadvantage, further adding to the deformity.

In cases of anterior vertebral disease, the deformity increases because of unrestricted growth of the posterior elements in the presence of collapse of involved vertebral bodies, anterior growth arrest, and tethering. The angle of kyphosis increases at 5–15 years by 10–30° in 12% of patients, by more than 30° in 3%, and does not progress significantly in the remainder.

When spinal decompression is undertaken for the neurological deficit associated with a kyphosis of 60° or more, removal of the internal gibbus (even if comprised of healthy bone) is mandatory, as this releases the cord anteriorly. Some neurological improvement occurs, although a complete cure is seldom observed. Attempted radical improvement of the severe gibbus is possible but involves anterior release, posterior instrumentation, and anterior bone graft. This is at least a two-stage and possibly a three-stage procedure. The improvement in the kyphosis is rarely worth the large risks involved, not least that a neurologically normal child may be rendered paraplegic.

Acknowledgment The first author of this chapter wishes to acknowledge the enormous help given by:

Dr. J. Cliff, Physician, Maputo Central Hospital and Department of Health, Mozambique Government.

For computer and graphics:

Ms. N. N. Ntuli, Economist, Johannesburg, South Africa.

Ms. H. Ntuli, Postgraduate student, University of Pretoria.

References

1. Girdlestone GR, Somerville EW, Wilkinson MC. Tuberculosis of Bone and Joint. 3rd ed. Oxford: Oxford University Press; 1955.
2. Fitzgerald JM. Management of adverse reactions to bacille Calmette-Guerin vaccine. Clin Infect Dis 2000; 31 (suppl.3): S75–S76.
3. Twine C, Coulston J, Tayton K. Bony lesions in BCG-vaccinated children: Consider BCG osteitis. J Paediatr Child Health 2007; 43(4):307–309.
4. Hodgson AR, Skinses OK, Leong JCY. The pathogenesis of Pott's paraplegia. J Bone Joint Surg Br 1967; 49A:1147–1156.
5. Tuli SM. Tuberculosis of the Skeletal System, 3rd ed. New Delhi: JP Bros; 2004.
6. Martini M. Tuberculosis of the Bones and Joints. Heidelberg: Springer; 1988.
7. Campbell JA, Hoffman EB. Tuberculosis of the hip in children. J Bone Joint Surg Br 1995; 77B:319–326.
8. Tuli SM, Srivastava TP, Verma BP. Giant cell tumour of bone – A study of natural course. Int Orthop 1978; 2:207–214.
9. Medical Research Council. A 10 year assessment of a controlled trial comparing debridement and anterior spinal fusion in the management of tuberculosis of the spine in patients on standard chemotherapy in Hong Kong. VIII Report. J Bone Joint Surg Br 1982; 64B:393–399.
10. Griffiths DL, Seddon HL, Roaf RO. Pott's Paraplegia. Oxford: Oxford University Press; 1956.

Chapter 12

Children's Orthopaedics in the Tropics

Sharaf B. Ibrahim and Abdul-Hamid Abdul-Kadir

Introduction

Objectives

In this chapter, an epidemiological and clinical survey of children's orthopaedics and trauma, as these relate to countries in the tropics, is presented. While there is a similarity with the majority of diseases encountered in the developed countries, there are certain defining characteristics in the incidence, the pattern, the severity or otherwise, and in the clinical presentation of many of these diseases. These peculiarities are the result of subtle influences exerted by changes in the environment and human behavior, wet and humid weather conditions coupled with changing weather patterns, poor socio-economic status, population density, population movement, low literacy and health awareness, and traditional, fatalistic, and mystical beliefs. The problems of accessibility to modern health-care facilities and services, compounded with a reluctance to seek treatment early and the fear of surgical intervention, also influence the outcome.

This chapter aims to highlight relevant aspects of the diseases in the above context, without delving systematically into details of their clinico-pathological presentations and management. Many conditions outlined in this section are dealt with in greater depth in other chapters in this book.

The Tropical Countries

The tropics lie between Tropics of Cancer and Capricorn bisected by the equator. It covers about one-quarter of the land surface of the earth. A large part of South and Central America, more than a third of the African land mass, the southern half of India, the whole of Southeast Asia, and the northern quarter of Australia fall into the region. Slightly more than one-third of the world's population of 6.7 billion lives within this zone.

Following World War II, many countries in the tropical belt entered a period of vigorous self-development. However, the socio-economic status achieved by these countries varies greatly. While some countries have successfully attained and maintained the social and health standards of developed countries, many are still economically poor and under-developed, compounded by socio-political upheavals. The manyfold increase in population in these countries with inadequate natural resources and the periodic occurrence of natural disasters like cyclones, floods, volcanoes, and earthquakes hamper development and progress.

Epidemiology

Diseases of tropical climates reach their highest incidence and present the greatest problems where high temperatures, humidity, and heavy rainfall prevail throughout the year. The low socio-economic status of the people, with poor standards of health care and overcrowding, leads to diseases which are peculiar to the area, as well as differences in the clinico-pathological presentations of "universal diseases."

Political upheavals, ethnic strife, and the resultant economic uncertainties of many of these many nations have led to the exodus of refugees and migrants across national borders (and seas), further straining the resources in these countries and seriously compromising the standard of living and health.

Demography

In Asia, life expectancy has increased from 41 years in 1950 to 67 years in 2005. Nonetheless, there is a wide discrepancy

S.B. Ibrahim (✉)
Departments of Orthopaedics and Traumatology, Hospital Universiti Kebangsaan Malaysia, Bandar Tun Razak, Kuala Lumpur, Malaysia

M. Benson et al. (eds.), *Children's Orthopaedics and Fractures*,
DOI 10.1007/978-1-84882-611-3_12, © Springer-Verlag London Limited 2010

between countries such as Papua New Guinea, where life expectancy is as low as 56 years, and Japan and Singapore, at 81 years. Acquired immunodeficiency syndrome (AIDS) has taken its toll in Africa resulting in the lowest life expectancy of 33–35 years in Swaziland, Botswana, and Lesotho. In many countries less than half the children reach the age of 15 years. Infant mortality rate (IMR) per 1,000 live births in 2005 is 160 in Sierra Leone, 109 in Nigeria, 30 in Guatemala, and 23 in Brazil, while it is 19 in Vietnam, 8 in Malaysia, and 3 in Singapore. The World Health Organization (WHO) has designated, among other criteria, IMR as one of the global indicators for monitoring progress toward health for all.

The ratio of people per doctor is also very variable. For example, in 2004 the number of physicians per 100,000 of the population was 17 in Africa and 45 in Southeast Asia compared with 327 in Europe. There is an inequitable distribution of doctors between urban (or developed) and rural (or undeveloped or inland) areas in most tropical countries [1].

Global Health Initiatives

In 1974, the WHO announced the Expanded Programme of Immunization, which decreed that infants should be immunized by the first year of life against six diseases: tuberculosis, diphtheria, pertussis, tetanus, poliomyelitis, and measles. The primary aim was the control of target diseases using immunization as the strategy; however, the program has only in part achieved its goal. Most unimmunized or partially immunized infants in developing countries are found in sub-Saharan Africa and South Asia. In 2004, the measles immunization rate was more than 90% in Latin America and the Caribbean and more than 80% in East Asia and the Pacific. In contrast, the rate for South Asia and sub-Saharan Africa was just over 60% [2].

In May 1977, the 30th World Health Assembly adopted a resolution which specified that the main social goal of governments and the WHO in the coming decades would be the attainment by all citizens of the world by the year 2000 of a level of health that will permit them to lead a socially and economically productive life. In 1978, at Alma-Ata, the resolution was further endorsed with the statement that the goal of Health for All by the year 2000 would be achieved through primary health care. In 2008, this resolution remains largely unfulfilled in many poor, tropical countries [3, 4].

Primary health care, besides providing curative care, more importantly embodies preventive, promotive, prophylactic, and rehabilitative medical care. It aims for poverty eradication, safe water and sanitation facilities, growth monitoring and surveillance, rehabilitation of malnourished children from poor families, school health

service and health services for children, and the development of a comprehensive infrastructure to provide an effective rural health service.

Orthopaedic Diseases in the Tropics

General

The pattern of orthopaedic diseases in Europe and North America has been considered to be different from those in tropical countries, particularly in relation to degenerative, auto-immune, congenital, and tumor-related conditions. While this may still be true in many countries, health education and awareness are altering the pattern of clinical practice in some of the countries with better developed healthcare facilities and services. Nevertheless, trauma remains the leading cause of orthopaedic admissions in developing countries [5, 6].

Musculo-skeletal trauma, acute osteomyelitis, and post-traumatic bone infection account for 20% of paediatric hospital admissions. Septic arthritis and tuberculous bone and joint infections are encountered less frequently than 20 years ago. Poliomyelitis has been totally eradicated in countries with strict immunization programs, for example, Singapore and Malaysia where no new cases have been diagnosed since 1992 [7]. In 2008, poliomyelitis remained endemic only in India, Pakistan, Afghanistan, and Nigeria [8].

Machinery and heavy tools used in industry and agriculture cause serious workplace limb injuries in children in countries where child labor continues to be practised. Burns and scalds from kerosene stoves and lamps in the home and injuries due to firecrackers and home-made explosive devices (mainly during festivals) continue to maim children.

Non-accidental injuries in infants are surfacing more frequently, though still probably under-reported. Malignant soft tissue and bone tumors are complicated by late presentation and radical or ablative surgery is often refused or considered of no value.

Traditional Beliefs and Treatment

In many countries, native or traditional healers and bone-setters provide first-line care for many ailments, including fractures, dislocations, and swellings in the limbs. This delays or complicates curative hospital care. Patients may present late for many reasons, which include living in the interior of a country, ignorance, and, sometimes, a fatalistic attitude toward illness and diseases generally. There is a general dislike for plaster casts because of skin sensitivity (partly due to the humid tropical climate), physical discomfort, and both emotional and physical intolerance. Bonesetters and traditional healers are well known to remove casts from the limbs of patients who seek their "second opinion." Gangrene following tight traditional splinting has been reported [9]. To minimize or overcome such eventualities, government health authority in some countries, like Ethiopia and Indonesia, conduct training sessions for traditional bonesetters. Recently a concerted attempt was made at integrating traditional treatment and complementary methods with Western medical practice in most countries in the region, particularly based upon clinical evidence that some of these local and cultural medical techniques are beneficial.

Parents are generally reluctant to subject their children to surgical intervention as they consider scarring the body or removing organs and limbs as being contrary to religious teachings. Voluntary organ donation and autopsy are also resisted because of a well-entrenched belief in the afterlife and the need for the body to be full and complete.

Children with club feet, radial club hand, webbed digits, severe idiopathic scoliosis, congenital hip dislocations, and chronic bone infections suffer these afflictions into adulthood because of the reluctance by parents to have them subjected to surgical procedures. In some sectors of the population a strong belief in fatalism and mysticism, whereby physical deformities in the newborns are divine punishment for worldly sins, compounds this reluctance to seek treatment early.

Drug Therapy

The emergence of strains of microorganisms resistant to standard drug therapy has affected the control of diseases like malaria, tuberculosis, and bone and joint infections. The lack of strict antibiotic control has also affected the management of many previously treatable infections. Patients are known to discontinue drugs that need to be taken on a long-term basis, such as in tuberculosis or leprosy. The lack of immediately apparent benefits or favorable outcome, and the deeply entrenched traditional beliefs that these drugs affect sex drive and life expectancy, lead to patient non-compliance. Quality control of drugs is also wanting in many countries, and the porous borders between nations encourage free flow of poor quality and untested medical products.

The easy availability of potentially toxic pharmaceutical preparations to street peddlers in many countries has added a new spectrum of diseases. Indiscriminate steroid therapy for quick pain relief brings in its wake serious side effects, and repeated intra-articular injection of steroid preparations leads to septic arthritis and neuropathic joints, particularly at the knee.

Congenital Disorders

Musculo-skeletal disorders in children accounted for 8% of all congenital anomalies seen in general hospitals in the region. The incidence of congenital musculo-skeletal malformations is estimated to be in the range of 4–10 per 1,000 live births [10, 11]. The entire spectrum of congenital disorders is often seen late in the clinics and hospitals.

Congenital Talipes Equinovarus

The most common congenital disorder seen in the tropics is congenital talipes equinovarus, with an estimated incidence of 1.25 per 1,000 live births. Children often present after the age of walking with painful, untreated clubfeet (Fig. 12.1). The Ponseti method of treating club foot has enabled many children to be treated in Malawi and Uganda without the need for major clubfoot surgery [12, 13]. In Brazil, the Ponseti method has been shown to be effective even in older children [14].

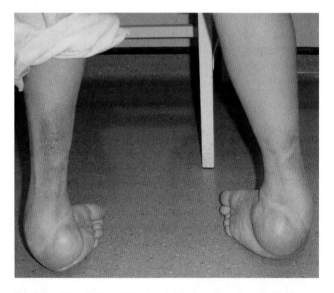

Fig. 12.1 Untreated clubfeet in a 30-year-old man who presented with pain on weight bearing. He was subsequently treated by triple arthrodesis

Developmental Dysplasia of the Hip

The incidence of dislocation of the hip in Malaysia is 0.7 per 1,000 live births [15], comparable to the incidence in other Asian and African countries. The low incidence of developmental dysplasia of the hip in some countries is ascribed to the mothers carrying their infants astride their hips or back as they go about their daily chores. The position keeps the hips flexed and abducted and the femoral heads in the acetabulum. In Saudi Arabia [16] and Singapore [17], the incidence of neonates with dislocated hips is much higher at 3.5 per 1,000 live births and 4.7 per 1,000 live births, respectively. In spite of clinical screening at birth, children still present after walking age with hip dislocation requiring open reduction with or without osteotomy.

Amniotic Deformity, Adhesion, and Mutilation Complex

The abnormalities of the amniotic deformity, adhesion, and mutilation (ADAM) complex occur as a result of intrinsic causes such as germ plasm defect and vascular disruption, and extrinsic causes such as amniotic membrane rupture and amniotic bands. In a multicenter epidemiological study from South America, 270 cases were identified from a total of 3,020,896 live and stillborn infants [18].

The condition may vary from simple ring constriction to those accompanied by massive lymphedema with gangrene of the foot (Fig. 12.2). Ring constriction may be accompanied by fusion of distal parts, with syndactyly of varying degrees, or intrauterine amputations. Facial abnormalities include cleft lip and palate.

Some mothers regard the defect as a visitation for cutting off crabs' legs while pregnant. Such beliefs and the reluctance by parents to accept physical imperfections in their children, hamper investigations into the etiology of this and other congenital disorders.

While newborns with severe forms of the condition are brought early for treatment, those with less severe forms and those with amputations often do not seek treatment until adult life and then only for cosmetic reasons.

Shallow rings with no distal lymphedema may not need treatment except for cosmetic reasons. Early surgery is indicated in deep rings in order to avoid auto-amputation. Traditionally, a two-stage excision with z-plasty of the constriction is carried out in stages 4–6 weeks apart. However, a single-stage excision is safe as the blood supply of the skin distal to the constriction is by musculocutaneous or cutaneous perforators [19, 20]. When associated with acrosyndactyly, separation of the digits is carried out with preservation of length. When there is congenital intrauterine amputation, there may be a need to refashion stumps to facilitate prosthetic fitting.

Congenital Insensitivity to Pain

Congenital insensitivity to pain is a rare disorder caused by a defect in the neurotropin signal transduction system. The diagnosis is based upon a history of recurrent fever, skin problems, insensitivity to pain, anhidrosis, infections,

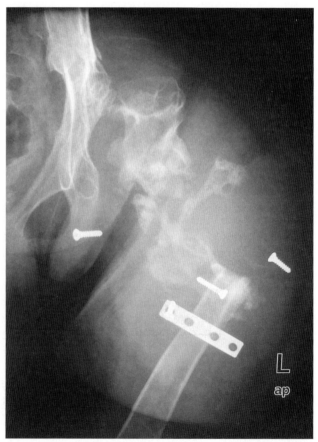

Fig. 12.3 A 16-year-old girl with congenital insensitivity to pain showing destruction of the left hip, non-union of the left proximal femur, and dislodgement of the plate and screws

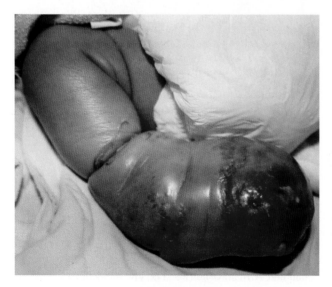

Fig. 12.2 Congenital constriction ring producing gangrene of the right foot in a neonate requiring an emergency below-knee amputation

malunion and non-union of fractures, and Charcot arthropathies (Fig. 12.3). Self-mutilating behavior and learning disabilities may be present [21, 22].

Infections

Acute and Chronic Osteomyelitis

The incidence of acute hematogenous osteomyelitis is higher than in countries with a moderate climate and occurs in children in rural environments and from poor socio-economic backgrounds. There is often a history of acute upper respiratory tract, otitis media, or skin infections. The bones typically involved are the growing ends of long bones like the femur, tibia, and humerus. The radiological appearance may mimic leukemia, osteosarcoma, Ewing's sarcoma, or tuberculosis, though clinically the child is usually febrile and toxic with septic foci elsewhere in the body.

Appropriate antibiotics are administered, parenterally for 10–14 days and then orally, for a total of 6 weeks. Surgical intervention is practiced with caution, to relieve subperiosteal pus collection, as aggressive sequestrectomy in the acute stage leads to excessive periosteal loss resulting in non-union (Fig. 12.4). There is a fairly high incidence (about 20–30%) of chronicity following acute osteomyelitis due to inadequate antibiotic therapy (Fig. 12.5), low dosage, and wrong route of administration, organism insensitivity, or failure of compliance. There is a 20–40% incidence of methicillin-resistant *Staphylococcus aureus* (MRSA) in Nigeria, Kenya, Cameroon, and India. The isolates are sensitive to vancomycin but the majority prove to be resistant to rifampicin, fusidic acid, and ciprofloxacin [23, 24].

Chronic osteitis due to open fractures treated by traditional bonesetters using herbal pastes or following vigorous massage with resultant skin reaction is also seen in children. Whole bone involvement often occurs in infants with acute osteomyelitis when it progresses to chronicity. Extensive bone defects, joint and muscle contractures, and loss of limb length due to epiphyseal damage are the inevitable sequelae, necessitating multiple corrective surgical procedures.

Septic Arthritis

Children with pyogenic or septic arthritis sometimes present late, having defaulted from treatment by general practitioners, or after management by traditional healers using massage and herbal foments based upon a "diagnosis" of twisted joints. The classical features of a septic joint, namely swelling, warmth, redness, tenderness, and loss of function, are invariably present and the child appears ill with a high fever (Fig. 12.6).

Management involves hospitalization, joint immobilization, and immediate parenteral antibiotic therapy, followed by decompression arthrotomy or arthroscopic joint lavage.

Septic arthritis, rare in children from developed countries, is fairly common in sub-Saharan Africa. In a study from Nigeria, 93 children with a mean age of 4.5 years presented with septic arthritis involving 104 joints. *S. aureus* was the commonest organism (50%). Approximately one-third of patients experienced complete resolution but many had varying degrees of joint destruction [25]. In Malawi, the commonest organisms cultured were *Salmonella typhimurium* and *Salmonella enteritidis*. Poor nutritional status, anemia, and malaria are endemic in sub-Saharan Africa, predisposing the children to salmonella infection [26].

Tropical Muscle Abscess

Pyogenic muscle infection is rare in temperate zones, but in the tropics is a fairly common accompaniment of staphylococcal bacteremia (Fig. 12.7). Children below the age of 4 years are more susceptible. Severe upper or lower respiratory tract infection may precede muscle involvement, although

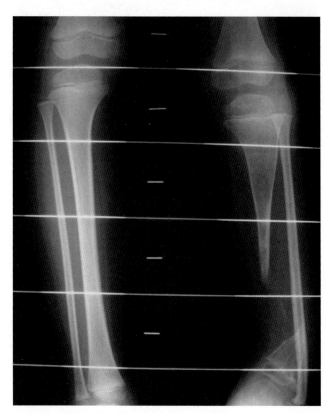

Fig. 12.4 Non-union of the tibia resulting from chronic osteomyelitis aggressive sequestrectomy in a 5-year-old child

Fig. 12.5 Chronic osteomyelitis of the fibula in a child. (**a**) A large sequestrum from the fibula has protruded through the skin. (**b**) Radiograph shows the sequestrum and thickened involucrum of the fibula

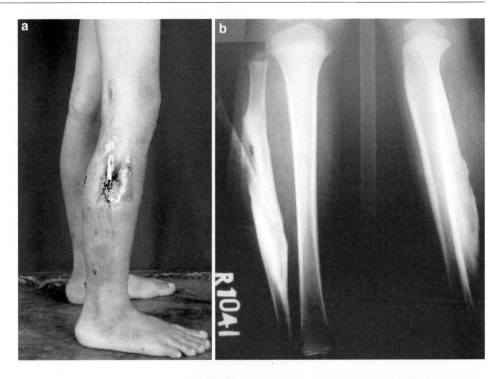

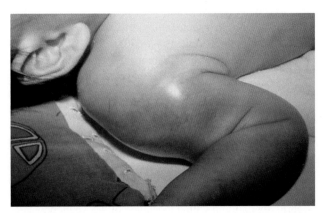

Fig. 12.6 Septic arthritis with gross swelling of the shoulder in an infant

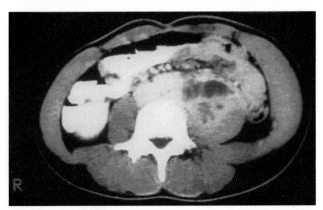

Fig. 12.7 A 14-year-old girl presented with fever and a painful left hip. The CT scan showed a left psoas abscess

quite often no other clinical source of infection may be evident. There is usually no history of trauma. The thigh is the commonest site of myositis, followed by the buttock, arm, leg, and groin. In the vast majority of cases, culture of purulent material yields *S. aureus* [27].

The formation of pus within the muscle does not cause destruction of muscle fibers. Healing is without fibrosis so there is little functional disability. Although the infection is a deep-seated pyogenic lesion in the extremities, it is rare to find clinical and radiological evidence of involvement of the underlying bone in this condition. However, sequestrum, probably because of initial periosteal involvement, has been occasionally encountered together with signs of chronic periostitis.

Neonatal Necrotizing Fasciitis

Necrotizing fasciitis is a grave condition which is seen infrequently in clinical practice. It has been highlighted as a "flesh-eating disease" in the lay press. It is a syndrome of progressive gangrenous infection of the soft tissues and was described by Meleney in 1924 as a severe bacterial infection of the skin, subcutaneous tissues, and fascia with edema, infarction, necrosis, and sloughing of the affected areas (Fig. 12.8). When the infection is unchecked, muscle involvement occurs.

The infection is most commonly caused by *Group A beta-hemolytic Streptococcus*. Some recent reports indicate involvement of *Group B Streptococcus*. In certain African

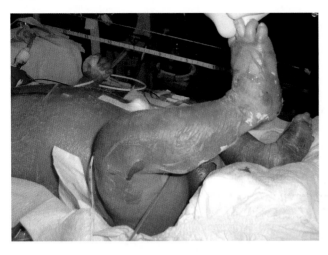

Fig. 12.8 A premature neonate with necrotizing fasciitis showing skin discoloration and bullous formation of both lower extremities

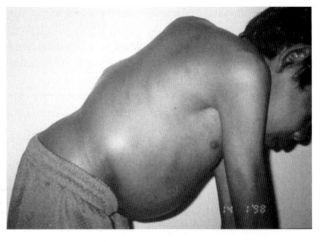

Fig. 12.9 Tuberculosis of the spine without neurological deficit causing kyphotic deformities over the thoracic and thoracolumbar regions in a 16-year-old boy

countries, necrotizing fasciitis is caused by *Clostridium tetani* infection.

The treatment of necrotizing fasciitis depends upon early recognition, aggressive fluid replacement and inotropes to treat shock, broad spectrum antibiotics, and prompt, if necessary repeated, debridement to remove all non-viable tissue [28]. Despite aggressive management, necrotizing fasciitis has a higher mortality in the developing countries than the 5% reported in the developed world [29].

Tuberculosis

There were 9.2 million new cases of tuberculosis in 2006, including 700,000 cases among people living with human immunodeficiency virus (HIV) and 500,000 cases of multidrug-resistant tuberculosis. An estimated 1.5 million people died from tuberculosis in 2006. In addition, another 200,000 people with HIV succumbed to HIV-associated tuberculosis. The highest incidence rate per capita of 363 per 100,000 population was in Africa. Africa, Southeast Asia, and the western Pacific accounted for 83% of the total new cases notified in 2006 [30].

The World Health Assembly had set targets of detecting at least 70% of all new sputum smear-positive cases and to cure at least 85% of these cases arising each year by 2005. The WHO estimated that 67 countries achieved the target detection rates and 57 countries achieved the target for treatment success, with 26 countries achieving both targets [31].

Spinal tuberculosis in children presents with angular kyphosis (Fig. 12.9), more commonly in the thoracic spine, particularly in patients below 10 years of age at the onset of disease. There is usually radiological evidence of collapsed vertebrae and paraspinal abscesses, possibly a "cold abscess"

in the back or thigh. Motor deficit occurs earlier than sensory loss and is also more severe. Tendon reflexes are the last to disappear. Healed tuberculous kyphosis in children may improve or deteriorate with growth [32]. Peripheral joint involvement occurs in 35% of all cases with skeletal manifestations and is usually monoarticular, mainly affecting the hip and knee (see Chapter 11).

Leprosy

Leprosy is a mildly contagious disease. Archeological and anthropological evidence indicates the Nile valley as the possible birthplace of the disease. There are Egyptian records from 1350 B.C. of leprosy among Negro slaves from Sudan and Darfur. In the Indian Vedas of about 1400 B.C., the word *kushta* (Sanskrit for leprosy) appears, and Chinese writings indicate the presence of the disease around 600 B.C.

The global registered prevalence of leprosy at the beginning of 2007 stood at 224,717 cases. During the past 5 years, the number of new cases detected has continued to decrease at an average rate of nearly 20% per year. Pockets of high endemicity still remain in some areas of Angola, Brazil, the Central African Republic, the Congo, India, Madagascar, Mozambique, Nepal, and Tanzania [33].

Mycobacterium leprae affects Schwann cells of superficially placed peripheral nerves in the limbs, as well as the facial nerve in the bony facial canal and the zygomatic branch of the facial nerve in the region of the zygoma. The nerves commonly involved, in decreasing order of frequency, are the ulnar nerve proximal to the elbow and proximal to the wrist, the median nerve proximal to the elbow, the common peroneal nerve at the neck of the fibula, the posterior tibial nerve proximal to the ankle, and the radial nerve proximal to the elbow. Typically, the nerves involved in leprosy, besides their superficial location, lie on the periosteum, proximal to an osteofascial tunnel and are subjected to alternating angulation and stretch in proximity to joints.

In children, upper limb involvement of median and ulnar nerves is more common than facial nerve involvement. Drop foot occurs but trophic ulcers are rare.

The drugs used are a combination of rifampicin, clofazimine, and dapsone for multibacillary leprosy patients. Clofazimine is omitted for paucibacillary patients.

The operation described by Brand in 1954—using the wrist extensors extended into four tails with tendon or fascia lata graft, drawn through the lumbrical canal volar to the deep transverse metacarpal ligament, and sutured to the extensor expansion in the fingers—produces excellent correction in supple Asian hands [34]. Both the extensor to flexor four-tailed tendon transfer and the palmaris longus four-tailed tendon transfer produce a similar clinical outcome [35].

Drop foot is treated by re-routing the tibialis posterior tendon (via the circumtibial or tibio-fibular interosseous membrane routes), then attaching it to the extensor digitorum longus and the extensor hallucis longus tendons on the dorsum of the foot [36].

Yaws

Yaws is a contagious and crippling, but not a killing, disease. It is endemic in Indonesia, Timor-Leste, and India. About 5,000 cases are reported annually with most of them occurring in Indonesia [37].

The condition is caused by *Treponema pertenue* and affects skin and bones. It is a childhood infection, contracted at 2–3 years of age, with the organism gaining entry through minor abrasions. The Wassermann reaction is strongly positive.

The skin lesions are papillomatous and serpiginous, and present as non-healing ulcers. When long bones, like the tibia, are affected, there is thickening and sclerosis, with anterior bowing similar to the saber tibia of syphilis. The late sequelae are contractures complicating ulcers close to the joints, spontaneous fractures, and absorption of bone leading to deformities. The skull may be affected and hyperkeratosis produces a Dupuytren's-like contracture. Treatment is with long-acting benzathine penicillin given in a single dose. The organism is highly sensitive to this preparation, which is safe and cost-effective. Yaws should be considered in the differential diagnosis of ulcers in the limbs of children living in poor rural areas [38, 39]. The WHO aims to eradicate yaws by 2010.

Syphilis

Congenital syphilis continues to be of concern in tropical countries, although its incidence is declining. The disease is an intrauterine infection, in which the spirochete, *Treponema pallidum*, crosses the placental barrier after the first trimester. In a 16-month survey from a hospital in Thailand, nine infants were diagnosed with congenital syphilis from a total of 64 mothers afflicted with syphilis [40]. Antenatal checkups in most tropical countries routinely include screening for syphilis.

The infant presents with pseudoparalysis and swollen joints in the first 4 months of life. Hepatosplenomegaly, anemia, desquamating skin lesions on the hands and soles, and systemic illness develop. The primary skeletal involvement is a bilateral, symmetrical poly-ostotic moth-eaten rarefaction of the diaphysis and erosions or exuberant callus in the metaphysis. Dactylitis of the hands and feet is also seen. Pathological fractures occur in the destructive lesions. The presentation is very similar to the "battered baby syndrome" [41].

Treatment of congenital syphilis in hospitals includes immobilization of fractures and antibiotic therapy with procaine penicillin.

Musculo-skeletal Tumors

In developing countries such as China, India, and Brazil between 20–30% of the population is less than 15 years of age. In contrast, the population below 15 years of age in developed countries like Japan and Germany is between 13 and 15%. The impact of malignant tumors is lessened by the high mortality due to serious infections, parasitic diseases, and malnutrition. Childhood tumors account for less than 10% of all malignancies in tropical countries. Accurate data are not available as only recent attempts have been made to establish tumor registries in these countries.

The most common childhood malignancies are leukemias, central nervous system tumors, and lymphomas. Together these malignancies make up 63% of cases. Soft tissue sarcomas and malignant bone tumors account for only 7 and 4.7%, respectively [42].

Osteosarcoma

Osteosarcoma ranks as the most common malignant bone tumor in children and adolescents; the distal femur accounts for 30% of cases. The cumulative incidence per million of the population in Nigeria, Uganda, Fiji, India, Hong Kong, and Singapore ranges from 37 to 128. The incidence of osteosarcoma per million of the population in the 0–14 age group is India 27, Philippines 36, Hong Kong 30, Singapore Chinese 48, and Singapore Malays 31. In an epidemiological study carried out in Malaysia, the incidence per 100,000 of the population per year was 0.11 for Malays, 0.23 for Chinese, and 0.23 for Indians. These figures were comparable to the incidence in Sweden of 0.28 per 100,000 [43].

Children with osteosarcoma frequently present late after traditional treatment with massage and herbal fomentation and spiritual exhortations. The tumors by then are considerably enlarged and sometimes ulcerate and fungate (Fig. 12.10). Patients come to hospitals very ill and even then may refuse what may just be palliative surgery, aimed at reducing the persistent discomfort and pain and to improve the quality of life remaining in these unfortunate children [44].

Ewing's Sarcoma

Ewing's sarcoma is a malignant small, round cell tumor of bone arising from medullary reticulo-endothelial supportive tissue. It affects both flat bones like the scapula and long bones. It is rare in blacks in Africa and in African-Americans, and in Chinese and Japanese. Seven to thirty-six percent of bone tumors in children aged under 14 years are Ewing's sarcomas. Although classically described as arising from the diaphysis of long bones, the tumor may develop at the metaphysis as well. Children present with a febrile illness and tissue biopsy is important to establish the diagnosis and to exclude acute osteomyelitis [45].

Soft Tissue Sarcoma

In an international study of childhood malignancy, soft tissue sarcomas comprised 4–8% of all malignancies between 0 and 14 years of age. Rhabdomyosarcoma and fibrosarcoma were the commonest subtypes. In Asia, the annual incidence rate for soft tissue sarcoma was below 6 per million. Among predominant white populations, the annual incidence rate for all soft tissue sarcoma was between 5 and 9 per million [46].

Hemophilic Pseudotumor

Hemophilic pseudotumors are rare and occur in 1% of patients with severe factor VIII or IX deficiency. These lesions are enlarging, encapsulated pseudotumors produced by recurrent bleeding, and may be purely within the fascial envelope of muscle or in the subperiosteal region, immediately adjacent to bone, causing bony erosion by interference with periosteal blood supply. The tumor may also develop within the bone itself, destroying its architecture (Fig. 12.11). The tumors often occur in the ilium and femur in adults, but in children there is a higher possibility of the lesion occurring in the small bones of the hands and feet [47, 48]. Early cases of hemophilic pseudotumor can be treated by compression, immobilization, and factor replacement therapy, but needle aspiration or evacuation of hematoma should be avoided as these may lead to wound breakdown, chronic fistula, or secondary infection. There is a risk of sarcomatous change and,

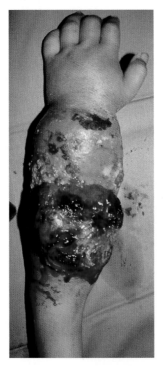

Fig. 12.10 Osteosarcoma of the distal radius in an 8-year-old girl. She presented with septicemia due to the infected, fungating tumor and required an emergency above-elbow amputation

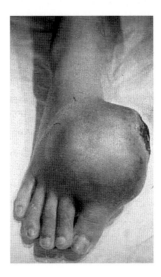

Fig. 12.11 Ten-year-old boy with hemophilic pseudotumor of the right foot due to poorly controlled hemophilia A. Skin necrosis over the medial aspect was due to pressure of the underlying hematoma

in children, growth plate damage. When necessary excision or amputation should be carried out with meticulous attention to surgical technique and hemostasis. Factor VIII level must be maintained at 100% or more during surgery and 50–60% until wound healing is complete.

Although there has been considerable progress in the management of hemophilia in developing countries, there is wide variability not only in the types of products used but also in the doses administered for similar indications [49].

Miscellaneous Conditions

Post-injection Fibrosis of Muscles

Post-injection fibrosis of muscles is an iatrogenic intramuscular complication from repeated injections administered during infancy or childhood [50] and is periodically seen in tropical countries. Contracture of the extensor mechanism of the knee causes restricted knee flexion or genu recurvatum and a variable degree of anterior tibial subluxation. There is often a history of repeated injections into the thigh, usually between the ages of 6 months and 2 years, for diseases like tuberculosis, poliomyelitis, enteritis, tetanus, or protracted febrile illnesses. The condition has to be distinguished from habitual dislocation of the patella and congenital conditions causing limitation of knee flexion. The degree of stiffness of the knee varies. Gross limitation of knee flexion to less than 30° is common. The child with contracture of the extensor mechanism compensates by lateral displacement of the patella to achieve flexion at the expense of knee stability.

The muscles affected are commonly the vastus lateralis and intermedius, less often the rectus femoris and the iliotibial band. The fibrotic change is maximal in the mid-thigh or just distal to it, but rarely proximally. Surgical release and excision of the fibrotic area is followed by intensive physical therapy. Flexion of up to 90° can be achieved in severe cases, sometimes after repeated operations. Post-operative extensor lag, however, may remain for some time.

Other muscles involved in post-injection fibrosis are the deltoid [51], which leads to abduction—internal rotation deformity of the shoulder, and the gluteal muscles, producing atrophic buttocks, abduction contracture of the hip, and sometimes pelvic tilt. These are also treated by excision of fibrotic muscle segments followed by stretching and intensive physical therapy.

Perthes' Disease

There is a significant ethnic and geographical variation in the incidence of Perthes' disease, influenced by socio-economic factors. In South Africa, the annual incidence in white children aged 14 years and under is 10.8 per 100,000, in colored children 1.7 per 100,000, and in black children 0.45 per 100,000. For all races, the incidence in urban areas is twice that in rural areas [52]. In a recent study from Korea, the mean annual incidence was 3.8 per 100,000 [53]. In Japan, the average annual incidence was lower at 0.9 per 100,000 [54]. An epidemiological study in South India found an incidence ranging from 4.4 per 100,000 children to 14.8 per 100,000 children [55]. This regional study in India concluded that Perthes' disease occurred more commonly in the southwest coastal plains of the Indian subcontinent, more in the rural than urban setting, and in children of an older age group. The incidence in southwest Scotland is 15.4 per 100,000 with the highest incidence in deprived areas [56]. This finding, however, does not explain the low incidence of Perthes' disease in many countries in the tropics (with the exception of south India) with low socio-economic status, and implies that other genetic and environmental factors are involved.

Scoliosis

Children in the tropics tend to present later with more advanced curves. Although the cost-effectiveness of school screening is debatable, its absence may be a contributing factor to late presentation [57]. A study in Nigeria reported an incidence of 1.2% in 410 children screened between the ages of 9 and 14 years old [58]. In India, the incidence of scoliosis among 25,376 students was 0.13%, with poliomyelitis as a main causative factor [59].

In a recent survey of 72,699 schoolchildren from Singapore, the prevalence rates were 0.05% for girls and 0.02% for boys at 6–7 years of age, 0.24% for girls and 0.15% for boys at 9–10 years of age, 1.37% for girls and 0.21% for boys at 11–12 years of age, and 2.22% and 0.66%, respectively, for girls and boys at 13–14 years of age [60]. Compared with the 1982 study [61], there was a significant increase in the prevalence rate in girls of 11–12 years of age.

Snake Bites

Snakes are cosmopolitan in distribution, other than in the Arctic and Antarctic regions. They thrive best in damp and humid areas of the world, such as the tropics. The venomous snakes seen in the tropics are cobras, kraits, mambas, and vipers. Their venoms are either neurotoxic or proteolytic causing severe illness and sudden death. Symptoms generally

Fig. 12.12 The dorsal aspect of the hand of an 11-year-old boy who was bitten by a snake, with bite marks at the middle finger, bullous eruptions, and ascending thrombophlebitis. Necrosis of the extensor compartment followed a few days later, requiring extensive debridement

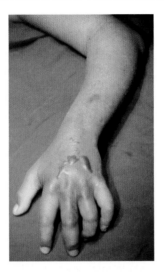

Fig. 12.13 A 37-year-old male with untreated Volkmann's ischemic contracture of the right upper extremity. He had sustained a supracondylar fracture of the humerus after falling off a tree at the age of 12 years, complicated by compartment syndrome

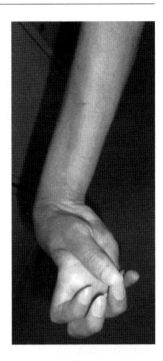

include swelling, discoloration, and severe pain at the site of the bite. Skin necrosis may occur eventually (Fig. 12.12).

A 10-year-study in Papua New Guinea reported 87 deaths among 722 snakebite admissions to the intensive care unit [62]. In a 5-year study from Kuala Lumpur, Malaysia, 126 snakebite cases were admitted. No deaths were reported [63].

Fig. 12.14 A 9-year-old girl with a non-union of a lateral condyle fracture of the humerus resulting in a cubitus valgus deformity. The injury was missed when it occurred at the age of 5 years

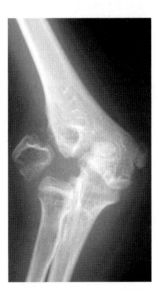

Orthopaedic Trauma

More children are injured in the home and its environs than on the road. The common supracondylar humeral fracture results from children falling at home or on the playing field, but in the tropics also from fruit trees, particularly the *rambutan* tree, which is too slender to take the weight of the child. Fractures in patients in rural areas are often treated by traditional bonesetters and healers using massage and herbal pastes, both of which may cause local skin reactions and increase the swelling, resulting in compartment syndrome and Volkmann's ischemic contracture (Fig. 12.13).

Neglected supracondylar and other fractures (Fig. 12.14) are frequently encountered, as are dislocations. Minimally displaced lateral humeral condylar non-union may be treated by in situ screw fixation. Cubitus valgus or varus deformity can be safely corrected by dome osteotomy combined with slight rotation of the distal fragment to reduce the prominence of one or other condyle [64, 65].

Neglected traumatic hip dislocation in children is uncommon. Open reduction is the only effective treatment as traction alone is rarely successful owing to soft tissue interposition and fibrosis [66, 67].

Face and hand injuries occur during festive seasons, when playing with fire-crackers or home-made explosive devices.

Child Abuse

Child abuse is a global phenomenon. In 1999, the WHO defined child abuse as all forms of physical and/or emotional ill-treatment, sexual abuse, neglect or negligent treatment, or commercial or other exploitation resulting in actual or potential harm to the child's health, survival, development, or dignity. It is estimated that worldwide nearly 53,000 children are murdered each year and sexual violence directed against those under the age of 18 years affects 150 million girls and 73 million boys [68].

Road Traffic Accidents

Morbidity and mortality resulting from road traffic accidents are a matter of serious concern in most developing countries because of the great increase in the number of vehicles, poor road conditions, careless and speeding drivers, and poor law enforcement. Motorcycles provide a cheap and convenient form of transport for laborers and workers. Though the minimum age for a motorcycle license is 16 years in Malaysia, children below that age are known to ride motorcycles and often suffer severe fractures and head injury, sometimes with loss of life.

Many countries have mandated the use of safety belts both in the front and back seat of vehicles. However, children are still seen sitting unstrapped beside their parents in the front passenger seat or unrestrained on an adult's lap.

It is also a common sight in the developing world to witness children and infants being carried sandwiched between parents on one motorcycle, although the law forbids more than two riders (Fig. 12.15). Despite the wearing of safety helmets being compulsory, the quality control of the helmets themselves is poor and riders often wear them insecurely fastened or not at all. The tropical heat and humidity discourage riders from wearing heavy protective gear and most wear slippers on their feet.

Road traffic injuries are the leading cause of death worldwide among young people aged 10–24 years. Globally, nearly 400,000 people under 25 die on the road each year, an average of more than 1,000 deaths a day. Most of these deaths occur in developing countries and among vulnerable road users, namely the pedestrian, cyclist, and motorcyclist [69].

Workplace Accidents

The International Labour Organization Convention 138 (1973) on the subject of child labor stipulated that the minimum age for employment should be 15 years. Despite laws in most developing countries on the minimum age for employment, enforcement by some governments is poor. The socio-economic status of families requires children to supplement the family's income; in many situations children are sole breadwinners. Working children are exposed to biological, chemical, physical, and psychosocial hazards.

The global number of child laborers aged 5–17 years was estimated at 218 million in 2004. The Asia–Pacific region has the largest number, 122 million, followed by sub-Saharan Africa at 49 million [70]. Rapid mechanization in urban and agricultural industries has been responsible for many injuries, not only among children, in family and cottage industries and workshops. In a recent study from Pakistan of 200 boys working in automobile workshops, 38% had received a major injury, 31% suffered from watery eyes, 29% had chronic cough, and 22% had diarrhea [71]. Long hours of work and exhaustion contribute to accidents in the workplace, and the injuries mainly involve the upper limbs and particularly the hand (Fig. 12.16). Children employed in construction and heavy industries suffer a variety of musculoskeletal injuries, including fractures and spinal injuries.

War Injuries

Under international law, the minimum age to join the military is 18 years. Yet there are nearly 300,000 children who have been forced to fight in some of the most brutal conflicts. There are more than 30 armed conflicts in the world today. In the last decade, 2 million children have died in wars, 6 million children have been disabled (Fig. 12.17), 12 million children have been left homeless, and 1 million children have been orphaned. Girls face a variety of threats including rape and forced prostitution [72].

Landmines, anti-personnel mines, or booby traps are often described as implements that cause death in slow motion and are primarily aimed to maim and mutilate rather than cause instant death. Landmines can remain active for almost 50 years, lying hidden in fields and paths. Globally, children

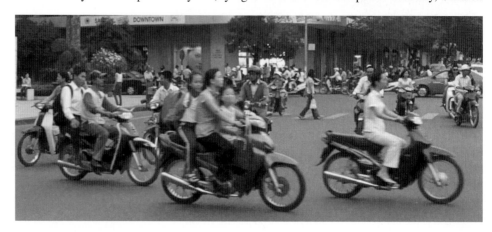

Fig. 12.15 A street scene in Vietnam with three riders on a motorcycle. Many are not wearing safety helmets

Fig. 12.16 A child's hand trapped in a coconut grinder (**a**) resulting in extensive injuries (**b**). This required multiple debridements and reconstruction of the hand. The index finger could not be salvaged. (**c**) The appearance of the hand 2 months after the injury

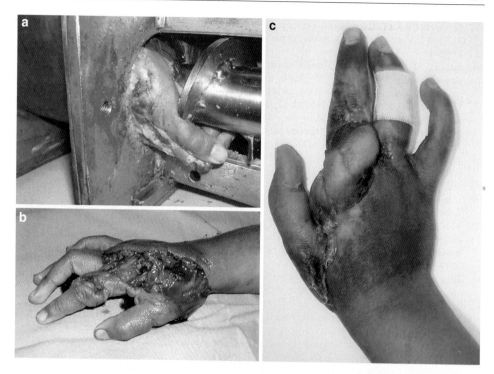

Fig. 12.17 (**a**) An 8-year-old Iraqi girl with bilateral below-knee amputation following a bomb blast during the 2003 Iraq war. (**b**) The radiograph shows shrapnel embedded in her below-knee stumps. (**c**) She was treated in Iraq and brought to Kuala Lumpur for rehabilitation and prosthetic fitting

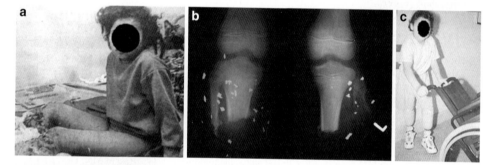

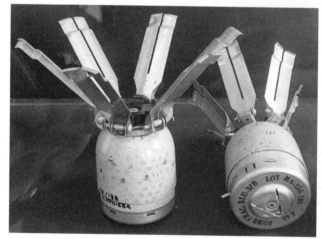

Fig. 12.18 The BLU-3/B pineapple bomblet, air-dropped during the Vietnam War, contains 200 steel pellets

With their natural curiosity, children are particularly vulnerable. While an adult may survive a detonation, even the smallest explosion can be lethal to a child [73].

Acknowledgment The authors acknowledge the provision of clinical material on fibular osteomyelitis by Professor Chairuddin Rasjad from the Department of Orthopaedics, Hasanudin University, Makassar, Indonesia.

in 87 countries live among 60 million landmines. Each year 10,000 children are maimed or killed by these landmines.

In addition to landmines, there are millions of bombs (Fig. 12.18) and grenades that failed to detonate on impact.

References

1. United Nations World Population Prospects: 2006 revision. At: http://www.un.org/esa/population/publications/wpp2006/WPP2006_Highlights_rev.pdf. Accessed March 18,2008.
2. World Development Indicators. At: http://devdata.worldbank.org/wdi2006/contents/Section1_1_4.htm. Accessed March 18,2008.
3. Shaikh BT, Kadir MM, Pappas G. Thirty years of Alma Ata pledges: is devolution in Pakistan an opportunity for rekindling primary health care? J Pak Med Assoc 2007; 57:259–261.
4. Hall JJ, Taylor R. Health for all beyond 2000: the demise of the Alma-Ata Declaration and primary health care in developing countries. Med J Aust 2003; 178:17–20.

5. Ahmed E, Chaka T. The pattern of orthopaedic admissions in Tikur Anbessa University Hospital, Addis Ababa. Ethiop Med J 2005; 43:85–91.

6. Sethi D, Aljunid S, Saperi SB, et al. Comparison of the effectiveness of major trauma services provided by tertiary and secondary hospitals in Malaysia. J Trauma 2002; 53:508–516.

7. Saraswathy TS, Khairullah NS, Sinniah M, et al. Laboratory acute flaccid paralysis surveillance in Malaysia: a decade of commitment to the WHO global polio eradication initiative. Southeast Asian J Trop Med Public Health 2004; 35:421–424.

8. World Health Organization. Poliomyelitis. 2008. At: http://www.who.int/mediacentre/factsheets/fs114/en/. Accessed March 19,2008.

9. Eshete M. The prevention of traditional bone setter's gangrene. J Bone Joint Surg 2007; 87B:102–103.

10. Fida NM, Al-Aama J, Nichols W, et al. A prospective study of congenital malformations among live born neonates at a university hospital in Western Saudi Arabia. Saudi Med J 2007; 28:1367–1373.

11. Bhat BV, Babu L. Congenital malformations at birth-a prospective study from South India. Indian J Pediatr 1998; 65:873–881.

12. Lavy CB, Mannion SJ, Mkandawire NC, et al. Club foot treatment in Malawi—a public health approach. Disabil Rehabil 2007; 29:857–862.

13. McElroy T, Konde-Lule J, Neema S, Gitta S; Uganda Sustainable Clubfoot Care. Understanding the barriers to clubfoot treatment adherence in Uganda: a rapid ethnographic study. Disabil Rehabil 2007; 29:845–855.

14. Lourenco AF, Morcuende JA. Correction of neglected idiopathic club foot by the Ponseti method. J Bone Joint Surg Am 2007; 89:378–381.

15. Boo NY, Rajaram T. Congenital dislocation of the hips in Malaysian neonates. Singapore Med J 1989; 30:368–371.

16. Mirdad T. Incidence and pattern of congenital dislocation of the hip in Aseer region of Saudi Arabia. West African J Med 2002; 21:218–222.

17. Ang KC, Lee EH, Lee PY, Tan KL. An epidemiological study of developmental dysplasia of the hip in infants in Singapore. Ann Acad Med Singapore 1997; 26:456–458.

18. Orioli IM, Ribeiro MG, Castilla EE. Clinical and epidemiological studies of amniotic deformity, adhesion, and mutilation (ADAM) sequence in a South American (ECLAMC) population. Am J Med Genet A 2003; 118:135–145.

19. Hall EJ, Johnson-Giebink R, Vasconez LO. Management of the ring constriction syndrome: a reappraisal. Plast Recon Surg 1982; 69:532–536.

20. Mutaf M, Sunay M. A new technique for correction of congenital constriction rings. Ann Plast Surg 2006; 57:646–652.

21. Shalimar A, Sharaf I, Farah Wahida I, Ruszymah BHI. Congenital insensitivity to pain with anhydrosis in a Malaysian family: a genetic analysis. J Orthop Surg 2007; 15:357–360.

22. Bar-On E, Weigl D, Parvari R, et al. Congenital insensitivity to pain. Orthopaedic manifestations. J Bone Joint Surg Br 2002; 84:252–257.

23. Kesah C, Ben Redjeb S, Odugbemi TO, et al. Prevalence of methicillin-resistant Staphylococcus aureus in eight African hospitals and Malta. Clin Microbiol Infect. 2003; 9:153–156.

24. Krishna BV, Patil A, Chandrasekhar MR. Methicillin resistant Staphylococcus aureus infections-implications in hospital infection control. Indian J Public Health 2007; 51:43–46.

25. Akinyoola AL, Obiajunwa PO, Oginni LM. Septic arthritis in children. West Afr J Med 2006; 25:119–123.

26. Lavy CB, Thyoka M, Pitani AD. Clinical features and microbiology in 204 cases of septic arthritis in Malawian children. J Bone Joint Surg Br 2005; 87:1545–1548.

27. Chauhan S, Jain S, Varma S, Chauhan SS. Tropical pyomyositis (myositis tropicans): Current perspective. Postgrad Med J 2004; 80:267–270.

28. Bingöl-Koloğlu M, Yildiz RV, Alper B, et al. Necrotizing fasciitis in children: diagnostic and therapeutic aspects. J Pediatr Surg 2007; 42:1892–1897.

29. Eneli I, Davies HD. Epidemiology and outcome of necrotizing fasciitis in children: an active surveillance study of the Canadian Paediatric Surveillance Program. J Pediatr 2007; 151:79–84.

30. World Health Organisation. A world free of tuberculosis. At: http://www.who.int/tb/en/. Accessed March 19,2008.

31. Dye C, Hosseini M, Watt C. Did we reach the 2005 targets for tuberculosis control? Bull World Health Organ 2007; 85:364–369.

32. Rajasekaran S, Prasad AS, Dheenadhayalan J, et al. Morphological changes during growth in healed childhood spinal tuberculosis: A 15-year prospective study of 61 children treated with ambulatory chemotherapy. J Pediatr Orthop 2006; 26:716–724.

33. World Health Organization. Leprosy today. At: http://www.who.int/lep/en/. Accessed March 19,2008.

34. Abdul-Kadir A. Correction of claw fingers in leprosy by the Brand four-tailed tendon graft operation. Med J Malaysia 1986; 41:264–268.

35. Taylor NL, Raj AD, Dick HM, Solomon S. The correction of ulnar claw fingers: a follow-up study comparing the extensor-to-flexor with the palmaris longus 4-tailed tendon transfer in patients with leprosy. J Hand Surg Am 2004; 29:595–604.

36. Ishida Y, Lwin S, Myint K. Follow-up of tibialis posterior transfer surgery (TPT) for drop-foot in leprosy. Nihon Hansenbyo Gakkai Zasshi 2007; 76:219–226.

37. World Health Organization. Eradicating Yaws. At: http://www.searo.who.int/en/Section10/Section2134.htm. Accessed March 20,2008.

38. Gip LS. Yaws revisited. Med J Malaysia 1989; 44:307–311.

39. Scolnik D, Aronson L, Lovinsky R, et al. Efficacy of a targeted, oral penicillin-based yaws control program among children living in rural South America. Clin Infect Dis 2003; 36:1232–1238.

40. Sangtawesin V, Lertsutthiwong W, Kanjanapattanakul W, et al. Outcome of maternal syphilis at Rajavithi Hospital on offsprings. J Med Assoc Thai 2005; 88:1519–1525.

41. Rasool MN, Govender S. The skeletal manifestations of congenital syphilis. A review of 197 cases. J Bone Joint Surg Br 1989; 71:752–755.

42. Linet MS, Ries LA, Smith MA, et al. Cancer surveillance series: recent trends in childhood cancer incidence and mortality in the United States. J Natl Cancer Inst 1999; 91:1051–1058.

43. Silva JF, Subramanian N. An epidemiologic study of osteogenic sarcoma in Malaysia. Incidence in urban as compared with rural environments and in each of three separate racial groups, 1969–1972. Clin Orthop Relat Res 1975; 113:119–127.

44. Pan KL, Zolqarnain A, Chia YY. Delay in treatment of primary malignant and aggressive musculoskeletal tumors. Med J Malaysia 2006; 61 Suppl A:53–56.

45. Rasit AH, Sharaf I, Rahman HA. Ewing's sarcoma of the talus in a four-year-old child. Med J Malaysia 2001; 56 Suppl C:86–88.

46. Stiller CA, Parkin DM. International variations in the incidence of childhood soft-tissue sarcomas. Paediatr Perinat Epidemiol 1994; 8:107–119.

47. Ibrahim S, Noor MA, Dhillon M. Hemophilic pseudotumor of the foot-a case report. J Orthop Surg 1994; 2:71–74.

48. Gupta AD, Bose A, Mahalanabis D. Hemophilic pseudotumor involving the right second metacarpal bone in a 5-year-old boy, treated by ray amputation. Hemophilia 2004; 10:408–409.

49. Srivastava A, You SK, Ayob Y, et al. Hemophilia treatment in developing countries: products and protocols. Semin Thromb Hemost 2005; 31:495–500.

50. Di Gennaro GL, Rossi R, Donzelli O. Injection-induced contractures of the quadriceps during childhood. Chir Organi Mov 2004; 89:35–43.

51. Ngoc HN. Fibrous deltoid muscle in Vietnamese children. J Pediatr Orthop B 2007; 16:337–344.

52. Purry NA. The incidence of Perthes' disease in three population groups in the Eastern Cape region of South Africa. J Bone Joint Surg Br 1982; 64:286–288.

53. Rowe SM, Jung ST, Lee KB, et al. The incidence of Perthes' disease in Korea: a focus on differences among races. J Bone Joint Surg Br 2005; 87(12):1666–1668.

54. Kim WC, Hiroshima K, Imaeda T. Multicenter study for Legg-Calvé-Perthes disease in Japan. J Orthop Sci 2006; 11:333–341.

55. Joseph B, Chacko V, Rao BS, Hall AJ. The epidemiology of Perthes' disease in south India. Int J Epidemiol 1988; 17:603–607.

56. Pillai A, Atiya S, Costigan PS. The incidence of Perthes' disease in Southwest Scotland. J Bone Joint Surg Br 2005; 87:1531–1535.

57. Oh KS, Chuah SL, Harwant S. The need for scoliosis screening in Malaysia. Med J Malaysia 2001; 56 Suppl C:26–30.

58. Jenyo MS, Asekun-Olarinmoye EO. Prevalence of scoliosis in secondary school children in Osogbo, Osun State, Nigeria. Afr J Med Med Sci 2005; 34:361–364.

59. Mittal RL, Aggerwal R, Sarwal AK. School screening for scoliosis in India. The evaluation of a scoliometer. Int Orthop 1987; 11(4):335–338.

60. Wong HK, Hui JH, Rajan U, Chia HP. Idiopathic scoliosis in Singapore schoolchildren: a prevalence study 15 years into the screening program. Spine 2005; 30:1188–1196.

61. Daruwalla JS, Balasubramaniam P, Chay SO, e al. Idiopathic scoliosis. Prevalence and ethnic distribution in Singapore schoolchildren. J Bone Joint Surg Br 1985; 67:182–184.

62. McGain F, Limbo A, Williams DJ, et al. Snakebite mortality at Port Moresby General Hospital, Papua New Guinea, 1992–2001. Med J Aust 2004; 181:687–691.

63. Jamaiah I, Rohela M, Ng TK, et al. Retrospective prevalence of snakebites from Hospital Kuala Lumpur (HKL) (1999–2003). Southeast Asian J Trop Med Public Health 2006; 37:200–205.

64. Tien YC, Chen JC, Fu YC, et al. Supracondylar dome osteotomy for cubitus valgus deformity associated with a lateral condylar nonunion in children. Surgical technique. J Bone Joint Surg Am 2006; 88 Suppl 1 Pt 2:191–201.

65. Pankaj A, Dua A, Malhotra R, Bhan S. Dome osteotomy for posttraumatic cubitus varus: A surgical technique to avoid lateral condylar prominence. J Pediatr Orthop 2006; 26:61–66.

66. Kumar S, Jain AK. Neglected traumatic hip dislocation in children. Clin Orthop Relat Res 2005; 431:9–13.

67. Aguilar JA. Treatment of neglected traumatic posterior hip dislocation in children. Techniques Orthop 2006; 21:143–149.

68. World Health Organization: prevention of child maltreatment. At: http://www.who.int/violence_injury_prevention/violence/activities/child_maltreatment/en/index.html. Accessed March 22, 2008.

69. World Health Organization: 10 facts on youth safety. At: http://www.who.int/features/factfiles/youth_roadsafety/en/index.html. Accessed March 22,2008.

70. International Labour Organization: Global child labour trends 2000–2004. At: http://www.ilo.org/dyn/declaris/DECLARATIONWEB.DOWNLOAD_BLOB?Var_DocumentID=6233-. Accessed March 22,2008.

71. Khan H, Hameed A, Afridi AK. Study on child labour in automobile workshops of Peshawar, Pakistan. East Mediterr Health J 2007; 13:1497–1502.

72. Canadian International Development Agency. War-affected children. At: http://www.acdi-cida.gc.ca/CIDAWEB/acdicida.nsf/En/REN-218125511-PX7. Accessed March 22,2008.

73. Wars against children: UN report calls for action to protect children from armed conflict. At: http://www.wcc-coe.org/wcc/what/jpc/echoes/echoes-20-03.html. Accessed March 22, 2008.

Chapter 13

Juvenile Idiopathic Arthritis

Günther E. Dannecker and Martin N. Arbogast

Part 1: Classification, Symptoms, and Medical Treatment

Günther E. Dannecker

Introduction

The term juvenile idiopathic arthritis (JIA) describes a heterogeneous group of several disease subtypes characterized by arthritis beginning before the age of 16 years and where symptoms persist for more than 6 weeks. All subtypes of JIA are of unknown cause. Although the pathogenesis for each subtype is likely to be different, JIA is generally regarded to be an autoimmune disease with the possible exception of systemic JIA. The causes are probably a combination of environmental (e.g., infectious) factors and immunogenetic (e.g., specific human leukocyte antigen [HLA] alleles) susceptibility. As there is no pathognomonic test for these disorders, the diagnosis is based upon the combined evaluation of the history, clinical presentation, and, to some extent, laboratory investigations.

A new classification was compiled in 2001 by the International League of Associations for Rheumatology (ILAR). The formerly used terms of "juvenile chronic arthritis" or "juvenile rheumatoid arthritis," used in Europe or North America, respectively, were substituted by the term "juvenile idiopathic arthritis" [1]. The new classification attempted not only to standardize different nomenclatures but also to define and identify as far as possible the homogeneous subtypes. This should allow a better understanding of pathogenesis and epidemiology and improve the quality of clinical studies. As with any clinical classification the new ILAR criteria have their limitations and will need further modification and redefining.

Classification

JIA is defined as arthritis of unknown etiology that begins before the 16th birthday and persists for at least 6 weeks. Other known conditions are excluded [1]. In this definition, arthritis means swelling within a joint or limitation in its range of joint movement with articular pain or tenderness unrelated to mechanical disorders or to other identifiable causes. As a consequence of the definition, the diagnosis of JIA cannot be made before 6 weeks from onset; the final classification into one of the following subgroups is usually possible after 6 months [1]. The seven currently recognized categories of JIA are shown in Table 13.1 and the major epidemiological features in Table 13.2 (modified according to Minden [2]).

The incidence of JIA is approximately 10/100,000 children per year among white children less than 16 years of age, and the prevalence varies between 16 and 150 per 100,000 children. Subtype distribution varies between different countries. Whereas oligoarthritis is the most common subtype in Europe, it occurs much less frequently in India and New Zealand, where polyarthritis is more common [3, 4].

Symptoms

The clinical manifestation of JIA is dependent upon the subtype. Different subtypes probably represent different diseases which have discrete causes which result in the final pathway of an inflamed joint.

Systemic Arthritis

In 1897, George Frederick Still published his observations on children with a systemic form of arthritis [5]. This category is

G.E. Dannecker (✉)
Department of Paediatrics, Olgahospital, Klinikum Stuttgart, Stuttgart, Germany

M. Benson et al. (eds.), *Children's Orthopaedics and Fractures*,
DOI 10.1007/978-1-84882-611-3_13, © Springer-Verlag London Limited 2010

Table 13.1 Classification of juvenile idiopathic arthritis [1]

Category	Definition	Exclusions
1. Systemic arthritis	Fever of at least 2 weeks' duration (daily for at least 3 days), arthritis in one or more joints, and one or more of the following: • Erythematous rash • Generalized lymph node enlargement • Hepatomegaly and/or splenomegaly • Serum alterations	a, b, c, d
2. Oligoarthritis	Arthritis affecting 1–4 joints during the first 6 months of the disease There are 2 subcategories: 1. Persistent = affecting ≤ 4 joints throughout the disease 2. Extended = affecting > 4 joints after the first 6 months	a, b, c, d, e
3. Polyarthritis, RF−	Arthritis affecting > 5 joints during the first 6 months and RF negative	a, b, c, d, e
4. Polyarthritis, RF+	Arthritis affecting > 5 joints during the first 6 months, with RF positive at least twice (tests at least 3 months apart)	a, b, c, e
5. Psoriatic arthritis	Arthritis and psoriasis or arthritis and at least 2 of the following: • Dactylitis • Nail pitting or onycholysis • Psoriasis in a first-degree relative	b, c, d, e
6. Enthesitis-related arthritis	Arthritis and enthesitis, or arthritis or enthesitis with at least 2 of the following: • Presence/history of sacroiliac joint tenderness and/or inflammatory lumbosacral pain • HLA-B 27$^+$ • Onset of arthritis in a male over 6 years of age • Acute (symptomatic) anterior uveitis • History of ankylosing spondylitis, enthesitis-related arthritis, sacroiliitis with inflammatory bowel disease, or acute anterior uveitis in a first-degree relative	a, d, e
7. Undifferentiated arthritis	Arthritis that fulfills criteria in no category or in 2 or more of the above categories	

One of the major aims of the ILAR classification is the mutual exclusivity of the subtypes. Therefore, the following list of possible exclusions for each category was defined:
a. Psoriasis or a history of psoriasis in the patient or first-degree relative
b. Arthritis in an HLA-B27$^+$ male beginning after the sixth birthday
c. Ankylosing spondylitis, enthesitis-related arthritis, sacroiliitis with inflammatory bowel disease, or acute anterior uveitis or a history of one of these disorders in the first-degree relative.
d. The presence of IgM rheumatoid factor on at least two occasions at least 3 months apart
e. The presence of systemic JIA in the patient

characterized by the classical triad of remittent fever, typical rash, and arthritis. The etiology is unknown but systemic JIA has been considered to belong to the auto-inflammatory syndromes rather than to the group of autoimmune diseases. In the inflammatory process the cytokines IL-1 and IL-6 seem to play crucial role [6, 7].

The systemic signs of fever and rash can precede the arthritis for weeks or even months. For a clear diagnosis, the presence of arthritis is necessary, accompanied by a fever over a minimum of 2 weeks, and one or more of the signs shown in Table 13.1. The febrile episodes are often accompanied by a characteristic macular, salmon-colored rash (Fig. 13.1) with circular or linear lesions of a transient nature. They are distributed most commonly over the trunk, are less than 10 mm in size, and are usually not pruritic. A possibly dangerous complication of systemic JIA is the macrophage activation syndrome (MAS), where an uncontrolled activation of macrophages leads to hemophagocytosis [8]. Arthritis can initially be oligoarticular but usually, if the disease persists, it becomes polyarticular. Joint

Table 13.2 Major characteristics of JIA and its categories

Category	Percentage of all JIA	Female (%)	Onset of disease (years)	ANA[a] (%)	HLA-B27+ (%)	Uveitis (%)
Systemic arthritis	6	50	5	14	5	1
Oligoarthritis	52	69	4	60	12	17
Polyarthritis, RF−	13	76	7	35	12	5
Polyarthritis, RF+	2	83	12	35	9	3
Psoriatic arthritis	8	64	7	41	20	10
Enthesitis-related arthritis	12	30	10	19	66	7
Undifferentiated	8	64	9	31	35	11
JIA total	100	64	6	46	22	12

The data shown are from the German registry for juvenile arthritis (3,510 patients, [2]).
[a]ANA = antinuclear antibodies

Fig. 13.1 Typical rash of systemic JIA

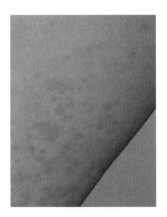

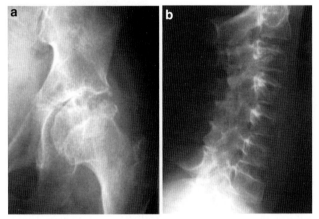

Fig 13.2 (**a**) Left hip of a 10-year-old male patient with inadequately treated systemic disease. (**b**) Cervical spine of the same patient with severe facet disease

destruction in systemic JIA can be very severe and leads to profound disability necessitating orthopaedic procedures like soft tissue release or joint replacement (Fig. 13.2).

The diagnosis of systemic JIA is always based upon clinical observation. The differential diagnosis includes the many causes of fever of unknown origin such as viral and bacterial infections, septicemia, malignancy, Kawasaki syndrome, rheumatic fever, and connective tissue diseases. Laboratory tests will demonstrate a leukocytosis, a raised erythrocyte sedimentation rate (ESR) and C-reactive protein (CRP), and clotting disorders. However, if MAS develops leucopenia and thrombocytopenia can occur accompanied by significantly elevated levels of ferritin, lactate dehydrogenase (LDH), and D-dimers.

Oligoarthritis

An arthritis that affects four or fewer joints during the first 6 months of the disease is termed oligoarthritis. According to the ILAR classification, two categories in this subtype can be distinguished [1]. The first is a persistent oligoarthritis which does not involve more than four joints. The second

is an extended oligoarthritis in which arthritis will involve more than four joints after 6 months. Oligoarthritis usually starts early in life, typically affecting children 2–3 years old. The arthritis is asymmetrical and predominantly involves the large joints of the lower extremities excluding the hip, which is rarely involved initially. The most frequently affected joints are, in decreasing order, the knees, ankles, elbows, and wrists. In approximately one-third of patients, only one joint is affected at the onset of the disease.

Oligoarthritis has a very strong female predilection and is sometimes difficult to diagnose. The signs of joint pain and swelling are not always recognized and a small child may not complain of pain but with easy fatigability and delay in development. Morning stiffness is typical and the involved joints are often warm, painful to move, and have a limited range of motion. Usually the affected joints are not erythematous but muscle atrophy and altered growth plate activity may be seen. A child with a unilateral knee arthropathy typically presents with a leg length discrepancy resulting in flexion and outward rotation of the affected knee (Fig. 13.3).

Fig. 13.3 Oligoarthritis affecting the left knee and right ankle. Note flexion/external rotation of the left knee

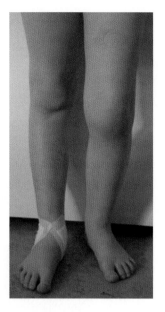

Polyarthritis, Rheumatoid Factor Negative

Rheumatoid factor negative (RF−) polyarthritis is defined as an arthritis that affects five or more joints in the first 6 months of the disease [1]. It is characterized by the absence of the immunoglobulin M-rheumatoid factor (IgM-RF), affects more girls than boys, and usually involves multiple large and small joints, often symmetrically. The etiology is unknown. The onset can be acute or insidious. Pain, limited movements, and morning stiffness are cardinal signs. Some patients with polyarthritis, especially if ANA positive, may actually belong to the oligoarthritis group, but just present with more joints involved. Others present with only small joint swelling, but pronounced stiffness and flexion contractions. Since the ESR is normal they prove to be especially hard to diagnose.

The acute phase reactants are normal or moderately increased, usually with a raised ESR. Antinuclear antibodies (ANA) can be detected in about 60% of the patients and represent a risk for the occurrence of iridocyclitis [9]. This is a typical feature of patients with oligoarthritis, affecting approximately 30%. While iridocyclitis may precede the arthritis, it usually manifests itself a few years later. Due to the insidious and often asymptomatic onset of iridocyclitis, children should be screened at regular intervals by slit-lamp examination, the frequency of these examinations depending upon the subtype of JIA. In high-risk patients such as those with oligoarthritis, the screening should be repeated every 8–12 weeks.

Polyarthritis, Rheumatoid Factor Positive

Rheumatoid factor positive (RF+) polyarthritis is defined as an arthritis affecting five or more joints, but here the IgM-RF can be demonstrated within the first 6 months of the disease on at least two occasions. The subtype is probably identical to the rheumatoid arthritis of adults. It is mainly seen in adolescent girls and usually presents as a symmetrical polyarthritis affecting small joints of the hands and feet. Very often the metacarpophalangeal and proximal interphalangeal, as well as metatarsophalangeal, joints are involved. Rheumatoid nodules on the extensor surfaces of the elbows may develop. This is the smallest group of JIA patients. In contrast to RF− polyarthritis, more joints are involved symmetrically. By definition, the presence of IgM-RF is mandatory, but other laboratory tests are non-specific.

Enthesitis-Related Arthritis

This is the only subtype of JIA which affects more males than females. It is characterized by a combination of enthesopathy and arthritis, the former being defined as tenderness at the insertion of a tendon, ligament, joint capsule, or fascia to the bone. Most of the patients are positive for HLA-B27, and this subtype comprises approximately 10–15% of all JIA patients. Although the association of HLA-B27 has been known for many years, the etiology of enthesopathy-related arthritis is still unknown [10].

The arthritis usually affects the joints of the lower limbs and the typical localization of the enthesopathy is the calcaneal insertion of the Achilles tendon (Fig. 13.4). Arthritis is frequently confined to four or fewer joints, but a polyarticular presentation is not uncommon. The hips may be involved and the disease may progress to affect the sacroiliac joints and other joints of the axial skeleton, leading to (juvenile) ankylosing spondylitis.

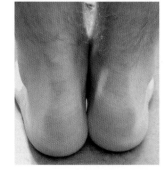

Fig. 13.4 Enthesopathy at the calcaneal insertion of the right Achilles tendon

Fig. 13.5 Dactylitis of the left middle finger

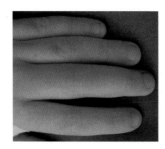

Psoriatic Arthritis

Psoriatic arthritis is defined as arthritis and psoriasis or as arthritis with typical signs (see also Table 13.1). In children arthritis may precede the psoriasis for many years. Larger joints are often affected, usually asymmetrically. Small joints may be involved, again in an asymmetrical pattern. By definition, the presence of dactylitis (Fig. 13.5), nail pitting, onycholysis, or a positive family history supports the diagnosis, but many children who are classified as psoriatic arthritis according to the ILAR criteria may belong to the oligoarticular group. The defining characteristics of juvenile psoriatic arthritis are therefore being questioned [11].

Undifferentiated Arthritis

This subgroup was created to include patients who do not fulfill the criteria of any of the described categories or who would fit in two or more of them. This category therefore does not represent a separate clinical subgroup.

Treatment

The treatment of children with JIA should aim not only to preserve joint function and mobility but also to nurture the child's general development and the health of the family. Therapy for the rheumatic diseases is challenging and complex. Both the patient and family may suffer from psychological problems. They need time and understanding to deal with the many different aspects of treatment and screening procedures, many of which are demanding and costly.

The rheumatic diseases of childhood are often neither benign nor short-lived [12]. Given the complex therapy that may be necessary for many years, it is essential that a multidisciplinary paediatric rheumatology team should be established. In addition to the paediatric rheumatologist, the orthopaedic surgeon, ophthalmologist, or oral surgeon should be consulted. Physical and occupational therapists, social workers, and psychologists should also be included. To ensure normal development and integration of the child into daily activities, close liaison with kindergarten and school should ensure that sport, play, and social interactions are encouraged. Inpatient hospital treatment should be minimized.

A combination of pharmacological interventions, physical therapy, and psychosocial support is the basis of managing JIA. Treatment should aim for complete control of the disease and the prevention of any long-term consequence. The risk of side effects must be constantly borne in mind. Although physical therapy and psychosocial support are as important as drug treatment, the main focus in this chapter is on pharmacotherapy.

Pharmacotherapy

There are no drugs available which cure the disease. However, treatment options have improved immensely for children within the last few years. Control of the disease is much more effective, faster, and with fewer side effects. This encouraging development is in part the result of modifying existing drugs or targeting them better and partly due to a new class of drugs, the so-called biologicals.

Non-steroidal Anti-inflammatory Drugs (NSAIDs)

NSAIDs control pain and inflammation by inhibition of the enzyme cyclo-oxygenase (COX). Most of the NSAIDs used in children are non-selective, inhibiting COX-1 as well as COX-2 inhibitors, the latter being more responsible for promoting inflammation. NSAIDs have been the mainstay of therapy for many years and in most children with JIA, therapy will be started with NSAIDs. The most commonly used are naproxen and ibuprofen. Both need to be administered in adequate doses for a sufficient length of time, usually for at least a month. There is no significant difference in effectiveness between the NSAIDs so that preferences depend upon availability and experience [13, 14]. Naproxen has the advantage of a longer half-life, with dosage required only twice a day. Most of the NSAIDs are well tolerated and demonstrate few side effects in children. When they do occur, the most frequent are nausea, abdominal pain, and decreased appetite. Mood changes and difficulties in concentration may develop, hence regular urine controls are necessary due to possible nephrotoxicity. One less well-known side effect is naproxen-induced pseudoporphyria, characterized by flat hypopigmented scars after minor skin trauma [15]. This side effect must lead to the discontinuation of naproxen, as scars can persist for many years.

Meloxicam, which inhibits COX-1 as well as COX-2, needs to be given only once daily and has proven to be as effective and safe as naproxen [16].

Intra-articular Steroid Injections

Intra-articular injections are used in children who have not responded to conventional parenteral therapy. They are used with increasing frequency as the initial therapy, especially in patients with oligoarthritis. Before recommending intra-articular steroids, Lyme disease arthritis has to be ruled out (see Chapter 25). Several studies have shown that triamcinolone hexacetonide appears to be the most effective agent, particularly in large joints. Children with polyarthritis may also benefit from steroid injections. The effect is usually noticed within a few days after the injection and the response rate is around 60–70%, lasting for several months. Contractures can be avoided or corrected and the development of leg length inequality is prevented. Although not proven scientifically, children seem to benefit from intensive physiotherapy and some restriction in physical activities after injection therapy. Subcutaneous atrophy and hypopigmentation are frequent side effects of injections especially in weight-bearing smaller joints (e.g., ankle, talocalcaneal, and talonavicular). Intra-articular steroid injections reduce symptoms but it has to be appreciated that they are not curative [17–20].

DMARDs (Disease-modifying Anti-rheumatic Drugs)

Although intra-articular steroid injections result in an improvement in approximately two-thirds to three-quarters of the patients, many children will have uncontrolled disease and need more aggressive treatment.

Methotrexate

Methotrexate (MTX) is an analogue of folic acid. It inhibits dihydrofolate reductase although this may not be the mechanism of action in JIA. MTX has become the second-line agent of choice for many children with persistent disease despite the combined use of NSAIDs, intra-articular corticosteroids, and adequate physical therapy. In 1992, a randomized study demonstrated the efficacy of 10 mg/m^2 once a week, where 63% of the patients demonstrated an improvement. The maximum effect of MTX is reached at a dose of 15 mg/m^2. If used parenterally, subcutaneous injections are preferable [21–23].

MTX is usually well tolerated; the most frequent side effects are liver enzyme elevations and gastrointestinal toxicity such as nausea and vomiting. In long-term use, the latter may become troublesome so that many children come to refuse their treatment. Supplements of folic acid may help and may also prevent elevation of liver enzymes. With MTX therapy, laboratory tests need to be performed regularly.

Sulfasalazine

Sulfasalazine lessens joint inflammation and laboratory parameters in children with JIA, especially in enthesitis-related arthritis. Long-term positive effects have been confirmed [24], but side effects develop in 30%. Many patients withdraw from treatment due to gastrointestinal toxicity and skin rashes.

Leflunomide

Leflunomide is a competitive inhibitor of the enzyme dihydroororat dehydrogenase and inhibits de novo synthesis of pyrimidines. In adult patients with rheumatoid arthritis, its effectiveness is similar to methotrexate. Experience in children is scarce, but one study compared its effectiveness with that of MTX. Leflunomide was almost as effective as MTX and has a role in polyarthritic patients who do not respond to MTX or do not tolerate it. The rate of side effects was comparable to MTX [25]. Due to possible hepatotoxicity, combination therapy with MTX is not recommended, although it is reported to be very effective. Close monitoring for hepatoxicity would be mandatory.

Glucocorticoids

Glucocorticoids are potent, fast-acting anti-inflammatory drugs, but their well-known side effects should limit their systemic use to severe or even life-threatening disease. Sometimes, a course of low-dose corticosteroids can be considered to control pain and morning stiffness while the patient awaits the therapeutic effects of MTX or other second-line agents (bridging agent). In severe disease, intravenous steroids (methylprednisolone) can be used alternatively in high doses (10–30 mg/kg) for up to 3 days, resulting in an immediate and profound anti-inflammatory effect.

Biologicals

The introduction of biological medications and especially the anti-tumor necrosis factor (TNF–) drugs has dramatically improved the treatment of rheumatic diseases in childhood. The key role of TNF in experimental and human arthropathies has been demonstrated and the successful clinical application of TNF– blockage demonstrates the central role of this cytokine in the pathogenesis of JIA. However, cytokine antagonists run the risk of immunosuppression (for example, in tuberculosis), and there is little information about long-term side effects. Therefore, at present, the use of biological drugs should be restricted to patients who fail to respond to conventional therapy or have intolerable side effects with other drugs. Paediatric rheumatologists should closely supervise therapy with biologicals and patients should be included in long-term registers.

Other Biological Modifiers

Anakinra is a recombinant interleukin-1-receptor antagonist which inhibits the pro-inflammatory mechanism of IL-1. The antagonist has shown some promising effects in patients with systemic JIA, as has also been demonstrated for an anti-interleukin-6 antibody [26, 27]. Other substances including abatacept, a fusion protein consisting of a T-cell activating antigen (CTLA-4) and IgG1 [28], and rituximab, an anti-B-cell antibody [29], are currently being evaluated for use in children with JIA. There is little doubt that more promising drugs will be available over the next few years.

Course and Prognosis

JIA is an important cause of short-term and long-term disability. It should not be considered a benign disease. The course of the disease in an individual child is impossible to predict but certain prognostic generalizations can be made. Children with oligoarthritis are at risk of developing uveitis, which can be a major complication with a correspondingly poor prognosis. Otherwise, patients with oligoarthritis can usually expect the best outcome. Even for these patients, however, the rate of remission after 10 years is still less than 50%. The outcome in polyarticular disease is much worse, especially in RF– polyarthritis, where the remission rate is as low as 6% [30]. The outcome of systemic JIA is variable in the long term. Approximately 50% of the patients have monocyclic or intermittent episodes of disease with a reasonable prognosis. In patients with no remissions, systemic inflammation eventually resolves, but chronic arthritis with substantial joint destruction may develop [31]. Despite the newer biological modifiers and the promise of stem cell therapy [32], these patients constitute the most severe and challenging form of JIA.

Acknowledgment The author would like to thank Dr. A. Hospach for providing Figs. 13.1, 13.3, 13.4, and 13.5.

Part 2: Surgery for Juvenile Idiopathic Arthritis

Martin N. Arbogast

Introduction

Surgical treatment for juvenile arthritis may be appropriate in pauci-articular disease. It is usually for those who fail to respond or are intolerant of medical therapy. In adults with rheumatoid arthritis operative treatment tends to be a final resort. In children with inflammatory disease surgery is often preventative. Operations in children are also necessary for those with polyarticular disease when deteriorating deformity develops in already badly damaged joints. A substantial discrepancy between clinical symptoms and subjective expressions of pain in children and young adults merits careful analysis if timely surgery is to be performed. Joint and soft tissue *retaining* procedures should be differentiated from joint *replacing* procedures. The aim of any operation is to modify and lessen the destructive course of the disease (Fig. 13.6).

Classification

The seven subtypes of juvenile idiopathic arthritis (JIA) have been described in Part 1 of this chapter. For orthopaedic surgeons it is useful to differentiate between pauci-articular disease and polyarthritis (Fig. 13.7). Each has a different prognosis and pattern of complications [28].

The likelihood of remission is greater in children than in adults with rheumatoid arthritis [29], particularly for those with mono- or pauci-articular disease. Research into the operative treatment of JIA can be classified only at level IIIa evidence.

Morphological and Pathological Changes

The synovial membrane produces essential substances for cartilage nutrition. These reach the cartilage cell by diffusion. Before epiphyseal closure the growth cartilage is also supplied by intraosseous vessels.

The histological changes in childhood inflammatory arthritic disease correlate well with those in the adult rheumatoid patient. The synovial surface cell layer thickens significantly, lymphocytes and plasma cells proliferate within the synovial stroma, while fibrin and proteases as well as collagenases reach the joint space as lysosomal enzymes which digest the surface layer of articular cartilage. After repeated inflammatory attacks, thickened inflammatory pannus grows from the collateral ligament recesses across the joint surfaces, injuring the articular cartilage layers. The first radiological changes of joint space narrowing are signs of this chondromalacia, heralding progressive degeneration.

Synovial thickening combined with recurrent or permanent effusion stretches the joint capsule and ligaments, leading to permanent joint instability. The swelling causes pain of varying severity in different joints: the shoulder, for example, tends to be less painful than the knee. As the arthritis progresses, muscles atrophy and joint contractures may develop. Persistent inactivity leads to decalcification of bone.

Tendons are damaged by intra- or epi-tendinous synovitis. Elongation may be followed by partial or even total tendon rupture, especially if mechanical irritants affect smooth tendon gliding (e.g., in the caput ulna syndrome).

Surgical Management

The decision to proceed with operative treatment must be preceded by discussions with the family and the whole paediatric rheumatology team. It is best if this occurs in an environment where all specialties can participate. Great care should be taken in describing realistic operative goals and detailing the postoperative course. Schooling, other siblings, and domestic concerns need to be considered. The risks and benefits must be balanced and explained.

Regional anesthesia is effective in the upper and lower extremities [30] both during surgery and for postoperative pain control (see Chapter 4).

Indeed, reduction of pain is usually the main goal of surgery, together with retaining joint movement, reducing deformity, and lessening muscular wasting and osteoporosis. Any operation should improve day-to-day functional activity.

Careful positioning of the patient on the operating table is necessary, especially when many joints are affected and there are severe contractures. As the cervical spine is often involved it is wise to check stability with flexion/extension radiographs preoperatively. If in doubt, the neck should be splinted during the operation. Intubation should be avoided whenever possible so the laryngeal mask may be appropriate.

Fig. 13.6 Progressive shoulder joint destruction over 2 years in a 16-year-old with JIA, despite specific anti-rheumatoid drug therapy **a**) and **b**): 2004 **c**) and **d**): 2006

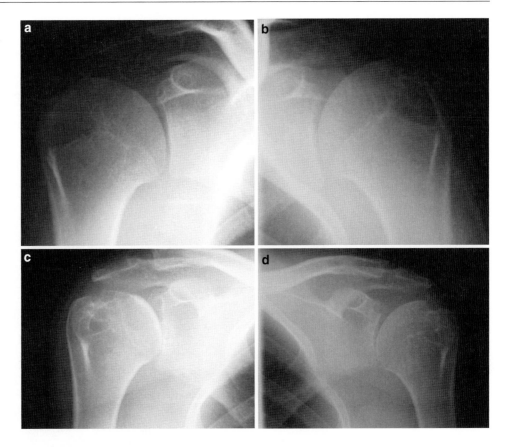

Drug treatment is usually continued until the time of the surgical procedure, particularly non-steroidal anti-inflammatories and low-dose corticosteroid medication. Immunosuppressants should be discontinued shortly before operation and resumed only after wound healing is complete. Drugs which influence blood clotting should be stopped some days before operation to avoid hemorrhage or hematoma formation.

Other causes of arthropathy should have been excluded before surgery. Ultrasonography combined with radiography allows the effusions and synovial changes to be graded. Larsen et al. [31] have grouped the radiological changes into six grades of severity. Supplementary investigation by magnetic resonance imaging (MRI) or computed tomography (CT) is sometimes of value in clarifying bone and soft tissue changes.

Surgical Procedures

Synovectomy

The German Rheumatology Society considers that one indication for synovectomy is persisting inflammation of a joint or tendon sheath for several months in spite of medication. Other indications include articular damage with stiffening, capsular laxity, tendon adhesion, and nerve compression.

If surgery is undertaken when radiographic changes are minimal and the joint surfaces relatively normal, pain and swelling will be reduced leading to functional improvement (Fig. 13.8). Furthermore the removal of inflamed tissue decreases the likelihood of joint and tendon destruction. Minimally invasive procedures with regional anesthesia limit surgical trauma and good postoperative analgesia, perhaps with continuous catheter infusion, encourages speedier rehabilitation. The shoulder, knee, and ankle joints can effectively be freed from pathological synovial tissue and lend themselves to arthroscopic synovectomy. Permanent reduction of pain with weight bearing and movement can be expected. Even in late-stage disease, reduced pain and improved function may still be expected. Minimally invasive procedures, however, are not yet routinely performed at the elbow, wrist, and hip, where open synovectomy is still more commonly undertaken.

Synovectomy of the elbow in Larsen's stages I and II usually leads to good pain relief and improvement in the activities of daily living [32]. In late-stage disease, functional improvement may follow if synovectomy is combined with radial head excision. The head should only be removed

Fig. 13.7 A 16-year-old boy with polyarticular JIA. He is unable to walk. (**a**) Clinical findings. (**b** and **c**) Destruction of both knee joints. (**d**) Destruction of femoral head. (**e**) Atlanto-occipital destruction with narrowing of the foramen magnum

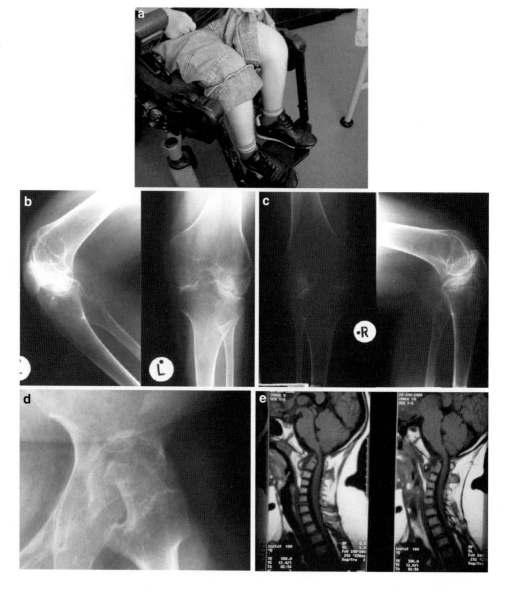

after skeletal maturity if valgus deformity and ulnar nerve irritation are to be avoided. In the hip joint, synovectomy is best performed if conservative measures, including joint aspiration and corticosteroid instillation, fail to prevent progressive stiffness and discomfort. Postoperative ankylosis may complicate synovectomy of the metacarpophalangeal joints: this is a greater problem in children than adults as the capsule lacks elasticity. This, therefore, should be reserved for special cases. Tenosynovectomy in the carpal tunnel and the palm leads to a better outcome than on the extensor surface of the hand, especially if there is accompanying nerve compression.

Inflammation of the ankle joint and its surrounding tendons is amenable to arthroscopic debridement of the ankle joint combined with open tenosynovectomy. The combined procedure is effective in improving walking.

Nerve Decompression

Nerves in close proximity to joints and tendon sheaths may be compressed by increased fluid production or thickened synovial tissue. The indication for surgery should be confirmed by nerve conduction studies. Most often the median nerve is affected at the palmar aspect of the wrist, causing pain and tingling in the classic distribution. The nerve is decompressed by carpal tunnel release and a limited flexor tenosynovectomy. At the elbow the ulnar nerve in the cubital tunnel can be affected by swelling or bony deformity. Early decompression of the ulnar nerve with anterior transposition and local synovectomy allows nerve recovery. The posterior tibial nerve may similarly be irritated behind the medial malleolus and benefit from decompression.

Fig. 13.8 (**a**) Palmar synovitis with extensor lag in a 14-year-old boy with polyarticular JIA. (**b**) Intra-operative removal of synovial tissue. (**c**) Intra-operative testing of tendon movement and inspection of the tendon sheath. (**d**) Four days postoperatively: full extension

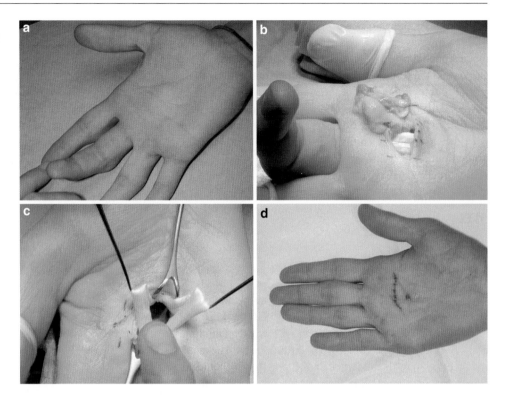

Tendon Lengthening, Shortening, and Transposition

Severely contracted joints, especially in the lower limb, which fail to improve with physiotherapy, serial splinting, or orthoses, may be re-aligned by tendon, bone, or joint procedures. Functional deficits and joint pain can be improved if contractures are overcome. This is most applicable to the adduction and flexion contractures of the hip and knee [33].

Extreme deformity may need to be managed in stages by distraction using an external fixator [38] combined with soft tissue release. The indications and methodology must be discussed thoroughly with the family as the procedures are time consuming and not without risk.

Corrective Osteotomy

Corrective osteotomies should be performed only for severe deformity, preferably before skeletal maturity. Bone healing and remodeling may be unpredictable but in rapidly progressing lower limb axial deformity corrective femoral osteotomy has a limited role. The ease of future joint replacement must be taken into account. Temporary relief can follow corrective osteotomy of the first metatarsal which helps to redistribute weight across the remaining toes.

Isolated bone shortening due to inflammation-induced growth deficiency occasionally merits bone lengthening by

an external fixation device but great care must be taken to ensure that compressive damage is not inflicted upon joints already stiffening from the rheumatoid process.

Resection Arthroplasty

After epiphyseal closure, painful destruction of the metatarsophalangeal joints may be seen occasionally in young adults. Resection arthroplasty of the first metatarsophalangeal joint may be helpful if insoles or orthopaedic shoes prove insufficient to relieve symptoms. As in adults, the operation described by Hueter and Mayo will not prevent later excision of the remaining metatarsal heads by the technique described by Hoffmann and Tillmann, which re-aligns the whole forefoot. Metatarsal arch supports should be prescribed additionally.

Resection arthroplasties in the upper limb are rarely indicated in the young, although the ulnar head can be partly or totally removed to regain painless forearm rotation in young adults.

Arthrodesis

After epiphyseal closure arthrodesis may be a sensible surgical option in some situations. Arthrodesis of the first metacarpophalangeal and proximal interphalangeal joints offer both stabilization and pain relief. Key-pinch and power grip may benefit, particularly by stabilizing the first metacarpophalangeal joint. Destruction and deformity of the carpus and the resulting limited hand function are helped by partial or total arthrodesis of the wrist, which improves grip power and corrects hand position. It may furthermore reduce the risk of spontaneous extensor tendon rupture. Chronic pain due to articular cartilage loss in the ankle, subtalar, or midfoot joints can be reduced by local arthrodesis. It is important to ensure that proper insoles and shoes are available following operation.

Joint Replacement

Arthroplasty has an important role to play in the adolescent with severe disability and pain, particularly at the knee and hip. A sensible compromise must be struck between minimal bone resection and stability of the arthroplasty. The quality of bone may dictate whether the prosthesis should be cementless or cemented. In these young patients it is likely that revision surgery will be required in future. Severe joint deformity combined with short stature may make custom-designed prostheses necessary.

Joint Specific Procedures

Upper Extremity

Shoulder

Joint-preserving procedures at the shoulder are best performed by minimally invasive techniques using the arthroscope. Operations can be performed easily using interscalene regional anesthetic blocks supplemented by propofol [35]. Three portals are used for complete synovectomy. Labrum or rotator cuff repair can also be carried out arthroscopically or by mini-open incision technique.

Joint replacement may be performed after epiphyseal closure when there is severe destruction in Larsen stages IV and V disease [33, 39]. Pain at rest and with movement may be much improved by humeral head replacement. In general, hemiarthroplasty is preferred in rheumatoid patients. Loosening of the glenoid component, which occurs early in 30%, can then be avoided. The range of movement is less after hemiarthroplasty than after total replacement [40, 41]. Preservation of the rotator cuff is important for active movement [42]. Even when only limited movement is regained, the reduction in pain is impressive.

Elbow

Synovectomy (Fig. 13.9) is successful in reducing pain and improving the range of motion in 74% of patients with Larsen stages I–III disease [43]. In end-stage disease with a significant flexion contracture, late synovectomy and arthrolysis may help to improve the activities of daily living. Only rarely in the young adult is joint replacement indicated.

Hand and Wrist

In the hand and wrist, palmar and dorsal tenosynovectomies should be differentiated from procedures at the carpus and the metacarpophalangeal and proximal interphalangeal joints.

Flexor tendon synovectomy in the carpal tunnel combined with nerve decompression is unusual in childhood. More commonly pain and limited movement are caused by epi- and intratendinous synovitis in the palm or the fingers (Fig. 13.10).

Carpal destruction is seen in polyarticular arthritis. Surgical options differ little from the adult. With severe disease, synovectomy of the wrist with resection of the ulnar head and partial or complete arthrodesis can be helpful (Fig. 13.11). Persistent pain due to deformity or secondary destruction usually occurs in early adult life.

Lower Extremity

Hip Joint

Synovectomy of the hip joint may be performed by open operation or arthroscopically [44, 45]. Neither allows a complete synovectomy, unless the femoral head is dislocated [46]. While newer techniques make dislocation safer, there remains the risk of femoral head necrosis [47]. This procedure is rarely performed early in the disease.

Polyarticular arthritis may lead to acetabular dysplasia, making joint replacement difficult (Fig. 13.7d). Custom-made prostheses with small heads and shortened stems may need to be fashioned. In polyarticular disease it is common for all four major lower limb joints to need replacement if reasonable mobility is to be regained.

Knee Joint

Arthroscopic synovectomy of the knee has considerable advantages over open surgery (Fig. 13.12). Trauma is less through three to six small portals; postoperative mobilization is quicker and easier and complications are reduced [32, 48–50]. Femoral and sciatic nerve blocks improve postoperative analgesia and allow early passive and actively assisted physiotherapy. While continuous passive motion devices speed up recovery, children still need time to regain their range of motion [37]. Disturbed proprioception in the growing joint may contribute to the slow recovery.

Metacarpophalangeal or proximal interphalangeal synovectomies should be performed only after careful monitoring of the radiographic changes as the postoperative

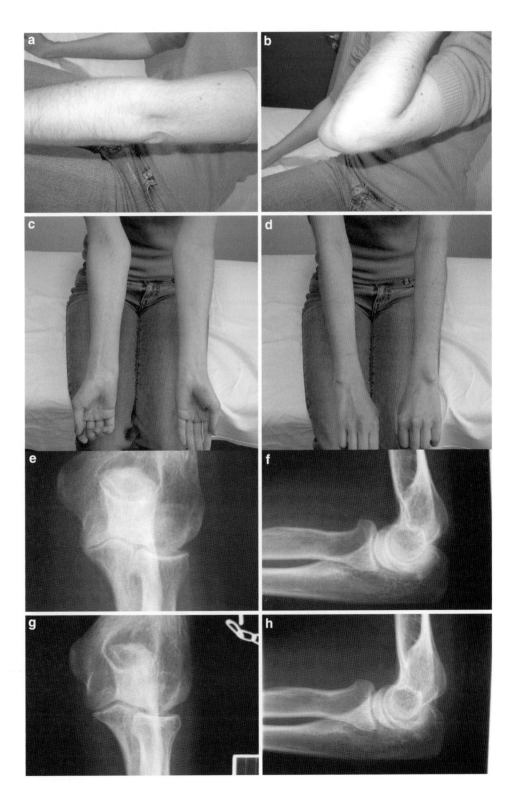

Fig. 13.9 Result of elbow synovectomy for pauci-articular disease 7 years postoperatively. No clinical or radiographic progression. (**a**) Extension; (**b**) flexion; (**c**) supination; (**d**) pronation; (**e** and **f**) preoperative; and (**g** and **h**) postoperative

Fig. 13.10 (**a** and **b**) Flexor
tendon synovitis with reduced
function in an 8-year-old with
polyarticular JIA;
(**c**) radiographic
changes—Larsen stage I; and
(**d**) intra-operative findings with
epi- and intratendinous synovitis

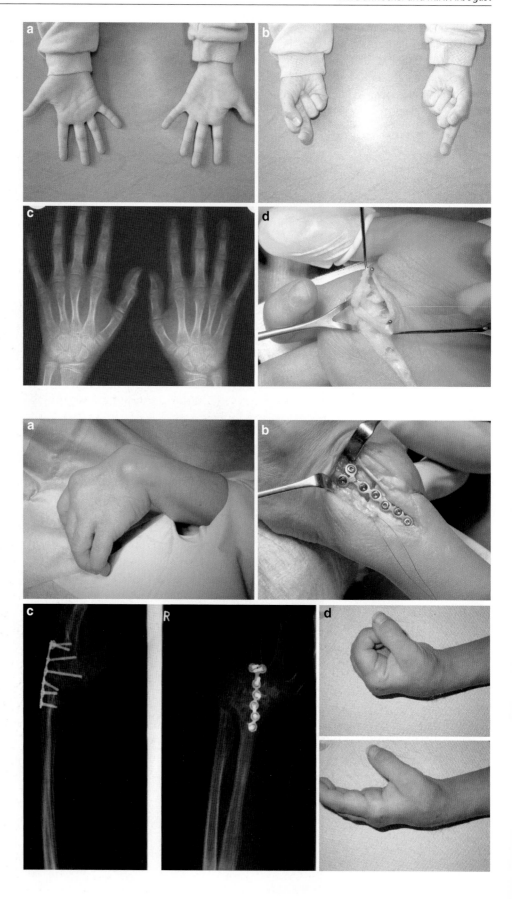

Fig. 13.11 (**a**) Bayonet
deformity preoperatively.
(**b**) Intra-operative
osteosynthesis.
(**c**) Wrist arthrodesis with
mini-titanium plate for bayonet
deformity. (**d**) Hand function 6
weeks later

Fig. 13.12 Arthroscopic knee synovectomy in a 16-year-old male with pauci-articular disease. (**a** and **b**) Clinical findings: drug-resistant swelling. (**c**) Radiographs: no destruction. (**d**) Ultrasonography: effusion and synovial thickening. (**e**) Operative findings: synovial pannus. (**f**) After arthroscopic synovectomy

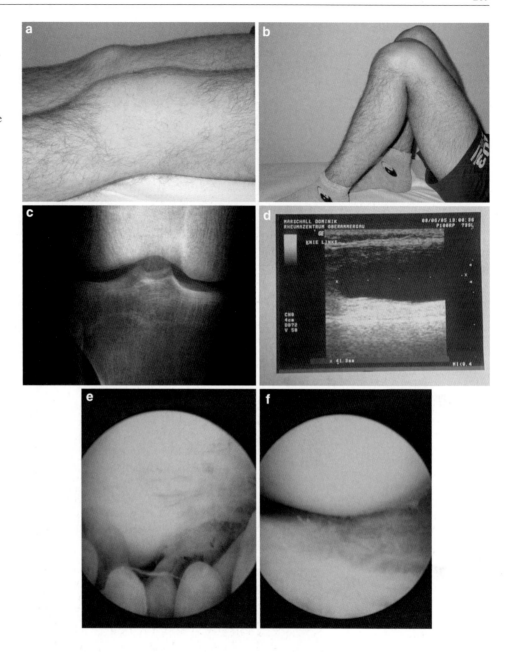

management is complicated and can lead to lost motion. Joint replacement is rare before maturity.

Joint replacement may be necessary in both poly- and pauci-articular arthritis [33, 42]. Skeletal growth should be complete. Planning for joint replacement must include assessment of all joints. Procedures in the young adult should spare as much bone as possible. Surface replacements are the implants of choice as they preserve bone stock for exchange operations in the future although some concern has been recorded about their use in young women. Contractures over 30° or significant collateral ligament laxity may dictate the need for semi-constrained implants. Joint replacement in the late teens or the early twenties allows the patient to

integrate properly into normal life (Fig. 13.13) including limited participation in gentle sports [42].

Ankle and Subtalar joints

Ankle joint synovectomy is possible arthroscopically. The procedure may be combined with open synovectomy of the posterior tibial and peroneal tendon sheaths. Early movement and partial weight bearing should be encouraged to ensure cartilage nutrition.

In Larsen stage IV or V disease, arthrodesis is worthwhile. Joint replacement has become more reliable but implant survival does not yet match that at the hip and knee joint.

Fig. 13.13 (**a**) Secondary degeneration of the knee after 17 years of pauci-articular JIA. (**b**) Radiograph after knee replacement. (**c** and **d**) Clinical result at 2 years (22-year-old female)

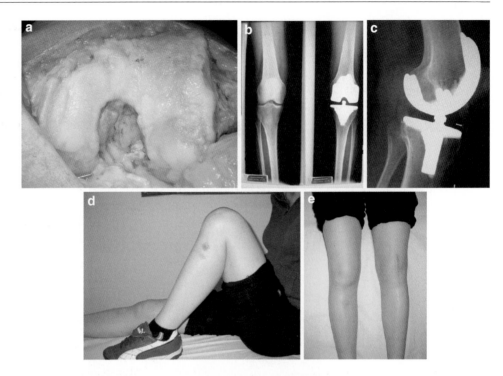

Fig. 13.14 An 18-year-old female patient with JIA. Corrective osteotomy of the first metatarsal with preservation of joint cartilage. (**a**) Clinical picture: second toe overlapping. (**b**) Radiographic picture. (**c**) After three-dimensional corrective osteotomy of the first metatarsal. (**d**) Repositioning the extensor hallucis longus tendon intra-operatively

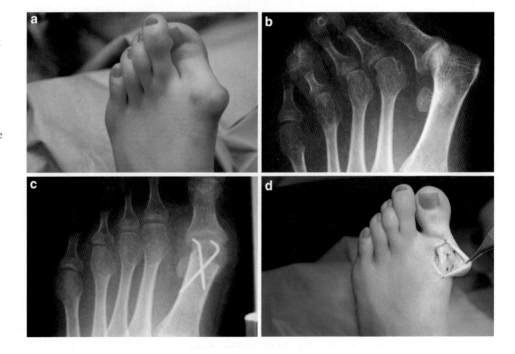

Foot

Surgery is mainly by corrective osteotomy or resection arthroplasty. Synovectomy is only rarely indicated. There is a tendency for joint ankylosis or tenodesis to develop with consequent loss of movement. When articular cartilage is preserved, corrective osteotomies are preferable to excision arthroplasty (Fig. 13.14). Resection procedures such as metatarsal head resection arthroplasty by Hoffmann and Tillmann's technique [51] may be postponed until a later date when insoles and orthopaedic shoes fail to offer sufficient support and comfort.

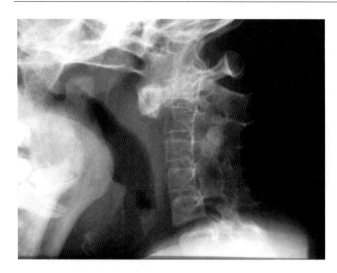

Fig. 13.15 Atlanto-axial instability and subaxial vertebral body fusion in polyarticular disease

Spine

When atlanto-occipital destruction causes neurological symptoms the spine needs to be stabilized by fusion. In JIA especially there may be a combination of atlanto-axial instability and subaxial spinal body fusion (Fig. 13.15). Careful neurological examination and imaging are necessary in the work-up of these patients. Multi-level instability must be carefully identified as localized fusion may otherwise be dangerous. Cervical collars may be necessary both before and after operation until fusion has occurred.

The thoracic and lumbar spine are rarely affected. Osteopenia resulting from inactivity or drug therapy may lead to vertebral deformity or fracture. Physiotherapy is the mainstay of treatment and it is rarely necessary to consider thoracolumbar spinal fusion or kyphoplasty in children.

Postoperative Management

Orthopaedic procedures in children with inflammatory joint disease should only be undertaken when careful postoperative physiotherapy is available. Best results follow physiotherapy at least once daily. Physical and occupational therapy complete the management strategy. Good orthoses are needed especially for the hand and foot.

Summary

Compliance is hard to achieve in children under 6 years of age but improves in the older child. This should be borne in mind when planning surgery. Elective surgery is best performed when the co-operation of both child and parents is assured. When considering surgery in children and young adults with JIA the systemic status of the disease must always be taken into account. No single joint should be considered in isolation; treatment must always be directed at the health and mobility of the whole child.

References

1. Petty RE, Southwood TR, Manners P, et al. International League of Associations for Rheumatology classification of juvenile idiopathic arthritis: second revision, Edmonton, 2001. J Rheumatol 2004; 31:390–392.
2. Minden K. Epidemiologie. In: Wagner N, Dannecker G, eds. Pädiatrische Rheumatologie. Heidelberg: Springer Medizin Verlag; 2007;179–181.
3. Manners PJ, Bower C. Worldwide prevalence of juvenile arthritis why does it vary so much? J Rheumatol 2002; 29:1520–1530.
4. Oen KG, Cheang M. Epidemiology of chronic arthritis in childhood. Semin Arthritis Rheum 1996; 26:575–591.
5. Still G. On a form of chronic joint disease in children. Medico-Chirurgical Trans 1897; 80:47–59.
6. de Benedetti F, Martini A. Targeting the interleukin-6 receptor: a new treatment for systemic juvenile idiopathic arthritis? Arthritis Rheum 2005; 52:687–693.
7. Pascual V, Allantaz F, Arce E, et al. Role of interleukin-1 (IL-1) in the pathogenesis of systemic onset juvenile idiopathic arthritis and clinical response to IL-1 blockade. J Exp Med 2005; 201: 1479–1486.
8. Behrens EM, Beukelman T, Paessler M, Cron RQ. Occult macrophage activation syndrome in patients with systemic juvenile idiopathic arthritis. J Rheumatol 2007; 34(5):1133–1138.
9. Ravelli A, Felici E, Magni-Manzoni S, et al. Patients with antinuclear antibody-positive juvenile idiopathic arthritis constitute a homogeneous subgroup irrespective of the course of joint disease. Arthritis Rheum 2005; 52:826–832.
10. Taurog JD. The mystery of HLA-B27: if it isn't one thing, it's another. Arthritis Rheum 2007; 56:2478–2481.
11. Ravelli A, Martini A. Juvenile idiopathic arthritis. Lancet 2007; 369:767–778
12. Minden K, Niewerth M, Listing J, et al. Long-term outcome in patients with juvenile idiopathic arthritis. Arthritis Rheum 2002; 46:2392–2401.
13. Giannini EH, Brewer EJ, Miller ML, et al. Ibuprofen suspension in the treatment of juvenile rheumatoid arthritis. Pediatric Rheumatology Collaborative Study Group. J Pediatr 1990; 117:645–652.
14. Leak AM, Richter MR, Clemens LE, et al. A crossover study of naproxen, diclofenac and tolmetin in seronegative juvenile chronic arthritis. Clin Exp Rheumatol 1988; 6:157–160.
15. Schad SG, Kraus A, Haubitz I, et al. Early onset pauciarticular arthritis is the major risk factor for naproxen-induced pseudoporphyria in juvenile idiopathic arthritis. Arthritis Res Ther 2007; 9:R10.
16. Ruperto N, Nikishina I, Pachanov ED, et al. A randomized, double-blind clinical trial of two doses of meloxicam compared with naproxen in children with juvenile idiopathic arthritis: short- and long-term efficacy and safety results. Arthritis Rheum 2005; 52:563–572.
17. Breit W, Frosch M, Meyer U, et al. A subgroup-specific evaluation of the efficacy of intraarticular triamcinolone

hexacetonide in juvenile chronic arthritis. J Rheumatol 2000; 27: 2696–2702.

18. Padeh S, Passwell JH. Intraarticular corticosteroid injection in the management of children with chronic arthritis. Arthritis Rheum 1998; 41:1210–1214.

19. Zulian F, Martini G, Gobber D, et al. Triamcinolone acetonide and hexacetonide intra-articular treatment of symmetrical joints in juvenile idiopathic arthritis: a double-blind trial. Rheumatology (Oxford) 2004; 43:1288–1291.

20. Sherry DD, Stein LD, Reed AM, et al. Prevention of leg length discrepancy in young children with pauciarticular juvenile rheumatoid arthritis by treatment with intraarticular steroids. Arthritis Rheum 1999; 42:2330–2334.

21. Giannini EH, Brewer EJ, Kuzmina N, et al. Methotrexate in resistant juvenile rheumatoid arthritis. Results of the U.S.A.-U.S.S.R. double-blind, placebo-controlled trial. The Pediatric Rheumatology Collaborative Study Group and The Cooperative Children's Study Group. N Engl J Med 1992; 326:1043–1049.

22. Ruperto N, Murray KJ, Gerloni V, et al. A randomized trial of par-enteral methotrexate comparing an intermediate dose with a higher dose in children with juvenile idiopathic arthritis who failed to respond to standard doses of methotrexate. Arthritis Rheum 2004; 50:2191–2201.

23. Alsufyani K, Ortiz-Alvarez O, Cabral DA, et al. The role of sub-cutaneous administration of methotrexate in children with juvenile idiopathic arthritis who have failed oral methotrexate. J Rheumatol 2004; 31:179–182.

24. Van Rossum MA, van Soesbergen RM, Boers M, et al. Long-term outcome of juvenile idiopathic arthritis following a placebo con-trolled trial: sustained benefits of early sulfasalazine treatment. Ann Rheum Dis 2007; 66:1518–1524.

25. Silverman E, Mouy R, Spiegel L, et al. Leflunomide or methotrex-ate for juvenile rheumatoid arthritis. N Engl J Med 2005; 352:1655–1666.

26. Verbsky JW, White AJ. Effective use of the recombinant inter-leukin 1 receptor antagonist anakinra in therapy resistant sys-temic onset juvenile rheumatoid arthritis. J Rheumatol 2004; 31: 2071–2075.

27. Yokota S, Miyamae T, Imagawa T, et al. Therapeutic efficacy of humanized recombinant anti-interleukin-6 receptor antibody in children with systemic-onset juvenile idiopathic arthritis. Arthritis Rheum 2005; 52:818–825.

28. Genovese MC, Becker JC, Schiff M, et al. Abatacept for rheuma-toid arthritis refractory to tumor necrosis factor alpha inhibition. N Engl J Med 2005; 353:1114–1123.

29. El-Hallak M, Binstadt BA, Leichtner AM, et al. Clinical effects and safety of rituximab for treatment of refractory pediatric autoimmune diseases. J Pediatr 2007; 150:376–382.

30. Oen K, Malleson PN, Cabral DA, et al. Disease course and out-come of juvenile rheumatoid arthritis in a multicenter cohort. J Rheumatol 2002; 29:1989–1999.

31. Singh-Grewal D, Schneider R, Bayer N, Feldman BM. Predictors of disease course and remission in systemic juvenile idiopathic arthritis: significance of early clinical and laboratory features. Arthritis Rheum 2006; 54:1595–1601.

32. Brinkman DM, de Kleer IM, ten Cate R, et al. Autologous stem cell transplantation in children with severe progressive systemic or polyarticular juvenile idiopathic arthritis: long-term follow-up of a prospective clinical trial. Arthritis Rheum 2007; 56:2410–2421.

33. Ansell B, Swann M. The management of chronic arthritis of children. J Bone Joint Surg 1983; 65B:536–543.

34. Häfner R, Truckenbrodt H, Michels H, von Altenbockum C. Therapie der juvenilen chronischen Arthritis. Dt Ärzteblatt 1991; 88:3622–3632.

35. Büttner J, Meier G. Kontinuierliche periphere Techniken zur Regionalanästhesie und Schmerztherapie-Obere und untere Extremität. Bremen: Uni-med; 1999.

36. Larsen A, Dale K, Eek M. Radiographic evaluation of rheumatoid arthritis and related conditions by standard reference films. Acta Radiol Diagn 1977; 18:481–491.

37. Arbogast M. Operative Therapie. In: Kinderrheuma—Wir können was tun, 1st ed. Garmisch-Partnkirchen: Deutsches Zentrum für Kinder- und Jugendrheumatologie; 2006.

38. Correll J, Truckenbrodt H. Correction of severe joint contractures and leg length discrepancies by external fixation (Ilizarov method). Rev Rheum Eng Ed 1997; 64(10 Suppl):163S–166S.

39. Eichinger S, Forst R, Kindervater M. Indikation zur Schulter TEP beim jüngeren Patienten. Orthopäde 2007; 36:311–324.

40. Schmidt-Wiethoff R, Wolf P, Lehmann M, Habermeyer P. [Physical activity after shoulder arthroplasty.] Sportverletz Sportschaden 2002; 16:26–30.

41. Ziegler J, Amlang M, Bottesi M, et al. [Results for endopros-thetic care in patients younger than 50 years.] Orthopäde 2007; 36: 325–336.

42. Arbogast M. Sports in rheumatic diseases and joint replacement. Acta Rheumatol 2008; 33:29–32.

43. Arbogast M, Häfner R, Michels H, Kremling E. Joint saving therapy of the elbow in juvenile idiopathic arthritis. Arthritis Rheumatol 2006; 26:364–368.

44. Gondolph-Zink B, Puhl W, Noack W. Semiarthroscopic synovec-tomy of the hip. Int Orthop 1988; 12:31–35.

45. Schraml A. Synovektomie des Hüftgelenkes bei juveniler chro-nischer Arthritis. In: Venbrocks R, ed. Neuroorthopädie und Rheumaorthopädie des Kindes. Berlin: Springer; 2000:123–131.

46. Morgensen B, Brattström H, Ekelund L, et al. Synovectomy of the hip in juvenile chronic arthritis. J Bone Joint Surg 1982; 64-B(3):295–299.

47. Heimkes B, Stotz S. Ergebnisse der Spätsynovetomie der Hüfte bei der juvenilen chronischen Arthritis. Z Rheumatol 1992; 51: 132–135.

48. Adamec O, Dungl P, Kasal T, Chomiak J. Knee joint synovec-tomy in treatment of juvenile idiopathic arthritis. Acta Chirur Orth Traum Checheslovaca 2002; 69(6):350–356.

49. Gschwend N. Synovectomy of the knee joint. In Gschwend N, Böni A. Surgical Treatment of Rheumatoid Arthritis. Stuttgart: Thieme; 1980:203–216.

50. Häfner R, Pieper M. Arthroskopische Kniegelenkssynovektomie bei juveniler chronischer Arthritis. Z Rheumatol 1995; 54: 165–170.

51. Gschwend N. Die operative Behandlung der chronischen Polyarthritis. Stuttgart: Thieme; 1977.

Chapter 14

Bone Tumors

Gérard Bollini, Jean-Luc Jouve, Franck Launay, Elke Viewheger, Yann Glard, and Michel Panuel

Introduction

Bone tumors and tumor-like conditions are uncommon in childhood and adolescence. They are difficult to manage because of their variable nature and accurate diagnosis cannot always be based on imaging appearance alone. However, a specific combination of clinical, biological, and radiological signs may suggest and sometimes confirm whether they will behave in an aggressive, latent, or indeterminate manner. Sometimes the radiological signs are easily recognized and many lesions require neither biopsy nor treatment. For others, however, management by clinicians, radiologists, and pathologists working as a multidisciplinary team in a specialized unit is necessary. It is important to bear in mind that children and adolescents are not just small adults. The lesions which affect them, the way they behave biologically, and the way they should be treated can be radically different.

Definition

A tumor may be defined as an abnormal mass of tissue that grows faster than normal and with an abnormal histology.

The term dystrophy or tumor-like dystrophy covers benign bone lesions that are neither overly aggressive nor neoplastic.

A benign tumor develops slowly and its cells are well differentiated. Metastases only occur in exceptional cases. The main features of a malignant tumor are that it develops rapidly and its cells do not differentiate normally. It is highly invasive, spreading to the neighboring tissues and metastasizing to other parts of the body.

Incidence

Benign tumors are fairly common, but most are asymptomatic and so their true frequency is unknown. Non-ossifying fibromas, osteochondromas, and isolated cysts are in this category.

Malignant bone tumors account for 5% of all paediatric malignancies. Their incidence varies according to age. They are rare in the under-5 age group, account for 4–6% of malignancies in the 0- to 14-year cohort, and rank third in the 10- to 24-year age group.

According to the World Health Organization (WHO) the incidence of bone tumors from 0 to 14 years is 6.6 per million people-years, standardized for the world population. The two commonest malignant tumors in children are osteosarcoma and Ewing's sarcoma which account for 50 and 40%, respectively, of bone malignancies in children [1].

Etiology

The etiology of most tumors is unclear. However, the frequency of bone tumors peaks during the second decade of childhood, suggesting that this period of rapid bone growth is important. Radiation exposure is reputed to be oncogenic for bone tumors. It is now recognized that osteosarcoma can develop after radiation therapy; as a result this type of treatment in children is now rarely indicated [2].

Some benign tumors such as osteochondromas, osteoblastomas, neurofibromas, and fibrodysplasia may become malignant but malignant transformation is rare and usually occurs in adult life. Viruses have been cited as a possible cause of tumors but this has not been formally demonstrated [3].

Some have a genetic predisposition. Multiple exostoses are inherited as an autosomal dominant. Family forms of osteosarcoma with mutations of the RB1 gene [4] and/or Li–Fraumeni syndrome [5] have been described. More recently

G. Bollini (✉)
Department of Paediatric Orthopaedics, Timone Children's Hospital, Marseille, France

M. Benson et al. (eds.), *Children's Orthopaedics and Fractures*,
DOI 10.1007/978-1-84882-611-3_14, © Springer-Verlag London Limited 2010

it has been demonstrated that some hereditary disorders are associated with a higher risk of developing an osteosarcoma [3]. Hilmann mentions 59 cases of osteosarcoma recorded in 24 families since 1930 [6].

Recent trauma is often described by families but has never been shown to be a significant factor.

Clinical Diagnosis

Bone tumors are frequently diagnosed incorrectly or late. There are usually two reasons for this: first, the warning signs are non-specific and second, because they are uncommon, they are rarely considered as the primary diagnosis by the attending physician. Sometimes they are found incidentally on a radiograph, usually taken for pain after an injury. Pain which occurs at night and affects the patient's physical activities can be suggestive. Less commonly a mass may be palpated or a pathological fracture occur.

Focal bone lesions can be due to infection. This differential diagnosis must always be considered and appropriate blood tests should be done to look for bacterial markers (see Chapter 10).

Investigations

A full history and examination should always be performed.

Imaging

Plain Radiograph

Good quality plain radiographs are important. They can provide information on the topography, morphology, and multiplicity of the lesions and whether there is a periosteal reaction. Based on their analysis a provisional diagnosis can usually be made and a management strategy devised, and in particular what further imaging is necessary. Previous radiographs, if available, may be helpful.

Now that digital radiology has become widespread it provides us with new tools such as electronic magnifiers for more accurate reading and archiving facilities.

Computed Tomography (CT)

A CT scan is better than plain radiographs for determining the "epicenter" of the lesion which may be medullary, cortical, or juxtacortical. It provides accurate morphological details of the bone anomaly, showing the tumor boundary, the adjacent bone tissue, the state of the cortical bone, and a detailed analysis of the matrix. It may also reveal micro-calcification in the lesion which is invisible on plain radiograph. CT scans complement plain radiographs, particularly in complex anatomical areas such as the pelvic and shoulder girdles, wrist, and spine.

A CT scan is indicated when a bone lesion has been identified on a bone scan although the plain radiographs appear normal. Lastly, a CT scan can help guide percutaneous cautery in treating lesions such as an osteoid osteoma or when injecting sclerosing agents into an aneurysmal bone cyst.

Magnetic Resonance Imaging (MRI)

MRI is not routinely indicated for clearly benign lesions which require no treatment (e.g., non-ossifying fibromas, benign bone islands, isolated cysts, or an incidentally discovered exostosis). However, it is the best form of imaging for an aggressive lesion suspected of malignancy or any lesion of uncertain nature. It allows a clear view of endosseous and extra-osseous tumor spread, contributing morphological details not visible on a plain radiograph. MRI should always be used before biopsy, which remains the only method of obtaining a precise tissue diagnosis [7–9].

MRI yields information on the spread of the tumor within the bone itself, in particular in relation to the growth plates, and it also shows up any cystic or necrotic areas that should be avoided when needle biopsy is performed [7, 9–12].

MRI is also useful in monitoring disease progress in patients undergoing chemotherapy or when local recurrence is suspected after surgery for benign or malignant tumors. However, the quality of the images obtained may be radically affected by local implants even if they are made of non-magnetic metal [13–16].

Scintigrams

Bone Scan

Bone scans use a phosphonate-derived agent labeled with ^{99m}technetium. A scintigram is a simple examination useful for exploring the whole skeleton. A scintigram cannot discriminate between a benign and malignant lesion. Its key asset is to confirm the presence of a lesion when plain radiographs are negative and to clarify the need for further imaging. If a lesion is visible on radiograph and seems benign, a scintigram is superfluous. A scintigram is often advised when there may be multifocal disease, e.g., Langerhans' histiocytosis, multiple chondromata, and polyostotic fibrous dysplasia.

Positron Emission Tomography (PET)

PET scan [17–19] is now used to assess the efficacy of chemotherapy in malignant tumors; however, it has little discriminatory value in the initial assessment as many tumors show increased uptake of the isotope [4, 20].

Other Examinations

While ultrasound and angiography are not used routinely in the assessment of bone tumors, an angiogram may be very helpful in certain circumstances such as operations involving risk to the spinal cord or a hypervascular tumor.

Case Analysis

Analysis of the information from imaging should aim at defining the number, site, and size of the lesions, their structure, and the reaction in the surrounding tissues.

The Number of Lesions

Whether a lesion is isolated or multiple can be important in making an accurate diagnosis. Multiple lesions may be found in enchondromatosis, multiple exostoses, eosinophilic granuloma in Langerhans' histiocytosis, or polyostotic fibrous dysplasia (Fig. 14.1).

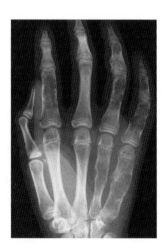

Fig. 14.1 Multiple enchondromas in a 13-year-old boy. Most of the radiolucent lesions are centrally located in the phalangeal diaphyses with a slow-growing appearance. There are also cortical lesions in the fourth and fifth metacarpals

The Site

The site of the lesion is an important factor in diagnosis. A distinction should be made between the flat, long, and short bones and the site of the lesion on or in the bone should be considered. It is essential to determine the "epicenter" of the lesion; this is particularly important when the lesion is bulky. The site must be accurately located both longitudinally and in the transverse plane: medullary, central or eccentric, cortical or juxtacortical. Some benign or malignant lesions have preferential or exclusive "epicenters" located in the longitudinal or transverse plane (Tables 14.1 and 14.2).

Size and Shape

The size and shape of the lesion may suggest a diagnosis but are rarely specific.

Reaction in the Adjacent Bone

The appearance of the adjacent bone is important, particularly the margin of the lesion, the state of the cortical bone,

Table 14.1 The locations of the main tumors and tumor-like conditions of the long bones

Condition	Epiphysis	Metaphysis	Diaphysis
Chondroblastoma	+	–	–
Chondroma	–	+	+/–
Fibrous dysplasia	–	+	+
Chondromyxoid fibroma	–	+	–
Non-ossifying chondroma and cortical defect	–	+	–
Osteofibrous dysplasia	–	–	+
Eosinophilic granuloma	+/–	+	+
Hemangioma	–	+	+
Benign bone island	+	+	–
Aneurysmal cyst	+	+	+/–
Simple or solitary bone cyst	–	+	+/–
Lymphoma	–	+/–	+
Osteoblastoma	–	+	+
Osteochondroma	–	+	–
Osteoid osteoma	+	+	+
Osteosarcoma	–	+	+/–
Ewing's sarcoma	–	+/–	+

Table 14.2 Preferential sites of tumors or tumor-like conditions within the bone

Intra-cancellous	Fibrous dysplasia
	Enchondroma
	Chondromyxoid fibroma
	Eosinophilic granuloma
	Simple or solitary bone cyst
	Conventional osteosarcoma
	Ewing's sarcoma
Intra-cortical	Non-ossifying fibroma and cortical defect
	Osteofibrous dysplasia
	Hemangioma
	Osteoid osteoma
	Superficial osteosarcoma

and possible periosteal reaction when considering whether it is an aggressive lesion or not. Many lesions create a void (lucency or cyst) in the bone structure. This cyst is created by the destruction of the cortical and/or cancellous tissue. The margin of the cyst and the type of osteolysis should be classified according to their site and whether they present a moth-eaten, permeative, or punctuate pattern in theoretical order of increasing aggressiveness.

Some benign lesions are also surrounded by a more or less well-marked peripheral osteoblastic reaction, for example, the sclerotic border seen around benign cystic lesions (Fig. 14.2) and the thickened bone that develops around an osteoid osteoma. The osteoblastic reaction shows that the ongoing process is developing slowly and suggests a benign lesion.

Edema around the lesion on the MRI is difficult to interpret because this occurs both in malignant lesions and infection.

The cortico-periosteal reaction is a fundamental part of the analysis because it is visible on plain radiograph. The periosteum reacts to aggression by ossification of its deepest layer. Benign processes can lead to a gradual erosion of the cortical bone which is replaced by a periosteal shell of varying thickness, smooth or lobular, which may or may not be visible on plain radiograph. The junction between the healthy cortical bone and the cortical bone abutting the lesion can also be thickened and present as a "flying buttress." Careful analysis of the cortical bone is a key point in the diagnosis of the sessile form of osteochondroma; the healthy cortical bone and the cortical part of the osteochondroma should form a continuum as should the cancellous bone. Different imaging slices will throw light on the doubtful case.

In the early development of a malignant tumor a periosteal reaction may sometimes be the only sign visible on plain

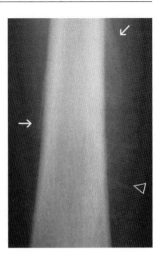

Fig. 14.3 Ewing's sarcoma of the femoral diaphysis. Several patterns of periosteal reaction related to the rapidly growing lesion are visible: interrupted lamellated reaction (*horizontal arrow*), Codman's triangle (*oblique arrow*), spiculated reaction (*arrowhead*)

radiograph; it will be thin and show up as a single layer. In other cases it may look quite different and be either continuous or have breaks, be spicular, or present in one or several thin layers. The border of the periosteal reaction often appears spur shaped—so called Codman's triangle—seen only in malignant tumors and some very aggressive infectious lesions (Fig. 14.3).

Imaging helps to analyze the structure and matrix of the lesion and contributes greatly to diagnosis. MRI remains the best tool for assessing its internal architecture, but is not in itself diagnostic.

Key Diagnoses

Once the plain radiographs and other imaging modalities have been analyzed there are three possibilities:

1. The lesion is aggressive and likely to be malignant. The child should be referred for further management to a hospital that manages malignant paediatric bone tumors (see below).
2. The lesion is obviously benign. The next step is to consider whether a biopsy is indicated and, if not, decide if the child may be discharged or clinical and radiological surveillance is necessary.
3. The diagnosis is uncertain. These cases should be managed as though they were malignant.

Biopsy

If the diagnosis remains uncertain or malignancy is suspected (types 2 and 3 above) a biopsy must be performed, preferably in the definitive treatment center. Selection of the biopsy site should be based on the imaging data.

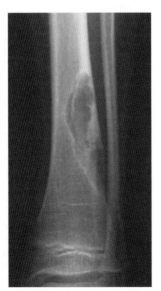

Fig. 14.2 Non-ossifying fibroma of the distal tibia in an 8-year-old child. There is an osteolytic lesion with an osteosclerotic margin arising from the lateral cortex of the tibia

The biopsy will be used for several tests and must be carefully planned. The samples must be adequate to allow proper histological interpretation:

- A smear should allow cytological examination. Frozen section analysis is helpful if expert histopathologists are available.
- Samples should be deep-frozen in liquid nitrogen for future molecular laboratory tests.
- Samples should be taken for bacteriological analysis.
- Decalcified samples should be prepared for morphological study. They may be used later for immunohistochemical tests.
- Samples should be taken for cytogenic examination.

Open Surgical Biopsy

A proper biopsy is essential for two reasons:

1. To confirm the diagnosis the surgeon must ensure that sufficient tumor is harvested, without compromising the subsequent resection.
2. The surgical approach for biopsy must be in line with the planned approach for surgical tumor resection. Once the skin and fascia have been incised the surgeon must access the tumor as directly as possible, bearing in mind the fact that this approach will be resected as part of the definitive operation. It must not interfere with neurovascular structures or open the joint capsule.

In the three most frequent locations—distal femur, proximal tibia, and humerus—the main issue may be gaining access to a tumor outside the compartment on the opposite side of the proposed surgical approach. In this situation the surgeon should not hesitate to drill through the bone and perform a "transosseous" biopsy. It is important to consider whether the biopsy has weakened the bone and if so, weight bearing should be restricted.

If the biopsy is at risk of severe bleeding, for example, in telangiectatic osteosarcoma, a tourniquet should be used if possible. Esmarch bandages must not be used as they risk crushing the tumor and encouraging its spread. A suction drain, aligned with the axis of the wound, should be used if bleeding is a problem.

Needle/Closed Biopsy

Biopsies may be performed with a core needle or a trocar under fluoroscopic or CT guidance.

Such needle or closed biopsies have become increasingly common. Skrzynski found their reliability to be 84% against 96% for open surgical biopsies [21]. Mitsuyoshi, an experienced musculoskeletal histopathologist, was able to differentiate malignant from benign tumors in 97% of cases (bone: 100%; soft tissue: 94%) and arrived at a specific diagnosis in 88% when adequate cores had been taken [22].

A biopsy taken with a core needle limits possible tumor spread but necessarily harvests limited material which may add to the diagnostic problems. The approach used to insert the core needle must be resected when the tumor is removed, so it must follow the anticipated surgical approach. Fluoroscopically guided transpedicular biopsy of a vertebral body tumor is a useful development of the technique. Any uncertainty in the result requires an open biopsy.

Benign Tumors and Tumor-Like Conditions

These cover a variety of conditions from benign or simple bone cysts and non-ossifying fibromas on the one hand to osteochondromas on the other. Tumors are usually classified into four groups: chondrogenic, osteogenic, fibrous, and miscellaneous.

Benign Chondrogenic Tumors

Osteochondromas

Also known as exostoses, these bony outgrowths have a normal histological structure. Their bases may be narrow (the pedicular form which appears to "grow" toward the diaphysis) (Fig.14.4) or broad (the sessile form) (Fig. 14.5). Their bony bases form a continuum with the cortex and adjacent cancellous bone. They are topped with caps of radiolucent cartilage with growth plates which allow continued growth. They are almost always located on the metaphysis and most frequently affect the distal femur, the proximal and distal tibia, and the proximal humerus [23]. Rare epiphyseal osteochondromas occur in epiphysealis multiplex congenita (Trevor's disease).

An isolated osteochondroma usually presents as a painless swelling. Sometimes the patient feels discomfort due to impingement on a tendon, an aponeurosis, a nerve, or blood vessel. When the lesion looks radiologically typical a biopsy is unnecessary. Surgical resection is indicated if discomfort is marked or the lesion lies in a potentially dangerous site, e.g., back of the knee, axillary fossa, or spine.

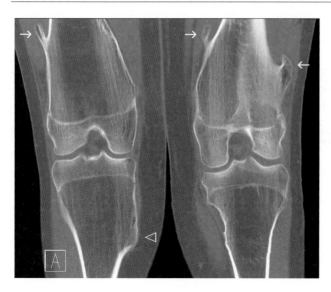

Fig. 14.4 Multiple osteochondromas around the knees in a 15-year-old (coronal reformatted CT-scan view). Sessile (*arrowhead*) and pedunculated (*arrow*) types are seen

Fig. 14.5 Sessile type of osteochondroma arising from the anterior aspect of the distal femoral metaphysis. The cartilaginous cap is outlined by a fatty pad (*arrow*)

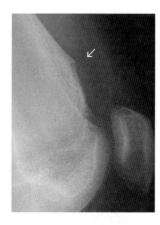

When the lesion is atypical on radiograph, an MRI and biopsy are useful. Patients with hereditary multiple exostoses (HME), an autosomal dominant, may have many osteochondromas on both sides of the body, often symmetrically.

Radiologically, each exostosis looks identical to the isolated lesion. In general only those lesions which cause symptoms should be resected. Exostoses can cause growth disorders, so the axial and appendicular skeleton should be regularly monitored clinically in affected patients.

An osteochondroma rarely becomes malignant (chondrosarcoma) before the age of 15 years and then usually when the child has multiple exostoses. Malignant transformation occurs most often in the pelvic and shoulder girdles. It should be suspected if the patient complains of pain or a thick, exuberant cap of cartilage appears on the osteochondroma. Cartilage cap thickness may be monitored by ultrasound and should not exceed 2 mm.

Chondroma

Still known as enchondroma this cartilage lesion mainly affects the limbs, particularly the feet and hands. Typically it creates a radiographic lucency or cyst with a clear border in the center of the bone, sometimes encroaching on the cortex; a thin rim of thickened bone can separate the lesion from the adjacent cancellous bone. Floccular or micro-calcification is often seen within the lesion. In adults the habitual form is located in the metaphysis of a long bone but this is rare in children as is malignant transformation [24].

Enchondromatosis or Ollier's disease is not a hereditary disorder: multiple chondromas affect the long bones of the limbs (Fig. 14.1). The chondromas are often elongated and eccentric and may cause considerable distortion of a bony segment.

Periosteal chondromas are an atypical form of chondroma, located under or in the periosteum. They are usually asymptomatic. They most commonly affect the bones of the hand, the femur, and the humerus. On the radiograph they appear as erosions on the cortical bone surface, very often surrounded by a thickened reactive zone not directly in contact with the periosteum. An MRI confirms that the lesion is cartilaginous.

Imaging is often sufficient to make the diagnosis, especially when the lesion is located in the finger bones. Curettage and grafting may be needed if there is a risk of pathological fracture.

In enchondromatosis most problems arise because of deformity and length discrepancy.

Chondroblastoma

Chondroblastomas usually develop in males aged 5–25 years. They are unusual as they develop in the epiphysis. They frequently affect the distal femur, the proximal tibia, the proximal humerus, and also "epiphyseal-equivalent" areas such as the greater trochanter [8, 25]. Chondroblastomas almost always present with pain.

The radiograph appearance is typical as a round epiphyseal lucency with a clearly defined margin, often surrounded by a thickened rim. The differential diagnosis on imaging should include other epiphyseal lucencies, which in children are mainly due to infection, or rarely, arise from joints (e.g., mucoid cyst), or pigmented villo-nodular synovitis. Giant cell tumors located in the epiphysis are very rare in children.

MRI is sufficient to make the diagnosis. Since the lesion is usually small, biopsy and curettage may be curative. Recurrences are frequent in chondroblastoma and the lesions are often difficult to remove safely as they are located between the joint cartilage and the growth plate. The aim is to curette the lesion completely but preserve sufficient growth plate for continued growth (Fig. 14.6a, b).

Fig. 14.6 Chondroblastoma of the proximal tibial epiphysis in an 11-year-old girl. (**a**) T1-weighted image after gadolinium administration: sagittal MRI at time of diagnosis shows a partially cystic epiphyseal lesion. (**b**) T1-weighted sagittal MRI 18 months after operation: autologous bone graft (*arrow*); cement between the physis and the bone graft (*asterisk*)

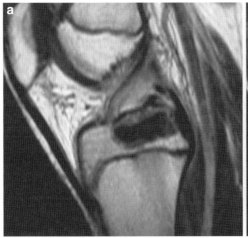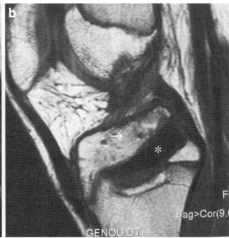

Chondromyxoid Fibroma

These rare tumors are made of fibrous, cartilaginous, and myxoid tissue. They are seen most often in the proximal tibial metaphysis. Radiologically they present as an eccentric, oval-shaped lucency in the diaphysis with a polycyclic thickened rim (Fig. 14.7). Sometimes the cortical bone is thinned and the lesion calcifies.

A biopsy is essential and they should be treated by surgical curettage and grafting. Careful monitoring is essential as recurrence is likely.

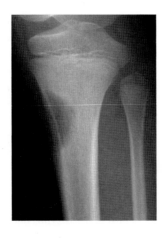

Fig. 14.7 Chondromyxoid fibroma of the proximal tibia in a 7-year-old boy. There is an osteolytic lesion with slightly sclerotic margin and a cortical erosion without periosteal reaction

Benign Osteogenic Tumors

Osteoid Osteomas

These benign tumors feature a nidus of osteoid tissue less than 2 cm in size, usually but not invariably surrounded by sclerotic bone. They frequently affect boys, causing pain, characteristically at night that is relieved by aspirin. When

the tumor is located close to a joint, the clinical picture may suggest arthritis although the blood tests are normal.

Any bone can be affected. The lesions usually appear on radiograph as a small lucency surrounded by sclerotic reactive bone. Micro-calcification in the nidus can be seen on a CT scan (Fig. 14.8). Multiple layers of periosteal new bone may abut the lesion in the periosteal form. When the lesion lies adjacent to a joint there is often a reactive effusion. The bone scan may be quite specific, picking up a hypersignal in all three examination phases which may prove very useful in doubtful cases. If the lesion looks typical on the CT scan, MRI is unnecessary.

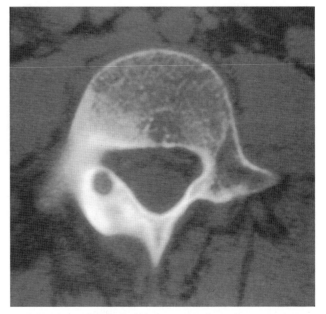

Fig. 14.8 Osteoid osteoma of a lumbar vertebra in a 10-year-old boy with a painful scoliosis. The nidus is the small, round, lucent lesion in the region of the right pars interarticularis. Note the marked sclerosis and enlargement of the right posterior elements

The differential diagnosis should include sub-acute focal osteitis, fatigue fracture, eosinophilic granuloma, and even Ewing's sarcoma.

For many years these lesions have been treated by en bloc surgical excision, but today CT-guided percutaneous drilling or laser cautery is preferred. These methods do not allow histological diagnosis so, although they are attractive techniques, they should not be used if the diagnosis is in doubt.

Osteoblastoma

Histologically osteoblastomas are very similar to osteoid osteomas, but they are much less common. Many authors believe the two lesions are the same, except that the nidus of the osteoblastoma exceeds 2 cm. The clinical symptoms are less distinctive than osteoid osteomas, and when discovered they are usually larger. They mainly affect the spine but can be found all over the body, although the epiphyses are never affected.

On radiograph an osteoblastoma appears as a lucency with a thickened margin, measuring over 2 cm along its main axis. A CT scan should be routine although, with less reactive sclerosis, MRI is more helpful than in osteoid osteomas and sometimes shows extensive edema around the lesion [26].

The differential diagnosis includes eosinophilic granuloma and aneurysmal bone cyst.

An osteoblastoma should be treated as benign although it is locally aggressive and recurrences occur. Its spinal location makes multidisciplinary planning important. When the lesion looks very typical on the imaging studies a biopsy is usually superfluous and a strategy for wide margin excision to remove the lesion as completely as possible should be considered. If the diagnosis is in doubt, especially if the lesion is in the appendicular skeleton a biopsy is justified.

Benign Bone Islands

Still sometimes known as an enostosis, a bone island is a condition that presents as a small area of compact bone in normal epiphyseal or metaphyseal cancellous bone. They are rarely seen in children. They are recognized incidentally on plain radiograph as a few millimeters of denser bone with a spicular edge extending into the adjacent cancellous bone. Only rarely—if there is diagnostic doubt or pain—is more detailed investigation necessary.

Osteomas

These benign tumors, sometimes called ivory osteomas, are very uncommon in children. They are outgrowths of compact bone which develop on the outer aspect of cortical bone (especially the mandible and the skull).

Fibrous Tumors and Tumor-Like Conditions

Benign Metaphyseal Cortical Defects and Non-ossifying Fibromas

These are more the result of errors in osteogenesis than true tumors.

Benign metaphyseal cortical lucencies or "cortical defects" are very common. They are often discovered incidentally in 5- to 12-year olds, affecting typically the distal femur, proximal tibia, proximal fibula, distal tibia, and proximal humerus, in order of frequency. They appear on radiographs as small (1–2 cm) cortical lucencies located close to the physis, which they do not modify in any way. They are sometimes bilateral. With growth the lucency migrates away from the physis. They may gradually disappear or present as non-ossifying fibromas. No treatment or surveillance is required.

Non-ossifying fibromas are similar but are seen at an older age and are usually larger. They are usually asymptomatic and are often discovered if a pathological fracture occurs. On radiograph the border between the lesion and cancellous bone is sclerotic. The cortical bone may be thin, with a polycystic appearance suggesting a wall-like internal structure (Fig. 14.2). Plain radiographs are usually diagnostic and a CT scan or MRI rarely justified. If there are several lesions it is important not to confuse a non-ossifying fibroma with type 1 neurofibromatosis or some of the rarer disorders encountered in polyostotic syndromes (e.g., Jaffé–Campanacci syndrome).

Biopsy is rarely indicated. As a rule no treatment is necessary for a non-ossifying fibroma, as it resolves with growth. Only if there is a risk of fracture, especially in the distal shaft of the tibia, should curettage and grafting be considered.

Periosteal Desmoplastic Fibromas

These lesions look like cortical defects. They present as cortical lucencies commonly located on the back of the distal femur where the medial head of the gastrocnemius or the adductor magnus insert. On radiograph the cortical lucency

Fig. 14.9 Periosteal desmoplastic fibroma with cortical irregularity of the postero-medial distal femur in a 12-year-old boy. This pseudotumor is related to a musculo-tendinous insertion site

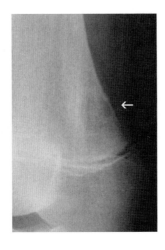

shows peripheral spicules (Fig. 14.9). If the lesion is discovered in a young athlete who complains of bouts of aching pain it should not be mistaken for an aggressive tumor.

Monostotic Fibrous Dysplasia

This may look very like a bone tumor. It is usually discovered in adolescence when a child complains of incidental pain, or occasionally if a spontaneous fracture occurs. It is caused by a disorder related to the mutation of a membrane protein (protein G) [27]. The monostotic form does not involve the signs and symptoms associated with polyostotic fibrous dysplasia (endocrine disorders and skin anomalies of the McCune–Albright syndrome). The lesion results from local fibro-osseous metaplasia. The preferred sites are the proximal femur, tibia, humerus, ribs, and facial bones. The pelvis, vertebrae, and extremities are more rarely affected. The long bone epiphyses are spared. The lesion is intramedullary.

Radiograph films are often equivocal and fibrous dysplasia may be suspected in any patient with a bone lucency or cyst. Typically the cyst has a "ground glass" appearance often with a sclerotic border. Small islands of osseous tissue are often visible within the lesion (Fig. 14.10). No periosteal new bone is seen unless a fracture occurs. CT scan and MRI are of little help. The differential diagnosis on plain radiograph should include simple bone cyst, aneurysmal cyst, chondroma, chondromyxoid fibroma, or even eosinophilic granuloma and low-grade osteosarcoma. Unless the lesion is asymptomatic or the radiological diagnosis is certain, a biopsy is necessary.

The treatment of the monostotic form is based on surveillance. Treatment is indicated only for threatened pathological fracture. Curettage and grafting are not recommended as recurrence is the rule. The best surgical treatment is to reinforce the bone by an intramedullary nail or pin.

Osteofibrous Dysplasia

Formerly known as non-ossifying fibroma, osteofibrous dysplasia or Campanacci's disorder usually develops in children under 10 years in the tibia or more rarely the fibula. The lower leg bows and is sometimes slightly painful. The x-ray film is very characteristic showing a long *intracortical* diaphyseal lucency often surrounded by an area of marked cortical sclerosis (Fig. 14.11). The differential diagnosis from fibrous dysplasia, which is more centrally placed in the bone, should be based on the transverse plane tomography. It is usually far more difficult to discriminate between osteofibrous dysplasia and adamantinoma, although the latter usually occurs after the age of 15. When in doubt, biopsy is essential.

Fig. 14.10 Monostotic fibrous dysplasia of the proximal femur in a 16-year-old boy. There is a slow-growing osteolytic lesion with sclerosis extending into the femoral neck. CT scan of the femoral neck shows the typical "ground-glass" appearance

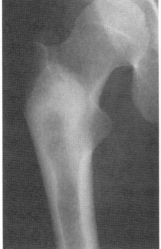
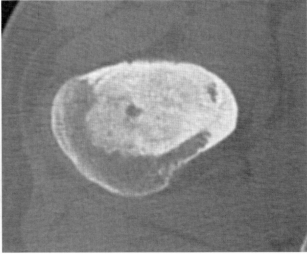

Fig. 14.11 Osteofibrous dysplasia of the tibia in a 15-year-old girl. The lesion is centered in the diaphyseal cortex and is partially osteolytic and partially sclerotic

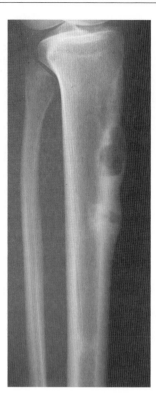

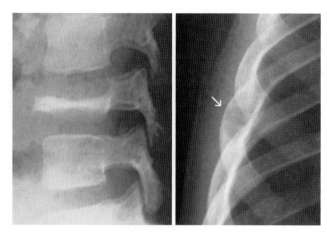

Fig. 14.12 Eosinophilic granuloma. There is a marked flattening of the vertebral body, "vertebra plana"; the intervertebral disc spaces are spared. There is a slow-growing osteolytic lesion in the rib (*arrow*)

with healing [28]. The differential diagnosis includes most causes of bone lucencies. When in doubt a biopsy should be performed.

Treatment depends largely on the severity of the lesion, its location, and the extent of the disease in general. In its local form it is reasonable to treat expectantly because spontaneous resolution is the rule [28]. When an eosinophilic granuloma is discovered in a child under the age of 2 the patient should be referred to a hematological oncologist for more detailed assessment and a search for extra-osseous lesions.

There is no mutation of protein G in osteofibrous dysplasia. Its management remains a subject of debate and there is no consensus on whether surveillance or wide resection is the better option.

Langerhans' Histiocytosis or Eosinophilic Granuloma

This form of eosinophilic granuloma affects bone tissue. The lesion may be single or multiple. Here we will discuss only those forms of histiocytosis which affect the skeleton where foci of normal bone marrow are replaced by a proliferation of histiocytes. Eosinophilic granuloma mainly affects boys aged 3–10 years and is rare after the age of 15. In almost 70% there is only one lesion which usually presents as a painful swelling. Any bone can be affected but the epiphyses of the long bones are rarely involved.

Radiologically the lesions appear as geographical lucencies of variable size (from a few millimeters to several centimeters) with borders that may be either sharp, irregular, or hazy according to their speed of development; a "motheaten" osteolytic picture is often seen (Fig. 14.12). Layered periosteal thickening is not uncommon. Some features are characteristic, especially vertebra plana, where the vertebral body collapses although the adjacent discs are intact. On MRI, the signal in the lesion and surrounding area varies with the stage of development. There is extensive edema in the surrounding bone and soft tissue which decreases

Tumors and Tumor-Like Conditions of Unknown Origin

Simple Bone Cyst

Sometimes called solitary or unicameral bone cysts, these are not tumors but a bone dystrophy of unknown origin. They are common in children, especially boys, over the age of 2 years. They may be discovered incidentally or when the child is seen for a fracture. Fifty percent are found in the proximal humerus. They develop in the metaphysis and only exceptionally encroach on the physis. (If they do they are more likely to be an aneurysmal bone cyst.) They develop in two phases: in their active period they increase in size, extending toward the diaphysis while remaining in contact with the physis. In their second, latent phase, their volume decreases and they appear to migrate away from the growth plate toward the diaphysis (Fig. 14.13).

Early radiographs show an oval-shaped central metaphyseal lucency, sometimes quite large, which encroaches upon and thins the cortical bone. The border on the diaphyseal side often looks like the bottom of an egg cup. MRI and bone

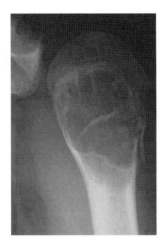

Fig. 14.13 Unicameral bone cyst of the proximal humerus in a 7-year-old boy. This is a slow-growing lytic and expansile lesion of the metaphysis abutting the growth plate with a cortical fracture

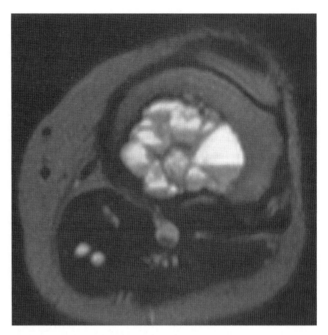

Fig. 14.14 Aneurysmal bone cyst of the proximal tibia. This T2-weighted transverse cut MRI shows a non-specific fluid level

scans add little. Once cysts have remodeled after fracture or treatment their radiograph appearance is more variable. When lesions are typical a biopsy is not necessary and radiograph surveillance is sufficient. They should be differentiated from aneurysmal bone cysts. MRI may help but only at least 2 months after a fracture. If in doubt, particularly if the radiographs are atypical, a biopsy is justified.

These lesions have been treated by a variety of methods ranging from simple observation to curettage and grafting and the intra-cystic injection of steroids or bone marrow. The best treatment remains controversial.

Aneurysmal Bone Cyst (ABC)

These benign lesions may present in two ways. They may be primary lesions (some have a genetic anomaly) or secondary to a pre-existing lesion (in one-third of cases) [29, 30]. ABCs have been described in association with solitary cysts, chondroblastomas, osteoblastomas, fibrous dysplasia, and giant cell tumors. In these cases they seem to represent a host reaction to the tumor process.

A past history of trauma is often reported. They are most common in youngsters but rare before the age of 5 years. They are always symptomatic. Apart from the spine, ABCs affect the metaphyses of long bones and the pelvis. When located in the epiphysis they may suggest a chondroblastoma. Cortical and even extra-osseous types occur.

On imaging, an expanding, often eccentric, osteolytic lesion is seen with scalloping of the cortical bone which sometimes disappears. The border with the adjacent normal cancellous bone is clear cut without reactive sclerosis. When located in the metaphysis, ABCs can encroach into the physis. A cyst divided by slender bony septa on plain radiograph or a CT scan should immediately suggest an ABC. On MRI the cystic components are clearly visible and the septa stand out, particularly after injecting contrast. Non-specific fluid levels are frequently observed (Fig. 14.14).

Two particular forms should be singled out: "solid" aneurysmal cysts, which are identical to giant cell reparative granulomas histologically, although the latter are seen in the small bones of the extremities, and the periosteal form, which presents with a rough, spicular edge that may suggest malignancy.

The main differential diagnosis of ABC is telangiectatic osteosarcoma. The two are sometimes difficult to differentiate even in the laboratory. Solitary bone cysts, chondromyxoid fibroma, and chondroblastoma usually present fewer radiograph dilemmas.

A biopsy guided by the imaging data should be performed before treatment.

It is important to bear in mind the high risk of local recurrence when considering treatment. The risk is as high as 30%. Three methods of treatment have been described: the injection of sclerosing agents, curettage and grafting, and complete extra-periosteal ablation. Sclerosants may cause embolic and fistula complications and are therefore usually reserved for surgically inaccessible lesions. When located in the spine these lesions are usually cervical and may require both anterior and posterior approaches. In this setting a preoperative angiogram may allow embolization of the main feeding vessels.

Giant Cell Tumor

It is rare to diagnose a giant cell tumor before the growth plates close. The diagnosis is made on the histology from a metaphysio-epiphyseal lytic lesion or a sacral tumor and must be checked by a pathologist who specializes in bone tumors.

Malignant Tumors

In the first two decades of life, osteosarcoma and Ewing's sarcoma are by far the most common malignant tumors. Before the age of 10 years, Ewing's sarcoma accounts for almost half the tumors; after this, osteosarcoma is much more likely.

Osteosarcomas produce an osteoid matrix, although sometimes only in small quantities. Several types have been described:

- The standard form of osteosarcoma is an intramedullary high-grade tumor. Distinction is made between osteoblastic, chondroblastic, and fibroblastic forms classified according to their type of matrix (Fig. 14.15).
- Telangiectatic osteosarcomas simulate aneurysmal cysts and are also high grade.
- Small cell osteosarcomas simulate Ewing's sarcomas.
- Rare forms reputed to be low-grade include juxtacortical, parosteal, and periosteal osteosarcomas (Fig. 14.16).

Ewing's sarcoma was believed to belong to the group of primitive neuro-ectodermal tumors (PNET). These are small, round cell tumors. However, recent papers consider Ewing's tumor to be of mesenchymal origin [31]. A translocation is frequently described on chromosome 11–22 (Fig. 14.17).

Other malignant tumors such as primary lymphoma, chondrosarcoma, fibrosarcoma, hemangioendothelioma, and adamantinoma are much rarer and are found only in exceptional cases.

When a malignant tumor is suspected on plain radiograph, a complete imaging assessment must be made (e.g., bone scan, MRI) before a biopsy is taken. The MRI will

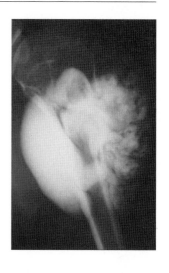

Fig. 14.16 Parosteal osteosarcoma of the proximal humerus in an 18 year-old girl. A huge sclerotic mass envelopes the humeral shaft

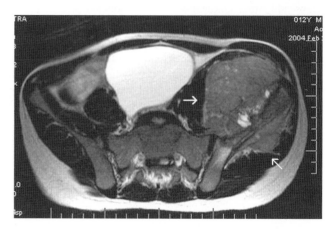

Fig. 14.17 Ewing's sarcoma of the left ilium in a 7-year-old boy. This T2-weighted transverse cut MRI shows a mass expanding anteriorly and posteriorly (*arrows*)

give details of the boundaries of the tumor within the bone segment and any extension into the soft tissues as part of the staging process. MRI will also allow a search for other lesions within the bone, so-called skip metastases. The bone scan should identify other skeletal involvement.

A full general assessment of the disease extent must include a search for lung metastases and medullary involvement in Ewing's sarcoma.

The current management of osteosarcoma and Ewing's sarcoma is based on neo-adjuvant chemotherapy, the goal being to treat micro-metastatic disease and reduce the bulk of the primary tumor before operation, making the procedure easier and safer. Surgery should be based on the imaging data [32]. The patient's response to chemotherapy is assessed by histological criteria, which are prognostically important in both osteosarcoma and Ewing's sarcoma. Good responders to chemotherapy have fewer than 5% of viable tumor cells for osteosarcoma and fewer than 10% for Ewing's sarcoma. After surgery a second course of chemotherapy is

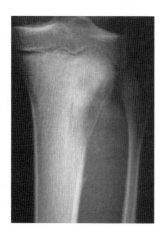

Fig. 14.15 Conventional osteosarcoma of the proximal tibia in an 8-year-old child. There is an aggressive lesion of the metaphysis with lytic and sclerotic areas and periosteal reaction (Codman's triangle and spiculated reaction)

started, based on a rationale that is closely linked to the tumor response to the initial chemotherapy regimen.

Staging the Lesions

Enneking [33] developed the concept of tumor "staging." He classified lesions as low- or high-grade malignancies by their clinical and histological features and their imaging appearance. This explains how tumors with the same diagnosis may be either low or high grade. There are three stages:

Stage I: low-grade malignancy with no metastases
Stage II: high-grade malignancy with no metastases
Stage III: lesion with regional or systemic metastases irrespective of its histological grade

This classification is made and then correlated with the anatomical compartment affected. By "compartment" Enneking meant a bone, joint, or a muscular chamber and its enveloping fascia. For our purposes, they are classified as:

A: Intracompartmental tumors that are contained fully within the cortical bone
B: Extracompartmental tumors that have encroached through the cortical bone and periosteum.

Using this tumor "staging" Enneking classified the types of tumor resection as shown in Fig. 14.18.

Enneking's classification was established on the basis of radiographic data. MRI has shown us its imperfections and Kawaguchi [34] has proposed a new method of evaluating resection margins based on MRI data. In his scheme the resection is classified as shown in Fig. 14.19.

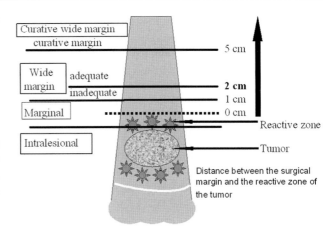

Fig. 14.19 Kawaguchi's bone tumor resection classification

In the transverse plane distances are converted into "tissue equivalents." Thus, a thin fascia is equivalent to 2 cm of normal tissue and a thick fascia the equivalent of 3 cm of normal tissue.

If there is healthy tissue, whatever its thickness, between tumor and fascia, and if the resection removes this fascia completely, the "equivalent distance" is 5 cm.

One difficulty in evaluating these distances is the natural trend of soft tissues to retract after resection. In his article Kawaguchi gets around this difficulty by asking surgeons to insert landmarks on the muscle fibers 5 cm from their insertion into bone before resection to assess this retraction.

Using this classification system for local lesions he found that in 86% of cases the tumor could be controlled by wide curative resection or wide adequate resection. The percentage fell to 66% if wide inadequate resection was performed and to 48 and 33% for marginal resection and intralesional resection, respectively.

The compartment-of-origin concept proposed by Enneking forms no part of Kawaguchi 's classification.

Tumor Resection

To remove the tumor completely, the resection plane must pass through healthy tissue. This is the principle underlying carcinological resection. Staging establishes the margins for safe excision of a malignant tumor. In practice, this evaluation should be made in close collaboration with the imaging and tumor teams. MRI has a key position in evaluating a tumor's boundaries. The two main steps in evaluating local tumor spread are the MRI performed before biopsy and the preoperative MRI after initial chemotherapy.

Intraosseous tumor extension should be assessed on the T-1 weighted sequences without contrast medium on the

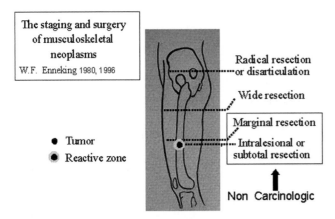

Fig. 14.18 Enneking's bone tumor resection classification

two sets of images. This will indicate whether local control has been achieved by chemotherapy or if the tumor has spread. When planning resection, the maximal tumor spread on either set of images should form the basis for planning resection.

Extension into the soft tissues should be carefully analyzed, together with the effect of therapy. On the initial MRI the signal changes show the tumor and reactive edema. Chemotherapy can change these values substantially, especially in Ewing's sarcoma.

Based on the margins described above we perform our resection at least 10 mm from the tumor's osseus and extraosseus boundaries, sparing the epiphysis if possible. The carcinological resection must be carefully planned preoperatively in great detail. It is essential to control the neurovascular structures first: the vascular and nerve sheaths must be opened and separated from the tumor sub-adventitiously. The bone must be resected under fluoroscopic control to ensure precision. The principles of cancer resection must be respected at all times. It must be through healthy tissue and the tumor must not be breached.

Reconstruction

After safe resection, two principles guide any reconstruction. The limb must be functional and continued growth should be possible to avoid future shortening.

Amputation and Rotationplasty

These are now rare following the progress made in chemotherapy. They are now reserved for tumors which have invaded the neurovascular structures, those located on the extremities, and for some local recurrences [35, 36].

Reconstruction with No Functional Joint

This method is based on arthrodesis. We use it for lesions of the shoulder when the rotator cuff has been removed or for the ankle where the limb functions well after fusion [37]. These reconstructions require large quantities of bone graft obtained from autografts or allografts. In our experience we often use a vascularized fibular graft sleeved onto an allograft for this type of reconstruction (Fig. 14.20a, b).

Reconstruction with a Functional Joint (without an Epiphysis)

This method is based on arthroplasty, using a prosthetic replacement. In our experience prosthetic reconstructions are

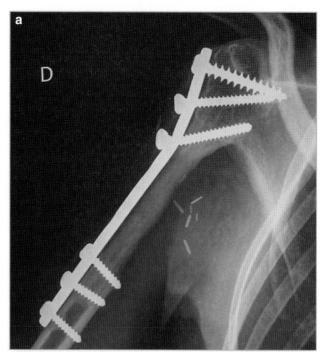

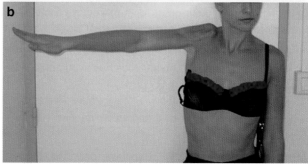

Fig. 14.20 Shoulder reconstruction with arthrodesis using a vascularized fibular graft. (**a**) Radiologic result at 3-year follow-up. (**b**) Clinical result

restricted to knee and hip replacement. The immediate result is satisfactory and some prostheses can be extended as the child grows. However, there are the long-term problems of loosening, wear, and loss of bone stock to consider [38–42]. The child and family must be warned of the possibility of having to resort to an arthrodesis later.

Reconstruction with an Epiphysis

This method uses intercalary bone grafts, which may be allograft, non-vascularized autograft, or vascularized autograft (Fig. 14.21). We have used one or two vascularized fibulas, combined sometimes with an allograft for over 10 years [20].

Masquelet's so-called induced membrane technique seems to be promising for intercalary bone reconstruction [43].

Fig. 14.21 Bone reconstruction for an osteosarcoma of the distal femur. The medial fibula graft is vascularized. The lateral fibula is non-vascularized. Radiological result 6 years later

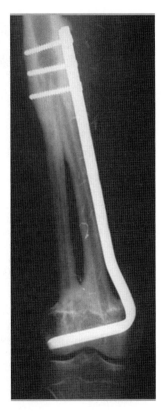

Post-operative Period—Prognosis

This is major surgery in a patient whose immune system is already compromised. After surgery chemotherapy must be resumed immediately and the regimen adjusted in light of the histological response. The complication rate is high and the family must be given a realistic prognosis [44].

In the short term, the most daunting complication is post-operative infection. If this is suspected and confirmed, careful bacteriological assessment is critical and surgical revision necessary. As a first line of treatment, prosthetic materials and osteosynthesis hardware should be left in place. The surgical wound must be thoroughly cleaned and drains inserted. "Second look" surgery is important.

An intravenous antibiotic regime is started and modified as bacteriological data become available. The antibiotics must be continued for 6 months, which means that the second and last phase of chemotherapy will be over once the treatment is finished.

Following antibiotic treatment, if infection recurs, all foreign materials should be removed, an antibiotic-impregnated spacer inserted, and systemic antibiotics recommenced. Re-implantation should only be undertaken when all inflammatory indices have returned to normal.

In the medium term the most serious complication is local tumor recurrence. Until recently local recurrence, if systemic disease was under control, justified amputation or excision of the joint. This position is not so clear-cut today as some favor further surgical tumor resection in an attempt to salvage the limb.

The relative impact of different factors on prognosis is not yet clearly established. The only known adverse factors are the failure of the tumor to respond to chemotherapy and the presence of trunk metastases. With new chemotherapy regimens the prognosis for malignant bone tumors has improved dramatically over the last 20 years. Since the beginning of the 1980s, 60–80% of children with non-metastatic osteosarcoma are alive and in remission 5 years after treatment [45, 46]. This rate seems to be stable. In non-metastatic Ewing's sarcoma the 5-year survival without recurrence is close to 70%. For those who present with metastases the prognosis is much poorer, with a 5-year survival rate of 20%.

Conclusion

Managing benign and malignant bone tumors is complex and requires a carefully coordinated approach based on a number of basic rules:

- Good quality imaging is essential as it indicates the host response to the tumor and often provides the diagnosis.
- A comprehensive imaging assessment must be done before biopsy.
- The team which manages the child should ideally perform the biopsy.
- Each stage of treatment, especially for malignant tumors, must be planned with a multidisciplinary team.

References

1. Stiller CA, Craft AW, Corazziari I. Survival of children with bone sarcoma in Europe since 1978: results from the EUROCARE study. Eur J Cancer 2001; 37:760–766.
2. Tucker MA, D'Angio GJ, Boice JD Jr, et al. Bone sarcomas linked to radiotherapy and chemotherapy in children. N Engl J Med 1987; 317:588–593.
3. Fuchs B, Pritchard DJ. Etiology of osteosarcoma. Clin Orthop 2002; 397:40–52.
4. Hansen MF, Koufos A, Gallie BL, et al. Osteosarcoma and retinoblastoma: a shared chromosomal mechanism revealing recessive predisposition. Proc Nat Acad Sc USA 1985; 82:6216–6220.
5. Carnevale A, Lieberman E, Cardenas R. Li-Fraumeni syndrome in pediatric patients with soft tissue sarcoma or osteosarcoma. Arc Med Res 1997; 28:383–386.
6. Hillmann A, Ozaki T, Winkelmann W. Familial occurrence of osteosarcoma: A case report and review of the literature. J Cancer Clin Oncol 2000; 126:497–502.

7. Hoffer FA, Nikanorov AY, Reddick WE, et al. Accuracy of MR imaging for detecting epiphyseal extension of osteosarcoma. Pediatr Radiol 2000; 30:289–298.

8. Leung JC, Dalinka MK. Magnetic resonance imaging in primary bone tumors. Semin Roentgenol 2000; 35:297–305.

9. Miller SL, Hoffer FA, Reddick WE, et al. Tumor volume or dynamic contrast-enhanced MRI for prediction of clinical outcome of Ewing sarcoma family of tumors. Pediatr Radiol 2001; 31:518–523.

10. Onikul E, Fletcher BD, Parham DM, et al. Accuracy of MR imaging for estimating intraosseous extent of osteosarcoma. AJR 1996; 167:1211–1215.

11. Norton KI, Hermann G, Abdelwahab IF, et al. Epiphyseal involvement in osteosarcoma. Radiology 1991; 180:813–816.

12. Panuel M, Gentet JC, Scheiner C, et al. Physeal and epiphyseal extent of primary malignant bone tumors in childhood. Correlation of preoperative MRI and the pathologic examination. Pediatr Radiol 1993; 23:421–424.

13. Ghanem N, Uhl M, Brink I, et al. Diagnostic value of MRI in comparison to scintigraphy, PET, MS-CT and PET/CT for the detection of metastases of bone. Eur J Radiol 2005; 55:41–55.

14. Goo HW, Choi SH, Ghim T, et al. Whole-body MRI of pediatric malignant tumors: comparison with conventional oncological imaging methods. Pediatr Radiol 2005; 35:766–773.

15. Panicek DM, Gatsonis C, Rosenthal DI, et al. CT and MR imaging in the local staging of primary malignant musculoskeletal neoplasms: Report of the Radiology Diagnostic Oncology Group. Radiology 1997; 202:237–246.

16. Panicek DM, Schwartz LH. MR imaging after surgery for musculoskeletal neoplasm. Semin Musculoskelet Radiol 2002; 6: 57–66.

17. Brisse H, Ollivier L, Edeline V, et al. Imaging of malignant tumors of the long bones in children: monitoring response to neoadjuvant chemotherapy and preoperative assessment. Pediatr Radiol 2004; 34:595–605.

18. Hawkins DS, Schuetze SM, Butrynski JE, et al. Fluorodeoxyglucose positron emission tomography predicts outcome for Ewing sarcoma family of tumors. J Clin Oncol 2005; 23:8828–8834.

19. McCarville MB, Christie R, Daw NC, et al. PET/CT in the evaluation of childhood sarcomas. AJR 2005; 184: 1293–1304.

20. Friedrich JB, Moran SL, Bishop AT, et al. Free vascularized fibular graft salvage of complications of long-bone allograft after tumor reconstruction. J Bone Joint Surg Am 2008; 90:93–100.

21. Skrzynski MC, Biermann JS, Montag A, et al. Diagnostic accuracy and charge-savings of outpatient core needle biopsy compared with open biopsy of musculoskeletal tumors. J Bone Joint Surg Am 1996; 78:639–43.

22. Mitsuyoshi G, Naito N, Kawai A, et al. Accurate diagnosis of musculoskeletal lesions by core needle biopsy J Surg Oncol 2006; 94:1–2.

23. Kricun M. Imaging of bone tumors. Philadelphia PA: WB Saunders; 1993.

24. Murphey MD, Flemming DJ, Boyea SR, et al. Enchondroma versus chondrosarcoma in the appendicular skeleton: differentiating features. Radiographics 1998; 18:1213–1237.

25. Unni KK, Dahlin DC. Dahlin's bone tumors. General aspects and data on 11,087 cases, 5th ed. Philadelphia: Lippincot–Raven; 1996.

26. Crim JR, Mirra JM, Eckardt JJ, Seeger LL. Widespread inflammatory response to osteoblastoma: the flare phenomenon. Radiology 1990; 177:835–836.

27. Dicaprio MR, Enneking WF. Fibrous dysplasia, pathophysiology, evaluation, and treatment. J Bone Joint Surg Am 2005; 87:1848–1864.

28. Azouz EM, Saigal G, Rodriguez MM, Podda A. Langerhans' cell histiocytosis: pathology, imaging and treatment of skeletal involvement. Pediatr Radiol 2005; 35:103–115.

29. Bollini G, Jouve JL, Cottalorda J, et al. Aneurysmal bone cyst in children: analysis of twenty-seven patients. J Pediatr Orthop 1998; B 7:274–285.

30. Mankin HJ, Hornicek FJ, Ortiz-Cruz E. et al. Aneurysmal bone cyst: a review of 150 patients. J Clin Oncol 2005; 23: 6756–6762.

31. Tirode F, Laud-Duval K, Prieur A, et al. Mesenchymal stem cell features of Ewing tumors. Cancer Cell 2007; 11:421–429.

32. Dyke JP, Panicek DM, Healey JH, et al. Osteogenic and Ewing sarcomas: estimation of necrotic fraction during induction chemotherapy with dynamic contrast-enhanced MR imaging. Radiology 2003; 228:271–278.

33. Enneking WF. A system of staging musculoskeletal neoplasms. Clin Orthop Rel Res 1986; 204:9–24.

34. Kawaguchi N, Matumoto S, Manabe J. New method of evaluating the surgical margin and safety margin for musculoskeletal sarcoma, analyzed on the basis of 457 surgical case. J Cancer Res Clin Oncol 1995; 121:555–563.

35. Agarwal M, Puri A, Anchan C, et al. Rotationplasty for bone tumors: is there still a role? Clin Orthop Relat Res 2007; 459:76–81.

36. Puri A, Agarwal M. Facilitating rotationplasty. J Surg Oncol 2007; 95:351–354.

37. Viehweger E, Gonzalez JF, Launay F, et al. Shoulder arthrodesis with vascularized fibular graft after tumor resection of the proximal humerus Rev Chir Orthop 2005; 91:523–529.

38. Marulanda GA, Henderson ER, Johnson DA, et al. Orthopedic surgery options for the treatment of primary osteosarcoma. Cancer Control 2008; 15:13–20.

39. Myers GJ, Abudu AT, Carter SR, et al. The long-term results of endoprosthetic replacement of the proximal tibia for bone tumors. J Bone Joint Surg Br 2007; 89:1632–1637.

40. San-Julian M, Duart J, de Rada PD, Sierrasesumaga L. Limb salvage in Ewing's sarcoma of the distal lower extremity. Foot Ankle Int 2008; 29:22–28.

41. Sim IW, Tse LF, Ek ET, et al. Salvaging the limb salvage: management of complications following endoprosthetic reconstruction for tumors around the knee. Eur J Surg Oncol 2007; 33:796–802.

42. Violas P, Kohler R, Mascard E, et al. Conservative surgical treatment of osteogenic sarcoma of the limb in children and adolescents. Rev Chir Orthop 2000; 86:675–683.

43. Masquelet AC, Fitoussi F, Begue T, Muller GP. Reconstruction of the long bones by the induced membrane and spongy autograft. Ann Chir Plast Esthet 2000; 45:346–353.

44. Sajadi KR, Heck RK, Neel MD, et al. The incidence and prognosis of osteosarcoma skip metastases. Clin Orthop Relat Res 2004; 426:92–96.

45. Arndt CA, Crist WM. Common musculoskeletal tumors of childhood and adolescence. N Engl J Med 1999; 341:342–352.

46. Bollini G, Kalifa C, Panuel M. Malignant bone tumors in children and adolescent. Arch Pediatr 2006; 13:669–671.

Part III
Neuromuscular Disorders

Chapter 15

Neuromotor Development and Examination

Robert A. Minns

Introduction

The adult nervous system is essentially a *static system* (or one which is in decline) and the clinical neurological examination is therefore cross-sectional. The paediatric neurologist, however, has to examine all of the various pathways of the nervous system, mindful of the timing of the appearance (and disappearance) of various developmental signs.

Most signs that are abnormal to the adult neurologist may, at some stage of development, be normal in the fetus and infant. For example, all of the signs that accompany an acute hemiplegic stroke in the adult can be normal in a healthy newborn baby. All infants have features of a double hemiplegia including apraxia, grasp reflex, brisk phasic reflexes, ankle clonus, and extensor plantar responses with extrapyramidal-type progression movement or neonatal athetoid movements. In a child with a later dense hemiplegia, no clinical abnormalities may be evident during the neonatal period; the neurological asymmetries and deficits develop later, so that by 3–5 years of age there are overt signs of a dense hemiplegia.

Similarly, at 13 months, when the child takes his or her first independent steps, the gait is broad based, the arms are held out from the side, and foot placement is pronated. This is really a physiological ataxia.

A number of clinical features are seen in normal children which, in the adolescent or adult would be regarded as representing neurological abnormality, but which are purely a reflection of maturation of the nervous system. These *maturational* (previously called "soft") *signs* in 6–8-year-olds include "mirror movements" to the opposite limb (arm to arm or arm to leg) and associated movements (opening the mouth or shoulder and elbow movements) in 52% of normal children; mirror dyspraxia (building blocks in reverse

fashion) occur in 13%; finger agnosia in 29%; inaccurate graphesthesia in 46%; ambilaterality (changing hands for the same and different tasks) in 23%; poor cross commands in 26% dynamic gesturing difficulties in 26%; and right–left discrimination in 9% [1].

Therefore it is important to not only be able to elicit these signs but to know the "plus and minus two standard deviations" of when they appear and disappear as a means of recognizing the pathological.

Brain Development

Brain development underpins all neurodevelopment and determines the effect of brain insults, occurring from early intrauterine life to approximately 5 years of age. Developmental assessment therefore depends upon the orderly programmed rate and sequence of brain development.

Stages of brain development include

1. Formation of the neural crest and closure of the neural tube. The neural folds and neural groove become evident at 22 days post-conception. Fusion of the neural tube commences in the middle of the neural fold and proceeds to "zip up" simultaneously in both proximal and distal directions. The proximal closure (anterior neuropore) is complete at 26 days and the rostral (posterior neuropore) at 28–30 days. By 21 days post-conception, cells at the side of the neural plate and normal ectoderm form the neural crest. Abnormalities at this stage result in neural tube defects (myelomeningocele and anencephaly), Arnold–Chiari malformation, Danny–Walker malformation, and caudal regression syndrome.
2. Primitive vesicle formation. The proximal neural tube dilates at about 28 days into three primitive vesicles: the prosencephalon, the mesencephalon, and the rhombencephalon. With lengthening, the cervical and

R.A. Minns (✉)
Department of Child Life and Health, University of Edinburgh, Edinburgh, UK; Royal Hospital for Sick Children, Edinburgh, UK

M. Benson et al. (eds.), *Children's Orthopaedics and Fractures*,
DOI 10.1007/978-1-84882-611-3_15, © Springer-Verlag London Limited 2010

pontine flexures occur. Abnormalities include holopros-encephaly, absence of corpus callosum, and septo-optic dysplasia.

3. Division of the telencephalon. The prosencephalon divides into the telencephalon and diencephalon. The telencephalon gives rise to the cortex. The telencephalon and the diencephalon give rise to the thalamus and the basal ganglia and the diencephalon also gives rise to the hypothalamus. The mesencephalon forms the mid-brain and the rhombencephalon the cerebellum, pons, and medulla. Each primitive division further divides into neuromeres under specific genetic control.

4. Cell division. Primitive stem cells arise in the germi-nal matrix adjacent to the ependyma of the telencephalic vesicle where they divide into two. One of these primi-tive neuroblasts will migrate and the other will continue to produce several generations of clone cells.

5. Cell migration along Bergmann fibers. Programmed neuroblasts migrate along invisible glial processes (Bergmann glial fibers) to form the future cortex. The cell migrates according to the "inside out rule" where the more recently migrating cell is more exter-nal. Cell division in the subependymal region remains active upto 28 weeks. Most neurones have migrated by 20 weeks and subsequently glioblasts (glial pre-cursors) migrate. With increasing cell numbers the previously smooth cerebral cortex before 22 weeks now infolds with gyral formation. Abnormalities at this stage include cortical dysplasias, neurofibromato-sis, tuberous sclerosis, effects of cocaine addiction, Zellweger syndrome, fetal alcohol syndrome, and lissencephaly.

6. Axonal and dendritic development. There are six dif-ferent neurone types in the cortex and they require to be correctly orientated, i.e., axons pointing downward. Connections are probably induced by chemical attrac-tants. Dendritic growth is maximal from 28 to 35 weeks with the formation of dendritic spines. Glial multiplica-tion (from 28 to 40 weeks) is responsible for the second DNA spurt.

7. Apoptosis. Redundant processes with no synaptic con-tact will dissolve; between 28 and 34 weeks the subependymal zone (germinal plate) undergoes rapid dissolution.

8. Synaptic pruning.

9. Angiogenesis.

10. Myelination. Myelin is produced by the oligodendroglial cells in the central nervous system and by Schwann cells in the peripheral nervous system. Each oligodendroglial cell can myelinate up to 15 axons. This allows rapid conduction down the axon and insulation from the ionic changes in the extracellular environment. As the brain weighs 350 g at birth and 1350 g at 4 years, much of this increase is due to myelination and the formation of dendrites, Nissl granules, and association pathways. It occurs rapidly in the first 6 months after birth, at a slower phase over the next 4 years, and then very slowly up to 16 years. Abnormalities at this stage include delayed myelination and dysmyelination.

11. Association fiber development. There are definite myel-ogenetic cycles [2]. The leg area of the cortex myelinates before the arm region, yet upper limb function is in advance of walking. Myelination of short association pathways such as the fronto-hypothalamic tract occurs during the first 12 years of life. These inhibit the nor-mal inhibitory pathway from the habenular nucleus to the pituitary, allowing puberty to develop. Association pathways are important for mental functions.

12. Dominance. The left side of the brain, particularly over the superior aspect of the temporal lobe, is anatomi-cally different from the right, with many more cells and with preprogramming for the learning of language. If a module is damaged on one side of the brain it can be taken over by the opposite lobe. Normally one side is inhibited, producing reciprocal cerebral inhibition or dominance so that there is no interference between one side of the brain and the other. These stages of devel-opment include the primary areas such as the motor strip, somatosensory and visual areas, and Heschl's gyrus.

13. Maturation of tertiary areas. Secondary association areas for vision, Wernicke's area, and motor association areas have connections across the corpus callosum and long intracortical connections. Maturation of the angular gyrus and frontal pole are the last to mature.

14. Psychogenesis. By this is meant the effect of the envi-ronment on brain development before and after birth. Prior to birth cerebral nutritive factors are paramount and following birth the external environment influ-ences development. The basic items of development (sitting, standing, walking, and crawling) are geneti-cally determined and therefore not learned or influenced by environment. However, the developmental skills are certainly influenced by environment, learning through walking, and in turn how to run, hop, skip, jump, and so on. Examples of this include infants in certain cultures who are swaddled until well into the second year of life. Since walking occurs within a few days of removal of the swaddling, nurture has been rather overstated with respect to these basic items of develop-ment. Adverse environmental influences, when reversed, can result in "catch up." For example, the previously institutionalized child shows quite retarded development emotionally and in speech and language but less retar-dation in the areas of posture and movement. When the child is removed to an optimal environment these

previously delayed items show "catch up." Measured intelligence may rise and brain size increase to the point of even splitting the cranial sutures. In severe psycho-social deprivation brain growth ceases, producing the clinical appearances of deprivation dwarfism. The child is floppy, pot-bellied, and manifests with poor visual and auditory responses along with poor responses to painful stimuli. Adrenocorticotropic hormones (ACTH) and growth hormone are low, giving the appearance of panhypopituitarism. Experimental animals stimulated through one eye only show increased myelination in the ipsilateral optic nerves. The practice of nursing a young infant prone results in earlier acquisition of crawling but no other developmental milestones. On the negative side, however, such babies often present with persistent toe walking. Babies nursed supine exclusively adopt a more "cowboy" pattern of ambulation.

15. Senescence.

Principles of Development Testing

Maturation is tested in young children by combining functional assessments of developmental items into groups such as gross motor skills (also called posture and mobility or locomotor); manipulation and vision; hearing, speech, and language; and social and emotional behavior.

Although all are functional items (e.g., reaching out for objects) they all involve many neurological pathways. Milestones reflect the acquisition of skills consequent upon neurodevelopmental maturation.

To commence an understanding of the neurodevelopmental examination one can build on the adult neurological examination which assesses muscle power, tone, coordination and truncal balance, phasic reflexes, sensation, cranial nerves, and higher cortical function. Posture and movement (as above) will therefore be assessing muscle power and tone.

Subcortical integrators of posture and movement are called "primitive reflexes," and in conditions where there is a delay or abnormality in posture and movement development these primitive reflexes persist.

Manipulation similarly involves pathways of muscle power, coordination, and praxic ability. Cranial nerves II–VI are concerned with vision, IX–XII with bulbar or feeding function, and VIII with acoustic and labyrinthine activity.

Social development requires conditioned learning rather than innate or cognitive learning; emotional development along with language represents aspects of higher cortical function. Speech is purely a motor act (articulation, phonation, and rhythm).

Major Influences on Development

Brain Damage

Acquired brain damage in the adult will result in hard neurological deficits such as hemiplegia, cortical blindness, and epilepsy. A similar insult to the developing brain not only results in these deficits but produces subsequent slowing of brain development either globally or focally. In general, global brain insults result in global delay and localized insults in specific delays. Acute system diseases have little effect upon the development of the nervous system but acute neurological disorders (affecting the organ of development) may produce substantial neurodevelopmental consequences. Chronic disease will retard optimal somatic growth but chronic neurological disease will impair neurological development as in chronic under-nutrition or hypothyroidism.

Gender

Males are delayed compared to females of a similar chronological age, presumably due to the retarding effect of the Y chromosome. Noxious influences at any particular time in development will therefore have more profound effects on the male, having the more immature nervous system.

Genetic Factors

Brain development is under genetic control and any ability would be expected to follow a normal distribution curve. Brain development continues until 17 or 18 years; however, the quicker the rate of early development, the earlier will be the completion of brain growth and development. Normal children who walk at 9 months will be no more proficient than those who walk at 14 months, and similarly with pubertal onset. In general fast achievers with a rapid rate of brain development ceiling earlier but do not continue with brain development for a longer period. Many developmental disorders such as dyslexia are proven to be genetic disorders and are not simply a slowing up of the normal rate of development (less than the third centile) because the deficit persists for life. It is important to differentiate a normal child with a slow rate of brain development from a developmental genetic disease or pathological brain insult slowing down brain development.

In general adverse genetic influences acting early in intrauterine life result in severe deficits such as anencephaly or spina bifida while those acting later affect migration and produce disorders such as tuberous sclerosis. Genetic deviants will be referred to later.

Neurodevelopment Examination (Concentrating on Posture and Movement/Mobility)

Figure 15.1 shows the normal development of posture and movement. It is essential to think of development in a longitudinal sense and not cross-sectionally, considering it from the most primitive through to the most normal. We have concentrated here on posture and movement/mobility because of the importance of this in orthopaedics although other aspects of development, manipulation, vision, hearing, speech, and language should also be considered in a longitudinal sense. The figure shows, at 12 weeks gestation, the first flexor phase of development, approximating to that of a spinal level. At 28 weeks a fetus is extended and this is equivalent to a lower

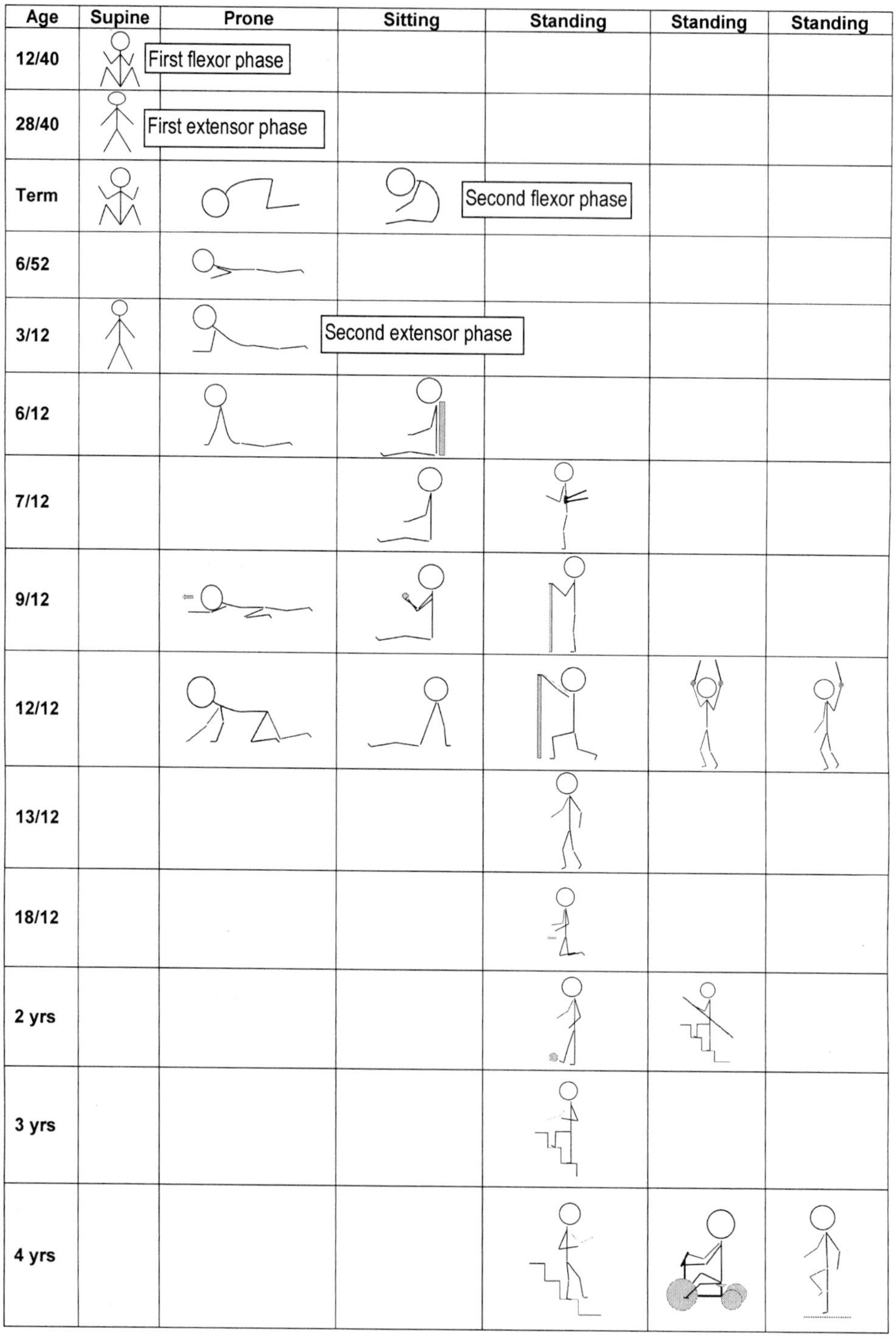

Age	Supine	Prone	Sitting	Standing	Standing	Standing
12/40		First flexor phase				
28/40		First extensor phase				
Term			Second flexor phase			
6/52						
3/12		Second extensor phase				
6/12						
7/12						
9/12						
12/12						
13/12						
18/12						
2 yrs						
3 yrs						
4 yrs						

Fig. 15.1 Schematic depiction of neuromotor development

brain stem level of functioning. The flexed term baby is functioning at a midbrain level. Thus the normal newborn has an impassive face with reptilian stare, quasi-athetoid hand movements, and oro-facial dyskinesia, which in the mature brain could indicate parkinsonism. By 3 months the baby is again in the second extensor phase where now, with cortical maturation, there is inhibition of lower centers. This changing pattern of first and second flexor and extensor phases does not represent a "change of mind" but rather increasing levels of hierarchical maturation.

In practical terms the infant's posture and movement are best assessed by looking at the child in four standard positions—supine, prone, sitting, and standing—first describing the posture that the child adopts and then the movements that he undertakes. After initial observations when supine, the child is pulled to sit (a traction response) and the degree of head lag or control is observed. The child is then observed in a sitting position. Again the child is pulled to stand and the posture and movements observed. Finally the child is placed prone by rotating the child through 180° (Fig. 15.2).

As the posture reflects tone and the movements reflect power this is truly a neurological assessment of a longitudinal (maturing) nervous system. Until 12 months of age the neurodevelopmental examination should consists of all these positions, but after 12 months all subsequent development of posture and movement occurs in the standing or vertical position.

When beginning to walk unaided, the infant frequently falls but immediately gets up and carries on and does this repeatedly. This is probably genetically "forced": there is a compulsion to use new developmental milestones when they come "on stream" to ensure that they are used. This is seen also in "forced grasping" at 3–4 months, forced visual pursuit, and forced utterances in early verbal communication.

These processes for learning skills must be differentiated from the appearance of basic items of development. For example, many of the later items of posture and movements/mobility *are* "true skills" and show a considerable variability in their age of acquisition in different developmental tests. Clearly the skills require the appropriate environment in order to advance.

Skills therefore depend upon the opportunity to practice and a lack of such skills in developmental histories should be carefully interpreted in the light of opportunity.

The learning of skills follows a very constant path, whether this is riding a bicycle, playing a piece of music on the piano, or learning to drive a car:

1. The movements are undertaken first in isolation.
2. They are made to involve both hands in sequence.
3. Speed is added to the skill.
4. When motor learning is complete and placed in the subconscious, dominant hemisphere expression takes over, producing fluidity of the skill with modulation from the non-dominant hemisphere.

Motor skills pathways involve the cerebellar hemispheres, red nucleus, dorsal nucleus, ophthalamus, motor strip, and premotor strip. The inability to sequence individual motor acts into a skill is *dyspraxia* and this is an abnormality which is an executive disorder of movement in the absence of hard neurological signs, producing clumsiness and an inability to learn certain skills. Praxis is necessary for skills involving movements of all types, not just gross motor skills. Similarly, dyspraxia may be seen as an axial dyspraxia, oculomotor dyspraxia, articulatory dyspraxia, ideomotor or ideational dyspraxia, or writing dyspraxia (dysgraphia). While many children of primary school age are reported to be clumsy, few adults admit to this because of subsequent maturation and also because, if there is a specific dyspraxic learning difficulty, the adult finds ways around this particular difficulty to achieve the task.

The progression in development in general occurs in a cephalocaudal direction and from mass function to discrete function, so that in the upper limb development proceeds from the shoulder first and then to the hand. Any diminution in function from a brain insult will result in a loss in the opposite direction, thus the hand is first involved. This

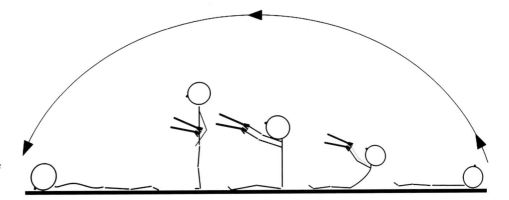

Fig. 15.2 Practical assessment of infant's posture and movements, through 180° change of position (including traction response)

can be seen, for example, with distal, severe praxic, and paralytic loss with the retention of proximal "fly-swatting" movements.

Until a new task becomes automatic it does require close attention by the child with sometimes an apparent lull in development of other areas. For example, at the commencement of independent walking upper limb function may appear to decline and thus one sees "fits and starts" in development.

Deviant Locomotor Development

Most children progress through posture and movement milestones in a common sequence: sitting, crawling, standing, and walking. However, 9% of the population are genetic deviants who have changed the order of this sequence. They frequently have an essential hypotonia, and this genetic trait is inherited in a dominant fashion. There are three distinct categories:

1. *Shufflers*, who represent 7% of the population. Their early motor milestones are delayed and they are hypotonic, shuffling on their bottoms rather than crawling in a standard way. They sit alone at 10 months, "shuffle" (i.e., are mobile) at 12 months, and walk alone at 19 months.
2. *Rollers* constitute 1% of children and they are mobile mostly by rolling but do crawl very briefly before walking. They are also hypotonic and roll at $8\frac{1}{2}$ months, sit at 9 months, and walk unaided at 16 months.
3. *Creepers* form approximately 1% of the population and sit at 10 months, creep in a commando crawling fashion at $12\frac{1}{2}$ months, and walk at about 20 months.

It is thought that there are two groups of children here, those who crawl and those who do not. Those who crawl and have normal muscle tone are the standard crawlers of the population. Those who crawl with hypotonia are the rollers and creepers. Children who do not crawl and are hypotonic are the shufflers and those who do not crawl and have normal muscle tone are the "fast" deviants in the population.

Clearly, "shuffle trait," which is inherited, can accompany acquired brain damage, probably altering the acquisition of some milestones. Its effect on pre-existing spasticity is not really known. Shuffle trait is frequently seen in children with Down's and other syndromes. The importance of this to the

Table 15.1 Primitive reflexes

Reflex	Elicitation
Cranial nerve reflexes, e.g.	
Rooting	Stimulus to the cheek results in the head and mouth turning to the stimulus
Sucking	Insertion of a teat in the mouth
Startle	1. Sudden noise or tapping elicits a similar response to Moro (see below), except the elbows and hands remain flexed
Extensor reflexes, e.g.	
Asymmetrical tonic neck reflex	Present from 1 to 3 months; on turning the child's head to one side, the child adopts a "fencing posture" with extension of both limbs on the side turned to
Moro	From 29 weeks onwards; the infant is held supine facing the examiner and the head is allowed to drop back (controlled) with resultant:
	(i) brief adduction of arms
	(ii) extension of arms with hands open
	(iii) adduction of arms
Progression reflexes, e.g.	
Walking	With the infant in a vertical position and the feet touching the surface, tilting the child results in high stepping
Placing	Stimulation of the dorsum of the foot on the edge of the table causes flexion of the leg and then extension and placement on the surface
Cutaneous reflexes, e.g.	
Palmar grasp	Introducing a finger into the palm from the ulnar side causes finger flexion
Plantar grasp	Stroking the plantar surface of the digits results in their flexion. This response is elicited in both hands and feet from 16 weeks' gestation to 3 months postnatally.

physician is the recognition of a normal genetic deviant, thus avoiding invasive investigations (muscle enzyme, muscle biopsy, and neurophysiology) and allowing parents to be reassured of eventual normality.

Primitive Reflexes

The mature child and adolescent can change posture and movements independently (e.g., can sit and write, lie prone and write, stand and write). The young infant, however, is unable to do so and there are subcortical integrators of posture and movement which ensure that if the child is placed in a certain position he will adopt a certain movement or posture. For example, the supine infant whose head is turned to one side will adopt a fencing posture. This is a *primitive reflex*. Some 70 or more of these have been described but should be considered as only one small facet of the neurodevelopmental examination of the infant. They can be grouped as cranial nerve primitive reflexes, extensor primitive reflexes, progression primitive reflexes, and cutaneous primitive reflexes. The important and easily recognizable progression reflexes are shown in Table 15.1.

These primitive reflexes are present early in development and disappear with maturation at a variable time. When brain insult causes cerebral palsy, by definition an abnormality of posture and movement due to an unchanging or static brain damage occurring during the period of brain growth or due to a congenital malformation of the brain, the integrators of posture and movement (primitive reflexes) persist, sometimes for life. Certain types of cerebral palsy are more frequently seen with persistent primitive reflexes. Their presence, however (e.g., primitive swimming reflex), does not signify potential future Olympic athletes.

Phasic Reflexes

Phasic reflexes must be differentiated from primitive reflexes. They are routinely assessed in the neurological examination and their absence signifies an interruption of the spinal reflex with denervation of either the afferent or the efferent pathway. Myopathic disorders with stretch receptors involved, or with severe myopathic weakness, will also result in reduced or absent phasic reflexes.

They are considerably uninhibited in infants compared to older children and are frequently elicited by means of a finger tap rather than conventional tendon hammer at that age. These reflexes are important in delineating neurosegmental levels in spinal cord lesions such as transverse myelitis or in

myelomeningocele. Their innervation is essential to know: ankle jerks S1–2 and knee jerks L3–4.

Signs of a pathological brisk phasic reflex include

- exaggerated response
- small amplitude stimulus
- wide afferent field
- crossed adduction
- clonus

A few beats of clonus are normal in early infancy. An extensor plantar response (Babinski sign) does not indicate pyramidal dysfunction and will normally be extensor until 12 months of age. Rarely, a flexor plantar response will be a false-negative finding with other signs of pyramidal dysfunction in the older child. Tendon reflexes in the upper limbs are normally less brisk than those in the lower limbs when elicited in a sitting position.

Examination of an infant or young child will often be less threatening and ensure more compliance if the child is examined sitting on the mother's lap and without the exposure of a tendon hammer.

Muscle Power

Movement reflects power and may be observed generally, although individual muscle groups often require an assessment of power in a more quantified way. The Medical Research Council (MRC) [3] developed the following scale:

0 = complete paralysis
1 = a flicker of contraction
2 = muscle can make normal movement with gravity eliminated
3 = normal movement against gravity but not additional resistance
4 = full normal power but overcome by resistance
5 = normal power

In the newborn it is important to distinguish hypotonia from weakness by observing volitional movement when the child is stimulated remote from the limbs (i.e., nose and anterior chest) and noting the resultant limb movements or crying or sucking.

There is an inherent relationship between muscle power and function in that a patient needs quadriceps power greater than MRC 3 for stance and good psoas activity for hip flexion during walking.

Proximal power in the upper limbs is assessed quickly and functionally by asking the child to raise the arms above the head, to touch the back of the neck, to stretch out the hands at the side, and to touch the base of the spine, the opposite knee, or hip. Distal power in the upper limb is readily assessed by grasp, finger abduction and adduction, and attempting to break opposition of thumb and index finger.

Muscle Tone Assessment

Muscle tone is a reflection of posture as mentioned above. It is assessed in quite discrete ways: by measuring resistance to passive movements, estimation of the joint angles, the feel of the muscles themselves, and by the posture.

1. Resistance to passive movements is generally assessed at the elbows, hips, knees, ankles, and wrists.
2. Joint angles are assessed clinically (rather than by using objective means such as goniometers) based upon a knowledge of the normal range of joint motion at different chronological ages:

   a. The elbow is assessed from a zero starting position with the arm straight; since this is a hinge joint natural movement is in flexion. Motion beyond the zero starting position is an unnatural one and is referred to as hyperextension. This may be evident in hypotonic children and is usually assessed in degrees beyond the zero starting point.
   b. Forearm pronation and supination are assessed from a vertical, zero starting, or "thumbs up" position with the forearms at the side of the body and the elbows flexed to 90°. Pronation ranges from 0 to 90° and supination from 0 to 90°. Excessive supination may enable the child to place the dorsum of his hands together when holding the arms extended and supinated (Fig. 15.3).

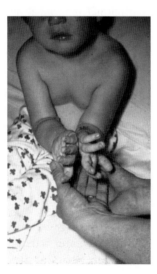

Fig. 15.3 Demonstrating hypersupination with elbows almost extended, indicative of exaggerated joint angles and hypotonia

i. Radial/ulnar deviations are not usually used for joint angle assessment of muscle tone, but the fingers of the hands are occasionally used.
ii. The *thumb* has a number of complex movements including abduction, adduction, flexion, extension, and opposition (circumduction). Extension of the thumb is undertaken parallel to the plane of the palm and is normally 90°. When it is excessive the thumb approximates to the radial forearm.
iii. The wrist may also be used as an indicator, particularly of hypotonia, with the forearm held upright and the hand allowed to fall forward. The hand normally makes an angle of 30° with the horizontal plane through the wrist. This is considerably less in hypotonic states (Holmes' sign) [4].

c. The shoulder has an almost complete range of global motion and indicators of hypotonia here are the "scarf sign," with the arms wrapped around the chest and the position of the olecranon assessed in relation to the nipple line (Fig. 15.4). In hypotonic states the elbows may approximate posteriorly. On lifting a hypotonic child under the axillae the examiner's hands may "slip through" the shoulder joint.
d. The spine may be assessed for exaggerated joint angles by looking at the degree of forward flexion and converting that angle to a measured distance such as inches from the floor to the fingertips, or in lateral movements of the spine, the distance the fingertips descend along the thigh.
e. The "straight leg raising" test, although not a record of spine motion, is carried out with the child lying supine on a firm, level examining table. The upward movement of the straight leg is a passive motion and measured in degrees from the zero starting position. The two sides may be compared (for more details, see Chapter 19).
f. The hip, which is a ball and socket joint, has a lesser range of motion than the shoulder. From a zero position and with the opposite leg held in maximum flexion (by the examiner or patient), thus flattening the lumbar spine, any hip flexion deformity of the other hip is demonstrated (Thomas' test). The examiner should place one hand on the iliac crest to note the point at which the pelvis begins to rotate. The normal range of active hip flexion is 110–120° [5]. Passive flexion may be as much as 140°+. Hip rotation in flexion and in extension is measured in angles. This gives an estimate of femoral anteversion, a cause for intoeing (along with diplegia and tibial torsion). Abduction and adduction of the normal hip are 45° and 40°, respectively, with knees extended and 45–60° with the knees flexed.

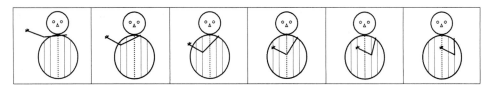

Fig. 15.4 The scarf sign is assessed by bringing one arm across the infant's chest until resistance is met. It tests passive tone in the flexors of the shoulder girdle. With increasing maturity (from 28 to 37 weeks post-conception or hypotonia) the elbow reaches from (i) the neck, (ii) opposite axillary line, (iii) opposite nipple line, (iv) xiphoid process, (v) ipsilateral nipple line, and (vi) ipsilateral axillary line

g. The knee is a modified hinge joint and the primary motion is flexion. It is examined looking for hyperextension and excessive flexion (i.e., greater than 135°). The "popliteal angle" is a useful joint angle particularly in newborns.

h. The ankle is another modified hinge joint, flexion, and extension occurring at the tibiotalar joint. It also has a slight degree of lateral motion when the ankle is plantarflexed. The zero point here is with the leg at right angles to the thigh and the foot at right angles to the shin. There is normally some 50° of combined tibiotalar and subtalar plantar flexion and 20° of dorsiflexion. Average ranges of joint motion may be found in various texts such as that published by the American Academy of Orthopaedic Surgeons 1965 [5].

3. The feel of the muscle is a rather subjective assessment of muscle tone but is applicable in states of gross hyper- and hypotonicity.

4. Posture. The "pithed frog posture" or round shouldered (slouching) posture may indicate poor tone. When the patient is examined on a firm examining couch there will be multiple points of contact between the body and the bed (i.e., no normal curvatures are evident). Disordered posture may indicate hypo- or hypertonia. Abnormal postures include

- Squint baby syndrome
- "Windsweeping" deformity
- "W sitting"
- Transient dystonia of prematurity
- "Sitting in air" (an elemental sensorimotor pattern, not a primitive reflex)

Hypotonia

Hypotonia may be of central or peripheral origin. If of central origin there will be preservation or exaggeration of phasic reflexes which are absent or diminished with peripheral causes. Increased joint angles may be due to hypotonia but may also be due to congenital ligamentous laxity. In this situation the joint angles *do not* reflect a reduced muscle tone as these individuals frequently do not have muscle hypotonia or weakness and may be contortionists or gymnasts. Various types of Ehlers–Danlos syndrome and congenital laxity of ligaments may give rise to a broad-based waddling gait, difficulty in rising from sitting, and an ability to assume abnormal postures such as placing the palms on the floor or make head-to-knee contact with knees extended. A further example of the ligamentous contribution to joint angles as a false-positive assessment of muscle tone can be demonstrated after a tendon lengthening for equinus deformity. No change in the muscle tone has been induced but the joint angle is increased. Likewise, exercise-induced muscle lengthening (the addition of sarcomeres) will result in some increase in joint angles.

In many conditions hypotonia and weakness may co-exist and in central core disease (a metabolic myopathy) hypotonia may be more obvious than weakness. With cerebellar hemisphere lesions abnormalities of coordination occur ipsilateral to the hemisphere involved with ipsilateral accompanying hypotonia. In the young infant with immature cerebellar and spinocerebellar pathways hypotonia may be the only sign of a cerebellar lesion. Ataxia must therefore enter the differential diagnosis of the "floppy baby."

The floppy infant will also present with delayed motor milestones and many severely learning disabled children are hypotonic.

Clinical Grades of Hypotonia

Hypotonia may be graded as follows:

0 = normal muscle tone
1 = decreased resistance to passive movement only
2 = decreased resistance to passive movement and joint hyperextensibility (i.e., increased joint angles)
3 = decreased resistance to passive movement and joint hyperextensibility causing postural effects in the lower limbs (e.g., valgus feet)
4 = decreased resistance to passive movement and joint hyperextensibility causing truncal postural effects (e.g., hyperlordosis)
5 = decreased resistance to passive movement and joint hyperextensibility causing postural effects in the shoulders and upper limbs (e.g., round shoulders)

Hypertonia

Spasticity is defined as stretch-dependent hypertonus which is abolished by posterior root section. There are two types, phasic and tonic. *Phasic spasticity* depends upon response to rapid stretch and is the earliest increase in muscle tone seen after cerebral lesions. This is often replaced with *tonic spasticity* which depends upon type 1 muscle fibers and does not vary with the velocity of stretch applied. The amount of lengthening of the muscle is reduced and the tonic muscle spindles fire for as long as the stretch is maintained. There is reciprocal inhibition of the antagonists and contractures occur in flexor, but not in the antigravity muscles. Tonic muscles are particularly geared to postural control. Occasionally there may be very little distal spasticity in combination with proximal tonic spasticity giving the appearance of a primary muscle disorder, the so-called proximal diplegia. In another group of children there is tonic paresis yet phasic spasticity with brisk reflexes, ankle clonus but a marked increase in muscle lengthening and joint ranges. This is often labeled ataxic diplegia or ataxic quadriplegia.

The original Ashworth Scale [6] is frequently used to assess increased muscle tone in adults:

1. No increase in muscle tone.
2. Slight increase in tone giving a "catch" when the affected part is moved in flexion or extension.
3. More marked increase in tone but the affected part is easily flexed.
4. Considerable increase in tone; passive movement difficult.
5. Affected part is rigid in flexion or extension.

Rigidity is an involuntary, sustained contraction of muscle but not muscle spindle dependent. It is driven by labyrinthine and proprioceptive systems and shows a constant resistance at varying angles. It is characterized by co-contraction of agonists and antagonists which may impose recognizably typical postures. There are two main types, *extensor dystonic rigidity* which produces clinical features depending upon whether there is labyrinthine or proprioceptive input which predominates. The muscle tone with rigidity is influenced by

1. contact with the surface
2. relationship of head to body
3. position in space
4. pressure through the long axis

The typical "prone/supine discrepancy" is an example of the dystonia seen in infancy from changing the head position. It is also influenced by anxiety, certain noises, lights, and esophageal reflux (Sandifer syndrome). These children have profuse primitive reflexes.

The second type is *flexor dystonia*. This is organized at the red nuclei/capsule. There are no progression or extensor reflexes in this pattern of deformity which is characterized by flexion at the arms, flexor recoil, and flexion of the legs but a normal lengthening reaction and a full range of movement. These types of deformity are therefore not fixed but dynamic deformities. These types of rigidity are clearly extrapyramidal and characteristically variable. They tend to affect all muscle groups—limb, axial, bulbar, and facial.

Mechanisms of Deformity in Children with Motor Disorders

The neurological examination attempts to understand the underlying mechanisms for the production of the dynamic, fixed, or structural deformity before the appropriate orthopaedic operation, drug, rhizotomy, or cerebellar stimulation. A further important fundamental is that positional deformities, whether intrauterine or postnatally acquired, may totally override the neurological picture which can make assessment of the etiology of the deformity difficult. Deformities may arise in several ways:

- Tonic spasticity
- Rigidity
- Paresis and muscle imbalance
- Growth
- Positional deformity
- Compensatory deformity
- Iatrogenic deformity
- Soft tissue contractural deformity
- Biomechanical muscle change

Positional deformities occur as a result of immobility plus the effect of growth and gravity. They may be seen in the neurologically normal child, in the neonatal physiological immobility of prematurity with resultant ballerina or cowboy postures, as mentioned previously, and in the "squint baby syndrome." They are seen in the neurologically abnormal child in its worst form with "wind sweeping," but also in "baby buggy spine" with knee flexion contractures from sitting in a wheelchair, and equinus feet from restrictive bed clothes covering the acutely ill child.

Contractures (to be distinguished from contractions) occur in many neurological conditions of childhood such as

1. Myopathies, especially:

   - Duchenne muscular dystrophy
   - Emery–Dreifuss sex-linked muscular dystrophy
   - Congenital fiber-type disproportion

2. Denervating conditions:

- Intermediate forms of chronic spinal muscular dystrophy
- Traumatic denervation
- Poliomyelitis
- Post-infective polyneuritis
- Prenatal denervation producing arthrogryposis

3. Spastic disorders:

- Cerebral palsy (hemiplegic, diplegic, and quadriplegic)
- Hereditary spastic diplegia

4. Extrapyramidal disorders:

- Athetoid/dystonic cerebral palsy
- Torsion dystonia
- Post-encephalitic athetosis
- Post-anoxic damage to the basal ganglia
- Genetically determined neurometabolic syndromes

Contractures may be dynamic (appearing during movement), fixed (independent of movement or immobility), and structural when secondary bone and joint changes have resulted from the persistent contracture.

Muscle Fasciculation

Muscle fasciculation, signifying lower motor denervation, is best seen in the tongue but also in the interossei along with fine, irregular tremor of the fingers in infants and young children with spinal muscular atrophy. Fasciculation may be elicited by tapping the muscle belly with the finger. It is seen particularly in the thenar and hypothenar muscles of the hand and in the shoulder muscles.

Muscle Wasting, Trophic, and Growth Changes

Muscle wasting or atrophy in childhood neurological conditions may result from central causes such as parietal (sensory) wasting in the affected limb and may also be due to trophic changes resulting from the autonomic dysfunction accompanying peripheral neuropathies. Other trophic effects will include changes to skin, hair, nails, and bone, characteristic of myelomeningocele, poliomyelitis, and arthrogryposis. Somatic growth changes frequently result from other generalized and functional limitations affecting feeding, weight bearing, and walking.

Muscle Wasting and Trophic Changes from Cerebral Lesions

Trophic limb changes may occur from a unilateral parietal lobe lesion. Aram et al. [7] found that there were corresponding contralateral shorter lengths of the hands and feet in children up to the age of 6 years who had no hemiplegia whereas there were no differences in normal children. If a unilateral brain lesion without hemiplegia can produce significant unilateral atrophy then this must at least contribute to the unilateral wasting in hemiplegia.

The pyramidal tract has a close relationship to the parapyramidal (autonomic) tracts which control vasomotor responses since movement inevitably requires an increase in blood flow to the muscle. Pyramidal lesions such as at the internal capsule or cortex can involve the parapyramidal tracts. This is evidenced by the fact that the wasted limb is often affected by abnormalities in vasomotor (vascular) control, with cold, blue limbs, prolonged capillary return, poor healing, and thickened nails.

Growth Failure in Cerebral Palsy and Other Neurological Conditions

In cerebral palsy the incidence of short stature and growth failure is high and the limbs are short and thin. This may be generalized in quadriplegic cerebral palsy with short stature (poor linear or skeletal growth) and wasting, or it may occur in a more localized fashion with a short limb (muscle and bone) that is thin (dwarfed or wasted) in hemiplegic or diplegic cerebral palsy.

In hemiplegia the disturbance is more likely to affect the leg than the arm and results in dwarfing of the lower limb or unequal leg lengths; a 2 cm difference between the lower limbs was found by Lin and Brown [8] (Fig. 15.5). In the upper limbs mean arm length is 5–8% less on the affected side. There is a decrease in limb circumference, muscle mass, bone mineral content, and density. The discrepancy in length of one lower limb has a potential to induce secondary changes such as a compensatory forefoot equinus or a pelvic tilt.

Other possible causes for muscle wasting in hemiplegia include

- "end organ resistance" to the hormonal control of growth
- reduced bone mineral density on the affected side from limited weight bearing, worse with severe neurological deficits

Fig. 15.5 Posterior view of the lower limbs during walking illustrating a right hemiplegic gait

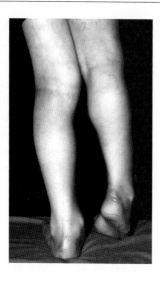

- spasticity reducing sarcomere number and size
- paralysis and disuse atrophy

In diplegia the pelvis is smaller and the lower limbs thinner and shorter than would be expected for the size of the trunk, with the net effect of reduced height and abnormality of posture.

In quadriplegia, growth failure occurs in some 52% [9] The causes are multifactorial and include nutritional contributory factors and bulbar palsy, resulting in generalized and localized growth failure (less than the third centile for height and weight) and markedly reduced muscle glycogen.

In myelomeningocele there is significant dwarfing of the lower limbs and short stature is frequent, especially with higher level lesions. Growth failure results from the neurosegmental motor and sensory level, from the hydrocephalus, from possible renal impairment, and from disordered autonomic control corresponding to the neurological level. Other factors include weight bearing and ambulatory status, vertebral anomalies and curvatures, and, rarely, growth hormone insufficiency.

Other neurological conditions with reduced muscle mass or growth failure include Duchenne dystrophy, Down's syndrome, Prader–Willi syndrome, and Sotos syndrome.

Disuse atrophy can occur very quickly and in one limb may confuse the diagnosis of an osteoid osteoma or other tumor. "Reflex" wasting is secondary to pain from a fracture or synovitis. Muscle wasting may be difficult to evaluate in an obese infant, and imaging (ultrasound or magnetic resonance imaging [MRI]) may be helpful to determine its true extent.

Limb hypertrophy may occur in association with hemihypertrophy of the brain or with the hemangioma of Klippel–Trénaunay syndrome, neurofibromatosis, or hypermelanosis of Ito.

Sensation

Primary sensation can be assessed even in the newborn, particularly with respect to pain. Testing in children is best carried out with a wooden "cocktail stick" or tooth pick rather than the more frightening needle. Dermatome levels are assessed simply in the lower limbs by proceeding anteriorly from the hip to the dorsum of the foot, to the plantar surface of the foot, and then—with the child prone—proceeding up the back of the leg to the buttocks and perianal area. Peripheral nerve lesions can also be identified in this way. The use of cotton wool for light touch and the testing of secondary sensory (proprioceptive) function require significant cooperation from the child and are usually possible only in those of school age or older. The effects of sensory loss are painless fractures, pressure sores and trophic ulcers, and chronic sensory arthropathy (Charcot joints). They are seen in children with myelomeningocele and spinal dysraphic states as well as the congenital sensory neuropathies (Fig. 15.6).

Fig. 15.6 Charcot's joint at the right ankle in a 6-year-old child with hereditary sensory neuropathy characterized by deficiency of small myelinated axons. Marked soft tissue swelling around the ankle joint masks extensive destruction (lytic/sclerotic) changes secondary to chronic trauma to a neuropathic joint

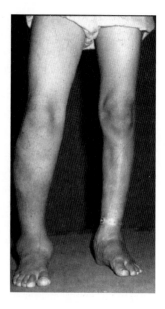

Ataxia

Ataxia means unsteadiness or incoordination and may be induced by cerebellar or spinocerebellar dysfunction, sensory loss, basal ganglia disorders, or spinal cord conditions. In Guillain–Barré syndrome there is a degree of truncal imbalance but no primary ataxia of cerebellar origin, so that all unsteadiness or incoordination is rightly called ataxia, not just that consequent upon cerebellar or spinocerebellar connections.

The development of balance follows a common pattern. While it takes the newborn infant some 12–18 months to be reasonably steady during stance, the newborn animal is steady a short time after birth. The first indication of cerebellar maturation is manifested by "righting reactions," either head-on-trunk righting or trunk-on-pelvis righting, best seen with the child held in a sitting position. These findings are present from 6 or 8 weeks to 3 months. The next level of balance control is seen at 6 months when the sitting child is tilted to either side, extends an arm in a parachute response (lateral parachutes), then an anterior parachute (forward extension of the upper limbs on forward tilting), and finally the posterior parachute at approximately 9 months, when the child extends the arms posteriorly to prevent falling backward. After this stage the child is readily able to change posture and movements independently and with stability. If he can sit and pivot his trunk with stability the primitive reflexes no longer operate and do not require to be tested.

The adult and older child will not use such protective reflexes unless involved in a major fall offsetting any force which attempts to alter the center of gravity and destabilize the trunk by contracting the antigravity muscles to maintain posture. These are dyssynergic movements which are equilibrial reactions and are the most sophisticated evidence of maturation of spinocerebellar connections.

Examination for ataxia is carried out in the upper limbs, trunk and neck, and lower limbs.

Upper Limbs

The finger–nose test is the conventional upper limb test for incoordination, looking for dysmetria and intention tremor (and more accurately disorderly, discontinuous, dysmetric, and off-direction components of the test). It is applicable in older children. As with a lot of paediatric neurology, different testing methods require to be used in order to test the same neurological pathways: for example, the repetitive and sequential finger movements (as standardized by Denckla [10]), rapid hand patting, diadoko- and dysdiadokokinesia, and piano-playing movements. Involuntary movements may be seen in the outstretched hands. Alternatively, in non-compliant younger children functional assessments of coordination can be made during writing, drawing, and coloring.

Truncal Ataxia

In the older child and adolescent this is best assessed with tandem walking where the child walks in a straight line with arms folded on the chest and feet placed heel to toe. Simple gait observation will also give an idea of truncal ataxia, as will standing on either leg or hopping forward, followed by hopping on the spot.

Observation of gait is discussed below but the features of a truncal ataxia are the variability in all gait parameters (speed, direction, step length, double support time, cadence, velocity of swing). The standard deviation of objective measures of these will give an index of ataxia.

Lower Limb Coordination

Many incorrectly think that standing on one leg or hopping is an index of lower limb coordination when in fact it represents truncal control. In the older patient the classical heel–shin test is applied but in the younger child alternative methods of testing are required such as asking the child to jump with both feet together, then both feet apart, and both feet together, repeatedly, and the more difficult jumping with an alternate foot forward. A toe–finger test can be the equivalent of a finger–nose test. The child can be asked to describe the figure 3 or 2 in the air with his big toe. Phasic reflexes in ataxic conditions may be "pendular."

Observational Gait Assessment

Observation of gait is a useful component of the neurological examination, reviewing at least six stride pairs in both the anterior–posterior and lateral direction during each walk. The gait should be at the child's self-selected walking speed. The examiner systematically looks at foot placement and whether this is with a heel–toe disposition with a triple rocker (heel strike, weight bearing, and heel raise/toe-off), flat-footed placement with inversion or eversion, toe-heeling placement, or persistent dynamic equinus. These represent degrees of increasing severity of a typical hemiplegic gait. Foot slapping, a wide base, or other types of foot placement are noted. On the second walk the observer records any change in knee position from extension to 90° of flexion and back again or whether there is any loss of terminal extension prior to heel strike. On the third walk the observer concentrates upon the hip and whether there is any obvious persistent flexion contracture or crouch gait and also whether there is circumduction or waddling. Finally the observer notes any truncal sway.

The important temporal and spatial parameters of gait include the step length, swing time, double support time, cadence (number of steps per minute), walking speed (meters per second), and the velocity of swing phase (See Chapter 6). All of these parameters will change with age and with height. The young child increases his walking speed by increasing cadence whereas the older adolescent increases speed by increasing stride length. Many toddlers have very little double support time. There is a normal asymmetry of gait, the left and right values differing by as much as 10% in any one individual. These asymmetries may relate to established laterality. Wheelwright et al. [11] showed the step length was equal to 43% of the height and that height and gender are major determinants of swing time and cadence, although height, leg length, and gender are independent determinants of double support time.

The normal process of walking involves forward progression of the hip flexors on one side and then heel strike and weight bearing. At this point the individual throws his weight on to the other hip as the other leg achieves heel raise and eventual toe-off. During the swing phase, the leg is similar to a pendulum starting with a zero velocity, increasing to maximum velocity at mid-swing and back to zero velocity at heel strike.

Pattern recognition allows one to distinguish many abnormal gait patterns, for example, the congenital or acquired hemiplegic gait, the diplegic gait, dyskinetic gaits, the gait of Duchenne muscular dystrophy and peripheral neuropathy, the ataxic gait, antalgic gait, festinating gait, and bizarre gaits. The congenital hemiplegic gait pattern (as above), with upper limb flexed and adducted and with flexion at the hip, heel cord and hamstrings, and internal rotation of the lower limb, is different from that of the acquired hemiplegic gait where there is external rotation and abduction in the upper limb and in the foot position. The diplegic gait is essentially a bilateral lower limb hemiplegic-type picture. Dyskinetic gaits show a florid amount of involuntary movements, often with crouch and sway so that it is surprising that upright ambulation is possible. The Duchenne gait is classically with equinus, waddling at the hips, and hyperlordosis. The peripheral neuropathic gait is high stepping and the ataxic gait has variability in all gait parameters as mentioned previously. In practice such children stand on a wide base, make several point turns, do not gauge the slowing down before obstacles, veer off-direction, and progress with variable step lengths and other phases of gait. The antalgic gait is protective against pain. Festinating gaits classical of parkinsonism do not occur in childhood but bizarre gait patterns are seen with psychological disorders, for example, with gross spinal flexion.

Fog Test

For this test the child is asked to walk on the outer borders of both feet and the observer looks for two features:

1. gross asymmetries, the sign of a minimal hemiparesis
2. immature flexion in the upper limbs, a maturation sign

Toe Walking

Toe walking may be normal in the young child who has recently learned to walk. It is often seen in children who are overactive and generally the heel can be brought to the ground in stance. If the habit persists, fixed equinus may develop. Signs of spasticity must be examined for. If a fixed contracture is present, underlying spasticity should be considered a cause although fixed contractures frequently override neurological features as is the case with all positional deformities.

Pes Cavus

In the common equinus deformity this may be at the forefoot or the hind foot (see Chapter 32). In the forefoot variety this may result from persistent toe walking (ballerina syndrome) and develop into a marked cavus foot with claw toes.

The hind foot equinus (Fig. 15.7) may result from paresis (and muscle imbalance), for example, with weak dorsiflexors or a tight calf (tonic spasticity or rigidity), or be consequent upon a short tendon or short leg.

In assessing the foot the Dick or Jack test is often used, passively extending the big toe to see the extent of elevation of the arch of the foot for mobile/structural pes planus. Pes cavus is a feature of diastematomyelia, syringomyelia, spinal intramedullary pathology, such as cysts and progressive conditions, such as Friedreich's ataxia, ataxia telangiectasia, and hereditary motor and sensory neuropathies.

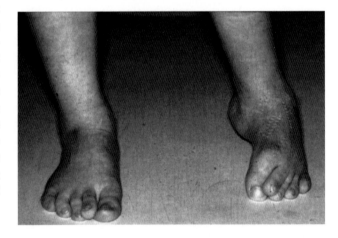

Fig. 15.7 Cavovarus deformity as part of a myelodysplastic limb

Spinal Curvatures

Idiopathic thoracic scoliosis is usually convex to the right; scoliosis to the opposite side is a feature of syringomyelia with Arnold–Chiari malformation (see also Chapter 36).

The spinal curvatures occur with a variety of neurological disorders including diastematomyelia, spinal congenital cysts, Sprengel's shoulder, and the Klippel–Feil deformity. Head tilt may be a manifestation of cerebellar hemisphere tumor before the classical cerebellar signs or signs of raised intracranial pressure occur.

The purpose of developmental screening and testing is to screen for pathology, relying upon a combination of reported developmental milestones and clinical examination. Such motor delay triggers a need for investigations such as creatinine phosphokinase levels, neurophysiology, and imaging, which clarify the diagnosis. The delay in neurodevelopmental acquisition of posture and movement milestones is noted. A fuller developmental assessment (e.g., Griffiths, test) will depict other aspects of development and will provide an indication of the effect that the motor disorder has had on other areas of the child's development. Following appropriate treatment or therapy a reassessment of the neurodevelopmental status will monitor the benefits of treatments.

Diseases Which Require Special Neurodevelopmental Examination of the Motor System

Neural Tube Defects

Newborn babies with myelomeningocele (see Chapter 17) require a detailed examination of the lower limbs shortly after birth in order to derive the neurosegmental motor sensory and reflex levels. Examination will also identify the features of the "isolated cord" which are

- isolated muscle spasticity
- loss of reciprocal inhibition
- reflexes elicited in toes, hamstrings, and tibialis anterior
- flexor withdrawal with oscillation
- no extensor activity
- flexor pattern of tone if long segment
- anal reflex preservation
- dermatome to myotome responses
- spastic pelvic floor and bladder neck
- deformity due to unopposed spastic muscles
- wide afferent field with crossed adductor responses
- spontaneous spinal myoclonus

In addition to these observations, detailed clinical examination of power, reflexes, sensation, and deformity is recorded at the ankle, foot, knee, hip, and spine.

The pattern of cord involvement can be deduced, such as the type 1 cord in which the myelomeningocele destroys the cord terminally to a variable height causing flaccidity, areflexia, and anesthesia in the distal segment. The lowest normally functioning neurosegmental level describes the lesion level. The neurological level is the functionally important level, not the lesion level or vertebral level.

In type 2 cord involvement, the myelomeningocele destroys a more proximal area of the spinal cord to a variable degree, leaving normal but isolated cord distally. The isolated cord here may be a short segment or a long segment which is akin to a transverse myelitic lesion.

Type 3 is where the myelomeningocele only partially destroys the cord, for example, in the thoracolumbar region, and some descending long tracks will be preserved and others halted at the upper level of the lesion. Only examination of the lower limbs will decide which are intact.

Type 4 is an incomplete conus lesion where the terminal part of the cord is incompletely involved and again some descending tracts descend the full length of the cord whereas others do not.

From a deformity point of view, the pattern of cord involvement is very important. In type 1 normal power muscle groups oppose flaccid muscle groups across joints; in type 2 flaccid muscle opposes spastic muscle groups. The mechanism of deformity in children with neural tube defects is due to

- an imbalance of muscle action across joints
- positional deformity either in utero or acquired postnatally

Examination of these infants involves ultrasound of the hips, bladder, and kidneys; ultrasound or MRI scanning of the spinal cord and spine; as well as imaging of the Chiari 2 malformation and hydrocephalus. The neurosegmental motor levels are particularly important for predicting subsequent walking, and children with MRC 3 power or better in the quadriceps (L3, 4) are generally ambulant with below-knee orthoses or aids. Children with higher motor levels require above-knee bracing and sticks or hip guidance or reciprocating gait orthoses. Hip dislocation is not a separate congenital malformation but a result of muscle imbalance occurring early in high-level and low-level lesions but not in mid-lumbar level lesions.

Chiari Malformation

The Chiari 1 malformation occurs where there is descent of the cerebellar tonsils through the foramen magnum. The Chiari 2 malformation occurs in association with myelomeningocele and the descent of the tonsils and vermis. The Chiari 3 malformation is an occipital or cervical meningocele with enclosed cerebral tissue and the Chiari 4 malformation is cerebellar hypoplasia.

It is of theoretical importance whether the descending tissue is the cerebellar tonsils or vermis, and on MRI a descent of 2 cm below the foramen magnum is considered significant. The appearance of descending cerebellar tissue is important and, if rounded, probably indicates that there is no significant impaction. The sharply contoured descending portion is more indicative of tightness at the craniocervical junction. T2 MRI images may exaggerate the amount of surrounding subarachnoid space available.

All children with spina bifida should be routinely checked for signs of impaction or cavitation (hydromyelia or syringomyelia) in the cervical cord as a result of Chiari malformation. They should be checked for muscle power distally in the upper limbs and be examined for wasting of the thenar/hypothenar muscle groups and fasciculation in the hands or shoulders. Reflexes (biceps and triceps) are tested and impaired bulbar function checked (difficulty with swallowing and speech or "strain"-type headaches on coughing or sneezing).

Brisk upper limb reflexes alone will indicate a degree of impaction, and cavitation will produce signs of lower motor neurone lesion in the upper limbs. Somatosensory potentials (although technically difficult to obtain in the infant and young child) from the upper limbs along with sequential imaging and clinical examination will help to decide whether occipital and cervical decompression are indicated.

Tethered Cord

The normal spinal conus terminates at L1 but may be considerably lower if tethered to a fatty lump (lipomeningocele) or paired myelomeningocele. Tethering of the cord or filum may occur at various levels and the child presents with a loss of acquired function which may be motor, sensory, or reflex, a change in bladder innervation, or pain in the back or lower limbs. Examination of the lower limbs will confirm a changed neurosegmental level (there may be a pre-existing myelodysplasia) and somatosensory evoked potentials from the lower limbs likewise show a changed pattern. Clinical and physiological changes will differentiate a radiological tethering from symptomatic tethering of the cord. The child may become symptomatic during periods of rapid linear growth; height is routinely measured at all outpatient visits. Spinal dysraphic states are suspected if there is a vascular pigmented nevus, hairy patch, pit, or lipoma near the distal midline of the spine.

Classically the myelodysplastic leg is thin with cavovarus deformity and autonomic (trophic) changes. With only one leg involved the child cannot develop a neuropathic bladder.

Duchenne and Other Muscular Dystrophies

Clinically muscular dystrophy is suspected because of a delay in the motor milestones of a young boy with calf hypertrophy and a positive Gower's sign. Ankle reflexes may be lost and the child walks on his toes with a waddling gait and a severe lordosis.

The clinical progress of Duchenne dystrophy may be monitored by following a scale to monitor the rate of progression of this regressive condition [12]:

1. walks and climbs stairs without assistance
2. walks and climbs stairs with aid of railing
3. walks and climbs stairs slowly with aid of railing (>25 s for eight standard steps)
4. walks unassisted and rises from chair but cannot climb stairs
5. walks unassisted but cannot rise from chair or climb stairs
6. walks only with assistance or walks independently with long leg braces
7. walks in leg braces but requires assistance for balance
8. stands in long leg braces but unable to walk even with assistance
9. remains in wheelchair or bed

Clinical slowing of progression is achieved by maintaining ambulation, by corrective scoliosis surgery, and by nocturnal continuous positive airways pressure (CPAP) ventilation. Cyclical steroids are also tried. This is further discussed in Chapter 16.

Congenital Motor Disorders (Cerebral Palsy)

Congenital motor disorders (cerebral palsy) are discussed in Chapter 19, but here are detailed: (1) the range of neurological abnormalities in a hemiplegia, (2) "cerebral palsy in evolution," (3) transient dystonia of prematurity, and (4) "minimal hemiplegia."

Components of Hemiplegia

Although a hemiplegia appears to be a homogeneous entity, it consists of a number of different components including dyspraxia, peripheral weakness, impaired proximal fly-swatting movements, spasticity/rigidity, brisk tendon reflexes, extensor plantar responses, abnormal limb posture, asymmetrical protective reflexes, involuntary movements (athetoid postures), abnormal sensation, vasomotor changes, unilateral primitive reflexes, retention of grasp reflex, excessive "associated" and "mirror" movements, and abnormal growth.

Recognition of cerebral palsy in evolution can be challenging for the neurologist. In early infancy hemiplegic signs may not be obvious and may take 6–9 months to evolve. A hint to the future motor pattern may be seen with asymmetry of the phasic reflexes, preference for voluntary movement on one side, asymmetrical parachute responses or delay in sitting, kicking one leg more than the other, and developing a strong hand preference in infancy.

Transient Dystonia Following Prematurity

This is often seen in mid-infancy with a prone/supine discrepancy, the child arching his back and extending the limbs when held vertical or placed prone and adopting a more flexor pattern when in supine. The transient rigidity picture is to be distinguished from the more florid evolution of dystonic or spastic diplegia or quadriplegia. It is said that cerebral palsy occurs during the phase of brain growth, in the first 4 years of life, but can be diagnosed when the motor features are present before this, for example, in dyskinetic cerebral palsy.

Minimal Hemiplegia

A minimal hemiplegia can be distinguished clinically only with difficulty by assessing distal fine finger movements (Denckla test [10]) or fastening buttons, a mild pronator catch, asymmetrical or associated movements on fog testing, mild weakness of grasp, failure to swing the arm during walking, or exaggerated asymmetry of nail breadths.

Hereditary Sensory Motor Neuropathies

There are a number of clinically and genetically distinct orders in which abnormalities of sensory motor nerves are prominent. They have to be distinguished from conditions in which peripheral neuropathy is part of a more generalized neuraxial abnormality such as Friedrich's ataxia or motor chromatic leukodystrophy, and from sensory neuropathies in which the motor nerves are spared but may produce neuropathic joints, fractures, and ulceration. Of the six types, the most important to the orthopaedic surgeon is type 1 Charcot–Marie–Tooth disease, an autosomal dominant disorder often presenting with pes cavus, equinus, and broadening of the forefoot. Kyphosis and scoliosis may present later. Tendon jerks are lost early and sensory impairment (joint position and vibration) may develop. The "champagne bottle" leg deformity is rarely seen in children. In this condition examination of the parents may be helpful.

Among sporadic cases 30% are new, dominant mutations and the remainder recessive. A few have gender-linked recessive inheritance. In type 2, axonal neuropathy is more slowly progressive and sensory impairment less obvious. Type 3 is more severe, with club feet, severe muscle wasting and weakness, and impairment of all sensory modalities. There is also proximal involvement with hip dislocation, and scoliosis is seen eventually. In this type there is hypertrophic interstitial neuropathy with onion skin formation seen microscopically and palpable thickening of subcutaneous nerves. Such patients do not tolerate prolonged immobilization, for example, after corrective surgery. Genetic counseling can be very helpful.

The Profoundly Handicapped Child

The neuromotor patterns of the profoundly handicapped child are illustrated in Fig. 15.8, and such children are prone to secondary positional deformity (wind sweeping deformity) where, for example, in side lying, the plane of the shoulder and hip is not aligned. The child corkscrews about a longitudinal access giving rise to scoliosis, pelvic obliquity, leg length discrepancy, plagiocephaly, bat ear, thoracic asymmetry, and a skew posture of the lower limbs. The deformation overrides the original neurological pattern. This is the most severe type of positional deformity and results from the effects of gravity upon a child who is unable to change position. Positional deformity may occur in normal infants, for example, following prematurity with the squint baby or molded baby syndrome. At 3 months of age assessment of positional asymmetries is at its most difficult, particularly in deciding whether there is an underlying neuromotor condition predisposing to it.

Children recovering from serious traumatic brain injury or meningitis are especially prone to developing positional deformities superimposed upon residual neurological deficits. Their care demands scrupulous attention to postural turning and nursing principles.

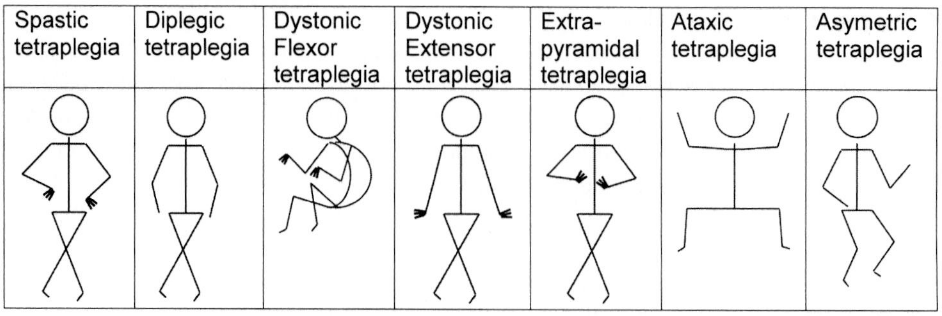

Fig. 15.8 Schematic of the different tetraplegic motor patterns seen in the profoundly handicapped child

Spastic tetraplegia	Diplegic tetraplegia	Dystonic Flexor tetraplegia	Dystonic Extensor tetraplegia	Extra-pyramidal tetraplegia	Ataxic tetraplegia	Asymetric tetraplegia

References

1. Minns RA, Sobkowiak CA, Skardoutsou A, et al. Upper limb function in Spina Bifida. Zeitschrift fur Kinderchirurgie 1977; 22:(4):493–506.

2. Yakovlev PI, Lecours A-R. The myelogenetic cycles of regional maturation of the brain. In: Minkowski A, ed. Regional Development of the Brain in Early Life. Oxford: Blackwell; 1967:3–70.

3. Medical Research Council. Aids to the investigation of peripheral nerve injuries. War Memorandum No 7 ed. London: HMSO, 1943.

4. Holmes G. The Croonian lectures on the clinical symptoms of cerebellar disease. Lancet 1922; 199:(5155):1177–1182.

5. American Academy of Orthopaedic Surgeons. Joint Motion. Method of measuring and recording. Edinburgh: Churchill Livingston, 1965.

6. Ashworth B. Preliminary trial of carisoprodol in multiple sclerosis. Practitioner 1964; 192:540–542.

7. Aram DM, Ekelman BL, Satz P. Trophic changes following early unilateral injury to the brain. Dev Med Child Neurol 1986; 28:(2):165–170.

8. Lin JP, Brown JK. Peripheral and central mechanisms of hindfoot equinus in childhood hemiplegia. Dev Med Child Neurol 1992; 34:(11):949–965.

9. Minns RA, Wong B, Brown JK, Fraser WI. Neuro-developmental study of profoundly mentally handicapped children in hospital care. J Ment Defic Res 1989; 33:(Pt 6):439–454.

10. Denckla MB. Development of speed in repetitive and successive finger-movements in normal children. Dev Med Child Neurol 1973; 15:(5):635–645.

11. Wheelwright EF, Minns RA, Elton RA, Law HT. Temporal and spatial parameters of gait in children. II: Pathological gait. Dev Med Child Neurol 1993; 35:(2):114–125.

12. Vignos PJ. Rehabilitation in the myopathies. In: Vinken PJ, Bruyn GW, eds. Handbook of Clinical Neurology. Amsterdam: North-Holland Pub. Co.; 1979.

Chapter 16

Hereditary and Developmental Neuromuscular Disorders

Eugene E. Bleck and James E. Robb

Introduction

This chapter considers those conditions characterized by weakness resulting from pathology primarily in the muscles or the anterior horn cells of the spinal cord. In their later stages these disorders have recognizable clinical features, but in the early stages all share a common set of symptoms and physical signs. Generally, motor disorders are either genetic or acquired. Children with the former tend to present with weakness and delayed motor skills whereas those with the acquired type usually have fairly rapid progression of weakness and loss of function. Children who are floppy at birth are likely to be evaluated initially by a paediatrician or paediatric neurologist but the orthopaedic surgeon may be the first specialist to assess a child with a walking difficulty caused by Duchenne's or Becker's dystrophy.

Assessment

Symptoms

The majority of children with a muscle disorder will present with delayed motor milestones. An experienced mother may recognize that her child has moved less than usual in utero. The history should confirm developmental milestones and, if the motor problem was not noticed in early development, at what age the deterioration in motor development occurred. After birth the affected child may be weak and floppy (Fig. 16.1) and unlike other children may present with delayed sitting, crawling, or walking. However, this is also seen in children with global developmental delay. Normally, a term infant will sit at 6 months, crawl at 9 months, stand at 10 months, and walk at 12–14 months. About 10% of

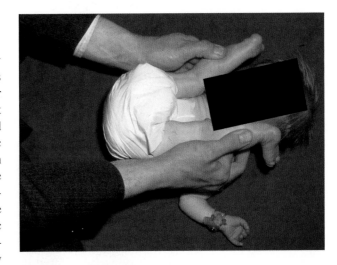

Fig. 16.1 Floppy baby. Courtesy of Dr P. Eunson

children bottom-shuffle rather than crawl, and 97% walk six steps unaided by 18 months.

The most common symptoms that cause parents to seek consultation are listed in Table 16.1. It is salutary to remember that Read and Galasko [1] reported a mean delay of 2 years in making the diagnosis of Duchenne muscular dystrophy (DMD), particularly on the part of orthopaedic surgeons.

Examination

A standard orthopaedic examination including a neurological assessment is required but will also focus on delayed motor milestones, muscle strength and tone, muscle fasciculation, and gait. Some conditions are associated with learning difficulties, for example, DMD. Sensation will be normal in muscular dystrophies, spinal muscular atrophy (SMA), myopathy, and myasthenia gravis but impaired in sensorimotor neuropathies such as Charcot–Marie–Tooth disease.

The presence of joint contractures at birth should alert the clinician to the possibility of arthrogryposis (Fig. 16.2)

E.E. Bleck (✉)
Department of Orthopaedic Surgery, Stanford University School of Medicine, Stanford, CA, USA

M. Benson et al. (eds.), *Children's Orthopaedics and Fractures*,
DOI 10.1007/978-1-84882-611-3_16, © Springer-Verlag London Limited 2010

Table 16.1 Common symptoms of neuromuscular disease

Infancy	Floppy baby
	Slow development; not sitting unaided at 9 months
	Muscles lack consistency and tone
Childhood	Tiptoeing (most common complaint in Duchenne muscular dystrophy)
	Clumsy; awkward
	Cannot keep up with other children
	Runs strangely
	Seems weak and fatigues easily
	Waddling gait
	Posture is poor; stands with "sway-back and pot-belly"
	Cannot cut with scissors in kindergarten
	Printing by hand or writing is slow and labored
	Is he/she "learning disabled?"

impairment. In some conditions, both central and peripheral hypotonia may coexist [2].

Posture

Slight degrees of shift of the spine from the midline may be noted in addition to a loin crease, both of which are early signs of scoliosis which can be an early manifestation of neuromuscular disease. Forward drooping of the shoulders, a prominent abdomen, or lumbar lordosis should arouse suspicion (Fig. 16.3). Winging of the scapula can be mistaken for a benign, slumped posture.

In the young infant a hypotonic posture may be noted (Fig. 16.4) and head lag seen when pulling the infant from supine to sitting (Fig. 16.5). "Slip through" at the shoulder girdle may occur when the infant is held vertically under

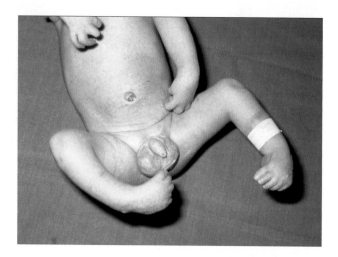

Fig. 16.2 Arthrogryposis. Courtesy of Dr P. Eunson

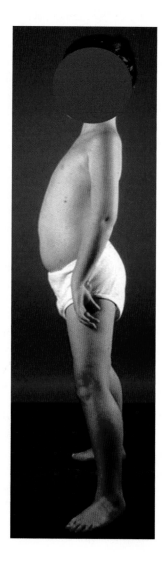

Fig. 16.3 Prominent abdomen and lumbar lordosis in DMD. Note the pseudo-hypertrophy of the calves

as well as neuromuscular disorders that are associated with low tone, muscle imbalance, or paralysis. This should be distinguished from "packaging disorders."

It may also be useful to determine if the infant has a central or peripheral type of hypotonia. Paralytic hypotonia with significant weakness suggests a peripheral neuromuscular problem such as SMA, neuropathy, myopathy, muscle dystrophies, or myasthenic syndromes. A non-paralytic hypotonia without significant weakness suggests a central cause, which may be neurological, genetic, syndromic, or metabolic. A peripheral problem may be associated with a delay in motor milestones but relatively normal social and cognitive development whereas a central problem may be associated with motor delay and social and cognitive

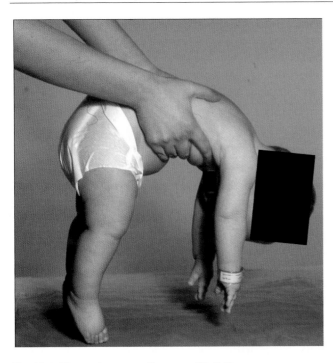

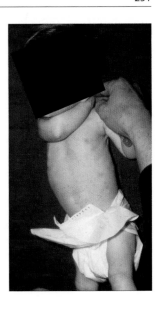

Fig. 16.6 Scarf sign. Illustration courtesy of Dr P. Eunson

Fig. 16.4 Hypotonic posture. Courtesy of Dr P. Eunson

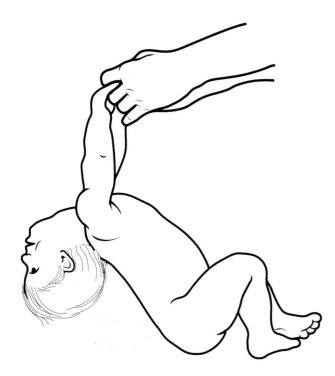

Fig. 16.5 Head lag

Muscular Testing and Observation

Activity Test

The child should be asked to walk on his heels, sit on the floor and then rise, stand on one foot, hop, step up and down from a stool, climb stairs, and walk on tiptoe. Gower's sign is when the child has to use the hands and arms to "walk" up the body from a squatting position due to lack of lower extremity muscle strength (Fig. 16.7). One-sided tiptoeing, while the examiner holds the child's hand for balance, is a useful way of demonstrating significant gastrocnemius–soleus weakness. Normally, a child should be able to rise on one foot 8–9 times in sequence. Trendelenburg sign may be difficult to elicit in a normal child younger than 6 or 7 years because of a lack of fully developed balance reactions.

the arms and the "scarf sign" also indicates shoulder girdle weakness (Fig. 16.6). The infant may not be able to bear weight through the legs when supported under the axillae. In older infants the ability to roll over, sit unaided, and to pull to stand should be noted.

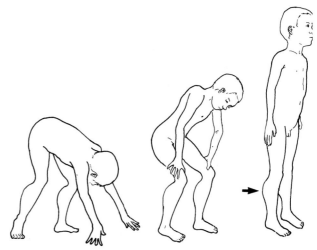

Fig. 16.7 Gower's sign

Manual Muscle Testing

Manual muscle testing can be difficult in younger children but in those who can cooperate manual muscle testing and Medical Research Council (MRC) grading should be performed (Table 16.2).

Table 16.2 Manual muscle testing (MRC grading)

Power 5 (normal)	The portion of the limb being tested moves through its full range against gravity and maximum resistance
Power 4 (good)	Moves against gravity and moderate resistance
Power 3 (fair)	Moves against gravity but not against resistance
Power 2 (poor)	Moves only with gravity eliminated
Power 1 (trace)	Flicker of contraction only
Power 0 (zero)	No movement

Muscle Tone

Although contemporary physiotherapists commonly use the term "tone," its meaning is poorly defined. The French use the terms *extensibilité*—the amount of lengthening permitted by the muscle—and "passivité"—denoting the lack of resistance to passive movement [3]. *Passivité* can be assessed by grasping the child's forearm and flapping the wrist up and down rapidly. The real value of the term is in the diagnosis of the "floppy" or hypotonic infant [4]; later in childhood, the sign is less useful. The presence of contractures at birth suggests a peripheral neuromuscular disorder such as congenital muscular dystrophy and may also be seen in any disorder that limits fetal movement such as spina bifida.

Atrophy and Hypertrophy

The degree of atrophy in lower motor neurone disease generally correlates with the amount of weakness, whereas in primary myopathies it does not. Hypertrophy is most noticeable in myotonia congenita, in which muscle strength is proportional to bulk. Early in DMD the calf, deltoid, and vastus lateralis muscles will appear hypertrophied. In later stages "pseudohypertrophy" occurs as the muscle fibers are replaced by fat (Fig. 16.3). Three myopathies are characterized by severe weakness but no atrophy: myasthenia gravis, polymyositis, and periodic paralysis. This observation is very important because these three myopathies are among the few that can be treated.

Fasciculations

Spontaneous twitching of the muscles, especially in the calf, the intrinsic muscles of the hand, and the tongue, characterizes a degenerating anterior horn cell disease. Even if fasciculations are not seen, anterior horn cell disease cannot be ruled out, as denervation fibrillation (arrhythmic "blips" that can be seen only on the electromyograph [EMG]) may still be present.

Reflexes

The deep tendon reflexes usually disappear early in the neuropathies and diminish in parallel with increasing muscle weakness in the myopathies. They are preserved in polymyositis and myasthenia gravis. The plantar responses are always flexor (negative Babinski sign) in the myopathies and neuropathies except in the rare case of spinal muscular atrophy with pyramidal tract involvement [5]. If extensor responses occur, an upper motor neurone disorder should be suspected.

Gait

Older children should be asked to walk, if possible, along a well-lit walkway or corridor and their gait observed to allow assessment of the stance and swing phases in the sagittal plane and rotation in the transverse plane (see Chapter 6). A waddling gait may not necessarily represent hip abductor weakness and hip dysplasia should be excluded radiologically. A high-stepping gait is associated with weakness of ankle dorsiflexion and a toe-drag gait with spasticity. When asked to run, a child with barely perceptible spastic hemiplegia will often flex the elbow and clench the fist on the involved side so attention should be paid to the upper limbs when observing a gait. A child with muscle weakness appears labored when running and may mimic ataxia. Three-dimensional gait analysis is useful in providing a baseline evaluation of gait for future reference.

Laboratory Investigations

Serum Enzymes

By far the most sensitive test in the diagnosis of DMD is the measurement of serum creatine kinase (CK). Very high levels occur before the onset of symptoms and signs and gradually decrease as the disease progresses because the muscle is replaced by fat. The concentration of serum aldolase is also elevated in DMD. Serum lactate and pyruvate should be obtained if a mitochondrial disease is suspected. If congenital hypothyroidism is suspected the infant should have the thyroid function checked. An edrophonium test is used to diagnose myasthenia gravis.

Electromyography

DNA testing is supplanting EMG studies in the diagnosis of muscle disorders and is used to support the diagnosis of a muscle disease. EMG features in peripheral hypotonia are shown in Table 16.3.

Table 16.3 EMG features in peripheral hypotonia

Neurogenic	Large amplitude action potentials, reduced interference pattern, increased internal instability
Myopathic	Small amplitude action potentials with increased interference pattern
Myotonic	Increased insertional activity
Myasthenic	Abnormal repetitive and single fiber studies

Adapted from Gowda et al. [2]

Muscle Biopsy

The surgeon should consult with the pathologist before undertaking a muscle biopsy to ensure that the specimen will be of adequate size, transported in the correct medium, and delivered at an appropriate time of day to allow processing. The surgeon should also check with the pathologist whether a core needle biopsy would suffice or whether an open biopsy is preferred. The muscle chosen for biopsy should be abnormal and a pre-biopsy magnetic resonance image (MRI) may help to identify areas of abnormality if there is doubt. Biopsies are usually obtained from the vastus lateralis or deltoid, as they are proximal and often affected early in myopathies and dystrophies. Generally, the labeled biopsy specimen is placed on a damp saline swab and needs to be sent fresh to the laboratory promptly to avoid desiccation. Examples of normal muscle and that seen in DMD are illustrated in Fig. 16.8.

Etiology and Inheritance

Most muscle disorders, except polymyositis, have defined patterns of inheritance: the dystrophies and myopathies are usually autosomal dominant or sex-linked, whereas the atrophies are generally autosomal recessive. A positive family history is not invariable, as spontaneous mutations may occur. The responsible gene in Duchenne and Becker muscular dystrophies has been identified on the xp21 region of the X-chromosome, and the genetic locus for SMA has been identified on chromosome 5q. Advances in genetic research offer the prospect of gene therapies for genetically determined muscle disease and now that the first trials of gene therapy for DMD are starting it is important to know the exact mutation for each boy. Families can also be counseled appropriately about the risk of future children being affected by a genetically based disorder.

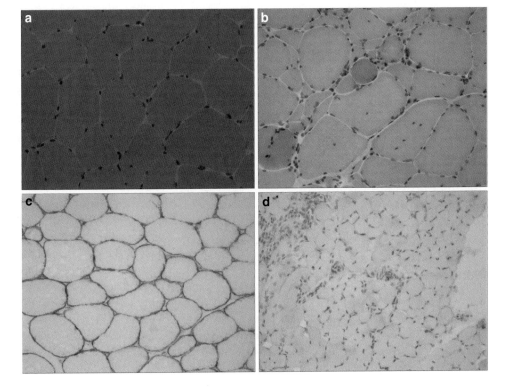

Fig. 16.8 (**a**) Normal muscle (H&E stain ×20 magnification). (**b**) Duchenne muscle showing fiber splitting and hypercontracted (red) fibers (H&E stain ×40 magnification). (**c**) Immunohistochemistry for dystrophin in normal muscle (×40 magnification). (**d**) Immunohistochemistry for dystrophin which is absent in Duchenne muscle (×40 magnification). Illustrations courtesy of Dr C. Smith

Differential Diagnosis

Figure 16.9 categorizes anatomically the most common neuromuscular disorders that need to be considered in children, showing the relevant clinical, hereditary, and laboratory details.

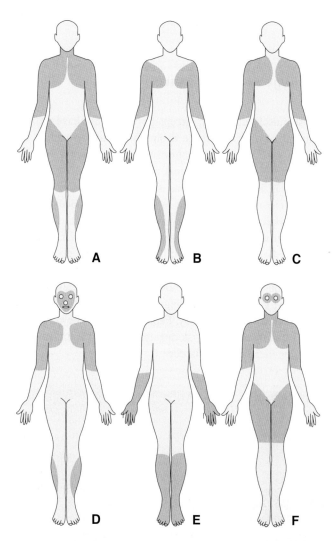

Fig. 16.9 General distribution of the muscle dystrophies (**a**) Duchenne and Becker. (**b**) Emery–Dreyfuss. (**c**) Limb-girdle. (**d**) Fascio-scapulo-humeral. (**e**) Distal. (**f**) Occulopharyngeal. *Shaded* = affected areas. After Emery AE [16]

Management

The child is best managed through a neuromuscular clinic offering care from a range of disciplines, typically paediatric neurology, orthopaedics, cardiology, respiratory medicine, physiotherapy, occupational and speech therapy, orthotic provision, and rehabilitation technology. The aims of management are summarized below (see also Chapter 3).

Physiotherapy and Occupational Therapy

The emphasis is upon mobility and independence. The child should be moved out of the seated position during the day and allowed to roll about and play on a mat. This may be more effective than passive stretching although every attempt should be made to counteract the remorseless development of contractures and the effects of gravity. Walking should be encouraged, but eventually proves impossible when the hip abductor and extensor muscles weaken to MRC grade III or less. Adaptive physiotherapy and wheelchair games seem to encourage respiratory exchange and avoid repetitive and tedious exercises. Standing frames are useful to give a child a different perception of the environment from that seen from a wheelchair and can also provide a passive stretch to joints of the lower limb. Swimming in a heated pool is ideal, as water allows the trunk and limbs to move as freely as possible and at the same time provides resistance to maintain muscle strength.

External supports should be used to maintain walking ability and transfer skills. When this is no longer possible, the child should be provided with a manual or powered wheelchair as appropriate.

Physiotherapy is also required for those children with respiratory impairment to maintain for as long as possible the child's ability to clear secretions and maintain an adequate tidal volume.

Aids to daily living and modification of the child's environment should include ground floor accommodation, bathroom alterations, and provision of a hoisting system. Powered wheelchairs that allow the patient to recline, sit up, and stand up are available. Electrically operated beds afford comfort when resting and sleeping. Electric toothbrushes and bath aids, alteration in shower cubicle entrances, and bidets that attach to toilet seats to obviate the need for laborious and often impossible paper cleansing have improved independence as well as eased the constant burden on the family and carers. Electronic environmental controls with sensitive pressure switches put the command of much of the household at the fingertips and can be used for communication devices. Patients with impaired breathing can be assisted by ventilatory systems powered from their wheelchair's batteries. Transport in adapted cars or vans has expanded the horizon of these children and increased the freedom of the family. Wheelchair-accessible residences, public buildings, streets, and pavements should provide freedom of movement and improved social contact.

Orthotics

Ankle–foot orthoses (AFOs) are useful in preventing equinus contracture, providing stability in stance and accommodating a foot or ankle deformity. AFOs are useful as long as the child has the hip muscle power to walk. Bracing at the knee, hip, and trunk is too cumbersome to permit efficient walking and knee–ankle–foot orthoses (KAFOs) and hip–knee–ankle–foot orthoses (HKAFOs) are not recommended. Orthoses do not prevent hip flexion contractures because the patient merely develops a greater compensatory lumbar lordosis. Hip flexion contractures greater than 45° lead to loss of standing ability.

Thoraco-lumbar-sacral orthoses (TLSOs) are ineffective in preventing the progression of a neuromuscular scoliosis and there may also be concerns that the orthosis will restrict chest wall expansion in a child who already suffers respiratory compromise. The Milwaukee brace, a cervical-thoracic-lumbar-sacral orthosis, is also contraindicated for the same reason and extensive bracing can interfere with comfortable sitting in a wheelchair. However, a TLSO may be used to stabilize the trunk to free the arms so the child can operate an electric wheelchair or eat, for example. The TLSO may also "hold" a scoliosis until the child is old enough to undergo spinal instrumentation and fusion [6]. Molded seating may be necessary to accommodate a scoliosis in those children for whom spinal surgery is contraindicated.

Cardiopulmonary Function

Cardiomyopathy occurs in muscle disorders, such as Becker muscular dystrophy (BMD) and in disorders of glycogen and lipid use. Screening and review by a paediatric cardiologist is desirable and also necessary before consideration of extensive surgery such as spinal stabilization and fusion.

Diaphragmatic and intercostal muscle weakness results in diminished respiratory function. It usually occurs insidiously and sleep apnea may be the first presenting sign; sleep studies are then required. As respiratory function deteriorates the child has difficulty in clearing secretions, which may also be compounded by a bulbar palsy resulting in an unsafe swallow and aspiration pneumonia.

Non-invasive mechanical ventilation can be considered in the later stages of deteriorating pulmonary function. Bi-level positive airway pressure may be helpful for sleep apnea. The decision to proceed to tracheostomy and formal ventilation is a difficult one in the face of incurable, progressive muscle disease and is a quandary for the child, parents, and carers.

Prevention of Infection and Nutrition

Children with impaired respiratory function are at risk of chest infection so an annual influenza vaccination and pneumococcus immunization are recommended. Adequate nutrition is required to ensure growth and short-term nasogastric feeding may be necessary in the acute stages of an infective illness to minimize catabolism. A bulbar palsy may necessitate percutaneous enteral feeding. For some children gastro-esophageal reflux is an associated problem that can be helped by endoscopic fundoplication. Surgery, if required, is best performed at an early stage because of the associated cardiopulmonary compromise.

Orthopaedic Surgery

Scoliosis occurs in 90% of the spinal muscular atrophies, DMD, and some of the myopathies. Fortunately, in the past 20 years the development of spinal instrumentation has allowed surgical correction before respiratory compromise becomes too great and the operative risk untenable. Transdiaphragmatic approaches to the spine for disc excision should be avoided in children with impaired cardiorespiratory function. The use of cell-saver devices and donor bone graft is widespread in these extensive spinal fusions. Although spinal fusion is generally successful in improving comfort for seating, patients and parents should be aware that the improved spinal alignment may impair the ability of the child to feed independently. When there is upper limb weakness, the loss of the ability to bring the mouth toward the hand when the spine was collapsed pre-operatively can be lost post-operatively.

Flexion contractures of the hip and knee and equinus and varus of the ankle and foot are common in neuromuscular disorders and are inevitable in the non-walking child whose limb alignment adapts to the shape of their wheelchair. Muscle and tendon lengthenings at the hip and knee in the non-walker are not generally effective. However, management of equinus of the ankle and varus of the foot are exceptions to this limited surgical perspective as equinovarus impairs proper foot contact with the child's immediate environment. This foot posture may produce areas of high contact pressure on the lateral border of the foot and/or toes, cause difficulty in shoe wear fitting and/or orthoses, and preclude a comfortable resting position of the foot on the footplate of a wheelchair for the non-walker.

Hip subluxation and dislocation occur frequently in the myopathies and may account for the failure to maintain reduction in some cases of presumed developmental dysplasia of the hip. The diagnosis of a myopathy should alert the surgeon and the family to a guarded prognosis and the likely development of contractures despite physiotherapy [7].

Spinal Muscular Atrophy

The incidence of SMA is approximately 1 in 15,000 to 1 in 20,000 live births [8]. All forms of SMA involve selective destruction of anterior horn cells and all patients have muscle weakness.

Classification and Clinical Features

SMA is a heterogeneous condition but for clinical purposes can be classified into three types according to the patient's age at the onset of the disease.

Type I—Acute Infantile (Werdnig–Hoffmann's) Disease

The onset of this form is from birth to 6 months and the infant presents with floppy limbs and trunk and paucity of limb movement. Affected infants appear alert and the facial muscles are initially spared. Weakness is progressive and infants experience swallowing and breathing difficulties. As the weakness progresses the upper and lower limbs may be positioned in the "pithed frog" posture with abduction and external rotation at the hips and shoulders. The mean survival is 6 months and 95% of affected infants are dead by 18 months. The use of long-term ventilation in severe SMA is controversial.

Type II—Chronic Infantile (Intermediate Group)

The chronic infantile form of spinal muscular atrophy has an onset from 6 months of age and usually manifests by the age of 2 years, after which it is slowly progressive. The infant usually attains head control and the majority of children achieve sitting balance but not independent walking. Life expectancy can extend into the third decade of life. Progressive scoliosis, limb contractures, and diminished vital capacity are the rule.

Type III—Chronic Proximal (Kugelberg–Welander)

Type III is usually diagnosed in later childhood between the ages of 2 and 15 years and commonly affects young adults. Their symptoms may be confused with DMD as the children often have an exaggerated lumbar lordosis, hip abductor and extensor weakness, and a positive Trendelenburg sign. Knee extensor weakness and hyperextension are also

seen. Walking deteriorates in late adolescence and most are wheelchair users in adult life although life expectancy is usually normal.

Further Investigations

Muscle biopsies reveal a typical neuropathic pattern and EMG shows characteristic fibrillation and fasciculation potentials.

The genetic locus for SMA has been identified on chromosome 5q [8]. In 96% of patients autosomal recessive SMA is caused by mutation of the survival motor neurone gene (SMN1). SMN1 can also be replaced by an almost identical gene, SMN2, also located on the same chromosome. Deletions within both copies of SMN1 result in Type 1 SMA (Werdnig–Hoffmann) and the milder forms of SMA result when SMN1 is replaced by SMN2 [9–12]. Boylan et al. [13] have described a rare form of SMA that is inherited in an autosomal dominant pattern.

Orthopaedic Management

Scoliosis in SMA develops early and invariably progresses to a severe degree. Posterior spinal fusion and instrumentation should be performed relatively early in the non-walker before the curve becomes too severe. Early post-operative management can be challenging because of respiratory compromise so anterior spinal surgery should be avoided. Spinal fusion in walkers may remove compensatory lumbar and pelvic movement and reduce their walking ability.

Contractures of the hip and knee are inevitable in the non-walker and there is no functional gain from surgical releases at the hip or knee as any improvement is difficult to maintain and recurrence of the deformities is the norm. Hip displacement is common in SMA and coxa valga is often seen radiologically. Attempts to relocate hips have not been very satisfactory and Zenios et al. [14] concluded that surgery for subluxation of the hip in SMA is not justified. Sporer and Smith [15] noted that a small number of patients had symptoms associated with dislocated hips and recommended observation rather than surgery in these patients.

Muscular Dystrophies

The general distribution of muscle weakness in the commoner dystrophies is shown in Fig. 16.9 [16].

Duchenne Type

The prevalence of this sex-linked, severe, and progressive dystrophy has been estimated at between 1.9 and 3.4 per 100,000 of the population. It is a disease almost entirely exclusive to males. Female carriers can be detected by an increased serum CK concentration in 70–75% of cases. Delay in motor milestones or clumsiness in a boy are the usual presentations of DMD.

Further Investigations

Dystrophin, the protein missing in DMD, is also expressed in the brain and occasionally the boys may first present with a delay in intellectual development, as their mean IQ is less than their peers [17]. Any boy not walking by 18 months, with global developmental delay, or with delayed speech development should have their serum CK level checked. The diagnosis is confirmed by genetic testing for the deletion in the Xp21 gene that encodes for dystrophin, which is absent in DMD, thus avoiding the need for muscle biopsy. Spontaneous mutations occur in approximately 30% of new cases of DMD.

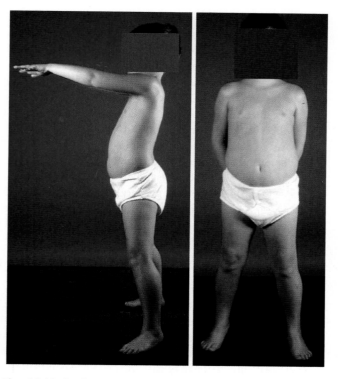

Fig. 16.10 Duchenne muscular dystrophy. Note the prominent abdomen and lumbar lordosis, calf pseudohypertrophy, and equinus at the ankles

Clinical Features

The earliest symptoms are clumsiness, impaired balance, and a tiptoe gait because of the muscle weakness (Fig. 16.10). Muscle hypotonia and pseudohypertrophy is usually seen and sometimes the boy first presents as a toe walker because of muscle weakness. Although present at birth, the disease does not normally manifest itself until the age of 3–4 years. Walking ceases at a median age of 10 years (range 7–11 years); fatal respiratory failure occurs between the ages of 19 and 21 years and occasionally up to 25 years. The intellect is affected, and approximately 30% of patients have an intelligence quotient (IQ) less than 75.

Orthopaedic Management

Obesity is common in the muscular dystrophies, probably as a result of immobility. The condition is incurable; attempts have been made to slow its rate of progress with steroid therapy, which has benefited some boys if used before the onset of weakness. However, the side effects of steroids such as weight gain, cataracts, and osteoporosis may outweigh the benefits. Although cardiac muscle is involved, symptomatic cardiomyopathy is unusual, unlike in BMD and Friedrich's ataxia. Survival is improving and advances in gene therapy may offer improved prospects for patients in the future.

Most boys with DMD develop scoliosis, typically a long C-shaped curve and associated pelvic obliquity. This is often associated with hyperlordosis due to hip flexion contractures. The pelvic obliquity may be associated with hip displacement [18]. The scoliosis deteriorates after cessation of walking and often causes difficulties in comfortable seating and skin pressure care where there is rib impingement against the iliac crest. It is generally considered that scoliosis should be treated surgically in DMD [19] although, to date, there are no randomized controlled clinical trials available to evaluate its effectiveness and thus no evidence-based recommendation can be made for clinical practice [20]. However, the clinical impression is that patients benefit from spinal surgery performed early, before the combination of a progressing deformity and deteriorating respiratory function becomes an unacceptable surgical risk. Surgery should be considered once the Cobb angle has reached 30° and before the forced vital capacity is less than 35% of age-matched normal values [21]. Pre-operative cardiac and pulmonary assessments are mandatory and the surgery should be carried out in a center where there is appropriate expertise. The surgery comprises posterior spinal fusion with instrumentation and segmental stabilization using either pedicle screw fixation or segmental sublaminar wiring, or a combination of both. Anterior surgical approaches that divide the diaphragm should be avoided because of impaired respiratory function. Fixation to the pelvis is recommended to provide a level pelvis for comfortable seating. Complications of spinal surgery in DMD are a concern; blood loss is generally higher than that for equivalent surgery in idiopathic scoliosis and Shapiro and Sethna [22] and Ramirez et al. [23]. have reported complication rates of 27%. Velasco et al. [24] showed that the rates of respiratory decline were 4% per year pre-surgery and decreased to 1.75% per year after posterior spinal fusion.

The extensive release of contractures to prolong walking beyond the usual age of 10 years (when it ceases in most boys who have DMD) must be very selective. Claims that boys of 14 or 15 years continue to walk after surgical treatment have to be questioned, because they may have had undiagnosed BMD. In addition, there is a variation in the age at which the ability to walk in DMD is lost so this is a confounding factor when considering the effect of surgery in prolonging the ability to walk. After surgery the period of walking is generally brief, as energy consumption is too great. Helping the patient achieve optimal function and independence in a powered wheelchair and with adaptations to other equipments is probably more appropriate in the longer term.

There is no indication to release hip and knee contractures in non-walkers with DMD. However, equino-varus deformities of the feet can be treated surgically when there is difficulty in the shoe fitting or pressure symptoms over the lateral border of the foot when it rests on the footplate of the wheelchair. This can be managed by lengthening of the tendo-Achilles and tibialis posterior. The equinus is not necessarily confined to the ankle and if a fixed plantaris deformity is present it requires bony surgery for correction. Usually this component of the equinus can be accepted and managed with an orthosis to avoid extensive surgery in a boy with respiratory compromise.

Although DMD affects the upper limbs they do not require surgical intervention.

Prognosis

Death from progressive respiratory failure usually occurs by the late teens to early twenties and once the vital capacity falls below 1 l the 5-year survival rate is only 8% [25]. Home ventilation has improved survival and Dreher et al. [26]. reported a median survival of 132 months after beginning mechanical home ventilation in 12 patients with DMD. Recent improvements in survival are probably due to better management of chest infections, correction of the scoliosis, and non-invasive ventilation. With advances in gene therapy it is possible that the life expectancy for boys with DMD will be further improved.

Benign X-Linked (Becker) Muscular Dystrophy

Clinical Signs

BMD is a sex-linked recessive muscle disease that differs from DMD by its later onset and relatively benign course. Only 10% of those affected cease to walk before the age of 40 years. Calf enlargement is the most frequent early sign of the disease and muscle cramps are more common than in the other dystrophies and myopathies. Leg pains and cramps are so prevalent in childhood that patients with BMD can be mistaken for having non-specific leg pains or cramp after exercise.

Diagnosis

Serum CK is high and a normal finding rules it out in boys who complain of persistent leg pains and cramps. Muscle dystrophin determination will differentiate BMD from DMD because dystrophin is present, albeit in smaller amounts than normal, in the former and absent in the latter. About 85% of males with BMD have an identifiable mutation in the DMD gene. Bushy, Thambyayah, and Gardner-Medwin [27] have shown that the prevalence rate of BMD is 2.38 per 100,000 compared to 2.48 per 100,000 for DMD. The cumulative birth incidence of BMD (at least 1 in 18,450 male live births) is about one-third that of DMD (1 in 5,618 male live births), suggesting that BMD is more common than previously thought.

Prognosis

Contractures are rare and do not occur until very late in the disease when the patient is already confined to a wheelchair. Life expectancy exceeds that of DMD (mean age of death 42 years, range 23–63 years) but patients are at risk of cardiomyopathy.

Emery–Dreifuss Muscular Dystrophy

Emery–Dreifuss muscular dystrophy (EDMD) was first described in 1966 [28] and its inheritance is usually X-linked but can also be autosomal dominant. The gene associated with EDMD is located in the distal Xq28 region of the X chromosome [29] and encodes for a nuclear membrane protein, emerin [30, 31]. Recent studies have shown that alterations in lamins, the principal component of the nuclear lamina, have been found in a phenotype resembling EDMD

[32], which may account for the cardiac conduction system disease seen in EDMD.

Clinical Signs

EDMD is characterized by a triad of features: (1) early contractures of the Achilles tendons, elbows, and post-cervical muscles; (2) slowly progressive muscle wasting and weakness with a predominantly humero-peroneal distribution in the early stages; and (3) cardiomyopathy with conduction defects and risk of sudden death [28, 29]. The initial presentation of EDMD is a non-specific muscle weakness in the first few years of life, with an awkward gait and, possibly, toe-walking. The dystrophy becomes fully developed in the second decade of life and, most importantly, these patients have bradycardia and eventually develop complete heart block which may be silent.

The serum CK concentration is only slightly to moderately elevated and levels are not as high as those seen in DMD or BMD. If the latter have been ruled out by dystrophin estimation the diagnosis of EDMD should be considered.

Prognosis

Muscle weakness is progressive but slow, so that walking is generally possible until the fifth or sixth decades of life. The ankle equinus can become severe. Elbow contractures appear as early as 7 years, whereas limited flexion of the neck caused by the extension contracture may be evident at 5 years and is clearly present by the twenties. The importance of defining this type of muscular dystrophy is the need for a cardiac assessment. Bradycardia and a first-degree atrio-ventricular heart block can result in sudden death between the ages of 25 and 60 years [33].

Orthopaedic Management

Lengthening of the Achilles tendon may be indicated for severe equinus. If varus of the foot is present, lengthening or transfer of the posterior tibial tendon may be indicated. Elbow flexion contracture, even if it is 90°, rarely limits function; consequently, no treatment is necessary as further flexion, pronation, and supination are usually preserved. If scoliosis develops, it generally stabilizes at an acceptable 40° after spinal growth has ceased, so that surgery is probably not indicated. The cervical extension contracture limits neck flexion and later there may be a restriction of lateral rotation as well.

Limb-Girdle Muscular Dystrophies

Limb-girdle muscular dystrophy (LGMD) is a descriptive term for a spectrum of inherited muscle disorders that have a fairly similar phenotype [34]. They are characterized by progressive muscle wasting and weakness of variable distribution and severity [16, 35]. These are distinct from DMD and BMD and the commoner types have an autosomal recessive inheritance but the spectrum also includes rare subtypes that have an autosomal dominant inheritance pattern. The molecular genetics of this spectrum of disorders is complex and numerous abnormalities have been identified but are beyond the scope of this chapter.

Clinical Signs

Two broad patterns are seen; those that affect the upper limbs in adolescence (scapulo-humeral type) and those that affect the lower limbs (limb-girdle type), without facial weakness, after the age of 20 years. In more severe cases, the distal muscles of the limbs are also affected. The presence of facial weakness changes the term to fascio-scapulo-humeral (FSH) muscular dystrophy. The hallmark of the scapulo-humeral type of LGMD is winging of the scapula (Fig. 16.11). Although the biceps and triceps are affected the deltoid seems to be preserved. Foot drop as a result of anterior tibial muscle weakness occurs in the FSH type, but is rare in the scapulo-humeral form. Contractures of muscles and joints are not a prominent feature.

An infantile form of FSH muscular dystrophy has been identified. It is more severe than the adult form and is inherited as an autosomal recessive. Facial diplegia and sensorineural hearing loss are usually diagnosed by the age of 5 years. Scapular winging is present but the most striking deformity is a marked lumbar lordosis, upon which

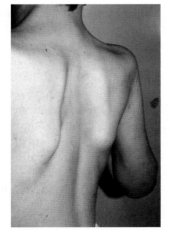

Fig. 16.11 Winging of the scapula in scapulo-humeral dystrophy. Courtesy of Dr P. Eunson

the patient depends to maintain balance. Walking ability is usually lost after the age of 20 years [33].

Diagnosis

The CK concentration is very high in the LGMDs and EMG confirms a general myopathy. A normal dystrophin assay will distinguish LGMD from DMD and BMD.

Orthopaedic Management

General measures include weight control, exercise to maintain mobility, and the prevention of contractures. Specifically, scapulothoracic fusion may be indicated for intractable pain, loss of range of shoulder movement, and scapular instability during upper limb tasks. Berne et al. [36] found that abduction increased by 25° and flexion increased 29° at a nearly 10-year average follow-up after scapulothoracic fusion in patients with FSH muscular dystrophy. However, Krishnan et al. [37] have reported complications in more than half of their 22 patients after scapulothoracic fusion.

Scoliosis rarely requires spinal fusion because the onset of the disease is later than that of DMD. Severe lordosis is more common than scoliosis and there may be no useful solution other than recommending a wheelchair if it causes intractable back pain. Attempts to correct the lordosis by spinal fusion will remove the ability to balance so that standing and walking will become impossible.

A leaf spring AFO may be useful in controlling a foot drop provided there is no fixed deformity at the ankle and it remains mobile.

Congenital Muscular Dystrophy

The congenital muscular dystrophies (CMDs) are a group of disorders almost all of which are inherited in an autosomal recessive manner. There are syndromic and non-syndromic types of CMD and in the former structural abnormalities of the brain are seen on an MRI scan. The infants are floppy at birth and may also have joint contractures. The serum CK is usually elevated and muscle biopsy shows a dystrophic or myopathic pattern. In contrast to DMD and BMD, no involvement of the dystrophin gene is found.

Merosin deficiency of the basement membrane has been shown to cause CMD linked to chromosome 6q2 and merosin CMD is prevalent in European populations. In Japan mutation of the fukutin gene has been identified in the majority of cases of Fukuyama CMD [38].

Muscle Myopathies

The myopathies are characterized by hypotonia at birth (the floppy infant) and by delay in motor development. In childhood and adolescence, joint contractures, foot deformities, and scoliosis are common as the disease progresses. The varieties of myopathy can be diagnosed only by muscle biopsy and histological studies. Serum enzymes are within normal limits, and EMG shows only the non-specific electrical activity of myopathies in general.

Central Core Disease

This has a wide spectrum of clinical presentation and is usually inherited as an autosomal dominant condition although autosomal recessive cases are also seen. In milder cases most children achieve independent walking and their life expectancy is usually normal. In severe cases children present with profound hypotonia, scoliosis, and hip dislocation, succumbing to respiratory failure early in life. This disorder may cause unexpected outcomes in children who are being treated for presumed developmental dysplasia of the hip as redislocation occurs in more than 50% of cases. Recurrent dislocation of the patella is resistant to surgical correction and pes planus is very common. Scoliosis can be managed with instrumentation and fusion.

The diagnosis is made on muscle biopsy where typical cores are seen and most cases are associated with a mutation in RYR1 that codes for ryanodine receptor 1. Surgeons and anesthetists should be aware that patients who have central core myopathy are prone to malignant hyperthermia [39].

Nemaline Myopathy

This is a rare disorder that can be inherited either in an autosomal dominant or recessive manner (Fig. 16.12). There is a wide spectrum of clinical presentation. Hypotonia is associated with unusually slender, but reportedly surprisingly strong, muscles. The distribution of weakness is seen mainly in the face, flexors of the neck, and proximal limbs. Facial weakness and nasal speech are the results of palatal muscle weakness. Scoliosis, hypermobility, and foot deformities are common but disability from muscle weakness is only moderate. Feeding difficulties and respiratory failure as a result of diaphragmatic involvement are seen. The diagnosis is made on muscle biopsy where nemaline rods are seen in the sarcoplasm of skeletal muscle fibers. No definitive correlation

Fig. 16.12 Nemaline myopathy. Courtesy of Dr P. Eunson

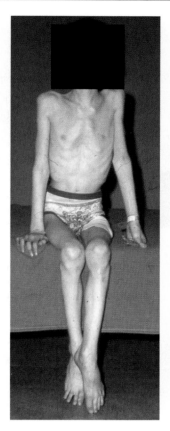

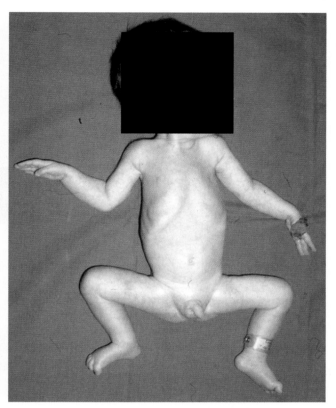

Fig. 16.13 Myotubular myopathy. Courtesy of Dr P. Eunson

has been found between the number of rods and severity or age of onset of the myopathy [40].

X-linked Myotubular Myopathy, Congenital Fiber-Type Disproportion, Multiminicore Disease, and Mitochondrial Disease

Congenital fiber-type disproportion is a genetically heterogeneous condition and mitochondrial diseases are a clinically heterogeneous group of disorders that arise as a result of dysfunction of the mitochondrial respiratory chain [41]. Multiminicore disease is inherited in an autosomal recessive manner and X-linked myotubular myopathy (Fig. 16.13) is associated with a mutation in MTM1. These myopathies have no distinctive clinical features other than hypotonia, muscle weakness, contractures, and scoliosis.

Myotonias

Clinical Signs

Myotonia is muscle contraction that persists after the voluntary effort has ended. The muscle relaxes slowly, so that a handshake, for example, gives the sensation of a lingering grip.

Diagnosis

Diagnosis is confirmed by the EMG pattern, which depicts the initial contraction of the muscle with a gradual trailing-off in activity (Fig. 16.14).

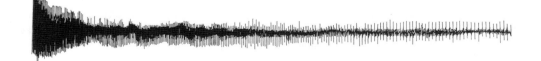

Fig. 16.14 Electromyograph showing classic myotonic discharge pattern on voluntary muscle contraction

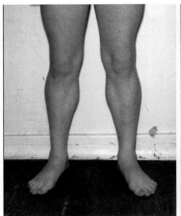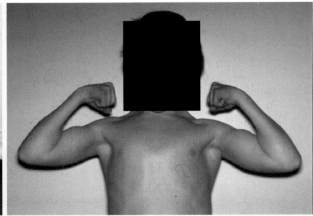

Fig. 16.15 Myotonia congenita.
Courtesy of Dr P. Eunson

Myotonia Congenita

Myotonia congenita usually affects infants. The symptoms of stiffness are made worse by rest and cold but are relieved by exercise. The patients are strong and have well-developed muscles (Fig. 16.15). Surgeons and anesthetists should be aware that these children are prone to malignant hyperthermia and depolarizing muscle relaxants should be avoided. Myotonia congenita is inherited both in an autosomal recessive manner (Becker disease) and in an autosomal dominant manner (Thomsen disease). The diagnosis is made on clinical examination, EMG (which shows myotonic bursts of activity), and a family history. A mutation of CLCN1 is associated with myotonia congenita [42].

Myotonic Dystrophy

Two forms are recognized: type 1, also known as Steinert disease, and type 2 or proximal myotonic myopathy. Both have autosomal dominant inheritance patterns. Rare, as muscle diseases are, type 1 has an incidence of 4.9–5.5 per 100,000 of the population. The genetic defect in type 1 is a mutation in chromosome 19 and in type 2 in chromosome 3 in some patients. There is a spectrum of phenotypes in type 1 from mild to severe and type 2 generally affects adults.

Congenital Myotonic Dystrophy

Infants with congenital myotonic dystrophy have severe hypotonia at birth, facial diplegia, a long narrow face, mental retardation, and a high incidence of severe clubfoot. Characteristically, they experience difficulty in breathing and feeding. All affected children present with delays in speech and motor development, but eventually walk. The clinical signs are fully developed by the time the child is aged 10 years, and some develop scoliosis in adolescence.

Polymyositis–Dermatomyositis

Polymyositis and dermatomyositis do occur in children and represent a spectrum of autoimmune disease [43]. Dermatomyositis is the most frequent inflammatory myopathy in children but polymyositis is rare. In dermatomyositis, a butterfly-shaped rash on the anterior neck and upper chest, hyperemia at the base of the fingernails, and shiny red skin at the pulps of the fingers are important clues to diagnosis. In late cases, radiographs of the limb may show tiny flecks and plaques of calcification in the muscles and under the skin. Polymyositis should be considered in children presenting with unexplained gradual muscle weakness and difficulty in elevating the arms or climbing stairs. It is important to exclude a muscle dystrophy and the diagnosis of polymyositis is one of the exclusion. Serum CK is markedly raised in polymyositis and may be elevated in dermatomyositis. EMG shows myopathic changes and MRI may show increased signal in affected muscles but is non-specific. Muscle biopsy will show degeneration, regeneration, and infiltration with inflammatory cells. The child should be referred to a paediatric rheumatologist.

Myasthenia Gravis

The characteristic presenting feature of myasthenia gravis is painless, fatigable weakness either developing or becoming more evident with exertion [44]. The condition is very rare in children and forms a heterogeneous group of diseases that are caused by an abnormality of neuromuscular transmission. This may be considered as pre-synaptic (e.g., an abnormality of choline acetyltransferase), synaptic, or post-synaptic (e.g., an abnormality of the acetylcholine receptor) [45]. In congenital myasthenia the infant may present with a bulbar palsy and respiratory distress.

In later life symptoms are generally insidious in onset and often variable. The patient may initially experience ptosis and diplopia from involvement of the facial muscles and then pharyngeal muscle weakness causes difficulties with speech and swallowing. The symptoms may progress to include general muscular weakness or the patient may present with respiratory arrest. The importance to surgeons and anesthetists is that myasthenic patients are sensitive to non-depolarizing muscle relaxants.

Acknowledgments We thank Dr Paul Eunson, consultant paediatric neurologist, Royal Hospital for Sick Children Edinburgh, for his helpful suggestions in the preparation of this chapter and for providing many of the clinical illustrations, and Dr Colin Smith, senior lecturer in pathology, University of Edinburgh, for providing the histological illustrations.

References

1. Read L, Galasko CSB. Delay in diagnosing Duchenne muscular dystrophy in orthopaedic clinics. J Bone Joint Surg Br 1986; 68:481–482.
2. Gowda V, Parr J, Jayawant S. Evaluation of the floppy infant. Paediatr Child Health 2008; 18:17–21.
3. André T, Chesni Y, St Anne-Dargassies A. The neurological examination of the infant. Little Club Clinics in Developmental Medicine No 1. Spastics Society 1960.
4. Dubowitz V. The Floppy Infant, 2nd ed. Clinics In Developmental Medicine. Mac Keith Press, London; 1980.
5. Gardner-Medwin D, Hudgson P, Walton JN. Benign spinal muscular atrophy arising in childhood and adolescence. J Neurol Sci 1967; 5:121–158.
6. Evans GA, Drennan J, Russman BS. Functional classification and orthopaedic management of spinal muscular atrophy. J Bone Joint Surg Br 1981; 63B:516–522.
7. Gamble JG, Rinsky LA, Lee JH. Orthopaedic aspects of central core disease. J Bone Joint Surg Am 1988; 70: 1061–1066.
8. Brzustowicz LM, Lehner T, Castilla LH, et al. Genetic mapping of chronic childhood-onset spinal muscular atrophy to chromosome 5q11.2–13.3. Nature 1990; 344:540–541.
9. Lefebvre S, Burglen L, Reboullet S, et al. Identification and characterization of a spinal muscular atrophy-determining gene. Cell 1995; 80:155–165.
10. Swoboda KJ, Prior TW, Scott CB, et al. Natural history of denervation in SMA: relation to age, SMN2 copy number, and function. Ann Neurol 2005; 57:704–712.
11. Yamashita M, Nishio H, Harada Y, et al. Significant increase in the number of the SMN2 gene copies in an adult-onset type III spinal muscular atrophy patient with homozygous deletion of the NAIP gene. Eur Neurol 2004; 52:101–106.
12. Sumner CJ. Molecular mechanisms of spinal muscular atrophy. J Child Neurol 2007; 22:979–989.
13. Boylan KB, Cornblath DR, Glass JD, et al. Autosomal dominant distal spinal muscular atrophy in four generations. Neurology 1995; 45:699–704.
14. Zenios M, Sampath J, Cole C, et al. Operative treatment for hip subluxation in spinal muscular atrophy. J Bone Joint Surg Br 2005; 87B:1541–1544.
15. Sporer SM, Smith BG. Hip dislocation in patients with spinal muscular atrophy. J Pediatr Orthop 2003; 23:10–14.
16. Emery AE. The muscle dystrophies. Lancet 2002; 359(9307): 687–695.
17. Zwelleger H, Hanson JW. Psychometric studies in muscular dystrophy type IIIa (Duchenne). Dev Med Child Neurol 1967; 9:576–581.
18. Chan KG, Galasko CSB, Delaney C. Hip subluxation and dislocation in Duchenne muscular dystrophy. J Pediatr Orthop Br 2001; 10:219–225.
19. Kinali M, Messina S, Mercuri E, et al. Management of scoliosis in Duchenne muscular dystrophy: a large 10-year retrospective study. Dev Med Child Neurol 2006; 48:513–518.
20. Cheuk DK, Wong V, Wraige E, et al. Surgery for scoliosis in Duchenne muscular dystrophy. Cochrane Database Syst Rev 2007; Jan 24(1):CD005375.
21. Miller RG, Chalmers AC, Dao H, et al. The effect of spine fusion on respiratory function in Duchenne muscular dystrophy. Neurology 1991; 41:38–40.
22. Shapiro F, Sethna N. Blood loss in pediatric spine surgery. Eur Spine J 2004; 13 Suppl 1:S6–S17.
23. Ramirez N, Richards BS, Warren PD, Williams GR. Complications after posterior spinal fusion in Duchenne's muscular dystrophy. J Pediatr Orthop 1997; 17:109–114.
24. Velasco MV, Colin AA, Zurakowski D, et al. Posterior spinal fusion for scoliosis in Duchenne muscular dystrophy diminishes the rate of respiratory decline. Spine 2007; 32:459–465.
25. Phillips MF, Quinlivan RC, Edwards RH, Calverley PM. Changes in spirometry over time as a prognostic marker in patients with Duchenne muscular dystrophy. Am J Respir Crit Care Med 2001; 164:2191–2194.
26. Dreher M, Rauter I, Storre JH, et al. When should home mechanical ventilation be started in patients with different neuromuscular disorders? Respirology 2007; 12:749–753.
27. Bushby KM, Thambyayah M, Gardner-Medwin D. Prevalence and incidence of Becker muscular dystrophy. Lancet 1991; 337:1022–1024.
28. Emery AE, Dreifuss FE. Unusual type of benign x-linked muscular dystrophy. J Neurol Neurosurg Psychiatr 1966; 29:338–342.
29. Yates JR, Warner JP, Smith JA, et al. Emery-Dreifuss muscular dystrophy: linkage to markers in distal Xq28. J Med Genet 1993; 30:108–111.
30. Manilal S, Nguyen TM, Sewry CA, Morris GE. The Emery-Dreifuss muscular dystrophy protein. Hum Mol Genet 1996; 5:801–808.
31. Ura S, Hayashi YK, Goto K, et al. Limb-girdle muscular dystrophy due to emerin gene mutations. Arch Neurol 2007; 64:1038–1041.
32. Maioli MA, Marrosu G, Mateddu A, et al. A novel mutation in the central rod domain of lamin A/C producing a phenotype resembling the Emery-Dreifuss muscular dystrophy phenotype. Muscle Nerve 2007; 36:828–832.
33. Shapiro F, Specht L. Current Concepts Review. The diagnosis and orthopaedic treatment of inherited muscular diseases of childhood. J Bone Joint Surg Am 1993; 75A:439–454.
34. Mathews KD, Moore SA. Limb-girdle muscular dystrophy. Curr Neurol Neurosci Rep 2003; 3:78–85.
35. Emery AEH. Fortnightly review: The muscular dystrophies. Br Med J 1998; 317:991–995.
36. Berne D, Laude F, Laporte C, et al. Scapulothoracic arthrodesis in facioscapulohumeral muscular dystrophy. Clin Orth Rel Res 2003; 409:106–113.

37. Krishnan SG, Hawkins RJ, Michelotti JD, et al. Scapulothoracic arthrodesis: indications, technique, and results. Clin Orthop Rel Res 2005; 435:126–133.

38. Tomé FM. The Peter Emil Becker Award lecture 1998. The saga of congenital muscular dystrophy. Neuropediatrics 1999; 30:55–65.

39. Treves S, Jungbluth H, Muntoni F, Zorzato F. Congenital muscle disorders with cores: the ryanodine receptor calcium channel paradigm. Curr Opin Pharmacol 2008; 8(3):319–326.

40. Ryan MM, Ilkovski B, Strickland CD, et al. Clinical course correlates poorly with muscle pathology in nemaline myopathy. Neurology 2003; 60:665–673.

41. Wallace DC. Mitochondrial diseases in man and mouse. Science 1999; 283:1482–1488.

42. Colding-Jørgensen E. Phenotypic variability in myotonia congenital. Muscle Nerve 2005; 32:19–34.

43. Ramanan AV, Feldman BM. Clinical features of juvenile dermatomyositis and other childhood onset myositis syndromes. Rheum Dis Clin N Am 2002; 28:833–857.

44. Vincent A, Palace J, Hilton-Jones D. Myasthenia gravis. Lancet 2001; 357:2122–2128.

45. Hantai D, Richard P, Koenig J, Eymard B. Congenital myasthenic syndromes. Curr Opin Neurol 2004; 17:539–551.

Chapter 17

Neural Tube Defects, Spina Bifida, and Spinal Dysraphism

H. Kerr Graham and Klaus Parsch

Introduction

Neural tube defects are a varied group of congenital spinal anomalies associated with abnormal closure of the neural tube. Anencephaly represents the most severe abnormality that may occur at the cranial end of the tube.

Spina bifida is the general term used to describe conditions caused by disturbance of the development of the vertebral arches. They are often associated with abnormalities of the structures derived from the neural tube and the meninges and may be associated with cyst formation.

Spinal dysraphism refers to a number of hidden abnormalities affecting the spinal cord or cauda equina which may produce occult or overt neurological disturbance. The diversity of these conditions suggests that causative factors exert their effects at different periods of fetal development.

The absence of the posterior elements of spine allows for the extrusion of the meninges (meningocele) and the spinal cord elements (myelomeningocele). Lesions in the cervical spine tend to be meningoceles and are often associated with other defects like the Arnold–Chiari malformation.

Myelomeningocele

The exposed cord and neurons seem to function early in gestation but are progressively destroyed (Fig. 17.1). This has prompted the development of intrauterine surgery to close the defect in an attempt to limit neurological deterioration. Some early results are encouraging. Myelomeningocele remains the form of neural tube defect which most commonly leads to spinal deformity with significant motor and sensory deficit in the lower limbs.

H.K. Graham (✉)
Department of Orthopaedics, The Royal Children's Hospital, Parkville, Victoria, Australia

In addition to the major spinal defect, other lesions are frequently present—the Arnold–Chiari malformation (cerebellum and brainstem displaced distally and compressed at the foramen magnum), cerebellar hypoplasia, hydrocephalus, hydromyelia, syringomyelia, and diastematomyelia. Many patients also have upper limb problems due to a variety of subtle neurological lesions which may prove progressive. Children with myelomeningocele generally have paralysis of the bladder, bowel incontinence, and a propensity to trophic ulceration in areas of insensate skin. Approximately 80% of affected children will develop hydrocephalus and as a group these children score 10–15 points below average on standardized intelligence tests. Neuropsychological testing reveals a consistent profile of learning difficulties and short-term memory problems, as well as deficits in visuospatial, perceptual, numerical, and executive skills.

Spina Bifida

Incidence

The incidence of spina bifida varies with the geographical area and ethnicity. There are also seasonal variations. During the past 20 years there has been a dramatic decrease in the number of births of children with spina bifida in developed countries and a less dramatic fall in the incidence of pregnancies with spina bifida. Peri-conceptual vitamin supplementation, maternal alpha-fetoprotein testing, routine antenatal ultrasound, and termination of affected pregnancies are some of the factors which have brought about this change.

The highest incidence in the world was reported in Ireland, Wales, and the north of England (up to 5 per 1000 live births), although this has now dropped precipitously. A high incidence has been reported in certain regions of China. In North America and Australia the incidence is less than 1 per 1000 live births.

M. Benson et al. (eds.), *Children's Orthopaedics and Fractures*,
DOI 10.1007/978-1-84882-611-3_17, © Springer-Verlag London Limited 2010

Fig. 17.1 (**a**) A newborn child with an open spina bifida lesion and dressing in situ. Evidence of congenital deformities and muscle imbalance can be seen and much gained by careful neonatal examination. (**b**) The sites of neurological involvement include hydrocephalus, the Chiari 2 malformation, syringomyelia, and the tethered cord. While the problems of hydrocephalus are generally seen neonatally, neurological deterioration secondary to the Chiari 2 malformation, syringomyelia, and cord tethering often present insidiously in later childhood

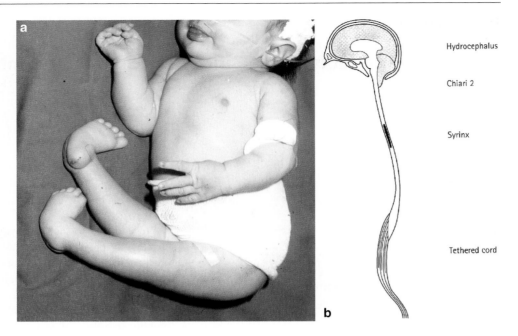

Etiology

This is thought to be multifactorial and both genetic and environmental factors have been implicated. It is believed that the spectrum of neural tube defects results from similar causes acting at slightly different times during embryogenesis.

Genetic Predisposition

Neural tube defects have been shown to follow a multifactorial pattern of inheritance. A number of genes are thought to have a small additive effect which may combine with environmental factors. When this compound effect passes a critical threshold the child is liable to be born with a neural tube defect. There is also an association with chromosomal disorders (trisomy 13, trisomy 18, triploidy, unbalanced translocations, and microdeletion of 22q11) as well as rare dominant and recessive disorders. Recently, substances that interfere with the GABA receptors have been implicated. The birth of a child with spina bifida predisposes to subsequent children being born with anencephaly, with extensive congenital vertebral abnormalities or with spinal dysraphism.

Diet and Drugs

The environmental factors which have been suggested as a cause of neural tube defects include folate deficiency, other vitamin deficiencies, absence of selenium from the regional soil and hence from the diet, poor maternal nutrition, a high maternal alcohol intake, maternal diabetes mellitus, fever at a critical stage of pregnancy, and a wide variety of other factors [1]. Drugs associated with an increased incidence of neural tube defects include anti-epileptic agents such as sodium valproate and carbamazepine, isotretinoin (for the treatment of acne), etretinate (for the treatment of psoriasis), thalidomide, and methotrexate.

Embryology and Pathology

Spina bifida may be subdivided into spina bifida cystica, when a cyst forms, and spina bifida occulta, when the defect is completely or largely hidden from the examining eye. The various forms of spina bifida are illustrated in Fig. 17.2.

Spina Bifida Cystica

This can occur in the following forms:

Myeloschisis or myelocele (Fig. 17.2a). The vertebral arches are deficient and neural plate material is spread out on the surface, sometimes in a shallow depression, more commonly over a cystic swelling of the meninges.

Myelomeningocele (Fig. 17.2b). There is a fluid-filled cystic swelling, lined by dura and arachnoid, protruding through a defect in the vertebral arches under the skin. The spinal cord and nerve roots are carried out into the fundus of the sac.

Meningocele (Fig. 17.2c). There is a cystic swelling of dura and arachnoid, protruding through a defect in the vertebral arches under the skin. The spinal cord is entirely confined within the vertebral arches but may exhibit abnormalities.

Fig. 17.2 Schematic diagrams of the major types of spina bifida. (**a**) Myeloschisis; (**b**) myelomeningocele; (**c**) meningocele; and (**d**) spina bifida occulta

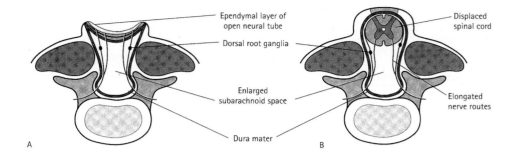

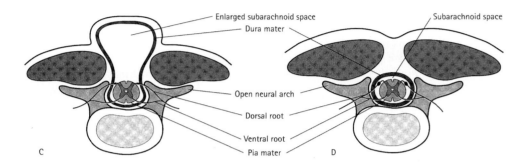

Spina Bifida Occulta

In this form (Fig. 17.2d), there is a localized defect in one or more of the vertebral arches, because the respective halves of the vertebral arches fail to meet and fuse in the third month of intrauterine life. The spinal cord and meninges remain within the vertebral canal. The skin overlying the spina bifida occulta may be normal or there may be a dimple which may be connected with the dura by a fibrous cord, a patch of hair, pigmentation, or a lipoma (possibly continuous with a similar intradural lipoma). All these and the rare intramedullary dermoid probably represent abnormalities of separation of presumptive skin from neural tissue, as both are ectodermal in origin, during the process of closure of the neural tube. These conditions will be considered under the heading "spinal dysraphism."

Causes of Deformity

Muscle Imbalance Due to Lower Motor Neurone Lesions

Muscle imbalance has been traditionally regarded as the major cause of deformity in patients with spina bifida. However, it is only one of many causes and may be less important than suggested by some earlier studies. The imbalance is due in large part to the defects in the nerve roots and spinal cord already present at birth. However, further neurological injury, associated with a change in neurosegmental level, may be produced by prenatal traction on the abnormally tethered cord, direct pressure and longitudinal shearing forces during delivery, and postnatal drying and infection of the neural plate [1]. There is some correlation between the lowest functioning neurosegmental level, the muscles acting, and the limb posture (Table 17.1). This correlation is most obvious at the foot and ankle but less so at the hip. Patients in whom L5 is spared almost invariably have a calcaneus deformity of the foot because of activity in the tibialis anterior, the peroneus tertius, and the extensor digitorum longus, and no activity in the soleus or gastrocnemius. Such muscle imbalance ultimately leads to fixed deformity.

More recent studies raise some doubt about the influence of muscle imbalance, especially on hip deformity. Flexion contracture at the hip is most severe and progressive in those patients with thoracic level lesions with no motor function at the hip [2]. In these children postural factors related to greatly reduced physical activity are probably the most important factor. There was, furthermore, no evidence of spasticity in the patients with the most severe flexion contractures at the hip. Further studies [3,4] raise additional doubts about the place of muscle imbalance as the most significant cause of deformity in spina bifida.

Muscle Imbalance Due to an Upper Motor Neurone Lesion

Two-thirds of infants with myelomeningocele have an additional upper motor neurone lesion. There is an interruption of long spinal tracts with preservation of reflex activity in isolated distal segments. Reflex activity can often be mistaken

Table 17.1 Effect of the neurosegmental level of the lesion on muscle activity and limb posture

Lowest neurosegmental level functioning	Muscle acting	Limb posture
T 12		Dictated by gravity
L 1	Sartorius	Flexion/external rotation
	Iliopsoas weak	(frog position)
L 2	As above plus	
	Iliopsoas strong	Flexion and adduction at hip
	Pectineus	
	Gracilis	
	Hip adductors	
	Rectus femoris	Hip flexed and adducted
L 3	As above plus	Hip flexed and adducted
	Quadriceps	Knee extended
L 4	As above plus	Hip flexed and adducted
	Tibialis anterior (post)	Knee extended
	Medial hamstrings weak	Foot in varus
L 5	As above plus	Hip flexion
	Tensor fasciae latae	Knee in some flexion
	Gluteus medius/minim.	Foot in calcaneus
	Peroneus tertius	
	Extensor digitorum long.	
S 1	As above plus	Hip in some flexion
	Gluteus maximus	Knee in some flexion
	Biceps femoris	
	Gastrocnemius	Flattening of the sole
	Soleus	Clawing of toes
	Flexor digitorum longus	
	Flexor digitorum brevis	
	Flexor hallucis longus	
	Flexor hallucis brevis	
Lower lumbar level	With spasticity in hamstrings	Knee flexion deformity
Spastic sacral segment	With spasticity calf peronei	Foot equines
		Foot vertical talus

by parents and clinicians as useful voluntary movement. Three subtypes can be recognized.

In the first, cord function is intact down to a certain level where there is flaccid paralysis with loss of sensation and reflexes; more distally there is isolated cord function as evident from exaggerated reflex activity.

In the second the "gap" in cord function is narrow, amounting virtually to a cord transection. There is no movement of the lower limbs when the infant is crying, but a wealth of purely reflex activity (including flexion withdrawal) can be elicited by direct stimulation.

In the third subtype transection of the long tracts is incomplete and the child will have a spastic paraplegia with preservation of some voluntary movement and sensation.

Thus the muscle imbalance producing deformity in spina bifida may be of three types:

1. Normal muscle versus flaccid antagonist
2. Spastic muscle versus normal antagonist
3. Spastic muscle versus flaccid antagonist.

The last type produces the worst deformity.

There is evidence that important upper motor neurone lesions occur around the time of birth. Deformities due to spasticity are therefore not present at birth but develop in the early months of life (Fig. 17.3).

Intrauterine Posture

Sometimes deformity is present at birth in totally paralyzed lower limbs. In some of these patients the deformity may be fixed, which suggests that muscle power and imbalance have been present in fetal life. In others, the pattern of deformity suggests that it has resulted simply from pressure on paralyzed limbs.

Habitually Assumed Posture After Birth

Deformity can develop after birth in flaccid legs that are allowed to lie in one particular posture, under the influence of gravity. For example, the classic "diamond posture" or "pithed frog position" of hip flexion, abduction and external rotation in combination with knee flexion, and equinus or equinovarus at the ankle and foot.

Coexistent Congenital Malformations

Arthrogryposis

Some limb deformities resemble those seen in arthrogryposis multiplex congenita. There is rigidity and lack of normal flexion creases thought to be associated with lack of movement in utero. Such deformities are very resistant to treatment.

Traction of Nerve Roots

Some children, who have had a myelomeningocele closed at birth, may present later with progressive foot deformity (usually cavo-varus). This may be associated with spinal cord tethering which should be surgically released before correcting the foot deformity. As a result, any foot deformity which develops for the first time in the growing child should prompt a careful search for spinal cord pathology including the various manifestations of spinal dysraphism.

Fig. 17.3 The neurological lesion in spina bifida is usually asymmetrical rather than symmetrical. (**a**) The 7-year-old girl shows flexion and abduction on the left leg, adduction in the right hip. There is also spasticity in the left leg. The function of the left arm is impaired. (**b**) After correction of the flexion deformity the girl is able to stand in a hip/knee/ankle/foot orthosis

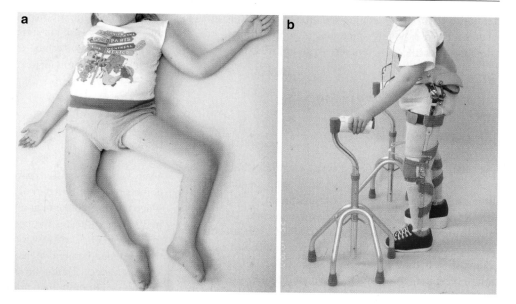

Special Risks

Pressure Sores and Chilblains

These are the result of skin insensitivity and poor circulation. If serial plasters are needed to correct deformity they should be very carefully padded because deficient pain sensation fails to warn the surgeon of pressure on the skin. In most instances, plaster casts should be used only to *maintain* the soft tissue surgical correction of deformity, not to *achieve* correction. Hip spicas should include paralyzed feet. Varus feet are always unacceptable and pressure sores inevitable. Parents should also be warned to protect their children from extremes of temperature.

Bone Fragility

Pathological fractures occur in approximately 20% of patients with paralysis in the lower limbs. Epiphyseal displacements and hyperplastic callus formation are common. Osteopenia, because of reduced muscle bulk and physical activity, is the most obvious reason for bone fragility.

Pathological fractures in patients with spina bifida are commonly mistaken for bone or joint infection (Fig. 17.4). The patient may present with a painless, red, hot, and swollen limb without a history of trauma. Radiographs will often disclose a fracture which has occurred days or weeks previously. In the later stages, if there is a delay in diagnosis and immobilization of a fracture, the florid callus may be misdiagnosed as a primary bone tumor.

The principle of treatment of pathological fractures is that immobilization of the child and the fractured limb should be kept to the minimum compatible with union in a satisfactory

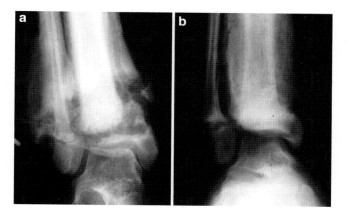

Fig. 17.4 (**a**) Pathological epiphyseal loosening of the distal tibia and fibula and exuberant callus formation in a 10-year-old girl, who did a lot of walking on her completely paralyzed feet. (**b**) After a year most of the changes have disappeared, an early closure of the growth plate must be expected

position. Well-padded hip spica casts applied with extended knees may permit early weight bearing in a standing frame, thus reducing the risk of osteopenia postoperatively [5,6]. Fractures in patients who are unable to walk can usually be adequately treated by simple closed methods avoiding invasive surgery.

Other Risks

Deficient peripheral blood flow, recurrent urinary tract infections, cognitive impairment, obesity, constipation, and respiratory problems all increase the rate of complications. So do wound dehiscence and secondary infections. Latex allergy is another potential problem: this ranges from simple contact dermatitis to bronchial edema and anaphylaxis. Care must be taken to avoid exposing spina bifida children repetitively to latex products like catheters, drips, and gloves.

Prevention and Counseling

Primary Prevention

Over the last three decades, a series of studies have demonstrated that the incidence of neural tube defects can be dramatically reduced by the administration of folic acid in very early pregnancy as neural tube closure takes place around the fourth week of gestation. Since 1998, all enriched cereals sold in the United States have been fortified with folic acid; the first time food has been fortified for the prevention of birth defects [7,8]. Despite uncertainties regarding the mechanism of action, dose, timing, and optimum method of administration, public health policy in all countries should be directed toward this simple and safe method of primary prevention of neural tube defects.

Genetic Counseling

Genetic counseling should provide the family with sufficient information on which to base a decision about further children and help them come to terms with the problems they face. Counseling should involve careful discussion of the recurrence risk for further pregnancies and the availability of antenatal diagnosis. A sympathetic understanding of the burden faced by the parents and the child and an explanation of the variability of the condition are essential.

Counseling aims to be non-directive: the family needs time to make decisions about the future. Such decisions should evolve slowly as the family learns to cope with the affected child.

Recurrence Risk

Over 90% of infants with spina bifida are born to women with no previously affected children; more than 90% have myelomeningoceles. Recurrence risk varies from area to area. Counseling should be based on local experience. The most detailed guidelines have been published in the United Kingdom. In general, the recurrence risk following the birth of an affected baby is approximately 1 chance in 25, of which half is for anencephaly and half for other neural tube defects. If the parents have had two affected children, the risk rises to approximately 1 in 10 and after three children to approximately 1 in 4. The birth of a child with anencephaly, multiple congenital vertebral anomalies, or spinal dysraphism gives

families the same predisposition to the occurrence of neural tube defects. Adult survivors with spina bifida who are contemplating a family face the same risk as the parents of a single affected child (1 in 25).

Antenatal Diagnosis

Ultrasound

Many countries offer parents screening for neural tube defects based on a maternal alpha-fetoprotein level more than twice the normal mean and associated with a risk of around 1 in 30. This indicates the need for detailed ultrasound screening. About 95% of myelomeningoceles are identifiable by the associated cranial signs which are more obvious than the spinal changes. Detection of lesions with no cranial signs is unreliable although they are likely to be less severe. Parental counseling with regard to prognosis should be guarded as although the anatomical upper level of the lesion can be estimated within one spinal level, the sensory level does not always correspond. Ultrasound at 12 weeks can virtually exclude anencephaly. Detailed morphological ultrasound can be undertaken at 18–24 weeks, but some recommend earlier transvaginal ultrasound at 14–16 weeks in severe cases although the sacrum is poorly seen before 17 weeks [9,10].

Amniocentesis

Amniocentesis for amniotic fluid alpha-fetoprotein levels and acetylcholinesterase banding is another method in addition to ultrasound but bears a risk if 1% of miscarriage from the procedure itself.

Secondary Prevention

Intrauterine diagnosis allows the abortion of babies with neural tube defects when this is acceptable to parents. Thus, antenatal diagnosis has the potential to reduce greatly the incidence of this disorder, and the recent fall in the frequency of neural tube defects in live births in England and Wales is in large part due to an effective antenatal diagnostic program.

It has been shown that there is a lower incidence of severe neurological deficit in those babies who have been delivered by caesarean section at the 36th week of pregnancy compared with those delivered vaginally at term. The parents who will not accept abortion may accept the possibility of a less severely disabled child by embracing this option. In 1998, successful fetal surgery for spina bifida was reported [11]. This approach may preserve neurological function and arrest or reverse the development of hydrocephalus and the Arnold–Chiari 2 malformation.

Prophylaxis in Subsequent Pregnancies

There is clear evidence that peri-conceptual vitamin supplementation will reduce the very high risk of a second child being affected after the birth of a child with a neural tube defect.

Coordinated Management—The Spina Bifida Clinic

A proper management program for affected children, involving as it does many disciplines and a variety of medical specialists and allied health professionals can only be properly carried out if there is a formal organization—the spina bifida clinic. The orthopaedic problems of these children cannot be managed in isolation from their numerous other problems, which should be dealt with by a minimum number of inpatient admissions and outpatient attendances by staff who have been trained in the special problems created by the condition.

The team for the clinic should include

- Coordinator
- Neurosurgeon
- Orthopaedic surgeon
- Urologist
- Psychologist and psychiatrist
- Social worker
- Physiotherapist
- Occupational therapist
- Orthotist

Adequate treatment and care of the multi-handicapped child depends upon recognizing him or her as an individual whose needs far exceed the range of the separate specialities listed above (see Chapter 3). The coordinator should be a doctor or health professional with training and expertise in managing children with multiple disabilities. The coordinator unites the clinic staff and is the person to whom parents may turn as their "general practitioner." The coordinator should possess a good working knowledge of all the specialist treatments and expertise in managing complex child and family interactions.

Such an organization offers maximum support to the family by ensuring that treatment is integrated and that attendances and admissions to hospital are properly coordinated.

Neonatal Management

The orthopaedic surgeon should examine every spina bifida child at birth or as soon as possible thereafter, not only to record basic information but to make it possible to monitor progress over the first few months and to plan orthopaedic treatment if survival seems likely. The only condition requiring orthopaedic treatment in the neonatal period is talipes equinovarus using very well-padded Ponseti serial casts (see Chapter 31) to protect the insensate skin.

Aims of Orthopaedic Management

The principal aim for those children who are thought to have the potential to stand is to establish a stable posture in extension by correcting fixed deformity. If such children are to stand for long periods and to remain on their feet in adult life, they must have their centers of gravity directly over their feet. This requires minimal flexion deformities at the hips and knees and it is ideal if there is some hyperextension at both hips and knees. About 60% of spina bifida children have neurological problems in their upper limbs and often need to use both hands for activities which other children manage with one hand. It is for this reason that we strive, where possible, to encourage them to stand for long periods without using their hands for support.

Orthopaedic surgery has different goals according to the level of the neurosegmental lesion. This level may be ill-defined because of skin lesions, other neurological deficits, or general disabilities. Furthermore, the neurosegmental level may change because of tethering of the cord. The implications of the level of the lesion with regard to walking are as follows:

- Children with thoracic lesions will not continue useful walking in adult life.
- Children with lumbar lesions may continue useful walking in adult life if they have strong quadriceps muscles and do not develop significant deformity at their hip joints. Those with strong quadriceps require not only below-knee orthoses, but may also need assistive devices (walking sticks or crutches).
- Children with sacral lesions can be expected to be useful walkers, without orthoses, into adult life. However, Bartonek et al. [12] in a 12-year follow-up study of 60 walking myelomeningocele patients at a median age of 22 years showed that 19 had deteriorated in walking ability. Important causes of this deterioration were deterioration in neurological level, development of spasticity, hip and

knee flexion deformities, low back pain, and lack of motivation. Medical problems such as strokes, sepsis, and lower limb edema were also factors.

The Functional Motor Scale (FMS) developed by Graham et al. is helpful in describing functional mobility [13]. It is meant to be uncomplicated and useful as a communication tool among health professionals. It is scored over 5, 50, and 500 m, distances thought to correlate well with mobility in the home, at school, and in the community, respectively. Dependence on walking aids is documented.

Those who will not continue walking require simple surgery to provide them with a stable posture in childhood, while those who will continue walking require more sophisticated surgery to meet the increased demands of their way of life. Because the surgery necessary in children with high lesions is relatively minor, it should if possible be performed at several levels and in both limbs under one anesthetic. Muscle imbalance must be corrected so that recurrent deformity does not occur. Radical surgery is necessary to correct rigid, arthrogryposis-like deformities especially in the feet and care must be taken to avoid pressure on insensitive skin. For this and other reasons operative correction of deformities is usually preferable to conservative methods. All management in spina bifida must involve immobilization of the child

Table 17.2 Orthopaedic management related to stage of development and age

Developmental stage	Management
Birth	Assessment begins with a view to determine realistic aims
	Ponseti manipulation of foot deformities
First year of life Head control	Developmental stimulation
	Encourage sitting balance
Second to fourth year of life Sitting	Encourage hand skills and coordination
	Encourage upper limb strength and coordination of hand function
	Sitting aids
	Continued assessment, increased social stimulation
Upright stance	Standing orthosis
	Physiotherapy and orthoses appropriate to the neurosegmental level
	Soft tissue releases hip deformity
	Reduction of hip dislocation if indicated
	Intertrochanteric and pelvic osteotomy if indicated
Upright mobility	Tendon release or transfer in deforming foot and knee tendons
Fourth to sixth year of life	Kyphosis surgery
	Correction of fixed flexion knees
	Pelvic osteotomy in hip dysplasia
Tenth to sixteenth year of life	Correction of neurogenic scoliosis
	Correction of recurrent hip or knee deformity

and of the uninvolved limbs for as short a time as possible so that the incidence of pathological fractures is minimized. It should be assumed initially that all these children, except those with limited cognitive ability or gross spasticity, have the potential to stand and walk if only for a limited time in childhood. Children should be taught to stand and walk as soon as this becomes practicable. The age at which various orthopaedic procedures are recommended is shown in Table 17.2.

Gait Analysis

While the principal goal of orthopaedic surgery is to correct deformity, there are frequently secondary goals such as improving gait and function. The impact of deformity on function and gait is not always obvious. For example, the impact of hip dislocation on gait has almost certainly been overstated in previous studies and the results of tendon transfers and hip reduction are therefore frequently disappointing. Conversely, the impact of torsional abnormalities on gait has probably been underestimated. Vankoski et al. [14] demonstrated the deleterious effect of excessive external tibial torsion in myelomeningocele patients who walked with solid ankle/foot orthoses (AFOs). At the same time the beneficial effect of AFOs on gait and energy expenditure was reported [15,16].

Three-dimensional gait analysis has been used in several studies to give a good description of the typical gait patterns in children with spina bifida. Not surprisingly, kinematic deviations are closely related to neurosegmental level. Children who have sacral level lesions have a mild crouch gait with reduced power generation from the calf muscle [17]. As the neurological level ascends, greater deviations are seen because of the compensations required for increasing paralysis. At the L3/L4 level, the trunk must be moved over the stance limb to compensate for paralysis of the hip abductors and extensors, and large pelvic rotations are required to advance the limb during swing phase. Understanding these gait deviations is not just of academic interest as there are many implications for the surgical management. An abnormally wide range of hip abduction is required for independent walking in children with spina bifida. Surgery to reduce a dislocated hip, which results in stiffness, may abolish independent walking, despite a satisfactory appearance on the radiograph. A mobile lumbar spine is also a prerequisite for independent walking at the midlumbar level. Spinal instrumentation and fusion may effectively correct deformity but adversely affect gait. Three-dimensional kinematics may be used to plan reconstructive surgery and to monitor outcomes.

Energy studies are very useful in spina bifida, explaining which gait deviations are energy expensive, identifying which children have sustainable community-walking potential, and measuring outcome after surgical or orthotic intervention [19].

Orthoses and Mobility Aids

Bracing is provided when the child shows some interest in pulling to stand. AFOs are provided at an early stage to control mobile ankle or foot deformities and provide a more stable base for standing and walking. The parapodium or a standing frame is also very useful for the younger child to introduce the experience of standing (Fig. 17.5).

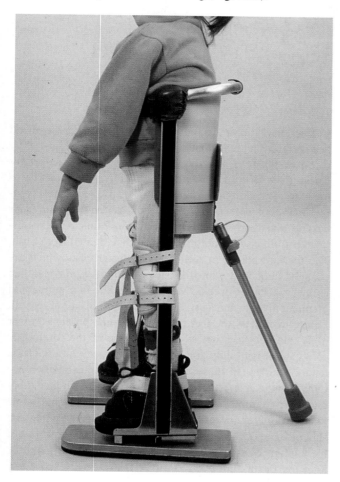

Fig. 17.5 A swivel-walker for a 3-year-old girl with high-level paraplegia to enable her stand upright

Ankle/Foot Orthosis

Floor reaction or ground reaction AFOs are ideal for the child with reasonably strong quadriceps and a paralyzed or weak calf. They provide control of the "plantar flexion–knee extension" couple, resisting the tendency to crouch gait by promoting knee and hip extension [15] (Fig. 17.6). Rotation cables may provide additional help against the tendency of internal rotation.

Knee/Ankle/Foot Orthosis (KAFO)

A greater degree of quadriceps weakness demands that KAFOs be employed. Children will not tolerate these above-knee orthoses for long periods until they have reached an age when they no longer prefer to crawl.

Hip/Knee/Ankle/Foot Orthosis (HKAFO)

For children with more extensive paralysis, bracing is required up to hip level and a number of options are available. The parapodium is useful for the younger child, but is an aid to standing rather than walking. The swivel walker or the hip guidance orthosis (HGO) is used in some centers. Those children with some hip flexor power and no significant fixed deformity obtain great benefit from the use of the reciprocating gait orthosis (RGO) or the para-walker. The RGO is the most effective and widely used form of high bracing and offers advantages in cosmesis and acceptable energy efficiency.

Wheelchairs

Very few children in high bracing will continue with braced walking in the second decade of life. They are much more functional in wheelchairs and can attend more easily to bladder management unencumbered by high-level bracing. Children with high-level lesions and their parents should be informed at a relatively early age that a wheelchair is likely to be preferred to walking and should not be regarded as inferior to walking. Those children who have considerable paralysis, with or without gross spasticity in their legs and with or without upper limb abnormality, may never walk and will be reliant upon a wheelchair from the age of 2 years.

Children with less severe disability will commonly walk during early childhood and then, generally between the ages of 10 and 16 years, find that they are more mobile and more integrated into society, e.g., at school, in a wheelchair, and seldom stand or walk subsequently. This transition should be anticipated, planned for, and conducted after detailed discussions involving the child, the physiotherapist, orthopaedic surgeon and, in the United Kingdom, the community paediatrician (see Chapter 3). In the final analysis, the child's wishes are paramount.

Fig. 17.6 (**a**) Crouch position of both legs in a lumbar lesion with knee flexion contracture and external rotation of feet. Standing and walking is difficult for the 8-year-old boy. (**b**) Two years after surgical correction of knee flexion and foot valgus standing upright

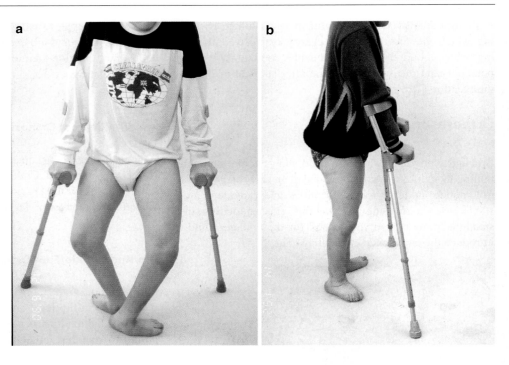

The cessation of braced walking should not be viewed as a failure but as a logical progression. It has been shown that children who have walked for a period, when compared with those who have never walked, have fewer deformities, fewer fractures, transfer more effectively, and are more mobile in the community. However, they spent longer in hospital and there were no major differences in the skills of daily living, function of the hands, and frequency and severity of obesity [19].

Management of Deformities

The Foot and Ankle

Fixed varus deformity invariably requires correction by operation, as complications from weight bearing on a small area of the sole or lateral border of the foot are otherwise inevitable. Under-correction must never be accepted since further surgery will almost certainly be required.

Valgus feet, while they remain mobile, can usually be controlled with appropriate footwear and orthoses until adolescence. Mobile valgus deformity of the subtalar joint is commonly complicated by torsional and valgus deformity of the ankle mortise: the deformity is difficult to control by bracing and surgery is often necessary to correct this complex deformity. Valgus deformity at the foot and ankle requires careful clinical and radiological evaluation including standing anteroposterior (AP) and lateral radiographs of the foot as well as a standing mortise view of the ankle (Fig. 17.7).

Correction of the valgus foot will fail if there is unrecognized and therefore untreated ankle valgus.

Equinovarus deformity. The rigidity of this deformity varies from that seen in idiopathic talipes equinovarus to the extreme rigidity of arthrogryposis. This is the most troublesome foot deformity because of its tendency to recur despite apparently adequate initial correction. Unless survival is unlikely, the deformity should be treated from birth. The feet are placed in well-padded plaster casts which are changed frequently while the baby is still in hospital and then at intervals of 4–6 weeks. More recently the Ponseti method of manipulation and cast application has been successful. Before treatment, the feet may appear to be purely varus or even calcaneovarus but as the adduction of the forefoot is corrected, it is usually apparent that there is tightness of the tendo-Achilles. In these circumstances percutaneous tenotomy is indicated. The rigid equinovarus foot will inevitably require posteromedial release (see Chapter 31) but some modifications are necessary. If the calf is not functioning, the skin incision does not need a vertical component. Portions of the tendons of the tendo-Achilles, tibialis posterior, and the long toe flexors are excised rather than just divided. Only occasionally will the degree of deformity be so mild that conservative treatment will correct the varus and adductus, leaving only equinus to be corrected by posterior release [20, 21].

Tendon transfers can play a part in children with muscular imbalance. Should the deformity recur then a repeat soft tissue release is performed. In addition a lateral wedge may be resected from the cuboid bone and fixed by K-wires.

Fig. 17.7 Paralytic talipes equinovarus. (**a**) Bilateral rigid clubfoot at 1 year of age. Manipulation and casts had failed to correct the position. (**b**) After peritalar release in both feet, satisfactory position at 2 years of age. (**c**) Both feet preserved their correction at follow-up at 12 years

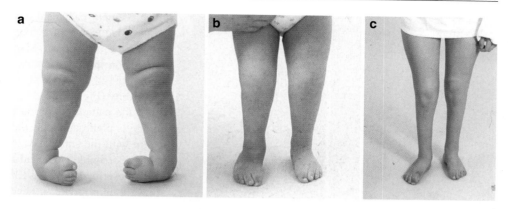

The majority of children who present with recurrent foot deformity have reduced or absent sensation. Occasionally the Ilizarov frame can help to achieve complete correction of deformity. Soft tissue releases, osteotomies, and occasionally talectomy can be used in conjunction with circular frame deformity correction (Table 17.3).

Table 17.3 Summary of talipes equino varus management in spina bifida

- Birth to 3 months: serial casting, well padded, and carefully monitored (Ponseti)
- 3–6 months: percutaneous tendo-Achilles tenotomy and serial casting
- 6–12 months: posteromedial release
- Late childhood: medial and lateral column surgery, heel and midfoot osteotomies, Ilizarov techniques
- Adolescence: heel and midfoot osteotomy

Cavus deformity. The management of this condition depends on the degree of rigidity of the deformity and the age of the child. Open division of the tight plantar structures may correct minor deformity in a young child. If the heel varus is flexible according to the Coleman block test (see Chapter 32), surgery to correct the pronated forefoot is indicated; however, if it is rigid osteotomy of the calcaneum at the age of 4 years or over is better. The efficacy of soft tissue and bony procedures may be improved by the use of an Ilizarov frame and fewer children will require salvage by triple arthrodesis at maturity.

Calcaneus deformity tends to be progressive, becomes fixed, and should be treated surgically. Transfer of the tibialis anterior to the calcaneus via the interosseous membrane is the best option. While mobile feet are preferable to stiff feet, triple arthrodesis at maturity has a useful place in the management of both varus and valgus deformity [22].

This deformity is generally left untreated until muscle power can be properly assessed at the age of 3–5 years. If the strength of the tibialis anterior is normal then this tendon is transferred through the interosseous membrane to the heel

[23]. Any other active ankle dorsiflexors are divided and, if there is fixed calcaneus deformity, an anterior ankle release is combined with this tenotomy. If the anterior muscles are spastic or if they are weak, they are divided and the tendo-Achilles is tenodesed to the fibular metaphysis [24]. The drill hole through the fibula stimulates growth at the lower end of the fibula and this may correct valgus deformity at the ankle mortise—a deformity which commonly occurs in combination with calcaneus deformity. The late-developing calcaneus deformity with a "pistol grip" heel (see Chapter 32) is best treated by osteotomy of the calcaneum, removing a wedge based posteriorly so that the tuberosity lies less vertically. At the same time restoration of muscle balance by tenodesis or tendon transfer achieves balance. More effective displacement of calcaneal osteotomies for calcaneus deformity may be achieved by using slow distraction in a circular frame.

Valgus deformity. This deformity may occur at the ankle mortise, the subtalar joint, or at both of these sites. Clinical examination and weight-bearing radiographs of the foot and ankle will clarify the site of the deformity.

Ankle valgus. Clinically the distal end of the fibula lies more proximal than the medial malleolus. Radiographs show that the lower fibular growth plate lies proximal to the ankle joint, while it should be at the same level. The lower tibial epiphysis is wedge-shaped with the medial portion of the epiphysis being wider than the lateral [25]. Under the age of 6 years this deformity may be reversed by arrest of the medial portion of the lower tibial growth plate. This arrest can be performed open using staples or by percutaneous screw hemiepiphysiodesis which is the least invasive and preferred method (Fig. 17.8).

Deformity at a later age and of a degree sufficient to present a problem should be corrected by a transverse osteotomy of the tibia with excision of a medially based wedge of lower tibia and an oblique osteotomy of the fibula. The tibial osteotomy should be approximately 1 cm proximal to the lower tibial growth plate. Any external tibial torsion that is present should be simultaneously corrected. The

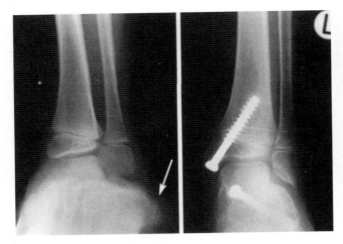

Fig. 17.8 Ankle valgus has been managed by screw epiphysiodesis through the medial malleolus and the subtalar valgus by a subtalar fusion using screw fixation and autogenous iliac crest grafting

osteotomy may be secured with a single staple or with two crossed K-wires. There is an incidence of wound breakdown and delayed union following this procedure. The Ilizarov frame is the best method of managing such complications and for revision surgery. This type of prolonged fixation, however, needs careful discussion as it is not tolerated by all children.

Subtalar valgus. If this is so gross that it cannot be controlled by an AFO under the age of 10 years then a medial displacement calcaneal osteotomy can be performed using a threaded K-wire for fixation [26]. Calcaneal lengthening should be considered. Many prefer an extraarticular subtalar fusion in which greater correction is traded for loss of mobility [27,28]. Care should be taken not to overcorrect the deformity (Fig. 17.9).

If the patient is approaching maturity then there is commonly a plano-abductus deformity of the forefoot in association with the subtalar valgus. If the deformity is mild and easily corrigible calcaneal lengthening by the method originally described by Evans [29] and popularized by Mosca [30] may be appropriate; it needs to be combined with peroneal tendon lengthening.

Severe plano-abducto-valgus is best corrected by triple arthrodesis. The most satisfactory form of triple arthrodesis for the myelomeningocele valgus foot which generally lacks any fixed deformity but sweeps into valgus on weight bearing is the lateral inlay arthrodesis [31].

Ankle and subtalar valgus. This requires surgery at two sites. Supramalleolar osteotomy of the tibia and fibula may be combined with either calcaneal osteotomy or lateral inlay triple fusion [32] depending on the nature of the foot deformity present.

Paralytic convex pes valgus (vertical talus). This complex deformity occasionally occurs in children suffering from myelomeningocele or from diastematomyelia. The neuromuscular form of this condition is often less rigid than the classical congenital form and may develop slowly in the

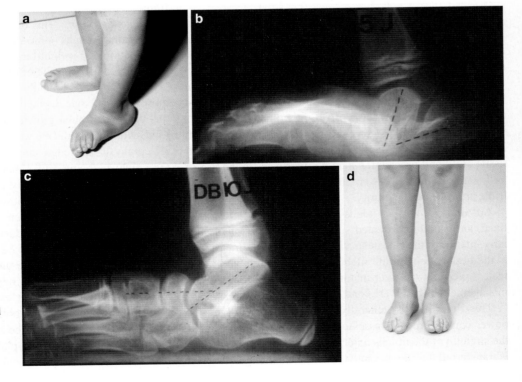

Fig. 17.9 (**a**) Rocker bottom foot in a 3-year-old girl, with problems standing on the everted foot. (**b**) Radiograph of the vertical talus. (**c**) Radiograph of the corrected foot at 10 years, 7 years after reduction of talus, and extraarticular arthrodesis after Grice. (**d**) Clinical appearance at 10 years. Full weight bearing is possible

Table 17.4 Summary of management of valgus foot

Distinguish ankle from subtalar valgus	
Young child	Ankle foot orthosis
Ankle valgus	Screw epiphysiodesis
Heel valgus—severe	Extraarticular arthrodesis (Grice); os calcis osteotomy
Heel valgus—mild	Extraarticular arthrodesis (Grice)
Abduction forefoot—mild	Os calcis lengthening
Ankle and subtalar valgus	Supramalleolar osteotomy and subtalar fusion

first years of life [33]. The management of vertical talus is described in Chapter 33.

Table 17.4 summarizes management of valgus.

The Knee

Flexion deformity and a limited range of flexion at the knee are most common in children with thoracic level lesions [3]. This suggests that muscle imbalance has been overrated as the cause of deformity in spina bifida since those with thoracic level lesions have no muscle imbalance at the knee.

The Flail Undeformed Knee

This is found in approximately 30% of those children who survive to an age at which walking may occur. Bracing is necessary to support the knees if the child is to stand and walk.

The Undeformed Knee with Quadriceps Weakness

This situation is common. Early in life bracing annoys these children because they wish to be able to crawl. Later a floor reaction orthosis may be useful. For some children a KAFO on one leg and an AFO on the other with alternate bracing on alternate days may provide an answer.

Fixed Flexion Deformity [18]

Fixed flexion deformity of up to 20° is commonly present at birth. Deformity of less than 20° can generally be ignored. If the deformity is greater than 20°, surgery in the form of a posterior release of all the hamstrings allows the child to be braced and to stand. A posterior capsular release may be needed if the tendon release fails to correct the deformity. Postoperatively the knee is immobilized in a well-padded cast enabling early standing to avoid osteoporosis as far as possible. Overzealous stretching may threaten the popliteal vessels and, if they are at risk, serial postoperative casting may be safer. Rarely, a supracondylar osteotomy of the femur is indicated (Fig 17.10).

Limited Flexion with Recurvatum

Some neonates have a recurvatum deformity, but this usually responds to serial well-padded casting. However, the knee that is rigid in extension may have the featureless appearance seen in arthrogryposis multiplex congenita. Such knees may be treated by subcutaneous tenotomy of the ligamentum patellae. This is usually performed at the age of 6 months to

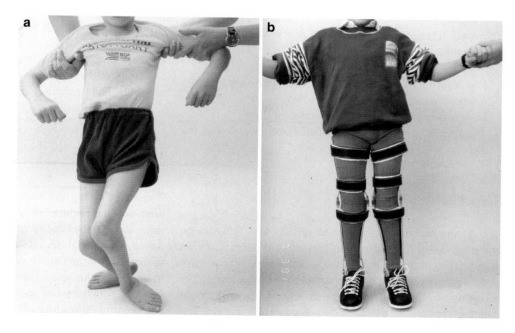

Fig. 17.10 (**a**) Flexion contractures in both knees of boy at 5 years. Inability to be braced for walking. (**b**) After tendon release of the hamstrings the boy is able to stand and walk with knee/ankle/foot orthoses

Fig. 17.11 (**a**) Fixed extension in both knees does not allow correct sitting in 3-year-old girl. (**b**) After quadriceps lengthening full flexion, good for sitting. For walking she needs knee/ankle/foot orthoses

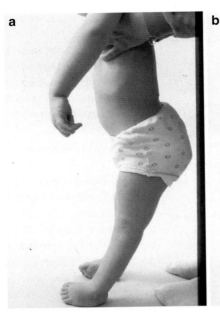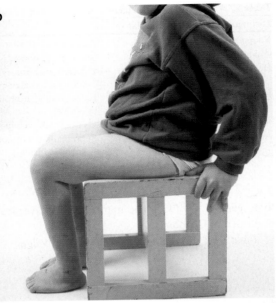

enable early crawling with flexible knees. If this is not done early at a later age when the legs are elongating they protrude when the child is seated in the classroom or a vehicle. If tenotomy is not done at an early age quadricepsplasty may be necessary (Fig. 17.11).

Valgus Deformity

This is not a common problem but may occur in children with lower thoracic or upper lumbar lesions; it may rarely require medial growth plate arrest or osteotomy.

The Hip

There are three indications to treat hip problems in spina bifida patients:

- Hip deformity which creates a problem during walking—usually a fixed flexion deformity
- Dislocation of the hip in certain circumstances
- The need to provide abductor and extensor power at the hip

Hip Deformity

The commonest deformity is fixed flexion. It is most severe and progressive in patients with flail hips [2] but is also seen in patients with lower-level lesions. Should the patient have good walking potential and the deformity is in excess of 20° and progressive, then a soft tissue release of all the tight structures in front of and lateral to the hip is performed. The

muscles are swept off both the inner and outer surfaces of the ilium, the psoas tendon is divided, sartorius and rectus femoris are released and, if necessary, the anterior capsule of the hip joint is divided transversely. At the conclusion of the procedure the anterior superior iliac spine and adjacent portions of the iliac crest will protrude anteriorly and should be trimmed.

Commonly, both hips require this procedure and both should be corrected under one anesthetic. Even if only one hip is operated upon, both should be draped to allow Thomas's test to be carried out intraoperatively. If this reveals a significant contracture, the second hip should also be released. Postoperatively the patient should be in a standing cast to prevent osteoporosis [5]. Rarely, extension osteotomy is necessary to correct gross flexion deformity in children over the age of 10 years. Proximal femoral osteotomy is a versatile procedure for the correction of multiplanar fixed deformity of the hip, using combinations of extension, varus or valgus, and derotation.

Hip Dislocation

The effect of hip dislocation on gait and function in children who have spina bifida is difficult to assess and despite many studies, the benefits of surgical reduction are difficult to define. Smith et al. [34] described and tested a questionnaire to evaluate the activities of daily living that are important to children with spina bifida and dislocated hips and their families which can be used reliably to evaluate treatment outcomes in these children.

Table 17.5 Indications for reduction of hip dislocation in spina bifida

Type of lesion	Bilateral	Unilateral
High lesions	Never	Seldom if asymmetry is no problem
Low lesions	Seldom if hip flexion contracture	Always

Reduction of the dislocated hip in spina bifida may not improve walking ability. Nevertheless some patients, particularly if the dislocation is unilateral, have a troublesome leg-length discrepancy if the hip remains dislocated. A guide to decision making is outlined in Table 17.5.

If the hip is to be reduced it is important to minimize the duration of plaster immobilization. Hip reduction should be stabilized by either Pemberton or Dega pelvic osteotomy (see Chapter 26). Six weeks only of immobilization in a standing hip spica which incorporates the feet minimizes the risk of osteoporotic fracture after operation.

Provision of Abductor and Extensor Power

The absence of functioning hip extensors and abductors at the lumbar level has been considered the main reason for hip dislocation and provides the logic for muscle and tendon transfer surgery. Sharrard [35] stressed the importance of providing abductor and extensor power and depriving the hip of the strong flexor power of the psoas muscle by performing iliopsoas transfer. It is now clear that dislocation of the hip is most common in patients with flail hips and there is doubt about the need to correct muscle balance at the hip in the prevention of hip dislocation. The iliopsoas transfer has proven advantageous in many children but has some practical and theoretical flaws [36]. Gait analysis studies suggest that the transfer continues to fire during the swing phase of gait, as a result it makes the key pelvic kinematic deviations worse and by inference it increases energy expenditure [37]. None of the tendon transfers described to stabilize the hip in spina bifida has been adequately studied objectively and the suspicion remains that they are all flawed by incorrect timing or inadequate strength. The percentage of hips reduced at follow-up is an inadequate measure of success; it is gait and function which are paramount. If a child can take steps upright but cannot climb a step the functional benefit is obviously not very good. The recurrence of flexion deformity is most often prevented by iliopsoas transfer. In addition to the posterior iliopsoas transfer (Fig. 17.12) other transfers include external oblique transfer to the greater trochanter or transfer of the adductor origin posteriorly [38].

Varus derotation osteotomy (VDRO) of the proximal femur may be used to stabilize an open or closed reduction of the hip. Given the current uncertainties regarding the value of individual operations in managing the unstable hip our current practice is pragmatic rather than scientific and based on whether there is evidence that relocating the hip will improve function and quality of life.

The unilaterally dislocated hip usually requires open reduction, psoas and adductor lengthening, Pemberton or Dega acetabuloplasty, and VDRO as a one-stage hip reconstruction. We no longer use tendon transfers (Fig. 17.13).

When there is long-standing subluxation and the acetabulum is bilocular it may not be possible to reduce the femoral head into the original acetabulum; stabilization can then be achieved by salvage, utilizing the Chiari osteotomy and/or shelf procedures.

Summary

A reducible hip subluxation is managed by VDRO. Acetabular dysplasia is managed in the younger child by a Pemberton or Dega acetabuloplasty and in the adolescent by a Chiari osteotomy or Staheli shelf.

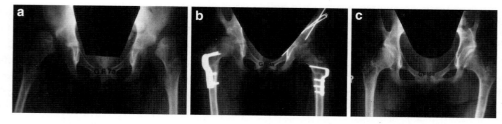

Fig. 17.12 (**a**) Bilateral hip dislocation in a 7-year-old girl, with fixed flexion and strong iliopsoas. (**b**) At 9 years after posterolateral iliopsoas transfer and reduction. After surgery the flexion contracture did not recur. (**c**) At 12 years the reduction of both hips was preserved. The girl was household-ambulatory with ankle/foot orthosis

Fig. 17.13 (a) Unilateral hip dislocation with asymmetry and leg-length discrepancy at 4 years. (b) After open reduction pelvic osteotomy and intertrochanteric osteotomy. (c) Pelvic radiograph at 5; 8 years symmetric hips provide equal leg length. Residual dysplasia is visible. (d) Symmetric standing of the patient using ankle/foot orthoses

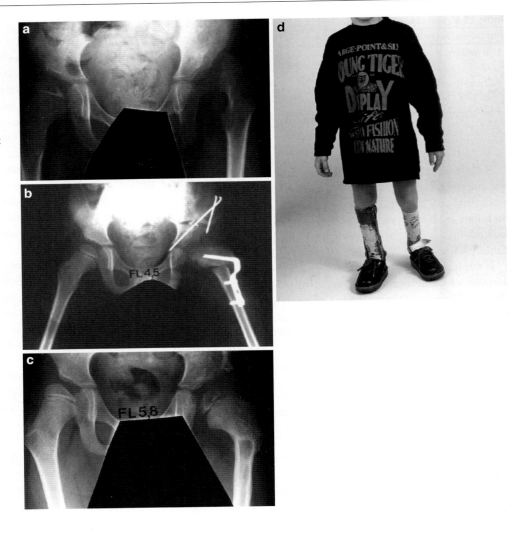

The Spine

Spinal deformity is frequently too disabling to be ignored, but conservative methods of treatment are seldom applicable.

Spinal deformity will not only impair walking but may make sitting difficult. If the child has poor sitting balance because of spinal deformity and has to use one hand to maintain upright posture, this can be a crippling impairment of function. Spina bifida patients commonly need to use both hands for functions which unaffected people can carry out with one hand because of subtle neurological disturbances in the upper limbs.

When treating the spinal deformity surgically (see Chapter 36) every effort must be made to avoid prolonged immobilization. Osteoporosis, fractures, genitourinary complications, and psychological disturbance are heavy prices to pay for a surgical complication such as infection or pseudoarthrosis. A child with spina bifida, off his feet for as little as 3 months, may never walk again.

Classification of Spinal Deformity

Spinal deformities in spina bifida patients may take one or more of the following forms:

- Defects of the neural arch and wide separation of the pedicles at the level of the neurological and meningeal lesion
- The full range of vertebral body anomalies seen in congenital scoliosis and occurring either at the level of the spina bifida or any other level of the spine. These anomalies include defects of segmentation, defects of formation, and mixed defects
- Diastematomyelia
- Spondylolisthesis
- Absence of the sacrum—partial or complete
- Kyphosis—paralytic and congenital forms
- Lordosis—commonly secondary to fixed flexion deformity of the hip and becoming fixed

- Scoliosis—the most common form of scoliosis occurring in myelomeningocele patients is paralytic in type, but congenital and mixed congenital and paralytic curves also occur. The curve may be a lordo-scoliosis or a kypho-scoliosis.

Kyphosis

Children who are born with kyphosis generally have hydrocephalus and are among the most severely affected: some do not survive. The kyphosis is generally in the lumbar spine and averages 80° at birth, increasing by an average of 8° per annum. Portions of the erector spinae muscles lie anterior to the axis of flexion and, by becoming spinal flexors, aggravate the tendency to kyphosis. Those children who are born with a lumbar kyphosis generally have complete paralysis of the leg muscles.

Management of kyphosis. The indication for correction is recurrent skin ulceration. A variety of surgical techniques are available and the choice will depend on the age of

the child and the severity of the kyphosis [39,40]. A long-term review of kyphectomy in 2004 [41] reported excellent clinical results in terms of improved sitting balance and independent use of the hands despite high postoperative rates of wound healing and skin breakdown; parent and patient satisfaction levels were high (Fig. 17.14).

Procedures available include

- kyphectomy with some form of segmental posterior instrumentation and fusion
- anterior strut graft/fusion
- combinations of anterior and posterior surgery

Scoliosis

While the curve is most commonly paralytic in origin it may be congenital or mixed [42]. Furthermore, patients who have hydrosyringomyelia may develop secondary scoliosis; drainage of the syrinx may prevent progression. All children with spina bifida therefore require magnetic resonance

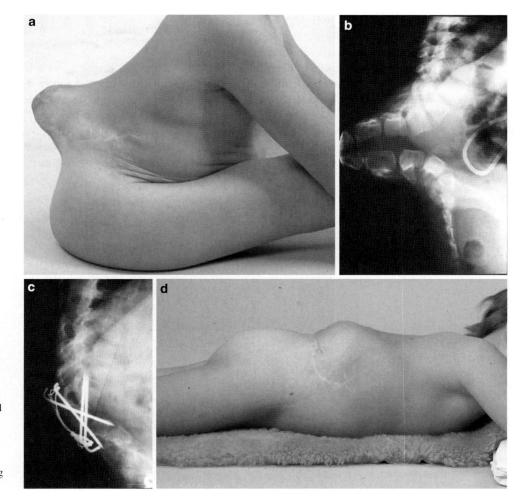

Fig. 17.14 (a) Fixed lumbar kyphosis in 4-year-old boy. (b) Radiographic view of the fixed kyphosis of 145°. (c) Radiographic view of the lumbar spine after excision of gibbus and tension band osteosynthesis. (d) Clinical appearance 2 years after surgery. There is residual kyphosis, which does not influence sitting upright and lying on the back

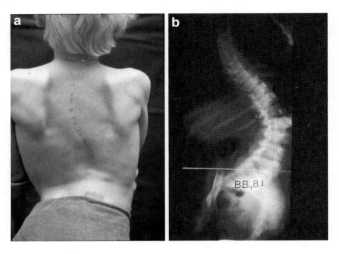

Fig. 17.15 (a) Severe scoliosis in a 7-year-old girl. (b) Radiographic appearance of the same patient shows 90° angle

imaging (MRI) of the entire cord before spinal surgery. If cord tethering is present release of the tether may help some curves smaller than 40°, but curves over 40° and thoracic curves will continue to progress [43] (Fig. 17.15).

Severe and progressive scoliosis is most common in patients with thoracic-level lesions. The incidence progressively diminishes with lesser degrees of neurological deficit.

There is a small place for bracing in children with rapidly progressive scoliosis who are considered too young for surgery.

Indications for operation include deformity increasing over 50° between the ages of 8 and 14 years, taking into consideration the child's size, the growth of the spine, and the

flexibility of the curve. Less commonly other circumstances provide an indication. The main aims of surgery are

- to produce a stable fusion which will prevent further deformity;
- to provide a stable posture for standing and sitting;
- to create a level pelvis and a vertical trunk, without the need for hand support;
- to maintain maximal trunk length and remove convexities which may lead to pressure sores;
- to preserve respiratory function and satisfactory cosmesis.

The principles of surgery. Stable fusion by both anterior and posterior approaches should be considered. Anterior instrumentation enables correction of the tight curve at the apex of the primary curve (usually at the thoraco-lumbar junction) and has a high fusion rate; posterior instrumentation increases the length of spine that can be fused and allows better correction of pelvic obliquity [44] (Fig. 17.16) (see Chapter 36).

Summary

Orthopaedic management of spina bifida patients must be tailored to meet the future demands of the child. In general, those with high-level lesions and weak quadriceps muscles will place minimal demands on their feet and legs during the period when they are walking and are best served by simple surgery. This simple surgery will generally take the form of soft tissue release to free the patient from fixed deformity.

Fig. 17.16 (a) Ten-year-old girl with severe right convex scoliosis before correction. (b) Two years after anterior fusion without instrumentation followed by posterior fusion with instrumentation (with permission from Parsch D et al. [44])

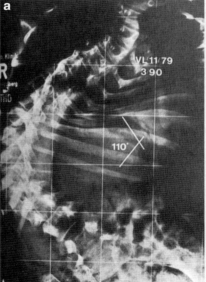
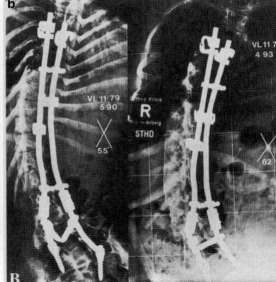

A proportion of children with low-level lesions and strong quadriceps muscles may walk throughout life or at least into adult life [12]. They put greater demands on their feet and legs [45] and benefit more from a good range of motion at the hip and knee. The role of tendon transfers to stabilize the hip and surgery for hip dislocation requires more objective study including gait analysis [46] and functional mobility scores such as that devised by Graham et al. (2004) for cerebral palsy [13] and is now being used in spina bifida patients. Plantigrade feet are essential.

Those with high-level lesions will be mobile in a wheelchair and are more likely to require radical surgery for severe spinal deformity such as scoliosis or kyphosis.

Spinal Dysraphism

This term is applied to a group of conditions in which the dorsum of the embryo forms abnormally. The condition is of importance to orthopaedic surgeons as a cause of foot deformity and leg weakness.

Definition

Spinal dysraphism refers to all forms of abnormality of formation of midline structures of the future dorsum of the embryo.

Incidence

Between 10 and 30% of the population have a degree of this abnormality be it only spina bifida occulta affecting one vertebral arch. Clinically significant spinal dysraphism is rare and the precise incidence is not known.

Embryology and Pathology

The condition may affect all or some of the primary embryonic layers to a varying degree. The type of dysplasia and the resultant conditions are illustrated in Table 17.6 [47]. Details of all aspects of the condition have been described by James and Lassman [48,49].

The commonest forms of pathology are the following:

- Diastematomyelia, where the spinal cord or filum terminale, or both, are split sagittally by a bony or fibrocartilaginous septum
- Lumbosacral lipoma

Table 17.6 Spina bifida, spinal dysraphism, or the spinal dysraphic state. Adapted from Lichtenstein (1940)

Embryonal origin	Type of dysplasia	Result condition
Cutaneous: Somatic Ectodermal	Cutaneous	Cutaneous defect Hypertrichosis Nevus Dermal sinus
Mesodermal	Vertebral	Split in spinous process Laminal defects Rachischisis
	Dural	Non-fusion of dura mater
Neural Neuroectodermal	Neural tube	Myelodysplasia Intramedullary and extramedullary growths associated with dysraphia
	Neural crest	Ectopia of spinal ganglia and of posterior nerve roots

- Meningocele manqué, in which a loop of nerve root or trunks emerges from the spinal cord, cauda equina, or filum terminale, becomes adherent to the dura, and then returns to the cauda equina or filum near to its point of origin
- Dermoid cyst
- Tight or tethered filum terminale: this may result in an abnormally distal conus (normally the conus lies at the following levels: in the fetus at the coccyx; at birth at the upper border of the third lumbar vertebra; at 5 years at the upper border of the second lumbar vertebra).
- Hydromyelia
- Atrophy meningocele
- Arachnoid cyst
- Various forms of myelodysplasia.

Frequently more than one of these abnormalities are present in combination.

Diagnosis and Differential Diagnosis

Patients may present to the orthopaedic surgeon at any age from birth to maturity. Most commonly they will present under the age of 5 years with one of the following:

- A short and often wasted leg
- A small foot
- A cavovarus foot deformity
- A paralytic valgus foot deformity
- Trophic ulceration (Fig. 17.17)

There may in addition be a cutaneous lesion in the form of a patch of hair, a nevus, a lipoma, a scarred area, or a sinus or

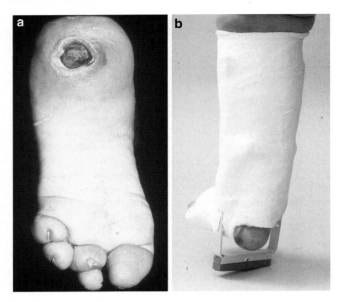

Fig. 17.17 (**a**) Perforating ulcer in a boy with spinal dysraphism with absent sensibility in this foot. (**b**) Weight relief in a walking cast and a window to take care of the trophic ulcer. The ulcer healed within 8 weeks

dimple. In a series of 200 patients [34] approximately one-quarter had no external cutaneous manifestation. Thus, it is imperative that the clinician has a high level of suspicion and carries out appropriate special investigations.

The differential diagnosis depends to some extent on the presenting features: If the child is seen with a short leg or small foot then the common differential diagnosis is hemi-hypertrophy or hemiatrophy. If neurological features are present then the following disorders must be excluded:

- Cerebral palsy in the form of a mild hemiplegia
- Spinal cord tumor
- Hereditary sensory and motor neuropathy
- Polyneuritis

Patients should be fully investigated, as described below, before accepting a diagnosis of "idiopathic" pes cavus (which is rarely unilateral).

Special Investigations

These will generally be performed in the following sequence (see Chapter 5):

1. *Plain radiographs.* These may disclose

   - Varying degrees and extent of spina bifida
   - A wide interpedicular distance

- Various anomalies of formation and segmentation of vertebrae
- A bony spur (if diastematomyelia is present)

It is important that the full length of the spine is radiographed in all patients.

2. *Ultrasound* (Fig 17.15). This investigation is useful antenatally and up to the age of 6 months. Diastematomyelia is more easily identified antenatally by ultrasound than by postnatal radiographs. Both bony and cartilaginous bars can be shown [10]. Should a patient present with a cutaneous lesion on the back or a foot deformity then this investigation can clarify the nature of the underlying lesion without the need for general anesthesia.

3. *Plain computed tomography(CT)* (Fig. 17.18). *MRI* has replaced myelography. These investigations have increased the sensitivity in defining the precise nature of the spinal defect.

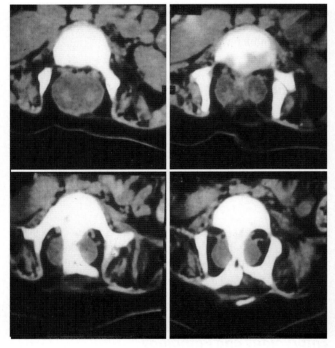

Fig. 17.18 Diastematomyelia. The CT scan of a 7-year-old girl. The spinal cord is split sagittally by a bony spur as seen on two cuts

Management of Dysraphism

The sequence of events to follow in managing a child with suspected spinal dysraphism is as follows:

1. Recognize that a neurological condition is present
2. Diagnose the cause of the condition to allow treatment of the causative spinal lesion and assessment of prognosis
3. Manage any foot deformity that is present

Recognize the Neurological Deficit

This depends on a high degree of suspicion in a child with any lower limb abnormality and in particular a foot deformity or discrepancy in foot and leg size. The clinician should look for muscle imbalance, carry out a careful neurological examination, and always examine the spine of the patient. Liaison with a paediatric neurologist is important in making a precise diagnosis and advising on appropriate investigations which should allow the neural tube defect to be accurately defined. Once clarified, the advice of a paediatric neurosurgeon should be sought.

Managing the Foot or Leg Abnormality

Cavus and other foot deformities that may be present are in general managed by

- Correcting muscle imbalance by tendon lengthening and transfer
- Soft tissue release between birth and age 5 years
- Metatarsal and calcaneal osteotomies between 5 and 10 years
- Wedge tarsectomy or triple arthrodesis at 12 years to maturity
- Circular frame correction may be used as an adjunct to conventional surgery

Complications

Deformity may recur after soft tissue releases due to persistence of the causative spinal lesion. Overzealous soft tissue release may result in reversal of the deformity.

Excessive lengthening of the tendo-Achillis may result in calcaneus deformity, which is worse than the original equinus deformity. It is generally wise to correct cavus deformity at one stage and equinus deformity at a second stage.

Postoperative casts should be carefully applied to avoid pressure on insensitive skin, particularly overlying prominent metatarsal heads.

Summary

Spinal dysraphism is one cause of abnormality in size, shape, or muscle power in the leg or foot. In the presence of such abnormalities the surgeon should always examine the lumbar spine, carry out a neurological examination, and be aware of the special investigations which are appropriate.

References

1. Shurtleff DB. Myelodysplasias and exstrophies: significance, prevention and treatment. Orlando, FL: Grune & Stratton; 1986.
2. Shurtleff DB, Menelaus MB, Staheli LT, et al. Natural history of flexion deformity of the hip in myelodysplasia. J Pediatr Orthop 1986; 16: 666–673.
3. Wright J, Menelaus MB, Shurtleff DB, et al. Natural history of knee contractures in myelocele. J Pediatr Orthop 1991; 11: 725–730.
4. Broughton NS, Menelaus MB, Cole WG, Shurtleff DB. The natural history of hip deformity in myelomeningocele. J Bone Joint Surg [B] 1993; 75: 760–763.
5. Parsch K. Origin and treatment of fractures in spina bifida. Eur J Pediatr Surg 1991; 1:298–305.
6. Dosa NP, Eckrich M, Katz DA, et al. Incidence, prevalence, and characteristics of fractures in children, adolescents, and adults with spina bifida. J Spinal Cord Med 2007; 30 Suppl 1:S5–S9.
7. Watkins ML. Efficacy of folic acid prophylaxis for the prevention of neural tube defects. Ment Retard Dev Disabil Res Rev 1998; 4: 282–290.
8. Brent RL, Oakley GP, Mattison DR. The unnecessary epidemic of folic acid-preventable spina bifida and hydrocephalus. Pediatrics 2000; 106: 825–827.
9. Broughton NS, Menelaus MB, eds. Orthopaedic Management of Spina Bifida Cystica, 3rd ed. London: WB Saunders; 1998.
10. Foster BK, Furness ME, Mulpori K. Prenatal ultrasonography in antenatal orthopaedics: a new subspecialty. J Pediatr Orthop 2002; 22: 404–409.
11. Sarwak JF. What's new in pediatric orthopaedics. J Bone Joint Surg[Am] 2003; 85A: 976–981.
12. Bartonek A, Saraste H, Samuelson L, Skoog M. Ambulation in patients with myelomeningocele: a 12 year follow up. J Pediatr Orthop 1999; 19: 202–206.
13. Graham HK, Harvey A, Rodda J, et al. The Functional Mobility Scale (FMS). J Pediatr Orthop 2004; 24: 514–520.
14. Vankoski SJ, Michaud S, Dias L. External tibial torsion and the effectiveness of the solid ankle foot orthosis. J Pediatr Orthop 2000; 20: 349–355.
15. Duffy CM, Hill AE, Cosgrove AP, et al. Three dimensional gait analysis in spina bifida. J Pediatr Orthop 1996; 16: 786–791.
16. Duffy CM, Graham HK, Cosgrove AP. The influence of ankle-foot orthoses on gait and energy expenditure in spina bifida. J Pediatr Orthop 2000; 20: 356–361.
17. Moen T, Gryfakis N, Dias L, Lenke L. Crouched gait in myelomeningocele: a comparison between the degree of knee flexion contracture in the clinical examination and during gait. J Pediatr Orthop 2005; 25: 657–663.
18. Snela S, Parsch K. Follow-up study after treatment of knee flexion contractures in spina bifida patients. J Pediatr Orthop part B 2000; 9:154–160.
19. Mazur J, Shurtleff D, Menelaus MB. Orthopaedic management of high-level spina bifida. J Bone Joint Surg [Am] 1989; 71A: 56–61.
20. de Carvalho Beto J, Dias LS, Gabrieli AP. Congenital talipes equinovarus in spina bifida: treatment and results. J Opediatr Orthop 1996; 16: 782–785.
21. Flynn JM, Herrera-Soto JA, Ramireu NF, et al. Clubfoot release in myelodysplasia. J Pediatr Orthop B 2004; 13: 259–262.
22. Olney BW, Menelaus MB. Triple arthrodesis of the foot in spina bifida patients. J Bone Joint Surg[B] 1988; 70B: 234–235.
23. Banta JV, Sutherland DH, Wyatt M. Anterior tibial transfer to the os calcis with Achilles tenodesis for calcaneal deformity in myelomeningocele. J Pediatr Orthop 1981; 1: 125–130.

24. Westin GW, Dugeman RD, Gausewitz SH. The results of tenodesis of the tendo Achilles to the fibula for paralytic pes calcaneus. J Bone Joint Surg[Am] 1988; 70A: 320–328.

25. Dias LS. Valgus deformity of the ankle: pathogenesis of fibular shortening. J Pediatr Orthop 1985; 5; 176–18.0

26. Torosian CM, Dias L. Surgical treatment of severe hindfoot valgus by displacement osteotomy of the Os calcis in children with myelomeningocele. J Pediatr Orthop 2000; 20: 226–229.

27. Gallien R, Morin F, Marquis F. Subtalar arthrodesis in children. J Pediatr Orthop 1989; 9: 59–63.

28. Bourelle S, Cottalorda J, Gautheron V, Chavier Y. Extraarticular subtalar arthrodesis. A long-term follow-up in patients with cerebral palsy. J Bone Joint Surg Br 2004; 86: 737–742.

29. Evans D. Calcaneovalgus deformity. J Bone Joint Surg[B] 1975; 57B: 270–278.

30. Mosca VS. Flexible flatfoot and skewfoot. J Bone Joint Surg[Am] 1995; 77A: 1937–1945.

31. Williams PF, Menelaus MB. Triple arthrodesis by inlay grafting: a method suitable for the undeformed or valgus foot. J Bone Joint Surg[B] 1977; 59B: 333–336.

32. Nicol RO, Menelaus MB. Correction of combined tibial torsion and valgus deformity of the foot. J Bone Joint Surg[B] 1983; 65B: 641–645.

33. Duckworth T, Smith TWD. The treatment of paralytic convex pes valgus. J Bone Joint Surg Br 1974; 56: 305–313.

34. Smith PL, Owen JL, Fehlings D, Wright JG. Measuring physical function in children with spina bifida and dislocated hips. J Pediatr Orthop 2005; 25: 273–279.

35. Sharrrard WJW. Posterior iliopsoas transplantation in the treatment of paralytic dislocation of the hip. J Bone Joint Surg[B] 1964; 46B: 426–444.

36. Parsch K, Dimeglio A. The hip in children with myelomeningocele. J Pediatr Orthop B; 1992; 1: 3–13.

37. Duffy CM, Hill AE, Cosgrove AP, et al. Energy consumption in children with spina bifida and cerebral palsy: A comparative study. Develop Med Child Neurol 1996; 38: 238–243.

38. Yngve DA, Lindseth RE. Effectiveness of muscle transfer in myelomeningocele hips measured by radiographic indices. J Pediatr Orthop 1982; 2: 121–125.

39. Fuerderer S, Eysel P, Hopf C, Heine J. Sagittal static imbalance in myelomeningocele patients: improvement in sitting ability by partial and total gibbus resection. Eur Spine J 1999; 8: 451–457.

40. Nolden MT, Sarwark JF, Vora A, Grayhack JJ. A kyphectomy technique with reduced perioperative morbidity for myelomeningocele kyphosis. Spine 2002; 15: 1807–1813.

41. Niall DM, Dowling FE, Fogarty EE, et al. Kyphectomy in children with myelomeningocele: a long term outcome study. J Pediatr Orthop 2004; 24: 37–44.

42. Guille JT, Sarwark JF, Sherk HH, Kumar SJ. Congenital and developmental deformities of the spine in children with myelomeningocele. J Am Acad Orthop Surg 2006; 14: 294–302.

43. Piez K, Banta J, Thompson J, et al. Effect of tethered cord release on scoliosis in myelomeningocele. J Pediatr Orthop 2000; 20: 362–365.

44. Parsch D, Geiger F, Brocai DR, et al. Surgical management of paralytic scoliosis in myelomeningocele. J Pediatr Orthop B 2001; 10: 10–17.

45. Duffy CM, Hill AE, Graham HK. The influence of flexed-knee gait on the energy cost of walking in children. Develop Med Child Neurol 1997; 39: 234–238.

46. Duffy CM, Hill AE, Cosgrove AP, et al. The influence of abductor weakness on gait in spina bifida. Gait Posture 1996; 4: 34–38.

47. Lichtenstein BW. Spinal dysraphism. Spina bifida and myelodysplasia. Arch Neurol Psych 1940; 44: 792–810.

48. James CCM, Lassman LP. Spinal dysraphism. Spina bifida occulta. London: Butterworths; 1972.

49. James CCM, Lassman LP. Spina bifida occulta. Orthopaedic, radiological and neurosurgical aspects. London: Academic Press/New York: Grune & Stratton; 1981.

Chapter 18

Poliomyelitis

Wang Chow, Yun Hoi Li, and Chi Yan John Leong

Introduction

Poliomyelitis is a highly infectious viral disease that mainly affects young children. It spreads through contaminated food and water. The virus may attack the central nervous system and cause paralysis and subsequent deformity. The first known description of poliomyelitis was given by Underwood in 1789 and it was not until 1855 that Duchenne described the pathological process in poliomyelitis involving the anterior horn cells of the spinal cord.

The disease had been endemic worldwide before the introduction of an effective vaccine and the launch of a global vaccination program. In 1988, the Global Polio Eradication Initiative was launched by the World Health Organization (WHO), Rotary International, the US Centers for Disease Control and Prevention (CDC), and UNICEF. The number of cases has fallen by 99% from an estimate of more than 350,000 cases in 1988 to only 1951 reported cases in 2005. The disease was widely endemic on five continents in 1988 and is now found only in parts of Africa and south Asia. At the time of writing, there are four countries, Nigeria, India, Pakistan, and Afghanistan with endemic polio, down from more than 125 countries in 1988 [1–3].

Etiology and Immunization

The disease is caused by one of the three types of poliomyelitis virus (Brunhilde, Lansing, and Leon) belonging to the enterovirus group, which includes Coxsackie C and the ECHO viruses. The last two viruses can produce a clinical picture indistinguishable from that of poliomyelitis. The lack of cross-immunity between each type of polio virus makes reinfection possible.

The virus is most commonly transmitted through the gastrointestinal tract from infected food or fecal matter, although the disease may also be contracted via the respiratory tract. The virus is blood-borne to the central nervous system. Epidemics used to occur during summer and autumn; however, with the widespread use of oral vaccine, epidemics are now unusual.

Two types of vaccines are available. The Salk vaccine, first introduced in 1954, is a killed vaccine given by injection, whereas the Sabin vaccine is a live, attenuated oral vaccine [4]. The latter type is cheaper, safer, and more effective against all three types of polio virus. Immunity conferred is usually lifelong. However, recent attention has been given to the vaccine-associated poliomyelitis caused by the oral vaccine. The risk of contracting poliomyelitis from the vaccine is extremely low, with a rate of 1 case per 2.5 million doses. The CDC has reported complete elimination of this vaccine-associated poliomyelitis in 2006 after a change of vaccination program. The child is now first inoculated with the inactivated vaccine, followed by the oral attenuated one.

Pathology

Acute Stage

Poliomyelitis starts as a systemic infection. The incubation period varies from 1 to 3 weeks. Initial extraneural involvement is mainly in the reticulo-endothelial system, with hyperplasia of the spleen and lymph nodes. Only 1–2% of those affected ultimately suffer from neural damage.

Neural involvement occurs chiefly in the brain stem and anterior horn cells of the spinal cord. However, inflammatory changes may occur in the posterior ganglia and nerve roots.

Initially, the spinal cord shows inflammatory changes, with polymorphonuclear cell infiltration, later replaced by lymphocytes. There are varying degrees of neuronal degeneration, with cell death and disintegration being the worst

W. Chow (✉)
Department of Orthopaedics and Traumatology, Hong Kong, China

M. Benson et al. (eds.), *Children's Orthopaedics and Fractures*,
DOI 10.1007/978-1-84882-611-3_18, © Springer-Verlag London Limited 2010

histological signs after a few days. Glial cell replacement occurs as the chronic stage of the disease appears. Because of anterior horn cell involvement, there is lower motor neurone paralysis, especially of muscles innervated by the cervical and lumbar enlargements. Flaccid paralysis is present, with normal sensation in the extremities. Intramuscular injection during the acute stage may lead to localization of paralysis in a certain segment of the cord. Similarly, surgery such as tonsillectomy may trigger the appearance of bulbar palsy.

Chronic Stage

Residual paralysis is of varying severity and combinations. The muscles of the lower limb are affected at least four to five times more often than those of the upper limb. The quadriceps, glutei, tibialis anterior, hamstrings, and hip flexors are involved, in descending order of frequency. The intrinsic muscles of the foot are sometimes affected. In the upper limb, the deltoid, triceps, and pectoralis muscles are commonly affected. Trunk muscles are weakened less often.

After the initial stage of muscle irritability and spasm, atrophy and fibrosis set in. Muscle imbalance leads to joint deformity and sometimes dislocation. This is often aggravated by gravity, posture, and subsequent growth of the child. Secondary contracture of the tendons, ligaments, joint capsule, and sometimes the skin, all add to the rigidity of the deformity. Because paralysis occurs in a growing limb, shortening will develop. The bones are thin and sometimes osteoporotic and prone to fracture. The joints may show restricted mobility with possible subluxation or dislocation. Osteoarthritis does not commonly occur unless there has been previous operation or trauma.

The respiratory system may be affected secondary to bulbar palsy or paralysis of the ventilatory muscles (intercostals or diaphragm). Bulbar palsy usually recovers fully.

Recovery Prognosis

Most functional recovery in muscle power occurs within the first few months and is complete by 6 months after the initial illness; theoretically, recovery is possible for up to 2 years. Good prognostic factors for recovery include young age, partial paralysis, and upper extremity involvement. Careful muscle charting, followed by serial assessment during the initial few months, is therefore important as a means of assessing the likelihood of recovery.

Clinical Features

Acute Stage

Acute symptoms include fever and malaise. Symptoms of encephalomyelitis appear within a week: severe headache, vomiting, neck rigidity, meningism, and backache are common. Simultaneously, paralysis of the extremities occurs. Asymmetrical involvement of the lower extremities is the most common pattern. Absence of progression of muscle paralysis heralds the end of the acute phase. Signs during the early stage include muscle spasm, with tenderness on palpation. With impending paralysis of the affected limb, the deep tendon reflex is either exaggerated or decreased. The superficial reflexes are usually absent initially. Irritation may be present, but sensation of the limb is normal.

Upper limb muscle paralysis affects the shoulder girdle more often than the arm. Particular attention must be paid to detecting paralysis of the intercostals and diaphragm. Neck muscle weakness may be associated with difficulty in swallowing. Lower limb muscle paralysis is invariably associated with back and abdominal muscle weakness and the quadriceps are most frequently involved [5]. The acute stage usually lasts 1–2 weeks.

Convalescent Stage

This is the stage in which muscle recovery occurs. It lasts for 2 years after the acute illness. Serial muscle charting is necessary, especially in the first few months, when most of the recovery is expected. Initial examination may be difficult because of muscle pain or spasm. Loss of recovery potential in some muscles may occur if excessive activity is allowed in the early convalescent stage. Contractures of fascia, muscle aponeurosis, and muscle itself begin during this period.

Chronic Stage

No muscle recovery is expected 2 years after the onset of the disease. By then, the orthopaedic surgeon is best placed to utilize residual motor activity. Deformities may be fixed or mobile: with time, some mobile deformities, if neglected, can become fixed. Growth and posture further aggravate the joint deformities. Initially, only the soft tissues are involved, but later secondary changes occur in bone and joint. The younger the patient, the greater the chance of significant deformity [6, 7]. Common deformities in the chronic phase are shown in Table 18.1.

Table 18.1 Common deformities in the chronic phase of poliomyelitis

Site	Lesion	Effect
Upper Limb		
Shoulder	Deltoid paralysis	Weakness of shoulder abduction
Elbow	Flexor paralysis	Inability to flex the elbow
Forearm	Fixed supination	Inability to pronate interfering with the position of the hand in daily activities
Wrist	Extensor weakness	Inability to dorsiflex the wrist
Hand	Intrinsic paralysis	Impaired hand function
Thumb	Thenar muscle loss	Lack of opposition of the thumb
Lower limb		
Hip	Relative overaction of the hip flexors and adductors	Paralytic dislocation
	Contracture of anterior and sometimes lateral structures	Flexion or flexion–abduction contracture
	Gluteal paralysis	Usually mixed extension–abduction weakness
	Extensive weakness of muscles around hip	Flail hip
Knee	Strong hamstrings and weak quadriceps	Flexion contracture
	Contracted ilio-tibial tract	Genu valgum and external tibial torsion
	Weak quadriceps and lax soft tissue at the back of knee	Genu recurvatum
	Extensive paralysis around the knee	Flail knee
Foot and ankle	Weak tibialis anterior and weak tibialis posterior	Equinovalgus contracture
	Weak tibialis posterior only (rare)	Eversion deformity
	Weak tibialis anterior, peronei, and toe extensors	Equinovarus deformity
	Weak triceps surae	Calcaneus deformity
	Overactive long toe extensors (with weak ankle dorsiflexors)	Claw toes
	Overactive long toe flexors (with weak triceps surae)	Pes cavus and calcaneus
	Imbalance between intrinsic and extrinsic foot muscles	Pes cavus
	Shortened muscles affect bone growth	Leg length discrepancy
Trunk		
Spine	Asymmetric paralysis of paraspinal muscles. Ilio-tibial tract contracture and pelvic obliquity	Scoliosis
	Ilio-tibial tract contracture (hip abductor contracture)	Pelvic obliquity
	Leg length discrepancy	
	Scoliosis	
	Weak abdominal muscles	

Diagnosis

The diagnosis of poliomyelitis is largely a clinical one. The prodromal phase is similar to other viral infections of the gastrointestinal or upper respiratory tracts. It may pass unnoticed, especially if it is not followed by neurological problems. The poliomyelitis virus may be found in the throat swab or stool. The diagnosis is usually made at the paralytic stage (see differential diagnosis below). Laboratory investigation shows nonspecific changes, such as a slight increase in the erythrocyte sedimentation rate and a leucocytosis. Lumbar puncture yields clear, pus-free fluid.

There may be an increase in cerebrospinal fluid pressure, together with an increase in the white blood cell count, initially neutrophils, but later lymphocytes. The protein content in the cerebrospinal fluid may increase. Attempts at culture of the poliomyelitis virus from the cerebrospinal fluid are rarely useful, and other sophisticated laboratory tests are impractical. Patients in the chronic stage cease to reveal these changes.

Differential Diagnosis

Acute Stage

- Any cause of meningitis or encephalitis
- Guillain–Barré polyneuritis
- Bone and joint infections
- Pseudoparalysis of whatever cause
- Myalgia or acute paraplegia of whatever cause
- Acute rheumatic fever

Chronic Stage

- Tuberculosis/spinal infection
- Transverse myelitis
- Spinal/spinal cord tumor
- Cerebral palsy
- Talipes equinovarus

Management

General

During the acute stage, the patient is usually under the care of a paediatrician. General, supportive treatment is necessary. Ventilatory failure requires active resuscitation and the prevention of complications. Tracheotomy, assisted ventilation, chest physiotherapy, and antibiotics may be needed, particularly for patients with bulbar involvement who need expert ventilatory monitoring. Bed rest and fluid replacement are necessary, but sedatives should be avoided because they cause further depressant effects.

The orthopaedic surgeon should be involved even in the acute stage. Muscle spasm is relieved by hot packs and contractures are prevented by early splintage of the joints in a functional position. Particular attention should be paid to prevent equinus contracture of the ankles by well-padded ankle–foot splints and deformity of the knees by support with a small roll behind the knees. The hips are protected by keeping the thighs in slight abduction and neutral rotation and the deltoids by holding the arms in mild abduction and neutral rotation. Physiotherapy should be started gently (especially while the irritable stage is subsiding), consisting of gradual gentle stretching of spastic muscles by passively putting the joints through the normal range of motion. In the later stage of the acute phase, assisted muscle exercises lead gradually to an active exercise program.

Management of Established Contractures

Basic Principles

Secondary factors frequently worsen the effects of a primary muscle imbalance, producing fixed contractures. These secondary factors consist of contractures of the joint capsule, aponeurosis, neurovascular bundle, and skin, and deformity of joint surfaces.

Gentle stretching of a joint contracture is very useful, but care must be exercised during manipulation because the osteoporotic bone is prone to fracture or the epiphysis may slip. When the contracture has been fully stretched, the joint is splinted in an overcorrected position but removed from the splint for mobilization every day.

Dynamic splintage is preferred to static splintage. If conservative treatment fails, consideration should be given to surgical correction. The following clinical factors must be taken into account:

- The degree of contracture in the adjacent joints of the ipsilateral limb
- The status of the contralateral limb
- Residual power of the lower limbs as a predictor of independent walking, with or without calipers
- Residual power of the upper limbs (especially triceps function, to enable the patient to use elbow crutches)

As a general rule, older patients with severe deformities respond poorly, but young patients with mild to moderate fixed deformity are suitable candidates for surgery.

Provision of motor power after correction of contractures is important in management. This requires the application of the basic principles of tendon surgery [8], sometimes in combination with bony stabilization procedures (preferably delayed until bone maturity).

Orthotic splintage is necessary not only to keep the manipulated joint in the overcorrected position to prevent recurrence of deformity but also to augment weak muscles and to protect paralyzed muscles from overstretching. Tendon transfers should also be protected from overstretching in the first few months after surgery.

Upper Limbs

Shoulder

The most common upper limb muscle that is paralyzed in poliomyelitis is the deltoid, followed by the elbow flexors and extensors. In the hand, the opponens pollicis is the most often involved [9]. Reconstructive procedures for the shoulder are not indicated unless there is good function of the arm, forearm, and hand [10].

Deltoid Paralysis

The deltoid and the clavicular head of the pectoralis major are the two prime movers of the shoulder joint. Paralysis of the deltoid results in the loss of abduction power. Deltoid paralysis is usually partial, with sparing of the posterior portion, and therefore transfer of trapezius is recommended [11]. However, multiple muscle transplantation in stages may be necessary (depending upon the remaining muscle power) using the clavicular fibers of pectoralis major, the remaining posterior portion of deltoid, the origin of the long head of triceps and the short head of biceps, latissimus dorsi, and teres major [12–15]. The possible transfers are detailed in Table 18.2.

Shoulder Arthrodesis

Extensive muscle paralysis around the shoulder causes subluxation or dislocation. When this becomes symptomatic, shoulder arthrodesis may be considered, provided that

- good scapulothoracic control by trapezius and serratus anterior compensates for the loss of glenohumeral movement
- the limb functions well distal to the shoulder

The exact position of shoulder arthrodesis is controversial; the position should allow the hand to reach the face for feeding and cleaning and the perineum for toileting.

Table 18.2 Possible substitute by transfer

Muscle paralyzed	Substitution
Subscapularis	Superior portion of serratus anterior
Supraspinatus	Levator scapulae or sterno-cleidomastoid
Subscapularis/infraspinatus	Latissimus dorsi or teres major
Serratus anterior paralysis	Pectoralis minor by posterior transfer

Excellent results are generally seen in patients with good elbow and hand function [12, 16–18]. The recommended position for children is 45° of abduction, 25° of flexion, and 25° of internal rotation [19]. Rowe recommended fusion in 20° of abduction, 30° of flexion, and 40° of internal rotation for adults. Major disability in any patient who has had an arthrodesis of the shoulder is related to the lack of internal rotation as it is important for the arm to reach the midline [20]. The angle of abduction should be determined by the angle between the shaft of humerus and the vertebral border of the scapula instead of the angle between the arm and the lateral thoracic wall.

Elbow

Flexor Paralysis

Loss of elbow flexion power is very disabling because the patient cannot bring the hand to the head and mouth. Treatment of elbow flexor paralysis is indicated only if the patient has good hand function. The spread of neurological involvement of the whole upper limb and the associated functional loss should be assessed in detail before planning any surgery. Reconstruction of the hand should precede procedures at the elbow. Weakness of the muscles around the shoulder and wrist are contraindications to reconstruction.

The most commonly used substitute for the elbow flexors is the wrist flexor mass (Steindler's flexorplasty) [21], in which the medial epicondyle and the origin of the wrist flexors are transferred proximally to the lower humerus. Possible complications include the development of a fixed pronation deformity and a mild flexion contracture of the elbow. Failure of the operation may be due to initially weak wrist flexors or poor fixation of the medial epicondyle to the humerus. A posterior bone block operation may prevent a weak elbow flexor from becoming overstretched.

When Steindler's flexorplasty is not feasible, other muscle transfers may be considered to reconstitute elbow flexion. The muscles that have been used include the whole group of pectoralis major (Brooks–Seddon procedure), sternal head of pectoralis major (Clark's procedure), latissimus dorsi (Hovnanian procedure), and triceps (Table 18.3) [22, 23].

Triceps Paralysis

Gravity assists elbow extension and thus partly compensates for loss of triceps function. However, when active, forceful elbow extension is needed, as in crutch walking or transferring from bed, strong extension is needed. Possible transfers include brachio-radialis or latissimus dorsi. The latissimus dorsi has a long neurovascular bundle, making mobilization of the muscle easy.

Table 18.3 Transfers to produce elbow flexion

Muscle transfer	Comment
All of pectoralis major muscle (Brooks–Seddon procedure)	Clavicular portion of pectoralis major must be strong. Used when the biceps brachii is completely paralyzed. Muscle control of shoulder and scapula must be good
Sternal head of pectoralis major (Clark's procedure)	Used when the clavicular portion of pectoralis major is paralyzed
Pectoralis minor	Used when pectoralis major and biceps are paralyzed. A fascia lata graft is necessary to bridge the gap
Sterno-clavicular head of sterno-cleidomastoid muscle	Fascia lata graft to bridge the gap; may cause webbing of the neck
Latissimus dorsi muscle (Hovnanian procedure)	Provides good cross-sectional area and strength for the transfer. Origin of latissimus dorsi transplanted into biceps tendon
Triceps anterior transfer	Indicated when other transfers are not feasible. Active extension of the elbow may be weakened

Forearm

Pronator Contracture

Supination is restored by transferring pronator teres and flexor carpi radialis around the ulnar border and the dorsum of the forearm to the radio-volar aspect of the radius.

Supinator Contracture

This is usually associated with a strong biceps. When there is insufficient power for tendon transfer, osteotomy of both forearm bones and stabilization in an overcorrected position are necessary. The alternatives for fixed deformity include interosseous membrane release, release of the radio-ulnar joints, and biceps lengthening.

Wrist

Wrist drop develops if the wrist dorsiflexors are involved; it can be controlled by a splint. If this improves finger function, a wrist arthrodesis may be indicated.

Fingers

Clawing of the fingers is the result of intrinsic muscle paralysis. The thumb lacks active opposition because of involvement of opponens and the short abductor muscles. The classical Bunnell transfer is sometimes helpful in providing opposition, but the flexor digitorum sublimis that is to be transferred from the middle or ring finger must have at

least Medical Research Council (MRC) grade 4 power. The remaining profundus muscle must be strong enough to flex the finger [24, 25].

Lower Limbs

The aim of surgery in the lower limb is to provide a stable, balanced gait, with or without a caliper. Muscle contracture and imbalance, contracture of intermuscular septa and fasciae, shortened tendons, and retardation of bone growth all contribute to difficulty in walking. The patient presents with an abnormal gait. Examination of the lower extremities should concentrate on the presence and extent of fixed or mobile deformity, the range of motion of the joints, residual muscle power, leg length discrepancy (both real and apparent), and concomitant pelvic obliquity. Lower limb deformities are usually multiple, so good initial documentation is necessary, followed by careful planning. In general, the hip problems, usually a contracture, should be dealt with first. Sometimes, deformities can inhibit a weakened muscle, and release of such deformities places the weakened muscle in a mechanically more advantageous position [26–28].

Hip

Flexion or Flexion–Abduction Contracture

The offending structure is usually a contracted ilio-tibial tract and lateral intermuscular septum. This tether is very often associated with an anterior soft tissue contracture (rectus femoris, tensor fasciae latae, sartorius, ilio-psoas, and the

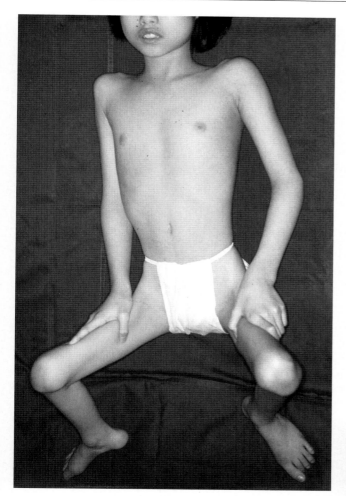

Fig. 18.1 A patient with flexion–abduction contractures of both hips

with hip extended and knee flexed. This method reduces the movement of the pelvis that may occur when the patient is lying on his side [30].

Unilateral or asymmetrical abduction contracture will produce a pelvic obliquity and lumbosacral scoliosis and the contralateral hip is prone to subluxate. In addition to this, a contracted ilio-tibial tract will also produce a flexion and valgus deformity of the knee joint in association with external tibial torsion (Fig. 18.2) [31, 32]. In severe cases, posterolateral subluxation of the knee joint may occur. Another sequel of the external tibial torsion is the compensatory varus deformity of the foot which will disappear after the tibial torsion is corrected [33]. If the soft tissue contractures and muscle imbalance are not treated, further secondary bony deformities will progress with growth.

Surgical release of anterior soft tissue contracture can be achieved proximally with Ober's fasciotomy and distally with Yount's procedure [29, 34]. In mild cases, distal release with sectioning of the ilio-tibial tract together with a portion of the lateral intermuscular septum alone is simple and effective. If adequate correction cannot be obtained with the distal release in more severe contracture, Ober's procedure can be performed at the same time. The contracted muscles that must be released include tensor fasciae latae, gluteus

hip capsule), further aggravated by weakness of hip extension (gluteus maximus) and hip abduction (gluteus medius) (Fig. 18.1).

The ilio-tibial tract lies anterior to the hip and posterior to the knee joint and therefore produces a flexion contracture of the hip and knee. The Ober test is performed to elicit an abduction contracture [29]. The patient lies on his normal side, with the thigh on the examination couch and the hip and knee flexed enough to obliterate any lumbar lordosis. The knee of the affected leg is flexed to a right angle and the hip initially in a flexed position. The examiner grasps the ankle lightly with one hand and steadies the patient's pelvis with the other. The affected leg is extended so that the thigh is in line with the body. If there is any abduction contracture, the leg will move into abduction. This tight band can be easily felt with the examining fingers between the crest of the ilium and the anterior aspect of the trochanter. The Ober test can be modified by putting the patient in the prone position; the amount of hip abduction tightness can be assessed

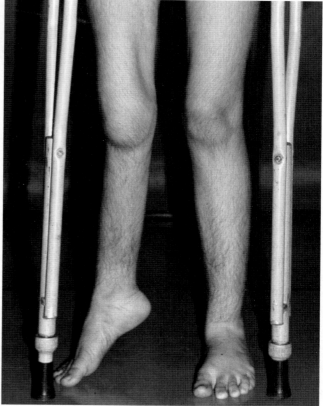

Fig. 18.2 External tibial torsion as a result of contracted ilio-tibial tract

medius and minimus, sartorius, rectus femoris, and the anterior hip capsule. Release must be followed by serial casting, with the hip in progressive adduction and extension and the knee straight.

Gluteal Paralysis

Weakness of hip abduction (gluteus medius and minimus) produces a positive Trendelenburg sign. This can be treated by the Mustard procedure [35]. When both gluteus medius and maximus are paralyzed, hip abduction and extension are weak. There is also forward tilting of the pelvis (backward body lurch) in addition to a Trendelenburg sign. Under such circumstances, the Sharrard transfer of ilio-psoas is preferred [36]. The ilio-psoas transfer forms part of the treatment of paralytic dislocation of hip in poliomyelitis. It should not be forgotten that hip flexion is weakened by the transfer.

Ilio-psoas transfer by the Mustard and Sharrard procedures is useful for patients with partial gluteal paralysis. It will improve stability during walking and thus the gait. Good abdominal muscle strength and a powerful sartorius, which becomes a primary hip flexor later, are important prerequisites.

The aim of the Mustard procedure is to transfer the ilio-psoas to augment hip abduction. The ilio-psoas, with its bony attachment, is isolated via a standard Smith–Peterson approach. The muscle is passed through a bony notch between the anterior superior and inferior iliac spines, to be attached to the greater trochanter. Post-operative immobilization of the hip in abduction is necessary.

In the Sharrard procedure, the ilio-psoas is transferred posterior and lateral to the hip joint through a large window in the ilium adjacent to the sacro-iliac joint [26, 27, 36]. The tendon is advanced through a tunnel in the greater trochanter to its anterolateral surface. This procedure is more extensive and technically more difficult than the Mustard procedure, but may be appropriate for patients with weakened hip extension. Prior anterior soft tissue release, abductor tenotomy and concomitant varus osteotomy of the hip may be required. From our experience, both transfers (Sharrard and Mustard) seldom produce strong abduction power but prevent the hip from redislocation by a tenodesis effect.

External Oblique Transfer

This muscle may be transferred to the greater trochanter in patients suffering from gluteus medius paralysis in whom the ilio-psoas is not suitable for transfer.

Tensor Fasciae Latae Transfer

This muscle can be transferred posteriorly for gluteus medius weakness and hip instability when no other muscles are suitable for transfer [27, 28].

Erector Spinae Transfer

This procedure is occasionally used for gluteus maximus weakness [37].

Paralytic Poliomyelitic Hip Subluxation and Dislocation

There are two groups of patients with subluxation or dislocation in poliomyelitis. The first group is due to muscle imbalance [38]. Initially, the hip adductors and flexors overpower the abductors and extensors. Subsequently, bony factors develop in the form of femoral neck valgus and increased anteversion. The acetabulum becomes shallow and oblique as the patient begins to bear weight, stretching the capsule, and allowing the femoral head to subluxate or dislocate. Pelvic obliquity aggravates this process, the hip on the higher side adducting and displacing (Fig. 18.3).

Both soft tissue and skeletal factors have to be dealt with. Concentric reduction of the hip is achieved by either closed or open reduction. Traction is often required for late cases before open reduction, especially after 3 years of age.

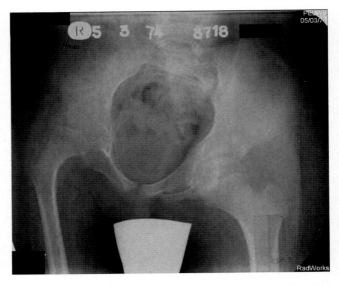

Fig. 18.3 Right hip subluxation. The right hip is adducted with resulting pelvic obliquity. Note the right hemipelvic and femoral hypoplasia

The muscle imbalance must be corrected by appropriate tendon transfers, but should be deferred until bony deformities have been corrected [38, 39]. Both upper femoral varus derotation osteotomy (sometimes with shortening of the femur to decrease the tension on the reduced femoral head) and acetabular reconstruction are required; alternatively, redirection by innominate osteotomy or increase in femoral head coverage by the use of a Chiari osteotomy may be indicated, depending upon the configuration of the acetabular defect. Acetabular reorientation procedures are often inappropriate because the acetabulum has "wandered" superiorly and laterally. Any associated predisposing cause of subluxation such as pelvic obliquity must be dealt with to prevent recurrence. Hip arthrodesis is seldom indicated for paralytic dislocation unless there is articular degeneration and painful impingement.

In the second group of patients, the hip subluxation or dislocation is provoked by pelvic obliquity with resulting poor coverage of the higher hip. Correcting the pelvic obliquity alone may improve the containment of the hip in some patients. Additional procedures to correct the excessive femoral anteversion and coxa valga and to improve the acetabular coverage may be needed if the reduction is still unsatisfactory after the pelvic obliquity is corrected.

The Flail Hip

Lack of muscle power around the hip is often associated with major paralysis distally. Multiple orthotic devices may be necessary to allow standing and walking. The flail hip seldom dislocates and is usually asymptomatic unless it is associated with pelvic obliquity, usually a sequel to paralytic lumbar scoliosis. Arthrodesis of a flail hip is associated with many disadvantages and is generally reserved as a salvage procedure. Sharp et al. [40] reported a high incidence of femoral fracture and pseudoarthrosis. Hallock showed good pain relief after hip fusion in poliomyelitic patients with arthritic hip subluxation or dislocation and improved stability in hips that have extensive muscle weakness [39, 41, 42].

Pelvic Obliquity

This can be produced by contracture above the pelvis when lumbar or thoraco-lumbar scoliosis is produced by asymmetrical paralysis of the quadratus lumborum and oblique abdominal muscles (Fig. 18.4). Below the pelvis, a contracture of the ilio-tibial tract causes ipsilateral downward tilting of the pelvis followed by contracture of the trunk muscles on the contralateral side. A lumbar scoliosis and hip subluxation are further aggravated by an adduction contracture with apparent shortening of the opposite leg. The

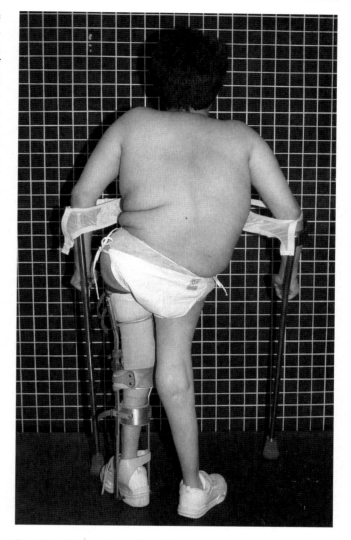

Fig. 18.4 This patient suffered from severe lumbar scoliosis with marked pelvic obliquity

treatment of pelvic obliquity is directed at the cause and any fixed secondary deformities, if present. [43] Lee, Choi, et al. [44] classified the pelvic obliquity in poliomyelitis into two major types and four subtypes depending upon the side of the shorter leg. In type I, the pelvis is lower on the side of the short leg and in type II it is raised. In type I, ipsilateral abductor release and contralateral lumbodorsal fasciotomy are recommended to correct the deformity. Type II deformities are less common. Contralateral abductor fasciotomy is undertaken first if an abduction contracture is present. This is followed by triple pelvic osteotomy with transiliac lengthening and ipsilateral lumbodorsal fasciotomy if the higher hip is not sufficiently stable or the correction of pelvic obliquity is inadequate.

The Knee

The most common deformity of the knee is fixed flexion deformity of varying severity. Other deformities are genu recurvatum, genu valgum, and, rarely, genu varum.

Knee Flexion Contracture

The causes of fixed flexion contracture include ilio-tibial tract contracture and quadriceps paralysis in the presence of normal hamstrings. Genu valgum and external rotation of the tibia coexist because of ilio-tibial tract contracture and a strong biceps femoris with weak medial hamstrings. Posterior subluxation of the tibia may also occur secondary to muscle imbalance. This is one of the factors limiting serial plaster correction of fixed-knee deformities so this technique should be used only in mild cases (Fig. 18.5) [45].

Knee flexion contracture places the knee at a mechanical disadvantage. The weak quadriceps fails to compensate for the loss of the locking mechanism that occurs in the slight knee hyperextension during the stance phase of gait. In order to prevent the knee buckling during walking, the patient may require a "hand on the knee" gait (Fig. 18.6). A Yount fasciotomy of the ilio-tibial tract may be necessary [34]. Flexion contracture of moderate to severe degree is difficult to treat. Secondary adaptive changes are present in the form of flattening of the articular surface and disproportionate increase in growth of the anterior portion of the tibia and femur compared with the posterior portion. This further increases the chance of posterior subluxation of the tibia upon the femur. Supracondylar osteotomy is preferred to soft tissue release in

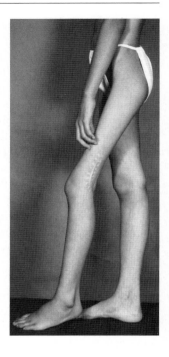

Fig. 18.6 Mild knee flexion contracture. The patient walked with a hand-on-knee gait

the presence of secondary bony changes; it can correct any valgus deformity that coexists [46].

Surgical correction of severe flexion contracture may require staged procedures; the results are usually better in children. Initial posterior capsulotomy and ilio-tibial tract release, including division of the posterior cruciate ligament, and skeletal traction or casting may be necessary. A supracondylar osteotomy with or without shortening of the bone is required in the second stage. A good range of knee flexion is important for success (Fig. 18.7) [46].

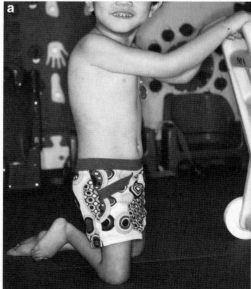
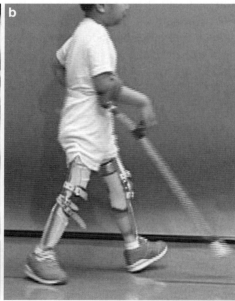

Fig. 18.5 (a) This boy had severe knee flexion contractures and had to walk on his knees. (b) He managed to walk with a pair of calipers after correction of the deformity

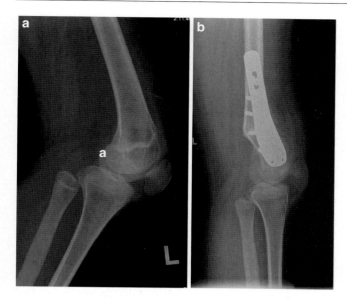

Fig. 18.7 (**a**) Knee flexion contracture was secondary to quadriceps weakness and was too severe to be corrected by soft tissue release alone. (**b**) Supracondylar extension osteotomy with plate and screws fixation to allow earlier mobilization. The knee is overcorrected to produce slight recurvatum which will improve the stability of the knee during stance

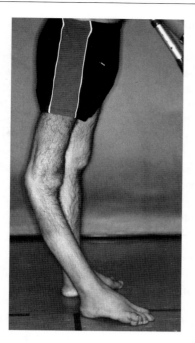

Fig. 18.8 Severe knee recurvatum

Genu Recurvatum

Mild genu recurvatum is common and is not disabling. In early cases, it results from overstretching of the posterior knee structures and later on, secondary bony changes occur with progressive flattening of the anterior aspect of both upper tibia and femoral condyles.

When the triceps surae is normal in the presence of paralysis of the quadriceps and hamstrings, the knee cannot be locked in neutral extension. The ground reaction force pushes the tibia posteriorly and the knee hyperextends in the stance phase of gait. The weight-bearing area of the knee joint is shifted anteriorly, and with time, the tibial plateau slopes downward and forward. This deformity can be corrected by wedge osteotomy of the proximal tibia. Mehta and Mukherjee [47] reported successful correction of the knee recurvatum with a distal femoral flexion osteotomy in patients with flattening of the anterior condyles.

When there is weakness in both the triceps surae and hamstrings, the knee hyperextends and the posterior structures stretch (Fig. 18.8). Gait is poor because of lack of push-off by the calf muscles. This type of recurvatum progresses more rapidly due to lack of dynamic support posteriorly, and early long-leg bracing is necessary [48]. Triple tenodesis, described by Perry et al. [49], utilizes the posterior capsule, semitendinosus, gracilis, biceps tendon, and the anterior half of ilio-tibial band and works well if the posterior soft tissues are protected until they are fully mature and any ankle equinus deformity corrected to the neutral position [49]. A posterior tenodesis may stretch if used alone to block hyperextension of the knee. An anterior bone block utilizing the patella can be used to prevent progressive increase of hyperextension. Men et al. [50] reported long-term good results with the anterior bone block. Knee arthrodesis is usually considered as a salvage procedure.

Quadriceps paralysis is common. With adequate power of the hamstring and triceps surae or the presence of mild ankle equinus, the knee will be locked and stabilized in hyperextension in the stance phase of gait. Lengthening of the contracted triceps surae in a patient with quadriceps paralysis should be done cautiously as it may result in loss of this stabilization mechanism. Anterior hamstring transfer is reserved for the potentially brace-free patient with good hip flexion and extension power. The presence of an adequate triceps surae is essential to prevent the development of knee recurvatum deformity after the transfer. Transfer of both biceps femoris and semitendinosus is the preferred combination, although other muscles such as adductor longus and sartorius have also been utilized. Lateral dislocation of the patella is a troublesome complication following the transfer of biceps femoris alone [51, 52].

Flail Knee

The knee is very unstable and can be supported with an above-knee orthosis and a drop-lock. Arthrodesis will free the patient from the additional weight of an orthosis and is indicated for skeletally mature patients whose work is strenuous [53].

Foot and Ankle

A stable, plantigrade foot is required for normal walking. The foot affected by poliomyelitis may be unstable and muscle imbalance produces various combinations of deformity, which become structural with time. Plantar flexion/dorsiflexion imbalance produces equinus/calcaneus deformity at the ankle joint, whereas invertor/evertor imbalance produces varus/valgus deformity at the subtalar joint. Tendon release or transfer is useful and is the main method of treatment for a flexible deformity before bony maturity [27, 28, 54]. Bony resection and stabilization are indicated after skeletal maturity and are often best performed just before tendon transfer.

Dorsiflexor and Invertor Insufficiency

This is caused by tibialis anterior paralysis. The foot assumes an equinovalgus posture in the swing phase (Fig. 18.9). The proximal phalanges hyperextend and the metatarsal heads depress with resulting cock-up deformity due to overactivity of the toe extensors attempting to compensate for the loss of ankle dorsiflexion power. The unopposed triceps surae becomes contracted with resulting equinus deformity. The tibialis anterior dorsiflexes the first metatarsal and the peroneus longus plantar flexes it. Unopposed peroneus longus action will pronate the first ray and result in cavus deformity, the hindfoot being driven into varus during standing.

Early equinus can be corrected with intensive stretching of the tight structures behind the ankle followed by night time splintage. In more severe equinus deformity, posterior ankle capsulotomy and release of the subtalar joint are effective.

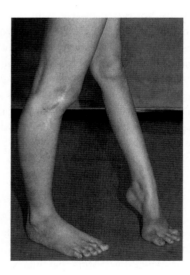

Fig. 18.9 Ankle equinus as a result of ankle dorsiflexor insufficiency

Lengthening of the Achilles tendon is best avoided whenever possible in order not to weaken the triceps surae. Loss of plantar flexion power results in major functional disability. Dorsiflexion power of the ankle can be restored with anterior transfer of the peroneus longus to the base of the second metatarsal. The peroneus brevis is sutured to the distal stump of peroneus longus to preserve its remaining tension on the first metatarsal. Active dorsiflexor power can be further improved by transferring the extensor digitorum longus to the dorsum of the midfoot or to the neck of the metatarsal for correction of claw toe deformity at the same time (Jones procedure).

Plantar release will improve the cavus deformity in early cases and first metatarsal or tarsal dorsal closing wedge osteotomy may be needed if secondary bony changes occur. If the deformity is associated with fixed hindfoot varus, it is corrected with a lateral closing wedge or lateral translation osteotomy of the os calcis. Joint fusion in the foot is avoided if possible to prevent the development of premature degeneration in adjacent joints. Good balancing of motor power across the joint by muscle transfer is important to achieve a good result and to prevent the recurrence of deformity. Triple arthrodesis (Lambrinudi modification) or subtalar joint fusion is needed if both peroneal tendons are utilized for transfer, thus avoiding subtalar instability.

Paralysis of tibialis anterior and tibialis posterior results in equinovalgus deformity. The peroneus longus is transferred to the base of the second metatarsal to replace the action of tibialis anterior. The flexor hallucis longus or flexor digitorum longus can be transferred to the tibialis posterior tendon.

Isolated tibialis posterior paralysis is rare. An eversion deformity results. Tendon transfer using flexor hallucis longus, flexor digitorum longus, or extensor hallucis longus has been successful.

Evertor Insufficiency

Isolated evertor insufficiency is rare. It usually occurs in association with paralysis of the long toe extensors and tibialis anterior.

In pure peroneal palsy, the hindfoot inverts and the forefoot adducts. The deforming force is the tibialis anterior which produces a dorsal elevation of the distal part of the first metatarsal and a dorsal bunion (Fig. 18.10). Lateral transfer of the tibialis anterior to the base of second metatarsal will correct a mild, flexible deformity. Fixed first metatarsal deformity requires osteotomy at its base, whereas hindfoot deformity requires a triple arthrodesis. Sometimes when the extensor hallucis longus overacts after tibialis anterior transfer, it may need transfer to the first metatarsal with interphalangeal fusion or tenodesis (Robert–Jones operation).

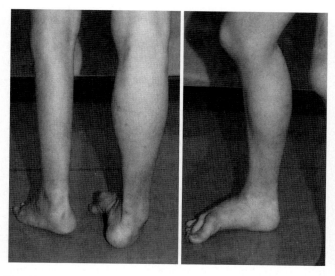

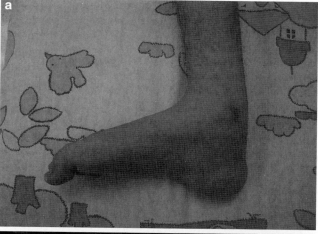

Fig. 18.10 Pes varus due to evertor insufficiency. The unopposed tibialis posterior inverts the hindfoot and the strong tibialis anterior elevates the first metatarsal and produces a dorsal bunion

Weakness of both peronei and long toe extensors produces a mild equinovarus deformity and treatment is the same as for pure evertor insufficiency. Paralysis of peronei, long toe extensors, and tibialis anterior produces a severe equinovarus deformity. The tibialis posterior and triceps surae are the deforming forces, and anterior transfer of the tibialis posterior to the base of the third metatarsal is effective. It may be augmented by prior soft tissue release of the cavus and anterior transfer of the long toe flexors.

Triceps Surae Paralysis

Triceps surae paralysis produces a calcaneus deformity. There is a lack of push-off during the gait cycle and the weight of the body cannot be transferred effectively to the metatarsal heads. Active ankle dorsiflexion, in the absence of a strong triceps surae, stretches the triceps surae and the posterior ankle capsule. The ankle joint is dorsiflexed with the head of talus and anterior part of os calcis displaced upward. The plantar flexors, namely, tibialis posterior, peronei, and long toe flexors, overact in an attempt to plantarflex the hindfoot, cause depression of the metatarsal heads, and produce a calcaneocavus deformity. The short toe flexors and plantar fascia will become contracted and act as a bowstring to pull the forefoot and os calcis together, resulting in further aggravation of the calcaneocavus deformity.

The posterior lever arm of the os calcis decreases as the os calcis become more dorsiflexed and vertical. This puts the weakened triceps surae in a mechanically unsounded position with further aggravation of dorsiflexion and plantar flexion imbalance. The loss of the normal contour of the heel results in a "pistol grip" deformity (Fig. 18.11).

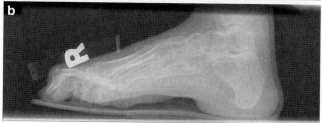

Fig. 18.11 (**a**) Calcaneal deformity with the typical "pistol grip" appearance due to weakness of triceps surae. (**b**) Radiograph of a calcaneal foot

Treatment of Calcaneus Ankle and Foot Deformities

Early splintage and a muscle exercise program are used to achieve maximal recovery of muscle power and to prevent the calcaneus deformity. An orthosis may be necessary to assist plantar flexion at the ankle and to limit dorsiflexion.

In the skeletally immature foot, "push-off" power can be helped by multiple tendon transfers such as tibialis posterior, the peronei and, rarely, tibialis anterior to the os calcis [55]. The plantar aponeurosis and intrinsic muscles should be released.

In the skeletally mature foot, bony resection and arthrodesis of the hindfoot are necessary before tendon transfer, usually after an interval of 6 weeks. With gross instability, a pantalar arthrodesis may be indicated. This is usually undertaken in patients with associated paralysis in order to eliminate the use of a caliper.

Tendon Transfer in Calcaneal Deformities

Invertor and evertor balance must be achieved during tendon transfer for calcaneal deformity. Calcaneocavus deformity is controlled by transfer of both peroneus brevis and tibialis posterior to the heel. Calcaneo-cavovalgus deformity requires transfer of both peronei. For the mobile calcaneal deformity, translocation of the peroneus longus into a groove on the posterior aspect of the os calcis is sometimes useful. The hamstrings have also been used to replace triceps surae function. Transfer of the tibialis anterior posteriorly through the interosseous membrane is advocated for younger patients with a flexible deformity [55].

Other Procedures for Calcaneal Foot Deformity

Calcaneal Osteotomy

Cavovarus deformity in a growing child may benefit from a calcaneal osteotomy. The os calcis can also be displaced posteriorly during the osteotomy [56].

Talectomy

This is indicated only when arthrodesis cannot be performed. The result is satisfactory for pain relief and cosmesis. Tibiocalcaneal fusion is necessary if talectomy fails [57, 58].

Elmslie's Procedure

This is a two-stage operation. Initially, soft tissue release and dorsal wedge excision of the talonavicular and calcaneocuboid joints correct the cavus deformity. This is followed by a second-stage posterior wedge excision of the subtalar joint, with the base of the wedge posteriorly to correct the calcaneal deformity. The Achilles tendon is shortened and tenodesed to the posterior aspect of the tibia. The long toe flexors are cut and sutured to the Achilles tendon.

Forefoot Equinus

A mobile forefoot equinus needs splintage only. Structural forefoot equinus deformity (plantaris) requires release of the plantar aponeurosis and wedge resection of the midfoot to enable the foot to be fitted with an orthosis.

Arthrodesis for Foot and Ankle Deformities

The most commonly practiced procedures are extra-articular subtalar arthrodesis and triple arthrodesis. Bone block procedures and ankle arthrodesis are now seldom performed.

Extra-articular Subtalar Arthrodesis

The Grice–Green extra-articular subtalar arthrodesis aims to correct hindfoot valgus in the supple foot (Fig. 18.12) [6, 59, 60]. The procedure was performed in young children to preserve the growth potential of the foot by avoiding injury to the preosseous cartilage. A tibial cortical graft was used as the strut in the sinus tarsi with good initial results. Graft complications and unsatisfactory later results led to the introduction of modifications of the original procedure with improved fixation and graft sources. A fibular graft inserted from the neck of talus through the sinus tarsi was devised by Batchelor, but a high rate of nonunion has been reported (Fig. 18.13) [61–65]. Dennyson and Fulford modified the Batchelor procedure by replacing the fibular graft with a screw and adding cancellous grafts into the sinus tarsi [66]. A combined Batchelor–Grice technique, using cancellous graft from the iliac crest with a fibular graft, was reported by Jaffray et al. [67] to achieve a 96% union rate and eliminated problems related to the presence of a screw (Fig. 18.14). The modified procedures reduced the occurrence of post-operative hindfoot varus deformity, which can produce a painful callosity over the lateral border of the foot.

Mosca has popularized the calcaneal lengthening osteotomy (first described by Evans in 1975) as an alternative for treatment of hindfoot valgus in neuromuscular patients [68]. However, in the authors' unpublished series of similar procedures, some loss of early correction was seen at mid-term follow-up. The procedure preserves the mobility of the subtalar joints and theoretically should reduce the

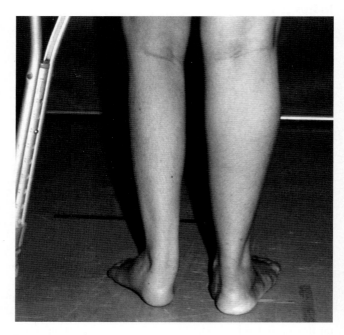

Fig. 18.12 Planovalgus deformity due to weakness of tibialis posterior

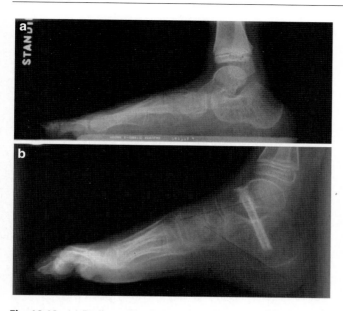

Fig. 18.13 (a) Radiographs of planovalgus foot. Note the increase of the talocalcaneal angle. (b) Batchelor type of extra-articular subtalar fusion. The fibular graft is inserted through the neck of talus

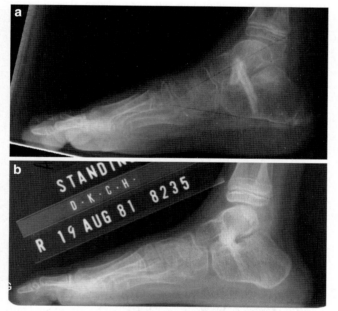

Fig. 18.14 (a) Combined Batchelor–Grice extra-articular subtalar fusion. Cortico-cancellous graft is inserted into the sinus tarsi in addition to the fibular graft. (b) Radiograph at 1 year after surgery. Note the fusion mass at sinus tarsi

incidence of adjacent joint degeneration. The procedure is not suitable in patients with complete paralysis or significant imbalance of the ankle invertors and evertors which cannot be corrected.

Standing radiographs of the foot and ankle are necessary to determine the site of the valgus deformity, which is occasionally present in the ankle.

Triple Arthrodesis

This operation is frequently performed for equinovalgus or varus deformity after the child has reached the age of 10 years [69]. The subtalar, calcaneocuboid, and talonavicular joints are resected and arthrodesed. Bony wedges are taken out to produce a plantigrade foot. Modifications of this procedure include posterior displacement of the foot to improve the mechanical advantage of the weakened triceps surae and the Lambrinudi arthrodesis for severe and rigid equinus deformity [70]. Any rotational malalignment of the limb must be considered before the triple arthrodesis in order to avoid malalignment of the foot during the procedure. The talonavicular joint is prone to nonunion and avascular necrosis of the talus may occur because of excessive resection [69]. The pseudoarthrosis rate has been reduced significantly in later reports because of improved fixation techniques. Residual deformity is not uncommon but does not result in significant symptoms. Late osteoarthritis of the ankle and midtarsal joints may develop secondary to stiffening of the hindfoot and ankle ligament laxity [71]. Although recurrence of hindfoot deformity is rare, secondary forefoot deformity may occur because of muscle imbalance. Nowadays, multiple osteotomies to correct the midfoot and hindfoot deformities are preferred to triple arthrodesis. The procedure is reserved for salvage in recurrent deformities and in chronic foot deformities associated with degenerative changes. For recurrent and severe deformities, gradual correction following osteotomies with the Ilizarov external fixation has been advocated [72].

Ankle and Pantalar Arthrodesis

Both procedures are seldom performed for poliomyelitis [69]. The flail foot is an indication for such a fusion and it will eliminate the need for an orthosis. A strong gluteus maximus (to extend the hip) and good hamstrings and posterior knee capsule (to prevent hyperextension of the knee) are prerequisites. The ankle has to be fused in 5° of equinus which will help to keep the knee in slight hyperextension during stance. A preoperative weight-bearing lateral radiograph will demonstrate talar subluxation in cases where pantalar arthrodesis is indicated.

Toes

There are three common causes for claw toe deformity (hyperextension of the metatarsophalangeal joint and flexion of the interphalangeal joints):

1. Loss of ankle dorsiflexion. The clawing is noticeable during the swing phase, as the long toe extensors try to compensate for the loss of ankle dorsiflexion power. Restoration of ankle dorsiflexion cures the clawing if it is still mobile.
2. Loss of ankle plantar flexion. The clawing is noticeable during stance phase, as the long toe flexors try to compensate for loss of ankle plantar flexion power. Restoration of active plantar flexion will eliminate the clawing.
3. Clawing associated with a cavus foot. The prime object is to treat the cavus. Intrinsic weakness is often present.

Clawing of the big toe can be dealt with by transferring the extensor hallucis longus tendon to the neck of the first ray (Jones operation). The interphalangeal joint of the big toe needs to be arthrodesed [73].

Clawing of the other toes as a result of the long toe flexors overacting may need a flexor to extensor transfer.

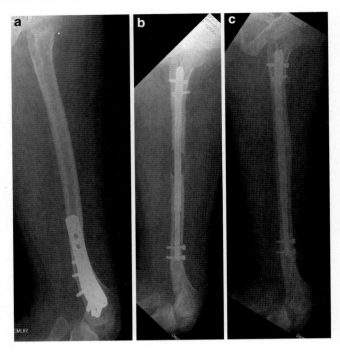

Fig. 18.15 (**a**) This patient had a previous supracondylar osteotomy for knee flexion contracture. She has 4.5 cm of left lower limb shortening (**b**) Femoral lengthening of 4 cm with intramedullary skeletal kinetic device in process. (**c**) Radiograph 1 year after surgery

Leg Length Discrepancy

Leg length discrepancy is common in patients with poliomyelitis [74, 75]. The limb shortening can be apparent due to pelvic obliquity and deformity of the limb. The treatment of apparent leg length discrepancy should be directed to the deformity and its correction should be carefully planned, taking into consideration the effects of the deformity upon gait. True leg length discrepancy is usually the result of asymmetric involvement of the lower limbs. From the authors' experience, leg lengthening in selected patients will improve the gait (Fig. 18.15). It is important to remember that the ankle equinus which originally compensated for the shortening should not be corrected past neutral if the quadriceps muscle is weak.

Post-poliomyelitis Syndrome

The post-poliomyelitis syndrome is characterized by the development of new muscle weakness, muscle fatigability, pain, and depression in patients who have recovered from paralytic poliomyelitis. The patients should have suffered from poliomyelitis with partial or complete neurological recovery but recovered sufficiently to enjoy good function and neurological stability for several decades (usually more than 20 years) [76]. The diagnosis is made after other medical, orthopaedic, and neurological conditions are excluded. The prevalence reported in the literature is 20–80%.

The exact pathogenesis of the syndrome is still not certain [77–80]. The most likely cause is distal degeneration of the enlarged post-poliomyelitis motor unit. Ageing, with motor neuron loss, overuse, and disuse could be the contributing factors. Viral replication and reactivation have been suggested but have never been confirmed.

There is no specific treatment for the syndrome. Drugs such as pyridostigmine and steroids have been tried in randomized studies with no proven effect on the improvement of the symptoms. A multidisciplinary approach with emphasis upon muscle strengthening, the use of assistive devices in daily activities, and control of body weight may help to manage the symptoms. Intermittent breaks can be introduced into daily activities. Physical training has been recommended to counteract fatigue but may itself worsen the weakness.

Spinal Deformity

Scoliosis is a common sequel of poliomyelitis [81, 82]. Kyphosis is relatively rare. Post-poliomyelitic scoliosis is due to imbalance between the trunk and the intercostal muscles in the growing child. Curvature can be due to asymmetrical paralysis of trunk muscles or extensive symmetrical paralysis resulting in a collapsing spine. Six types of curves are commonly seen:

1. High thoracic curve: this is extremely unsightly and the prognosis is poor.
2. Thoracic curve: this is usually a long curve associated with an angular rib hump.
3. Lumbar curve: this is usually associated with pelvic obliquity, impaired sitting balance, and asymmetric ischial pressure. The hip on the high side may subluxate.
4. Double major curve: this is uncommon.
5. Long C curve: the entire trunk is involved, with the apex at the thoraco-lumbar junction.
6. Collapsing spine: the entire trunk sags because of extensive muscle involvement and the effect of gravity. The patient supports himself on the upper limbs holding onto the bed. Pelvic obliquity may be present.

Indications for Surgical Treatment

Most moderate to severe curves require surgery. Bracing is poorly tolerated and acts as a passive holding device only. Patients with profound weakness of the lower limb manage to walk with trick movement of the trunk. Patients have to be alerted to the possibility that the walking ability may deteriorate after the spine is fused. Before surgery, the following should be considered.

Age

The ideal time for surgery is just before the adolescent growth spurt, when most progression is expected. An extensive fusion is usually necessary because of the nature of the curve.

Curve Pattern

High thoracic curves need early fusion. The collapsing spine tends to remain flexible but should be fused when flexibility decreases or if upper limb function is grossly impaired and is no longer able to support the trunk. A mild thoracic, thoraco-lumbar, lumbar, or double major curve should be treated according to the same principles as idiopathic curves.

Progression

Curves of more than 40–50° that progress despite adequate bracing require surgical correction and fusion.

Pelvic Obliquity

Obliquity of more than 30° disturbs sitting balance and causes hip dislocation and asymmetrical ischial pressure. Surgical correction and fusion are indicated.

Method of Treatment

Preoperative casting has largely been abandoned because it is uncomfortable and causes further pulmonary impairment. The results of spinal surgery in poliomyelitis without internal fixation showed considerable loss of correction at final follow-up and a high pseudoarthrosis rate. Multiple operations were usually required. By contrast, the use of internal fixation has markedly improved correction and maintenance of correction at long-term follow-up. The most popular posterior instrumentation 30 years ago was the Harrington system, with or without sublaminar wiring, followed by 3–6 months of casting until radiological fusion was achieved. This was associated with high rate of pseudoarthrosis so that subsequently techniques of combined anterior and posterior instrumentation were developed with significant improvement in fusion rates [81–86]. Nowadays, segmental instrumentation with wires, hooks, and screws has become the standard procedure for paralytic scoliosis, giving a more stable fixation. This allows better correction of the curve with increased fusion rates; post-operative bracing is usually unnecessary. Combined anterior and posterior instrumentation is used in severe and rigid curves, especially with severe pelvic obliquity [44, 81, 82, 84, 87].

Preoperative halo-pelvic/halo-femoral traction can be useful in the treatment of the poliomyelitic spine undergoing corrective surgery, especially when staged anterior and posterior surgery are contemplated. This combined method is useful for long lumbar C curves, collapsing spines, and severe long thoracic curves (89). Combined anterior and posterior fusion down to the sacrum reduces the chance of pseudoarthrosis. Anterior instrumentation down to L5 provides maximum correction of pelvic obliquity. Curves above 100° or between 80° and 100° with rigidity will benefit from preoperative halo-pelvic traction. Long C curves, collapsing spines, and lumbar curves with pelvic obliquity should always be fused to the sacrum.

References

1. Anonymous. Poliomyelitis in 1977, Notes and News. WHO Chron 1979; 33:63–70.
2. World Health Organization. Poliomyelitis. Fact sheet #114. At: http://www.who.int/mediacentre/factsheets/fs114/en/index.html. Accessed 19 Sep. 2008.

3. Strebel PM, Sutter RW, Cochi SL, et al. Epidemiology of poliomyelitis in the United States one decade after the last reported case of indigenous wild virus-associated disease. Clin Infect Dis 1992; 14:568.

4. Sabin AB. Oral poliovirus vaccine. History of its development and prospects. Eradication of poliomyelitis. JAMA 1965; 194:872–881.

5. Diveley RL. Anterior poliomyelitis: A study of the acute stage with special reference to the early diagnosis and treatment. J Bone Joint Surg Am 1929; 11:100–122.

6. Green WT, Grice DS. The management of chronic poliomyelitis. AAOS Instr Course Lect 1952; 9:85–90.

7. Lenhard RE. Prognosis in poliomyelitis. J Bone Joint Surg Am 1950; 32:71–79.

8. Mayer L. The physiologic method of tendon transplants. Reviewed after forty years. AAOS Instr Course Lect 1956; 13: 116–121.

9. Kumar K, Kapahtia NK. The pattern of muscle involvement in poliomyelitis of the upper limb. Int Orthop 1986; 10:11–15.

10. Bennett JB, Allan CH. Tendon transfers about the shoulder and elbow in obstetrical brachial plexus palsy. J Bone Joint Surg 1999; 81-A:1612–1627.

11. Kotwal PP, Mittal R, Malhotra R. Trapezius transfer for deltoid paralysis. J Bone Joint Surgery Br 1998; 80-B:114–116.

12. Saha AK. Surgery of the paralysed and flail shoulder. Acta Orthop Scand Supplement 1967; 97:7–90 .

13. Saha AK. Surgical rehabilitation of paralyzed shoulder following poliomyelitis in adults and children. J Int Coll Surg 1964; 42:198.

14. Brockway A. An operation to improve abduction power of the shoulder in poliomyelitis. J Bone Joint Surg Am 1939; 21:451–455.

15. Harmon PH. Anterior transplantation of the posterior deltoid for shoulder palsy and dislocation in poliomyelitis. Surg Gynecol Obstet 1947; 84:117.

16. American Orthopaedic Association—Research Committee: A survey of end results on stabilization of the paralytic shoulder. J Bone and Joint Surg 1942; 24:699–707.

17. May VR Jr. Shoulder Fusion. A Review of Fourteen Cases. J. Bone and Joint Surg 1962; 44-A:65–76.

18. De Velasco Polo G, Monterrubio AC. Arthrodesis of the Shoulder. Clin Orthop 1973; 90:178–182.

19. Mah JY, Hall JE. Arthrodesis of the shoulder in children. J Bone Joint Surg Am 1990; 72:582–586.

20. Rowe CR. Re-evaluation of the Position of the Arm in Arthrodesis of the Shoulder in the Adult. J Bone and Joint Surg Am 1974; 56:913–922.

21. Steindler A. Muscle and tendon transplant at the elbow. AAOS Instr Course Lect Reconstr Surg 1944; 2:276–282.

22. Carroll RE, Hill NA. Triceps transfer to restore elbow flexion. J Bone Joint Surg Am 1970; 52:239.

23. Clark JMP. Reconstruction of biceps brachii by pectoral muscle transplantation. Br J Surg 1946; 34:180.

24. Irwin CE, Eyler DL. Surgical rehabilitation of the hand and forearm disabled by poliomyelitis. J Bone Joint Surg Am 1951; 33:825–835.

25. Schnute WJ, Tachdjian MO. Intermetacarpal bone block for thenar paralysis following poliomyelitis: An end-result study. J Bone Joint Surg Am 1963; 45:1663–1670.

26. Sharrard WJW. Distribution of permanent paralysis of lower limbs in poliomyelitis—a clinical and pathological study. J Bone Joint Surg 1955; 37 B:540.

27. Sharrard WJW. Paediatric Orthopaedics and Fractures. 2nd ed. Oxford, London: Blackwell Scientific; 1979:889.

28. Watts HG. Orthopedic techniques in the management of the residua of paralytic poliomyelitis. Techn Orthop 2005; 20(2):179–189.

29. Ober FR. The role of iliotibial band and fascia lata as a factor in the causation of low-back disabilities and sciatica. J Bone Joint Surg Am 1936; 18:105–110.

30. Green NE, Griffin PP. Hip dysplasia associated with abduction contracture of the contralateral hip J Bone Joint Surg Am 1982; 64:1273–1281.

31. Asirvatham R, Watts HG, Rooney RJ. Rotation osteotomy of the tibia after poliomyelitis. J Bone Joint Surgery Br 1990; 72-B:409–11.

32. Irwin CE. The iliotibial band: Its role in producing deformity in poliomyelitis. J Bone Joint Surg Am 1949; 31:141.

33. McNicol D, Leong JCY, Hsu LCS. Supramalleolar Derotation Osteotomy for Lateral tibial torsion and associated equinovarus deformity of the foot. J Bone Joint Surg Br 1983; 65: 166–170.

34. Yount CC. The role of the tensor fasciae femoris in certain deformities of the lower extremities. J Bone Joint Surg. 1926; 8:171–177.

35. Mustard WT. A follow-up study of iliopsoas transfer for hip instability. J Bone Joint Surg 1959; 41B:289–293.

36. Sharrard WJW. Posterior iliopsoas transplantation in the treatment of paralytic dislocation of the hip. J Bone Joint Surg 1964; 46B:426–434.

37. Hogshead HP, Ponseti IV. Fascia lata transfer to the erector spinae for the treatment of flexion-abduction contractures of the hip in patients with poliomyelitis and meningomyelocele: Evaluation of results. J Bone Joint Surg Am 1964; 46:1389.

38. Lau JHK, Parker JC, Hsu LCS, Leong JCY. Paralytic hip instability in poliomyelitis. J Bone Joint Surg 1986; 68B:528–533.

39. Hallock H. Surgical stabilization of dislocated paralytic hips: End-results study. Surg Gynecol Obstet 1942; 75:742.

40. Sharp NN, Guhl JF, Sorensen RI, et al. Hip fusion in poliomyelitis in children: A preliminary report. J Bone Joint Surg Am 1964; 46:121–133.

41. Hallock H. Arthrodesis of the hip for instability and pain in poliomyelitis. J Bone Joint Surg Am 1950; 2:904.

42. Hallock H. Hip arthrodesis in poliomyelitis. Bull N Y Hosp 1958; 2:18.

43. O'Brien JP, Dwyer AP, Hodgson AR. A paralytic pelvic obliquity. J Bone Joint Surg 1975; 57A:626–632.

44. Lee DY, Choi IH, Chung CY, et al. Fixed pelvic obliquity after poliomyelitis. J Bone Joint Surg 1997; 79:190.

45. Hughes RE, Risser JC. The correction of knee-flexion deformity, after poliomyelitis, by wedging plasters. J Bone Joint Surg Am 1934; 16:935–946.

46. Leong JCY, Alade CO, Fang D. Supracondylar femoral osteotomy for knee flexion contracture resulting from poliomyelitis. J Bone Joint Surgery 1982; 64-B:198–201.

47. Mehta SN, Mukherjee AK. Flexion osteotomy of the femur for genu recurvatum after poliomyelitis. J Bone Joint Surg Br 1991; 73:200.

48. Heyman CH. Operative treatment of paralytic genu recurvatum. J Bone Joint Surg Am 1962; 44:1246.

49. Perry J, O'Brien JP, Hodgson AR. Triple tenodesis of the knee: a soft-tissue operation for the correction of paralytic genu recurvatum. J Bone Joint Surg 1976; 58-A:978–985.

50. Men HX, Bian CH, Yang CD, et al. Surgical treatment of the flail knee after poliomyelitis. J Bone Joint Surg Br 1991; 73-B:195–199.

51. Broderick TF, Reidy JA, Barr JS. Tendon transplantations in the lower extremity: A review of end results in poliomyelitis II. Tendon transplantations at the knee. J Bone Joint Surg Am 1952; 34:909–914.

52. Crego Jr CH, Fischer FJ. Transplantation of the biceps femoris for the relief of quadriceps femoris paralysis in residual poliomyelitis. J Bone Joint Surg 1931; 13:515.

53. Cleveland M. Operative fusion of the unstable or flail knee due to anterior poliomyelitis: A study of the late results. J Bone Joint Surg Am 1932; 14:525–534.

54. Emmel HE, Le Cocq JF. Hamstring transplant for the prevention of calcaneocavus foot in poliomyelitis. J Bone Joint Surg Am 1958; 40:911–917.

55. Hsu LCS, Swanson L, Leong JCY, Low WD. Telemetric electromyographic analysis of muscles transferred to the os calcis in paralysed limbs. Clin Orthop 1985; 201:71–74.

56. Pandey AK, Pandey S, Prasad V. Calcaneal osteotomy and tendon sling for the management of calcaneus deformity. J Bone Joint Surg Am 1989; 71:1192–1198.

57. Legaspi J, Li YH, Chow W, Leong JCY. Talectomy in patients with recurrent deformity in club foot. A long-term follow-up study. J Bone Joint Surg 2001; 83B:384–387.

58. Nicomedez FPI, Li YH, Leong JCY. Tibiocalcaneal fusion after talectomy in arthrogrypotic patients. J Pediatr Orthoped 2003; 23(5):654–657.

59. Grice DS. An extra-articular arthrodesis of the subastragalar joint for correction of paralytic flat feet in children. J Bone Joint Surg Am 1952; 34-A:927–940.

60. Seymour N, Evans DK. A modification of the Grice subtalar arthrodesis. J Bone Joint Surg Br 1968; 50-B:372–375.

61. Hsu LCS, O'Brien JP, Yau ACMC, Hodgson AR. Batchelor's extra-articular subtalar arthrodesis: A report on sixty-four procedures in patients with poliomyelitic deformities. J Bone Joint Surg Am 1976; 58-A:243–247.

62. Hsu LCS, O'Brien JP, Yau ACMC, Hodgson AR. Valgus deformity of the ankle in children with fibular pseudarthrosis. J Bone Joint Surg Am 1974; 56-A:503–510.

63. Bhan S, Malhotra R. Subtalar arthrodesis for flexion hindfoot deformities in children. Arch Orthop Trauma Surg 1998; 117:312–315.

64. Brown A. A simple method of fusion of the subtalar joint in children. J Bone Joint Surg Br 1968; 50-B:369–371.

65. Hsu LCS, Yau ACMC, O'Brien JP, Hodgson AR. Valgus deformity of the ankle resulting from fibular resection for a graft in subtalar fusion in children. J Bone Joint Surg Am 1972; 54-A: 585–594.

66. Dennyson WG, Fulford GE. Subtalar arthrodesis by cancellous grafts and metallic internal fixation. J Bone Joint Surg Br 1976; 58-B:507–510.

67. Jaffray D, Hsu L, Leong JCY. The Batchelor-Grice extra-articular subtalar arthrodesis. J Bone Joint Surg 1986; 68-B:125–127.

68. Mosca VS. Calcaneal lengthening for valgus deformity of the hindfoot. Results in children who had severe, symptomatic flatfoot and skewfoot. J Bone Joint Surg Am 1995; 77:500–512.

69. Crego CH, McCarroll HR. Recurrent deformities in stabilized paralytic feet: A report of 1100 consecutive stabilizations in poliomyelitis. J Bone Joint Surg Am 1938; 20:609–620.

70. Tang SC, Leong JCY, Hsu LCS. Lambrinudi triple arthrodesis for correction of severe rigid drop-foot. J Bone Joint Surg 1984; 66B:66–72.

71. Saltzman CL, Fehrle MJ, Cooper RR, et al. Triple arthrodesis: Twenty-five and forty-four-year average follow-up of the same patients. J Bone Joint Surg 1999; 81-A:1391–1402.

72. Kong KFJ, Li YH, Kwok HY. Treatment of foot deformities in children by Ilizarov method. Proceedings, the 19th Annual Congress of the Hong Kong Orthopaedic Association. 1999: 61

73. Jones R. The soldier's foot and the treatment of common deformities of the foot. Part III Claw foot. Br Med J 1916; I:749.

74. Aldegheri R. Distraction osteogenesis for lengthening of the tibia in patients who have limb-length discrepancy or short stature. J Bone Joint Surg Am 1999; 81:624–634.

75. Macnicol MF, Catto AM. Twenty-year review of tibial lengthening for poliomyelitis. J Bone Joint Surg 1982; 64B:607–610.

76. Perry J, Fontaine JD, Mulroy S. Findings in post-poliomyelitis syndrome. Weakness of muscles of the calf as a source of late pain and fatigue of muscles of the thigh after poliomyelitis. J Bone Joint Surg Am 1995; 77:1148–1153.

77. Farbu E. Post-polio syndrome—diagnosis and management. ACNR 2005; 5:10–11.

78. Lin KH, Lim YW. Post-poliomyelitis syndrome: Case report and review of the literature. Ann Acad Med Singapore 2005; 34:447–449.

79. Nollet F. Post-polio syndrome. Orphanet Encyclopedia; 2004:2–8. At http://www.orpha.net/data/patho/GB/uk-PP.pdf. Accessed 02 October 2008.

80. Trojan DA, Cashman NR. Post-poliomyelitis syndrome. Muscle Nerve 2005; 31:6–19.

81. Leong JCY, Wilding K, Mok CK, et al. Surgical treatment of scoliosis following poliomyelitis. J Bone Joint Surg 1981; 3A:726–732.

82. Leong JCY, Hsu LCS. Poliomyelitis of the spine. In: McCollister Evarts C, ed. Surgery of the Musculoskeletal System, 2nd ed. New York: Churchill Livingstone; 1990:2049–2072.

83. Eberle CF. Failure of fixation after segmental spinal instrumentation without arthrodesis in the management of paralytic scoliosis. J Bone Joint Surg Am 1988; 70:696.

84. Hsu LCS, Cheng CL, Leong JCY. Treatment of severe poliomyelitis spinal deformity after failed posterior fusion. J West Paci Orthop Assoc 1985; 22(2):27–33.

85. Mayer PJ, Dove J, Ditmanson M, et al. Post-poliomyelitis paralytic scoliosis. A review of curve patterns and results of surgical treatments in 118 consecutive patients. Spine 1981; 6:573.

86. Pavon SJ, Manning C. Posterior spinal fusion for scoliosis due to anterior poliomyelitis. J Bone Joint Surg 1970; 52-B:420–431.

87. O'Brien JP, Yau AC, Gertzbein S, Hodgson AR. Combined staged anterior and posterior correction and fusion of the spine in scoliosis following poliomyelitis. Clin Orthop Rel Res 1975b; 110:81–111.

Chapter 19

Orthopaedic Management of Cerebral Palsy

James E. Robb and Reinald Brunner

Definition

Ingram has provided a suitable description:

> Cerebral palsy is used as an inclusive term to describe a group of non-progressive disorders occurring in young children in which disease of the brain causes impairment of motor function. Impairment of motor function may be the result of paresis, involuntary movement, or incoordination, but motor dysfunctions which are transient, or are the result of progressive disease of the brain, or attributable to abnormalities of the spinal cord, are excluded. [1].

All children with cerebral palsy (CP) are "brain-damaged" and have associated disabilities such as epilepsy (33%), mental handicap (19–50%), speech disorders (25–80%), behavioral disturbances, specific learning difficulties, or abnormal visual perception (34–58%) [2]. The likelihood of significant visual deficits is greater in children with higher gross motor function classification system (GMFCS) scores, independent of gestational age [3]. Sensory deficits are also present and Sanger and Kukke have shown that children with secondary dystonia and diplegia due to CP have deficits of tactile sensation [4]. An appropriate sensory input is a prerequisite for an adequate motor control. While the neurological damage may be non-progressive, CP is certainly a progressive orthopaedic condition, which may be influenced by growth or intervention. The condition is rarely manifest at birth but presents later as developmental delay.

Classification

This may be

1. Topographical: hemiplegia, diplegia, and total body involvement (tetraplegia).
2. Neurological: spastic, athetoid, ataxic, rigid, or mixed.

Classification based on severity is difficult because of the inaccuracy of quantifying the severity of spasticity, athetosis, or ataxia. Some children fit into typical patterns, but others do not and often there is an overlap. The term "total body involvement" is preferred to tetraplegia as it embraces the concept of impaired head and trunk control.

Incidence

Cerebral palsy occurs in approximately 0.25% of all live births and in the majority no cause can be identified. It was commonly thought that the disorder resulted from brain asphyxia due to problems during labor, but despite advances in obstetric care, the incidence has remained constant in the recent past. However, the pattern of CP has changed in that there has been a notable decrease in athetosis due to erythroblastosis fetalis. In a multicenter study which involved approximately 54,000 births, Nelson and Ellenberg found that only 21% of the 189 children who developed CP had any sign of intra-partum asphyxia and 9% had evidence of asphyxia in the absence of congenital malformation [5]. Maternal mental retardation, a birthweight below 2 kg, and fetal malformation were the leading predictors. Breech presentation was also a predictor, but breech delivery was not. This study showed that a large proportion of the cases of CP remain unexplained. Bejar et al. observed periventricular leukomalacia (PVL, multifocal necrosis of the white matter) on echo encephalography in utero. Their study suggested that there were prenatal antecedents of CP rather than intra-partum and post-natal factors [6]. Ultrasound of the brain is a useful noninvasive procedure that can demonstrate PVL and hemorrhagic brain lesions [7]. Magnetic resonance imaging (MRI) of the brain can also demonstrate hypoxic ischemic brain injury and can be used for the fetus, neonate, and infant [8].

Pathology

In general terms the areas of the brain which control movement are the motor cortex, basal ganglia, and cerebellum;

J.E. Robb (✉)
Department of Orthopaedic Surgery, Royal Hospital for Sick Children, Edinburgh, UK; University of Edinburgh, Edinburgh, UK; University of St. Andrews, Edinburgh, UK

M. Benson et al. (eds.), *Children's Orthopaedics and Fractures*,
DOI 10.1007/978-1-84882-611-3_19, © Springer-Verlag London Limited 2010

therefore, spastic CP is due to cerebral cortical damage, dyskinesia from basal ganglia damage, and ataxia from abnormalities of the cerebellum [2]. It is important to distinguish between spasticity, which is an increasing muscle contraction in response to stretch [9] and can be abolished by posterior root section, and rigidity, which is not affected by posterior root section. There are two clinical types of spasticity: phasic and tonic. In phasic spasticity the muscle does not produce a permanent contracture, whereas the tonic system is adapted to postural control and the muscle always resists stretching. This can induce shortening of the muscle and a joint contracture. In rigidity there is an involuntary, sustained contraction of the muscle, which is neither dependent on a stretch being applied to the muscle nor abolished by posterior root section. A clinical example of this is dystonic CP, which may be flexor or extensor. In clinical practice one sees "dynamic deformities" and an associated full range of movements under general anesthesia or slow and gentle examination. Although it is helpful to define tone patterns, many patients have a mixed neurological picture. Muscle weakness occurs in CP and may arise for several reasons, e.g., from underlying brain damage, immobility, and imbalance in musculotendinous lengths. The problem of muscle weakness in spastic conditions is increasingly gaining attention as part of maintenance of function. Reciprocal innervation of joint agonist and antagonist muscle groups provides a mechanism where one relaxes, while the other contracts. If only one group is weakened, a secondary and worse deformity may be produced by the unopposed action of the antagonist. Grading by the Medical Research Council (MRC) scale of strength in CP is difficult for the above reasons but is still useful clinically.

The brain develops despite the damage and adopts strategies to compensate for the deficits and to optimize function. The peripheral expression of the underlying central damage often changes as the patient grows. Compensatory mechanisms may, at first, be advantageous but later may result in secondary deformities. During growth, muscle has to keep pace with skeletal lengthening. In spastic paralysis there is relative shortening of the musculotendinous unit during growth and often little stretching of muscle during daily activities in some muscle groups. Ziv et al. have shown experimentally that muscle adds sarcomeres in response to constant stretch, but when muscles are spastic this mechanism does not occur [10]. Tardieu et al. believed that the major factor causing contracture was the maintenance of the muscle in a shortened position, either passively or by sustained contraction [11]. Deformity in CP may arise in several ways: as a result of brain damage, as an aberration of growth, and as a result of positional deformity. Compensatory mechanisms may produce deformity that results from management.

Deformities in CP may be mobile or fixed and arise from disorganized posture, balance, and movement.

Developmental delays cause retarded motor skills and the persistence of infantile reflexes. Delay in acquiring motor skills means that these appear later than normal and may be fewer than those in the normal child. There may also be variations and abnormal patterns in the motor skills that are subsequently acquired. There may be other reasons for motor delay such as visual handicap or learning difficulties. Immobility may be a result of multiple handicaps, blindness, and learning difficulties [12]. Postural mechanisms are an intrinsic part of motor skills and are linked to voluntary movement mechanisms. If equilibrium is poor, a child may not be able to initiate movement even though voluntary motion is possible. Retarded postural mechanisms may lead to lack of trunk and head control. Postural control and equilibrium dysfunction may be more pronounced if a potential compensation is impaired by a visual deficit. Abnormal reflexes may manifest as automatic stepping or the asymmetric tonic neck reflex, and recurring stimulation of abnormal reflexes may result in deformity. Abnormal postures develop from deformities as muscles shorten, or as a compensation to maintain equilibrium or its loss. They may also result from asymmetry of muscle function or from limb length inequality. Spasticity may also be used as a compensation, and the child relies on this to stand erect. Established contractures of one joint can have a subsequent effect on other joints, for example, a hip flexion contracture may cause equinus on the affected side. Isolated muscle groups are not spastic, but there is co-contraction of agonists and antagonists at any given joint. Usually it is the effect of the weaker antagonist that results in the deformity. This can be seen at the hip where abnormal forces cause joint subluxation or dislocation and the acetabulum then develops a deformity.

Physical Assessment

Static Examination

The patient lies supine on a couch, which can be replaced by mother's lap in young children. If the patient is positioned with the pelvis on the end of the couch, the legs are not supported. This position allows assessment of the range of motion of all joints of the lower extremities without moving the patient. The child can then be brought into the sitting position to observe head control, spinal deformity, and pelvic obliquity. In a walking child, the upper limbs are examined while the child sits. The assessment should include passive and active movements of the shoulder, elbow, wrist, and hand. Stance and gait need to be observed in a walker, appropriately undressed. Coordination and balance can be assessed by asking the child to stand or jump on one leg.

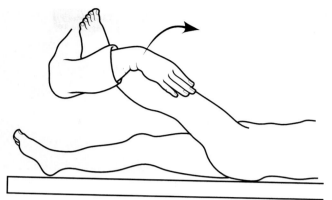

Fig. 19.2 Straight leg raising test to assess hamstring length

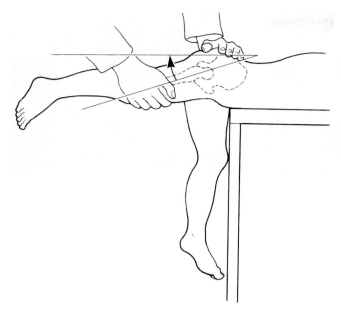

Fig. 19.1 Staheli hip extension test

Thomas's test is traditionally carried out and is accurate enough for clinical purposes but is less accurate than measuring hip flexion contractures as described by Staheli in the prone position (Fig. 19.1) [13]. The patient is placed so that the pelvis lies off the examining table and one hand is placed on the posterior superior spines, while the hip under examination is extended. The point of contracture is when the pelvis begins to tilt posteriorly. While supine, internal and external rotation and abduction and adduction can be measured. This is assessed with the hips in extension for a walker and with the hips in flexion for a nonwalker as these are the positions of function in these two circumstances. When assessing abduction and adduction it is essential to observe and palpate the anterior superior spines to allow an accurate assessment of the amount of abduction. If the spines are not visualized and felt, it is possible to show a "satisfactory" range of abduction when in reality on one side there may be only 5 or 10° of abduction and 30–40° on the opposite side. The knee is assessed for range of movement and capsular contracture. Straight leg raising assesses hamstring spasticity and contracture (Fig. 19.2). An alternative is to use the popliteal angle, which is found by flexing the hip to a right angle and extending the knee to the point of resistance. The popliteal angle lies between the vertical and the tibia at the point of resistance (Fig. 19.3).

The range of dorsiflexion of the ankle is measured with the heel held in inversion; this stabilizes the talonavicular joint and prevents lateral bow-stringing of the tendo-Achilles (escape valgus) when the heel is valgus thus producing a pseudo-correction. By holding the foot in varus, dorsiflexion of the mid-tarsal joints is prevented. In a varus deformity,

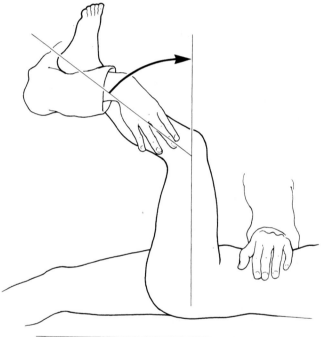

Fig. 19.3 Popliteal angle

however, the heel has to be kept in valgus. Traditionally Silverskiöld's test is used to differentiate between contracture of the gastrocnemius and soleus. The knee is flexed to 90° and the ankle/foot dorsiflexed, while the foot is held in inversion as far as possible, and an assessment is made of the foot–shank angle. This is then repeated with the knee fully extended. The amount of dorsiflexion when the inversion is released represents the overall mobility and instability of the hind- and mid-foot joints (Fig. 19.4). Subtalar and mid-tarsal movements can then be assessed along with toe deformities.

The patient is then moved up the couch and lies prone. Femoral anteversion is determined by palpation of the greater

Fig. 19.4 Dorsiflexion with the foot inverted (**a**) and everted (**b**)

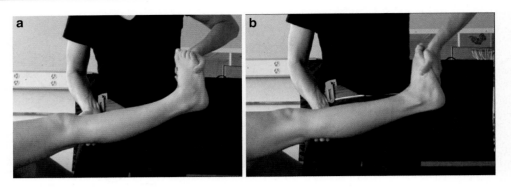

trochanter at its maximally prominent site and by measuring the angle between the tibia and the vertical [14]. The thigh–foot angle [15] is then assessed, giving an indirect clinical measurement of tibial torsion. The knee is flexed to 90° and the ankle is dorsiflexed into neutral, but without everting or inverting the foot. The relationship of the heel to the thigh is assessed visually or with a goniometer. The foot–thigh angle is invalid after hindfoot surgery. The examination so far will determine torsions between the femoral shaft and the calcaneus. There may be torsions within the foot itself. Because most patients have a mobile hindfoot, it may be more accurate to assess tibial torsion by measuring the angle between the transmalleolar axis and the femoral condyles or by using the footprint method [16]. The knee needs to be flexed to 90° for this measurement.

Traditional stretch tests are inaccurate in CP and have limited specificity. The Duncan Ely test (rectus stretch test) also generates action potentials in iliopsoas [17] and the Thomas test generates similar electrical activity in rectus and iliopsoas. Phelp's (gracilis) test and straight leg raising induce the same amount of electrical activity in the medial hamstrings. The specificity of Silverskiöld's test has been questioned by Perry et al., because on electromyography both gastrocnemius and soleus showed increased action potentials irrespective of the position of the knee [18].

Evaluation of Gait

Walking is a complex activity, and events occur in the coronal, sagittal, and transverse planes. Descriptions of the gait cycle have been traditionally made in the sagittal plane. The goals of gait are stability and progression. The prerequisites are stance phase stability, swing phase clearance, foot preposition in terminal swing, adequate step length, and energy conservation [19]. The upper body must be supported in both double and single supports and may be challenged by two factors: first by body weight and second by the alterations of the body segments during walking.

Smooth progression depends upon the maintenance of forward velocity, clearance of the leg in swing, and absorption of energy before and at foot contact. During single support there are two main progressional forces: first, there is the input of energy to stabilize the lower limb and to assist the upward and forward motion of the hip and upper body. This is then followed by a controlled and downward fall of the body from a high point and represents the conversion of potential to kinetic energy assisted by gravity.

Visual observation of gait is used traditionally to assess aberrations in walking patterns. In practice it is difficult to perform this accurately when there are abnormalities at several anatomical levels—trunk, pelvis, hip, knee, ankle, and foot, and in three planes. One effective way of improving gait observation is to employ video recordings and a freeze-frame playback facility or to use a visual gait score such as the Edinburgh Gait score [20]. Gait analysis (Chapter 26) has become an important investigative tool in CP and in some centers is regarded as essential before surgery for the walker. Gait analysis certainly provides a means of objective audit after intervention, but not all have access to this complex type of investigation. A comprehensive gait evaluation in CP would include kinematics, kinetics, energy consumption, and dynamic electromyography (EMG).

Although ungainly, abnormal walking patterns may represent the most efficient method of progression for the child and result from a variety of factors. The walking pattern may be a compensation for deficient control of equilibrium, joint contracture, or muscle spasticity. Many children with CP are effectively in a state of "collapse" and cannot support their body weight on one leg thus walking rapidly to avoid falling over. Patients with CP may also have an excessive forward lean of the trunk when walking to control extension at the knee. The common pattern in hemiplegia and diplegia is internal rotation, flexion, and adduction of the hip (Fig. 19.5). There may also be flexion of the knee and an equinus posture of the ankle. The knee may extend fully passively but may tend to be in valgus when walking, although there may not be a fixed valgus deformity. Secondary deformities may ensue, such as external tibial torsion distal to

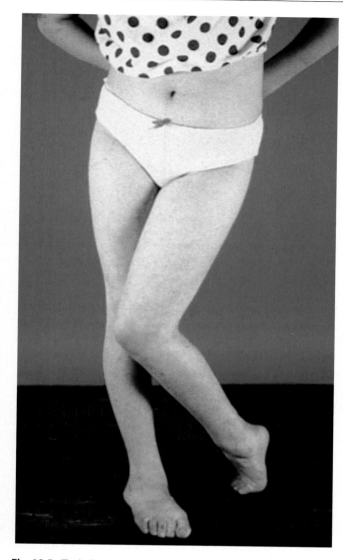

Fig. 19.5 Typical posture of adduction and internal rotation at the hip, and flexion at the knee and ankle

Principles and Aims of Management

In general, the shape of the locomotor system depends upon function, which depends upon use. This explains why a joint can lose motion if its range is not used. One aim in the management of patients with CP therefore involves control of posture and daily activities, during which the available range of joint movement and muscle length should be used.

It is important to distinguish between disturbances of function due to the underlying condition, useful adaptations, which may look abnormal, and functional difficulties secondary to deformity. Compromises may have to be made between the balance of benefit from an intervention and the disadvantages. For example, standing with the knees bent places a load on the quadriceps, which is tiring. Straightening the knees can solve this stance phase problem for the patient but may cause difficulties in the swing phase of gait.

Dynamic instability, or lever arm dysfunction, is a major factor interfering with movement and can result in bony deformity and joint dislocations. For example, in diplegia many patients have increased femoral anteversion and initially walk on tiptoe. Pes valgus then commonly develops and the foot becomes externally rotated with respect to the tibia but is also functionally plantigrade. External tibial torsion may then develop as a consequence of the pes valgus and increased femoral anteversion produces the so-called miserable malalignment. Joints can be stabilized with orthoses or by arthrodesis. Absolute stability at a given joint may be a disadvantage in the longer term and can remove some compensatory movement for a deformity at a more proximal level.

Some patients with CP appear to have strong muscles but spasticity often masks an underlying muscle weakness. The imbalance of muscle action across a joint may be managed by lengthening or weakening the agonist to restore the imbalance between agonist and antagonist. Force and length are related to each other physiologically. Lengthening results in a reduction of force and is used to gain length or to reduce force. Muscle tension may decrease after tendon transfers and a reduction of force is seen as a secondary phenomenon. Thus reduction of muscle force is a regular consequence of nonoperative and operative managements. The effect is transient after casting or aponeurotic (intramuscular) lengthening [21] but longer lasting after tendon lengthening [21–23]. Force reduction may give the impression of being advantageous, because spasticity seems to be reduced. In reality, however, the output from the central nervous system remains unchanged although spasticity may be less noticeable due to the decrease in muscle force. The advantage of reduction of spasticity may be counteracted by the disadvantage of muscle weakness for postural control and function. Hence muscle strengthening exercises may help to improve function despite

excessive internal femoral torsion. A valgus calcaneus and pes valgus are common associated deformities.

One way of compensating for muscle weakness is to control the center of gravity to unload a weak muscle. For example, in Duchenne type of gait pattern (lateral trunk lean toward the affected hip) the lateralization of the center of mass minimizes the commonly present external hip adduction moment which requires hip abductor activity to avoid contralateral pelvic drop. Similarly, knee extension can be controlled by forward lean of the trunk which reduces the load on the knee extensors.

The aim of clinical examination and gait analysis is to define a list of biomechanical problems apart from the neurological disorder, having considered muscle length, strength, bony lever arms, and alignment.

concerns about possibly increasing spasticity [24]. The aims of management have to take into account the overall function of the patient and the existence of a deformity which does not necessarily merit treatment.

Orthotic Management

The general aims of orthoses are to provide stability in dynamic and static conditions, to control the position and shape of body segments, and to guide motion. Hence they are used to control function, to correct and prevent deformities, and to substitute for missing muscle activity and strength. They can be used as aids worn during function or as positional devices such as night splints. However, as function is impaired by malposition of joints, instability, and deformity, the efficacy of functional orthoses is generally superior to a positional device. Orthoses should only be used if benefits outweigh disadvantages.

Ankle–foot orthoses (AFOs) may be prescribed for several reasons: to maintain posture, to prevent deformity, and to obtain a biomechanical effect. They may be used for walkers and nonwalkers. The manufacture of an orthosis depends upon an accurate, positive plaster cast of the child's foot and calf, from which a lightweight thermoplastic splint is manufactured. Apart from static functions, such as preventing deformity and maintaining posture, the orthosis can be used to alter the biomechanical forces acting upon joints.

When the foot is applied to the ground, an equal and opposite ground reaction force is generated in response to this load (Newton's third law). The ground reaction force has magnitude in three directions and can be measured with a force plate (see Chapter 26). Knowledge of the orientation of the vertical component of the ground reaction force to any given joint is helpful when changing orthotic prescription. In the case of the child with crouch gait, where the vertical component of the ground reaction force is flexor in relation to the knee, the goal is to change the direction of the ground reaction force to pass through the knee joint. During normal walking there is a smooth progression of the ground reaction force origin from the heel at foot contact to the metatarsal heads at foot-off. In the case of crouch gait, the origin of the ground reaction force remains at the heel throughout stance, and forward progression of the upper body over the stationary foot occurs by an excessive amount of tibial progression over the foot, resulting in knee flexion. The AFO prevents excessive tibial progression in relation to the foot (Fig. 19.6) [25]. This then re-orientates the vertical component of the ground reaction force so that it passes through or near to the knee joint center, and thus the patient walks in a more upright posture. AFOs are a powerful tool, not just a piece of plastic, and can have dramatic and reversible effects upon

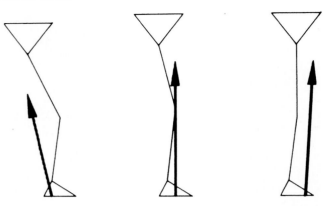

Fig. 19.6 Effect of an ankle–foot orthosis on crouch gait. Diagrammatic representation of the pelvis, thigh, shank, and foot in the sagittal plane. The arrow indicates the vertical component of the ground reaction force

the biomechanics of gait as well as standing posture. They are usually worn in normal shoewear, and these shoes always have a slight heel raise. The shank axis needs to be perpendicular to the floor as in normal standing and the height of the heel on the shoe needs to be taken into account when setting the foot–shank angle of the AFO. A little plantar flexion (or equinus) of about 5° is often left in the AFO so that the AFO–shoewear combination gives a satisfactory orientation of the shank to the vertical. If this is not taken into account, standing is comparable to standing in a ski boot with a slight anterior tilt.

Orthoses can be used to modify different phases of the gait cycle. The goal of foot contact is to bring the heel down first on the ground. An orthosis can be used here to control a drop foot, to permit heel contact rather than toe contact with the ground, or to control varus or valgus alignment of the foot. An analogy would be an aircraft landing on its main wheels, not on the nose wheel. During the loading response the orthosis can substitute for pretibial muscle function and prevent excessive inversion or eversion, and an orthotic modification for this phase would be the provision of a solid ankle cushion heel. The aircraft analogy in this case would be to prevent the wheels buckling on landing. During the first phase of single support the goal is tibial progression over the stationary foot with control of the ground reaction force in relation to the hip and knee. Here excessive tibial progression can be prevented by the use of an AFO or a floor reaction orthosis. An externally applied rocker to the shoe may also allow a smoother progression of the foot along the floor. In terminal stance the goal is to provide acceleration of the limb before pre-swing. There is no orthotic solution for problems in this phase of the gait cycle at present. In CP the main use of the AFO is to substitute for tibialis anterior and gastrocnemius and soleus activity. In swing the prerequisites are limb clearance and step length so in this phase the orthosis will compensate for a foot drop and preposition the foot in terminal swing. Orthoses should not interfere with knee motion. These various demands are best achieved with mobile, flexible orthoses, which improve gait more than rigid ones in the walker [26]. Resting orthoses may be used at night to minimize future deformity or to stretch contracted muscles. However, stretching can be an uncomfortable sensation and interfere with sleep. For this reason, orthoses are often poorly tolerated at night or are tolerated if no stretch is applied. The orthosis is then no longer functioning as intended.

A knee–ankle–foot orthosis (KAFO) may be indicated to stretch short hamstrings. This orthosis is applied during rest, but not at night, under full tension for 1–2 h during the daytime. The KAFO can also be used post-operatively and has the advantage over plaster of being removable. This helps to prevent neurological compromise or skin pressure problems. There is increasing interest in using dynamic orthoses in the management of knee contractures [27] but their efficacy in the longer term is unknown.

Thoraco-lumbar orthoses are used to control trunk posture in the nonwalker but only have a minor effect, compared to surgery, on the natural history of spinal deformity progression in neuromuscular scoliosis which is independent of the adolescent growth spurt [28, 29]. Early onset of conservative treatment and good correction by the brace are essential factors for a good postural effect [28]. Progress is monitored by radiographs taken with the patient erect in the brace (Fig. 19.7). If used in a walker who has a spinal deformity, the brace should allow some spinal motion when this is being used to compensate for a stiff leg gait. Stabilizing the spine in a nonwalker can substitute for weak paraspinal muscles, thereby improving head control and hand function.

Surgery

Abnormal tone, muscle imbalance, contractures, and bony deformity are amenable to surgery. Bony deformities and contractures are typical indications for orthopaedic intervention. Muscle balancing procedures, however, can be done for an imbalance of strength or length but muscle strength will be diminished as a result of muscle or tendon lengthening, which may not always benefit the patient. Problems resulting from excessive tone, rather than muscle shortening, require tone management. The fundamental injury to the central nervous system, namely loss of selective control and persistent reflex activity, is incurable. There are two important steps in assessing a patient for surgery: clinical examination and assessment of gait in the walking patient. An examination under anesthesia can be carried out separately but is usually unnecessary if a gentle and slow technique of assessment is used during clinical examination.

Orthopaedic operations may involve muscle or tendon lengthening (Fig. 19.8), tendon transfers, tenotomy, bony operations to improve rotational problems or to relocate joints, and neurectomy. Although surgery to the muscles and tendons will weaken the muscle, soft tissue surgery alone will not correct a fixed skeletal deformity. There is a trend now to perform surgery at one stage where possible, and operations in the walking child can be designed for both swing and stance phase problems. In the presence of mobile deformity the surgeon should think of balancing procedures around joints, whereas rotational and fixed bony deformities require bony surgery.

Tone Management

Selective posterior rhizotomy for reduction in spasticity has been popularized by Peacock et al. [30]. Its objective is to obtain a better balance between facilitatory and inhibitory control of the anterior horn cells. They have reported encouraging data in predominantly spastic diplegic patients where spasticity of muscle was reduced even to the point of flaccidity. The procedure entails selective sectioning of approximately one-quarter to one-half of the L2-S1 nerve rootlets that demonstrate abnormal responses to electrical stimulation at the time of surgery. This does not abolish primitive motor reflexes or fixed contractures of musculotendinous units or joints.

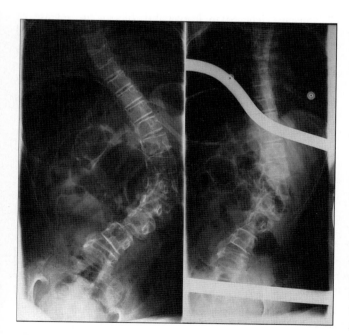

Fig. 19.7 Spinal alignment in and out of a thoraco-lumbar-sacral orthosis

The ideal patient for rhizotomy is a walking spastic diplegic who has minimal fixed contractures, but the approach may also be helpful for the nonwalker with total body involvement. Other favorable criteria include prematurity, pure spasticity, good trunk control and strength, minimal contractures, motivation, and the availability of physiotherapy. Poor indicators are hemiplegia, weakness of antigravity muscles, rigidity, dystonia, athetosis, marked flexion contractures, and fixed spinal deformity [31]. One concern after rhizotomy is the possibility of producing later spinal deformity, which could result from post-operative hypotonia and the laminectomy. Spiegel et al. found that after selective dorsal rhizotomy (SDR) using a laminoplasty technique, 12% of children developed a spondylolisthesis and 17% a scoliosis [32]. Greene et al. reported rapid progression of hip subluxation in six patients during the year after SDR, which was explained by the reduced sensory input from the joint, necessary for dynamic control [33]. Normally the L1 root is preserved, so the hip flexors may not be as denervated as their antagonists, thus predisposing to dysplasia. Steinbok has confirmed the benefits of SDR in spastic diplegia and a more limited role in spastic quadriplegia [34]. He found very strong evidence that SDR results in improvements in lower limb spasticity, an increase in the range of movement in the lower limb joints, and either no change or improvement in lower limb strength. There is moderate certainty that improvements in impairment are maintained up to 5 years after SDR and some weaker evidence that the improvements are maintained in the longer term. There is good evidence from prospective case series that there are improvements in self-care and performance of activities of daily living after SDR. The advantage of SDR is that the procedure is definitive, and the patient is not dependent upon lifelong medication as is the case with a baclofen pump [35]. The functional benefit of SDR seems to be even greater than after multi-level surgery [36]. SDR, however, may have significant and persistent complications such as muscle weakness and sphincter incontinence.

Oral baclofen has been used for many years to reduce spasticity, but often therapeutic doses cause drowsiness and excessive drooling. The intrathecal route delivers the drug close to its site of action at the spinal cord and much lower doses are needed to produce a therapeutic tone-reducing effect. The pump is inserted in the subcutaneous or subfascial layer of the anterior abdominal wall and a catheter is routed subcutaneously into the intrathecal space. Intrathecal baclofen (ITB) reduces tone and pain thus easing care and improving function [37, 38]. The main advantages of ITB are that the dose can be tailored to the patient's requirements and that the effects are reversible. The main disadvantages are a 5% risk of infection, the need to renew the batteries of the pump after about 5 years, and the fact that the therapy is not definitive. Albright has concluded that ITB is an effective treatment for children with hypertonicity secondary to spasticity and dystonia and often results in dramatic improvements in quality of life and in easier care [39]. In spite of the complications, most families and patients ask to continue ITB therapy at the end of pump battery life. There has been concern about the risk of spinal curvature increasing after ITB. For example, Ginsburg and Lauder found a significant increase in spinal deformity if trunk control was reduced [40]. However, Senaran et al. have shown that the procedure did not have a significant effect on spinal curve progression, pelvic obliquity, or the incidence of scoliosis when compared with an age, gender, and GMFCS score-matched control group of patients with spastic CP without an ITB pump [41].

Intramuscular botulinum toxin A is another drug which has gained increasing importance in the management of spastic muscles. The toxin irreversibly blocks the release of acetyl choline from the neuromuscular end plate causing a flaccid paralysis of the muscle but muscle activity recovers as new end plates form after about 3 months. Cosgrove et al. reported a beneficial effect on muscle growth in spastic mice [42]. Good, but often temporary, functional improvements

Fig. 19.8 Techniques of musculotendinous lengthening. (**a**) Z-lengthening, (**b**) intramuscular tendon lengthening, and (**c**) aponeurotomy

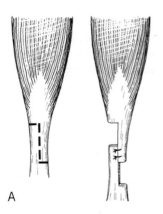

A

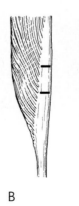

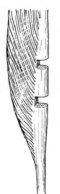

B

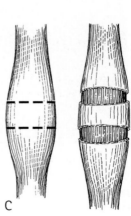

C

Fig. 19.9 Before and after soft tissue releases for seating and perineal access

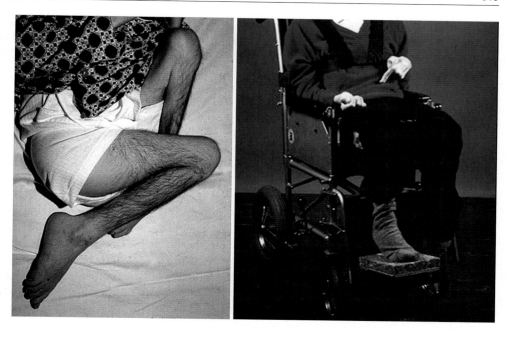

are seen in younger patients where muscle tone is the dominant problem [43]. Molenaers et al. found that botulinum toxin A treatment delayed and reduced the frequency of surgical procedures in children with CP who were able to walk [44]. Target muscles can be identified from gait analysis and apart from delaying the need for muscle surgery the botulinum toxin A can also give an indication of the possible functional outcome of muscle surgery by weakening the target muscle. The injections are often combined with casting and/or physiotherapy to stretch a shortened muscle. Botulinum toxin A injections have also been used in post-operative management following multi-level surgery in CP.

Surgery to a muscle may also reduce spasticity. Tardieu et al. have shown that tendon lengthening results in a persistent loss of muscle strength [23]. However, muscle strength is only temporarily reduced after intramuscular or aponeurotic lengthening procedures [21] (Fig. 19.8).

Surgery for the Nonwalker

It can be very difficult to assess a patient's functional ability in the presence of severe impairment. Often the clinician has to rely on the parents, carers, or therapists for further information. Assessment of "hip" pain can be difficult as, in the total body-involved patient, gastrointestinal pain can present as pain in the hip region. Severe handicap of itself should not prevent treatment.

The major cause of restricted function in severely affected patients is the lack of coordination and muscle control. One

of the major goals for a nonwalker is to acquire the ability to transfer either independently or with a helper. Any intervention which may interfere with lower limb joint stability, for example, proximal femoral resection for hip dislocation, may be disadvantageous for the patient who is capable of an assisted transfer. Management of severe secondary deformities should not affect existing function.

Goals in this group are different from those in walking patients, and mostly orientated toward a pain-free existence, balanced seating or, if the patient is capable of transfers, plantigrade feet, and the reduction of knee and hip flexion contractures. Adduction deformities of the hip can be particularly troublesome for seating and nappy (diaper) changing (Fig. 19.9).

Spinal Deformities

The cause of spinal deformity is the lack of dynamic muscle control to counteract the deforming force of gravity. The greater the deformity, the greater the lever arm for the deforming force and the faster the progression. Thoracolumbar orthoses can stabilize the trunk in an upright position and reduce progression of the spinal deformity, although they are less efficient than surgery [28]. They may also be used to assist trunk control during feeding or to provide trunk stability for arm function.

The spine should not be viewed in isolation. Hip dislocation, subluxation, and pelvic obliquity often coexist with scoliosis. James found that muscle release operations beneath the iliac crest did not alter the scoliosis [45], and Lonstein and Beck failed to find any association between hip dislocation, pelvic obliquity, and scoliosis in CP; the scoliosis developed regardless of the pelvic position [46]. Although single and double thoraco-lumbar curves occur in CP, the single C-type curve occurs more frequently in the total body-involved patient, who usually has absent truncal equilibrium reactions and pelvic obliquity. Curve progression is inevitable, and Madigan and Wallace found that the greatest progression was in the most severely involved groups [47]. Curves continue to progress even after skeletal maturity [48]. If the curve is progressive and threatens the child's ability to sit in spite of wheelchair modifications and bracing, surgical stabilization of the spine should be considered. Recently there has been greater interest in performing spinal fusion, even in the severely handicapped child who is a permanent wheelchair user. Indications include a severe sagittal plane deformity, loss of sitting ability or balance, back pain and pain from impingement of the ribs against the hemipelvis, and inefficacy of a spinal brace. Surgical stabilization of the spine can either extend to the sacrum, thereby removing any possibility of compensatory movement, or leave the L5-S1 segment free, allowing some mobility but the risk of subsequent lumbosacral pain. If there is fixed pelvic obliquity, the fusion should extend to the sacrum. This is major surgery, and severe learning difficulties or handicap may present a quandary for the parents or caregivers. Technical details of this type of surgery using a unit rod have been reported by Dabney et al. [49]. Studies have confirmed parental and carer satisfaction with spinal stabilization but functional benefits for the individual have been less easy to define [29, 50]. However, relieving the patient of discomfort due to pelvic obliquity and rib impingement on the iliac crest is likely to be an advantage and the patient with a straighter spine is easier to nurse and seat.

Kyphosis is also seen and usually begins as a postural problem in patients who have poor trunk and head control. It is flexible initially but can become fixed during subsequent growth. Severe kyphosis is a disabling deformity. In severe cases surgical correction including anterior release and posterior correction and fusion is indicated. Hyperlordosis is usually indicative of hip flexion contractures. The sacrum becomes almost horizontal and back pain often ensues. Because severe and persistent hyperlordosis can become painful a persistent lordotic posture should be avoided.

The Hip

The windswept deformity (adduction contracture and increased internal rotation of one hip and displacement of the other hip in abduction and external rotation) is a typical finding in the nonwalker and causes difficulties with perineal hygiene and seating. The incidence of hip displacement varies but in a recent study the risk of displacement was found to be directly related to gross motor function as graded by the GMFCS [51]. The risk was 0% in children in GMFCS level I and 90% in GMFCS level V. Bracing is not effective in spastic hip displacement. Graham et al. studied the combined effect of intramuscular injection of botulinum toxin A and abduction hip bracing in the management of spastic hip displacement in a randomized trial and found that progressive hip displacement continued to occur in the treatment group. They did not recommend this treatment [52].

In the absence of hip flexion contracture, myotomy of gracilis and an intramuscular adductor tenotomy of adductor longus are usually sufficient, provided symmetry of abduction can be obtained (Fig. 19.10). A more extensive procedure, including an anterior obturator neurectomy or more extensive myotomy, should not be carried out as an extreme abduction deformity and loss of dynamic control of the hip may result and cannot be remedied. The latter is especially a concern for patients who are almost, or just able, to transfer as this capability will be lost after excessive adductor lengthening.

The cause of hip dislocation in CP is not clear, but some assumptions are possible. The hip is, as a rule, normal at birth but acetabular enlargement gradually ensues as result of lack of dynamic control and may result in dislocation. Another factor may be positioning [2, 53] and many children with severe CP rest in the same position particularly at night, such as side-lying where one hip remains in adduction. The role of spasticity remains unclear, but is probably

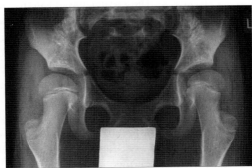 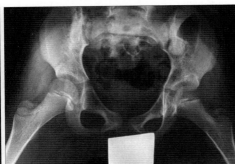

Fig. 19.10 Uncovering of the femoral heads improved with abduction of the hips

Fig. 19.11 Reimer's migration index is the part of the femoral epiphysis extending beyond Perkins' line (P) expressed as a percentage of the entire width of the epiphysis measured in the horizontal plane

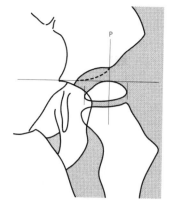

overestimated, because hip dislocations occur in hypotonic as well as hypertonic conditions. Another factor may be impaired proprioception which results in inadequate muscle control [4].

Clinical signs are unreliable in making the diagnosis of a hip dislocation, as contractures are common and restrict motion. The diagnosis is made from radiographs. Although standard radiological criteria can be used, a critical assessment of the patient and radiograph is important as geometric indices such as the Reimer's migration index [54] (Fig. 19.11) or the Wiberg center–edge angle depend upon the position of the joint at any given moment and are influenced by rotation and adduction. Faraj and colleagues have recently questioned the reliability of Reimers' index for clinical purposes as they found significant inter-observer errors that could be outside clinical acceptability [55]. A better early indicator is the lateral acetabular edge [56]. A progressive convexity indicates excessive pressure from the femoral head against the acetabular edge and progression to femoral head displacement with time. In this instance the risk of dislocation remains despite normal geometry.

Arthrographic findings show that progressive deformation of the cartilaginous acetabulum and femoral head occurs in some cases before obvious hip instability [57]. The hip develops a typical deformity during this dislocation process which consists of a unidirectional enlargement of the acetabulum, unidirectional joint instability, and then joint decentering. On the femoral side increased anteversion and/or valgus and muscle contractures are seen [58]. As 91% of the hips dislocate cranio-laterally this deformity is seen on antero-posterior radiographs of the pelvis. Other directions of dislocation exist, however (anterior 8%, posterior 1%), and are sometimes only visible on 3D-computed tomography (CT) scans.

Treatment for hip dislocation is indicated for three reasons: instability, which cannot be controlled by the patient; restriction of motion, which predisposes to pathological fractures; and pain, which may already be present in mild subluxations [59, 60]. There is controversy, however, as to whether a dislocated hip is painful, but Cooperman et al. suggested that 50% of a small group of institutionalized patients with CP complained of pain in the dislocated hip [61]. They concluded that a dislocation should be reduced. Noonan et al. found that the incidence of hip pain was low and not associated with hip displacement or osteoarthritis in their study of 77 adults with CP [62]. They recommended that surgical treatment of the hip in severely affected patients should be based upon the presence of pain or contractures and not on radiographic signs of hip displacement or osteoarthritis. In many centers children with severe CP have a hip surveillance program consisting of an annual pelvic radiograph after the age of 5 until skeletal maturity [63]. Under the age of 5 years progressive lateral displacement of the head is managed in some centers by adductor longus intramuscular tenotomy, gracilis myotomy, and psoas tenotomy. This is only likely to be effective in the longer term if hip abduction can be maintained. Progressive uncovering of the femoral head requires the addition of varus derotation osteotomy [64]. A varus osteotomy of the femur has the same effect as passive hip abduction but has the advantage that its effect is independent of passive movement. The femoral deformity is either excessive anteversion or valgus, or both. It should be remembered that coxa valga is often a radiographic artefact due to femoral torsion, so that a corrected view of the proximal femur should be obtained. An antero-posterior radiograph with the femur in internal rotation to neutralize anteversion is a prerequisite to show the true femoral pathology and the neck–shaft angle. The aim of surgery is to restore the neck–shaft angle and an AO blade plate provides excellent fixation for this purpose. Significant re-operation rates have been reported after early soft tissue or proximal femoral procedures when performed at an average age of 4 years, as acetabular remodeling did not reliably occur post-operatively [65]. In practice many nonwalking children with CP present to the orthopaedic surgeon with established radiological signs of hip displacement. Where there is acetabular dysplasia or a dislocation, the femoral osteotomy needs to be supplemented by an acetabular procedure such as a Pemberton [66] or Dega pelvic osteotomy [67]. These procedures bend down the elongated part of the acetabulum over the reduced femoral head. It is also possible to perform a Dega osteotomy after closure of the triradiate cartilage in patients with severe CP as the pelvic bone is often osteoporotic [68]. Procedures to redirect the acetabulum or to enlarge femoral head cover are less effective and are indicated for other acetabular pathologies. An open reduction of the hip is not always necessary but when needed should include resection of the ligamentum teres and division of the transverse acetabular ligament. Sufficient shortening of the femur at the time of femoral osteotomy is most important to lengthen, relatively, the contracted muscles and to avoid pressure on the femoral head; additional soft tissue procedures are rarely necessary. This complex operation has a success rate of about 95% in experienced hands for lateral or posterior dislocations, but for anterior dislocation there is a failure rate of up to 30%. Even severe deformity of the femoral head is not necessarily a contraindication to reduction since the risk of subsequent arthritis appears to be small. If the femoral head is unreconstructable, there is a choice of procedures to obtain reasonable abduction. The demand on the hip in these severely handicapped patients is low and osteoarthritic changes seen radiologically can remain asymptomatic for many years. A subtrochanteric abduction osteotomy can be carried out which will give sufficient abduction for perineal hygiene and seating [69]. Proximal femoral resection has been plagued by ectopic bone formation but may be prevented by the technique of interposition arthroplasty described by Castle and Schneider using the gluteus medius and minimus and vastus lateralis between the resected femur and the acetabulum [70].

The Knee

In the nonwalker the goals of treatment for the knee are to obtain a comfortable posture when sitting in a chair, lying in bed, and standing in a standing frame, if such a device is used. Excessive knee flexion causes skin problems on the edge of the chair. Fractional hamstring lengthening rarely brings complete correction but may be enough to improve hamstring length sufficiently. If the result is insufficient, a closing wedge supracondylar extension osteotomy can be added. This will not give the patient any further range of motion but will change the arc of available movement to a more useful one.

Foot and Ankle Deformity

In the nonwalker, the goals are a well-shaped foot for shoewear, for the foot to rest on the footplate of the wheelchair, and for it to be plantigrade when standing in a standing frame. Severe equinus is undesirable. Fixed bony deformity may have to be corrected by bony surgery. Joint fusions are well tolerated and provide long-lasting results, whereas there is a high risk of the deformity recurring after soft tissue procedures alone.

Surgery for the Walker

One prerequisite for normal gait is to be able to use as little energy or muscle force as possible, compatible with efficient locomotion. Ideally the ground reaction force should pass behind the hip joint center and in front of the knee joint center thereby creating passive external knee and hip extensor moments. Mild hyperextension at the knee and hip helps to stabilize these joints in stance as the patient can use their ligaments and capsule as a "backstop" to counteract the external extension moment. The position of the shank relative to the floor is critical for the triceps surae to control the ground reaction forces with respect to the proximal joints. The position of the foot relative to the floor is less critical, but to increase stability the heel should contact the floor. This can be achieved by adding a heel raise to the shoe if there is equinus. During swing the leg must shorten functionally to pass the opposite leg. The knee must extend again in terminal swing before the foot next contacts the ground.

There are surgical solutions for both the stance and the swing phases of gait. Correction of deformities should be considered in the sagittal, coronal, and transverse planes. Only a small percentage of patients with total body involvement are mobile, and the following section relates mainly to those with diplegia and hemiplegia. Multi-level surgery based on pre- and post-operative gait analysis has been shown to be effective for the walking child with CP [71, 72] and health-related quality of life outcomes also improve post-operatively [73].

The Hip

Loss of extension of the hip is a problem and will also influence the position of the knee and ankle. It is of less importance, however, if the patient can only walk with aids, resulting in a flexed position of the trunk when standing or walking. Although intramuscular psoas tenotomy has been advocated this has to be balanced against the possible risk of post-operative hip flexor weakness that could affect forward propulsion of the lower limb. Preservation of hip flexor strength is important for patients with CP and there is now a trend away from psoas lengthening. Adduction contracture of the hip may be manifested by short stride length, approximation of the knees, and, in severe cases, scissoring. In walking patients who have a functional adduction deformity shown by gait analysis, intramuscular adductor longus tenotomy and gracilis myotomy are the procedures of choice, but it is important to be sure that the "adducted" posture of the knees is not due to internal femoral rotation. If there is asymmetry of abduction, the adductor longus tendon and gracilis may be tenotomized on one side and the gracilis only on the other. Anterior branch obturator neurectomy is contraindicated in the walking patient because the adductor brevis muscle, a hip stabilizer, is denervated.

Internal rotation deformity can be corrected by derotation femoral osteotomy. Biomechanical analysis has shown that the level of correction, subtrochanteric or supracondylar, does not affect the end result [74]. The site of osteotomy is chosen with regard to concomitant procedures such as correction of a knee flexion contracture or femoral neck–shaft angle. A blade plate can be used either proximally or distally and gives excellent fixation. In general it is better to delay derotation osteotomy until 7 or 8 years of age as femoral torsion does not change significantly in children after the age of 9 and may recur if performed in younger children [75, 76]. When assessing rotational deformity in the leg, it is important that a compensatory external tibial torsion is not made more obvious after femoral derotation osteotomy and is recognized and corrected at the same time.

Dislocated or subluxed hip joints are treated as in the nonwalker by joint reconstruction including open reduction, if necessary, femoral and pelvic osteotomy, and, rarely, additional soft tissue procedures. It is preferable to shorten the femur enough to reduce pressure within the joint and hence avoid femoral head necrosis than to preserve leg length. Residual leg length discrepancy can be corrected toward skeletal maturity by a contralateral epiphysiodesis at the knee.

Internal rotation is a common deformity in walkers but is not necessarily functionally disabling. Patients may have difficulties in controlling their legs which may give way and flex at the knees. An internally rotated position of the lower limbs places the flexed legs under the center of mass and requires less compensatory movement to rebalance the trunk. In external rotation, however, the patient must still position the trunk over the lower limb to attempt to align the center of mass, which often results in a Duchenne type of gait pattern (lateral lean of the trunk toward the stance lower limb). For this reason there is now a trend toward leaving some residual internal rotation of not more than 10° when improving internal femoral rotation surgically.

The Knee

There may be extension or flexion deformities at the knee. A flexed knee posture may have several causes, for example, spasticity of the hamstrings, weakness of the quadriceps, a hip flexion contracture, spasticity of the gastrocnemius, or a combination of these factors. The joints above and below the knee should be examined as the knee should not be considered in isolation. Fractional lengthening of the medial hamstrings is the procedure of choice if the hamstrings are to be lengthened and allows some choice over the degree of lengthening. The problem with co-spasticity of the quadriceps has been addressed by Gage et al., who recommended a medial transfer of the distal part of the rectus femoris to reduce the spasticity of the quadriceps after fractional hamstring lengthening [77]. The rectus femoris tendon is transferred medially to sartorius or semitendinosus or semimembranosus. The effect on rotation, however, is

minimal, and hence a lateral transfer is not recommended. This procedure increases the dynamic range of motion at the knee by about 15–20° [78] and is recommended in conjunction with fractional hamstring lengthening provided that co-spasticity of the hamstrings and rectus has been demonstrated. Knee hyperextension may result from previous surgery if the knee flexors become too weak. The hamstrings also control the position of the pelvis and excessive weakening may result in an increased anterior pelvic tilt and a compensatory lumbar hyperlordosis. If the knee hyperextension is due to spastic quadriceps, one solution is to perform a distal rectus tenotomy. Persisting crouch gait associated with patella alta, elongation of the patellar tendon, short hamstrings, and a knee capsular contracture can be managed by a supracondylar femoral extension osteotomy, patellar tendon shortening (or distal transfer of the tibial tuberosity if the tibial apophysis has closed), and fractional hamstring lengthening.

Foot and Ankle

These are common deformities. Equinus may be primarily caused by a contracture of the gastrocnemius or the soleus or be secondary to hip or knee flexion contractures. Whereas compensation for a knee flexion contracture requires hip flexion and vice versa, the position of the ankle is independent of the position of the hip and knee, provided the entire foot can make contact with the ground, either directly or indirectly via shoewear or a splint. Normal individuals can wear shoes of varying heel height and still maintain normal alignment of the hip and knee. Because hip and knee flexion results in a functional shortening of the leg, a compensatory equinus position is often used to allow foot contact. Therefore, the ankle should not be examined in isolation. The aim of treatment of an equinus deformity is to obtain full contact between the plantar aspect of the shoe and the ground and ensures that the shank is perpendicular to the floor in the standing position. Thus equinus can be accepted but requires a heel raise for compensation. In this situation additional stabilization by shoewear or an orthosis may be necessary. An AFO is especially helpful to compensate for drop foot deformity, as this is difficult to improve surgically.

If the equinus deformity is too severe or conservative treatment is not acceptable, the aim of management is to produce a plantigrade foot. Mild contracture of the calf muscles may respond to serial casting. Resting AFOs are widely used at night, but if tension is applied to improve dorsiflexion, there is usually poor compliance. Serial casting requires diligence and skill and may postpone the need for surgery. Applied injudiciously, serious damage can result

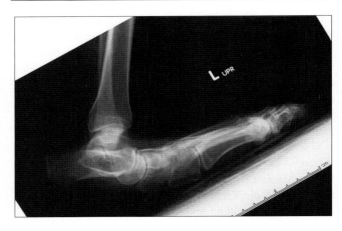

Fig. 19.12 Mid-foot break

if the foot is used as a lever to dorsiflex the ankle, producing a pseudo-correction at the expense of a mid-tarsal or hindfoot break (Fig. 19.12). To apply true stretch to the triceps surae muscle the subtalar joint must be locked by adduction–inversion in cases of valgus–abduction feet or the opposite in varus–adduction feet. If surgical lengthening of the triceps surae (Achilles tendon lengthening in hemiplegia or aponeurotic or gastrocnemius tendon lengthening or tenotomy in diplegia) is performed at an early age there is a likelihood of repeat surgery before skeletal maturity. Botulinum toxin injections can be used to lower tone and delay surgery. This has to be balanced against the disadvantages and social inconvenience of multiple visits for serial casting. Secondary deformities in the proximal lower limb, and the risk of iatrogenic overlengthening of the triceps muscle, are recognized risks. Flexible AFOs worn during function can maintain or even slightly improve dorsiflexion if plantar flexion is blocked and dorsiflexion is left free. These orthoses are superior to walking barefoot or with stiff orthoses [21].

In the assessment of equinus it is essential to distinguish, if possible, between tonic and phasic spasticity because the former is more capable of producing fixed contracture. Most operations are designed for muscle shortening resulting from tonic spasticity. Calf muscle force should be preserved as much as possible as the triceps surae controls standing posture, and its force is necessary for running, jumping, and stair climbing. Weakening this muscle might improve gait and heel posture relative to the floor but interferes with many other functions. Most centers now are cautious about lengthening the soleus in diplegia for fear of defunctioning the triceps. It is now considered safer to lengthen the gastrocnemius only in diplegia and to accept, if necessary, some residual equinus from a short soleus which can be compensated for by shoewear or a small heel raise. The gastrocnemius tendon can be divided using the Vulpius [79] or

Strayer [80] technique. In hemiplegia, however, there is often coexisting shortening of the gastrocnemius and soleus and so Achilles tendon lengthening here is permissible. Although the muscle itself is short, most surgeons perform an elongation of the tendo-Achilles and this may be done open or closed. A percutaneous Hoke technique is effective assuming that this is a primary procedure and that no other lengthenings in that region are required. Care must be taken, however, to prevent overlengthening as control of heel cord length may be difficult with this procedure. If a concomitant intramuscular tibialis posterior lengthening is required, the Achilles tendon procedure can be done by an open technique using a Z-lengthening. Repeated Achilles tendon lengthening can also be done percutaneously, providing the skin is not adherent to the underlying tendon. The tendon is tenotomized at three sites: one-half medially and distally, one-half medially and proximally, and one-half laterally between the two medial cuts. The tendon slides apart as the foot is dorsiflexed to no more than a right angle when holding the hindfoot in varus. A below-knee cast is then applied while the foot is held at a right angle, but not beyond, to avoid producing calcaneus. If less correction is required, aponeurotic lengthening, the Baumann procedure [81], is sufficient: the aponeuroses of the gastrocnemii and, if necessary, of the soleus are exposed in the middle third of the shank and are divided at three or four sites perpendicular to the fiber direction. This procedure does not produce a direct gain in muscle length, and hence post-operative physiotherapy is mandatory. The advantage of this procedure is the preservation of muscle strength [21, 22].

There are three common causes for pes varus: spasticity of the tibialis posterior, tibialis anterior, or of the gastrocnemius–soleus, or a combination of these. Gastrocnemius–soleus causes inversion of the ankle, whereas the tibialis posterior causes hindfoot varus, and tibialis anterior mid-foot varus. Indications for surgery in this group are failure of an orthosis to control the foot deformity, which is especially difficult if the deformity is produced during swing. Subsequent bony changes need to be prevented. A variety of procedures has been advocated. If there is no fixed joint deformity, the aim should be to balance the foot by procedures on the deforming musculotendinous units. Inversion at the ankle is corrected by judicious elongation of the tendo-Achilles in hemiplegia and of the gastrocnemius in diplegia. Inversion of the hindfoot can be corrected by either an intramuscular tibialis posterior lengthening [82] or a split tibialis posterior transfer [83]. The former can be accomplished through the same incision used for Achilles tendon or gastrocnemius surgery, which usually has to be performed as well. Simple tibialis posterior tenotomy is contraindicated for fear of producing a flat foot and valgus deformity. Inversion of the mid-foot is corrected by a split tibialis anterior tendon transfer [84, 85]. Alternatively, the whole tendon can be transferred to the dorsum or lateral side of the foot depending upon the correction required. The object is to balance muscle action across the medial and lateral sides of the foot. Fixed bony deformity requires a combination of soft tissue surgery and bony correction. For a fixed varus hindfoot a lateral closing wedge osteotomy of the calcaneus in addition to soft tissue surgery is indicated. For a fixed hind- and mid-foot a triple fusion may be indicated after soft tissue release, but it should be noted that patients with stiff feet can have difficulty walking on uneven ground. Pes valgus may be due to spasticity of the peroneal muscles or triceps surae, but a major factor is pathological torsional moments during gait. Unless treated, the deformity will progress from flexible to rigid and produce secondary hallux valgus. The foot deformity can be managed either conservatively by an AFO or surgically. The procedure of choice is a calcaneal lengthening (Evans procedure) which is effective as long as the foot is flexible. An alternative is the extra-articular subtalar fusion, and the Dennyson and Fulford modification of the Grice–Green technique [86] has proved very reliable. Should hallux valgus occur, this may be treated by a metatarsal osteotomy or metatarso-phalangeal fusion. The foot should not be considered in isolation and it is essential to check that the underlying cause for a foot or toe deformity does not lie more proximally.

In older children a flexion deformity of the great toe can be troublesome, producing pressure sores on the metatarso-phalangeal joint (MTPJ), interphalangeal joint (IPJ), or on the pulp of the toe. This deformity is best managed by Z-lengthening of the muscle causing the deformity, and in severe cases by fusion of the IPJ or MTPJ depending on the site of the deformity.

Upper Limb Surgery

Conservative Management

Indications for orthotic provision in the upper limb are rare. There are, however, two groups of patients who benefit from orthoses. In the first, spasticity of the muscles controlling wrist posture may position the hand out of the patient's direct field of vision which makes use of the hand difficult and in some patients finger and thumb function can be improved by stabilizing the wrist with a splint. In the second, patients present with progressive flexion deformity of the fingers and wrist, which interferes with care and nursing. These muscles often respond to stretching by a positional splint worn during the day. The splint needs to be adjusted regularly to maintain any gain in range of motion. Splinting for elbow and shoulder is difficult and cumbersome, and the rare successes hardly justify its use.

Surgery

Some patients, especially when older, develop severe flexion deformities in the upper limb at the wrist, elbow, and sometimes the shoulder. These contracted muscles can respond to injections of botulinum toxin A combined with stretching and positional orthoses.

Only a small number of patients are suitable for upper limb surgery. Assessment should be considered with the overall disability of the child and realistic goals set. Surgical procedures usually consist of positioning the arm in a more functional or cosmetic position. Important criteria for intervention include the intelligence, motivation, motor function, sensibility, and age [87]. As with the lower limb, muscle weakness, fixed deformity, dynamic deformity, and contractures need to be assessed. Similarly, a distinction should be made between phasic and tonic spasticity. Rigidity may produce either flexor or extensor dystonia. There is no reciprocal inhibition associated with dystonia so both agonists and antagonists grow normally and tendon transfers in this situation can produce the opposite and equally disabling posture. Poor sensibility does not exclude surgery, but poor stereognosis, two-point discrimination greater than 15–20 mm, and an inability to position the hand in space when the eyes are closed are relative contraindications to procedures designed to improve fine coordination [87]. Athetosis may make tendon transfers unreliable.

Operations in the upper limb include joint stabilization, release of contractures, musculotendinous lengthening, and tendon transfer. The usual deformity in the shoulder is adduction and internal rotation. Where there is a fixed contracture, derotation humeral osteotomy can improve elbow and forearm positions. Painful subluxation due to untreated shoulder deformity is rare. Elbow flexion contractures can cause severe functional problems. Loss of 30° of extension may not require treatment on its own, but if loss of elbow extension prevents efficient use of crutches or if the patient, who is usually hemiplegic, dislikes the appearance, surgical release can be effective. An anterior elbow release (Z-lengthening of biceps tendon, fractional lengthening of brachialis, and release of the flexor–pronator origin) can improve the contracture but care should be taken to avoid a fixed extension deformity. For daily activities it is usually more important for the patient to have sufficient flexion at the elbow to be able to reach the head and mouth than to have full elbow extension.

The following deformities may occur distal to the elbow: pronation of the forearm, wrist and finger flexion, and thumb adduction or "thumb-in-palm." In the forearm, pronation can be dealt with by pronator teres tenotomy if this is an isolated problem or can be combined with a flexor–pronator release [88] if there is a severe flexion deformity of the wrist and fingers. This operation produces an unselective release of all the flexors and should be reserved for severe deformity with no prospect of useful hand function; otherwise selective flexor lengthenings and transfers should be considered.

Excessive wrist flexion is a common deformity and inhibits hand grasp. Zancolli et al. have provided guidelines on the surgical management of wrist and finger flexion deformities, summarized below [89]. Wrist flexion is often associated with ulnar deviation, and tendon transfers can improve extension. Where there is mild spasticity, a tenotomy of the flexor carpi ulnaris and musculo-aponeurotic release of the flexor origins are recommended. If the wrist extensors are weak the flexor carpi ulnaris is transferred to extensor carpi radialis brevis.

Musculo-aponeurotic release of the flexors may also be necessary and where finger extension is only possible with the wrist flexed beyond 50°, an additional pronator release is recommended. Severe flexion of the fingers and an inability to extend the fingers in full wrist flexion may be treated by multiple tendon lengthenings in the forearm. Transfer of flexor carpi ulnaris to extensor digitorum communis has the advantage over the Green and Banks [90] transfer to extensor carpi radialis brevis in that it may not result in extension contractures of the fingers. Wrist arthrodesis is indicated for cosmesis in the nonfunctional hand and is usually requested by hemiplegics, for degenerative changes at the wrist with associated pain, or where there is functional finger flexion and extension when the wrist is immobilized in neutral. One technique is to use a contoured one-third tubular plate for aligning the third metacarpal with the radius after the articular surfaces have been denuded. One pitfall of arthrodesis in a functional hand is in those patients who rely on crutches or a wheelchair for mobility. They may not be able to use crutches efficiently once the wrist has been fused in the "optimum" position because they are unable to transfer body weight to the palm of the hand. Adduction contracture of the thumb can be treated by myotomy of the adductor muscle in the palm. This is preferred to tenotomy as it releases the first metacarpal but does not allow hyperextension of the metacarpo-phalangeal joint [91]. The thumb-in-palm deformity is complex and often difficult to treat. The main deforming force is the flexor pollicis longus but there may also be spasticity of the adductor pollicis, flexor pollicis brevis, or abductor pollicis brevis. To confirm that the flexor pollicis longus is the principal deforming force, thumb flexion should decrease on wrist flexion and conversely wrist extension will exaggerate the deformity. Several procedures are necessary to deal with the deformity: release of adductor pollicis, flexor pollicis brevis, and abductor pollicis brevis; arthrodesis of the metacarpophalangeal joint if unstable; lengthening of flexor pollicis longus; and re-routing of extensor pollicis longus [53, 87, 92].

Post-Operative Management and Complications

Immediate post-operative management will depend upon the type of procedure performed. Bony and tendon surgery will require a period of immobilization to allow tissue healing and to lessen the effects of muscle spasm. In the lower limb, calf muscle or tendon surgery can be undertaken as a day case and immediate weight-bearing in a below-knee plaster cast begun within the limits of comfort. Isolated hamstring and rectus femoris surgery requires the use of either a long leg cast or a lightweight removable splint. If the hamstrings are particularly tight, the knee is not extended to its limit but left in a slightly flexed position. A new cast is applied with the knee extended under general anesthesia 2 weeks later, after wound healing. Excessive stretch of the flexed knee has been reported to produce persistent neural damage [93]. Alternatively, a positional orthosis with an extendible knee mechanism can be used. The advantage is that stretch can be applied while the patient is conscious and adjustments made as necessary. The splint needs to be fitted before surgery and is worn 23 out of 24 h per day until the desired extension has been achieved. A hip spica or equivalent orthosis may be used after hip relocation surgery in the nonwalker.

In the immediate post-operative period careful consideration should be given to the relief of pain and spasm and the maintenance of the desired position of the limb. In the lower limb post-operative epidural anesthesia is highly desirable as it addresses these two main immediate problems and can be maintained for several days. The child should be mobilized as soon as is practicable.

Rehabilitation after surgery is lengthy, time consuming, and involves both the therapist and parents or carers. Recovery after even a minor procedure can take many months because of the new demands made on the neuromuscular system. It may take over a year to achieve maximum benefit after multiple-level surgery in the lower limb and the patient, parents, therapist, and surgeon can be frustrated by the apparent lack of progress after such procedures.

It should not be forgotten that CP is an incurable condition, and careful preoperative assessment is essential to avoid exchanging one problem for an even worse one. Therefore goals must be realistic. The need for surgery may coincide with unfavorable events occurring in the natural history of the child's development, such as diminishing efficiency of walking, and an indifferent outcome does not necessarily result from surgery but may appear to. The present trend toward multiple-level surgery at one sitting is justifiable provided that excellent preoperative assessment is made but does increase the possibility of error.

There are several pitfalls in the surgical management of CP apart from complications common to any surgical procedure. The most serious penalties result from inadequate assessment, performing operations at the wrong level, and failing to allow for the action of muscles that cross two joints. An example of this type of error is an Achilles tendon lengthening for an equinus attitude that is caused by a hip flexion contracture. Overlengthening of musculotendinous units may produce an even worse deformity; examples include calcaneus after excessive Achilles tendon lengthening, an excessively broad-based gait or, even worse, an abduction contracture at the hip after excessive adductor surgery. In principle it is better to correct proximal deformities first and to reassess the influence of this distally. Incorrect assessment of bony deformity can give poor results; for example, significant uncovering of the femoral head is unlikely to be remedied by muscle releases alone, and if relocation is contemplated it should be done before the appearance of significant femoral head deformity. Equally, in considering torsional deformity, neither the femur nor the tibia should be viewed in isolation; correction of excessive femoral internal torsion by external derotation osteotomy in the presence of compensatory external tibial torsion will exaggerate the clinical appearances of an externally rotated lower limb. Unpredictable results follow surgery for rigidity or phasic spasticity and after soft tissue procedures in the presence of fixed bony deformity.

Assessment of the child with CP is challenging, and surgery can be effective but should be seen as only one aspect in the comprehensive management of the patient.

References

1. Ingram TT. Paediatric aspects of cerebral palsy. Edinburgh: Livingstone; 1964.
2. Brown JK, Minns RA. Mechanisms of deformity in children with cerebral palsy. Sem Orthop 1989; 4:236–255.
3. Ghasia F, Brunstrom J, Gordon M, Tychsen L. Frequency and severity of visual sensory and motor deficits in children with cerebral palsy: gross motor function classification scale. Invest Ophthalmol Vis Sci 2008; 49:572–580.
4. Sanger TD, Kukke SN. Abnormalities of tactile sensory function in children with dystonic and diplegic cerebral palsy. J Child Neurol 2007; 22:289–293.
5. Nelson KB, Ellenberg JH. Antecedents of cerebral palsy. New Eng J Med 1986; 315:81–86.
6. Bejar R, Wozniak P, Ailard M , et al. Antenatal origin of neurologic damage in newborn infants. Preterm infants. Am J Obstet Gynecol 1988; 159:357–363.
7. Padilla-Gomes NF, Enríquez G, Acosta-Rojas R, et al. Prevalence of neonatal ultrasound brain lesions in premature infants with and without intrauterine growth restriction. Acta Paediatr 2007; 96:1582–1587.
8. Zimmerman RA, Bilaniuk LT. Neuroimaging evaluation of cerebral palsy. Clin Perinatol 2006; 33:517–544.
9. Sherrington C. The integrative action of the nervous system. New Haven CT Yale University Press; 1947.
10. Ziv I, Blackburn N, Rang M, Korerska J. Muscle growth in normal and spastic mice. Dev Med Child Neurol 1984; 26:94–99.
11. Tardieu C, Lespargot A, Tabary C, Bret MD. For how long must the soleus muscle be stretched each day to prevent contracture? Dev Med Child Neurol 1988; 30:3–10.
12. Levitt S. Treatment of Cerebral Palsy and Motor Delay, 4th ed. Oxford: Blackwell; 2004.
13. Staheli LT. The prone hip extension test. Clin Orthop Rel Res 1977; 123:12–15.
14. Ruwe PA, Gage JR, Ozonoff MB, DeLuca PA. Clinical determination of femoral anteversion. J Bone Joint Surg Am 1992; 74A:820–830.
15. Staheli LT, Engel GM. Tibial torsion. A method of assessment and a survey of normal children. Clin Orthop Rel Res 1972; 86:183–186.
16. Hazlewood ME, Simmons AN, Johnson WT, et al. The footprint method to assess transmalleolar axis. Gait Posture 2007; 25:597–603.
17. Perry J, Antonelli D, Plur J, et al. Electromyography before and after surgery for hip deformity in children with cerebral palsy. J Bone Joint Surg Am 1976; 58A:201–208.
18. Perry J, Hoffer MM, Giovan P, et al. Gait analysis of the triceps surae in cerebral palsy. J Bone Joint Surg Am 1974; 56A:511–520.
19. Gage JR. Gait analysis in cerebral palsy. Clinics in developmental medicine, no. 121. Oxford: MacKeith Press; 1947.
20. Read HS, Hazlewood ME, Hillman SJ, et al. Edinburgh Visual Gait Score for use in cerebral palsy. J Pediatr Orthop 2003; 23:296–301.
21. Brunner, R. Die Auswirkungen der Aponeurosendurchtrennung auf den Muskel. Habilitation-Dissertation, University of Basel, Basel, Switzerland, 1998.
22. Jaspers RT, Brunner R, Pel JJ, Huijing PA. Acute effects of intramuscular aponeurotomy on rat gastrocnemius medialis: force transmission, muscle force and sarcomere length. J Biomech 1999; 32:71–79.
23. Tardieu G, Thuilleux G, Tardieu C, Huet, et al. Tour E. Long term effects of surgical elongation of the tendo calcaneus in the normal cat. Develop Med Child Neurol 1979; 21:83–94.
24. Damiano DL, Kelly LE, Vaughn CL. Effects of quadriceps femoris muscle strengthening on crouch gait in children with spastic diplegia. Phys Ther 1995; 75:658–667.
25. Hullin MG, Robb JE, Loudon IR. Ankle-foot orthosis function in low-level myelomeningocele. J Pediatr Orthop 1992; 12: 518–521.
26. Brunner R, Meier G, Ruepp T. Comparison of a stiff and a spring-type ankle-foot orthosis to improve gait in spastic hemiplegic children. J Pediatr Orthop 1998; 18:719–726.
27. Farmer SE, Woollam PJ, Patrick JH, et al. Dynamic orthoses in the management of joint contracture. J Bone Joint Surg 2005; 87B:291–295.
28. Terjesen T, Lange JE, Steen H. Treatment of scoliosis with spinal bracing in quadriplegic cerebral palsy. Dev Med Child Neurol 2000; 42:448–454.
29. Tsirikos AI, Chang W-N, Dabney KW, Miller F. Comparison of parents' and caregivers' satisfaction after spinal fusion in children with cerebral palsy. J Pediatr Orthop 2004; 24:54–58.
30. Peacock WJ, Arens LJ, Goldberg MJ. Cerebral palsy spasticity. Selective posterior rhizotomy. Paediatr Neurosci 1987; 13:61–66.
31. Oppenheim WL. Selective posterior rhizotomy for spastic cerebral palsy. Clin Orthop Rel Res 1990; 253:20–29.
32. Spiegel DA, Loder RT, Alley KA, et al. Spinal deformity following selective dorsal rhizotomy. J Pediatr Orthop 2004; 24:30–36.
33. Greene WB, Dietz FR, Goldberg MJ, et al. Rapid progression of hip subluxation in cerebral palsy after selective posterior rhizotomy. J Pediatr Orthop 1991; 11:494–497.

34. Steinbok P. Selective dorsal rhizotomy for spastic cerebral palsy: a review. Childs Nerv Syst 2007; 23:981–990.

35. Farmer JP, Sabbagh AJ. Selective dorsal rhizotomies in the treatment of spasticity related to cerebral palsy. Childs Nerv Syst 2007; 23:991–1002.

36. Buckon CE, Thomas SS, Piatt JH Jr, et al. Selective dorsal rhizotomy versus orthopedic surgery: a multidimensional assessment of outcome efficacy. Arch Phys Med Rehabil 2004; 85:457–465.

37. Krach LE, Kriel RL, Gilmartin RC, et al. GMFM 1 year after continuous intrathecal baclofen infusion. Pediatr Rehabil 2005; 8:207–213.

38. Hoving MA, van Raak EP, Spincemaille GH, et al. Dutch Study Group on Child Spasticity. Intrathecal baclofen in children with spastic cerebral palsy: a double-blind, randomized, placebo-controlled, dose-finding study. Dev Med Child Neurol 2007; 49:654–659.

39. Albright AL. Intrathecal baclofen for childhood hypertonia. Childs Nerv Syst 2007; 23:971–979.

40. Ginsburg GM, Lauder AJ. Progression of scoliosis in patients with spastic quadriplegia after the insertion of an intrathecal baclofen pump. Spine 2007; 32:2745–2750.

41. Senaran H, Shah SA, Presedo A, et al. The risk of progression of scoliosis in cerebral palsy patients after intrathecal baclofen therapy. Spine 2007; 32:2348–2354.

42. Cosgrove AP, Graham HK. Botulinum toxin A prevents the development of contractures in the hereditary spastic mouse. Dev Med Child Neurol 1994, 36:379–385.

43. Koman LA, Mooney JF 3rd, Smith BP, et al. Management of spasticity in cerebral palsy with botulinum-A toxin: report of a preliminary, randomized, double-blind trial. J Pediatr Orthop 1994, 14:299–303.

44. Molenaers G, Desloovere K, Fabry G, De Cock P. The effects of quantitative gait assessment and botulinum toxin a on musculoskeletal surgery in children with cerebral palsy. J Bone Joint Surg Am 2006; 88A:161–170.

45. James JIP. Paralytic scoliosis. J Bone Joint Surg Br 1956; 38B:660–685.

46. Lonstein JE, Beck K. Hip dislocation and subluxation in cerebral palsy. J Pediatr Orthop 1986; 6:521–526.

47. Madigan RR, Wallace SL. Scoliosis in cerebral palsy: short term follow-up and prognosis in untreated institutionalized patients. Orthop Trans 1986; 10:17.

48. Thomas KJ, Simon SR. Progression of scoliosis after skeletal maturity in institutionalized adults who have cerebral palsy. J Bone Joint Surg Am 1988; 70A:1290–1296.

49. Dabney KW, Miller F, Lipton GE, et al. Correction of sagittal plane spinal deformities with unit rod instrumentation in children with cerebral palsy. J Bone Joint Surg Am 2004; 86A:156–168.

50. Miller F. Spinal deformity secondary to impaired neurologic control. J Bone Joint Surg Am 2007; 89A:143–147.

51. Soo B, Howard JJ, Boyd RN, Reid SM, Lanigan A, Wolfe R, Reddihough D, Graham HK. Hip displacement in cerebral palsy. J Bone Joint Surg [Am] 2006; 88A:121–9.

52. Graham HK, Boyd RN, Carlin JB, et al. Does botulinum toxin A combined with bracing prevent hip displacement in children with cerebral palsy and 'hips at risk'? A randomized, controlled trial. J Bone Joint Surg Am 2008; 90A:23–33.

53. Bleck EE. Orthopaedic management in cerebral palsy. Clinics in Developmental Medicine, no. 99/100. London: Mac Keith Press; 1987.

54. Reimers J. The stability of the hip in children. A radiological study of the results of muscle surgery in spastic cerebral palsy. Acta Orthopaedica Scandinavica (Supplement) 1980; 184:1–97.

55. Faraj S, Atherton WG, Stott NS. Inter- and intra-measurer error in the measurement of Reimers' hip migration percentage. J Bone Joint Surg Br 2004; 86B:434–437.

56. Howard CB, Williams LA. A new radiological sign in the hips of cerebral palsy patients. Clin Radiol 1984; 35:317–319.

57. Heinrich SD, MacEwan GD, Zembo MM. Hip dysplasia, subluxation and dislocation in cerebral palsy: an arthrographic analysis. J Pediatr Orthop 1991; 11:488–493.

58. Brunner R, Picard C, Robb JE. Morphology of the acetabulum in hip dislocations due to cerebral palsy. J Pediatr Orthop Part B 1997; 6:207–211.

59. Brunner R, Baumann JU. Clinical benefit of reconstruction of dislocated and subluxated hip joints in patients with spastic cerebral palsy. J Pediatr Orthop 1994; 14:290–294.

60. Brunner R, Döderlein L. Pathological fractures in patients with cerebral palsy. J Pediatr Orthop Part B 1996; 5:232–238.

61. Cooperman DR, Bartucci E, Dierrick E, Millar EA. Hip dislocation in spastic cerebral palsy: long-term consequences. J Pediatr Orthop 1987; 7:268–276.

62. Noonan KJ, Jones J, Pierson J, et al. Hip function in adults with severe cerebral palsy. J Bone Joint Surg Am 2004; 86A:2607–2613.

63. Dobson F, Boyd RN, Parrott J, et al. Hip surveillance in children with cerebral palsy. Impact on the surgical management of spastic hip disease J Bone Joint Surg Br 2002; 84B:720–726.

64. Kalen V, Bleck EE. Prevention of spastic paralytic dislocation of the hip. Dev Med Child Neurol 1985; 27:17–24.

65. Schmale GA, Eilert RE, Chang F, Seidel K. High reoperation rates after early treatment of the subluxating hip in children with spastic cerebral palsy. J Pediatr Orthop 2006; 26:617–623.

66. Pemberton PA. Pericapsular osteotomy of the ilium for treatment of congenital subluxation and dislocation of the hip. J Bone Joint Surg Am 1965; 47A:65–86.

67. Mubarak SJ, Valencia FG, Wenger DR. One-stage correction of the spastic dislocated hip. Use of pericapsular acetabuloplasty to improve coverage. J Bone Joint Surg Am 1992; 74A:1347–1357.

68. Robb JE, Brunner R. A Dega-type osteotomy after closure of the triradiate cartilage in non-walking patients with severe cerebral palsy. J Bone Joint Surg Br 2006; 88B:933–937.

69. Hogan KA, Blake M, Gross RH. Subtrochanteric valgus osteotomy for chronically dislocated, painful spastic hips. J Bone Joint Surgery Am 2007; 88A:2624–2631.

70. Castle ME, Schneider C. Proximal femoral resection-interposition arthroplasty. J Bone Joint Surg Am 1978; 60A:1051–1054.

71. Rodda JM, Graham HK, Nattrass GR, et al. Correction of severe crouch gait in patients with spastic diplegic with use of multilevel orthopaedic surgery. J Bone Joint Surg Am 2006; 88A:2653–2664.

72. Schwartz MH, Viehweger E, Stour J, et al. Comprehensive treatment of ambulatory children with cerebral palsy. An outcome assessment. J Pediatr Orthop 2004; 24:45–53.

73. Cuomo AV, Gamradt SC, Kim CO, et al. Health-related quality of life outcomes improve after multilevel surgery in ambulatory children with cerebral palsy. J Pediatr Orthop 2007; 27: 653–657.

74. Pirpiris M, Trivett A, Baker R, et al. Femoral derotation osteotomy in spastic diplegia: proximal or distal? J Bone Joint Surg Br 2003; 85B:265–272.

75. Fabry G. Torsion of the femur. Acta Orthop Belg 1977; 43:454–459.

76. Brunner R, Baumann JU. Long term effects of intertrochanteric varus-derotation osteotomy on femur and acetabulum in spastic cerebral palsy. J Pediatr Orthop 1997; 17:585–591.

77. Gage JR, Perry J, Hicks RR, et al. Rectus femoris transfer to improve knee function of children with cerebral palsy. Dev Med Child Neurol 1987; 29:159–166.

78. Abel MF, Damiano DL, Pannunzio M, Bush J. Muscle-tendon surgery in diplegic cerebral palsy: functional and mechanical changes. J Pediatr Orthop 1999; 19:366–375.

79. Vulpius O, Stoffel A. Tenotomie der Endsehnen der Mm. gastrocnemius et soleus. Orthopädische Operationslehre. Stuttgart: Verlag von Ferdinand Enke; 1913:29–31.

80. Strayer LM. Recession of the gastrocnemius. An operation to relieve spastic contracture of the calf muscles. J Bone Joint Surg Am 1950; 32A:671–676.

81. Baumann JU, Koch HG. Ventrale aponeurotische Verlängerung des Musculus gastrocnemius. Operative Orthop Traumatol 1989; 1:254–258.

82. Ruda R, Frost HM. Cerebral palsy spastic varus and forefoot adductus, treated by intramuscular posterior tibial lengthening. Clin Orthop Rel Res 1971; 79:61–70.

83. Green NE, Griffen PP, Shiavi P. Split posterior tibial tendon transfer in spastic cerebral palsy. J Bone Joint Surg Am 1983; 65A:748–754.

84. Hoffer MM, Barakat G, Koffman M. 10-year follow-up of split anterior tibial tendon transfer in cerebral palsied patients with spastic equino-varus deformity. J Pediatr Orthop 1985; 5: 432–434.

85. Barnes MJ, Herring JA. Combined split anterior tibial-tendon transfer and intramuscular lengthening of the posterior tibial tendon. J Bone Joint Surg 1991; 73A:734–738.

86. Dennyson WG, Fulford GE. Subtalar arthrodesis by cancellous grafts and metallic internal fixation. J Bone Joint Surg Br 1976; 58B:507–510

87. Koman AL, Gelberman RH, Toby EB, Poehling GG. Cerebral palsy: management of the upper extremity. Clin Orthop Rel Res 1990; 253:62–74.

88. Page CM. An operation for the relief of flexion-contracture in the forearm. J Bone Joint Surg 1923; 5:233–234.

89. Zancolli EA, Goldner JL, Swanson AB. Surgery of the spastic hand in cerebral palsy; report of the committee on spastic hand evaluation. J Hand Surg 1983; 8:766–772.

90. Green WT, Banks HH. Flexor carpi ulnaris transplant and its use in cerebral palsy. J Bone Joint Surg Am 1962; 44A:1343–1352.

91. Matev I. Surgical treatment of spastic 'thumb-in-palm' deformity. J Bone Joint Surg Br 1963; 45B:703–708.

92. Goldner JL, Koman AL, Gelberman R, et al. Arthrodesis of the metacarpophalangeal joint in children and adults. Adjunctive treatment of thumb in palm deformity in cerebral palsy. Clin Orthop Rel Res 1990; 253:75–89.

93. Aspen RM, Porter RW. Nerve traction during correction of knee flexion deformity. A case report and calculation. J Bone Joint Surg Br 1994; 76-B:471–473.

Chapter 20

Arthrogryposis multiplex congenita

John A. Fixsen

Introduction

Arthrogryposis multiplex congenita literally means multiple curved joints, occurring as a congenital anomaly in the newborn. The first description is ascribed to Otto in 1841 [1]. Sheldon in 1932 published the first detailed description in the United Kingdom and called the condition "amyoplasia congenita" emphasizing the lack of muscle development in this condition [2]. It is important to realize that arthrogryposis is a descriptive term and not an exact diagnosis. Hall who has made a special study of the genetics of the disorder pointed out that there are at least 150 possible diagnoses that can result in multiple curved joint deformities in the newborn child [3]. The reader is referred to Hall for a comprehensive discussion of the disorder [4].

The features of the condition are multiple rigid joint deformities with defective muscles but normal sensation (Fig. 20.1). In the classical form, called amyoplasia congenita by Sheldon, all four limbs are involved, but the condition can also occur only in the upper limbs or only in the lower limbs. Hall et al. described a distal form in which the hands and feet are severely deformed with only minor contractures more proximally, although the spine may develop scoliosis [5]. This form is important, as it can be inherited as an autosomal dominant, whereas the majority of forms of classic arthrogryposis do not have a genetic background. At birth, the children can look terribly deformed and the parents are often horrified by the appearance of their child. In addition to the multiple rigid joint contractures, the skin lacks creases and deep dimples over the joints are very characteristic (Fig. 20.2). The limbs are tubular and featureless, but the trunk may be affected, giving a characteristic "wooden doll" appearance. Other congenital anomalies such as cryptorchidism, hernias, gastroschisis, and bowel atresia may also occur.

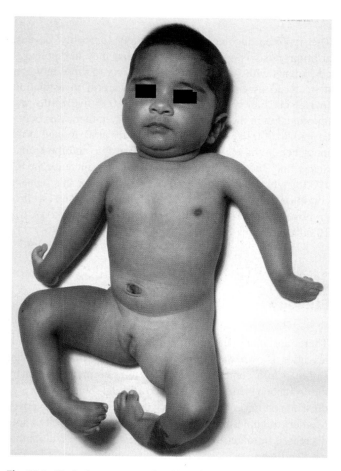

Fig. 20.1 Typical appearance of a child with four-limb arthrogryposis. Note adduction and internal rotation at the shoulders, extension at the elbows and flexion of the wrists, fixed flexion of the knees, and severe equinovarus feet

J.A. Fixsen (✉)
Orthopaedic Department, Great Ormond Street Hospital for Sick Children, London, UK

M. Benson et al. (eds.), *Children's Orthopaedics and Fractures*,
DOI 10.1007/978-1-84882-611-3_20, © Springer-Verlag London Limited 2010

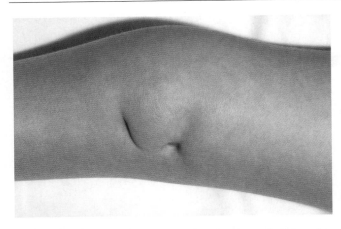

Fig. 20.2 Clinical photograph of the knee showing typical deep skin dimples

Incidence

The reported incidence varies widely, probably because arthrogryposis is a descriptive term that may be applied to all patients with stiff curved joints or only to those in whom there is no ascertainable cause after careful investigation. In Helsinki, an incidence of 3 per 10,000 live births was reported, but in the Edinburgh birth register, there was only 1 case in 56,000 live births. Wynne-Davies et al. looked at the incidence in the United Kingdom, Australia, and the United States and showed there was an apparent increase in the 1960 s, which suggested an infective cause for this unusual condition [6]. Hall quotes an incidence of classical arthrogryposis multiplex congenita (amyoplasia congenita) of 1 in 10,000 live births [4].

Etiology

There are many causes of arthrogryposis. Animal studies have shown that limitation of intrauterine movement can lead to a contracture at birth. Intrauterine infection by the Akabane virus in sheep, cows, and horses can produce a condition very similar to classical arthrogryposis. Mothers of babies born with multiple contractures often note decreased intrauterine mobility of the fetus. The factors that predispose to decreased intrauterine mobility include neuromuscular and connective tissue disorders, fetal crowding, oligohydramnios, multiple pregnancy, and malposition such as breech presentation.

An interesting case is reported of a pregnant mother treatment with curare for severe tetanus who gave birth to an arthrogrypotic baby. Wynne-Davies et al. concluded that

the best description of the etiology was "an environmental disease of early pregnancy associated with one or more unfavorable intrauterine factors" [6].

Diagnosis

The paediatrician or orthopaedic surgeon presented with a child with arthrogrypotic features must first try to establish the diagnosis. The parents of the child are, not surprisingly, often extremely upset by the appearance of their child and want immediate answers to the cause of their child's deformity. However, parental counseling should be approached with care, particularly with regard to prognosis and possible treatment, until the etiology has been elucidated. It is not uncommon for anxious parents to be given an extremely pessimistic prognosis before the diagnosis is fully understood. Conversely, an overoptimistic prognosis can also be misleading if the child subsequently proves to have a severe underlying cause for the arthrogrypotic deformities.

The following investigations should be considered:

- Radiographs of the whole spine and computed tomography (CT) of the head
- Chromosome analysis
- Collagen biochemistry
- Plasma creatine kinase estimation to exclude myopathic disorders
- Electromyography (EMG) and nerve conduction studies
- Muscle and nerve biopsy

Possible *differential diagnoses* can be considered under the following headings.

Neurological Disorders

1. Spina bifida and spinal dysraphism in all its forms
2. Myelodysplasia
3. Sacral and lumbar agenesis (Fig. 20.3)
4. Spinal muscular atrophy
5. Fetal neuropathy

Muscle Disorders

1. Dystrophia myotonica
2. Congenital muscular dystrophy
3. Fetal myopathy
4. Fetal myasthenia

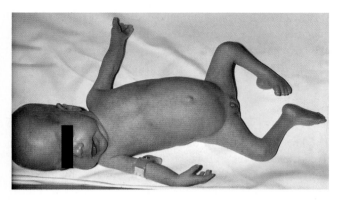

Fig. 20.3 Infant with sacral agenesis. Note how similar the lower limbs are to those in the arthrogrypotic child in Fig. 20.1

Connective Tissue Disorders

1. Marfan's syndrome
2. Ehlers–Danlos syndrome

Miscellaneous Syndromes

1. Freeman–Sheldon syndrome (cranio-carpo-tarsal dystrophy)
2. Turner's syndrome
3. Edward's syndrome (trisomy 18)
4. The pterygium or popliteal web syndrome
5. Diastrophic dwarfism

Bevan et al. suggests a multi-disciplinary team including a geneticist, paediatric orthopaedic surgeon, paediatric physiotherapist, and paediatric occupational therapist is very important both in establishing the diagnosis and the subsequent successful management of the child [7].

In general, classic amyoplasia congenita is not inherited, except for the distal form [5] affecting the hands and feet, which is commonly inherited as an autosomal dominant.

Orthopaedic Management

From the orthopaedic point of view, it is important to see these patients as soon as possible. Although it will take some time to establish the exact diagnosis, it is important to start treating the deformities early, as some of them will respond remarkably well to physiotherapy, stretching, and splintage. Some of the patients may be born with fractures and need treatment. However intractable a deformity may appear, it

is worth trying gentle manipulation and simple splintage, much of which can be done by the parents under the supervision of the physiotherapist in the first few months of life [8]. This strategy can also be very helpful in coping with the understandable parental concern. The parents must be told, however, that simple conservative treatment with stretching and splintage is unlikely to correct the deformities completely. Significant gains are especially likely in the hands, and often the knees and elbows.

In general, the limb deformities tend to be more severe distally. The feet and hands are nearly always involved, but the hips and shoulders may be quite mobile. None the less, if the hips are involved this is often with irreducible dislocation. The application of early splintage to such hips should be avoided, as it may cause avascular necrosis and increase the child's disability. Many of these children are rather weak and floppy in the first few months of life. Robinson has pointed out that they have significant problems with feeding, swallowing, sucking, weight gain, and recurrent chest infections in the first year of life [9]. Corrective surgery should be delayed until it is clear that the child is thriving and is developing trunk and sitting balance.

If orthopaedic deformities are corrected early, they must be rigorously splinted. There is a very strong tendency for recurrent deformity unless the corrected position can be adequately held by splintage. This can be very difficult in the small, tubular, featureless limbs that characterize this condition. Lower limb deformities that inhibit or prevent standing and walking by the time the child shows evidence of wanting to do so should be corrected if possible by the age of 18 months to 2 years.

In the upper limb, a careful assessment of overall function should be made before any decision regarding surgery. This usually means waiting until the age of 4 or 5 years, and a considerable period of observation and assessment. The use of special tools and utensils, assessment, and education by an experienced paediatric occupational therapist are often preferable to a complex operation, which may improve one joint but introduce other problems for the child because of the overall nature of the disorder [10, 11].

Orthopaedic Management of the Lower Limbs

The Foot

The foot is usually in fixed severe equinovarus (Fig. 20.1). Less commonly, a congenital vertical talus deformity is present. Serial stretching and strapping or splintage using the Ponseti method (see Chapter 31) may sometimes correct the deformity. However, frequently the foot is completely incorrigible and shows no response to conservative treatment. Once it is clear that conservative treatment will not be successful, surgery should be considered, preferably when the child is ready to walk. The foot is likely to require an extensive soft tissue release involving the medial, posterior, and lateral structures, which is best performed through the Cincinnati approach. If the foot fails to correct fully with even the most extensive soft tissue release or relapses quickly within 2–3 years, talectomy may have to be considered.

Talectomy has produced good results in these stiff, rigid feet [12–14]. The talus is best approached through a lateral incision, as for a triple arthrodesis. The important details are as follows. First, the entire talus must be removed. This can be difficult, because the normal tissue planes are poorly developed and the anatomy distorted, particularly if previous extensive soft tissue surgery has been performed. Second, it is important to find the ankle joint early during the operation and work round the talus, avoiding cutting into the talus itself or the tibia and malleoli. The posterior structures form an inextensile tether, and it is sensible not simply to lengthen the tendo-Achilles but to excise a 1-cm length of the fibrous cord that represents the tendo-Achilles posteriorly. Once the talus has been removed, the os calcis should be stabilized below the tibia by a K-wire, driven up through the heel pad and calcaneus into the tibia and retained for 6 weeks. Talectomy produces a plantigrade foot that is inevitably stiff and requires long-term splintage.

Recurrent deformity after talectomy is difficult to treat. The flexor hallucis longus is often tight, and it should be divided distally at the level of the metatarso-phalangeal joint of the big toe to prevent troublesome flexion of the toe. Talectomy cannot influence forefoot adduction, and if this persists and is symptomatic, a lateral calcaneocuboid fusion can be considered. Spontaneous fusion of the calcaneus to the tibia occurs in some patients but does not cause problems provided the calcaneus is in a satisfactory neutral position.

The Ilizarov technique and apparatus offer the opportunity of correcting complex foot deformities in three dimensions. Grill and Franke [15] reported the use of the Ilizarov apparatus in nine severely deformed feet, with satisfactory results in terms of function and appearance; one of their patients suffered from arthrogryposis [9]. More recently Reinke and Carpenter reported that Ilizarov application in the paediatric foot achieved satisfactory results in 21 of 24 feet; three of their patients suffered from arthrogryposis [16].

The rarer congenital vertical talus (see Chapter 33) is approached through a Cincinnati incision, allowing a posterior release, reduction of the talo-navicular dislocation, and lengthening of the tight lateral structures. The corrected position is held with K-wires. This operation produces a satisfactory stiff plantigrade foot for walking. Again, there is no urgency to rush into operation because the child can stand

very well on a rocker-bottomed foot and, if necessary, the operation can be deferred until other procedures on the hip and knee have been carried out.

The Knee

The knee presents with one of two problems: either severe fixed flexion (Fig. 20.1) or fixed extension (Fig. 20.4). Both deformities should be treated initially by repeated stretching and splintage, supervised by the physiotherapist. Surprisingly good results can be obtained in apparently rigid deformities. If the deformity does not respond to soft tissue stretching, surgery must be considered [17]. It is most important to plan surgery for the knee in relation to treatment of the foot. If the foot requires immobilization with the knee flexed, then attempts to straighten a flexed knee should wait until the foot has been treated. Conversely, if the knee is in fixed extension, it is often better to correct the knee

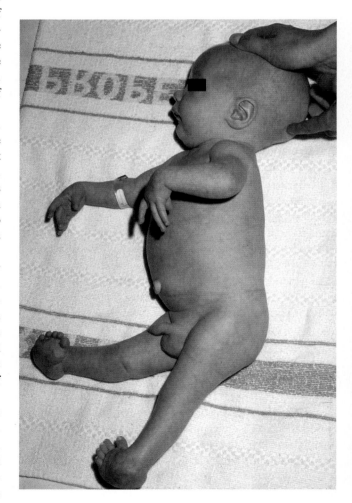

Fig. 20.4 Infant with arthrogryposis and fixed extended knees

extension before operation on the foot, so that the foot can be immobilized with a flexed knee.

In general, most joints in arthrogryposis have a relatively fixed arc of movement, and the aim of surgery is to transfer that arc into the most useful range rather than hoping to gain a significant improvement. Although occasionally there is a very gratifying improvement in the overall range, the main aim of treatment is to convert, for instance, a range of movement at the knee from fixed flexion of 90° with further flexion to 130°, to a range of flexion from 5 to 45°— a much more useful range for walking and acceptable for sitting. The operation for fixed flexion involves an extensive posterior release of all the soft tissue structures except the neurovascular bundle at the back of the knee. Usually it is not possible to use a tourniquet because of the small size of the child's leg. It is essential to divide all the structures that are tight. Medial and lateral incisions, rather than a midline longitudinal incision, should be used to minimize problems with wound healing when the knee is extended. The heads of the gastrocnemii and the posterior capsule of the knee joint are usually a significant part of the contracture and should be divided. Sometimes the posterior cruciate has to be released. Instability is rarely a problem because these joints are inherently stiff and the patient will have to wear an orthosis for many years to maintain correction. It is often impossible to extend the knee fully immediately because of the tightness of the neurovascular bundle; serial plasters over a period of weeks can slowly improve the range of extension. Once this is gained, splintage for many years is necessary to maintain knee extension (Fig. 20.5). Sometimes, in older children who have not had early soft tissue surgery, it is not possible to extend the knee without jeopardizing the blood supply to the lower leg. In this situation an extension and shortening osteotomy of the distal femur to produce relative lengthening of the soft tissues can be used to obtain full extension at the knee. Occasionally if there is gross bony deformity at the knee, fusion to correct the deformity may be considered. It is extremely tempting to consider supracondylar osteotomy to obtain correction and to ease the problem of the soft tissues. Unfortunately unless this is delayed until near maturity, the patient may develop, with growth, an extremely ugly and awkward angular deformity at the site of the osteotomy (Fig. 20.6). In general, osteotomies for the correction of deformity in arthrogryposis should be delayed until near maturity to avoid progressive or recurrent deformity.

Fixed hyperextension of the knee may respond remarkably well to serial stretching and splintage [17]. If there is no response to conservative treatment, a quadricepsplasty comprising an extensive dissection of the scarred and fibrotic quadriceps muscle is necessary to obtain some flexion at the knee. Long-term splintage is likely to be necessary to protect and support the knee after this type of surgery unless

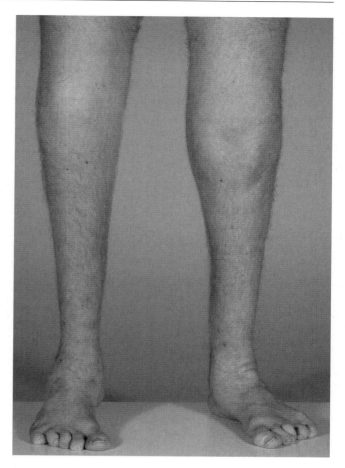

Fig. 20.5 Child after treatment for fixed flexion of the knees and several years splintage.

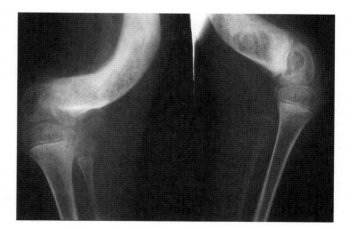

Fig. 20.6 Lateral radiographs of both knees showing severe posterior angulation of the femur above the knee following supracondylar osteotomies several years earlier

there is at least quadriceps power of grade 3 or more [18]. For this reason Parsch and Pietrzak prefer not to lengthen the quadriceps if the muscle is too weak to stabilize the knee post-operatively without braces [19].

The Ilizarov apparatus would appear to be an attractive alternative to difficult surgery with a high recurrence rate in the knee. However, Damsin and Trousseau [20] and Brunner et al. [21] point out the difficulties and high recurrence rate, particularly in young children, with this method. Nevertheless, it provides a useful alternative to surgery after failed physiotherapy, particularly in the older patient or the patient in whom previous surgery has failed.

The Hip

Frequently, one or both hips are dislocated. The clinical diagnosis can be very difficult. The general stiffness of the joints may make it impossible to perform the clinical tests for hip instability. There is often marked limitation of abduction, and a radiograph or ultrasound of the hips is necessary to decide whether they are displaced. If the hips are dislocated, they are rarely reducible on abduction and should not be splinted if irreducible. Splinting an unreduced hip is liable to cause avascular necrosis. If one hip is reduced and the other dislocated, it is worth surgically reducing the dislocated hip. If both hips are dislocated, Lloyd-Roberts and Lettin advised that they should be left alone, as it was rarely possible to get a satisfactory result on both sides, and the complication rate, particularly stiffness and recurrent dislocation, was high [22]. In 1987, Staheli et al. reported a small series of patients in whom reduction through the medial approach was performed in 25 hips, 7 of which were unilateral and 9 bilateral [23]. The majority of these operations were undertaken in children younger than 1 year. In a 5–6 year follow-up of these patients Szoke et al. reported only one redislocation and two cases of increased stiffness [24]. In contrast, Akazawa et al. recommended an extensive anterolateral approach to the hip and reported satisfactory results in a small series of patients followed for a mean of 11.8 years [25]. In the author's small experience of the medial approach, when successful, this does not appear to cause increased stiffness, but redislocation can occur, particularly if the hip is very dysplastic. Experience of extensive open reduction with femoral shortening has not always produced a stable, mobile hip. Yau et al. reported a 20-year follow-up of hip problems in arthrogryposis showing that open reduction was successful in stabilizing the hip but the hips were usually stiffer [26]. Adult patients with arthrogryposis and bilateral stable but completely dislocated hips tend to manage very well. If surgery is undertaken for bilateral dislocation and is not successful on both sides the result for the patient is often worse than if the hips had been left untreated

Apart from dislocation, the hips may be fixed in a very awkward frog or "Buddha" position of abduction and external rotation (Fig. 20.7). Fortunately, the conservative measures for the deformities in the lower limb distal to the

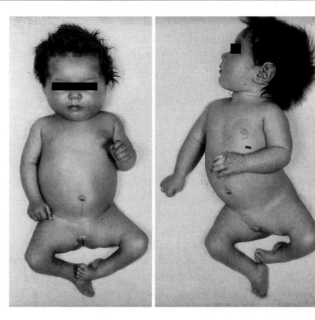

Fig. 20.7 Child showing the flexed abducted hips and flexed knees of the so-called Buddha position

hip, such as the plasters and splintage necessary for treating the feet and knees, help to stretch the hips, making it usually unnecessary to perform soft tissue release or corrective osteotomies to bring the hips into a neutral position. Fixed flexion of the hips is very common. It may require release, but when combined with some flexion at the knee it is often best left alone. As always in arthrogryposis, it is important to consider the treatment of the whole limb and not a single joint in isolation.

Orthopaedic Management of the Upper Limbs

As stated in the introduction, because of the complex interactions of all the deformities in the upper limb and the child's ability to develop remarkable trick movements, surgery should be considered very carefully and probably delayed at least until the child is aged about 4 years [27]. Physiotherapy has a major role in obtaining as much movement as possible at all the joints, especially in the fingers and wrists, where stretching and night splintage in the first year of life can be very helpful. Careful assessment by a skilled physiotherapist or occupational therapist should always be undertaken before making decisions about surgery.

The Shoulder

Weakness around the shoulder is very common. The characteristic position is adduction and internal rotation (Fig. 20.1).

Surgical intervention is rarely indicated although a simple external rotation osteotomy of the upper humerus will bring the hand and forearm into a more useful functional position.

The Elbow

At the elbow, the two common positions are fixed extension with little or no flexion (Fig. 20.8) and fixed flexion with little or no extension. Both deformities respond quite well to physiotherapy, but surgery may have to be considered once the child is established in walking. Activities such as using crutches and reaching the perineum for toileting require active extension of the elbow. The same applies to the ability to push oneself out of a chair, and so it is very important not to jeopardize active extension in the elbows by surgery designed to improve active flexion. If it is clear, once the child is walking, that it would be valuable to increase flexion in the elbow, there are three methods of gaining active flexion once passive flexion has been achieved.

Passive flexion is achieved by a posterior release of the elbow, lengthening the triceps, and releasing the posterior capsule and the collateral ligaments. This can be a very rewarding procedure and produces a useful arc of movement that allows the child to get hand to mouth without losing too much extension. Many children find that they can use passive flexion extremely well and do not particularly want to have an operation to provide active flexion if it means that they will lose active extension.

Once a reasonable range of passive flexion has been established, active motor power can be provided in the following ways:

1. If the forearm flexors and extensors are sufficiently strong, a Steindler flexorplasty advancing the flexor origin up the humerus, and reinforcing this if necessary by advancing the extensor origin, is satisfactory. The problem with this operation is that, often, the muscles are not sufficiently strong to give useful flexion, and it may adversely affect the function of the fingers and wrist.

2. Triceps transfer was initially popularized by Williams [10]. In this operation, the triceps tendon is transferred to the radius and is a very strong active flexor. However, there is loss of active extension, which could be devastating for those patients requiring crutches or to push out of a wheelchair. Another troublesome complication is increasing fixed flexion, which may develop with time after this transfer, so that it is now rarely, if ever, used.

3. Pectoralis major transfer into the biceps tendon can be used but unfortunately the reported results deteriorate with progressive flexion deformity as the child grows [28]. If the biceps tendon is not present a modified Clark type of transfer will be necessary [22]. This requires mobilizing the pectoralis major low down on the chest wall and produces an extensive and unsightly scar.

The Wrist and Hand

The wrist is frequently fixed in flexion and the fingers curved and relatively immobile (Fig. 20.9). Manipulation and splintage in the first year of life can produce remarkable improvement in the range of movement. The thumb is often adducted and should be stretched out of the palm. Operations to correct wrist deformity have been described, such as partial or complete carpectomy or a dorsal wedge carpectomy. However, with growth, recurrence is very common. Fortunately, the flexed position of the wrist is very functional in these children, and often an advantage rather than a disadvantage.

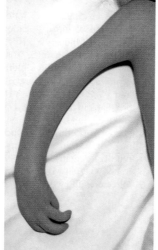

Fig. 20.8 Upper limb in arthrogryposis showing fixed extension of the elbow with only 20° flexion, flexion of the wrist and fingers

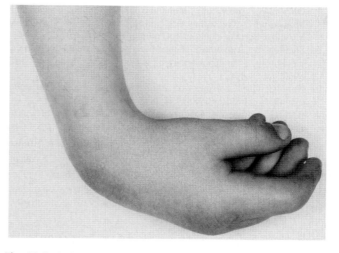

Fig. 20.9 Arthrogrypotic wrist and hand showing typical wrist and finger flexion and adducted thumb

It is extremely difficult to improve finger function because of the basic stiffness of the fingers, and operations are rarely indicated. Release of the thumb adductors and enlargement of the first web space can be useful to correct the "thumb-in-palm" deformity. These patients become extremely adept at using their stiff, flexed fingers and hands as hooks and "hangers," on which articles can be hung and manipulated.

At or near maturity, wrist arthrodesis can be considered both for functional and cosmetic gain but, as in rheumatoid arthritis, it is usually wise to fix the wrist in a slight degree of flexion rather than extension.

Conclusion

These patients cause great distress to their parents when they are born because of their appearance. It is important in the early stages to counsel parents carefully and to be cautious about prognosis until the possible causes of the condition have been elucidated. Those patients who have the classical type of arthrogryposis (amyoplasia congenita) are usually delightful children who are a pleasure to treat because they try so hard and are so adept at finding ways around their physical disabilities. There is a tendency for deformity to recur throughout growth and, as a result, long-term splintage and orthosis are frequently necessary. However, the classical form of the condition is nonprogressive and there is no disorder of sensation, so that the children can benefit significantly from carefully planned surgery and will remain active in adult life.

References

1. Otto AW. Monstrum humanum extremitatibus incurvatus. Monstorum sexcentorum description anatomica in Vratislaviae Museum. Breslau: Anatomico-Pathologieum; 1841:322.
2. Sheldon W. Amyoplasia congenita (multiple congenital articular rigidity: arthrogryposis multiplex congenita). Arch Dis Child 1932; 7:117–136.
3. Hall JG. Genetic aspects of arthrogryposis multiplex congenita. Clin Orthop Rel Res 1985; 194:44–53.
4. Hall JG. Overview of arthrogryposis. In: Staheli LT, Hall JG, Jaffe KM, Pahoike DE, eds. Arthrogryposis: A Text Atlas, Cambridge: Cambridge University Press; 1998:1–25.
5. Hall JG, Reed SD, Green G. The distal arthrogryposis; delineation of new entries: review and nosologic discussion. Am J Med Gen 1982; 11:185–239.
6. Wynne-Davies R, Williams PF, O'Connor JCB. The 1960's epidemic of arthrogryposis multiplex congenita. A survey from the United Kingdom, Australia and the United States of America. J Bone Joint Surg 1981; 63B:76–82.
7. Bevan WP, Hall JG, Baushad M, Strakeli LJ, et al. Arthrogryposis multiplex congenita (amyoplasia) (An orthopaedic perspective). J Pediatr Orthop 2007; 27:594–598.
8. Palmer PM, MacEwan GD, Bowen JR, Matheus PA. Passive motion therapy for infants with arthrogryposis. Clin Orthop Rel Res 1985; 194:54–59.
9. Robinson RO. Arthrogryposis multiplex congenita: feeding, language and other health problems. Neuropaediatrics 1990; 21: 177–178.
10. Williams PF. Management of upper limb problems in arthrogryposis. Clin Ortho Rel Res 1985; 194:60–67.
11. Robinson RO, Cartwright R, Fixsen JA, Jones M. Arthrogryposis. In: McCarthy GT, ed. Physical Disability in Childhood. Edinburgh, London, New York: Churchill Livingstone; 1992.
12. Green ADL, Fixsen JA, Lloyd-Roberts GC. Talectomy for arthrogryposis multiplex congenita. J Bone Joint Surg 1984; 66B: 697–699.
13. Hsu LCS, Jaffray D, Leong JC. Talectomy for club foot in arthrogryposis. J Bone Joint Surg 1984; 66B:694–696.
14. D'Souza H, Aroojis A, Chawara GS. Talectomy in arthrogryposis: analysis of results. J Pediatr Orthop 1998; 18:760–764.
15. Grill F, Franke J. The Ilizarov distractor for the correction of relapsed or neglected clubfoot. J Bone Joint Surg 1987; 69B: 593–597.
16. Reinke KA, Carpenter CT. Ilizarov applications in the pediatric foot. J Pediatr Orthop 1997; 17:796–802.
17. Murray C, Fixsen JA. Management of knee deformity in classical arthrogryposis multiplex congenita (amyoplasia congenita). J Pediatr Orthop 1997; B6:186–191.
18. Fucs PWWB, Svartman C, Cesar de Assumpcao RM, et al. Quadricepsplasty in arthrogryposis (amyoplasia): Long term follow-up. J Pediatr Orthop 2005; B14:219–224.
19. Parsch K, Pietrazak S. Arthrogryposis multiplex congenital. Orthopade 2007; 36:281–292.
20. Damsin JP, Trousseau A. Treatment of severe flexion deformity of the knee in children and adolescence using the Ilizarov technique. J Bone Joint Surg 1996; 78B:140–144.
21. Brunner R, Hefti F, Tgetgel JC. Arthrogrypotic joint contracture of the knee in children and adolescence using the Ilizarov technique. J Bone Joint Surg 1997; 78B:140–144.
22. Lloyd-Roberts GC, Lettin AWF. Arthrogryposis multiplex congenita. J Bone Joint Surg 1970; 52B:494–508.
23. Staheli LT, Chew ED, Elliott JS, Mosea VS. Management of hip dislocation in children with arthrogryposis. J Pediatr Orthop 1987; 7:681–685.
24. Szoke G, Staheli LT, Jaffe K, Hall JG. Medial approach open reduction of hip dislocation in amyoplasia type arthrogryposis. J Pediatr Orthop 1996; 16:127–130.
25. Akazawa H, Mitani S, Yoshitaka T, et al. Surgical management of hip dislocation in children with arthrogryposis multiplex congenita. J Bone Joint Surg 1998 80B:636–640.
26. Yau PWP, Chow W, Li YH, et al. Twenty year follow-up of hip problems in arthrogryposis multiplex congenital. J Pediatr Orthop 2002; 22:359–363.
27. Axt MW, Niethard FU, Doderlein L, Weber M. Principals of treatment of the upper extremity in arthrogryposis multiplex congenita type 1. J Pediatr Orthop 1997; B6:179–185.
28. Lahoti O, Bell MJ. Transfer of pectoralis major in arthrogryposis to restore elbow function. J Bone Joint Surg 2005; 87B:858–860.

Part IV
Regional Disorders

Section 1
The Upper Limb

Chapter 21

Developmental Anomalies of the Hand

Peter D. Burge

Incidence

A large study of limb reduction defects in British Columbia reported an incidence of 5.97 per 10,000 live births, with 75% affecting the upper limb [1]. Half the cases had associated abnormalities, mostly in the musculoskeletal system, but defects of other organ systems were also common.

Limb Development

The upper limb bud appears toward the end of the fourth week of intrauterine life and is fully differentiated by the end of the seventh week. Digits become separated at just over 50 days. The developing limb bud comprises a core of mesenchymal tissue covered with ectoderm and its three orthogonal axes are proximo-distal, anteroposterior (i.e., radio-ulnar), and dorso-ventral. The distal outgrowth of the limb bud requires the activity of members of the fibroblast growth factor (Fgf) family that are synthesized in the apical ectodermal ridge (AER), a signaling center at the tip of the limb bud. Removal of the AER results in truncation of the limb. Fgf signaling also maintains the expression of sonic hedgehog (Shh) which is produced by a second signaling center, the polarizing zone, in the posterior margin of the limb bud. Shh provides positional information across the anterior–posterior limb axis and also acts to maintain the expression of several Fgfs in the overlying AER [2]. Transplantation of the polarizing zone to the anterior aspect of another limb bud produces a symmetrical duplication that imitates the rare human malformation of mirror hand. The Wnt signaling pathway may control dorso-ventral development. Much work remains to characterize fully the molecular basis of limb development, which may eventually explain the wide phenotypic expression of congenital anomalies of the upper limb. For the present, the cause of most malformations is unknown.

Identification of genes associated with inherited upper limb anomalies is increasing rapidly (e.g., Holt–Oram syndrome, triphalangeal thumb) [3]. However, many anomalies that are sporadic and unilateral presumably result from vascular or other insults to the limb at a crucial stage of development. The developing limb bud is sensitive to teratogenic agents, but the variety of defects that can be produced by a single agent probably reflects the critical effects of timing and concentration upon the interactions between components of the limb bud during development. Conversely, defects that are superficially similar, such as transverse deficiencies, may have differing causes.

Classification

The classification adopted by the International Federation for Societies for Surgery of the Hand (IFSSH) is widely used [4], although some malformations do not sit easily in a system that attempts to give embryological explanations for abnormalities that at present have only morphological descriptions. The classification divides malformations into seven categories. The list below shows how the anomalies described in this chapter fit into the classification.

I. Failure of formation of parts

Transverse arrest
    Proximal forearm
    Digital absence
    Symbrachydactyly
Longitudinal arrest
    Radial dysplasia
    Ulnar dysplasia
    Cleft hand
    Intercalated defects (phocomelia)

P.D. Burge (✉)
Hand Surgery Unit, Nuffield Orthopaedic Centre, Oxford, UK

M. Benson et al. (eds.), *Children's Orthopaedics and Fractures*,
DOI 10.1007/978-1-84882-611-3_21, © Springer-Verlag London Limited 2010

II. **Failure of differentiation (separation) of parts**

> *Soft-tissue involvement*
> > Syndactyly
> > Clasped thumb
> > Absent finger extensors
> > Windblown hand
> > Camptodactyly
> > Trigger digits
>
> *Skeletal involvement*
> > Radio-ulnar synostosis
> > Radial head dislocation
> > Clinodactyly
> > Kirner deformity
> > Triphalangeal thumb
>
> *Congenital tumorous conditions*
> > Neurofibromatosis
> > Hereditary multiple exostoses

III. **Duplication**

> Thumb
> Post-axial polydactyly

IV. **Overgrowth**

> Macrodactyly

V. **Undergrowth**

VI. **Congenital constriction band syndrome**

VII. **Generalized abnormalities and syndromes**

> Madelung's deformity

General Principles of Management

Aims of Treatment

Treatment of congenital hand anomalies is directed at achieving the best possible function. Cosmesis may be an indication for operation but it should not be achieved at the expense of function.

The main requirements for function of the hand are *control of its position* in space, *sensate skin*, and motor activity sufficient for *power grasp* and *precision handling*. The function of congenitally deficient hands is remarkable when compared with hands that have suffered anatomically similar defects as a result of trauma because the developing brain "grows up" with the anomalous hand and learns the most effective pattern of control. But the functional needs of the small child are not those of the adult. Decisions about treatment need to consider the future needs of the patient and should aim to maximize the function and options for employment in the longer term. In unilateral defects, the presence of a normal limb ensures that most daily activities can be completed without assistance, regardless of the deficiency of the anomalous limb. However, the presence of a simple pinch or grasp in the abnormal limb confers the great benefit of *bimanual* activity and should be provided if possible. Bilateral defects impair function much more severely and consequently justify more extensive procedures.

A sympathetic approach to parents and a realistic prognosis are important aspects of general management. An early consultation with the team that will be responsible for management can do much to allay anxiety and reduce feelings of guilt [5]. Genetic counseling may be required and parents should be informed about support groups that exist for patients and their families. Referral to a paediatrician for exclusion of anomalies in other organ systems may be appropriate. Parents should be helped to understand the limitations of surgical reconstruction; it is seldom possible to replace what is missing, only to rearrange what remains. Videotapes of post-operative cases or, even better, meeting a patient with a similar problem may help them to understand what surgery will achieve.

Timing

Reconstruction of congenital hand anomalies should be completed before school age, if possible, bearing in mind that more than one operation is required in some cases. There is an increasing trend to operate between the ages of 1 and 2 years. Edema distal to a constriction band may require operation during the neonatal period. Early surgery (between 6 and 12 months of age) is needed in conditions that are liable to cause progressive deformity such as radial dysplasia or syndactyly between digits of different length.

Failure of Formation

Transverse Absence

Proximal Forearm

The commonest site of terminal transverse absence is the upper third of the forearm. It is usually sporadic, not associated with other anomalies, and more common on the left side. The high prevalence of digital nubbins suggests that many transverse absences are types of symbrachydactyly [6]. A light plastic prosthesis fitted in the first few months of life improves cosmesis and accustoms the child to wearing a prosthesis. At about 18 months of age a gripping device such as a split hook operated by a motivating cord and loop from the opposite shoulder can be fitted. Training in its use by a therapist, regular review, and support of the parents are essential at this stage. At the age of 3.5 years a myoelectric prosthesis operated by electrical impulses generated in the forearm muscles may be fitted. Small children can learn to make excellent functional use of a myoelectric prosthesis.

Transverse absence at the level of the carpus is consistent with useful manipulative function using the mobile proximal carpal row which is usually present. A prosthesis interferes with sensibility and impairs function but may be worn for cosmesis on social occasions.

Digital Absence

Transverse absence of digits is seen in three situations:

1. Transverse absence
2. Symbrachydactyly
3. Congenital constriction band syndrome

The term symbrachydactyly has been used to denote a type of terminal absence characterized by digital nubbins containing rudimentary nails that may retain connections to tendons, causing the nubbins to retract with active movement (Fig. 21.1). The appearance suggests an intercalary defect in which the skeleton has failed to develop, leading to secondary failure of development of the soft tissues. Whether this anomaly is truly different to simple transverse absence is unknown. Symbrachydactyly shows a teratogenic sequence that ranges from simple shortness of the middle phalanges to absence of all phalanges with short metacarpals. The index,

middle, and ring fingers are most severely affected and the thumb least affected. Absence of the central digits gives the appearance formerly termed atypical cleft hand.

Four types of symbrachydactyly are recognized:

1. Short finger type
2. Cleft hand type
3. Monodactylous type; a hypoplastic thumb is the only digit
4. Absence of all five digital rays

Most cases are unilateral and sporadic. Tendons and arteries that are useful for reconstruction are usually present in the more distal lesions.

Absence of one or two fingers is consistent with good function. In more extensive anomalies, the aim should be the provision of a basic type of grasp. This requires a minimum of two digits, at least one of which must be mobile. Therefore, if a single digit is present, every attempt should be made to provide another digit or "post" for opposition. Lengthening of a short metacarpal or deepening of the first web may give side-to-side pinch. Short digits may be lengthened by transfer of toe phalanges, which are more likely to grow if they are transferred extraperiosteally as nonvascularized grafts before the age of 15 months. This transfer is indicated if a modest increase in length will improve function and the recipient ray has functioning tendons. Microvascular transfer of a second toe is feasible if suitable nerves and tendons can be found in the hand. Loss of the second toe is functionally and cosmetically acceptable. Transfer of one or both second toes can greatly improve function of the severely deficient hand [7].

Longitudinal Absence

Radial Dysplasia

Radial dysplasia is the commonest form of longitudinal deficiency. This ugly deformity results from complete or partial absence of the radius, but the deficiency affects other tissues in the limb. Although many cases are sporadic, there are important associations with anomalies in different organ systems, especially the hemopoietic and cardiovascular systems (Fig. 21.2), that influence decisions about surgical management (Table 21.1). The thumbs are present in the thrombocytopenia-absent radius (TAR) syndrome but often absent in other forms of severe radial dysplasia. Thrombocytopenia is usually transient in this autosomal recessive disorder. Fanconi anemia is an autosomal recessive, progressive pancytopenia of childhood in which the cells exhibit extreme chromosomal instability.

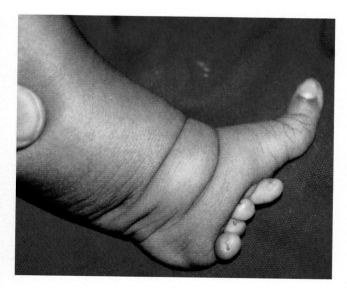

FIG. 21.1 Symbrachydactyly

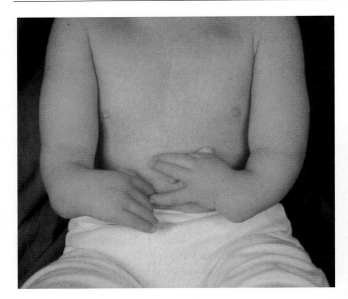

Fig. 21.2 Bilateral radial absence with floating thumbs. Note the median sternotomy scar

Table 21.1 Anomalies commonly associated with radial dysplasia

Thrombocytopenia—absent radius (TAR) syndrome
Fanconi anemia
Holt–Oram syndrome
VACTERL association

Holt–Oram syndrome is an autosomal dominant disorder that includes radial dysplasia (often comprising triphalangeal thumb) and cardiac anomalies such as septal defects and Fallot's tetralogy. VACTERL is a mnemonically useful acronym for vertebral anomalies, anal atresia, cardiac malformations, tracheoesophageal fistula, renal anomalies, and limb anomalies (humeral hypoplasia and radial aplasia). There are many rare syndromes that may be associated with radial dysplasia [8].

Skeletal deficiency ranges from mild shortening to absence of the radius (Table 21.2). In complete absence, the ulna is bowed and typically grows to 60% of the length of the normal forearm (Fig. 21.3). The carpus articulates with the radial aspect of the distal ulna. The scaphoid and trapezium may be absent. Muscle anomalies tend to be proportional to the skeletal deficiency and chiefly affect the radial side of the limb. The radial flexor and extensor muscles of the wrist are often fused and inserted into the carpus via a short tendon. Extensor tendons of the index and middle fingers may be absent or show abnormal insertions. The superficial radial nerve is absent, being represented by a radial branch of the median nerve. The median nerve itself is abnormally situated and at risk of operative injury, lying just beneath the deep fascia on the radial side of the forearm. The radial artery

Table 21.2 Classification of radial dysplasia

Type 1.	Short distal radius
Type 2.	Hypoplastic radius
Type 3.	Partial absence of radius
Type 4.	Absent radius

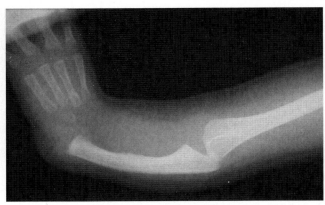

Fig. 21.3 Radiograph of radial absence. The ulna is bowed and the thumb is absent

is absent; the hand is supplied by the ulnar artery, which is usually normal, and by the anterior interosseous artery.

The thumb may be absent or hypoplastic. The index and middle fingers often show hypoplasia, contractures, and stiffness, reflecting the deficiency that extends widely across the radial side of the limb. The ring and little fingers usually have normal movement and may be preferred by the patient for manipulative activity. The elbow may lack passive flexion at birth but the range usually improves with growth. However, bilateral lack of elbow flexion is a contraindication to centralization, as the hands may then fail to reach the mouth.

The deformity of radial absence is unsightly. The power of the finger muscles is dissipated by instability at the wrist. Centralization of the carpus gives a marked esthetic improvement and also increases function [9].

The management of the newborn child comprises exclusion of other anomalies and prevention of fixed contracture until centralization can be performed at the age of 6–12 months. In most cases of radial absence, the deformity is correctable at birth. Regular passive stretching should be instituted as soon as possible. After each feed, gentle traction and ulnar deviation are applied. Splintage is difficult to maintain in the neonate but may have place in the older infant. If the deformity is not correctable, distraction lengthening may be needed prior to centralization.

The surgical treatment of radial absence has a long history but modern efforts have centered on placement of the carpus on the ulna. Two operations are in common use.

Centralization places the distal ulna in a slot cut into the carpus [9]. (Fig. 21.4a). In radialization, the carpus is mobilized extensively and the ulna is placed beneath the radial aspect of the carpus so as to maximize the moment arm of muscles on the ulnar side (Fig. 21.4b) [10]. Re-balancing of the deforming forces by shortening of the extensor carpi ulnaris tendon and transferring of the deforming radial wrist muscles to the ulnar side of the wrist are essential components of each procedure. In every case, the position is maintained by a longitudinal pin (Fig. 21.5). Osteotomy of a bowed ulna may be performed at the same time. Great care must be taken to avoid damage to the distal ulnar epiphysis and its blood supply. Radialization requires that the deformity is correctable and is best performed between 6 and 12 months of age. It retains some useful wrist motion from the neutral position into flexion (Fig. 21.6). The skeletal shortening of centralization allows correction of fixed deformities and is more applicable to older children or those with fixed deformity. Although centralization aims to maintain some motion

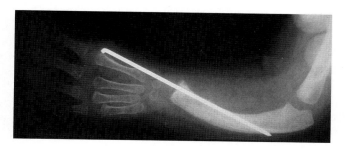

Fig. 21.5 Radiograph after radialization of the carpus

Fig. 21.6 Appearance of the forearm 3 years after radialization

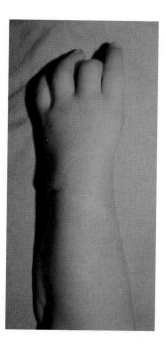

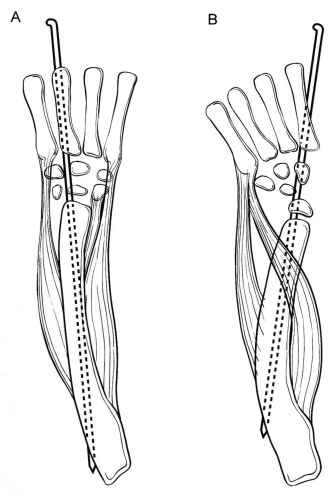

Fig. 21.4 (**a**) "Centralization" of the carpus. (**b**) "Radialization" of the carpus, preserving carpal bone

between carpus and ulna, long-term maintenance of correction is often associated with spontaneous ulno-carpal fusion. The wrist is stiff but there may be a little motion at the carpometacarpal joints. Skeletal distraction with an external fixation device is being used increasingly to correct fixed deformities prior to radialization or centralization [11].

The pin is removed some months later. If necessary, pollicization of the index finger is performed at a later stage. The wrist is splinted full time for several months and at night until skeletal maturity. There is a tendency to recurrent radial angulation in many cases [12], although seldom to the original position. Complications of centralization and radialization include premature closure of the distal ulnar epiphysis, pin breakage, and recurrent deformity.

Ulno-carpal fusion may be needed at or near skeletal maturity for persistent deformity or instability. Distraction lengthening of the ulna has been used but it is questionable whether the gain in length justifies the high-complication rate [13].

Ulnar Dysplasia

Ulnar dysplasia is several times less common than radial dysplasia. Most cases are sporadic but may be associated with lower limb anomalies such as fibular ray deficiency [14]. Absence of the ulna may be associated with radiohumeral synostosis (Table 21.3). Unlike radial dysplasia, associated anomalies in other organ systems are uncommon.

Table 21.3 Classification of ulnar dysplasia

Type 1.	Hypoplastic ulna
Type 2.	Partial absence of ulna
Type 3.	Absent ulna
Type 4.	Absent ulna and radiohumeral synostosis

Hypoplasia of the ulna is associated with bowing of the radius and dislocation of the radial head, but the carpus is supported by the radius and does not show the acute angulation that characterizes radial dysplasia (Fig. 21.7).

Deficiencies in the hand tend to be more extensive in ulnar dysplasia than in radial dysplasia [15]. Multiple digital absence, syndactyly, and camptodactyly are common, but there is no correlation between the extent of hand deformity and the degree of ulnar deficiency.

The main determinants of functional impairment are the extent of hand deformity and stiffness of the elbow rather than bowing of the forearm. Management of the hand deformities may include release of syndactyly and correction of

first web space contractures. Progressive bowing of the forearm has been treated by excision of the fibrous anlage of the ulna but its value is unclear. Severe instability of the forearm can be corrected, at the expense of rotation, by creation of a one-bone forearm, fusing the ulna proximally to the radius distally. Some patients with radiohumeral synostosis have a severe internal rotation or adduction posture that may be improved by osteotomy of the humerus.

Cleft Hand

Cleft hand is characterized by a central V-shaped cleft with absence of one or more digits. Unlike radial and ulnar dysplasia, it is not accompanied by deficiency in the forearm. In the past, cleft hand has been grouped with other causes of central deficiency such as symbrachydactyly. True cleft hand is often familial, bilateral, and associated with cleft feet. Inheritance is autosomal dominant with variable penetrance. Cleft hand may be part of syndromes such as EEC (ectrodactyly, ectodermal dysplasia, and cleft lip/palate) and the split hand/split foot malformation (SHSM) [16].

The depth of the cleft varies from absence of the phalanges only to a deep cleft extending into the carpus. Syndactyly between the border digits (thumb/index and ring/little) and contracture of the thumb web are common (Fig. 21.8). Skeletal remnants of the missing rays may be aligned transversely or fused with adjacent bones. The term "lobster claw hand" is disliked by patients and their families; *cleft hand,* which is neutral and more accurate, is preferred

Flatt has stated that typical cleft hand is "a functional triumph and a social disaster" [17]. Functional impairment results more from syndactyly and thumb web contracture than from the cleft itself. Border syndactyly should be released by the age of 6 months, before unequal growth can produce angular deformity of the longer digit. Early

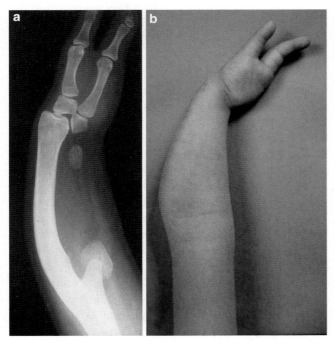

Fig. 21.7 Ulnar dysplasia. (**a**) Absent ulna and radiohumeral synostosis (type IV). (**b**) The forearm is bowed to the ulnar side in a type III case

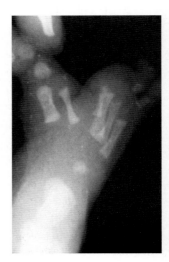

Fig. 21.8 Cleft hand with complex syndactyly

removal of transverse bones that are causing deformity may also be needed. In a typical case of first web contracture and absence of the middle ray, simultaneous closure of the cleft and widening of the thumb web are performed at around 18 months.

Failure of Differentiation

Syndactyly

Syndactyly is a common congenital anomaly of the hand. It is an example of incomplete differentiation of digital rays, which normally occurs by programmed cell death (apoptosis) of interdigital tissue. The process begins distally and proceeds proximally; its failure leads to partial or complete syndactyly.

Simple syndactyly involves skin and soft tissue; in *complex* syndactyly, the digits are also connected by bone. *Complete* syndactyly extends to the fingertips, *partial* syndactyly does not. In *acrosyndactyly,* which occurs in congenital constriction band syndrome and in association with craniofacial deformities such as Apert's syndrome, short digits are fused at the tips and are often separated proximally by fenestrations.

Syndactyly may occur in association with other hand anomalies, such as ulnar dysplasia, cleft hand, or as a feature of a syndrome (Poland's syndrome, craniofacial syndromes, constriction band syndrome). Simple syndactyly is inherited in at least 10% of cases, usually as an autosomal dominant trait. In half the cases it is bilateral. The distribution of syndactyly between the digital rays is shown in (Fig. 21.9).

Syndactyly *always* represents a shortage of skin [18]. Although it might appear that there is *additional* skin joining the digits, simple geometry shows that 22% *less* skin covers the syndactylized digits than surfaces two separate fingers. Skin is also deficient transversely in the interdigital web, as may be seen by measurement of the distance along the web from the tip of one finger to the tip of its neighbor.

Syndactyly between digits of unequal length (thumb–index, ring–little) should be released by the age of 6 months, before unequal growth deforms the longer digit. Otherwise, the timing of release is not critical but is generally before the age of 3 years. Successful release of syndactyly requires the use of acute zigzag incisions, local flap skin for reconstruction of the web, and full-thickness skin grafts. Skin grafts are taken from the groin crease, lateral to the femoral pulse (to avoid growth of hair at puberty). If a finger is joined to the digits on each side, only one surface should be released at one operation.

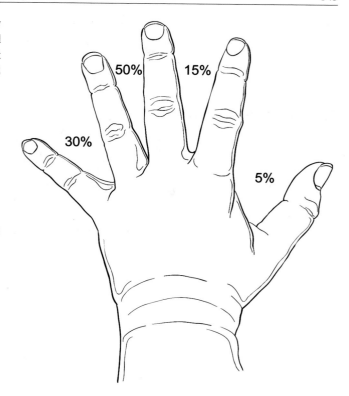

Fig. 21.9 The frequency of syndactyly of digital clefts

Congenital Clasped Thumb

A congenital clasped thumb lies flexed across the palm and cannot be extended actively. Two types of clasped thumb can be recognized [19].

Supple clasped thumb is due to isolated deficiency of the thumb extensor tendons. It is often bilateral and is more common in males. Passive extension is usually normal at birth but may be lost if the disorder is untreated. Clasped thumb may present as loss of extension at the interphalangeal (IP) joint, at the metacarpophalangeal (MP) joint, or at both joints. Differentiation from trigger thumb is straightforward if there is no loss of passive extension. In cases of clasped thumb with flexion contracture, the contracture usually affects the MP joint and other soft tissues, whereas the contracture of trigger finger is confined to the distal joint.

Supple clasped thumb frequently responds to continuous and prolonged splintage in extension if treatment is started soon after birth. A plaster cast extending to the thumb tip is changed every few weeks to accommodate growth and retained for 3–6 months. If active extension is not regained, tendon transfer is required.

Complex clasped thumb refers to disorders in which the thumb is part of a more extensive anomaly such as arthrogryposis, thumb hypoplasia, or Freeman–Sheldon (windblown hand) syndrome. The skin, thumb web, adductor pollicis, and flexor pollicis longus may require lengthening, in addition to chondrodesis of the MP joint and augmentation of extension by tendon transfer.

The Windblown Hand

Congenital flexion deformity of the fingers takes several forms and probably has several causes. Less severe types resemble the supple clasped thumb, affecting one or more fingers with deficient active extension but normal passive extension. They are probably due to congenital deficiency of the extensor mechanism and may respond to prolonged splintage in extension. Reconstruction by tendon transfer is required in some cases.

The combination of flexion contracture of the fingers, ulnar deviation at the MP joints, and a flexion/adduction contracture of the thumb is known as windblown hand. It is a feature of distal arthrogryposis and the Freeman–Sheldon (whistling face) syndrome.

Splintage can improve contractures or hold them stable until the child is fit for surgery. Correction of the thumb web contracture is valuable; surgery can improve the fingers but does not provide full movement. Each component of the deformity requires correction. Releases of skin and fascia at the base of the digits are closed with full-thickness skin grafts. Centralization of the extensor mechanism at the MP joint requires release of tight ulnar sagittal bands and plication or reconstruction of elongated radial sagittal bands, as well as crossed intrinsic transfer in some cases [20]. Release of the thumb web contracture generally creates a defect that requires a transposition flap from the dorsoradial aspect of the index. An unstable thumb MP joint may be stabilized by ligament reconstruction or by chondrodesis. Tendon transfers may augment thumb extension.

Thumb Hypoplasia

Hypoplasia of the thumb is frequently associated with radial dysplasia and may, therefore, be accompanied by visceral malformations. The classification of Blauth is widely used (Table 21.4) [21].

Type I hypoplasia is consistent with normal function and requires no treatment. In type II (Fig. 21.10), function is impaired by instability of the MP joint, contracture of the thumb web, weakness of opposition, and limited motion of the IP joint. Release of the web usually requires lengthening of the web skin by Z-plasty or by a transposition flap from the dorsum of the thumb or index finger. If the ring superficialis tendon is employed as an opposition transfer, it may be

Table 21.4 Classification of thumb hypoplasia

I	Minor hypoplasia, normal function
II	Thumb web contracture; thenar muscle hypoplasia MP joint instability; anomalous flexor tendon
III	A severe skeletal and muscle hypoplasia
B	+ deficient basal joint
IV	Floating thumb
V	Absent thumb

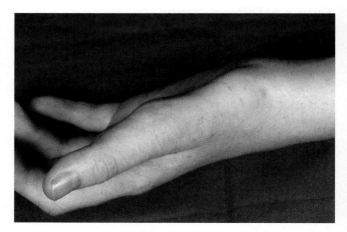

Fig. 21.10 Type II hypoplasia of thumb showing hypoplasia of the thenar muscles

passed through the metacarpal neck and used to reconstruct the ulnar collateral ligament of the MP joint. Anomalous connections between the long flexor and the extensor tendons may limit IP joint flexion or lead to abduction deformity (pollex abductus).

It may be difficult to decide whether a type III hypoplastic thumb is worthy of reconstruction (Fig. 21.11) and even more difficult to convince parents that it is not. Much depends upon the tissues that are available. However, if the basal joint is unstable, pollicization of the index finger is likely to provide better function.

Attempts at reconstruction of the floating thumb (type IV) are fruitless; the digit contains no useful skeleton or tendons and it is attached too far distally and dorsally to be functional (Fig. 21.12). Pollicization of the index finger provides much better function [22]. Pollicization is also the appropriate treatment for the absent thumb (type V) (Fig. 21.13). Current techniques of pollicization are based on the work of many surgeons over the last 50 years, notably Buck-Gramcko [22]. In essence, the index finger is mobilized on the intact digital neurovascular bundles and dorsal veins, excising the shaft of the metacarpal and placing the metacarpal head anterior to the base of the metacarpal. The metacarpal head is sutured into place with the MP joint extended, otherwise the new thumb may exhibit excessive hyperextension at its basal joint. The digit is rotated 160° into opposition. The first dorsal and first palmar interosseous muscles are sutured

Fig. 21.11 Type III hypoplasia of thumb with deficient basal joint

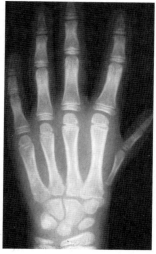

Fig. 21.12 Floating thumb (type IV hypoplasia) is not capable of useful reconstruction. It should be excised and replaced by pollicization of the index finger

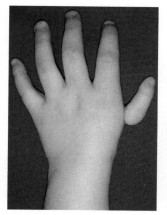

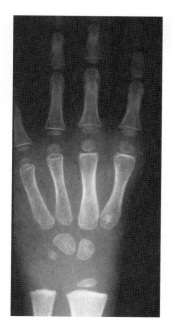

Fig. 21.13 Absent thumb

into the lateral bands at the level of the proximal interphalangeal (PIP) joint, becoming the short thumb abductor and the adductor pollicis, respectively. It is necessary to shorten the extensor tendons, but the flexor tendons will in time accommodate to the shorter skeleton. For the index finger to look like a thumb, skin flaps must be designed so that the new thumb web reaches the digit at the level of the PIP joint (the new MP joint) (Fig. 21.14). When the absent thumb is accompanied by a normal radius, the index finger usually has good musculature and supple joints; it will make a satisfactory thumb. The decision to pollicize the index finger should take into account the pattern of prehensile function that the child shows. Children who lack thumbs employ a "cigarette" grip between adjacent fingers. When the thumb is missing as part of severe radial dysplasia, the index frequently lacks good motion. Nevertheless, it may still make a satisfactory thumb provided that the child uses the index–middle cleft for prehension. If the child excludes the index finger from hand function, the digit may be ignored after pollicization.

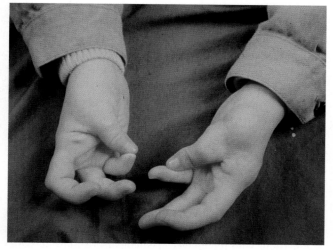

Fig. 21.14 Pollicization of the index fingers for bilateral absent thumb

Camptodactyly

Camptodactyly describes a common, painless, nontraumatic flexion deformity of the PIP joint, usually affecting the little finger. An autosomal dominant pattern of inheritance is frequently present. Camptodactyly occurs in two age groups that coincide with periods of rapid growth of the hand. In *infants,* it may affect any finger; it is equally common among males and females, and it may be associated with other anomalies. In *adolescents,* camptodactyly is more frequent in females and almost invariably affects the little finger. It

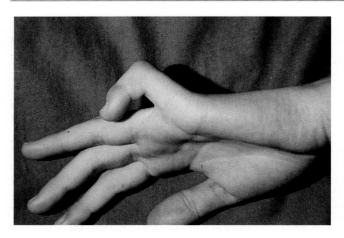

Fig. 21.15 Camptodactyly

appears as a fixed flexion contracture of the PIP joint which is usually at least 30° at the time of presentation (Fig. 21.15). The little finger may adopt the intrinsic-minus posture of hyperextension of the MP joint with increased flexion of the PIP joint when the fingers are extended actively. Involvement of more than one finger suggests one of the many syndromes associated with camptodactyly.

Camptodactyly may be distinguished from post-traumatic boutonnière deformity by the absence of swelling and by the presence of full distal joint movement. Ulnar nerve palsy is excluded by the absence of neurological signs.

In an established case of adolescent camptodactyly, examination will demonstrate tightness of the volar PIP joint capsule, the superficialis tendon, and the skin. It is not surprising, therefore, that almost every structure which crosses the palmar aspect of the PIP joint has been implicated in the etiology of camptodactyly. Imbalance between the extrinsic and intrinsic muscles of the little finger during the periods of growth is the most plausible mechanism. This explanation is consistent with recognized mechanisms of musculoskeletal deformity and is supported by the frequent finding of an abnormal insertion of the lumbrical muscle into the capsule of the MP joint, the superficialis tendon, or the extensor expansion of an adjacent finger [23]. Shortening of the superficialis muscle is a common and probably secondary feature that may be demonstrated by the effect of wrist and MP joint position on deformity of the PIP joint.

Treatment

Infancy

As much correction as possible should be obtained by splintage. Static splints such as serial plaster casts are easier to manage at this age than dynamic splints. Persistent

contractures may be managed by the release of tight volar soft tissues and tendon transfer to augment extension. However, it may be difficult to restore normal movement. Long-term extension splintage is often required.

Adolescence

It is difficult to restore full extension in adolescent camptodactyly. Static and/or dynamic splintage may produce useful improvement but splintage must be continued until skeletal maturity [24]. Since a moderate flexion deformity is consistent with good function and less disabling than loss of flexion, most patients should be advised to use a splint and accept the deformity unless it is severe or the patient has a specific requirement for good extension. The results of operative treatment of fixed contracture are unpredictable and the chief risk is loss of flexion [25]. Soft tissue release is contraindicated if there is bony deformity of the PIP joint (Fig. 21.16); dorsal angulation osteotomy through the neck of the proximal phalanx will improve extension at the expense of flexion. The rare patient who exhibits inadequate active PIP joint extension but who has full passive extension may be improved by transfer of a superficialis tendon or extensor indicis proprius into the extensor mechanism over the PIP joint.

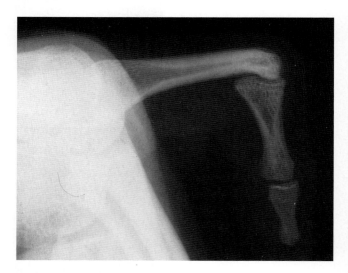

Fig. 21.16 Long-standing camptodactyly with secondary deformity of the head of the proximal phalanx, precluding soft tissue release

Clinodactyly

Clinodactyly is angulation of a digit to the radial or ulnar side. It is a manifestation of a variety of syndromes, but the common isolated form is bilateral radial angulation of the little finger with autosomal dominant inheritance. Clinodactyly is the result of abnormal growth, usually of the middle phalanx, which may have many causes.

Three types of clinodactyly are encountered:

1. Minor angulation, normal length
2. Minor angulation, short phalanx
3. Marked angulation, delta phalanx

Minor degrees of clinodactyly are common and consistent with normal function. Corrective osteotomy is indicated if the finger overlaps the adjacent digit on flexion, using a closing wedge osteotomy if the length of the phalanx is normal and an opening wedge if it is short.

Although delta phalanx is named after the triangular Greek letter, the bone is usually trapezoidal. It is a curious anomaly in which the proximal epiphysis extends beyond its normal transverse position to pass along the shorter side of the bone to its distal end (Fig. 21.17). The C-shaped epiphysis effectively constitutes a bony bridge that restricts longitudinal growth and causes progressive angulation. Delta phalanx is frequently found in association with triphalangeal thumb and with polydactyly.

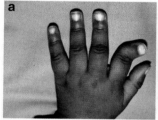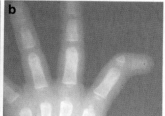

Fig. 21.17 Angular deformity of the index finger resulting from a delta phalanx

Division of the longitudinal bar and interposition of a free fat graft may permit more normal growth. For later cases, reverse wedge or opening wedge osteotomy is the best option. Great care must be taken to avoid damage to the joint surfaces and to divide the small bone cleanly. The osteotomy is transfixed with a Kirschner wire for 4–6 weeks.

Kirner Deformity

In 1927 Kirner described a curvature of the distal phalanx in a radial and palmar direction. It affects females more commonly than males and may be inherited as an autosomal dominant trait. The onset is between 8 and 12 years, beginning with painless swelling of the distal phalanx followed by progressive radio-palmar deviation of both little fingers. The age of onset, the presence of swelling, and the radiographic

appearance of lysis within the growth plate (Fig. 21.18) suggest that the disorder is acquired rather than congenital. Its nature is unknown. A similar deformity may follow epiphyseal damage by frostbite or by an infected open fracture. Severe deformity may be improved by osteotomy of the distal phalanx.

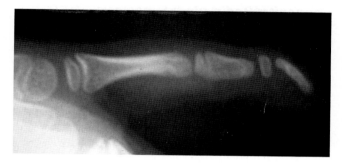

Fig. 21.18 Kirner deformity with palmar angulation in the distal phalanx

Trigger Digits

Trigger thumb is the most common hand disorder in children. It presents with painless loss of passive extension of the interphalangeal (IP) joint. The clicking which characterizes trigger thumb in adults is uncommon in children. A nodule may be palpable at the proximal (A1) flexor tendon pulley at the level of the metacarpophalangeal (MP) joint. It should be distinguished from congenital clasped thumb (see above), in which the deformity usually affects the MP joint.

Trigger thumb is seldom present at birth; no cases were found in a screening study of 1116 neonates [26]. The normal infant tends to hold the thumb flexed into the palm and it may be sometime before the problem is noticed. Approximately 30% of trigger thumbs presenting in infancy resolved spontaneously within 12 months [27]. Of those presenting between 6 and 36 months, 12% resolved within 6 months of presentation. A period of observation is appropriate in children presenting in the first year. Extension splintage appears to cure a proportion of trigger thumbs [28]. If the condition persists, division of the A1 pulley is curative. Permanent IP contracture does not seem to occur provided that the digit is released by the age of 4 years. The skin is incised transversely at the proximal MP joint crease, avoiding the digital nerves which lie immediately beneath the skin. The A1 pulley is incised longitudinally under direct vision, revealing a nodule (Notta's node) or thickening of the flexor tendon. The oblique pulley should be preserved so as to avoid bowstringing of the flexor tendon.

Trigger finger is much less common than trigger thumb in children. In contrast to adult cases, some cases in children may occur at the flexor digitorum superficialis (FDS)

decussation rather than at the A1 pulley [29]. These cases may need excision of one of the slips of the FDS tendon in addition to A1 pulley release.

Congenital Radio-ulnar Synostosis

Synostosis may be longitudinal (e.g., humeroradial synostosis in type-IV ulnar dysplasia) or transverse. Radio-ulnar synostosis is the most common form (Fig. 21.19), resulting from the failure of completion of the distal-to-proximal separation of the forearm mesenchyme. It may be unilateral or bilateral and is usually at the proximal end of the forearm. Some compensatory rotation occurs at carpal level.

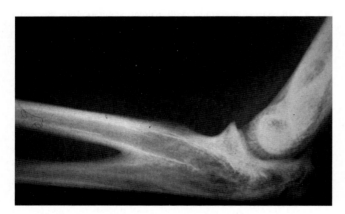

Fig. 21.19 Radiograph of congenital radio-ulnar synostosis at the typical proximal site

Disability depends upon the rotational alignment of the forearm. Internal rotation and abduction of the shoulder can bring a supinated hand into the palm-down position. Shoulder motion compensates less readily for fixed pronation. Unilateral synostosis causes little disability and seldom requires treatment. Bilateral synostoses are often fixed in marked pronation, causing difficulty with accepting coins and holding a glass.

Until recently, attempts to restore rotation had been unsuccessful and operative correction was confined to rotational osteotomy, generally through the fusion mass. The technique of Green and Mital [30] controls alignment with a longitudinal intramedullary pin and rotation with a transverse trans-ulnar pin incorporated in a cast. The method allows the correction to be undone easily in the event of neurovascular compromise post-operatively. Further experience is required to determine if rotation can be restored reliably by excision of the synostosis, interposition of a vascularized fat-fascia flap, and relocation of the dislocated radial head by radial shortening osteotomy [31].

Congenital Radial Head Dislocation

Dislocation of the radial head may be congenital, traumatic, or secondary to diminished growth of the ulna (e.g., ulnar dysplasia, multiple hereditary exostoses). Congenital dislocation is posterior in two-thirds of cases; the remainder is lateral or anterior. Differentiation between traumatic and congenital dislocation is sometimes difficult since deformity of the radial head and hypoplasia of the capitellum are features of both types. Dislocation is likely to be congenital if it is bilateral, familial, associated with other malformations, or present in infancy. A healed fracture of the ulna or heterotopic ossification suggests that dislocation was the result of injury.

Congenital dislocation of the radial head is a feature of numerous malformation syndromes, which should be sought during examination. The dislocation causes remarkably little loss of function during childhood, although radial head excision after skeletal maturity may be indicated for pain and prominence of the radial head if these symptoms are clearly attributable to the dislocation.

Dislocation of the radial head is liable to occur whenever growth of the ulna is diminished and radial growth continues. It may be possible to prevent dislocation if the length of the ulna can be maintained by distraction lengthening, with or without radial shortening or epiphyseal stapling. Parents may ask that the radial head be relocated. However, the indication for operative reduction of established congenital radial head dislocation has not been defined. The procedure may involve osteotomy of a bowed ulna and radial shortening in addition to reconstruction of the annular ligament. Considering the minimal symptoms experienced by most patients, such surgery is seldom justified.

Duplication

Duplication may be *radial* (preaxial), *ulnar* (post-axial), or, rarely, *central*. It is probably the commonest congenital anomaly in the hand. Ulnar polydactyly is common as an autosomal recessive condition in African-Americans, in whom it is seldom associated with other abnormalities. It is 8–10 times less common in Caucasians but is more likely to be part of a syndrome.

Radial polydactyly is usually sporadic. Wassel [32] described a logical classification based upon the level of duplication (Fig. 21.20). Almost half the cases are type IV (Fig. 21.21). In types I and II, where the duplication is symmetrical, a central wedge may be excised and the defect closed by apposition of the outer halves of the distal phalanges (Bilhaut–Cloquet procedure). Nail bed deformity

Fig. 21.20 Wassel classification of thumb duplication. Type IV accounts for almost 50% of cases

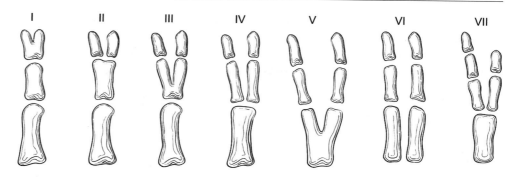

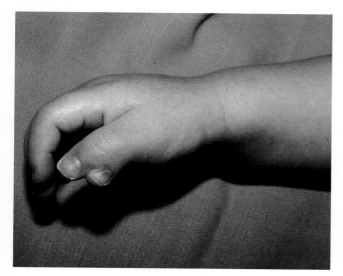

Fig. 21.21 Wassel type IV duplication of the thumb

and premature epiphyseal closure may mar the final result. Instead of splitting the nail, the entire nail bed may be taken from one thumb and the nail bed of the other discarded.

In considering operative treatment of types III–VII, it is vital to regard the procedure as a reconstruction of a split thumb and not excision of an extra thumb. A decision on which thumb should be discarded is based upon size, deviation, passive joint mobility, stability, and anomalous tendon insertions of the parts. The principles of reconstruction include zigzag incisions (to avoid later scar contracture), preservation or reconstruction of ligaments, alignment of the skeleton, and alignment of tendon insertions. It may be necessary to augment the remaining thumb with tissues from the excised segment.

Triphalangeal Thumb

Triphalangeal thumb may be part of type VII duplication, when it is an autosomal dominant condition, or an isolated anomaly. The additional bone is interposed between the distal and proximal phalanges. It may be a normal phalanx, a

short phalanx, or a delta phalanx; as a result, the thumb may be too long, angulated, or both. The metacarpal may also be too long.

Triphalangeal thumb is consistent with good function but many fine precision activities are hampered by excessive length. Excision of a delta phalanx should be performed as early as possible and the soft tissues of the IP joint reconstructed. For cases presenting later in childhood it may be necessary to fuse the distal phalanx to the proximal phalanx after excision of the intervening delta phalanx. Correction of thumb web narrowing and thenar muscle hypoplasia may also be required.

Overgrowth

Macrodactyly

Macrodactyly is congenital enlargement of a digit. It is very rare and is not inherited; 90% of cases are unilateral. In 70% of patients, more than one digit is affected and the involvement corresponds with the territory of one or more peripheral nerves, most frequently the median. The enlargement may be present at birth and grow in proportion with other digits but more commonly it progresses during childhood. Macrodactyly affects all tissues in a digit and should be distinguished from other causes of enlargement such as hemangioma, arteriovenous malformations, and lymphedema.

Three types of macrodactyly are seen. *Nerve territory orientated macrodactyly* is associated with enlargement or lipofibromatous hamartoma of a peripheral nerve. The peripheral nerve is thickened by infiltration with fat and fibrous tissue; these changes may extend well proximal to the enlargement of other tissues and, in the case of the median nerve, may lead to its compression within the carpal canal. Skin, nerve, and bone are affected more than tendon or blood vessels. Less frequently, macrodactyly is associated with *neurofibromatosis*. In the rare *hyperostotic macrodactyly,* osteocartilaginous protuberances arise around the digital joints and limit motion. In addition to the serious cosmetic impairment, these large digits are likely to be stiff, deformed, and prone to ulceration.

Treatment of macrodactyly is difficult. Amputation may be appropriate for digits that are severely deformed, stiff, painful, or ulcerated. In childhood, cosmetic considerations often demand attempts at reduction procedures, which should be staged to avoid vascular impairment [33]. The blood supply of the skin is relatively poor and necrosis of skin flaps is a common complication. Longitudinal growth may be controlled by fusion of the phalangeal epiphyses when the digit has reached its expected adult length; however, circumferential growth may continue.

Constriction Band Syndrome

Constriction band syndrome (also known as amniotic band syndrome and Streeter's dysplasia) occurs sporadically at the rate of around 1:15,000 live births. Amniotic disruption leading to constricting intrauterine amniotic bands is currently thought to be the mechanism. The abnormalities are asymmetrical and present at birth. Four types of lesion occur.

1. Simple constriction bands
2. Constriction rings with distal deformity and/or lymphedema
3. Soft tissue fusion of distal parts (acrosyndactyly)
4. Amputation

Constriction band syndrome is distinguished from other types of congenital deformity and amputation by the presence of constriction bands, by the multiple asymmetrical defects, and by the normality of the part proximal to the band. Deep constriction bands may seriously impair vascular supply and innervation; a temperature gradient across the band and distal lymphedema are signs of vascular impairment.

Circular constricting bands are excised and the circular scar broken up by Z-plasties. Bands that produce severe distal lymphedema in the neonate may require urgent release. Syndactyly and intrauterine amputations may also need treatment. The normality of proximal nerves, vessels, and tendons is a distinct advantage during reconstruction.

Miscellaneous Abnormalities and Syndromes

Madelung's Deformity

Madelung's deformity is a congenital disorder that affects growth of the distal radius. It is seldom evident before the age of 8 years. Females are affected more often than males and it is usually bilateral. The primary abnormality is failure of normal growth of the ulnar and palmar halves of the distal radial physis, leading to curvature in an ulnar and palmar direction (Fig. 21.22). A localized area of radiolucency may appear on the ulnar edge of the distal radius and the ulnar part of the physis fuses prematurely. The ulna is relatively long and becomes prominent dorsally. The carpus sinks, along with the ulnar half of the distal radial articular surface, into the gap between the two forearm bones. Rotation of the forearm is limited by incongruity of the distal radio-ulnar joint.

The cause of Madelung's deformity is unknown. It may be inherited as part of dyschondrosteosis (Leri–Weill disease). Similar deformities may occur in multiple hereditary exostoses, multiple epiphyseal dysplasia, and dyschondroplasia (Ollier's disease), or after damage of the distal radial physis by trauma or infection.

Many patients with Madelung's deformity function well and the problem is chiefly cosmetic. Pain may develop at the wrist or distal radio-ulnar joint as the patient approaches skeletal maturity. Pain may improve after skeletal maturity.

During growth, deformity may be controlled or reduced by physiolysis of the volar/ulnar part of the distal radial physis [34]. Unfortunately, patients tend to present at an age when there is little possibility for correction with further growth. Excision of the volar ligament and dome osteotomy of the radius reduced pain and improved the appearance of 26 wrists [35]. The Ilizarov method has also been used successfully [36]. Wrist fusion and operations such as ulnar head excision and the Sauve–Kapandji procedure are salvage options.

Multiple Hereditary Exostoses

Hereditary multiple exostosis is an autosomal dominant condition resulting from mutations in the EXT family of tumor suppressor genes [37]. It should probably be classed as a familial neoplastic trait rather than as a skeletal dysplasia.

Involvement of the forearm may cause swelling, pain, loss of motion, and unequal longitudinal growth. Exostoses that affect the radius seldom produce severe angular deformity. However, exostoses of the distal ulna are associated with restricted ulnar growth, leading to bowing of the forearm and frequently to dislocation of the radial head. The end result is a short, bowed forearm with loss of rotation. The range of forearm rotation is related to the length of the ulna and the number of exostoses [38]. The dislocated radial head is prominent and may be painful.

Excision of exostoses may be indicated to improve appearance and forearm rotation. Since exostosis size is inversely correlated with ulnar length [37], it would be logical to remove the exostoses as early as possible. However, the effect on growth is not known.

Fig. 21.22 Madelung deformity. (**a**) Anteroposterior view: inadequate growth of the ulnar half of the distal radial epiphysis allows the lunate to sink between the forearm bones. (**b**) Lateral view: the distal radius is angulated palmarward and the distal ulna is prominent dorsally

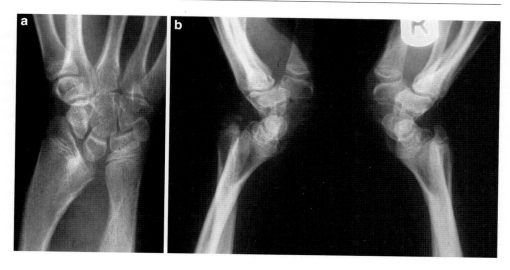

Distraction lengthening of the ulna can help to correct the length discrepancy, to improve bowing, and to maintain length. Monoaxial fixators or small circular frames can be used [39]; concomitant angular correction may also be required.

Management of established radial head dislocation associated with multiple exostoses is difficult. Relocation of the radial head requires extensive surgery and may fail to provide a congruent joint or satisfactory forearm rotation. If instability of the forearm is a problem, creation of a one-bone forearm by fusing the ulna proximally to the radial shaft distally may be appropriate.

Evidence of neurofibromatosis is present in most cases. Untreated, it produces progressive deformity, instability, and loss of rotation. Failure of ulnar growth may lead to dislocation of the radial head.

Conventional orthopaedic techniques such as nonvascularized bone grafts and internal fixation have generally failed to achieve union. Thorough excision of abnormal tissue, free vascularized fibular grafting, and stable osteosynthesis offer the best chance of healing. Creation of a one-bone forearm, providing stability at the expense of rotation, is an alternative when only the distal part of the ulna is affected.

Congenital Pseudarthrosis of the Forearm

Congenital pseudarthrosis of the forearm bones is very rare. In many respects it resembles congenital pseudarthrosis of the tibia. One or both bones may be affected (Fig. 21.23).

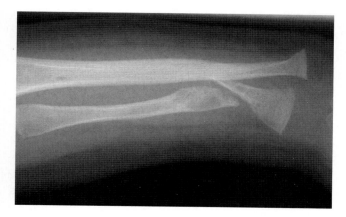

Fig. 21.23 Congenital pseudarthrosis of the radius in a 3-year-old with neurofibromatosis

Finger-Sucking Deformities

Radial deviation and supination deformities of the index finger may occur as a result of prolonged finger sucking (Fig. 21.24) [40]. Deformity is unlikely if the habit ceases by the age of 6 years. Moderate deformities may correct spontaneously once the deforming force is removed. A period of observation of 1–2 years seems appropriate, followed by osteotomy if deformity persists.

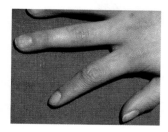

Fig. 21.24 Rotational deformity of the index finger caused by finger sucking

Arthrogryposis Multiplex Congenita

Arthrogryposis is derived from the Greek, meaning "curved joint." It is a syndrome of multiple, nonprogressive joint contractures which are present at birth. The *etiology* is unknown; in about 90% of patients, the disorder appears to be due to an underlying neuropathic process affecting the motor unit. A myopathic process has been postulated in the remaining cases.

The typical *clinical* picture comprises multiple contractures of joints in the upper and lower limbs. The limbs are atrophic, the skin is waxy, and joint creases are absent. Skin dimples may be found over contracted joints. The characteristic postures of the upper limbs are shoulder adduction, elbow extension, flexion/ulnar deviation at the wrists, and flexion deformity of the fingers with flexion/ adduction of the thumb (Fig. 21.25).

The *treatment* of arthrogryposis is difficult. As soon as possible after birth, attempts should be made to correct contractures by serial splintage and to maintain the correction by static splintage. Correction is usually incomplete. When considering operative correction, provision of independent walking should generally take priority over the upper limbs.

Loss of active and passive flexion of the elbow is a common problem in arthrogryposis. Restoration of active flexion of one hand to the mouth is desirable, but strong extension at the opposite elbow should be preserved for pushing up from the sitting position and for personal hygiene. If passive flexion of the elbow is good or can be restored by serial splintage, an elastic harness will encourage hand–mouth function until the child is old enough for tendon transfer. Posterior soft tissue release and triceps lengthening may be necessary. The pectoralis major, which is nearly always in good condition, may be transferred into the biceps tendon or into the proximal ulna, but the results tend to deteriorate with growth [41].

Flexion deformity of the wrist is managed by splintage. Soft tissue release or proximal row carpectomy may be necessary in severe cases. The aim of treatment of the flexed and adducted thumb is provision of a simple pinch, but the combined deficiency of extensors, abductors and web skin, together with contracture of adductor pollicis and flexor pollicis longus requires extensive surgery and the results may be disappointing. Function of the fingers may be impaired by flexion and ulnar deviation deformities, but their function is seldom improved by surgery.

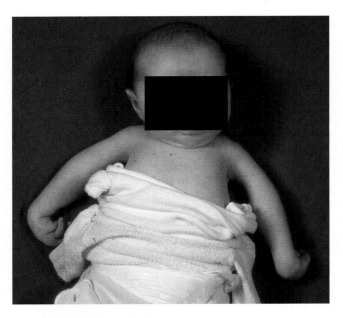

Fig. 21.25 The typical posture of arthrogryposis: elbow extension and wrist flexion

References

1. Froster-Iskenius UG, Baird PA. Limb reduction defects in over one million consecutive livebirths. Teratology 1989; 39(2):127–135.
2. Tickle C. Making digit patterns in the vertebrate limb. Nat Rev Mol Cell Biol 2006; 7(1):45–53.
3. Daluiski A, Yi SE, Lyons KM. The molecular control of upper extremity development: implications for congenital hand anomalies. J Hand Surg Am 2001; 26(1):8–22.
4. Swanson AB, Swanson GD, Tada K. A classification for congenital limb malformation. J Hand Surg Am 1983; 8(5 Pt 2):693–702.
5. Kay SPJ. Pyschosocial aspects of the child with a congenital hand anomaly. In: Green DP, Hotchkiss RN, Pederson WC, eds. Operative Hand Surgery. 4th ed. New York: Churchill Livingstone; 1999.
6. Kallemeier PM, Manske PR, Davis B, Goldfarb CA. An assessment of the relationship between congenital transverse deficiency of the forearm and symbrachydactyly. J Hand Surg Am 2007; 32(9):1408–1412.
7. Kay SP, McCombe D. Absence of Fingers. In: Green DP, Hotchkiss RN, Pederson WC, Wolfe SW, eds. Green's Operative Hand Surgery. 5th ed. Philadelphia: Elsevier/Churchill Livingstone; 2005:1415–1430.
8. Online Mendelian Inheritance in Man. at www3.ncbi.nlm.nih.gov/omim/
9. Lamb DW, Scott H, Lam WL, et al. Operative correction of radial club hand. A long-term follow-up of centralization of the hand on the ulna. J Hand Surg Br 1997; 22(4):533–536.
10. Buck-Gramcko D. Radialization as a new treatment for radial club hand. J Hand Surg Am 1985; 10(6 Pt 2):964–968.
11. Goldfarb CA, Murtha YM, Gordon JE, Manske PR. Soft-tissue distraction with a ring external fixator before centralization for radial longitudinal deficiency. J Hand Surg Am 2006; 31(6):952–959.
12. Damore E, Kozin SH, Thoder JJ, Porter S. The recurrence of deformity after surgical centralization for radial clubhand. J Hand Surg Am 2000; 25(4):745–751.
13. Peterson BM, McCarroll HR Jr, James MA. Distraction lengthening of the ulna in children with radial longitudinal deficiency. J Hand Surg Am 2007; 32(9):1402–1407.
14. Schmidt CC, Neufeld SK. Ulnar ray deficiency. Hand Clin 1998; 14(1):65–76.
15. Cole RJ, Manske PR. Classification of ulnar deficiency according to the thumb and first web. J Hand Surg Am 1997; 22(3):479–488.

16. Kay SP, McCombe D. Central Hands Deficiencies. In: Green DP, Hotchkiss RN, Pederson WC, Wolfe SW, eds. Green's Operative Hand Surgery. 5th ed. Philadelphia: Elsevier/Churchill Livingstone; 2005:1404–1415.

17. Flatt AE. The Care of Congenital Hand Anomalies. 2nd ed. St. Louis: Quality Medical Publishing; 1994.

18. Eaton CJ, Lister GD. Syndactyly. Hand Clin 1990; 6(4):555–575.

19. McCarroll HR Jr. Congenital flexion deformities of the thumb. Hand Clin 1985; 1(3):567–575.

20. Kalliainen LK, Drake DB, Edgerton MT, et al. Surgical management of the hand in Freeman-Sheldon syndrome. Ann Plast Surg 2003; 50(5):456–462. discussion 463–470.

21. Manske PR, McCarroll HR Jr. Reconstruction of the congenitally deficient thumb. Hand Clin 1992; 8(1):177–196.

22. Buck-Gramcko D. Pollicization of the index finger. Method and results in aplasia and hypoplasia of the thumb. J Bone Joint Surg Am 1971; 53(8):1605–1617.

23. McFarlane RM, Classen DA, Porte AM, Botz JS. The anatomy and treatment of camptodactyly of the small finger. J Hand Surg Am 1992; 17(1):35–44.

24. Miura T, Nakamura R, Tamura Y. Long-standing extended dynamic splintage and release of an abnormal restraining structure in camptodactyly. J Hand Surg Br 1992; 17(6):665–672.

25. Smith PJ, Grobbelaar AO. Camptodactyly: a unifying theory and approach to surgical treatment. J Hand Surg Am 1998; 23(1):14–19.

26. Kikuchi N, Ogino T. Incidence and development of trigger thumb in children. J Hand Surg Am 2006; 31(4):541–543.

27. Dinham JM, Meggitt BF. Trigger thumbs in children. A review of the natural history and indications for treatment in 105 patients. J Bone Joint Surg Br 1974; 56(1):153–155.

28. Lee ZL, Chang CH, Yang WY, et al. Extension splint for trigger thumb in children. J Pediatr Orthop 2006; 26(6):785–787.

29. Bae DS, Sodha S, Waters PM. Surgical treatment of the pediatric trigger finger. J Hand Surg Am 2007; 32(7):1043–1047.

30. Green WT, Mital MA. Congenital radio-ulnar synostosis: surgical treatment. J Bone Joint Surg Am 1979; 61(5):738–743.

31. Kanaya F, Ibaraki K. Mobilization of a congenital proximal radioulnar synostosis with use of a free vascularized fascio-fat graft. J Bone Joint Surg Am 1998; 80(8):1186–1192.

32. Wassel HD. The results of surgery for polydactyly of the thumb. Clin Orthop 1969; 64:175–193.

33. Tsuge K. Treatment of macrodactyly. J Hand Surg Am 1985; 10(6 Pt 2):968–969.

34. Vickers D, Nielsen G. Madelung deformity: surgical prophylaxis (physiolysis) during the late growth period by resection of the dyschondrosteosis lesion. J Hand Surg Br 1992; 17(4):401–407.

35. Harley BJ, Brown C, Cummings K, et al. Volar ligament release and distal radius dome osteotomy for correction of Madelung's deformity. J Hand Surg Am 2006; 31(9):1499–1506.

36. Houshian S, Schroder HA, Weeth R. Correction of Madelung's deformity by the Ilizarov technique. J Bone Joint Surg Br 2004; 86(4):536–540.

37. Porter DE, Emerton ME, Villanueva-Lopez F, Simpson AH. Clinical and radiographic analysis of osteochondromas and growth disturbance in hereditary multiple exostoses. J Pediatr Orthop 2000; 20(2):246–250.

38. Watts AC, Ballantyne JA, Fraser M, et al. The association between ulnar length and forearm movement in patients with multiple osteochondromas. J Hand Surg Am 2007; 32(5):667–673.

39. Ip D, Li YH, Chow W, Leong JC. Reconstruction of forearm deformities in multiple cartilaginous exostoses. J Pediatr Orthop Br 2003; 12(1):17–21.

40. Srinivasan J, Hutchinson JW, Burke FD. Finger sucking digital deformities. J Hand Surg Br 2001;26(6):584–588.

41. Lahoti O, Bell MJ. Transfer of pectoralis major in arthrogryposis to restore elbow flexion: deteriorating results in the long term. J Bone Joint Surg Br 2005; 87(6):858–860.

Chapter 22

The Shoulder and Elbow

John A. Fixsen

Congenital and Acquired Dislocation of the Shoulder

Congenital dislocation of the shoulder is very rare. It is usually associated with other significant anomalies in the upper limb, such as absence of the radius and deficiency or absence of part of the humerus. On examination, the humerus is unstable in all directions and the condition is normally painless. The shoulder is small, with deficiency of the deltoid, the pectorals, and other periscapular muscles. Radiographs show a small scapula, with an underdeveloped glenoid. The proximal portion of the humerus may be deficient. There is no satisfactory surgical treatment for this condition, but function of the rudimentary shoulder and abnormal upper limb is often surprisingly good, despite the inherent instability.

Acquired dislocation of the shoulder occurring at birth in association with obstetrical brachial plexus palsy is more common, but frequently remains unrecognized for several months. The arm is flail, and only when the fixed abduction deformity persists is the diagnosis of an anterior subglenoid dislocation made, as pointed out by Babbitt and Cassidy [1]. The clinical findings were reported as fixed abduction of the shoulder with winging of the scapula. The humeral head was palpable in the subglenoid position. Closed reduction failed and open reduction was necessary to reduce the dislocation. Dunkerton [2] reported four patients who presented late with posterior dislocation and associated birth palsy. In the past, this has been considered to be the result of abnormal muscle pull after birth [3] or subscapularis contracture [4]. However, Dunkerton felt that true posterior dislocation at birth was due to the brachial plexus injury (see Chapter 23).

Recurrent dislocation, although common in adults, is rare in children, but may be seen in association with marked familial joint laxity in those younger than 2 years. The child is usually brought to the clinic by the parents who are alarmed by the shoulder apparently "slipping" or "snapping" in and out of joint when the child is being dressed or undressed. The condition is usually pain-free and the shoulder reduces spontaneously. Carter and Sweetnam [5] reported this type of joint dislocation in association with familial joint laxity. Fortunately, the shoulder usually stabilizes with time. Maneuvers that cause the shoulder to displace should be avoided. Recurrent dislocation is also seen in other conditions with excessive joint laxity, such as osteogenesis imperfecta and the Ehlers–Danlos syndrome, and should be treated conservatively if possible. More recently, Hamner and Hall [6] reported two patients with multidirectional shoulder instability in association with Sprengel's deformity, which they believed was caused by repetitive stretching of the shoulder capsule as a result of the relative immobility of the scapula in this condition. Wood et al. [7] reported progressive instability of the shoulder in Apert's syndrome, which could occur both at the shoulder and at the elbow: they suggested it was due to ligamentous laxity leading to progressive bony dysplasia.

Traumatic dislocation of the shoulder in the newborn with normal musculature is extremely rare, if it occurs at all. Bateman [8], in experimental attempts to produce traumatic dislocation, showed that epiphyseal separation occurs rather than dislocation of the joint. The capsule forms a stout protective layer over the joint which is continuous with the periosteum of the humerus. The epiphyseal plate or physis is the weakest zone and as a result traumatic epiphyseal separation, as in the hip joint, is more likely than dislocation to occur in the normal child (see Chapter 41).

Congenital Pseudarthrosis of the Clavicle

This condition is rare: approximately 100 cases have been reported [9]. It presents as a nontender lump lateral to the midpoint of the clavicle (Fig. 22.1), usually at or soon after birth. It is almost invariably on the right side and has been

J.A. Fixsen (✉)
Orthopaedic Department, Great Ormond Street Hospital for Sick
Children, London, UK
e-mail: jafixsen@btinternet.com

M. Benson et al. (eds.), *Children's Orthopaedics and Fractures*,
DOI 10.1007/978-1-84882-611-3_22, © Springer-Verlag London Limited 2010

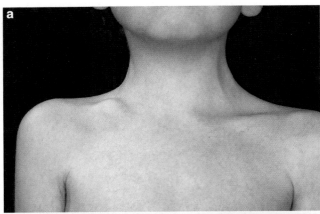

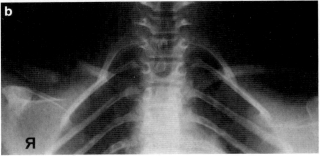

Fig. 22.1 (**a**) Clinical photograph of a child with pseudarthrosis of the right clavicle. Note the prominent lump. (**b**) Anteroposterior radiograph of the same patient showing the pseudarthrosis and the prominent lateral end of the sternal half of the clavicle

ossification. This is believed to start in membrane but, subsequently, cartilaginous growth areas develop at both acromial and sternal ends. Alldred [11] suggested that pseudarthrosis of the clavicle was the result of failure of the two centers of ossification to fuse. Lloyd-Roberts et al. [12] suggested that pressure attrition from the subclavian artery may be responsible for the pseudarthrosis. They noted that the right subclavian artery normally lies higher than the left and that this may explain the condition's right-sided predominance. They also noted that one of the very rare left-sided cases was associated with dextrocardia and an abnormally high left subclavian artery. A significant proportion of their patients also had abnormally high first ribs or cervical ribs. In the bilateral deficiencies seen in cleido-cranial dysostosis, abnormal elevation of the upper ribs is characteristic of the condition (Fig. 22.2).

Spontaneous union of the pseudarthrosis does not occur. Radiologically, there is an established pseudarthrosis, with a bulbous lateral end of the sternal half of the clavicle overlying a tapering medial end of the acromial half (Fig. 22.1). Shoulder and upper limb function is good on the affected side, but the prominent lump is unsightly. Unlike congenital pseudarthrosis of the tibia, the condition normally responds well to excision of the pseudarthrosis and bone grafting, using a block of iliac bone to bridge the gap and internal fixation with an intramedullary threaded pin to prevent migration. Alldred [11] suggested that union was easier to obtain before the child was 8 years of age and that operation was best performed around the age of 4 years. Grogan et al. [9] reported excellent results in eight children in whom the fibrous pseudarthrosis was resected early, carefully preserving the continuity of the periosteal sleeve and approximating the bone ends without grafting. All their patients healed solidly by 14 weeks after operation. They were aged from 7 months to 6 years at the time of surgery. After the age of 8 years, it appears to be more difficult to obtain fusion, and an alternative to bone grafting is excision of the prominent

described on the left side only in association with dextrocardia [10]. It may be mistaken for a clavicular fracture at birth, but it is not associated with birth injury or obstetrical palsy and, unlike a fracture, does not form callus. It should be differentiated from cleido-cranial dysostosis, in which all or part of both clavicles are deficient and associated anomalies are seen in the skull, facial bones, pelvis, and upper femora (Fig. 22.2). The clavicle is the first bone to undergo primary

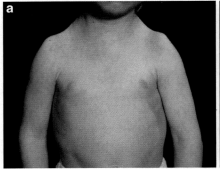

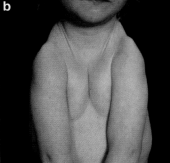

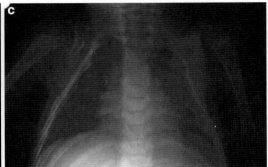

Fig. 22.2 Clinical photographs of a child with cleido-cranial dysostosis. (**a**) With the shoulders in the normal position. (**b**) With the shoulders approximated. (**c**) Anteroposterior radiograph of the chest and shoulders showing only rudimentary clavicles and abnormal elevation of the upper ribs

lateral end of the sternal half of the clavicle. This addresses the major cosmetic deformity, but ignores the pseudarthrosis, which rarely impairs function.

Congenital Elevation of the Scapula (Sprengel's Shoulder)

The limb bud for the arm appears during the fourth week of intrauterine life, between the fifth cervical and first thoracic vertebra. The scapula develops within the limb bud during the fifth week of intrauterine life and descends over the next 3 weeks to its normal position alongside the second to the seventh thoracic vertebrae. Failure to descend fully during this period gives rise to congenital elevation of the scapula, so-called Sprengel's deformity [13]. Occasionally the condition is familial, inherited as an autosomal dominant. Clinically, the scapula is elevated and rotated so that the superomedial angle is high and prominent, and the glenoid and acromion are rotated downward and forward (Fig. 22.3). In the past, the scapula was believed to be hypoplastic, but a recent 3D study by Cho et al. [14] has shown that affected scapulae have a characteristic shape, with a decrease in the height–width ratio, but were larger than the contralateral normal scapulae. The condition may be bilateral and is often associated with brevicollis and cervical abnormalities in the Klippel–Feil deformity (see Chapter 34).

The superomedial angle of the scapula may be joined to the cervical spine by a fibrous or bony omovertebral bar, first described by Willet and Walsham in 1880 [15]. The bar arises from the superomedial angle or upper one-third of the medial border of the scapula, to which it may be fused by bone or joined by a fibrous band, cartilage, or even a true joint. The medial end is attached to the spinous process, lamina, or transverse process in the lower half of the cervical spine between C4 and C7. The muscles of the shoulder girdle are often weak and defective, particularly the trapezius, which may be absent. The rhomboids and levator scapulae are hypoplastic and often partially fibrotic. The serratus anterior, pectorals, latissimus dorsi, and sternomastoid may also be affected. Other bony anomalies are frequently seen, in particular: absent or fused ribs, cervical ribs, brevicollis with vertebral anomalies, and spina bifida occulta in the cervical and upper thoracic region. The arm itself may also be short and hypoplastic. The condition is not always noticed at birth but usually becomes obvious when the child starts to stand. In bilateral cases, the neck appears unusually short and the shoulders hunched. The sexes are equally affected. When the condition is unilateral it is more commonly left sided. Abduction and external rotation of the arm are limited on the affected side, partly because of scapular immobility on the thorax and partly because the scapular position rotates the glenoid downward and forward. An anteroposterior radiograph showing both shoulders confirms the diagnosis (Fig. 22.4). Radiographs of the cervical spine and chest should be taken because of the commonly associated spinal and rib anomalies.

Treatment

The major concern is usually the cosmetic appearance rather than the limitation of shoulder movement. This is

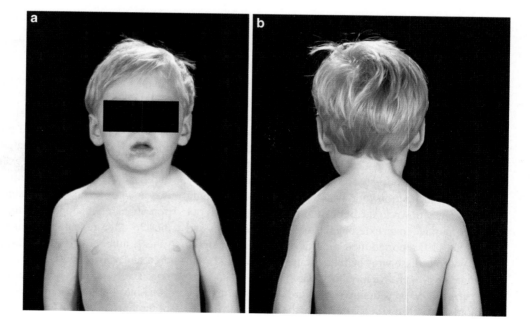

Fig. 22.3 Clinical photographs of a child with a left Sprengel's shoulder. (**a**) Anterior view. (**b**) Posterior view. Note the elevation and rotation of the left scapula

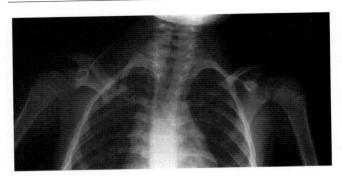

Fig. 22.4 Anteroposterior radiograph of the chest and shoulders showing congenital elevation of the right shoulder. Note anomalies in the lower cervical and upper thoracic spine and prominence of the lateral process of C7 on the right suggesting the presence of an omovertebral bar

the basis of the well-known Cavendish classification of the deformity [16], whereas the classification by Rigault et al. [17] is based on the radiographic level of the superomedial angle of the scapula at diagnosis. A program of exercises develops the maximum range of movement but does not alter the position of the scapula. From the surgical point of view, the surgeon may simply confine himself to a cosmetic procedure in which the prominent superomedial angle of the scapula is removed, together with the omovertebral bar if present. The bone should be removed extra-periosteally to avoid reformation. The patients and family must be warned that the extensive soft tissue dissection needed leaves an extensive posterior scar. The surgeon should be aware of the close proximity of the superomedial corner of the elevated scapula to the brachial plexus. This type of surgery produces an acceptable cosmetic result, but in no way alters the position of the scapula or the range of movement of the shoulder.

A more radical approach is to try to alter the position of the scapula and pull it down into its normal position. Green [18] described an extensive procedure in which the muscles connecting the scapula to the trunk are divided at their insertion along the medial border and spine of the scapula through a long posterior incision. The omovertebral bar and the superomedial angle of the scapula are removed extra-periosteally. The attachments of the latissimus dorsi muscle to the scapula are divided extra-periosteally and, by blunt dissection, a large pocket is created deep to the superior part of the latissimus dorsi. The scapula is displaced distally and secured by a traction wire, which passes from the scapula subcutaneously down to the opposite iliac crest and then out to be incorporated in an external plaster spica. Bellemans and Lamoureux [19] reported their modification of Green's procedure without dissection of the serratus anterior and with immediate post-operative mobilization; this gave satisfactory results in six of seven patients. Woodward [20] suggested that the scapular muscles be separated from the spinous processes

rather than the scapula itself, and the deformity corrected by moving the muscle origins downward. This procedure also requires a long posterior incision and may be modified by excision of the medial border of the scapula and part of its supraspinous portion [21]. Both procedures involve extensive dissection and can leave large and ugly scars. There is a well-reported incidence of damage to the brachial plexus if the scapula is displaced downward too forcefully.

Campbell and Wilkinson [22] popularized an attractive procedure, originally described by Konig in 1914 [23], in which a vertical osteotomy of the scapula 2 cm from its medial border is performed. This is combined with excision of the superomedial angle and the omovertebral bar, together with any fibrous tethering bands. The portion of the scapula lateral to the osteotomy is then rotated, correcting the abnormal downward inclination of the glenoid, improving the range of abduction at the shoulder, and the two portions are sutured together through offset drill holes, pre-drilled before the osteotomy, to maintain the corrected position.

This is a less extensive procedure than either the Green or the Woodward operations. Despite this, among the 11 patients reported, one developed mild brachial plexus palsy, but recovered, and slight winging of the scapula occurred in another patient.

Farsetti et al. [24] in a long-term study of 22 patients, 14 of whom were observed and 7 treated surgically, reported that shoulder abduction and cosmesis did not alter in the simply observed patients, but all except one were satisfied with the situation. In those treated surgically abduction was improved by an average of 38°. However, only four of the seven were satisfied, two were neither satisfied nor dissatisfied, and two were dissatisfied despite improvement in the Cavendish grade and range of abduction.

Abduction Contracture of the Shoulder

Bhattacharyya [25] reported three patients with abduction contracture of the shoulder resulting from fibrosis of the intermediate part of the deltoid. Clinically, the skin was indrawn over the contracted portion of the muscle and the arm was held in approximately 30° of abduction. In two patients this was bilateral; excision of the fibrotic muscle improved the range of movement in all three patients. There was no definite history of trauma or injection, but the condition appeared analogous to that described in the quadriceps muscle after repeated intramuscular injections. Since that time, a number of further cases have been reported in children and young adults [26–28]. The cause of the fibrosis is not usually known, but it seems likely that it follows injections into the muscle and responds satisfactorily to excision of the fibrous contracted area.

Congenital Anomalies of the Elbow

Supracondylar Humeral Spur

This is a palpable bony prominence or tubercle on the antero-medial surface of the distal humerus above the elbow. It is associated with a fibrous band extending to the medial epicondyle and was described by Struthers in 1849 [29]. Such a spur is normal in climbing mammals such as lemurs and in the cat family as a bony foramen through which the neurovascular bundle passes. It is rare but can be important as a cause of vascular and or nerve compression symptoms in the forearm and hand of a child [30]. The diagnosis can be confirmed by plain radiographs (Fig. 22.5) and, if it is clear that the symptoms are caused by it, exploration and decompression by removal of the spur and band are indicated.

Congenital Ankylosis of the Elbow

This rare condition may involve the whole elbow joint or only the humero-ulnar or humero-radial joints in which case the uninvolved bone is commonly absent (Fig. 22.6). It may occur in isolation in which case it is usually bilateral or with other anomalies such as absent radius or ulna or cranio-facial disorders, e.g., Crouzon's syndrome (Fig. 22.7). McIntyre and Benson [31] published a useful etiological classification which highlighted the pitfalls of phenotypic variability when using a simple morphological classification and provided information on associated anomalies and syndromes. Function for activities of daily living is often surprisingly good even in bilateral cases. Attempts to construct a mobile elbow joint are unrewarding. Osteotomy to reposition the forearm and hand in a more functional position can be helpful. It should be remembered, particularly in bilateral cases,

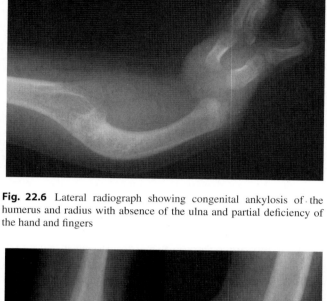

Fig. 22.6 Lateral radiograph showing congenital ankylosis of the humerus and radius with absence of the ulna and partial deficiency of the hand and fingers

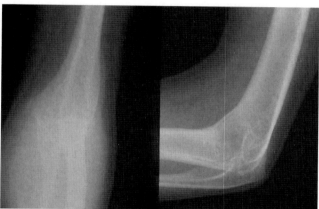

Fig. 22.7 Lateral radiograph showing congenital ankylosis of the elbow in a patient with Crouzon's syndrome

that one hand should reach the mouth and the other the perineum.

Bilateral Congenital Pseudarthrosis of the Olecranon

This was first reported in the English literature in 1987 by Burge and Benson [32] who described a child born with fixed flexion of both elbows. Early radiographs showed the olecranon separated from the ulnar shaft in both arms. When this gap failed to ossify and he was suffering from weakness of extension at the age of 6 years the pseudarthroses were operated upon sequentially by excision of the fibrous and fibrocartilaginous tissue and bone grafting stabilized by tension band wiring. The results were satisfactory clinically and radiologically. This condition appears to be different from congenital pseudarthrosis of the forearm (see Chapter 21).

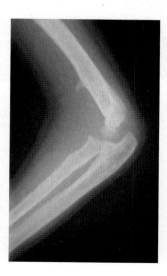

Fig. 22.5 Lateral radiograph of the elbow showing a humeral supracondylar spur. The patient presented with symptoms of vascular and median nerve compression in the forearm

Osteochondritis of the Capitellum (Panner's Disease)

This condition in which changes similar to those of Legg–Calve–Perthes' disease are seen in the capitellum was first described by Panner in 1927 [33]. More rarely the radial head may be similarly affected [34]. It is commoner in boys and usually occurs between the age of 4 and 10 years [35]. The patient presents with elbow pain and stiffness. On examination there is limitation of full extension and local tenderness over the capitellum. Sometimes there is local swelling and evidence of an effusion. Radiographs show irregular areas of increased density and fragmentation in the capitellum similar to the changes seen in Legg–Calve–Perthes' disease. Treatment consists of rest in a sling or cast in the acute phase followed by gentle mobilization. Spontaneous recovery normally occurs in 1–3 years. However, there may be some permanent loss of full elbow extension, permanent deformation of the capitellum, and occasionally of the radial head [35].

The Carrying Angle of the Elbow (Cubitus Valgus/Varus)

The term carrying angle of the elbow refers to the angle between the humerus and the forearm and hand in the antero-posterior plane with the elbow fully extended and supinated. In children there is usually around 5° of cubitus valgus. The commonest cause of abnormal angulation is malunion following a humeral supracondylar fracture associated with a cubitus varus deformity (Fig. 22.8) or cubitus valgus

following nonunion of a lateral humeral condylar fracture (see Chapter 44). However, a number of inherited disorders such as the nail-patella and Turner's syndrome (45X0) are associated with an increased carrying angle (cubitus valgus). In an interesting study relating the carrying angle to sex chromosome anomalies Baughman et al. [36] showed that there appears to be a spectrum of the "carrying angle" in relation to the sex chromosome anomaly from maximal cubitus valgus X0 (Turner's syndrome) to minimal cubitus valgus or even varus in patients with supernumerary sex chromosomes as in XXY (Klinefelter's syndrome) and XXXXX (Penta X syndrome) which can also be associated with radial head dislocation and radio-ulnar synostosis. In these congenital conditions, unlike those following malunion, operative treatment is rarely indicated.

Congenital dislocation of the radial head, and congenital radio-ulnar synostosis are described in Chapter 21.

References

1. Babbitt DP, Cassidy PH. Obstetrical paralysis and dislocation of the shoulder in infancy. J Bone Joint Surg 1968; 50A:1447–1452.
2. Dunkerton MC. Posterior dislocation of the shoulder associated with obstetric brachial plexus palsy. J Bone Surg 1989; 71B: 764–766.
3. Wickstrom J, Haslam ET, Hutchinson RH. The surgical management of residual deformities of the shoulder following birth injuries with a brachial plexus injury. J Bone Joint Surg 1955; 37A:27–36.
4. Narakas AO. Obstetrical brachial plexus injuries. In: Lamb DW (ed). The paralysed hand. The hand and upper limb, vol 2. Edinburgh: Churchill Livingstone; 1987:116–135.
5. Carter C, Sweetnam R. Recurrent dislocation of the patella and shoulder: their association with familial joint laxity. J Bone Joint Surg 1960; 42B:721–727.

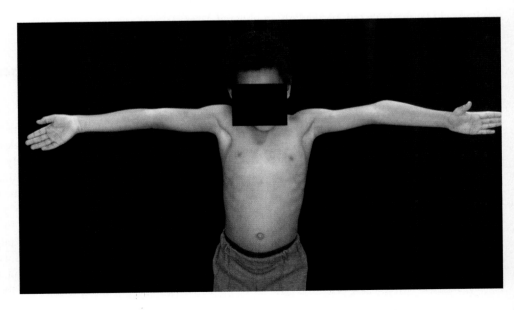

Fig. 22.8 Clinical photograph of a child with left cubitus varus following malunion of a supracondylar fracture

6. Hamner DL, Hall JE. Sprengel's deformity associated with multi directional shoulder instability. J Pediatr Orthop 1995; 15: 641–643.

7. Wood DE, Sauser DD, O'Hara RC. Shoulder and elbow in Apert's syndrome. J Pediatr Orthop 1995; 15:648–651.

8. Bateman JE. The shoulder and neck, 2nd ed. Philadelphia: WB Saunders; 1978:37.

9. Grogan DP, Love SM, Guideria KJ, Ogden JA. Operative treatment of congenital pseudarthrosis of the clavicle. J Pediatr Orthop 1991; 11:176–180.

10. Gibson DA, Carroll N. Congenital pseudarthrosis of the clavicle. J Bone Joint Surg 1970; 52B:629–643.

11. Alldred AJ. Congenital pseudarthrosis of the clavicle. J Bone Joint Surg 1963; 45B:312–319.

12. Lloyd-Roberts GC, Apley AG, Owen R. Reflections upon the aetiology of congenital pseudarthrosis of the clavicle. J Bone Joint Surg 1975. 57B:24–29.

13. Sprengel O. Die angeborene Verschiebung des Schulterblattes nach oben. Langenbeck Arch Klin Chir 1891; 42:545–549.

14. Cho T-J, Choi IH, Chung CY, Hwang JK. The Sprengel's deformity. J Bone Joint Surg 2000; 82B:711–718.

15. Willet A, Walsham WJ. An account of the dissection of the parts removed after death from the body of a woman the subject of congenital malformation of the spinal column, thorax and left scapular arch with remarks on the probable nature of the defects in development producing the deformities. Med Surg Trans London 1880; 63:256.

16. Cavendish ME. Congenital elevation of the shoulder. J Bone Joint Surg 1972; 54B:395–408.

17. Rigault P, Pouliquen JC, Guyonvarch G, Zujovic J. Congenital elevation of the scapula in childhood. Rev Chir Orthop 1976; 62:5–26.

18. Green WT. The Surgery correction of elevation of the scapula (Sprengel's deformity). J Bone Joint Surg 1957; 39A: 1439.

19. Bellemans M, Lamoureux J. Results of surgical treatment of Sprengel deformity by a modified Green's procedure. J Pediatr Orthop B 1999; 8:194–196.

20. Woodward JW. Congenital elevation of the scapula: correction by release and transplantation of the muscle origin. J Bone Joint Surg 1961; 43A:219–228.

21. Borges KLP, Shah A, Cobo Torres B, Bowen JR. Modified Woodward procedure for Sprengel's deformity of the shoulder. J Pediatr Orthop 1996; 18:508–513.

22. Campbell D, Wilkinson JA. Scapular osteotomy for the treatment of Sprengel's shoulder. J Bone Joint Surg 1979; 61B:514.

23. König F. Eine neue Operation des angeborenen Schulter blatthochstandes. Beitr Klin Chir 1914; 94:530–537.

24. Farsetti P, Weinstein SL, Caterini R, et al. Sprengel's deformity: Long term follow-up study of 22 cases. J Pediatr Orthop B 2003; 12:202–210.

25. Bhattacharyya S. Abduction contracture of the shoulder from contracture of the intermediate part of the deltoid. J Bone Joint Surg 1966; 48B:127–131.

26. Hill NA, Leibler WA, Wilson JH, Rosenthal E. Abduction contractures of both glenohumeral joints and extension contracture of one knee secondary to partial muscle fibrosis. J Bone Joint Surg 1967; 49A:961–964.

27. Goodfellow JW, Wade S. Flexion contracture of the shoulder joint from the anterior part of the deltoid muscle. J Bone Joint Surg 1969; 51B:356–358.

28. Wolbrink AJ, Hsu Z, Bianco AJ. Abduction contracture of the shoulders and hips secondary to fibrous bands. J Bone Joint Surg 1973; 55A:844–846.

29. Struthers J. On a peculiarity of the humerus and humeral artery. Monthly J Med Sci 1849; 9:264.

30. Kessel L, Rang M. Supracondylar spur of the humerus. J Bone Joint Surg 1966; 48B:765–769.

31. McIntyre JD, Benson MKD. An aetiological classification for developmental synostoses of the elbow. J Pediatr Orthop B 2002; 11:313–319.

32. Burge P, Benson M. Bilateral congenital pseudarthrosis of the olecranon. J Bone Joint Surg 1987; 69B:460–462.

33. Panner HJ. An affection of the capitulum humeri resembling Calve-Perthes disease of the hip. Acta Radiologica 1927; 8:617.

34. Trias A, Ray RD. Juvenile osteochondritis of the radial head. J Bone Joint Surg 1963; 45A:576–582.

35. Smith MGH. Osteochrondritis of the humeral capitulum. J Bone Joint Surg 1964; 46B:50.

36. Baughman FA Jr, Higgins JV, Wadsworth TG, Demaray MJ. The carrying angle in sex chromosome anomalies. J Am Med Assoc 1974; 280:718.

Chapter 23

Brachial Plexus Injuries
Peripheral Nerve Injuries

Alain L. Gilbert and Rolfe Birch

Part 1: Management of the Injury

Alain L. Gilbert

Introduction

Evolving microsurgical techniques have significantly changed our attitude to surgical reconstruction of peripheral nerve lesions, including those of the brachial plexus. However, because of the considerable distance the nerves have to regenerate after restoring anatomical continuity in the brachial plexus, the results in adults have been modest, despite the more sophisticated methods available. In contrast, similar methods in children give better results because of their superior capacity for regeneration and the shorter distances involved. The potential for regeneration diminishes gradually after birth, remaining fairly good until adolescence and then deteriorating rapidly after the cessation of growth. Obstetrical lesions occurring at birth are best considered separately, because they represent a uniform group for patient's age and type of lesion, whereas lesions occurring during childhood are more heterogeneous.

Etiology and Pathogenesis

Obstetrical birth palsy has been recognized since the late 19th century, but modern series reporting operative exploration have clarified the pathological changes.

The etiology is always a tearing force caused by traction on the head or arm. There are two basic types of lesion, which relate to presentation and birth weight:

1. overweight babies (over 4 kg) with vertex presentation and shoulder dystocia who require excessive force using traction, often with forceps or ventouse extraction, for delivery. This results in an upper plexus injury, most commonly of the C5 and C6, and occasionally the C7 roots. Sometimes a complete plexus injury occurs, involving rupture of the upper roots and lower root avulsions (Fig. 23.1).
2. Breech presentation, usually of small babies (under 3 kg) requiring hyperextension of the head and neck and, in many cases, manipulation of the hand and arm in a fashion that exerts traction on both the upper and the lower roots. This often causes an avulsion injury of the upper roots, or occasionally all of the roots (Fig. 23.2).

Clinical Presentation

The initial diagnosis is obvious at birth. After a difficult delivery of an obese baby by the vertex presentation or a small baby by the breech, the upper extremity is flail and dangling. A more detailed analysis of the pattern of paralysis of the various muscles of the upper extremity is now necessary, as the picture will change rapidly. Examination of the other extremities is important, to exclude neonatal quadriplegia or diplegia. Occasionally, birth palsy may be bilateral. Forty-eight hours later, a more accurate examination and muscle testing can be performed. At this stage it is usually possible to differentiate two types of paresis:

1. The *Erb-Duchenne* type paralysis of the upper roots. The arm is held in internal rotation and pronation. There is no active shoulder abduction or elbow flexion. The elbow may be slightly flexed (lesion of C5–C7) or in complete extension (lesion of C5–C6). The thumb is in flexion

A.L. Gilbert (✉)
Institut de la Main, Clinique Jouvenet, Paris, France

R. Birch (✉)
Peripheral Nerve Injury Unit, Royal National Orthopaedic Hospital, Stanmore, UK

M. Benson et al. (eds.), *Children's Orthopaedics and Fractures*,
DOI 10.1007/978-1-84882-611-3_23, © Springer-Verlag London Limited 2010

Fig. 23.1 C5/C6 brachial plexus lesion: paralyzed fibers are shaded (Reproduced with permission from Narakas [34])

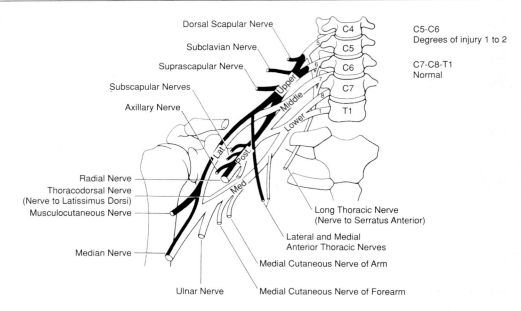

Fig. 23.2 Entire brachial plexus lesion. Rupture of the upper trunk, supraganglionic avulsion of C7 and C8, severe damage to T1 (Reproduced with permission from Narakas [34])

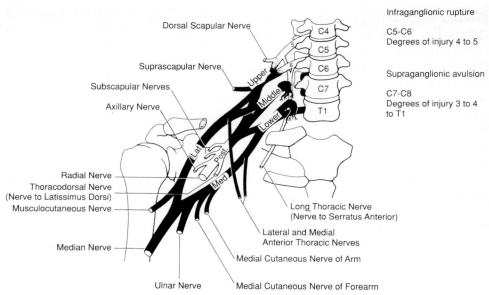

and sometimes the fingers will not extend. As a rule, the thumb and the finger flexors are functioning. The pectoralis major is usually active, giving an appearance of forward flexion of the shoulder. There are no vasomotor changes or gross alterations of distal sensation.

2. Complete paralysis (*Dejerine-Klumpke*). The entire arm is flail and the hand clenched. Sensation is diminished, and there is vasomotor impairment, giving a pale or even "marbled" appearance to the extremity. Often, Horner's sign is present on the affected side.

A shoulder radiograph should be taken to eliminate fracture of the clavicle or the upper humerus, which can occur

in association with the paresis. Occasionally, phrenic nerve palsy can be detected by diaphragmatic fluoroscopy.

The clinical development during the first month is variable, and many pareses will lessen during this stage [1]. However, Wickstrom et al. [2] reported that only 10% of total palsies recover to any useful extent. These patients should be carefully evaluated at the age of 3 months, clinically, electromyographically, and by cervical myelography. Gentle physiotherapy should be ensured during this recovery period to minimize the development of contractures while awaiting spontaneous recovery. At this stage, a complete paralysis with Horner's sign will remain unchanged so that early operation at 3 months of age should be considered for these babies.

Paralysis of the upper roots may show spontaneous recovery during the first 3 months. These babies should be treated with physiotherapy and assessed clinically and electromyographically by the age of 3 months.

Spontaneous Recovery

The literature reports varying rates of spontaneous recovery, from 7 to 80%. Useful guidelines are given in the thesis of Tassin [3] who came to the following conclusions:

Complete recovery is seen in those infants showing some contraction of the biceps and the deltoid by the end of the first month and a normal contraction by the second month. An infant in whom neither the deltoid nor the biceps contract by the third month cannot be expected to obtain a good result. Testing the deltoid can be difficult. As a result, assessment of the biceps is the most reliable indicator for operative intervention. If there is no evidence of any recovery in the biceps by the end of the third month, operation is indicated. Clinical assessment is more reliable than electrical testing. If surgery is not undertaken, some recovery will continue to take place spontaneously, but it is likely to be less satisfactory than that after surgery.

Indications for Operation

If recovery of the biceps has not begun by 3 months, the prognosis is poor and surgical repair of the plexus is indicated [4–6]. The following clinical situations pose particular problems:

1. Complete palsy with a flail arm after 1 month, particularly with a Horner's syndrome, does not recover spontaneously and is a prime candidate for surgery. These babies are best treated by early operation at the age of 12 weeks.
2. Complete palsy of C5 and C6 occurring after breech delivery with no sign of recovery by the third month should also be considered for surgical treatment.
3. The most common C5, C6, and sometimes C7 palsies almost always show some sign of recovery, which can be misleading, and which has in the past encouraged a conservative approach. If, however, after careful examination, recovery of the biceps (and not elbow flexion) is completely absent at 3 months, surgery should be considered. Great difficulty arises when infants are seen late, by the 6–8th month, and show minimal recovery of biceps function. The parents are often encouraged by the early signs of recovery and will not accept the idea of an unsatisfactory final result. Under these circumstances, it is difficult for the surgeon to advise an operation that cannot promise a definitive result. In order to avoid this situation, it is important to try to make decisions by the third month.

Several centers have been unable to show good correlation between electromyographic changes and the final outcome. Frequently, the pre-operative electromyogram (EMG) gives cause for over-optimism, because it takes only a few fibers to provoke an electrical response which is not associated with subsequent clinical recovery. However, a negative EMG with complete absence of signs of regeneration at the age of 3 months almost invariably signifies root avulsion.

Myelography has been used extensively in the past, but is unpredictable and associated with false-negative and false-positive results. Computed tomography with myelography has improved the quality of the results considerably.

The recent use of magnetic resonance imaging (MRI), although promising, does not always offer precise information for routine use. Both MRI and myelography need general anesthesia for the baby and should be used only if there is uncertainty about the condition of the roots (breech presentation, lower root avulsion).

Surgical Intervention

Operation is performed under general anesthesia. Usually a supraclavicular approach is sufficient, but this can de extended transclavicularly to expose the lower plexus if necessary. The neuroma usually lies between the C5 and the C6 roots and the divisions of the upper trunk at the level of the clavicle. The nerves may be ruptured totally or avulsed. The neuroma is resected back to normal tissue and one or two sural nerves are used as grafts between the sectioned nerve ends. The nerve anastomoses can be performed by fibrin glue (Tissucol). If avulsions are present, reconstruction must be tailor-made to the situation and the expertise of the surgeon. The reconstruction of the hand is a priority. Our results show that a major part of the remaining roots should be used to reconstruct C8–T1, even if the shoulder is weakened. Additional neurotizations may be used to compensate.

Neurotizations

For several years neurotizations have become increasingly popular and their usefulness confirmed. This can be used in desperate cases such as an avulsion of C5/C6 in a breech delivery where double (accessory spinal on suprascapular [7] and ulnar on musculocutaneous [8]) or triple (adding triceps branch on axillary [9]) neurotizations can give very satisfactory function at the shoulder [10]; they can also be used to complement a difficult repair if the roots are small and of doubtful quality. More classical (intercostal nerve) or more specific (phrenic nerve [11], contralateral C7 [12], and brachialis) neurotizations have been advocated by some surgeons but are not widely accepted. The outcome following end-to-side suture has not proven reliable in our hands and has not been scientifically substantiated.

Anatomical Lesions

The anatomical lesions observed at operation correspond to those described by Taylor in 1920 [13]. These include rupture at the level of the primary trunk or root, or avulsion of the roots. Unlike the reported lesions in the adult, we have never seen a double-level lesion or lesions of the secondary trunk of two branches of the plexus. Associated vascular lesions are exceptional, and we have seen only one rupture of the axillary artery, which was treated by vein graft. The upper roots are more often ruptured and the lower roots avulsed. The results in 436 surgical cases up to 1996 showed the following distribution of root lesions [14, 15]:

1. C5 and C6: 48%
2. C5–C7: 29%
3. Complete involvement: 23% (of which almost all were avulsions).

Post-Operative Care

Stretching the reconstructed region must be avoided for the first three post-operative weeks. This is best achieved by splintage. Physical therapy is then resumed by gentle passive exercises and the encouragement of voluntary movement. Every effort should be made to counteract retraction and internal rotation of the shoulder and encourage flexion of the elbow. Physiotherapy should be continued throughout the recovery period, usually for 2 years, when regular physiotherapy may be discontinued. Recovery is slow. It can be seen 4–6 months after direct suture and at 6–10 months after graft reconstruction. It can continue in upper plexus lesions for over 2 years and in complete lesions for over 3 years.

Results of Surgery

Since 1976, we have seen more than 4,330 cases. Up until April 2008, 996 have been operated upon. From this total we

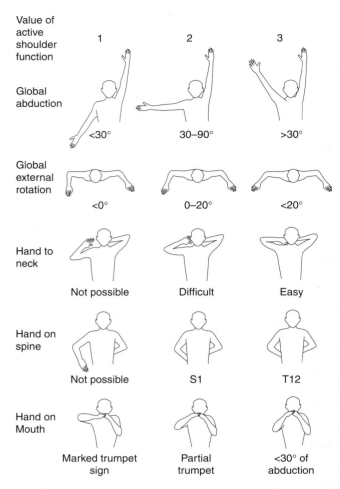

Fig. 23.3 The Mallet system of measuring function at the shoulder

have reviewed 436 patients with a minimum 4-year follow-up operated on between 1976 and 1995. The results in the shoulder, using the Mallet scale (Fig. 23.3) [16] are

C5 C6
at 2 years

>Grade IV (good–excellent)	52%
Grade III	40%
Grade II	8%

After 2 years one-third of the patients had secondary surgery:

13 subscapularis releases
33 latissimus dorsi transfers
6 trapezius transfers

and a new evaluation was completed at 4 years (after tendon transfers). The results were as follows:

Grade IV   80%
Grade III   20%
Grade II   0%
C5 C6 C7

At 2 years the results were

Grade IV   36%
Grade III   46%
Grade II   18%

After 2 years, one-quarter of the patients had secondary surgery:

7 subscapularis releases
24 latissimus dorsi transfers
1 trapezius transfer

and the results were evaluated again at 4 years.

Complete Paralysis

The results in the shoulder in complete paralysis are less satisfactory because part of the upper roots destined for the shoulder and elbow must be sacrificed in order to obtain function in the hand. The shoulder results at 4 years are as follows:

class IV: 22.5%
class III: 42%
class II: 35.5%

In the hand, however, for which the prognosis is very poor for spontaneous recovery, the results showed some function in 83% and useful function in 75% of patients, 8 years after neurotization.

Complications

In the series reviewed, there have been no operative deaths. The overall complication rate was 1%, including phrenic nerve lesions, lesions of the thoracic duct, wound infections, and vascular lesions, all of which have been managed satisfactorily, without late sequelae.

Recommendations

On the basis of the results of the author's series of patients, the following recommendations can be made:

1. Babies who do not recover biceps function by the age of 3 months should be considered for immediate operation.
2. Primary suture without tension is rarely possible. Nerve grafting is usually necessary for root or trunk ruptures.
3. In the presence of root avulsions, an internal neurotization should be attempted between different roots, particularly as children seem to have a far greater capacity to accommodate to differential neurotizations.
4. When it is not possible to perform an internal neurotization, an external neurotization can be performed, using one or more of the following donor nerves in the following order of preference: the spinal accessory nerve, the ulnar or median nerve, and the intercostal nerves.
5. The reconstruction should be protected from excessive motion for the first 3 weeks.
6. Physiotherapy should be continued up to 2 years of age, but then continued by the parents in the form of play and activities of daily living.
7. Secondary surgery can be considered when it is clear that recovery after reconstruction has failed.

Late Cases

When the patient is seen late the indications for surgery are difficult to define. It is not easy to convince a family that in order to recover some potential hand function it is necessary to scar the shoulder region and imperil natural recovery. Sometimes it is possible to use neurotizations and avoid losing existing function.

How Late Can Reconstruction Be Considered?

Children can be operated upon after several years as the muscles may stay alive much longer than in the adult, even 9 years after injury. It is necessary to record a good EMG showing fibrillations or some re-innervated fibers. Outcome is adversely affected by technical difficulties resulting from fibrosis at the sites of the lesions and by inadequate brain readjustment.

Part 2: Birth lesions of the brachial plexus Peripheral nerve injuries

Rolfe Birch

Etiology

The causes, characteristics, and consequences of this lesion were established during the latter part of the 19th century from work undertaken, for the most part, by French neurologists and surgeons (Fig. 23.4). The first reports of plexus repairs appeared in 1903, from Glasgow, Manchester, and London. Since that time the field has been plagued by controversy about causation, incidence, and natural history; about the cause and treatment of consequent deformity; and about the indications for and results of nerve repair. In 2003 Evans-Jones, Kay, and colleagues [17] published the findings of the first ever national census of the disorder. As they point out "most cases are due to trauma at delivery which is not necessarily excessive or inappropriate." The incidence, risk factors, and course to recovery during the first 6 months of life were recorded. Of 723,000 live births in the United Kingdom and the Republic of Ireland, there were 323 new cases of birth lesions of the brachial plexus (BLBP) in a period of 12 months; 143 of the 255 incomplete lesions had recovered fully by the age of 6 months. There was partial recovery in the remainder. None of the 98 complete lesions had fully recovered by 6 months. In six babies there was no recovery at all. Significant associated risk factors in comparison with the normal population included shoulder dystocia (60% vs. 0.3%), high birth weight, and instrument-assisted delivery. Evans-Jones et al. [17] point out that there was a significantly lower risk of BLBP in infants delivered by caesarean section. Breech delivery occurred in only 10 of the 323 confirmed cases which suggests that obstetricians in the United Kingdom take the matter of breech presentation rather more seriously than in some other countries. A total of 74 infants entered into the national census were followed for a minimum of 24 months after birth [18]. Recovery was full in 39 children. Operation for repair of the nerves was undertaken in nine children and for open reduction of posterior dislocation (PD) of the shoulder in 20 more.

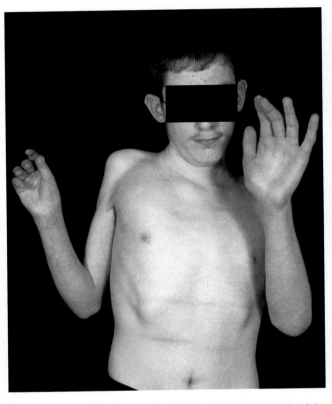

Fig. 23.4 Bilateral lesion complicating breech delivery. On the right, avulsion of C5, C6, and C7; on the left, avulsion C5, rupture of C6. The shoulders are flail; there is severe growth disturbance

The significance of risk factors has been clarified in two studies. The earlier report of 230 consecutive cases [19] found that the mean birth weight of affected babies was 4.5 kg, against the regional mean of 3.88 kg. Heavy babies had more serious nerve injuries. Shoulder dystocia was recorded in over 60% of deliveries. There was no significant correlation with social class. The later report comes from Tavakkolizadeh [20] who analyzed risk factors in over 1,000 consecutive cases. The relative risk of a baby suffering BLBP is as high as 180 when delivery is complicated by shoulder dystocia and about 10 in cases of neonatal asphyxia or maternal gestational diabetes. The relative risk of failure to perform cesarean section comes close to nine as does birth weight in excess of 3.4 kg. Tavakkolizadeh [20] confirms that increased maternal body mass index (BMI) is a significant risk factor. Anatomical variations, such as a cervical rib, may account for the 5% of cases where no obvious cause can be found [21].

Outcomes

Valuable long-term studies have been contributed by Strombeck et al. [22, 23]. Many young adults showed persisting deficits in function, exacerbated by deformity at the elbow and shoulder, and, perhaps, by continuing loss of motor neurones in the anterior horn of the spinal cord. Yang [24] found that "only 17% of children affected by right obstetric brachial plexus palsy prefer the right upper limb for overall movement." A significant correlation between defects in personal and social behavior and the extent of the lesion [25] reminds us that operations, hospitalization, and continuing dependence upon "health professionals" do the child no good.

Pathology

The nerve lesion in BLBP differs from the high-energy transfer adult injury in two important respects: traction and compression forces are expended upon the nerves for hours during a protracted and difficult delivery, and the response of the immature nervous system is very different from that seen in the adult. In the infant the spinal cord fills the cervical canal, the spinal rootlets emerging at, or close to a right angle from it. Fraher [26] states that "during development the CNS–PNS interface oscillates and continually changes its form and position as the two tissue classes establish their mutually exclusive territories." Myelination is incomplete, particularly at the junction between the roots of the spinal nerves and the spinal cord, so that conduction velocity in the neonate is only one-half that of the adult. It is even slower in premature babies. The density of nerve fibers in the neonate is higher than in the adult because of the paucity of connective tissue. Nerve blood flow is highest in the first weeks of life and thereafter declines [27]. Immature nerve fibers are more susceptible to ischemia and anoxic conduction block. Groves and Scaravilli [28] demonstrate that many neurones in the neonatal dorsal root ganglion die after axonotomy and the immature neurones of the anterior horn of the spinal cord are similarly vulnerable. Decisive evidence about defective regeneration in the immature nervous system is provided by Fullertan et al. [29, 30] who found "a selective failure of regeneration in the largest diameter fibers. . . .it seems more likely that the failure of recovery of fine movements is due to the fact that the proprioceptive pathway involving 1-α [alpha], 1-β [beta] and group 2 fibers on the afferent side and

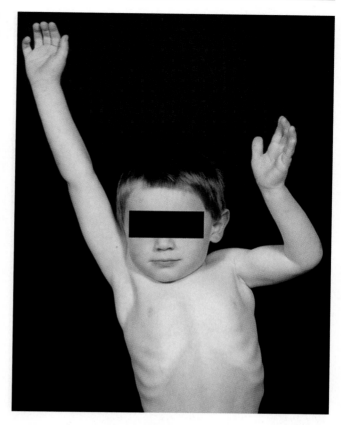

Fig. 23.5 Co-contraction of the muscles acting across the glenohumeral joint

the process of α and γ co-activation on the efferent side, is lost." These findings may account for the simultaneous activity in antagonistic muscles seen in so many children with BLBP and explain many of the disappointing results of nerve repair (Fig. 23.5).

The injury to the spinal nerves is different from that encountered in the adult. Combined, post-ganglionic rupture and intradural lesion are common; avulsion of the roots without displacement of the dorsal root ganglion (DRG) is frequent; rupture confined to the ventral or dorsal root has been confirmed [31]. Intra-operative neurophysiological investigation (NPI) of central and of peripheral conduction is valuable in analysis of the adult case: it is essential in the infant.

Clinical Assessment

Diagnosis is usually straightforward (Fig. 23.6). Lesions complicating breech delivery are frequently bilateral and often complicated by phrenic nerve palsy requiring plication of the hemi-diaphragm as a matter of urgency [32]. Records [33] made at first attendance include the risk factor chart,

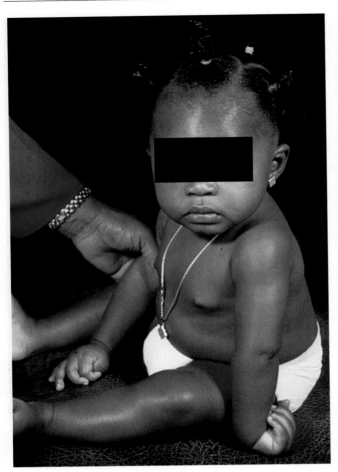

Fig. 23.6 Group 2 lesion (C5, C6, C7)

the Mallett shoulder system, and charts for operated and non-operated cases (Figs. 23.7 and 23.8). The active and passive ranges at the thoraco-scapular, the gleno-humeral, and the radio-ulnar joints are recorded. The charts are completed at every attendance in the clinic. The inferior scapulo-humeral (ISH) angle is measured between the long axis of humerus and the lateral border of the scapula. The active and the passive ISH angle is measured and recorded: the angles indicate the contributions to elevation of the thoraco-scapular and gleno-humeral joints and reveal weakness or contractures of those muscles acting across these joints. The posterior scapulo-humeral (PSH) angle subtends between the axis of the humeral shaft and the line of the spine of the scapula. The examiner holds the arm parallel to the ground and the child's hand rests on the opposite shoulder. If the PSH angle is wide, but active medial rotation is reduced, then the medial rotator muscles are defective (Fig. 23.9). Retroversion of the head of the humerus or less commonly contracture of the posterior capsule and lateral rotator muscles accounts for the narrowing of both active and passive PSH angles. Yang [24] analyzed the correlation between the different scoring

systems and function within the upper limb. The Mallett score strongly correlated with both gross and fine movements showing "the first significant correlation between actual task performance and two of the three tested obstetrical brachial plexus palsy outcome measures based on the extent of movement at different joints of the upper limb." Closer analysis of hand function requires functional assessment appropriately modified to the age of the child.

Parents should be involved in the treatment of the child from the outset. Regular and gentle exercises may prevent fixed deformity (Fig. 23.10). There is no place for vigorous manipulation. If gentle stretching movements cause pain, then there must be either a fracture or a posterior dislocation of the shoulder. The role of the therapist and the attending doctor is to teach and then to monitor progress.

The extent of nerve injury is graded using the classification of Narakas [34] in cases born by cephalic presentation. This system is not applicable to the special case of the breech lesion.

Group 1

The fifth and sixth cervical nerves are damaged. There is paralysis of supraspinatus, infraspinatus, deltoid, and biceps muscles. Good recovery is seen in 90% of cases.

Group 2

The fifth, sixth, and seventh cervical nerves are damaged. About 70% of these children make a good spontaneous recovery, but there are serious residual defects in the shoulder in the remaining 30%. Recovery of the shoulder abductors and the biceps is slower than in group 1 and these muscles often remain paralyzed or weak for the first 3 months of life.

Group 3

The paralysis is virtually complete. There is some flexion of the fingers at, or shortly after, birth. Full recovery occurs in less than one-half of these children. Defective function at the shoulder, elbow, and forearm is common. Wrist and finger extension does not recover in about one-quarter.

Group 4

The paralysis is complete. The limb is flaccid together with Bernard–Horner syndrome. Few children make a good overall recovery but we have observed useful spontaneous recovery in the hand in about one-half (Fig. 23.11).

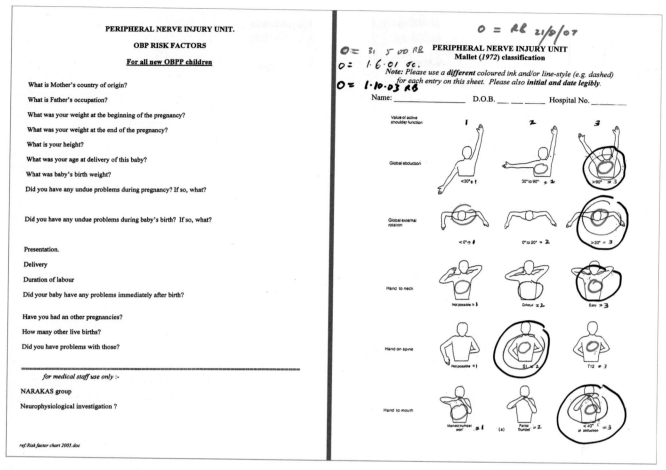

Fig. 23.7 On the left, the risk factor chart; on the right, the peripheral nerve injury Unit's modification of the Mallett system. Each entry is dated and signed by the clinician. Different colors record the dates of entry. The maximum score is 15

The Narakas classification does not recognize the rare lesion confined to C8 and T1. It may become clear that the middle nerves, C6, C7, and C8, have been severely damaged [35].

Prognosis

In favorable lesions, the parents report active grasp at 2 weeks and flexion at the shoulder and the elbow at 6–8 weeks. Return of grasp at 4 weeks virtually guarantees a useful hand. The methods of neurophysiological investigation (NPI) developed and applied by Smith [36, 37] are particularly helpful but the clinician using such information must understand the method. Nerve action potentials (NAPs) are measured from the median and ulnar nerves by stimulating at the wrist and recording at the elbow. The deltoid (C5), biceps (C6), triceps and forearm extensors (C7), forearm flexors (C8), and the first dorsal interosseous (T1) muscles are assessed by electromyography. The lesion is graded for each spinal nerve according to the degree of demyelination and axonopathy. NPI are usually pessimistic in the first weeks of life when Wallerian degeneration is at its height (Fig. 23.12). Serial NPI are reserved for cases of postganglionic injury of C8 and of T1 and also for some lesions of C5 where there is real doubt about progress. Bisinella [38] analyzed findings in over 350 spinal nerves in 126 children with groups 1, 2, and 3 lesions in whom elbow flexion had not recovered by the age of 3 months. Operation was undertaken in the 53 babies where poor progress was associated with unfavorable NPI grades. In these, rupture or avulsion was confirmed in at least one spinal nerve. No operation was performed in 73 children (199 nerves) with late recovery of biceps function, but with favorable NPI findings (type A or type B favorable) [38]. The predictions for recovery were matched against the clinical outcome at a mean of 4.3 years: they were confirmed in 92% of C6 and in 96% of C7 lesions. The predictions for C5 were confirmed in a smaller proportion (78%). The inability to record NAP and the high incidence of posterior dislocation (33 of 73 children) probably account for this.

Fig. 23.8 The document used for recording progress by the Peripheral Nerve Injury Unit at the Royal National Orthopaedic Hospital

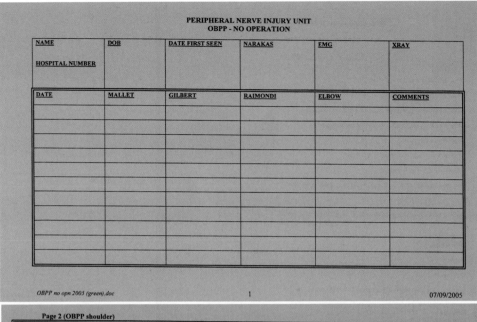

The tempo of recovery is important. Failure of biceps recovery by 3 months threatens a poor outcome [39]. Nehme et al. [40] showed that the prognosis is reliably predictable from three factors, namely birth weight, involvement of C7, and the tempo of recovery in biceps. Clark et al. [41] described a helpful scoring system which measures recovery of different segments of the limb. Combining the scores for return of elbow flexion with extension of the elbow, wrist, thumb, and fingers provides an accurate prediction of recovery. Those clinicians who rely solely on recovery of elbow flexion as a guide to prognosis for the whole limb risk serious error. Prolonged conduction block accounts for at least 15% of cases of delayed recovery of biceps function and the tearing of the muscle itself at birth explains more (Fig. 23.13) [42].

It is difficult to overstate the importance of recovery in the fifth cervical nerve. Shoulder movement is the key to function in the upper limb: far too many cases of posterior dislocation (PD) remain undetected for months or even years! The clinical appreciation of C5 recovery is greatly hindered by PD. It may be impossible to say how much lost movement is caused by the nerve injury and how much by mechanical obstruction. Operation for diagnosis and repair of the nerve lesion is justified in the following circumstances:

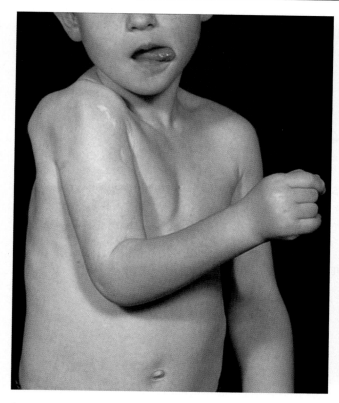

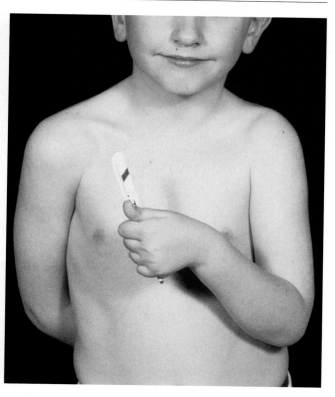

Fig. 23.9 Narrowing of the posterior scapulo-humeral angle caused by weakness of the medial rotator muscles at the shoulder

Fig. 23.11 Group 4 lesion. There was no recovery for 12 months. His parents declined operation offered at another hospital. At the age of 5 years he still has a Bernard–Horner sign. Hand function is excellent

- when failure of recovery of elevation and lateral rotation of the shoulder and of elbow flexion in groups 1, 2, and 3 by 3 months of age is accompanied by unfavorable NPI;
- group 4 lesions in which NPI and radiological evidence suggests avulsion;
- in breech lesions where there is damage to the upper cervical nerves associated with phrenic nerve palsy.

The Operation

Exposure of the brachial plexus in the infant requires a sure touch. Blunt dissection is dangerous. Scarring in the infant neck is often more severe than that seen after a closed traction lesion of the brachial plexus in the adult. After induction

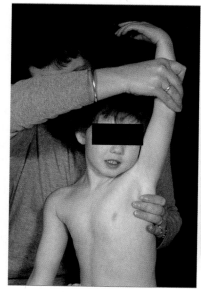

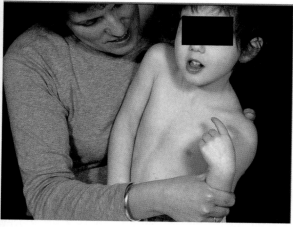

Fig. 23.10 Assiduous gentle stretching by this child's mother cured impending contractures of the shoulder and elbow. She uses one hand to block the scapula and moves the arm to open out the inferior and posterior scapulo-humeral angles

Fig. 23.12 The pre-operative analysis of lesion by Dr. Shelagh Smith was confirmed at later operation: avulsion of C5 and C6 and rupture of C7

Mixed NAP Study

	Ample (uV)	Peak Latency (ms)
Median		
Right	21	2.5
Left	24	2.4
Ulnar		
Right	5	2.6
Left	Nil seen (artefact ++)	

EMG (CNE)

Right Deltoid, Right Biceps – Small numbers of fibrillations sparse units, normal morphology, 0.2-0.5 mV.

Right Forearm extensor group – fibrillations ++. Reduced pattern, broad units firing in isolation at high rates, 1 mV.

Right Forearm flexor group, Right IDIO – No spontaneous activity. Normal units and pattern, 1-2mV.

Comments:

Median nerve action potentials are symmetrical. The right ulnar NAP is small (unfortunately, comparison with the unaffected nerve is not possible for technical reasons).

EMG findings in deltoid and biceps suggest severe axonal injury for C5 and C6, likely be pre-ganglionic in the context of the normal median NAP.
Similar EMG findings are seen in forearm extensor group, but early recover is evident.
The pattern in C8 and T1, myotomes is relatively normal.

Prediction

C5 and 6 - type C, pre-ganglionic.
C7   - unfavourable type B.
C8 and T1 - recovering.

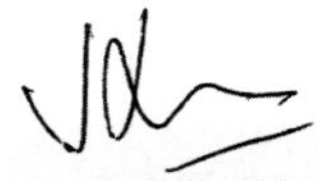

Dr S.J.M. Smith
Consultant in Clinical Neurophysiology

of anesthesia, recording electrodes are attached to the skin of the scalp and the neck. Somatosensory evoked potentials (SSEP) are recorded from the median and ulnar nerves at both wrists. The whole of the upper limb and one lower limb are prepared. A transverse supraclavicular incision is made, and the platysma is reflected with the skin flaps. The exposure is developed in the plane between the external jugular vein (medial) and the supraclavicular nerves (lateral). The omohyoid muscle and the fat pad are reflected. The external jugular, suprascapular, and transverse cervical veins are ligated with great care because of the proximity of the subclavian vein. The phrenic nerve is often deviated laterally and involved in the neuroma of the upper and middle trunks: it must be protected. The fifth and sixth cervical nerves are traced, then the middle trunk is displayed. Transection of scalenus anterior is needed to expose C8 and T1 and the subclavian artery requires careful handling. The clavicle should not be cut because of the risk of nonunion, instead the bone can be drawn up or down by a nylon tape. The findings for each spinal nerve are recorded and classified. Their

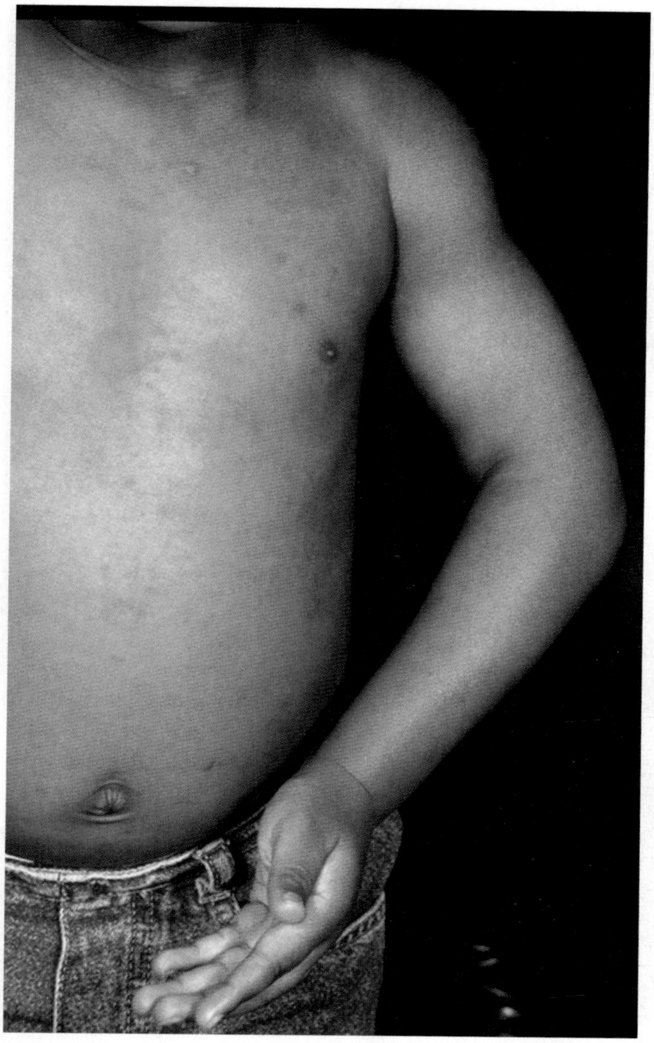

Fig. 23.13 A 9-year-old boy presenting with posterior dislocation of the shoulder and "pseudotumor" of the biceps muscle

It is worth emphasizing that the outlook for avulsed spinal nerves has been transformed by two important ideas from Gilbert [43]. In cases where rupture of the upper nerves is associated with avulsion of the lower nerves, the avulsed C8 and T1 nerves are re-innervated by one or two of the post-ganglionic stumps at C5 and C6 (intra-plexal transfer). The second concept is particularly elegant. Selective re-innervation of the ventral root of an avulsed spinal nerve is achieved by transfer of a healthy nerve, the spinal accessory, or lateral or medial pectoral nerve. I first used extraplexal transfer to an avulsed ventral root in an adult case in 1992 [33] and adopted the method in BLBP at the suggestion of Gilbert [43].

Results of Repair of the Nerves

Striking recovery of sensation and proof of central plasticity were demonstrated in a study of 24 group 4 cases [44]. The lesions to the spinal nerves included 47 avulsions, 58 ruptures, and 12 lesions in continuity. Recovery of sensibility greatly exceeded that of skeletal muscle and cholinergic sympathetic function. There was perfect localization in the dermatomes of avulsed spinal nerves which had been re-innervated by transfer of the intercostal nerves from remote spinal segments. Useful hand function was seen in just over one-half of the repaired cases. This degree of plasticity in the immature central nervous system may be a factor in the remarkable absence of neuropathic pain in BLBP, quite unlike the situation after a traction lesion in the adult. The results following grafts of ruptures are variable. In a prospective study of 100 repairs [31], a strong correlation between the pre-operative NPI and the findings at operation was found. The prediction of type C was confirmed in 177 of 191 spinal nerves. These nerves were ruptured or avulsed. Results were good in more than one-half of repair of the avulsed eighth cervical and first thoracic nerves. Extension of the wrist and fingers was regained in only one-third of the repairs of the seventh cervical nerve. A good result was seen in only one-third of repairs of the fifth cervical nerve. The outcome was worse in the 30 children who came to open reduction of PD.

It is futile to attach grafts onto poor stumps. Combined lesions of post-ganglionic rupture with an intradural component are better treated by extraplexal transfer. Every reasonable effort must be made to display avulsion, so allowing selective re-innervation of the ventral root and of the dorsal component of the spinal nerve. The undisplaced avulsion remains an enigma. Some of these recover. We leave them alone.

appearance and texture are noted. Evidence of conduction is gathered by stimulating proximal to the lesion and recording from the scalp, by proximal stimulation and noting muscle response, and by stimulation distal to the lesion and recorded from the scalp, again noting muscle response. Ruptures are repaired by nerve grafting; the small proportions of the infant make it a difficult matter to secure adequate donor nerve. The injured upper limb provides the medial and lateral cutaneous nerve of the forearm and the superficial radial nerve, which is sufficient for repairs of two ruptured spinal nerves. The sural nerve is needed for more extensive repairs and sometimes both are required. After closure of the wound the repair is protected by a plaster of Paris jacket which immobilizes the head and the affected arm.

Fig. 23.14 A 17-year-old girl who required open reduction of PD at the age of 2 years. The left clavicle is 10 cm in length and the right 13 cm. The left vertebral border of scapula is 10 cm in length, the right, 11 cm

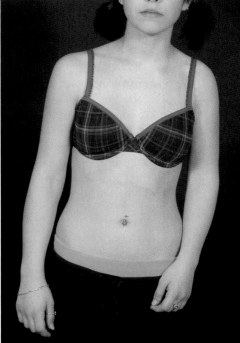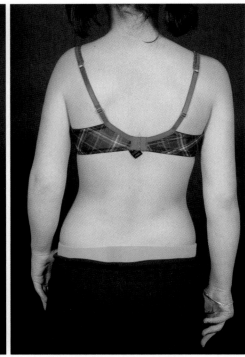

Fig. 23.15 On the left, the radiograph of the shoulder in a 10-year-old boy who had a forcible attempt at closed reduction under general anesthetic 8 years previously in another hospital. On the right, radiographs of dislocation of the elbow after over-zealous proximal advancement of the flexor origin performed in another institution

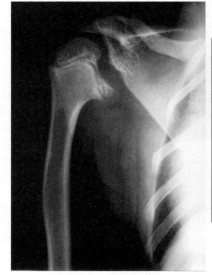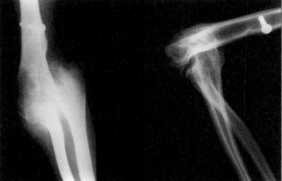

Deformity

There are four chief causes of deformity associated with BLBP:

(1) Direct damage to the skeleton and soft tissues is inflicted during a protracted and difficult delivery. Much fibrosis about the shoulder is caused during such deliveries and damage to the biceps muscle is not uncommon.

(2) There is atrophy of denervated target organs. Bone growth is impaired in all but the mildest cases of BLBP. Shortening of the clavicle, probably caused by paralysis of the clavicular head of pectoralis major may lead to serious problems at the shoulder (Fig. 23.14). The clavicle is the tie beam of the forequarter and when it is shortened it pulls the scapula forward; this pulls the acromion downward and forward and elevates its supero-medial border. The coracoid and coraco-acromial ligaments are displaced dorsally and impinge on the anterior aspect of

the head of humerus. The acromio-clavicular joint may dislocate.

(3) There is persisting muscular imbalance from incomplete neurological recovery. Imbalance between the weak lateral and the strong medial rotator muscles contributes to many shoulder dislocations. Poor medial rotation of the shoulder, a supinated forearm, ulnar deviation at wrist, and adduction of the thumb are common after a middle segment (C7, C8) lesion. Paralysis of the small muscles of the hand leads to an intractable extension deformity of the metacarpophalangeal joints.

(4) Then come the deformities provoked by treatment. Over-zealous manipulation of the incongruent shoulder damages the head of humerus and the glenoid. Incorrect muscle transfers replace one imbalance with another. Damage to the medial epicondyle during proximal advancement of the flexor muscles leads to dislocation of the elbow (Fig. 23.15). It must be restated that arthrodesis in a growing skeleton must never be performed until muscle imbalance has been corrected. The normal course of maturation of hand function and the development of limb dominance have been well described [45, 46].

Posterior Dislocation of the Shoulder

More than 500 cases have been operated upon in our unit over the last 20 years and we estimate that 100 new cases of PD occur in association with BLBP each year in the British Isles. Although the deformity may progress from a medial rotation contracture to subluxation and from there to dislocation, about one-quarter of dislocations occur at or shortly after birth. Another 50% develop during the period of neurological recovery. It is difficult to account for those cases presenting after recovery has stabilized. Fairbank [47] described the deformity and offered a logical operation which involved osteotomy of the coracoid, division of the subscapularis tendon, and anterior capsulotomy. Scaglietti [48] reported Putti's work. He considered that epiphysiolysis was common and that this contributed to retroversion of the head upon the shaft of humerus; Putti [49] also drew an analogy between the shoulder and the hip joint: "the aplasia of the glenoid corresponds exactly to that of the acetabulum in cases of congenital dislocation of the hip joint."

Valuable recent studies confirm the high incidence of incongruity at the gleno-humeral joint and the early onset of deformity of the glenoid [50–54]. Our prospective study [55] of 183 consecutive cases of PD in children with good neurological recovery, operated upon in the years 1995–2000 recorded 47 dislocations occurring at or soon after birth.

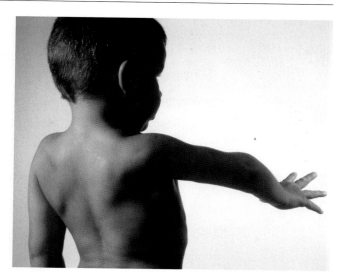

Fig. 23.16 Posterior dislocation in a 3-year-old boy

Dislocation occurred while the children were under observation in 25 shoulders and seven more children had been discharged with normal or near normal function.

Diagnosis is straightforward for the alert clinician. Palpation of the shoulder reveals dislocation in the infant. The posture of the limb, the awkward elevation of the shoulder with fixed medial rotation tells all in the older child (Fig. 23.16). Antero-posterior and axial radiographs confirm the diagnosis. Magnetic resonance imaging (MRI) is reserved for cases of unusual complexity.

It is useful to distinguish between subluxation and dislocation. In subluxation the articulation is between the head and the postero-inferior facet of the glenoid, which is lined with hyaline cartilage. In dislocation, the head lies in a distended capsular pocket adherent to the dorsal face of the scapula, and the articulation is between the hyaline cartilage of the head, the intervening capsule, and the underlying cortex of the scapula. "Telescoping" of the head of the humerus from subluxation to dislocation during forward flexion at the shoulder is a frequent finding in older children.

The Operation

The skin of the shoulder is infiltrated with local anesthetica before incisions. Interscalene block of the brachial plexus is forbidden because of the risk to the spinal cord. The shoulder is exposed through a delto-pectoral incision, which may be extended to permit exposure of the anterior shaft of humerus. Although the deltoid and pectoralis major muscles usually appear well innervated, it is common to find scarring between and deep in them. The coracoid, which is long,

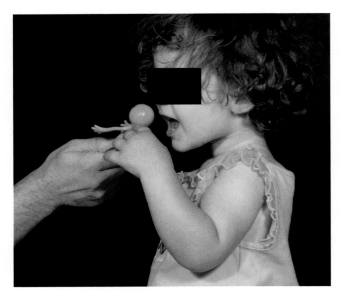

Fig. 23.17 Function 18 months after reduction of posterior dislocation with glenoplasty

rotation of the distal fragment is indicated when retroversion exceeds 40° and it is done with two objects in mind:

1. to improve stability at the shoulder after reduction
2. to ensure an adequate range of medial rotation.

The shaft of the humerus is exposed between the deltoid and the pectoralis major, preserving the upper one-quarter of the pectoralis tendon as guardian of the growth plate. A small plate is applied, the angle of rotation planned and marked by appropriate screw holes. The plate, held by one proximal screw, is rotated out of the way and the bone divided. The distal fragment is rotated medially and fixed to the plate with the planned medial rotation.

We now add glenoplasty if the head is still unstable after reduction. The posterior face of the scapula is displayed between the infraspinatus and the teres minor. The reduced head of humerus leaves behind redundant capsule which is elevated from the posterior face of the scapula. A radial incision permits identification of the posterior labrum and the edge of the hyaline cartilage of the inferior (false) facet. The posterior and the inferior rim of the glenoid is elevated by fine osteotomes and molded against the reduced humeral head. The gap is wedged open with the excised piece of the coracoid. The flap consists of the posterior inferior labrum, the inferior socket of the glenoid, and the overlying capsule. (Figs. 23.17 and 23.18) After wound closure the shoulder is protected by a plaster of Paris jacket which holds the arm in no more than 30° of abduction and no more than 45° of lateral rotation at the shoulder. The splint is retained for 6 weeks. Radiographs are taken 1 year and again 3 years after operation.

and lies vertically, is shortened to its base after releasing the coraco-acromial and coraco-humeral ligaments. A step elongation of the subscapularis muscle is done preserving as much of the anterior capsule as possible. This muscle is often fibrosed, especially in birth dislocations or after an earlier subscapularis slide. The head of humerus is now re-located. The subscapularis flaps are repaired as strongly as possible.

Retroversion of the head upon the shaft of the humerus is measured. This is the angle subtended between the coronal plane of the head and that between the lateral and medial epicondyles. Osteotomy of the shaft of the humerus with medial

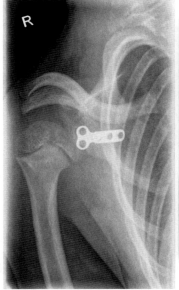

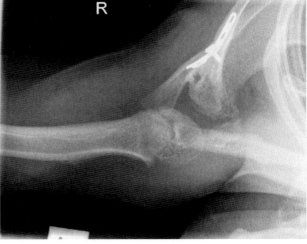

Fig. 23.18 AP and axial radiographs of the child shown in Fig. 23.17

Prolonged follow-up is essential. Dislocation recurred in 20 of the 183 children. These failures were seen in older children who showed advanced secondary deformities of the head of humerus, of the glenoid and, also of the acromio-clavicular arch. The surgeon presented with a long-standing dislocation may feel justified in advising the child, by now an adolescent, and his or her parents that it is better not to intervene. Set against this is the pain and rapid deterioration of function which led to the presentation of 24 young adults with untreated PD.

Clinicians engaged in work with these children must treat the whole child and must be alert to the significance of contractures at the shoulder, above all to restriction of lateral rotation, which usually signifies an incongruent gleno-humeral joint. These children must be observed to skeletal maturity. The early onset of a glenoid abnormality casts a shadow over the attractive idea of temporary paralysis of the medial rotators by botulinum toxin. The impressive work of Pearl et al. [56] opens the prospect of correcting medial rotation contracture and even early subluxation by arthroscopic release and muscle transfer. Nath and Paizi [57] have developed an elegant operation to deal with the deformity of the acromio-clavicular joint: the spine of the scapula and the clavicle are divided, so that the bone flap migrates upward and backward, opening out the acromio-clavicular arch. This method may contribute to the successful reduction of complex dislocations in children up to the age of about 7 years.

Lesions of the Peripheral Nerves

Most children's nerve injuries occur in the upper limb (Table 23.1). Too many are caused during treatment, usually during operation for fracture and joint injury, for "cysts" or other tumors, or during operations to correct fixed deformity. It is particularly disappointing to see cases of avoidable post-ischemic fibrosis. These iatrogenic cases account for one-third of the whole; the number of such cases continues to increase. Although the results of repair of distal nerves are generally fairly good, those following repair of the brachial plexus are rather worse than those seen in the adult. Young children ignore the insensate hand. The effect on foot posture of irreparable tibial or common peroneal nerve lesions is severe. (Fig. 23.19)

Table 23.1 Number of nerves operated in children in age from 6 months to 15 Years 1979–2007

Upper limb		Lower limb	
Cause	Number of operated cases	Nerve	Number of operated cases
Fractures and dislocations	274	Lumbosacral plexus	4
Tidy wounds	103	Femoral	3
Brachial plexus lesions	34	Sciatic	12
Cutaneous sensory nerves	39	Common peroneal	35
–	–	Tibial	9
–	–	Cutaneous sensory	26
TOTAL	450	–	89

Data assembled by Mr. Hesham Al-Khateeb, FRCS. Some of this is discussed elsewhere [69, 70]. More than 150 other children coming to operation for correction of fixed deformity or for palliation by musculo-tendinous transfer are excluded. The lesions were inflicted during treatment in one third of cases

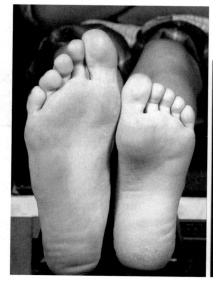
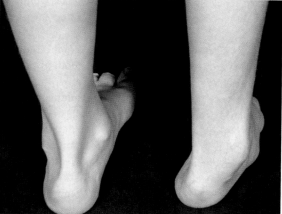

Fig. 23.19 On the *left*, the foot of a 9-year-old boy 5 years after failed repair of the tibial nerve. The painful cavus deformity was corrected by posterior transfer of tibialis anterior. On the *right*, equinovarus deformity seen 4 years after repair of sciatic nerve in a 7-year-old girl. Recovery for the common peroneal division of the sciatic nerve was poor

The surgeon must be alert to the need for muscle rebalancing operations to prevent fixed deformity in the growing skeleton and look out for progressive deformity caused by such transfers.

Diagnosis

Examination of the distressed child is not easy and is restricted if the limb is encased in plaster of Paris or other splint. It is helpful for the clinician to try to distinguish between lesions of conduction block (neurapraxia) from cases where Wallerian degeneration is occurring, the degenerative lesions of axonotmesis, or neurotmesis. The history is all important. Violent injury produces deep nerve lesions. If a nerve is not working and if there is a wound over the course of that nerve, then it is probably divided. If a nerve stops working after a surgeon has been near it with knife, scissors, or drill in hand, then that probability becomes near certainty.

A diagnosis of conduction block (neurapraxia) should be made with caution and reserved for cases where light touch sensation and the sudo- and vasomotor functions of the postganglionic sympathetic efferent fibers are preserved. One almost infallible sign is present in the first 24 h after transection of a nerve with a cutaneous sensory component: because the small as well as the large fibers are affected, the skin in the distribution of the affected nerve is warm and dry. This is particularly helpful in the diagnosis of severe lesions of the tibial, the median, and the ulnar nerves and also of the cutaneous branches of those nerves. Neuropathic pain is the most important symptom. It can be distinguished from fracture pain by irradiation into the territory of the nerve and by spontaneous abnormal or unpleasant sensory symptoms. Allodynia is a cardinal sign of serious nerve injury. It usually indicates that the noxious agent is still at work. A stimulus which is not normally painful produces pain: the child flinches when the hand or the foot is gently touched. In extreme cases, no examination of the affected part is tolerated.

Tinel's sign, when properly elicited and monitored, is an invaluable aid to the diagnosis of the depth of the injury and to the extent of regeneration. Children from the age of 4 years are very good witnesses. The examiner should explain to the child what is being done, emphasizing that it is not painful. The child is asked to say when the percussing finger, which moves from distal to proximal along the course of the nerve to be examined, induces "funny feelings" or "tingles" or "pins and needles" into the distribution of that nerve. The level of the Tinel sign is measured from a fixed bony point and recorded in the case notes. A positive Tinel sign advises

the clinician that the axons have been torn. The clinician is now in a position to ascertain the prognosis for recovery by repeating the examination at regular intervals over the next 4 weeks. If the Tinel sign remains static, recovery is unlikely. If the centrifugally progressing Tinel sign is stronger than that at the level of lesion, recovery will probably be good. If the static Tinel sign remains stronger than the advancing sign then partial transection of the nerve or the presence of an agent which is impeding regeneration is likely. In favorable degenerative lesions (axonotmesis) Tinel's sign progresses by at least 3 mm a day in the proximal part of the limb and by about 2 mm a day in the forearm and leg.

Many fracture services are poorly supported by neurophysiological investigative work, but it has to be said that timely studies of nerve conduction provide useful evidence. Electromyography is rarely necessary in the child. Conduction block (neurapraxia) is confirmed by the demonstration of persisting conduction in the nerve trunk distal to the level of the lesion at an interval of 2 weeks or more from injury. Demonstration of conduction across the lesion at any time from the day of injury proves that at least some nerve fibers are intact. I have no personal experience with ultrasound examination of the injured limb but suspect that this investigation will prove valuable to the clinician seeking confirmation of rupture or continuity of a nerve trunk or adjacent axial vessel within hours of injury.

Seddon [58] offered sound advice about the treatment of nerves injured in the arm and at the elbow. Recovery may be awaited if two conditions are met: "the first is reasonable apposition of the bony fragments and the other is *complete certainty that there is no threat of ischemia of the forearm muscles*" (original italics). The prognosis for spontaneous recovery for nerves injured in the lower limb is worse than it is in the upper limb. Of injuries to the sciatic nerve Seddon said "it is wise always to explore the nerve." Kato [59] found that spontaneous recovery was good in most cases of lesions of median and ulnar nerves caused by closed fractures or dislocations but that spontaneous recovery was very much worse for the common peroneal nerve damaged by closed injuries to the knee. The clinician will usually find it necessary to use nerve grafting in the repair of trunk nerves which have been ruptured by traction. The gaps between the stumps of the common peroneal and tibial nerves may be so reduced by flexion of the knee joint that direct suture is possible but the suture line must be protected for up to 12 weeks, gradually restoring extension at the knee by serial plaster of Paris splints.

It seems best to expose nerves damaged by fractures or by dislocations in the following circumstances: the injury requires open reduction and internal fixation; there is associated vascular injury; wound exploration of an open fracture is necessary; the nerve lesion deepens while under observation; and the nerve lesion has occurred during operation for open reduction and internal fixation. Many iatrogenic nerve lesions will be prevented or corrected urgently, if these principles are followed. Nerves and arteries become entrapped within fractures or dislocations; they are displaced by the fracture hematoma. The ulnar nerve is vulnerable to compression from hematoma in the cubital tunnel, the common peroneal nerve is similarly vulnerable at the neck of the fibula.

The Arterial Lesion

"The catastrophe of tissue necrosis after injury or surgery need never occur if complaints of undue pain in an extremity are investigated," wrote Harkess (Figs. 23.20 and 23.21) [60] Some clinicians persist in the belief that oxygenation of muscle and nerve enclosed within rigid osseo-fascial compartments can be assessed by noting return of circulation to the nail bed. Others persist with the notion that compartment syndrome is a distinct entity from the anoxia caused by interruption of flow through an axial artery. Both of these ideas are false; both were, or should have been, confined to dishonorable rest many years ago. In ischemia the final common pathway is the same: anoxia causes break down of homeostasis across the membrane of the cells of the capillaries, muscles, Schwann cells, and axons. Klenerman's [61] annotation on compartment syndrome is compulsive reading. The earliest symptom of peripheral ischemia is pain, often so intense that it does not respond to morphine. Alteration in sensibility in the extremity soon follows. The earliest fibers to suffer are the largest, those conveying proprioception and vibration sense. Deepening of sensory loss and the first signs of muscle weakness are proof positive of critical ischemia. One effect of anoxia is to increase the permeability of the capillary membrane, so that the true ischemia caused by cessation of arterial supply is added to the one caused by the rising pressure within the fascial compartments.

Perhaps it is time to replace the much misused term "critical ischemia" with the grading system for ischemia developed by The Society for Vascular Surgery and the International Society of Cardiovascular Surgery [62]. Class 2A describes a limb which is threatened, in which symptoms are limited to a mild sensory loss. Class 2B limbs are immediately at risk: there is pronounced sensory loss, mild-to-moderate motor loss and for these delay is unacceptable even with audible Doppler signals.

Those surgeons inclined to a complacent view of the loss of peripheral pulses complicating supracondylar fracture in child might care to consider Poiseuille's law which describes the volume of flow through a cylindrical tube. Among other factors volume is governed by the radius of the tube to the

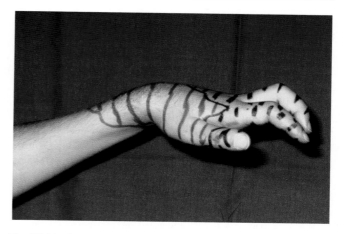

Fig. 23.20 Volkmann's ischemic contracture 10 weeks after supracondylar fracture in a 7-year-old boy. The fracture was "fixed" by Kirschner wires without exposing the brachial artery and median nerve which were entrapped within the fracture. His post-operative pain was ignored. All three nerves were involved. Black indicates complete loss of sensation; red indicates partial loss of sensation

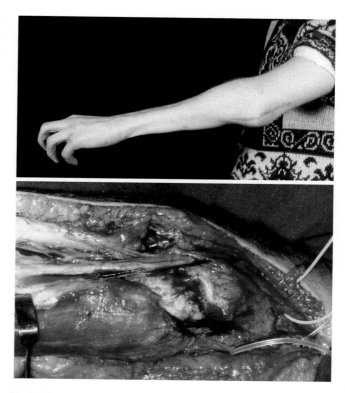

Fig. 23.21 Above: Recurrence of deformity 4 years after flexor muscle slide when the boy was aged 8 years. Below: The ulnar nerve exposed during this operation is narrowed and ischemic as it enters the infarcted muscle

power of 4 (R^4). The diameter of the brachial artery in 10-year-old children has been measured at 2.5–3 mm and resting flow is 200 ml per minute. If arterial flow is restricted to the collateral vessels running with the radial and ulnar nerves at the elbow, of a diameter of about 1 mm, then flow to forearm and hand may drop to as low as 20 ml per minute [63]. The pressure gradient is very important: Burton and Yamada [64] advise that "At a transmural pressure well above the critical closing pressure, the flow is proportional to the driving pressure but as the pressure is lowered, the flow decreases quite abruptly, to become zero at the critical closing pressure." The best advice comes from Atholl Parkes [65]: "in the absence of peripheral arterial pulses take immediate steps to relieve possible pressure on the main artery by reducing any displaced fracture or dislocation and, if still necessary, exploring the artery. With failing nerve or muscle function in a tensely swollen limb, do not be deceived by the presence of a good peripheral pulse—consider immediate decompression." Exposure of the brachial artery and of the median nerve at the elbow is, or should be, a simple enough matter. I have performed this in over 50 cases of supracondylar fracture in children. No brachial artery was ruptured, instead, they were entrapped in the fracture or compressed by hematoma. After decompression of the artery it is bathed in papaverine. It is gratifying to see the vessel dilating with the return of pulsatile flow after an interval of a few minutes. However, there have been reports of transection of the artery or of thrombosis after tearing of the intima. Repair of the brachial artery in a child is a very testing operation. Faulty technique fails. The wisest course is to involve an experienced arterial surgeon for the operation.

Pain

Neurostenalgia [66] is that pain caused by persistent compression, distortion, or ischemia and it is not uncommon in children (Fig. 23.22). The nerve is intact but is afflicted by an active, noxious agent. It is common when nerves are entrapped within fractures or joints, or when they are strangled in a swollen compartment. Causalgia is rare in children and this may account for the erroneous diagnosis of the so-called complex regional pain syndrome (CRPS) which leads to some children being subjected to protracted courses of treatment by medication or by various forms of nerve block which do not relieve the pain and which inflict physical and psychological harm (Fig. 23.23). The pathophysiological basis of CRPS is unsound. CRPS type 1 assumes no injury to a peripheral nerve. This has been discounted by Oaklander [67] who demonstrated extensive axonopathy and demyelination in cases so labeled. These findings have been confirmed by other investigators. CRPS type 2 is deeply unsatisfactory, for it is so wide-reaching as to be meaningless. The cardinal diagnostic features of causalgia include severe, intractable pain expressed throughout the limb; worsening of that pain by examination, by noise, and

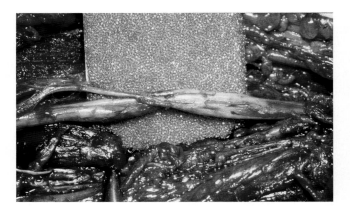

Fig. 23.22 Neurostenalgia. Mr. James MacLean (Perth) extricated this median nerve, which was entrapped in a distal fracture of humerus. The operation was done after 2 days because of pain complicating a deep median palsy. Pain was abolished; there was full recovery of the nerve

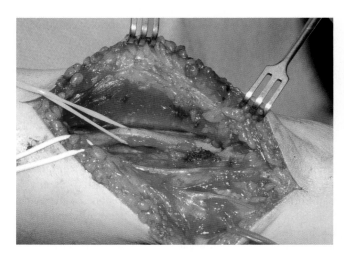

Fig. 23.23 Post-traumatic neuralgia. A branch of the dorsal cutaneous ulnar nerve was damaged during arthroscopy of the wrist in a 12-year-old girl. She developed intense pain which did not respond to a protracted course of analgesic and anti-depressant drugs. Psychological assessment revealed deterioration in cognitive skills, spatial skills, information processing accuracy, and auditory and working memories. Her reading and spelling skills declined. A request for further opinion from her educational psychologist and her mother was met with resistance but her family practitioner insisted on an urgent review. She was seen at 14 months after her first operation and the nerves were exposed 2 days later. The ulnar nerve was decompressed and a damaged branch of the dorsal cutaneous branch of the ulnar nerve was implanted into muscle. There was early relief of pain, improvement in hand function, and improvement in her psychological health

by other disturbance; vaso- and sudo-motor instability; and intense mechanical allodynia [68].

Causalgia follows incomplete transection of the lower trunk or the medial cord of the brachial plexus or the median and ulnar nerves in the upper limb, or of the tibial division of the sciatic nerve in the lower limb and is frequently associated with arterial injury or hematoma. Cure is almost always achieved by correcting the lesion of the nerve and artery. The clinician presented with a child with severe neuropathic pain must take every reasonable step to exclude a continuing provocation of that nerve before consigning that child to a pain clinic.

References

1. Bennet GC, Harrold AJ. Prognosis and early management of birth injuries to the brachial plexus. Br Med J 1976; 1:1520–1521.
2. Wickstrom J, Haslam ET, Hutchinson RH. The surgical management of residual deformities of the shoulder following birth injuries of the brachial plexus. J Bone Joint Surg 1958; 47A:27–36.
3. Tassin JL. Paralyses obstétricales du plexus brachial, evolution spontanée, resultats des interventions reparatrices precrées. Thése 1984, Université Paris VIII.
4. Gilbert A, Tassin JL. Réparation chirurgicale du plexus brachial dans la paralysie obstétricale. Chirurgie 1984; 110:76–75.
5. Gilbert A, Brockman R, Carlioz H. Surgical treatment of brachial plexus birth palsy. Clin Orth 1989; 264:39–47.
6. Gilbert A, Whitaker I. Obstetrical brachial plexus lesions. J Hand Surg 1991; 16B:489–491.
7. Dailiana ZH, Mehdian H, Gilbert A. Surgical anatomy of spinal accessory nerve: is trapezius functional deficit inevitable after division of the nerve? J Hand Surg Br 2001; 26(2):137–141.
8. Oberlin C, Beal D, Leechavengvongs S, et al. (1994). Nerve transfer to biceps muscle using a part of ulnar nerve for C5-C6 avulsion of the brachial plexus: anatomical study and report of four cases. J Hand Surg [Am] 19(2): 232–237.
9. Witoonchart K, Leechavengvongs S, Uerpairojkit C, et al. Nerve transfer to deltoid muscle using the nerve to the long head of the triceps, part I: an anatomic feasibility study. J Hand Surg Am 2003; 28(4):6.
10. Chuang DC, Lee GW, Hashem F, Wei FC. Restoration of shoulder abduction by nerve transfer in avulsed brachial plexus injury: evaluation of 99 patients with various nerve transfers. Plast Reconstr Surg 1995; 96(1):122–128.
11. Yang Y, Gu YD, Hu SN, Zhang H. Long-term impact of transfer of phrenic nerve on respiratory system of children: a clinical study of 34 cases. Zhonghua Yi Xue Za Zhi 2006; 86(17):1179–1182.
12. Gu YD, Chen DS, Zhang GM. Long term functional results of contralateral C7 transfer. Reconstr Microsurg 1998; 14:57– 59.
13. Taylor AS. Brachial birth palsy and injuries of similar type in adults. Surg Gynecol Obstetr 1920; 30:434–502.
14. Gilbert A, Razaboni R, Amar-Khodja S. Indications and results of brachial plexus surgery in obstetrical palsy. Orthop Clin North Am 1988; 19:91–105.
15. Gilbert A. Long-term evaluation of brachial plexus surgery in obstetrical palsy. Rand Clin 1995; 11:583–587.
16. Mallet J. Paralysie obstetricale. Rev Chirurgie Orthaped 1972; 58(suppl 1):115.
17. Evans-Jones G, Kay SPJ, Weindling AM, et al. Congenital brachial palsy: incidence, causes and outcome in the United Kingdom and Republic of Ireland. Arch Dis Fetal Neonatal 2003; 88 F185–F189.
18. Bisinella G, Birch R. Obstetric brachial plexus lesion: A study of 74 children registered with the British Surveillance Unit. J Hand Surg Br 2002; 28B:1:40–45.
19. Giddins GEB, Birch R, Singh D, Taggart M. Risk factors for obstetric brachial plexus palsies. J Bone Joint Surg 1994; 76B:Supps. II and III 156.

20. Tavakkolizadeh A. Risk factors associated with obstetric brachial plexus palsy. Dissertation. University of Brighton for degree of M Sc. 2007.
21. Becker MHJ, Lassner F, Bahm J, et al. The cervical rib. A pre disposing factor for obstetric brachial plexus lesions. J Bone Joint Surg 2002; 84:740–743.
22. Strömbeck C, Rehmal S, Krum Linde-Sundholm L, Sejersen T. (a) Long term functional follow up of a cohort of children with obstetric brachial plexus palsy: I; Functional aspects: Dev Med Child Neurol 2007; 49:198–203.
23. Strömbeck C, Rehmal S, Krum Linde-Sundholm L, Sejersen T. (b) Long term functional follow up of a cohort of children with obstetric brachial plexus palsy: II: Neurophysiological aspects. Dev Med Child Neurol 2007; 49:204–209.
24. Yang LJ, Anand P, Birch R. Limb preference in children with obstetric brachial plexus palsy. Paediatr Neurol 2005; 33:46–49.
25. Bellew M, Kay SPJ, Webb F, Ward A. Developmental and behavioural outcome in obstetric brachial plexus palsy J Hand Surg 2000; 25B:49–51.
26. Fraher JP. The CNS PNS transitional zone. In: Dyke PJ, Thomas PK, eds. Peripheral Neuropathy, 4th ed. Philadelphia: Elsevier Saunders; 2005:67–91.
27. McManis PG, Low PA, Lagerlund TD. Nerve blood flow and microenvironment. In: Dyke PJ, Thomas PK, eds. Peripheral Neuropathy, 4th ed. Philadelphia: Elsevier Saunders; 2005:67:1.
28. Groves MJ, Scaravilli F. Pathology of peripheral neurone cell bodies. In: Dyke PJ, Thomas PK, eds. Peripheral Neuropathy, 4th ed. Philadelphia: Elsevier Saunders; 2005:683–732.
29. Fullarton AC, Lenihan DV, Myles LM, Glasby MA. Obstetric brachial plexus palsy: a large animal for traction injury and its repair. Part 1: the age of the recipient. J Hand Surg 2000; 25B:52–57.
30. Fullarton AC, Myles LM, Lenihan DV, et al. Obstetric brachial plexus palsy: a comparison of the degree of recovery after repair of 16 ventral root avulsions in newborn and adult sheep. Brit J Plas Surg 2001; 54:697–704.
31. Birch R, Ahad N, Kono H, Smith S. Repair of obstetric brachial plexus palsy. Results in 100 children. J Bone Jt Surg 2005; 87B:1089–1095.
32. Blaauw G, Slooff ACJ, Muhlig S. Results of surgery after breech delivery. In: Gilbert A, ed. Brachial Plexus Injuries. London: Martin Dunitz; 2001: 217–224.
33. Birch R, Bonney G, Wynnparry CB. Surgical Disorders of the Peripheral Nerves, 1st ed. Edinburgh: Churchill Livingstone; 1998.
34. Narakas AO. Obstetrical brachial plexus injuries. In: Lamb DW, ed. The Paralyzed Hand. Edinburgh: Churchill Livingstone; 1987:116.
35. Brunelli GA, Brunelli GR. A fourth type of brachial plexus lesion: the intermediate (C7) palsy. J Hand Surg 1991; 16B:492–494.
36. Smith SJM. The role of neurophysiological investigation in traumatic brachial plexus injuries in adults and children. J Hand Surg 1996; 21B:145–148.
37. Smith SJM. Electrodiagnosis. In: Birch R, Bonney G, Wynn Parry C. Surgical Disorders of the Peripheral Nerves. Edinburgh: Churchill Livingstone; 1998:467–490.
38. Bisinella G, Birch R, Smith SJM. Neurophysiological predictions of outcome in obstetric lesions of the brachial plexus J Hand Surg 2003; 28B:148–152.
39. Gilbert A, Tassin JL. Réparation chirurgicale de plexus brachial dans la paralysie obstétricale. Chirurgie (Paris) 1984; 110:70–75.
40. Nehme A, KANY J, Sales-De-Gauzy J, et al. Obstetrical brachial plexus palsy, predictions of outcome in upper root injuries. J Hand Surg 2001; 27B:9–12.
41. Clarke HM, Curtis C. Examination and prognosis. In: Gilbert A, ed. Brachial Plexus Injuries. London: Martin Dunitz; 2001:159–172.

42. MacNamara P, Yam A. The false tumour of the biceps—a birth injury. An analysis of 40 cases. Manuscript in preparation: data kindly released by Mr. MacNamara. 2008

43. Gilbert A. Indications et résultats de la chirurgie du plexus brachial dans la paralysie obstétricale. In: Alnot JY, Narakas A, eds. Les Paralysie du Plexus Brachiale. Monographies du groupe d'étude de la main. Paris: Expansion Scientifique Française; 1995.

44. Anand P, Birch R. Restoration of sensory function and lack of long-term chronic pain syndromes after brachial plexus injury in human neonates. Brain 2002; 125:113–122.

45. Iyer VG. Developmental maturation of the nervous system In: Gupta A, Kay SPJ, Scheker LR, eds. The Growing Hand. London: Mosby; 2000:47–52.

46. Erhard RP, Lindley SG. functional development of the hand. In: Gupta A, Kay SPJ, Scheker LR, eds. The Growing Hand. London: Mosby; 2000:71–82.

47. Fairbank HAT. Subluxation of shoulder joint in infants and young children. Lancet 1913; I:1217–1223.

48. Scaglietti O. the obstetrical shoulder trauma. Surg Gynae Obstet 1938; 66:868–877.

49. Putti V. Analisi della triada radiosintomatica degli stati di prelus-sazione. Chir Organi Mov 1932; XVII:453–459.

50. Waters PM, Smith GR, Jaramillo D. Gleno humeral deformity secondary to brachial plexus birth palsy. J Bone Jt Surg 1998; 80A:668–677.

51. Pearl ML, Edgerton BW. Glenoid deformity secondary to brachial plexus birth palsy. J Bone Jt Surg 1998; 80A: 659–667.

52. Sluijs JA, Van Ouwerkerk WJR, De Gast A, et al. Retroversion of the humeral head in children with obstetric brachial plexus lesion. J Bone Jt Surg 2002; 84B 583–587.

53. Sluisz JA, van Ouwerkerk WJR, de Gast A, et al. Deformities of the shoulder in infants younger than 12 months with an obstetric lesion of the brachial plexus. J Bone Jt Surg 2001; 83B: 551–555.

54. Hoeksma AF, Steeg AMT, Dijkstra P, et al. Shoulder contracture and osseous deformity in obstetrical brachial plexus injuries. J Bone Jt Surg 2003; 85A:316–322.

55. Kambhampati SLS, Birch R, Cobiella C, Chen L. Posterior sub-luxation and dislocation of the shoulder in obstetric brachial plexus palsy. J Bone Jt Surg 2006; 88B:213–219.

56. Pearl ML, Edgerton BW, Kazimiroff PA, et al. Arthroscopic release and latissimus dorsi transfer for shoulder internal rotation contractures and glenohumeral deformity secondary to brachial plexus birth palsy. J Bone Jt Surg 2006; 88A:564–574.

57. Nath RK, Paizi M. Improvement in abduction of the shoulder after reconstructive soft tissue procedures in obstetric brachial plexus palsy. J Bone Jt Surg 2007; 89B:620–626.

58. Seddon HJ. (a) Common causes of nerve injury. In: Seddon HJ, ed. Surgical Disorders of Peripheral Nerves, 2nd ed. Edinburgh: Churchill Livingstone; 1975:67–88.

59. Kato N, Birch R. Peripheral nerve palsies associated with closed fractures and dislocations. Injury 2006; 37:507–512.

60. Harkess JW. Acquired deformities of the upper extremity. In: Gupta A, Kay SPJ, Scheker LR, eds. The Growing Hand. London: Mosby; 2000:725–752.

61. Klenerman L. The evolution of the compartment syndrome since 1948 as recorded in the JBJS (B). J Bone Jt Surg 2007; 89B:1280–1282.

62. Barros D'Sa AAB, Harkin DW. Pathophysiology of acute vascular insufficiency. In: Barros d'Sa AAB, Chant ADB, eds. Emergency Vascular and Endovascular Surgical Practice, 2nd ed. London: Hodder, Arnold; 2005:19–27.

63. Wajcberg E, Thoppil N, Patel S, et al. Comprehensive assessment of post-ischemic vascular reactivity in Hispanic children and adults with and without diabetes mellitus. Paediatr Diabetes 2006; 7: 329–335.

64. Burton AC, Yamada S. Relation between blood pressure and flow in human forearm. J. Applied Physiol 1951; 4:329–339.

65. Parkes AR. Ischemic effects of external and internal pressure on the upper limb. Hand 1973; 5:105–112.

66. Birch R, Bonney G. Pain. In: Birch R, Bonney G, Wynn Parry CB. Surgical Disorders of the Peripheral Nerves. London: Churchill Livingstone; 1998:373–404.

67. Oaklander AL, Rismiller JG, Gelman LB, et al. Evidence of focal small-fibre axonal degeneration in complex regional pain syndrome-1 (reflex sympathetic dystrophy). Pain 2006; 120:235–243.

68. Barnes R. Causalgia: a review of 48 cases. In: Seddon, HJ, ed. Peripheral Nerve Injuries by the Nerve Injuries Committee of the Medical Research Council. Medical Research Council Special Report series 282. London: HMSO; 1954:156–185.

69. Ramachandran M, Birch R, Eastwood D. Clinical outcome of nerve injuries associated with supracondylar fractures in of the humerus in children. J Bone Jt Surg 2006; 88B:90–94.

70. Birch R, Achan P. Peripheral Nerve Repairs and their Results in Children. Hand Clin 2000; 16:579–597.

Section 2
The Lower Limb

Chapter 24

Leg Deformity and Length Discrepancy

John A. Fixsen, Robert A. Hill, and Franz Grill

Part I: Classification and Management of Lower Limb Reduction Anomalies

John A. Fixsen and Robert A. Hill

Introduction

Congenital limb deficiencies or reduction anomalies in the lower limbs are the result of failure of formation of parts in the first trimester of pregnancy. They can also result from the constriction band syndrome sometimes known as Streeter's dysplasia.

Two types of abnormal development can occur, causing transverse or longitudinal deficiency. In *transverse deficiency*, the proximodistal development is normal until the level of the deficiency, although there is nearly always some attempt at the development of rudimentary digits (digital buds) on the end of the limb, which may vary from puckering of the skin to small but formed digits (Fig. 24.1). In *longitudinal deficiency,* there is a reduction or absence of a bone or bones in the long axis of the limb. However, there are often normal or near normal elements distal to the affected bone or bones. It is most important to remember that the deficiency is not simply of bone, but also of muscle and soft tissue.

Classification

In the past, many classifications have been suggested, often using Greco-Latin terms, such as fibular hemimelia,

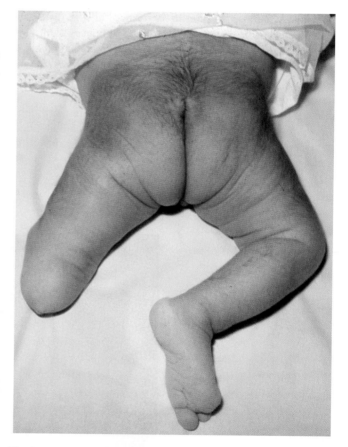

Fig. 24.1 Clinical photograph of a below-knee transverse deficiency. Transverse deficiency upper third leg (ISPO/ISO classification)

J.A. Fixsen (✉)
Orthopaedic Department, Great Ormond Street Hospital for Sick Children, London, UK

R.A. Hill (✉)
Orthopaedic Department, Great Ormond Street NHS Trust, London, UK

F. Grill (✉)
Department of Pediatric orthopaedics, Orthopaedic Hospital Vienna, Vienna, Austria

dysmelia, or amelia [1]. However, in 1989, the International Standards Organization published ISO 8548/1, "Method of Describing Limb Deficiencies Present at Birth" [2]. This has now been generally accepted by the International Society for Prosthetics and Orthotics (ISPO) and other national

M. Benson et al. (eds.), *Children's Orthopaedics and Fractures*,
DOI 10.1007/978-1-84882-611-3_24, © Springer-Verlag London Limited 2010

organizations. It uses a simple anatomical system based on whether the deficiency is transverse or longitudinal.

Transverse deficiencies in the lower limb are described by the segment at which the limb terminates and then the level within that segment beyond which there are no skeletal elements, disregarding digital buds. The segments defined in the lower limb are the pelvis, thigh, leg, tarsal, metatarsal, and phalangeal. (Note metatarsal and phalangeal can be combined when they are termed a "ray".) Thus a transverse deficiency at upper third tibial level would be termed "transverse leg upper third" (see Fig. 24.1).

Longitudinal deficiency is described by naming the affected bones in a proximodistal sequence and whether each affected bone is partially or totally absent. If a bone is partially absent, its position and the approximate fraction missing can be described. The bones are named as ilium, ischium, pubis, femur, tibia, fibula, tarsals, metatarsals, and phalanges; the last two can be described together as a ray. Thus a case of proximal femoral focal deficiency with partial absence of the fibula and a four-ray foot (Fig. 24.2) would be described as femur, partial upper two-thirds, fibula, partial upper quarter, ray 5 total. This gives an accurate description of the whole deficiency but is clumsy to use in clinical practice. The simple terms congenital femoral deficiency, congenital fibular deficiency, and congenital tibial deficiency are simple, clear, and focus on the major site of the deficiency [3].

Etiology

The orthopaedic surgeon dealing with children should be familiar with the three main forms of congenital shortening of the lower limb:

1. Congenital femoral deficiency in all its forms, encompassing idiopathic coxa vara, congenital short femur, and proximal femoral focal deficiency (PFFD).
2. Congenital fibular deficiency associated with shortening and deformity of the tibia. Also known as congenital short tibia with absent or hypoplastic fibula or fibular hemimelia.
3. Congenital tibial deficiency. Also called congenital dysplasia or absence of the tibia with intact fibula or tibial hemimelia.

The lower limb bud appears at 28 days of intrauterine life and major development of the limb is complete in 10–14 days, after which growth and enlargement occur. A number of agents, of which the drug thalidomide is the best known, can cause abnormalities of development during this early vital period. The majority of major congenital limb deficiencies occur sporadically: a few, such as tibial dysplasia and some instances of idiopathic coxa vara, have an unequivocal genetic background. In the chick embryo, it has been possible to reproduce all the various limb deficiencies by insults

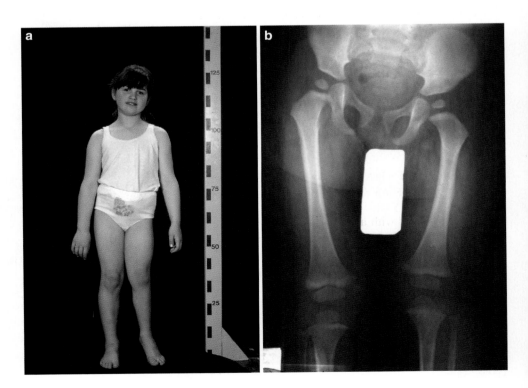

Fig. 24.2 (**a**) Eight-year-old with left congenital short femur. Note the bulky thigh, external rotation of the leg, the four-ray foot in equinus and that she can reach the floor by tilting the pelvis. (**b**) Anteroposterior radiograph of both femora and pelvis in the same patient. Note the left femur is shortened, slightly laterally bowed with some sclerosis in the diaphysis

to the limb bud: however, the cause in the great majority of children remains unknown. Abnormality in development of the normal vascular pattern in the limb has been suggested by Morgan and Somerville [4], Hootnick et al. [5] and more recently by Szeizel et al. [6], who looked at the association between smoking during pregnancy and congenital limb deficiency. Although the major deficiency is usually in one segment of the limb, a lesser degree of shortening in the other segments of the limb, which adds to the overall length discrepancy is extremely common and must be recognized. From the orthopaedic point of view particularly if limb lengthening and reconstruction are being considered it is important to remember that the bone of the major affected segment is not only short but also deformed and frequently has a sclerotic portion. A skin dimple is common over the affected bone and a degree of instability of the joints at each end of the segment must be expected

The parents of a child with a major limb deficiency are always extremely upset by the deformity and want to know the cause and the treatment as soon as possible. The advent of prenatal ultrasound screening means that parents may know before the child is born that it has a major limb anomaly and will require counseling and advice before the child is born and before the surgeon can actually examine the child. This type of counseling can be very demanding as the parents want clear and definite advice which is difficult for the surgeon to give until he has actually examined the child and apart from the few inherited forms, the cause is almost invariably unknown. Treatment should never be rushed, and it is most important to reassure parents that their children will be able to walk despite the major limb deficiency. It is usually most unwise to rush into any surgical treatment in the first year of life, although physiotherapy and splintage to stretch and mobilize deformities may be useful. Many of these children will require an extension prosthesis, extensive surgical reconstruction, and occasionally amputation. It is important to introduce the parents gently to the ideas of an extension prosthesis, extensive surgery, and possible amputation, as most will find this very hard to accept in the first instance. A visit to the prosthetic surgeon and the prosthetic unit where they can see another child with the same or similar condition is very helpful in reassuring them with regard to the child's future walking ability and function with a prosthesis. Contact with another family with a similarly affected child through a parent support group can also be very useful. An important report by the working party of the Amputee Medical Rehabilitation Society on recommended standards of care for the child with congenital limb deficiency was published in 1997 [7] and reviews the subject, recommending that there should be special limb deficiency clinics to which the child and the parents could be referred as soon as possible after birth—certainly within 3 months of birth. This would be a

major advance in the management of these children and their families.

Congenital Femoral Deficiency

Idiopathic Coxa Vara (Developmental Coxa Vara, Infantile Coxa Vara)

This condition is the most minor form of femoral deficiency. It involves the inferior portion of the capital femoral epiphysis and adjacent metaphysis. It is rarely diagnosed at birth but may cause confusion with neonatal ultrasound hip examination. It usually becomes apparent as the child grows and the leg appears short, with the development of a Trendelenburg gait, limitation of abduction, and increased external rotation of the affected side. The cause is unknown, although there are reports of families in which there appears to be a genetic influence. The child normally presents after walking age with a limp and shortening. On examination, there is limitation of abduction and usually an increased range of external rotation at the affected hip. The majority of cases are unilateral, but the condition can occur bilaterally. Its incidence is not clearly known. When first noticed clinically, idiopathic coxa vara is often mistaken for developmental dysplasia of the hip (DDH) (Chapter 26) and it is important to consider other causes of coxa vara such as trauma, infection, bone dysplasia, metabolic disease, osteogenesis imperfecta, and the common association with other forms of femoral and lower limb deficiency. The important point in idiopathic coxa vara is that the radiograph changes are confined to the femoral neck.

Radiological Changes

Radiological changes are typical once they appear. In the first year of life, they may be difficult to distinguish: until proximal femoral ossification occurs, the femur may appear relatively normal. As the femoral head and neck ossify, the classical triangular fragment (Fairbanks' triangle) on the inferior surface of the femoral neck becomes apparent, together with varus deformity of the femoral neck. The epiphyseal plate lies vertical and appears irregular. An inverted Y delineates the triangular fragment in the inferior part of the femoral neck (Fig. 24.2). If the condition is untreated the dysplasia of the femoral neck and the varus increases with proximal migration of the greater trochanter relative to the femoral head, giving rise to the so-called shepherd's crook deformity. When considering differential diagnoses it is important to remember cleidocranial dysostosis, which can give rise to bilateral coxa vara associated

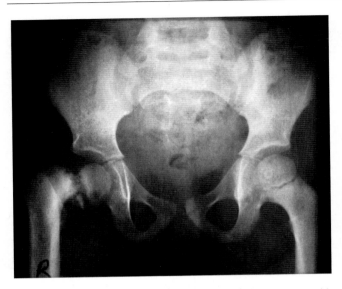

Fig. 24.3 Anteroposterior radiograph of the pelvis of a patient with idiopathic coxa vara affecting the right hip. Note the reduction in the head–neck/shaft angle, the "Fairbank's Triangle" and the inverted Y appearance of the epiphyseal plate

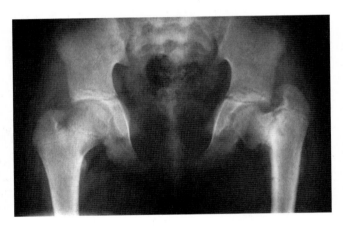

Fig. 24.4 Anteroposterior radiograph of the pelvis of a patient with cleidocranial dyostosis. Note left coxa vara with a "shepherd's crook" deformity and absence of ossification of the symphysis pubis

with absence or poor development of the clavicles, and delayed fusion of the skull suture lines and symphysis pubis (Fig. 24.4)

Management

Once the condition has been diagnosed, correction of the coxa vara should be considered. A neck–shaft angle greater than 110° should be observed as it may resolve. However, once the varus of the neck has decreased to less than 110° progression of the deformity is likely to occur. In the early

stages a simple shoe raise can be used, but if varus progresses to less than 100°, surgery should be considered to prevent inevitable deterioration. The aim of surgery is to correct the neck–shaft angle to 140° by an abduction osteotomy. Femoral retroversion can be an important part of the deformity also requiring correction [8]. Many techniques have been described including external fixation [9] but provided the operation achieves 140° of neck–shaft angle and a more horizontal position of the epiphyseal plate, the changes in the femoral neck should heal and recover. Bone grafting is not necessary. Repeat valgus osteotomy may be necessary, particularly if the initial osteotomy is performed early in childhood. Leg length discrepancy is rarely sufficient to require leg lengthening. Occasionally, in a neglected case, there is significant overgrowth of the greater trochanter and trochanteric transfer may be necessary.

Congenital Short Femur and Proximal Focal Femoral Deficiency (PFFD)

On the basis of the data from the Edinburgh birth register, Hamanishi [10] suggested that the incidence of this condition was around 1 in 50,000 live births.

The cause of this disorder is unknown. It can be associated with abnormalities not only in the lower limb but also in the upper limb and with facial anomalies as in the congenital short femur/abnormal facies syndrome.

Embryologically the hip and upper femur develop from the same anlage and so it is not surprising that the more dysplastic the upper end of the femur, the more dysplastic the hip joint. Clinically the leg appears short although minor degrees of congenital femoral deficiency (congenital short femur) may not be noticed at birth. Subsequently with growth the shortening becomes obvious. It is always associated with flexion and external rotation of the hip as a result of retroversion of the femoral neck. Early radiographs show a shortened femoral shaft or, in the most severe forms, no femoral shaft. The acetabulum may vary from virtually normal in mild cases to absent in the most severe.

It is customary to classify major congenital shortening of the femur into congenital short femur (CSF) and proximal focal femoral deficiency (PFFD). In reality, when one looks at the entire spectrum of the disorder, there is a steady progression from CSF (the femur is almost normal but short) to almost total absence of the femur with only the distal femoral condyles appearing in bone some years after birth. The first classifications by Amstutz and Wilson [11], Aitken [12], Hamanishi [10] (Fig. 24.5), and Pappas [13] were based on plain radiological appearances. Fixsen and Lloyd-Roberts in 1974 [14] pointed out the significance of the appearance

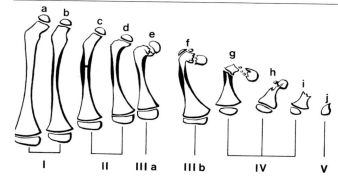

Fig. 24.5 Classification of femoral deficiency (dysplasia) as described by Hamanishi in 1980. Reproduced with permission and copyright © of the British Editorial Society of Bone and Joint Surgery. Hamanishi [10]

of the acetabulum and upper femur in early radiographs to the subsequent development of the hip and its importance in surgical treatment (Fig. 24.6). More recently, with the rapid advances in limb lengthening and reconstruction techniques, the classifications of Gillespie [15] and Paley [16] relate radiological appearance to both the hip development and the possibility for surgical reconstruction. In the Gillespie classification group A the hip is stable and if the femoral length is more than 60% of the contralateral side leg, equalization is possible. If the femoral length is less than 60%, the risks associated with lengthening increase and some surgeons would recommend a Van Nes rotationplasty [17] or fusion of the knee and amputation through the ankle joint rather than leg lengthening. In Gillespie group B the femoral length is less than 50% of the contralateral side and the hip is unstable as defined by Fixsen and Lloyd-Roberts [14]. The surgeon should aim for the best possible function with a prosthesis. In group C the femur is virtually absent or only a distal fragment is present and treatment is with a prosthesis.

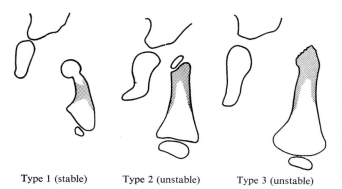

Type 1 (stable)   Type 2 (unstable)   Type 3 (unstable)

Fig. 24.6 Classification of PFFD as described by Fixsen and Lloyd-Roberts relating the appearance of the acetabulum and the upper end of the femur in the early radiograph to the future development and stability of the hip and upper end of the femur. (**a**) Type 1 (stable); (**b**) type 2 (unstable); (**c**) type 3 (unstable). Reproduced with permission and copyright © of the British Editorial Society of Bone and Joint Surgery. Fixsen and Lloyd-Roberts [14]

Paley's classification is based on what he considered necessary for reconstruction by limb lengthening with particular reference to the dysplasia and mobility of the knee as well as the hip. His type 1 is similar to Gillespie group A but with three sub-groups dependent on the state of the hip and knee. Type 2 has a mobile femoral pseudarthrosis which must be stabilized if lengthening is to be considered. Type 3 is again similar to Gillespie group C and lengthening is unlikely to be helpful. Ring [18, 19] made the important observation that the proportional shortening remains the same throughout growth, provided further displacement as a result of the coxa vara or hip subluxation does not occur. Therefore if the femur is 20% short at birth, it is likely to be 20% short in the adult, and so a reasonable estimate of the overall shortening at maturity can be made in the first year of life. In 2000, Paley et al. [20] published their multiplier method, which is very useful for predicting limb-length discrepancy at skeletal maturity in both congenital and developmental limb-length discrepancy. It is important to remember that the abnormality is not confined to the femur. The knee is nearly always to some extent unstable and there may be congenital absence of both cruciates [21, 22]. The lower leg is nearly always to some degree short, and there may be absence or hypoplasia of the fibula. The foot is often remarkably normal.

Congenital Short Femur

Congenital short femur is the milder form of congenital femoral deficiency. The femur is short with an average growth retardation of about 10%. Affected patients (see Fig. 24.2) typically have a bulky thigh with a fixed external rotation deformity at the hip and a mildly valgus and unstable knee.

Management

Congenital short femur is the most difficult of the major bone deficiencies to treat by lengthening because of the morphology of the bone, difficulty in placement of the external fixator, poor regenerate formation, and soft tissue complications particularly at the knee. Post frame removal, there is a significant risk of fracture and knee stiffness (Table 24.1). There are differing opinions as to the limits of lengthening. An individual patient's suitability may not just depend on the severity of the shortening but also on other factors including associated deformities. In general, lengthening is considered appropriate for an anticipated discrepancy at maturity of 5–20 cm. Discrepancies greater than this are probably better managed by a prosthesis although surgery may be indicated to facilitate fitting and to correct deformity.

Table 24.1 Complications of limb reconstruction for congenital limb deficiencies

Bony

1. Poor bone formation
2. Deformity and fracture after fixator removal
3. Loss of alignment during lengthening

Soft tissue

1. Joint contractures
2. Subluxation and dislocation of joints
3. Muscle weakness
4. Nerve palsy

Table 24.2 Bony abnormalities in congenital short femur

At the hip

1. Femoral neck retroversion (externally rotated leg)
2. Acetabular dysplasia
3. Coxa vara

In the femoral shaft

1. Proximal sclerosis—poor regenerate formation at this level
2. "Rib-like" shape of the bone—difficulty with fixation

At the knee

1. Hypoplasia of the lateral condyle–valgus deformity
2. Patella subluxation or dislocation

The femur is not only short but also abnormal in shape (Table 24.2). These abnormalities have to be taken into account and preferably corrected before or during lengthening. Reconstruction is a more appropriate description of management than simply lengthening as it recognizes a more comprehensive approach to the whole limb abnormality. Many patients will require more than one episode of reconstruction depending on the severity of the case. In practice, reconstruction of the congenital short femur demands the anticipation and avoidance of complications, particularly knee subluxation and stiffness, related to insufficiency of the anterior cruciate ligament and tight hamstrings. As with reconstruction for all major congenital deficiencies, management is best undertaken by an experienced surgeon working with a multidisciplinary team who can offer an expert care throughout treatment from pre-assessment and pre-admission to ongoing support for a prolonged period.

A monolateral external fixator is easier to apply and less cumbersome but may not offer sufficiently stable fixation to cope with the deforming force of the tight soft tissues which can result in bending of the regenerate bone. It is therefore a common practice to use a circular fixator but proximally to use half rings or arches for access reasons. It is also much easier to bridge the knee with a circular fixator. Correction of the associated bony abnormalities should be considered either prior to lengthening or at the time of frame application. Knee protection by extending the frame to the tibia

is almost mandatory when lengthening a congenital short femur. In order to maintain movement in a controlled manner but to avoid subluxation, the frame is provided with a hinge at the knee. There is controversy as to whether a simple or multi-axial hinge is best. Knee stiffness is a common complication following femoral lengthening despite the use of a hinge. Care must be taken with distal pin placement to try to avoid impaling the quadriceps muscle which should be on the stretch when the wires are inserted. Knee stiffness after frame removal may improve for several months with regular physiotherapy. Quadricepsplasty can be helpful in resistant cases [23].

The osteotomy should be carried out in the least damaging manner to enhance regenerate formation. A distal osteotomy has the advantage of being through more normal bone and potentially distal valgus can be corrected at the same time but the quadriceps muscle may adhere to the regenerate and become stretched and fibrotic. A proximal osteotomy above the bulk of the quadriceps does not have these disadvantages but the bone may be less normal and regenerate formation less good (Fig. 24.7).

The risk of complications after frame removal such as fracture and knee stiffness is higher after lengthenings over 5–6 cm and the surgeon should not be too ambitious when lengthening the congenital short femur.

Proximal Femoral Focal Deficiency (PFFD)

PFFD was described by Aitken [12] in 1969. He defined four types (A–D) (Fig. 24.8). He pointed out the importance of the appearance of the acetabulum with reference to the appearance of the femoral head and the increasing coxa vara that occurs with increasing severity. These patients are likely to have major shortening (Gillespie group B) and in the most severe cases the foot will be at the level of the opposite knee (Gillespie group C) (see Fig. 24.2). In those patients who develop a reasonable femoral head it seems logical to improve the range of abduction by a valgus osteotomy with internal fixation. This will also usually induce the pseudarthrosis, if present to heal thereby stabilizing the femoral head on the femoral shaft. The timing of surgery depends on the appearances and size of the bone but is not usually undertaken before the age of 3 years.

Goddard et al. [24] reviewed the natural history and treatment of instability of the hip in PFFD in 67 patients. These patients all have a degree of shortening which requires an extension prosthesis when they start to walk. Lengthening even by modern methods is very difficult and fraught with problems because of the severe shortening and abnormalities at the hip and knee (Gillespie groups B, C, and Paley types

Fig. 24.7 (**a**) Long leg standing radiograph of a patient with left congenital short femur prior to lengthening. Note blocks under the left foot. (**b**) Radiograph at the end of lengthening in the circular frame. Note lengthening over a Rush pin; the knee was controlled with a hinge and the staple across the medial growth plate of the distal femur to correct distal femoral valgus. (**c**) Postlengthening long leg standing radiograph

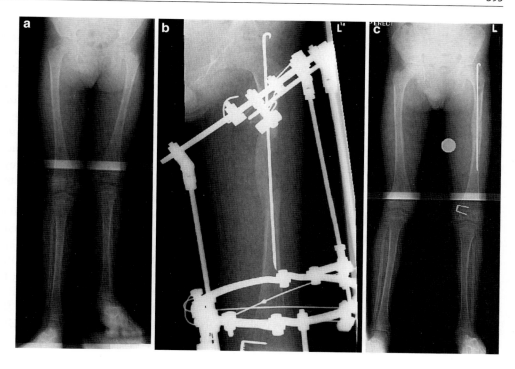

Fig. 24.8 (**a**) Child aged 1 year with severe left PFFD. Note the very short femoral segment which is flexed and externally rotated. The foot is remarkably normal and is almost at the level of the opposite knee. (**b**) Anteroposterior radiograph of a similar patient in early infancy. Note the short femoral segment, bulbous proximal end, and reasonable acetabulum suggesting this will become a stable hip despite the severe shortening

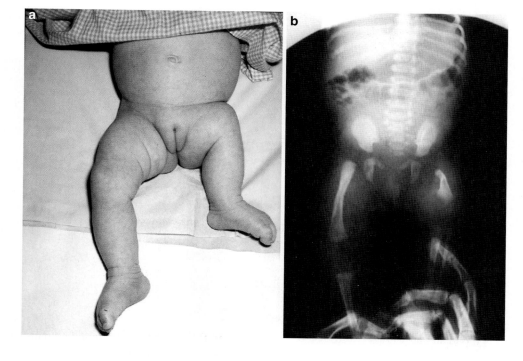

2b, 3a,b). Damsin et al. [25] published an excellent review of the problems of management of major congenital limb shortening. If the foot is at the level of the opposite knee, two possible approaches are advocated. The knee may be fused and the foot amputated to provide an adequate above-knee stump so that a good above-knee prosthesis can be fitted [26]. It is important to remember that through-joint amputations in children, unlike through-bone amputations, do not normally require revision during growth. Alternatively the Van Nes rotationplasty described by Borggreve in 1930 [27] and reviewed by Gillespie and Torode [17] may be advised. In this procedure the limb is rotated 180° and the knee fused. The foot faces backward and the ankle functions as the knee so that a below-knee prosthesis can be worn. There is considerable controversy regarding these two approaches. However, the Van Nes rotationplasty is suitable only if the foot and ankle are virtually normal and the foot will plantarflex to 180°.

In the most severe forms, where there is no satisfactory formation of the hip, it has been suggested that fusing the remnant of the femur to the ilium and using the knee as a primitive hinge hip may be useful [28]. However, in our own experience, most prosthetists find fitting and function better if the femoral remnant remains mobile.

Congenital Fibular Deficiency (or Hypoplastic Fibula)

This condition, like femoral deficiency, can vary in severity from complete absence of the fibula, with a short bowed tibia and a major reduction deformity of the foot, to simple shortening of the tibia and fibula, with no reduction deformity in the foot and a relatively minor shortening at maturity.

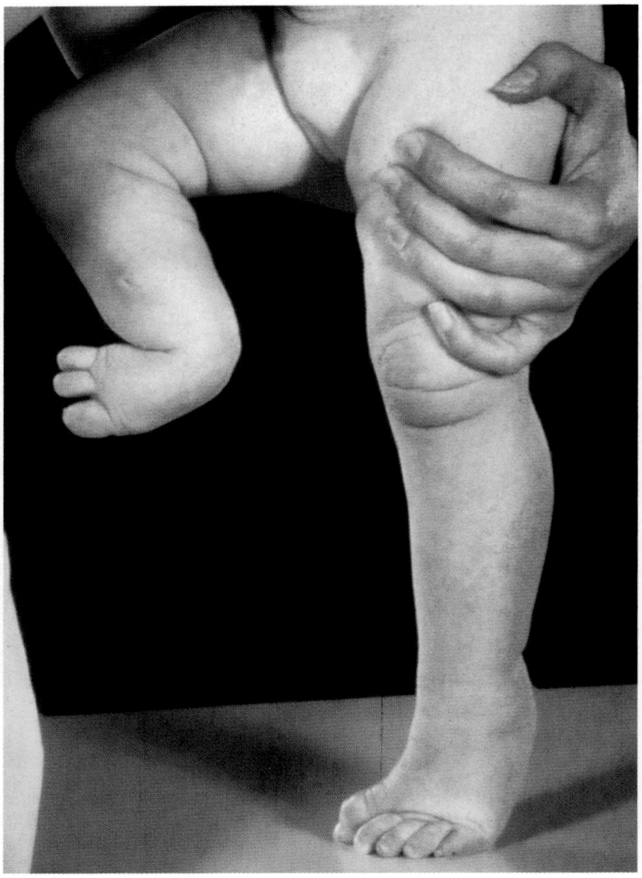

It is the most common form of major congenital shortening in the lower limb, occurring in approximately 1 in 25,000 live births. It does not appear to be inherited, but may be associated with other abnormalities in the same limb or the upper limb.

The clinical appearance in the classical form is typical, with marked anterior bowing of the tibia, and a dimple over the skin at the apex of the tibial kyphosis (Fig. 24.9); this dimple is also seen over the lateral side of the femur in congenital femoral deficiency. The foot is usually in valgus, with absence of one or more of the lateral radiographs. Radiographs show marked anterior bowing of the tibia with some sclerosis (Fig. 24.10). It is important not to mistake this condition for congenital pseudarthrosis of the tibia, which also shows sclerosis at the site of the bowing, but not the other features of this condition. The fibula may be totally absent or hypoplastic, being represented by a short or very small distal remnant of ossification. For many years the classification of Achterman and Kalamchi [29] (Fig. 24.11) was widely used. More recently Birch et al. [30] (Table 24.3) and Stanitski [31] have suggested classifications more closely related to modern reconstruction possibilities. The anterior bowing of the tibia often corrects spontaneously and usually does not require correction by osteotomy. If, however, the

Fig. 24.9 Clinical appearance of a right congenital fibular deficiency (Achterman and Kalamchi Type II). Note the anterior bowing of the tibia with a dimple over the kyphus, severe valgus of the foot with deficient lateral two rays

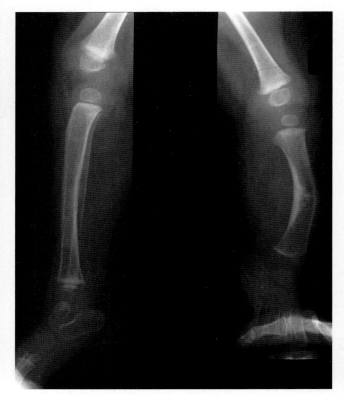

Fig. 24.10 Lateral radiographs of both lower legs showing a left congenital fibular deficiency (Achterman and Kalamchi Type II). Note the tibia is short, anteriorly bowed with complete absence of the fibula

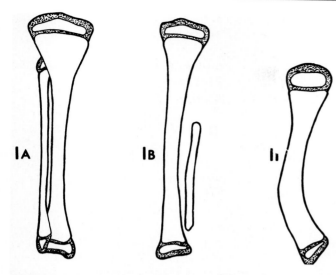

Fig. 24.11 Classification of congenital short tibia with absent or hypoplastic fibula (congenital fibula deficiency) as described by Achterman and Kalamchi. Reproduced with permission and copyright © of the British Editorial Society of Bone and Joint Surgery. Achterman and Kalamchi [29]

Table 24.3 Birch et al. classification of congenital fibular deficiency

Type based on state of foot treatment	
Type	
I	Functional foot reconstruction
IA	Leg 5% or less short orthosis/epiphysiodesis
IB	6–10% short epiphysiodesis or lengthen
IC	11–30% short 1 or 2 lengthenings or amputation
ID	>30% short >2 lengthenings or amputation
Type II Nonfunctional foot	
IIA	Functional upper limbs early amputation
IIB	Nonfunctional upper limbs retain foot

tibia is osteotomized, it will, unlike congenital pseudarthrosis, heal satisfactorily. The position of the foot in severe cases is nearly always in valgus. If the fibula is completely absent, a fibrous Thompson's band may be found. It is important to realize that, in addition to having a deficient ray or rays in the foot, there is frequently tarsal coalition, and so release of the lateral structures will not completely correct the valgus deformity of the foot. The knee often shows both cruciate deficiency and a valgus deformity associated with a hypoplastic lateral femoral condyle. Hootnick et al. [32] showed that the proportional shortening of the lower limb obeyed the same rules as that described by Ring in 1959 [18] and so it is possible in the first year of life to estimate the expected shortening at maturity. Subsequently, Hootnick et al. [5] demonstrated vascular abnormalities as a possible cause of the deformity.

Management and Limb Reconstruction

A patient's suitability for limb reconstruction is determined by the condition of the foot and the severity of the associated abnormalities especially the condition of the knee and the severity of the tibial shortening and deformity (Table 24.4). A three-ray foot is usually considered to be the minimum for reconstruction and it must be in a suitable position for weight bearing or be surgically realignable. The preliminary soft tissue realignment surgery is often carried out at around 12–18 months of age and the foot splinted until leg lengthening is commenced. If there is severe foot deformity then early treatment by amputation either through the ankle joint, a modified Syme's amputation, or retaining the calcaneum as in the Boyd amputation will facilitate prosthetic fitting and give an excellent result. It should be remembered that even patients treated by amputation may require further realignment surgery when they are older to correct, for example, progressive genu valgum due to distal femoral valgus.

The associated tibial deformities should be corrected at the time of tibial lengthening. The Taylor Spatial frame offers considerable advantages over the Ilizarov as it is easier to simultaneously correct the valgus, kyphosis, and rotation as well as lengthening (Fig. 24.12). Attention must be paid to any distal femoral valgus as this too will need correction. It is a mistake to try to correct a femoral deformity in the tibia and vice versa. Proper assessment of the whole deformity is essential prior to starting reconstruction.

Table 24.4 Abnormalities associated with congenital fibula deficiency

Foot and ankle
1. Lack of lateral support as fibula short or absent—tendency to valgus
2. Tarsal coalition
3. Ball and socket ankle joint
4. Abnormal triangular shape of distal tibial epiphysis—tendency to valgus
5. Absent rays
6. Equinovalgus or equinovarus of foot and ankle
Tibia
1. Short
2. Kyphotic
3. Internally rotated
4. Valgus
5. Diaphyseal sclerosis
Knee
1. Absence or hypoplasia of anterior cruciate ligament–knee subluxation
2. Distal femoral valgus—persistent valgus even after tibial correction.

Fig. 24.12 (**a**) Taylor spatial frame in use to correct both length and deformity in congenital fibular deficiency. (**b**) Anteroposterior radiograph after correction of length and deformity

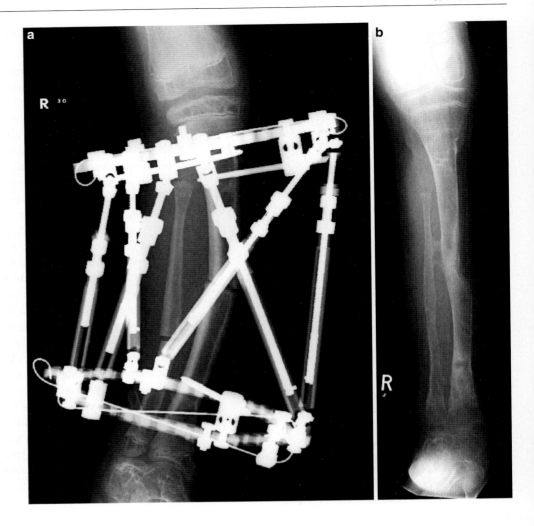

The general complications of limb reconstruction in congenital deficiencies are set out in Table 24.1 and apply to fibula deficiency. Equinovalgus of the ankle and foot are a particular problem even if the frame is extended to the foot. If the fibula appears absent on the radiograph, there may be a fibrous anlage (Thompson's band) which should be sought and resected at the time of frame application. Talocalcaneal coalition which may not be apparent on early radiographs is very common and can contribute to progressive heel and foot valgus. Late valgus of the foot and ankle may also be due to the abnormal shape of the distal tibia, lack of support from the absent or dysplastic fibula, and tightness of the tendo Achilles following lengthening. Ankle arthrodesis or an opening wedge subtalar fusion (if there is a subtalar joint) is sometimes required. Unfortunately stiffness of the foot and ankle is common and difficult to avoid.

In its more minor form, the condition may not be recognized because the fibula is present and the most obvious anomaly is the reduction deformity in the foot (Fig. 24.13). These patients are often believed to have simply a reduction deformity in the foot, and only present later with variable shortening of the lower leg. Radiographs confirm the reduction deformity in the foot, and also tarsal coalition. With the latter, there may be a ball and socket ankle joint. The fibula is present, though it may be slightly hypoplastic and, interestingly, the foot deformity is usually one of equinovarus rather than valgus. These children may present as a recalcitrant club foot. Careful scrutiny of the radiograph will show that the growth plate of the distal fibula is above the level of the ankle joint. These feet sometimes need treatment with limb reconstruction techniques as they do not always respond to conventional soft tissue surgery. Sometimes they require leg equalization, either by epiphysiodesis or by leg lengthening [33].

Congenital Tibial Deficiency or Absence of the Tibia with Intact Fibula

This is the rarest of the major congenital anomalies of the lower leg. It occurs in 1 in 1,000,000 live births. It may be inherited and associated particularly with medial duplication of both the hands and the feet (Table 24.5). Jones et al. [34] proposed a classification into four groups, based on the initial radiograph (Fig. 24.14). This was subsequently modified

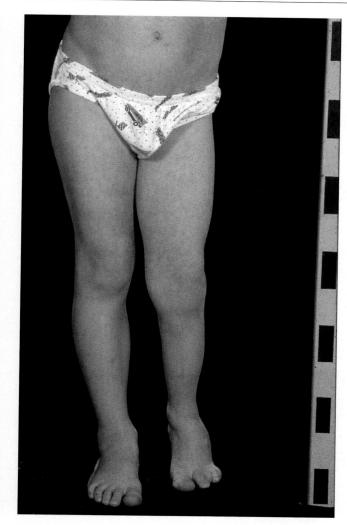

Fig. 24.13 Clinical photograph of the minor form of congenital fibula deficiency in the left leg. Note absence of the fifth ray, slight valgus at the knee, and shortening of the tibia and fibula which was present but mildly hypoplastic

Congenital Aplasia of the Tibia
Radiological Types

Type	Radiological Description	No. of limbs
1 a	• Tibia not seen • Hypoplastic lower femoral Epiphysis	6
1 b	• Tibia not seen • Normal lower femoral Epiphysis	12
2	• Distal Tibia not seen	5
3	• Proximal Tibia not seen	2
4	• Diastasis	4

Fig. 24.14 Classification of congenital tibial deficiency by Jones et al. Reproduced with permission and copyright © of the British Editorial Society of Bone and Joint Surgery. Jones et al. [34]

into three types by Kalamchi and Dawe [35] (Fig. 24.15). However, Schoenecker et al. [36], in a major review of 71 limbs in 57 patients, felt that the Jones classification into four groups was preferable.

Table 24.5 Abnormalities associated with congenital tibial deficiency

1. Polydactyly—sometimes also in the hands
2. Severe equinovarus
3. Tarsal abnormalities
4. Talus articulates with enlarged distal fibula

Tibia

1. Variable degree of absence (Jones' classification)
2. Deformity of shaft when present

Fibula

Overlong relative to tibia and prominent proximally

Knee

Instability

The clinical appearance is typical, with gross equinovarus deformity of the foot, which may show medial duplication (Fig. 24.16). The fibula is intact and there may be severe varus at the knee. As in femoral deficiency the radiograph at 1 year gives a clearer picture of the dysplasia than the radiograph at birth.

Management and Limb Reconstruction

Reconstruction for Jones Type 1a Tibial Dysplasia

In type 1a deformity, with complete absence of the tibia and no quadriceps apparatus, the best treatment is through knee amputation and a prosthesis. If this is not acceptable to the parents the alternative is the procedure described by Brown [37] in which the intact fibula is moved under the femoral condyles to replace the absent tibia. The results are usually poor because of inherent knee instability and lack of the quadriceps, requiring an orthosis, and a tendency to

Fig. 24.15 Classification of
congenital tibial deficiency as
modified by Kalamchi and Dawe.
Reproduced with permission and
copyright © of the British
Editorial Society of Bone and
Joint Surgery. Kalamchi and
Dawe [35]

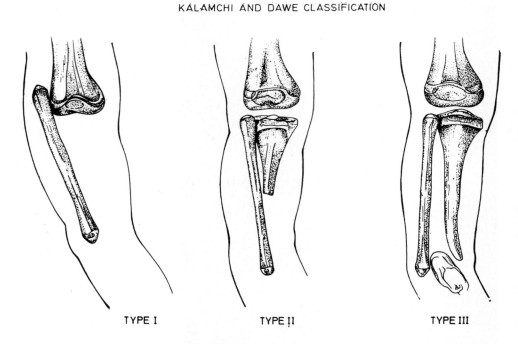

KALAMCHI AND DAWE CLASSIFICATION

TYPE I   TYPE II   TYPE III

Fig. 24.16 (**a**) Child with Jones'
type 2 congenital deficiency of
the right leg. Note the severe
equinovarus foot and duplication
of the hallux. (**b**) Anteroposterior
radiograph of the right showing
the proximal end of the tibia is
present in bone, the fibular is in
marked varus with severe
equinovarus of the foot and
duplication of the hallux

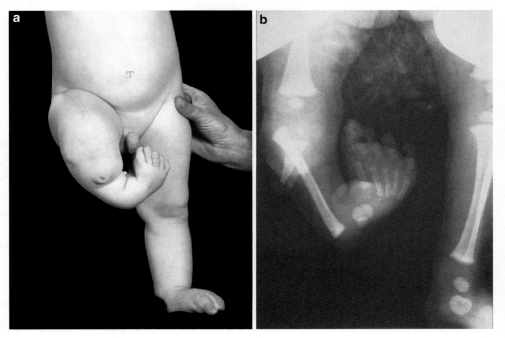

develop a knee flexion deformity. There are anecdotal reports of subsequent lengthening of the hypertrophied fibula.

Reconstruction for Type 1b Tibial Dysplasia

In type 1b the proximal tibia is present in cartilage and not visible on the early radiograph but can be seen on ultrasound and magnetic resonance imaging (MRI). The quadriceps

apparatus is also present and these patients can be treated as type 2 patients.

Reconstruction for Type 2 Tibial Dysplasia

In type 2 patients the upper end of the tibia and the quadriceps apparatus are present. Reconstruction is possible depending on the condition of the foot and ankle. If there is severe deformity then a below-knee amputation at

Fig. 24.17 (**a**) Anteroposterior radiograph of a patient with congenital tibial deficiency Jones type 2. (**b**) Anteroposterior and lateral radiographs following reconstruction by fusion of the fibula to the tibia using a screw. Note how the fibula is bowed and has hypertrophied. The foot has been stabilized on the distal end of the fibula. Further lengthening and deformity correction will be necessary later

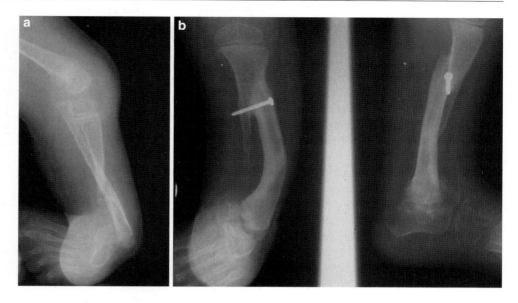

the level of the distal end of the tibia is probably the best option. As this is a through-bone amputation, stump revision, particularly for overgrowth of the fibula, is usually necessary. If the foot deformity is not too severe and the foot can be positioned by surgery for weight bearing then satisfactory reconstruction may be possible. As the distal tibia is absent the talus articulates with the fibula. It is usually necessary to explore the ankle and foot to correct an equinovarus deformity and position the talus under the fibula. Accessory toes may need excision. Later a one bone leg has to be created fusing the distal fibula to the tibial remnant usually with resection of the proximal fibula as this can be prominent and cause problems at the knee (Fig. 24.17a, b). Bone lengthening of the one bone leg can be carried out when the child is older together with adjustment of alignment either using an Ilizarov or using a spatial frame. These patients often have significant shortening and several lengthenings including femoral lengthening may be necessary. Knee and foot deformities can be troublesome [38].

Reconstruction for Type 3 Tibial Dysplasia

This is the rarest type of tibial dysplasia in which the tibia is represented by an amorphous segment of bone more distal than proximal. An MRI scan can be very helpful to assess the extent of the dysplasia as occasionally the proximal tibia is present in cartilage particularly if the femoral condyles appear normal. True type 3 cases are best treated by amputation which gives a good result and there is insufficient experience to recommend reconstruction.

Reconstruction for Type 4 Tibial Dysplasia

The tibia is present but short and there is a diastasis between the lower end of the tibia and fibula. The fibula is long relative to the tibia and is prominent proximally. The foot is usually in equinovarus. The talus may articulate with the tibia, fibula, or both bones. Although type 4 dysplasia is of variable severity, it is overall the mildest form of tibial dysplasia and reconstruction is often feasible. The foot position needs early correction at about 1 year of age. A decision has to be made at the time of surgery whether the talus is best positioned under the tibia or the fibula. The foot is then splinted until the patient is old enough for lengthening. It is important to control the foot in the frame and to consider differential lengthening of the fibula and the tibia to restore their normal relationship proximally. It is often necessary to include the foot in the frame to protect the ankle and most patients will have a stiff foot.

Congenital Pseudarthrosis of the Tibia

Congenital pseudarthrosis of the tibia is rare with an estimated incidence of 1 in 140,000 live births. Its etiology is unknown and its management difficult. The name is confusing, in that fracture at birth is rare; the condition is better called infantile pseudarthrosis of the tibia. Fracture commonly occurs in the first 2 years after birth, but may be delayed until very much later.

Clinical and Radiological Appearances

The tibia is bowed anteriorly, and commonly laterally, often with shortening (Fig. 24.18). The most common site of the deformity is at the junction of the proximal two-thirds with the distal one-third of the tibia. A number of classifications based on the clinical and radiological appearances have been described, of which the best known is that of Boyd [39], who describes six different types. Radiologically, however, there are two main types of deformity. The more common shows narrowing, and often obliteration, of the marrow cavity, with surrounding sclerosis related to the apex of the anterior bowing, usually at the junction of the middle and lower thirds of the tibia (Fig. 24.19). The less common type shows a cystic lesion at the site of the deformity in the tibia; it is important not to confuse this with fibrous dysplasia, which can cause a similar deformity and fracture, but responds much better to treatment in the form of curettage, grafting, and intramedullary rodding. The fibula is often involved in the disease process (Fig. 24.19). Isolated congenital pseudarthrosis of the fibula (CPF) is very rare and has a generally more benign prognosis [40]. Between 40 and 80% of patients will show neurofibromatosis, and it is important to look for the

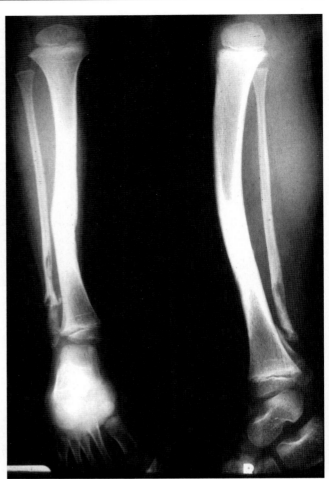

Fig. 24.19 Anteroposterior and lateral radiographs of a patient with congenital pseudarthrosis of the tibia which has not yet fractured. Note the anterior bowing, sclerosis and loss of the marrow cavity; the fibula is also affected and has already fractured in its distal third

stigmata of this condition, which may be present when the pseudarthrosis is diagnosed, or may develop later. The characteristic "cafe au lait" spots of pigmentation in the skin often do not appear until the age of 2 years. Other members of the family should be examined, because relatives very reasonably do not relate their child's bowed tibia to the occurrence of skin nodules, pigmentation, or nerve tumors in other members of the family.

Management

Management is complex. Once fracture has occurred union is very difficult to achieve. It is most important to recognize the condition in the pre-pseudarthrosis stage and not to osteotomize the bowed tibia and precipitate nonunion. Prophylactic bracing from the time the child is first diagnosed seems to be very worthwhile if compliance can be maintained. Murray and Lovell in 1982 [41] reported

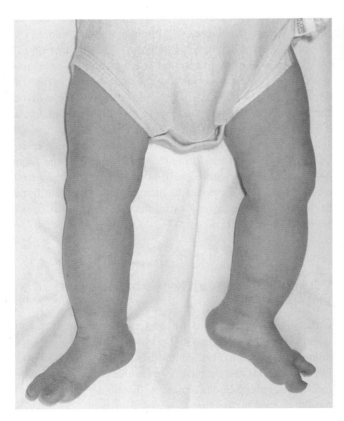

Fig. 24.18 Child aged 9 months with congenital pseudarthrosis of the left tibia. Note the anterior bowing and slight shortening. The tibia has not yet fractured and he was treated with a protective orthosis

good long-term results in a small group of patients treated by bracing alone. Fibular bypass grafting was described by McFarland in 1951 [42] and subsequently prophylactically by Lloyd-Roberts and Shaw [43] and Strong and Wong-Chung [44]. Once a pseudarthrosis becomes established it is extremely difficult to heal. Many methods of grafting have been advocated in a condition that is so rare that most experience is of small numbers and therefore anecdotal. In two large reviews by Hardinge [45] and Baker et al. [46] amputation rates of 29 and 22% were reported.

Three methods have emerged as useful in obtaining union in this difficult condition:

1. Intramedullary rodding and grafting as described by Charnley in 1956 [47] (Fig. 24.20). Anderson et al. [48] reported union in 10 out of 10 patients, but subsequent re-fracture required further grafting or re-rodding in 5. Paterson and Simonis [49] used electrical stimulation from an implanted stimulator (Osteostim) in addition to intramedullary rodding and obtained union in 20 of 27 tibiae. They emphasized the importance of retaining the intramedullary rod until maturity to avoid re-fracture.

2. Free vascularized fibula graft. Gilbert [50], Pho et al. [51], and Simonis et al. [52] have reported satisfactory results using a free vascularized fibula graft from the contralateral leg.

3. Bone transport. Grill [53] reported good results with a modification of the Ilizarov technique [54] in nine patients, seven of whom had failed several previous operations.

In view of its rarity it is important that in any one geographical area a particular surgeon or group of surgeons undertakes the management of this rare disorder to gain sufficient numbers and experience in its treatment. To try to overcome the problem of small anecdotal series the European Paediatric Orthopaedic Society (EPOS) set up a European multicenter study of treatment and published the results in 2000 [55]. They obtained detailed validated data from 172 patients and drew the following conclusions regarding management:

1. Prophylactic splintage in the pre-pseudarthrosis stage was very useful.

2. There was a clear correlation between the age of surgery and the final outcome with better results being achieved with increasing age.

3. Intramedullary rodding could be used to manage early fracture together with an orthosis.

4. The two most successful surgical treatments in the survey were the Ilizarov technique and the free vascularized fibula graft with union rates of up to 75%. Both methods gave better results if delayed until at least 4–6 years of age. An important observation, which has been supported by a more recent publication in 2006 [56], was that despite union of the tibia, function was often severely limited by residual problems such as valgus deformity and degenerative change in the ankle joint.

Reconstruction Techniques with a Circular Fixator

Treatment with the Ilizarov technique is more likely to be successful after the age of 6 years [55]. In the infant and young child the question of management before definitive treatment at the age of 6 years arises. It is undoubtedly easier to attempt limb reconstruction in a relatively straight tibia with well-aligned foot. If the foot and ankle have been neglected in this condition a troublesome valgus deformity

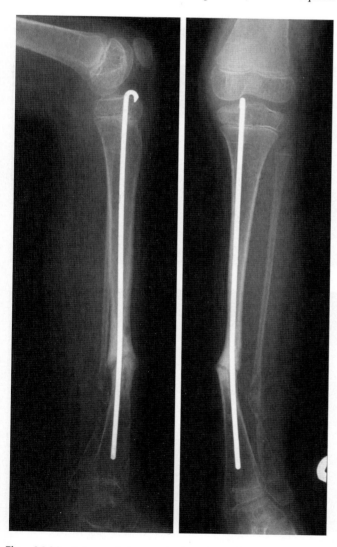

Fig. 24.20 Anteroposterior and lateral radiographs showing intramedullary rodding with a Rush pin for congenital pseudarthrosis of the tibia. Note a valgus deformity of the distal fragment has already developed

may develop. If the tibia has fractured or there is a significant deformity it is worthwhile correcting the deformity and stabilizing the tibia by a simple osteotomy (without attempting to resect the pseudarthrosis) and rodding the tibia. The lower leg and foot should then be splinted. Unfortunately, particularly with a very distal pseudarthrosis, replacement of the rod will be required at regular intervals. Some surgeons have tried telescopic or extending rods to obviate the need for frequent exchange. Occasionally the pseudarthrosis will heal with rodding alone.

Once the child reaches 6 or 7 years (although the older the child the better), definitive treatment can be attempted with a circular external fixator. The options are resection of the pseudarthrosis and bone transport or resection of the pseudarthrosis, acute compression, and lengthening above in as normal bone as possible. If an intramedullary rod (Rush pin) is still in situ it is useful to leave it in place to protect against fracture when the frame is removed. The principles of fixator

treatment include correction of the mechanical axis, a very stable frame, and apposition of viable bone. With a distal pseudarthrosis it is frequently necessary to extend the frame to the foot to gain adequate stability.

Tibia Recurvatum (Posteromedial Angulation of the Tibia)

This is a very rare deformity. The tibia is bowed posteriorly and, commonly, medially at the junction of the middle and lower thirds. It occurs in association with marked calcaneus of the foot (Fig. 24.21). The appearance is alarming, but the prognosis benign. The majority of cases respond readily to stretching and splintage of the foot into equinus. If the surgeon is prepared to wait long enough, probably all cases will correct with time. Pappas [57] reviewed a large group of 33 patients with this rare condition. He pointed out

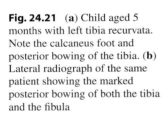

Fig. 24.21 (**a**) Child aged 5 months with left tibia recurvata. Note the calcaneus foot and posterior bowing of the tibia. (**b**) Lateral radiograph of the same patient showing the marked posterior bowing of both the tibia and the fibula

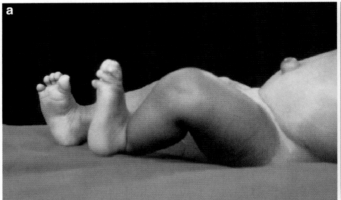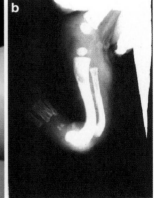

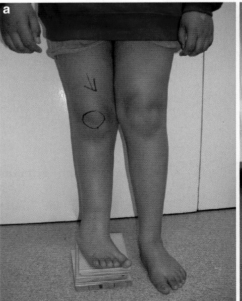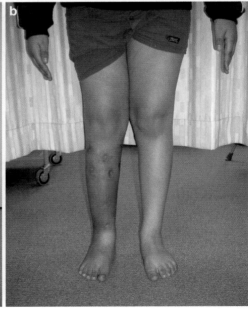

Fig. 24.22 (**a**) Patient with right tibia recurvata showing shortening and inward rotation of the foot. (**b**) Clinical photograph after correction using a Taylor spatial frame

that, in general, the greater the initial bowing the greater the ultimate leg length discrepancy and that the proportionate length differences between the normal and the bowed tibiae remain stable after the child had reached 12 months of age. The maximum leg length discrepancy seen in this series of patients was 6.9 cm. However, if there is persistent deformity when the child starts to walk, corrective osteotomy can be undertaken. Unlike congenital pseudarthrosis of the tibia, the osteotomy will heal, despite the sclerosis at the site of the angulation. However, union may take some time and an intramedullary rod is a useful way of splinting the tibia while awaiting union. Once the deformity has corrected, the child normally manages extremely well, but should be followed up as he or she is liable to be left with some residual shortening, which may require leg equalization procedures near maturity [58]. Any persistent deformity may be corrected at the time of lengthening near maturity using a spatial frame (Fig. 24.22).

Part II: Leg Length Inequality

Franz Grill

Introduction

Leg length discrepancy (LLD) is defined as a condition in which the lower extremities are noticeably unequal.

LLDs are relatively common. Knutson reports a prevalence of 90% in normal adults, with a mean inequality of 5.2 mm. LLD exceeding 20 mm affects at least one in every 1000 individuals [59].

The etiology of LLD may be subdivided into two categories: *anatomical leg length discrepancies* are caused either by shortening of bone structures, angular deformities, or by functional disorders. *Functional length discrepancies* usually result from joint contracture. At hip level, a contracture of the adductor muscles leads to functional shortening, while abduction contracture causes functional lengthening in the standing position. A fixed pelvic obliquity may also be due to a deformity of the lumbar spine. Additionally, flexion contracture of the hip and the knee joint may cause functional shortening, leading to foot deformities such as the equinus [60].

The question as to how much limb-length inequality creates a significant impact on the locomotor system is controversial [59].

According to gait studies in the laboratory, the crucial magnitude is between 2 and 3 cm [61–64]. The authors state that the body is well able to compensate for minor LLD below 2 cm.

Any greater difference in leg length will cause postural imbalance in standing and uneven gait. A common effect of anatomic LLD is rotation of the pelvis. Walsh found that pelvic obliquity was the most common method of compensation for LLD below 22 mm [65]. This compensation mechanism is not without consequences. When LLD exceeds 15 mm the prevalence of chronic back pain is 5.3 times that in the normal population [66].

In addition, an association was found between the LLD and the development of osteoarthritis in the knee and hip joint. Osteoarthritis was found to occur more commonly in the hip of the longer (84%) than the shorter (16%) leg [67, 68]. This conclusion was supported by Golightly, who also reported a higher rate of osteoarthritis in the knee joint of the longer leg [69].

Patellar apicitis in athletes is much more common in the longer leg because of the significantly increased quadriceps activity [70].

Children usually compensate for discrepancies by pelvic obliquity, flexion of the knee on the longer side, or equinus on the shorter side, resulting in significantly greater plantar flexion in the shorter limb.

Etiology of Limb-Length Inequality and Malalignment

Structural causes of limb-length discrepancy and malalignment are numerous. The etiology may be congenital or acquired. The natural course depends upon the degree of inhibition or acceleration of growth and varies according to etiology. In cases of congenital defects, LLD can be calculated and predicted more easily because growth remains proportional. The growth rate in vascular, infectious, traumatic, or neoplastic disorders, however, is variable (Table 24.6) [71].

Deformity

Deformities of part or all of the lower extremity are frequently associated with LLDs. Deformities may be present in the frontal, sagittal, or coronal planes. They may be single level, multilevel, uniplanar, or multiplanar. The biomechanical effect of malalignment exerts a negative impact on the function as well as the longevity of a joint.

Genu varum occurring at the age of 2–3 years is physiological and has an excellent prognosis. Mild bow-leg is common in many adult athletes. Genu valgum is physiological up to the age of 8 or 10 years and persists in mild degree in many adults, particularly women (Table 24.7).

Table 24.6 Etiologies of limb-length discrepancies

	Inhibition of growth	Acceleration of growth
Congenital	Proximal femoral focal deficiency	Klippel Trenaunay syndrome
	Tibial/fibular deficiencies	Proteus syndrome
	Coxa vara congenita	Hemihypertrophy
	Congenital hip dislocation	Hemophilia
	Silver–Russel syndrome	Arteriovenous malformation
	Hemiatrophy	–
	Ollier's disease	–
	Clubfoot	–
Infection/ inflammation	Osteomyelitis (metaphyseal), septic arthritis with growth plate damage	Osteomyelitis (diahyseal)
	–	Juvenile rheumatoid arthritis
Neurological Diseases	Poliomyelitis	–
	Myelomeningocele	–
	Cerebral palsy	–
Posttraumatic	Traumatic growth plate lesson	Metaphyseal fracture, diaphyseal fracture
	Slipped capital femoral epiphysis	Postoperative (osteotomy)
Tumor	Osteochondroma	Neurofibromatosis, malalignment
	Neurofibromatosis	Bone tumors
Other	Legg–Calvé–Perthes disease	Fibrous dysplasia
	Irradiation	–

Table 24.7 Different etiologies of malalignment

Cause	Genu valgum	Genu varum
Congenital	Fibular hemimelia	Tibial hemimelia
	Skeletal dysplasia	Skeletal dysplasias
Trauma	Partial physeal arrest	Partial physeal arrest
Arthritis	Juvenile rheumatoid arthritis	–
Infection	Partial growth arrest	Partial growth arrest
Metabolic	Rickets	Rickets
Others	Burns	Blount's disease

Assessment of the Patient

History

Eliciting a careful past medical history is essential when dealing with acquired discrepancy. A positive family history may indicate a syndrome.

Clinical Assessment

It is fundamental to distinguish between true and apparent shortening and to bear in mind the fact that some patients may have both.

As the causes of LLD are numerous, a meticulous, standardized clinical assessment must be performed to determine all associated abnormalities.

Discrepancies are commonly compensated for by altered function. Limping, circumduction, varus and valgus deformity, equinus on the shorter side, and knee flexion or hyperextension on the longer side may be present, depending upon the magnitude of the LLD.

Height, the relationship between the trunk and the extremities, thigh and lower leg proportions, as well as alignment and posture must be evaluated in the standing position. Pelvic obliquity is present in any LLD and the physician must determine by clinical examination whether this is due to a fixed deformity of one or more of the three lever arms attached to the pelvic ring, or secondary to structural spinal deformity.

In the supine position, joints have to be clinically tested in respect of instability or restriction of motion.

Measurement of Discrepancy

In the absence of fixed joint deformities, two methods for measurement of LLD provide reliable results:

- Assessment in the standing position by placing blocks of known height under the short leg to level the pelvis: each segment should be assessed visually by this method. Forward flexion of the spine allows the pelvic alignment to be reviewed from behind, along with rotation and tilting of the back.
- Tape measurement in the supine position of the distance between the anterior superior iliac spine and the medial or lateral malleolus: this method may be misleading in cases of pelvic asymmetry or hind foot deformity or if the legs are not positioned parallel to the pelvis and spine.

Clinical assessment of minor length inequalities may be difficult and imprecise when performed before the child begins to walk. Standing with blocks under the foot of the shorter leg is the best measurement in the older child.

Imaging

Radiography has long been considered the gold standard for LLD measurement and will determine any associated bone or joint deformities.

Radiographs in standardized reference planes are necessary to analyze deformity and obtain reproducible measurements. Angular deformities are better analyzed by the use of radiographs in the standing position. For the antero-posterior (AP) radiograph in the frontal plane, the knee is positioned with the patella exactly centered and pointing forward, regardless of the foot position [72]. In cases of fixed dislocation or subluxation of the patella, the tibial tuberosity is used to align the limb. A further option is to assess the knee flexion–extension axis and position the knee perpendicular to this axis. For a more accurate assessment of the impact of ligament laxity or joint laxity, a radiograph in single-leg stance may be obtained.

The knee must be exactly positioned in order to obtain a projection in the same plane as that used for the initial analysis. A long focal distance is necessary in order to visualize the hip, knee, and ankle joint on a single film. The advantage of the long distance is that magnification is minimized so that measurements and planning of the hardware can be performed more accurately. The majority of the digital radiograph systems currently in use permit digital synthesis of two or more separate images, enabling reconstruction of a full standing radiograph. Sagittal view films are particularly important to evaluate abnormal or diminished range of motion in the joint (flexion contracture or hyperextension). For the full standing lateral radiograph, the patient is positioned with the pelvis of the contralateral side rotated posteriorly by about 35° and the knee in full extension. However, in most instances a lateral radiograph of the femur and a lateral view of the tibia are sufficient to evaluate the respective joint alignment in the sagittal view. Full standing radiographs cause significantly greater radiation exposure than do ordinary ones because of the long film focus. They should be performed only if additional information about the femur and the tibia is needed to decide appropriate treatment, such as preoperative planning or fine-tuning of the final alignment when performing gradual correction of a deformity using an external fixator.

Assessment of LLD can be performed by the use of long, standing films or orthoradiography (Fig. 24.23). Orthoradiography is performed with the patient lying supine with a full scale between the legs on the table [73, 74]. Three separate sequential exposures with the central ray directed successively over the hip, knee, and ankle joints are necessary. As the scale is magnified by approximately the same factor as the bones, the true length of the femur and tibia can be calculated. However, this method does not provide any information about functional LLD or pelvic obliquity, or the role of foot height as a contribution to total LLD. A second imaging technique to assess LLD is the long, standing radiograph with extra-long film cassettes. Extra-long films of 51 in. in length (more than 1 m) are widely available in the United States, while smaller long films of 90 cm are available in most European countries. These provide images of the entire lower extremity including the foot and pelvis in adolescents as well as adults.

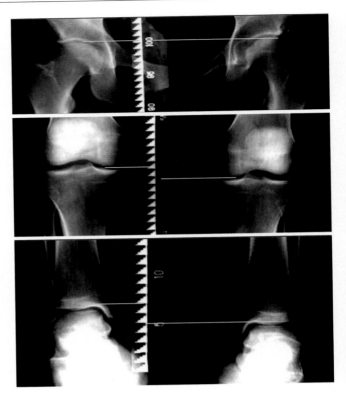

Fig. 24.23 Orthoradiography for measurement of LLD

Digital radiography imaging systems are increasingly used and usually offer a software solution to paste together two or more exposures, combining them into a single, continuous image. The advantage of such films is the ability to calculate precisely leg length, foot height, and the magnitude of a potential functional shortening.

Deformity Analysis

Deformity analysis and preoperative planning should be performed to compare the anatomy of the patient with the mean values of a normal population, to assess the exact location and magnitude of the deformity, and to predict the outcome in respect to the osteotomy and correction. In the past, the femorotibial angle was used to describe varus or valgus alignment of the knee and the Mikulicz line was used to assess the position of the mechanical axis. While the Mikulicz line is still used to describe the mechanical axis deviation (MAD), the center of rotation of angulation (CORA) planning method permits exact analysis of angular deformities of the lower limbs (Fig. 24.24) [75–77].

CORA can be analyzed for every angular deformity. A basic understanding of the nomenclature is necessary to plan the treatment. Alignment refers to the colinearity of the hip,

Fig. 24.24 Normal values for joint orientation according to Paley and Tetsworth

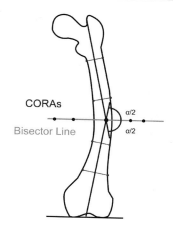

CORAs

Bisector Line

α/2

α/2

- if the osteotomy line and the ACA pass through the same CORA, the bones will angulate relative to each other without translation.
- when the ACA passes through a CORA but the osteotomy is at a different level, the ends of bone at the osteotomy level will angulate and translate to each other. The proximal and distal axis lines will realign fully when the correction is complete.
- if the ACA does not pass through the CORA, the proximal and distal axes of the bone will be parallel but will translate to each other. The same principles are applicable for multi-apical deformities or deformities of the upper extremity or the foot (Fig. 24.25).

Prediction of growth is a prerequisite prior to epiphysiodesis or distraction lengthening of a shortened extremity

knee, and ankle joints. Joint orientation refers to the position of an articular surface in relation to the axis of the limb segment. In mid-diaphyseal deformities it is relatively intuitive to draw a line along the axes of the respective segments. However, in deformities close to the joint or in juxta-articular deformities, the line for the short segment has to be constructed using predefined angles. The angles can be determined by drawing the axis of the long segment and the joint orientation line. Average figures based upon values for the normal population have been provided for all joint lines of the lower extremity.

Two modes of planning have been proposed for the frontal plane. For anatomical planning one uses the anatomical axis of the femur, the mid-shaft axis, and the anatomical axis of the tibia; the respective joint lines define the CORA. Mechanical planning is based upon the mechanical axis of the femur which is inclined 7° to the anatomical axis and usually connects the center of the femoral head with the center of the knee joint. In the tibia the mechanical axis is nearly identical to the anatomical axis; there is no difference here between the two planning modes. However, the two modes should never be mixed.

The CORA is the most important assessment for the correction of an angular deformity. The line that runs through the CORA and bisects the lateral and medial angle formed by the proximal and distal axes at the bone is named the transverse bisector line.

The other two important factors are the angulation correction axis (ACA) and the osteotomy level. ACA is the axis line around which the deformity is corrected. While the CORA is determined by deformity analysis and cannot be selected by the surgeon, the ACA and the osteotomy level can be freely selected. However, if ACA is not on the bisector line of CORA, a secondary translational deformity will occur. Paley and coworkers formulated three osteotomy rules to describe the relationship between the CORA, the ACA, the osteotomy level, and the result of correction:

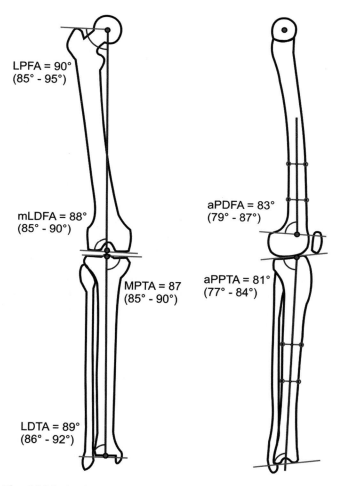

LPFA = 90°
(85° - 95°)

mLDFA = 88°
(85° - 90°)

MPTA = 87
(85° - 90°)

LDTA = 89°
(86° - 92°)

aPDFA = 83°
(79° - 87°)

aPPTA = 81°
(77° - 84°)

Fig. 24.25 Analysis of malalignment; determination of CORA. CORAs along the bisector line. Correcting around CORA on the convex side will result in shortening of the bone; the magnitude of lengthening increases in direct proportion to the distance of CORA from the bone and the concave side. This is particularly important in correction using unilateral fixators in the immature patient. Various methods have been proposed to calculate the magnitude of the remaining growth. The majority of these methods are not based upon chronologic age but on bone age, which can be estimated using specific indicators.

Calculation and Determination of Bone Age

Several disorders are associated with a delay in bone age, such as Perthes' disease, cerebral palsy, or Ollier's disease. The atlas of Greulich and Pyle uses gender-specific details of anteroposterior radiographs of the left hand to determine bone age [78]. However, the radiographs used for this atlas were obtained from children born between 1917 and 1942. An atlas produced by the French authors Sempé and Pavia provides similar data [79]. However, changes on radiographs may not be obvious during puberty, thus raising the likelihood of inaccurate interpretations.

The Sauvegrain method employs a scoring system to evaluate the AP and lateral views of the elbow. This method has been evaluated by Diméglio and coworkers [80] and was found to provide more details than the atlas of Greulich and Pyle [78, 81]. However, the method is restricted to the growth spurt during puberty, which occurs between the age of about 10 and 13 years in girls and between 12 and 15 years in boys.

The Tanner and Whitehouse system uses 20 indicators on the AP hand radiograph [82]. It is very time-consuming and cumbersome despite being available in computerized form on the Internet.

Prediction of the Progression of Deformity

In cases of posttraumatic hemiepiphysiodesis secondary to a bone bridge, the margin of the growth plate can be calculated. The width of the physis, the percentage of growth in relation to the growth of the entire bone, bone length, and age-specific multipliers must be determined. However, the proportion of growth from the distal femur and the proximal tibia is not the same at all ages [71]. As a temporary hemiepiphysiodesis by staples or a plate is recommended to correct angular deformities in the growing child, the prediction may only be necessary at the end of growth in order to ensure that the remaining growth is adequate to bring about full correction of the deformity.

Remaining Growth

The Green and Anderson method is based upon growth data [73, 74]. These longitudinal data include the length of the

femur and the tibia for females and males from the age of 1 year to maturity. A total of 700 children, 87% of whom had residual paralysis in one lower extremity and a normal extremity on the other side, and 158 normal children were included in this study.

The patients were Irish children from South Boston; the majority of them had poliomyelitis. It should be noted that the study did not account for differences in ethnicity, height, or socioeconomic status.

Straight Line Graph

The straight line graph was introduced by Moseley [83] and is based upon data provided by Green and Anderson. Moseley transformed the normal growth curve of Anderson data into a straight line by adapting the data points on the x- and y-axis of the chart. The result is a 45° line that represents normal growth and can be used to predict geometric growth and the effects of an epiphysiodesis. However, the straight line graph should ideally be used by performing three separate measurements at different ages, not always possible if the patient reports to the surgeon in later childhood or adolescence.

Minimum requirements for the calculation are the length of the long leg and the short leg, and skeletal age. The greatest difficulty associated with this method is to determine the percentile of the patient within the skeletal age range. This determination is improved by taking skeletal rather than chronological age into account.

Arithmetic Method

The arithmetic method was introduced by Westh and Menelaus and is used for the purpose of timing epiphysiodesis [84]. The method employs chronologic age and the difference in leg length by blocks. It should not be used when chronologic age and bone age differ by more than 1 year. As a rule of thumb, distal femur growth is 0.95 cm and proximal tibial growth 0.64 cm per year. However, this assumption does not account for growth spurts or the fact that the growth plates at the knee joint increase their percentage of total bone growth when approaching the end of growth.

Paley's Multiplier Method

Paley and coworkers introduced the multiplier method to predict bone length, adult height timing of epiphysiodesis, and even prenatal prediction of LLD at maturity

[20]. The multiplier method is a simple arithmetic formula. The data for this formula have been derived from the Anderson and Green growth data [73, 74] and compared with multipliers calculated from 19 other databases, including radiographic, clinical, and anthropological information from a variety of different populations. In all of these calculations, the same multipliers were established for the different data sets and populations. The method appears to be independent of percentile groups and is the same for the prediction of femoral, tibial, and total limb lengths.

The multiplier method can also be employed to calculate adult height. It is simpler to use than the percentiles of Bailey and Pinneau [85].

Error in Using Growth Charts

Little et al. [86] compared eight methods of predicting limb-length discrepancy, including those of Anderson [87] and Moseley [83]. They found that the methods using skeletal age were no more accurate than those based on chronological age. They evaluated the techniques for timing epiphysiodesis as described by Green and Anderson [73, 74], Moseley [83], and Westh and Menelaus [84] and registered similar accuracies for all, independent of whether chronologic or skeletal age was used.

All of these methods are valid only when there is constant growth inhibition of the short limb. Thus, they cannot be used in patients with conditions involving accelerations and decelerations of growth, such as rheumatoid arthritis.

Management of LLD

The goals of any treatment of LLD are to level the pelvis and avoid secondary problems such as low back pain or early osteoarthritis.

Treatment guidelines for limb-length equalization are well established. There is general consensus that no treatment is required in adults with discrepancies less than 2 cm unless these are symptomatic. Only about 10% of adults with a length discrepancy of up to 2 cm use a shoe lift.

In discrepancies of more than 2 cm, a shoe raise is indicated. The shoe raise should be about 1 cm less than the actual discrepancy. Adjustments can be applied inside or outside the shoe or as a combination of both. A shoe raise is generally not well accepted. Children as well as adults feel awkward when asked to use one and usually opt for surgical correction.

Surgical management of LLD depends upon age, basic pathology, severity, projected height at the end of growth, and associated deformities. Equalization can be achieved surgically either by shortening the longer limb or by lengthening the shorter limb, or both.

In a growing child, a prerequisite for any intervention is exact preoperative planning based upon the estimation of skeletal age, calculation of discrepancy, and body height at maturation. Ideally, relevant growth data should be collected over a number of years prior to surgery, permitting precise calculation.

In principle, correction of LLD should remain at the same level as the deformity. The two knees should be at the same level and the pelvis should be balanced after correction.

Surgical Limb Equalization

Shortening the Long Leg in Children

The pros and cons of shortening as a means of leg length equalization have to be discussed with the patient and the parents. In a child of normal height at maturation and an anticipated discrepancy of 2–5 cm, shortening should be the method of choice. It is safe and effective if there is sufficient growth left to effect a correction. The preferred method is epiphysiodesis, which is defined as surgical interruption of the growth of the physis of the longer leg. Epiphysiodesis of the distal femoral epiphysis is used to shorten the femur, while shortening of the tibia is best achieved by epiphysiodesis of the proximal tibia, including the fibula if there are more than 2 cm of expected skeletal growth. Using different techniques, epiphysiodesis can be either temporary or permanent. In case of valgus or varus deformity, the surgeon may perform a gradual correction by means of hemiepiphysiodesis (unilateral medial or lateral). When remaining growth is inadequate to achieve full correction by epiphysiodesis, surgical shortening by bone reSection may be indicated.

Epiphysiodesis

This is a simple method for equalizing leg lengths but is frequently neglected or not undertaken at the appropriate time. As it is a biological method, the final outcome is not entirely predictable. Nevertheless, the method is important not only for LLDs of 2–5 cm predicted at skeletal maturity but also in cases of severe LLD in congenital limb deficiencies as an adjunct to lengthening procedures. Parents tend to feel anxious when the healthy leg of their child is suggested as the site for operation. The surgeon must explain the method accurately so that the parents comprehend its benefits for their child. They should be made aware that procedures that lengthen the leg, or a shortening operation after skeletal maturation, are more complex and carry greater risk. An epiphysiodesis or hemiepiphysiodesis can be performed relatively simply by different techniques that bring about a permanent or temporary arrest of the physis [88]. The impact on final height is moderate, nevertheless the method should be avoided in patients of short stature

Permanent Growth Plate Arrest by Mini-invasive Techniques [92]

Under image intensifier guidance, a K-wire or small Steinmann pin is inserted through the middle of the physis from the medial aspect of the distal femur or proximal tibia using the Canale technique [89] or the lateral side using the Macnicol technique [90, 91]. The latter approach allows the proximal fibular physis to be ablated if appropriate. After performing a 10 mm skin incision directly over the epiphyseal guide wire, the epiphysis is entered using a cannulated drill [89]. The size of the drill bit is gradually increased from 6 to 12 mm (Fig. 24.26). The growth plate is drilled out along the K-wire to the opposite side. After withdrawing the K-wire, the drill bit is used to destroy the growth cartilage. The tubesaw method allows access from the lateral side [91], with removal of a 1 cm diameter core of the growth plate and neighboring bone followed by thorough removal of the physis which can be accessed by small curettes. The bone plug is reinserted transversely at the end of the operation, thus controlling postoperative hemorrhage. A plaster cast is unnecessary but crutches

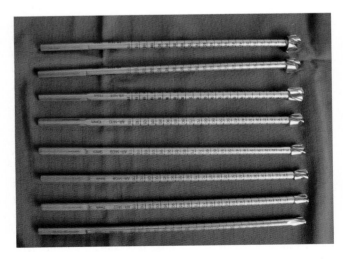

Fig. 24.26 Special design for drill bits used for Canale mini-invasive technique of epiphysiodesis. Diameters from 6 to 12 mm

are provided initially, with full activity permitted after 6 weeks.

Permanent Growth Plate Arrest—Phemister's Open Surgery Technique

A longitudinal 3-cm incision is made both medially and laterally over the physis. Using an osteotome, a cortical bone block (2 cm × 2.5 cm), centered over the physis, is removed on each side. A curette is used to excise part of the growth plate, especially in the central area of the physis. The bone blocks are then rotated 90° or 180° and impacted into the respective defects medially and laterally.

Postoperative immobilization with a knee immobilizer and partial weight bearing is advised for 4 weeks. Full activity is permitted after 6 weeks. However, postoperative morbidity is greater after the Phemister method than following the less invasive methods described [90]. Complications include postoperative hemorrhage or hematoma, under- and overcorrection of the discrepancy and angulatory deformity.

Permanent Hemiepiphysiodesis

These techniques can be used for permanent hemiepiphysiodesis although the rate of correction of angulation is unpredictable.

Temporary Arrest of the Growth Plate: Stapling

Physeal stapling consists of placing 2–3 staples medially and laterally across the physis (distal femur, proximal tibia) extraperiosteally. As long as the staples are in place, growth is inhibited. The staples should be left in position until the scheduled correction has been performed. They should not remain for more than 18–24 months because of the potential risk of permanent damage to the physis.

Several complications may be associated with this procedure, such as extrusion and breakage of staples, permanent arrest, overcorrection, growth abnormality (axial deviation), or rebound of longitudinal growth after removal of staples.

Temporary Arrest of the Growth Plate—Epiphysiodeses and Hemiepiphysiodeses—The 8-Plate Technique

Under C-arm control, the growth plate is identified. A small skin incision is made. Either from the lateral (varus deformity) or from the medial (valgus deformity) aspect, an

8-plate is fixed strictly extraperiosteally using two self-tapping cannulated screws, one fixed distally and one proximally to the growth plate. The plate should be perfectly positioned on the AP as well as lateral views. Inserted medial and lateral to the physis, the 8-plate can also be used to achieve a temporary growth arrest (Fig. 24.27).

The postoperative course is usually uneventful. The patients are able to walk the same day and clinical follow-up investigations must be performed every 3 months. The 8-plate (or staples) must be removed on time in order to avoid overcorrection.

The 3-month follow-up investigation is mandatory to identify overcorrection or any other disturbance of growth. In general, the staples or the 8-plate should not remain for longer than 18–24 months since exceeding this may lead to definitive damage of the physis.

The 8-plate is superior to conventional staples in several respects. A longer skin incision is required for stapling.

Usually the surgeon has to insert two or three staples. Postoperative rehabilitation takes longer and the technique is associated with greater risk.

Shortening Osteotomies

Acute shortening is indicated in patients with a discrepancy of 2–5 cm in adolescence with an absence of sufficient residual growth, or in young adults. The magnitude of shortening should not exceed 4 cm.

Femoral Shortening Techniques

From the lateral aspect, a segment of bone is resected at the proximal femoral level either at the subtrochanteric level or by a z-shaped interochanteric approach. After resection of the bone segment the osteotomy is coapted, compressed, and fixed by the use of a blade plate (Fig. 24.28) or a dynamic hip screw. Shortening should not exceed 10–15% of the total femoral length. Acute shortening is mainly indicated in patients with a discrepancy of 2–4 cm. Postoperatively the patient has to use crutches for at least 3 months until bony consolidation of the osteotomy has occurred.

A further technique is closed femoral shortening. By placing a saw in the intramedullary canal from proximally, a segment of the femur is excised and displaced by splitting the separated fragment. The femur is fixed with an intramedullary nail.

Tibial Shortening

The magnitude of the shortening should not exceed 3 cm. Resection is performed proximally, and fixation is achieved by the use of a plate or an interlocking nail.

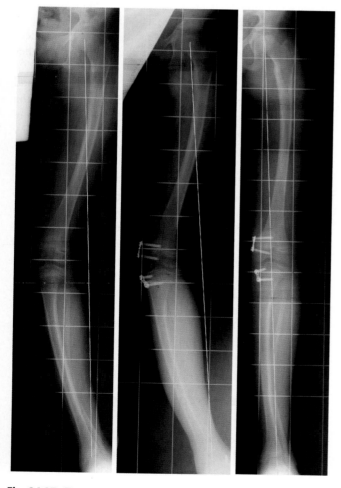

Fig. 24.27 Temporary arrest of growth plate in a 9-year-old female with valgus knee deformity treated by hemiepiphysiodesis at the distal femoral and proximal tibial level using 8-plates

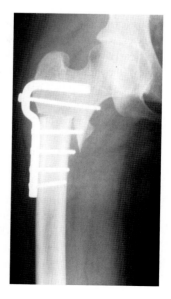

Fig. 24.28 Shortening osteotomy in a case of LLD secondary to poliomyelitis. The Wagner technique was used to preserve the lesser trochanter. Fixation used an AO-blade plate

In general, shortening of the femur is preferred to shortening of the tibia because the latter is associated with a greater risk of compartment syndrome, persistent muscular weakness, and delayed bone union.

Leg Lengthening

History

Long bone lengthening has been undertaken for more than 100 years, dating back to Codivilla who performed femoral lengthening in several steps using traction after femoral osteotomy, with a Steinmann pin placed in the calcaneus [93]. Codivilla reported on 26 patients whose femora had been lengthened by 3–8 cm.

Modern lengthening techniques have evolved and been refined gradually [72, 94–99]. The Wagner technique is now historical. It consisted of fixing a monolateral external fixator with a distraction unit on the bone, then performing a diaphyseal osteotomy followed by distraction. After having achieved the desired lengthening, the gap was filled with cancellous bone grafts and stabilization was achieved by inserting an AO plate.

The principle of distraction osteogenesis for bone healing during lengthening was described by Abbott, Anderson, and by Ilizarov [96, 100, 101].

Biology of Lengthening—Distraction Osteogenesis—Bone Regenerate

As in any fracture, after osteotomy bone healing starts by callus formation. Gradual distraction of living tissues creates stresses which stimulate and maintain active regeneration. This early reparative tissue is distracted by lengthening and followed by intramembranous ossification with the formation of a bone regenerate. Ossification occurs on both sides of this structure and columns or osteoid appear, a process known to occur in membrane bone formation as well. On radiographs these columns look striated in the line of the distraction force.

Callus formation is enhanced by performing a low-energy osteotomy (corticotomy). This minimally invasive procedure preserves blood supply and causes less damage to soft tissues and bone marrow. Under ideal conditions, distraction should start 5–7 days after corticotomy. Delays of 2–3 weeks are associated with a high risk of premature bone consolidation. On the other hand, unstable mechanical fixation and a distraction rate of more than 2 mm daily lead to poor bone formation and eventual nonunion.

The rate of lengthening for optimal bone formation is 1 mm per day. Lengthening is best achieved in increments of 0.25 mm.

The mechanical lengthening device must ensure stability in order to produce the distraction stress phenomenon. Undesirable angular or shearing movements will result in the formation of fibrous tissue and not fibrocartilage. Smoking delays bone healing, so patients should refrain from smoking at least during the period of their treatment, failing which they should be regarded as unsuitable candidates for lengthening [102].

There is good reason to believe that axial micromovements are beneficial or even essential for producing the correct tissue response. Axial micro motion signifies that the bone is dynamized throughout the lengthening process.

After the desired lengthening has been achieved, the external fixator is kept in place until full bone consolidation is evident. The fixator may be removed as soon as cortical bone has appeared.

Usually the index healing period for full consolidation per centimeter of lengthening biologically normal bone is around 25–35 days, depending upon the patient's age.

Up to 20% of any given bone can be safely lengthened. Larger magnitudes can be achieved at the expense of a higher complication rate.

The Gigli saw or the De Bastiani corticotomy method permit a more controlled bone cut [95]. When using the De Bastiani technique the cortical bone is predrilled using several circumferentially applied drill holes and the bony bridges between the drill holes are cut using a chisel or osteotome.

Chondrodiatasis lengthens by growth plate distraction. It can be achieved without rupture of the growth plate by increasing growth through the hypertrophic zone, between the proliferating cells and the zone of provisional calcification. Currently this procedure is only indicated in exceptional cases confined to individuals approaching skeletal maturity.

The results of Ilizarov's research and clinical work provide a clear understanding of the basic principles of bone lengthening, deformity correction, and treatment of bone defects [96, 97, 100, 101]. Such knowledge is mandatory for the surgeon performing limb lengthening.

Mechanical Devices for Leg Lengthening

Mechanical methods of lengthening include external fixation, external fixation in combination with an intramedullary nail (lengthening over nail), and intramedullary distraction devices.

A perfect device should allow for lengthening, permit simultaneous accurate correction of deformities in all planes and dimensions, provide stability of the bone regenerate, be user-friendly, painless for the patient, devoid of complications, and acceptable to the patient. The ideal device has not yet been developed. However, a large number of systems are available, depending upon the pathology and the respective anatomical conditions.

The Ilizarov Ring Fixator

The fixator consists of rings connected by threaded rods. Tensioned Kirschner wires are fixed to the ring and cross within the bone. The K-wires are made of either titanium or stainless steel. The wire tip is shaped like a bayonet and measures 1.5 or 1.8 mm. Smooth and olive types of wires are available. They have to be tensioned in the full ring to 130 kg and in the half ring to 70 kg. Fixation is not secure unless the rings are positioned in pairs. Two wires are used at each level. For maximum stability the two wires should cross at right angles. Anatomical limitations must be taken into account. It is mandatory for the surgeon to always remain in an anatomical safe zone. The advantages of wires are that they can be placed in tight spots, permit micro motion in axial loading, and stable fixation in porotic bone. A combination of wires and half pins increases stability and avoids the risks of limb transfixion.

The Ilizarov system consists of numerous items that permit the surgeon to construct a tailored device for any deformity, including those of the foot and the knee. The rings are connected by threaded rods. If angular deformities have to be corrected, the surgeon may include hinges in the construct. Hinge placement is performed according to the rules of deformity correction [72]. Angular, rotational, and translational deformities can be corrected by this procedure.

Extending the frame across a joint will protect it and permit progressive correction to occur either before or during lengthening. An equinus deformity can be corrected by placing hinges at the level of the ankle joint.

Lengthening can be combined with multilevel correction using proper ring and hinge placement. In bifocal lengthening both metaphyses within the segment may be lengthened simultaneously.

Other conditions that can be treated with the Ilizarov ring fixator are bone defects and pseudarthrosis. In these conditions a segmental bone transport is an effective technique for achieving bone consolidation and healing.

Lengthening Over a Nail

Lengthening over a nail is an option to shorten the duration of external fixator support. When using this technique in conjunction with an Ilizarov device or a monolateral fixator, an intramedullary locking nail is inserted. As soon as the desired lengthening has been achieved the nail is locked and the fixator can be removed.

Taylor Spatial Frame

The Taylor spatial frame is a hexapod system consisting of two rings connected with six telescope struts at universal joints. By adjusting only strut length, one ring can be repositioned in relation to the other. Simple or complex deformities are treated using the same frame. The multiple angles and translations of a given deformity are addressed by adjusting the length of struts only. The Taylor spatial frame fixator is capable of correcting 6-axis deformity, guided by a web-based software program. Six deformity parameters, three frame parameters, and four mounting parameters are required to achieve correction using the program. In the event of failure the program can be restarted by entering new and more accurate parameters [98]. The system permits correction of complex foot deformities using special foot applications and a foot correction computer program and can also be combined with Ilizarov items (Fig. 24.29). Joints can be bridged with the Ilizarov system. Multiple-plane correction can be achieved at three levels in the same limb segment. The Taylor spatial frame is much easier to handle than the conventional Ilizarov system, especially for correction of rotational and translational deformities. The Taylor spatial frame produces more accurate corrections of deformity than those achieved with the Ilizarov device. Patients find the system easy to use because a daily adjustment schedule is provided. The strut exchanges are listed and explained in chronological sequence (Fig. 24.30).

Monolateral Devices

The first widely used monolateral fixator was the Wagner device, which was designed for diaphyseal lengthening followed by cancellous grafting and plating. Unlike the Wagner technique, the earlier Abbott/Anderson method recognized the biological importance of gradual distraction, thus avoiding the use of bone grafting, but these early, double frames were torsionally weak and therefore did not allow walking. The Wagner device was replaced by the Orthofix fixator, a much more sophisticated monolateral system allowing bone lengthening, axial correction, segmental transport, and multilevel correction.

A new device (Multi-Axial Correction MAC Biomet) now makes it possible to obtain optimized multiplanar deformity correction by the use of a unilateral system. The latter is highly modular, can be integrated into a rail system and

Fig. 24.29 A Taylor spatial frame for lengthening in an 8-year-old boy at the proximal tibial metaphysis. Hybrid mounting with conventional Ilizarov items to avoid knee dislocation by bridging the knee and ankle joint to avoid equinus. (**a**) AP view. (**b**) Lateral view

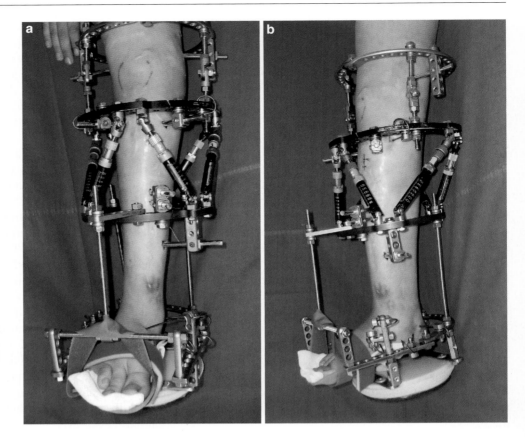

Fig. 24.30 (**a**) Twelve-year-old boy with posttraumatic shortening and valgus deformity of the left knee, treated using a TSF shortening of 5 cm with valgus knee deformity. (**b**) TSF in situ after deformity correction. (**c**) Radiograph showing perfect alignment, correction of valgus deformity, and shortening. (**d**) Final outcome after removal of the external fixator

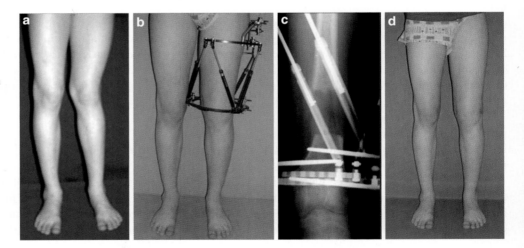

a hybrid ring construct, and also offers the possibility of articulated joint distraction.

The advantage of monolateral fixators is that they are less bulky. Their main indications in paediatric orthopaedics are trauma, lengthening of small bones such as metatarsals or metacarpals, as well as lengthening of the humerus. A further common indication is articulated distraction of the hip and elbow joint using dynamic monolateral fixators (Fig. 24.31).

Intramedullary Bone Lengthening

Patients with a discrepancy in limb length as well as short stature generally prefer to undergo a lengthening procedure that does not involve the use of external fixators. The disadvantage of external fixators is that the activities of daily life are severely limited. Painful pin site infection occurs in

Fig. 24.31 Monolateral fixator for hip joint distraction

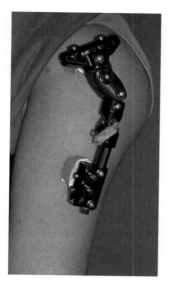

Fitbone

Fitbone is a further innovative concept that recognizes the biological importance of callus distraction. It consists of a fully implantable computer-controlled motor-driven distraction device. The internal drive system is provided with an electromechanical segment and an integrated electronic module that receives electric power through high-frequency transmission from outside the limb. There is no connection between the implant and the surface of the human body. The nail is very well accepted by patients because elongation occurs continuously and very slowly without rotational movements. It is also painless and does not limit joint movement. The metal is removed approximately 2 years after lengthening has been concluded and tibial or femoral bone union is assured (Fig. 24.32).

nearly all cases if skin is allowed to tent and is not regularly cleansed. Furthermore, the risk of fracture after removal of the fixator remains a concern. The development of an intramedullary bone lengthening implant was achieved in Germany by Götz and Schellmann in 1975 [103], Baumann and Harms [104], and Witt and Jäger [105]. Bliskunov in Russia has also developed a system [106–108]. The most recent innovations in this regard are the Albizzia nail developed by Guichet [109], the intramedullary skeletal kinetic distractor (ISKD) nail by Cole [110], and the Fitbone by de Baumgart et al. [111].

The implants can only be used if the medullary cavity is wide enough and the growth plates are about to close.

Albizzia Nail

Gradual lengthening is achieved by efforts of the patient who is required to produce rotational movements of 20° to lengthen the nail together with the bone. Manual rotation of this sort is painful and poorly tolerated by a large number of patients.

ISKD Nail

The ISKD was developed by Orthofix. Small rotational movements of 3–9°, effected by the patient, cause the telescopic nail to be lengthened. Analogous to Ilizarov's method, the ISKD nail is associated with gradual lengthening of callus. The rate of distraction depends on how frequently the patient rotates the limb. A monitor enables the patient to follow the progress of distraction.

Up to 8 cm of lengthening can be achieved but patients may overlengthen the limb and produce problems in bone regeneration.

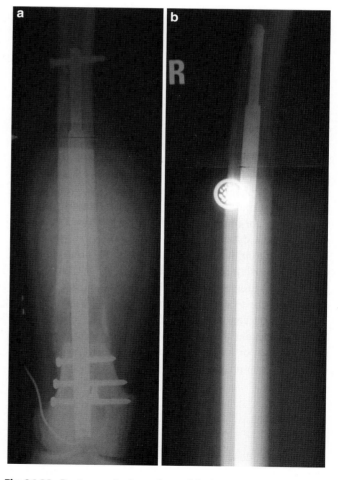

Fig. 24.32 Posttraumatic shortening and flexion deformity of the right femur due to partial growth arrest. Fitbone in situ with lengthening achieved. Correction of distal femoral malalignment performed using the placement of two bollar screws to achieve deformity correction. (**a**) AP projection. (**b**) Lateral projection

Obstacles in Limb Lengthening

Limb lengthening is a demanding surgical procedure and should be performed by experienced orthopaedic surgeons. As the entire treatment may take several weeks or even months, a number of minor or major complications may occur [112].

Minor Complications

Proper pin care is essential. The pin sites must be cleaned and disinfected on a daily basis; a regular shower is recommended. Pin site infections are usually painful as long as bone lengthening is in progress.

In case of early osseous consolidation of the bone regenerate, the osteotomy has to be repeated.

Major Complications

Severe stiffness as well as dislocation of the hip and knee joints may occur and may be difficult to treat.

Equinus deformity is common when physiotherapy is not performed on a regular basis. Support for the foot during distraction may be of value.

Nerve lesions, particularly those of the peroneal nerve, are a risk during treatment of congenital deficiencies and valgus deformities of the knee.

During lengthening, fractures may occur proximal or distal to the external fixator. After removal of the fixator, fractures may occur through the lengthened segment. Therefore, particularly in dysplastic bone and poor bone regenerate, it is advisable to protect the lengthened bone from fracture by inserting a Rush pin or Kirschner wire.

Axis deviation should not be overlooked and must be corrected prior to consolidation of the lengthened segment. The deviation can be corrected by new data input and an adjusted program for deformity correction using the Taylor spatial frame, or by hinge adjustment when Ilizarov frame distraction is in progress.

Prostheses

In congenital deficiencies with an anticipated LLD of more than 25 cm at maturity, equalization by surgery is not advisable because the patient may require repeated operations and prolonged hospitalization and because of the high risk of complications such as joint dislocation, stiffness, bone regenerate fracture, and psychological problems.

Treatment should be orientated toward maintaining a good function during childhood. This should be achieved by a combination of surgical procedures which allow optimal fitting of the prosthesis. Amputation may be an option in some instances, but leads to loss of proprioception, sensitivity and function. Modern orthoprosthetic technology increasingly provides nearly normal function and quality of life, and children usually tolerate prostheses well.

References

1. Frantz CH, O'Rahilly R. Congenital skeletal limb deficiencies. J Bone Joint Surg 1961; 43A:1202–1224.
2. Day HJB. The ISPO/ISO classification of congenital limb deficiency. Prosthetics Orthotics International 1991; 15:67–69.
3. Fixsen JA. Major limb congenital shortening: a mini review. J Pediatr Orthop B 2003; 12:1–12.
4. Morgan JD, Somerville EW. Normal and abnormal growth at the upper end of the femur. J Bone Joint Surg 1960; 42B:264–272.
5. Hootnick DR, Levinsohn EM, Randall PA, Packard DS Jr. Vascular dysgenesis associated with skeletal dysplasias of the lower limb. J Bone Joint Surg 1980; 62A:1123–1129.
6. Szeizel AE, Codaj I, Lenz W. Smoking during pregnancy and congenital limb deficiency. Brit Med J 1994; 308:1473–1476.
7. Amputee Medical Rehabilitation Society. Congenital Limb Deficiency. Recommended Standards of Care. A report by the working party of the Amputee Medical Rehabilitation Society published December 1997. Available from the Amputee Medical Rehabilitation Society c/o of the Royal College of Physicians, 11 St Andrew's Place, Regents Park, London NW1 4LE, UK.
8. Kim MT, Chambers HG, Mubarak SJ, Wenger DR. Congenital coxa vara: Computed tomographic analysis of femoral retroversion and the triangular metaphyseal fragment. J Pediatric Orthop 2000; 20:551–556.
9. Subharwal S, Muttal R, Cox G. Percutaneous triplantar femoral osteotomy correction for developmental coxa vara: A new technique. J Pediatr Orthop 2005; 25:28–33.
10. Hamanishi C. Congenital short femur: clinical, genetic and epidemiological comparison of the naturally occurring condition with that caused by thalidomide. J Bone Joint Surg 1980; 62B:307–320.
11. Amstutz HC, Wilson PD Jr. Dysgenesis of the proximal femur (coxa vara) and its surgical management. J Bone Joint Surg 1962; 44A:1.
12. Aitken GT. Proximal femoral focal deficiency. A congenital anomaly. Symposium held in Washington, 3 June 1968. Washington DC: National Academy of Sciences; 1969:1–22.
13. Pappas AM. Congenital abnormalities of the femur and related lower extremity malfunction: classification and treatment. J Pediatr Orthop 1983; 3:45–60.
14. Fixsen JA, Lloyd-Roberts GC. The natural history and early treatment of proximal femoral dysplasia. J Bone Joint Surg 56B; 1974 86–95.
15. Gillespie R. Classification of congenital abnormality of the femur. In: Herring JA, Birch JG, eds. The Child with a Limb Deficiency. Rosemont IL: American Academy of Orthopaedic Surgeons; 1998:63–72.
16. Paley D. Lengthening reconstruction surgery for congenital femoral deficiency. In: Herring JA, Birch JG, eds. The Child with a Limb Deficiency. Rosemont IL: American Academy of Orthopaedic Surgeons; 1998:113–132.

17. Gillespie R, Torode IP. Rotationplasty of the lower limb for congenital defects of the femur. J Bone Joint Surg 1983; 65B: 569–573.

18. Ring PA. Congenital short femur. J Bone Joint Surg 1959; 41B:73–77.

19. Ring PA. Congenital abnormalities of the femur. Arch Dis Child 1961; 36:410.

20. Paley D, Bhave A, Hertzenberg JE, Bowen JR. Multiplier method for predicting limb-length discrepancy. J Bone Joint Surg 2000; 82A:1432–1446.

21. Thomas MP, Jackson AM, Aichroth PM. Congenital absence of the anterior cruciate ligaments. J Bone Joint Surg 1985; 67B: 572–575.

22. Sanpera I Jr, Fixsen JA, Hill RA. The knee in congenital short femur. J Pediatr Orthop B 1995; 4:159–163.

23. Hosalkar HS, Jones S, Chowdhury M, et al. Quadricepsplasty for knee stiffness after lengthening in congenital short femur. J Bone Joint Surg 2003; 85B:261–264.

24. Goddard NJ, Hashemi-Nejad A, Fixsen JA. Natural history and treatment of instability of the hip in proximal femoral focal deficiency. J Pediatr Orthop B 1995; 4:145–149.

25. Damsin JB, Pous JG, Ghanem I. Therapeutic approach to severe congenital lower limb length discrepancies, surgical treatment versus prosthetic management. J Pediatr Orthop B 1995; 4: 164–170.

26. Panting AL, Williams PF. Proximal femoral focal deficiency. J Bone Joint Surg 1978; 60B:46–52.

27. Borggreve J. Kniegelenkersatz durch das in der Beinlangsachse um 180 Grad gedrehte Fussgelenk. Archiv der orthopadischen und Unfallchirurgie 1930; 28:175–178.

28. King RE. Some concepts of proximal femoral focal deficiency. In: Aitken GT, ed. Proximal femoral focal deficiency. A congenital anomaly. Symposium held in Washington, 3 June 1968. Washington DC: National Academy of Sciences; 1969: 23–49.

29. Achterman C, Kalamchi A. Congenital deficiency of the fibula J Bone Joint Surg Br 1979; 61B:133–137.

30. Birch JG, Lincoln TL, Mack PW. Functional classification of fibular deficiency. In: Herring JA, Birch JG, eds. The child with a limb deficiency. Rosemont IL: American Academy of Orthopaedic Surgeons; 1998:161–171.

31. Stanitski DF, Stanitski CL .Fibular hemimelia: A new classification. J Pediatr Orthop 2003; 23:30–34.

32. Hootnick DR, Boyd NA, Fixsen JA, Lloyd-Roberts GC. The natural history and management of congenital short tibia with dysplasia or absence of the fibula. A preliminary report. J Bone and Joint Surg 1977; 59B:267–271.

33. Maffuli N, Fixsen JA. Fibular hypoplasia with absent lateral rays of the foot. J Bone Joint Surg 1991; 73B:1002–1004.

34. Jones D, Barnes J, Lloyd-Roberts GC. Congenital aplasia and dysplasia of the tibia with intact fibula. J Bone Joint Surg 1978; 60B:31–39.

35. Kalamchi A, Dawe RB. Congenital deficiency of the tibia. J Bone Joint Surg Br 1985; 67B:581–584.

36. Schoenecker PL, Kapelli AM, Miller EA, et al. Congenital longitudinal deficiency of the tibia. J Bone Joint Surg 1989; 71A:278–287.

37. Brown FW. Construction of a knee joint in congenital total absence of the tibia (paraxial hemimelia tibia)—a preliminary report. J Bone Joint Surg 1965 47A:695–704.

38. De Sanctis N, Nunziata Rega A. New rationale in management of tibial agenesis type II: a maturity review of its functional, psychological and economic value. J Pediatr Orthop B 1996; 5:1–5.

39. Boyd HB. Pathology and natural history of congenital pseduarthrosis of the tibia. Clin Orthop 1982; 166:5–13.

40. Choi T-J, Choi IH, Chung CY, et al. Isolated congenital pseudarthrosis of the fibula. J Pediatr Orthop 2006; 26: 449–454.

41. Murray HH, Lovell WW. Congenital pseudarthrosis of the tibia, a long term follow-up study. Clin Orthop 1982; 166: 14–20.

42. McFarland B. Pseudarthrosis of the tibia in children. J Bone Joint Surg 1951; 43B:36–46.

43. Lloyd-Roberts GC, Shaw NE. The prevention of pseudarthrosis of the tibia and congenital kyphosis of the tibia. J Bone Joint Surg 1969; 51B:100–105.

44. Strong ML, Wong-Chung J. Prophylactic bypass grafting of the prepseudarthrotic tibia in neurofibromatosis. J Pediatr Orthop 1991; 11:757–764.

45. Hardinge K. Congenital anterior bowing of the tibia. Ann Royal Coll Surg Engl 1972; 51:17–30.

46. Baker JK, Cain TE, Tullos HS. Intramedullary fixation for congenital pseudarthrosis of the tibia. J Bone Joint Surg 1992; 74A:169–178.

47. Charnley J. Congenital pseudarthrosis of the tibia treated by the intramedullary nail. J Bone Joint Surg 1965; 38A:283–290.

48. Anderson DJ, Schoenecker PL, Sheridan JJ, Rich MM. Use of an intramedullary rod for treatment of congenital pseudarthrosis of the tibia. J Bone Joint Surg 1992; 74A:161–168.

49. Paterson DC, Simonis RB. Electrical stimulation in the treatment of congenital pseduarthrosis of the tibia. J Bone Joint Surg 1985; 67B:454–462.

50. Gilbert A. Vacularised fibular transfer for treatment of congenital pseudarthrosis. Annual Meeting of the American Academy of Orthopaedic Surgeons, Anaheim, California, 14 March 1983.

51. Pho RWH, Levack B, Satku K, Patradul A. Free vascularised fibulograft in the treatment of congenital pseudarthrosis of the tibia. J Bone Joint Surg 1985; 67B:64–70.

52. Simonis RB, Seirali HR, Mayou B. Free vascularised fibular grafts for congenital pseudoarthrosis of the tibia. J Bone Joint Surg 1991; 73B:211–215.

53. Grill F. Treatment of congenital pseudarthrosis of tibia with the circular frame technique. J Pediatr Orthop B 1996; 5:6–16.

54. Ilizarov GA. Basic principles of transosseous compression and distraction osteosynthesis. Ortopedia Travmatologiial i Protezirovanie 1971; 32:7–15.

55. Grill F, et al. Results of the EPOS multicentre study of congenital pseudarthrosis of the tibia. J Pediatr Orthop B 2000; 9:1–15, 69–102.

56. Muharrem I, El-Rasi G, Riddle EC, Kumar SJ. Residual deformities following successful initial bone union in congenital pseudarthrosis of the tibia J Pediatr Orthop 2006; 26:393–399.

57. Pappas AM. Congenital posteromedial bowing of the tibia and fibula. J Pediatr Orthop 1984; 4:525–531.

58. Heyman CH, Herndon CH, Keiple KG. Congenital posterior angulation of the tibia with talipes calcaneus. J Bone Joint Surg 1959; 41A:476–488.

59. Knutson GA. Anatomic and functional leg-length inequality: A review and recommendation for clinical decision-making. Part I, anatomic leg length inequality: prevalence, magnitude, effects and clinical significance. Chiropractic Ostopath 2005; 13:11.

60. O'Toole GC, Makwana NK, Lunn J, et al. The effect of leg length discrepancy on foot loading patterns and contact times. Foot Ankle Int 2003; 24:256–259.

61. Gurney B. Leg length discrepancy, Gait Posture 2002; 15: 195–206.

62. Kakushima M, Miyamoto K. The effect of leg length discrepancy on spinal motion during gait: three-dimensional analysis in healthy volunteers. Spine 2003; 28(21):2472–2476.

63. Song KM, Halliday SE. The effect of limb-length discrepancy on gait. J Bone Joint Surg Am 1997; 79(11):1690–1698.

64. Goel A, Loudon J, Nazare A, et al. Joint moments in minor limb length discrepancy: a pilot study Am J Orthop 1997; 26(12): 852–856.

65. Walsh M, Connolly P, Jenkinson A, O'Brien T. Leg length discrepancy—an experimental study of compensatory changes in three dimensions using gait analysis. Gait Posture 2000; 12(2):156–161.

66. Friberg O. Clinical symptoms and biomechanics of lumbar spine and hip joint in leg length inequality. Spine 1983; 8(6): 643–651.

67. Tallroth K, Ylikoski M, Lamminen H, Ruohoncn K. Preoperative leg length inequality and hip osteoarthrosis: a radiographic study of 100 conservative arthroplasty patients. Skeletal Radiol 2005; 34:136–139.

68. Gofton JP, Trueman GE. Studies in osteoarthritis of the hip: Part II. Osteoarthritis of the hip and leg length disparity. C M A J 1971; 104:791–799.

69. Golightly PT, Allen KD, Renner JB, et al. Relationship of limb length inequality with radiographic knee and hip osteoarthritis, Osteoarthritis Cartilage 2007; 15:824–829.

70. Kujala UM, Osterman K, Kvist M, et al. Factors predisposing to patellar chondropathy and patellar apicitis in athletes. Int Orthop 1986; 10(3):195–200.

71. Pritchett JW. Longitudinal growth and growth-plate activity in the lower extremity. Clin Orthop 1992; 275:274–279.

72. Paley D. Principles of Deformity Correction. Berlin: Springer; 2003.

73. Green WT, Anderson M. Epiphyseal arrest for the correction of discrepancies in length of the lower extremities. J Bone Joint Surg 1957; 39A:853–872.

74. Green WT, Anderson M. Experiences with epiphyseal arrest in correcting discrepancies in length of the lower extremities in infantile paralysis: A method of predicting the effect. J Bone Joint Surg Am 1947; 29:659–678.

75. Herzenberg JE, Paley D. Leg lengthening in children (Review). Curr Opin Pediatr 1998; 10(1):95–97.

76. Paley D, Tetsworth K. Mechanical axis deviation of the lower limbs. Preoperative planning of uniapical angular deformities of the tibia or femur. Clin Orthop Relat Res 1992; 280: 48–64.

77. Paley D, Herzenberg JE, Tetsworth K, et al. Deformity planning for frontal and sagittal plane corrective osteotomies. Orthop Clin North Am 1994; 25(3):425–465.

78. Greulich WW, Pyle SI. Radiographic atlas of skeletal development of the hand and wrist, 2nd ed. Stanford CA: Stanford University Press; 1959.

79. Sempé M, Pavia C. Atlas de la maturation squelettique: ossification séquentielle du poignet et de la main. Paris: SIMEP; 1979.

80. Diméglio A, Charles YP, Daures JP, et al. Accuracy of the Sauvegrain method in determining skeletal age during puberty. J Bone Joint Surg Am 2005; 87(8):1689–1696.

81. Greulich JW, Pyle SI. Radiographic Atlas of Skeletal Development of the Hand and Wrist, 2nd ed. Stanford: Stanford University Press; 1959.

82. Tanner JM, Whitehouse RH. Clinical longitudinal standards for height, weight, height velocity, weight velocity and stages of puberty. Arch Dis Child 1976; 51(3):170–179.

83. Moseley CF. A straight line graph for leg length discrepancies. J Bone Joint Surg Am 1977; 59:174–179.

84. Westh RN, Menelaus MB. A simple calculation for the timing of epiphysial arrest: a further report. Bone Joint Surg Br 1981; 63-B(1):117–119.

85. Bailey N, Pinneau SR. Tables for predicting adult height from skeletal age, revised for Greulich and Pyle hand standards. J. Pediatr 1952; 40:423–441.

86. Little DG, Nigo L, Aiona MD. Deficiencies of current methods for the timing of epiphysiodesis. J Pediatr Orthop 1996; 16: 173–179.

87. Anderson M, Green WT, Messner MB. Growth and predictions of growth in the lower extremities. J Bone Joint Surg Am 1963; 45:1–14.2.

88. Timperlake RW, Bowen JR, Guille JT, Choi IH. Prospective evaluation of fifty-three consecutive percutaneous epiphysiodeses of the distal femur and proximal tibia and fibula. J Pediatr Orthop 1991; 11:350–357.

89. Canale ST, Christian CA. Techniques for epiphysiodesis about the knee. Clin Orthop Rel Res 1990; 255:81–85.

90. Macnicol MF, Gupta M. Epiphysiodesis using a cannulated tube-saw. J Bone Joint Surg Br 1997; 97B:307–309.

91. Macnicol MF. Tubesaw epiphysiodesis. In: Tachdjian MO, ed. Atlas of Pediatric Orthopaedic Surgery. Philadelphia: WB Saunders; 1994.

92. Phemister DB. Epiphysiodesis for equalizing the length of the lower extremities and for correcting other deformities of the skeleton. Mem Acad Chir Paris 1950; 76(26–27): 758–763.

93. Codivilla A. On the means of lengthening in the lower limbs, the muscles and the tissues which are shortened through deformity. Am J Orthop Surg 1905; 2:353–369.

94. Bastiani G, Aldegheri R, Renzi-Brivio L, Trivella G. Chondrodiatalsis—controlled symmetrical distraction of the epiphyseal plate: limb lengthening in children. J Bone Joint Surg 1986; 688:550–556.

95. De Bastiani G, Aldegheri R, Renzio-Vrivio L, Trivella G. Limb lengthening by callus distraction (callotasis). J Pediatr Orthop 1987; 7:129–134.

96. Ilizarov GA. Clinical application of the tension-stress effect for limb lengthening. Clin Orthop Rel Res 1980; 258:8.

97. Ilizarov GA, Deviatov A. Operative elongation of the leg. Ortopedica Travmatologiia Prpteptezirovanie 1971; 32:20–25.

98. Taylor JC. Taylor spatial frame. In: Rozbruch SR, Ilizarov S, eds. Limb Lengthening and Reconstruction Surgery. Informa Healthcare USA; 2007: 613–637.

99. Baumgart R, Betz A, Schweiberer L. A fully implantable motorized intramedullary nail for limb lengthening and bone transport. Clin Orthop Rel Res 1977; 343:135–143.

100. Ilizarov GA. The tension-stress effect on the genesis and growth of tissues. Part I: The influence of stability of fixation and soft-tissue preservation. Clin Orthop Rel Res 1989; 238: 249–281.

101. Ilizarov GA. The tension-stress effect on the genesis and growth of tissues. Part II: The influence of the rate and frequency of distraction. Clin Orthop Rel Res 1989; 239: 263–285.

102. Baig MR, Rajan M. Effects of smoking on the outcome of implant treatment: a literature review. Indian J Dent Res 2007 Oct-Dec, 18(4):190–5.

103. Götz J, Schellmann WD. Continuous lengthening of the femur with intramedullary stabilisation. Arch Orthop Unfallchir 1975; 82(4):305–310.

104. Baumann F, Harms J. The extension nail. A new method of the femur and tibia. Arch Orthop Unfallchir 1977; 90(2):139–146.

105. Witt AN, Jäger M. Results of animal experiments with an implantable femur distractor for operative leg lengthening. Arch Orthop Unfallchir 1977; 88(3):273–279.

106. Bliskunov AI. Implantable devices for lengthening the femur without external drive mechanisms. Med Tekh 1984; (2): 44–49.

107. Bliskunov AI. Lengthening of the femur using implantable appliances. Acta Chir Orthop Traumatol Cech 1984; 51(6): 454–466.

108. Bliskunov AI. Intramedullary distraction of the femur (preliminary report). Ortop Travmatol Protez 1983; 10:59–62.

109. Guichet J, Deromedis B, Donnan L, et al. Gradual femoral length-ening with the Albizzia intramedullary nail. J Bone Joint Surg Am 2003; 85-A:838–848.

110. Cole J, Justin D, Kasparis T, et al. The intramedullary skeletal kinetic distractor: first clinical results of a new intramedullary nail for lengthening of the femur and tibia. Injury 2001; 32 Suppl 4:SD1229–1239.

111. Baumgart R, Zeiler C, Kettler M, Weiss S, Schweiberer L (1999) Der voll implantierbare Distraktionsmarknagel bei Verkürzungen, Deformitäten und Knochendefekten. Indikationsspektrum. Orthopäde 28: 1058–65.

112. Paley D. Problems, obstacles, and complications of limb length-ening by the Ilizarov technique. Clin Orthop 1990; 250: 81–104.

Chapter 25

The Limping Child

F. Stig Jacobsen and Göran Hansson

Introduction

Evaluating a limp in a growing child is a problem often faced by paediatricians, accident and emergency department doctors, general practitioners, and orthopaedic surgeons. There are many causes, ranging from surgical emergencies to children who need observation only [1]. It is often not possible to know with certainty how serious the condition is at the initial examination, and so it is important to adopt a systematic approach to evaluation.

The aim of this chapter is to give an overview of the limping child, to discuss the important points in the history and physical examination, to suggest appropriate imaging and laboratory tests, and to describe the most common causes. Treatment will be dealt with in the relevant chapters.

History

The history of a limp is just as important as the findings on physical examination. If the right questions are asked a provisional diagnosis can be made in most cases at the primary examination. Although the history may be difficult to obtain from a toddler it is usually possible to identify the specific anatomical area involved at the initial examination. The commonest site for symptoms in the limping child is the hip (34%), followed by the knee (19%), the remainder of the leg (18%), and the spine (fewer than 2%) [2]. Most children presenting with a limp have pain [2]. The likelihood of referred pain is greater in children than in adults [3]: pain from the spine may be referred to the thigh or the abdomen and hip pain is very often referred to the thigh or the knee.

The patient's age is important. Fractures and infection are seen in all age groups but some conditions are more age-specific (Table 25.1). Child abuse is most commonly seen in children under the age of 2 years, Legg–Calvé–Perthes' disease between 4 and 8 years, and a slipped capital femoral epiphysis is in adolescence.

A family history, past medical history, and details of previous treatment must be obtained together with an assessment of the child's general health.

The onset of fever should be noted, when it started, its variability, and whether the child is receiving any antipyretic medication or antibiotics. A preceding illness was found by Fischer and Beattie [2] in about 40% of children who presented with an acute limp.

It is important to determine whether the onset of the limp was sudden, as in trauma, or whether it came on gradually,

Table 25.1 Age-Specific Diagnosis of a Limp

Age	Condition
1–3 years	Developmental dysplasia of the hip
	Child abuse
	Tumor
	Neuromuscular disease
	Juvenile idiopathic arthritis
	Leg length discrepancy
	Infections
4–10 years	Transient synovitis
	Legg–Calvé–Perthes disease
	Leg length discrepancy
	Tumor
	Juvenile idiopathic arthritis
	Infections
	Köhler's disease
Greater than 10 years	Slipped capital femoral epiphysis
	Overuse syndrome such as
	Anterior knee pain: Osgood–Schlatter's disease
	Shin splints
	Tarsal coalition
	Heel pain
All age groups	Trauma
	Tumor
	Infection

F.S. Jacobsen (✉)
Orthopaedics Department, Marshfield Clinic, Marshfield, WI, USA

M. Benson et al. (eds.), *Children's Orthopaedics and Fractures*,
DOI 10.1007/978-1-84882-611-3_25, © Springer-Verlag London Limited 2010

which is typical of chronic disease. A history of trauma or a change in activity may prompt suspicion of a fracture or stress reaction. It is essential to ask about the duration of the limp and any aggravating factors. Juvenile idiopathic arthritis usually presents with limp and stiffness which are more marked in the early morning when the child gets out of bed. Neuromuscular problems are usually worse toward the end of the day because of muscle fatigue. Constant pain during the entire day and night should raise concern about a possible tumor.

Gait

Physical examination should start by observing the child's gait. The physician must therefore be familiar with normal gait patterns and motor development in children (Chapter 6).

Most children under 1 year are able to stand unassisted and cruise and are able to walk before 18 months. The toddler, however, has an immature gait that differs from that of the adult [4] and walks on a broad base in an abrupt and choppy fashion, with a faster cadence (steps/minute) but a slower velocity (cm/second) than the adult.

Fully mature gait is usually attained by 4 years and all subsequent changes in gait are related to change in height [4].

When examining gait the child should be wearing a minimum of clothing and must walk barefooted. Where possible the patient should be seen walking and running unassisted in a large room or a corridor which accentuates any pathological features of gait. To detect muscle weakness it is important to watch the child getting up unaided from the floor and climbing stairs.

The different components of the gait cycle should each receive attention with focus placed sequentially on the feet, the knees, and the hips. Often the child tries to walk normally and the abnormality of gait is seen only when the child thinks he or she is unobserved.

Pathological Gait

A child's limp may be caused by *pain, stiffness, structural change, weakness*, or a combination of these.

Antalgic Gait

The most common limp is antalgic (anti-pain), when the child "hurries off" the affected leg, so limiting the time spent upon it in the stance phase [5]. This is associated with a shorter swing phase on the opposite leg and a decreased stride length [6]. An antalgic gait can be due to any painful condition such as trauma, transient synovitis, and infection.

If the spine is affected the child walks carefully and slowly avoiding trunk rotation that exacerbates pain.

Leg Length Discrepancy Gait

The patient with a leg length discrepancy compensates either by walking on tiptoe on the short side or with slight hip and knee flexion on the long side, in an endeavor to balance leg length.

Trendelenburg Gait

A Trendelenburg gait is a painless limp in a patient with either weak hip abductor muscles or an unstable hip fulcrum. In the stance phase, the opposite side of the pelvis drops. To compensate, the child leans over the affected hip. Bilateral involvement causes a waddling gait with a bilateral lurch. The time spent in the stance phase on the affected leg is normal, as pain is often absent. A typical Trendelenburg gait is seen in developmental dysplasia of the hip or in those hip problems in which overgrowth of the greater trochanter weakens the hip abductors.

Gait in Cerebral Palsy

The gait pattern in cerebral palsy depends on the specific brain lesion, secondary muscle contractures, and compensatory movements (see Chapters 6 and 19). Tightness in the gastrocnemius–soleus complex and the hamstrings often causes toe walking and secondary flexion of the knee during stance. Rotational malalignment of femur or tibia leads to in or out toeing and tight adductors to scissoring. Relative weakness of the gastrocnemius–soleus complex causes a typical crouched gait, with increased flexion of the hips and the knees. A spastic rectus femoris muscle can give rise to a stiff knee gait, with difficulties of foot clearance during the swing phase.

Gait in Muscular Dystrophy

The muscle weakness in many muscular dystrophy patients causes a very characteristic posture and gait (see Chapter 16). Duchenne's muscular dystrophy, with early and striking proximal hip extensor weakness, causes hip flexion contractures and a secondary lumbar lordosis which brings the centre of gravity over the hip. The child tiptoes because of tightness and early contracture of the gastrocnemius–soleus complex with a wide, waddling Trendelenburg gait.

Physical Examination

Standing

With the patient standing the back should be examined for scoliosis, local tenderness, and range of motion. The whole spine must be visible. If a pelvic tilt is present it can be corrected by placing blocks under the shorter leg until the pelvis is level. A positive Trendelenburg test may indicate hip dysplasia, the sequelae of Legg–Calvé–Perthes' disease, or slipped capital femoral epiphysis. Spine motion should be tested as it will be limited with discitis and extension will be painful with spondylolysis.

Cutaneous changes such as skin dimples and hairy patches over the lumbar spine, erythema, or heat over joints should be noted. Café au lait spots, particularly in the axillae, should lead to the suspicion of neurofibromatosis or fibrous dysplasia.

Supine

With the patient supine each joint should be examined separately. Look for swelling, feel for tenderness, and assess movement. Hip flexion contracture can be judged by Thomas's test. The abdomen should always be examined, as conditions such as appendicitis can occasionally present as a limp [7].

A full neurological examination should be performed to assess atrophy, muscle strength and tone, sensation, and reflexes. Atrophy of the quadriceps muscle is often associated with a painful hip or knee and correlates with the duration of symptoms.

The examiner should check for leg length discrepancy by measuring the distance from the anterior superior spine to the medial malleolus, in addition to examining the patient standing to look for a pelvic tilt. A short leg must be distinguished from apparent shortening that is caused by scoliosis with pelvic obliquity or joint contracture. Rarely the longer leg, whether true or apparent, is the abnormal one.

Prone

Hip rotation in extension is best tested with the patient prone. The knees are flexed to 90 and the tibiae used as lever arms. The amount of internal and external rotation can easily be measured and any asymmetry detected. Limited painful internal rotation of the hip suggests synovitis of the hip joint or a slipped capital femoral epiphysis. Further, with the patient prone, femoral anteversion can be measured and tibial torsion evaluated by measuring the foot–thigh angle.

Diagnostic Investigations

Blood Tests

Most of these are nonspecific. Appropriate tests depend on the patient's history and physical examination. Any patient with fever or possible infection should have a complete blood count, white blood count, erythrocyte sedimentation rate (ESR), and C-reactive protein (CRP) tests performed. Blood cultures are important and should ideally be taken at fever peaks.

An ESR of 50 mm/h or more strongly suggests serious disease in children who present with a limp [8]. The C-reactive protein concentration usually increases and subsequently decreases more rapidly than the ESR. It is, therefore, more useful for assessing the efficacy of treatment [9]. In children in whom an arthritic etiology is suspected, rheumatoid factor, antinuclear antibodies, HLA B27, and Lyme titre should be checked, although many of these may be negative in the early stages of the disease.

Joint Aspiration

Joint effusions should always be aspirated when infection is suspected. The aspirate should be sent for Gram staining, aerobic and anaerobic culture, a cell count, and glucose determination (compared with blood glucose levels).

Diagnostic Imaging

Plain Radiographs

These are readily accessible, inexpensive, and specific for a whole range of disorders such as tumor, infection, or fracture [10] (see Chapter 5). Although they give information on bone pathology they may not show early changes and give limited information about soft tissue and cartilage. There are many conditions, therefore, not detectable by radiograph alone [11].

Simple radiological examination should be undertaken first. An anteroposterior and a lateral view are always necessary. A comparative view of the contralateral limb is often useful. Specific radiographs may be necessary (e.g., oblique radiographs of the lumbar spine may show a pars interarticularis defect; a lateral view of the hip is always necessary in suspected slipped capital femoral epiphysis; a tunnel view for osteochondritis dissecans of the knee; oblique radiographs of the foot to show calcaneonavicular coalition).

Bone Scintigraphy

This uses a tracer, technetium-99m-labeled methylene diphosphate, which is concentrated in areas of osteoblastic activity. It is a nonspecific test that highlights areas of increased bone metabolism.

Bone scintigraphy may detect subtle abnormalities such as stress fractures before they are evident on plain radiograph. It cannot differentiate between different diseases but helps to indicate the anatomical area involved [12]. Aronson et al. [13] found bone scans of great value in a group of limping children in whom the diagnosis was in doubt.

A bone scan need not always show increased activity to be positive. A photon-deficient (cold) scan may be seen in osteomyelitis, particularly in the neonate. The rapid progression of bacterial infection in bone and subperiosteum can cause increased intraosseous pressure and decreased blood flow. Affected patients have aggressive osteomyelitis and need urgent treatment [14].

Ultrasound Imaging

Ultrasound of the hip shows the relationship of the cartilaginous femoral head to the acetabulum. It also offers dynamic evaluation of hip stability without irradiation. The child does not require sedation.

Ultrasound is invaluable in assessing hip effusions and synovitis, as seen in transient synovitis, Legg–Calvé–Perthes' disease, or juvenile idiopathic arthritis. The normal hip capsule appears concave but, with an effusion, it balloons out and becomes convex. A 2-mm separation between the femoral neck and the joint capsule is diagnostic (Fig. 25.1) [15].

Ultrasonography is very useful in checking for an effusion in all limb joints. Early subperiosteal collections of fluid or pus in osteomyelitis are detectable well before lamellar new bone can be seen on radiograph. It also helps to guide aspiration.

Computed Tomography (CT)

This determines more precisely the anatomy of an area involved and is particularly useful in osteoid osteoma, in evaluating a tarsal coalition or the patellofemoral joint and, of course, in some tumors.

Magnetic Resonance Imaging

Magnetic resonance imaging (MRI) is an expensive and highly sophisticated tool capable of providing a great deal of information. It can be useful in the early diagnosis of Legg–Calvé–Perthes' disease, avascular necrosis, and in the assessment of tumors and infections. However, most young children will require sedation or anesthesia.

Causes of Limping

Trauma is by far the most common reason for a child to limp. The etiology of non-traumatic causes of limping varies, but is often inflammatory (Table 25.2). In one review, 23% of

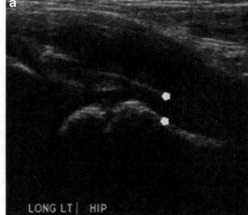
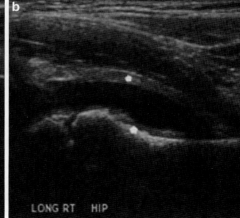

Fig. 25.1 Ultrasonography of the hips in a 3-year-old with a right antalgic limp.**(a)** The left hip shows a normal hip joint space between the two markers. **(b)** The right (painful) hip shows an effusion with a distended bulging joint capsule between the two markers compatible with *transient synovitis*

Table 25.2 Differential diagnosis of acute atraumatic limp after Fischer & Beattie [2]

Cause	Frequency in %
Inflammatory	
Tansient synovitis	39,5
Juvenile arthritis, viral illness	3,2
Infection	3,6
Developmental or acquired (LCP, SUFE etc)	4,1
Neoplasia	0,8
Muscle strain, overuse	17,7
Others (torsion of testis, orchitis etc)	1,2
No definite diagnosis made	29,9
	100,0

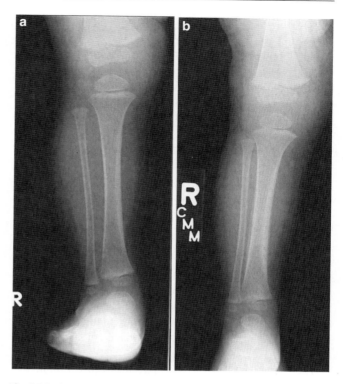

Fig. 25.2 (a) Normal radiograph of an 18-month-old boy with a limp and slight tenderness of the lower tibia. He was treated in a cast on suspicion of a fracture. (b) Radiograph 2 weeks later showing the periosteal elevation typical of a healing *toddler's fracture*

children younger than 5 years who presented with a limp or refusal to bear weight proved to have a severe bacterial infection [16].

In the differential diagnosis of acute limp without obvious trauma the majority is caused by transient synovitis. In almost 30% of children a definite diagnosis could not be found. (Table 25.2)

Trauma

Fractures

They are usually apparent clinically and radiologically. They require appropriate treatment by reduction if necessary and immobilization.

A toddler tibial fracture is a common reason for limping. It is a low energy, usually non-displaced, fracture of the tibia without concomitant fibula fracture. The parents often do not recall trauma. The child presents with a limp or refusal to weight bear. The initial radiograph is often negative but follow-up radiographs a week or two later usually show the fracture or periosteal elevation (Fig. 25.2). Treatment consists of a cast immobilization. Similarly in the toddler a fracture of the calcaneus may be difficult to diagnose and to see on plain radiographs unless an axial view is taken.

Stress Fractures

These are a common cause of limping in children, especially in adolescence. When seen in otherwise normal bone they are the result of increased or repetitive muscle action rather than direct impact [17]. Bone responds to excessive stress by remodeling and resorption and eventually by increased bone formation. A stress fracture develops when the fatigue process exceeds the bone repair process.

Fractures may also occur as a result of normal physiological stresses in bones with deficient elastic resistance [17]. These insufficiency fractures may occur in bone tumors,

osteogenesis imperfecta, rickets, or the osteoporosis associated with immobilization or cerebral palsy. Anatomical conditions may also predispose to stress fracture; for instance a rigid cavus or flat foot may fail to absorb energy normally.

The most common site for a stress fracture is the tibia, which accounts for up to 50% of all cases [18]. The fractures, which occur most frequently in 10–15-year-olds, are usually located between the metaphysis and diaphysis of the proximal tibia, either on the posteromedial or on the posterolateral corner. The fibula is the second most common site of stress fracture, usually in a younger age group. Stress fractures also occur in the metatarsals, calcaneum, pelvis, and femur (see Chapter 38).

Stress fractures are most common in younger children in spring, when activity levels increase after an inactive winter. In the adolescent, when the bone elasticity of the young is decreasing, stress fractures develop during or after athletic activities.

Symptoms depend on the stress fracture site but the most common complaint is pain related to activity, relieved by rest, and associated with an antalgic gait. Local swelling and tenderness may be present. There is often a history of increased or changed activity or a change of shoes or running surface. Radiographs initially show a small cortical lucency followed by a gradual increase in periosteal and endosteal bone formation. These findings may take up to 3 weeks to appear depending on the patient's age.

A bone scan is useful in the early detection of a stress fracture before other radiological changes occur. MRI and CT may help to establish the diagnosis in difficult cases. The differential diagnoses include tumors such as osteoid osteoma and Ewing's sarcoma. Biopsy can be misleading because the changes of fracture repair may be hard to differentiate from a tumor.

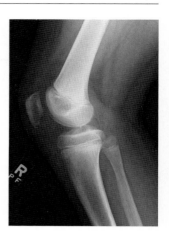

Fig. 25.3 Lateral knee radiograph of 12-year-old boy with a painful limp and tenderness over the distal patellar pole. The small avulsion at the inferior pole represents *Sinding–Larsen–Johansson disease*

Overuse Syndromes

Increasing numbers of children now participate in organized sport. This increase is matched by the numbers who present with overuse syndromes, often with a painful limp. Overuse injuries often occur where tendons, ligaments, muscles, and bone adjoin. Children who have recently undergone a significant growth spurt have less flexibility and are more prone to injury.

The following overuse syndromes may cause a limp:

1. *Spondylolysis* is a stress fracture of the pars interarticularis common in sports such as gymnastics, rowing, diving, weightlifting, bowling, and throwing.
2. *Iliac apophysitis* may be seen in adolescent runners. It is also called a "hip pointer" and presents with pain over the iliac crest one hands breadth behind the anterior superior iliac spine [19]. Avulsion of a pelvic apophysis may follow violent contraction of the hamstrings, adductors, or the iliopsoas and is common in jumping and sprinting. Pain and tenderness are localized in the groin or buttock and the diagnosis is confirmed by radiograph. Non-weight-bearing with crutches is usually the only treatment necessary.
3. *Osgood–Schlatter's disease* is the most common condition around the knee. It is a stress-related partial avulsion injury of the tibial tubercle, with inflammatory changes and swelling. It occurs most commonly in boys between 10 and 15 years, with symptoms of local pain, swelling, and discomfort with activity. Radiographs show soft tissue swelling and fragmentation of the tibial tubercle.
4. *Sinding–Larsen–Johansson disease* causes anterior knee pain and is probably caused by excessive and repetitive traction on the inferior pole of the patella. It is also seen in patients with cerebral palsy and a "crouch gait." There is usually striking tenderness of the inferior pole of the patella (Fig. 25.3).

5. *Patellofemoral pain* is common in girls and often occurs in association with increased femoral anteversion, knee valgus, external tibial torsion, etc. It may or may not be associated with patellar instability and tracking needs to be carefully checked.
6. *Sever's disease* (Haglund's disease) is characterized by pain and tenderness at the tendo Achilles insertion into the calcaneal apophysis. It is usually chronic and related to activity. Although plain radiographs may show fragmentation of the calcaneal apophysis this may be a normal finding in this age group and is nonspecific.

When an overuse syndrome is correctly diagnosed, treatment is usually pain control and activity modification followed by rehabilitation.

Child Abuse

This must be considered when a child is in pain or limps with no clear cause, particularly if the child is younger than 2 years. It should be considered in a child with a questionable history of trauma or a delay in presenting to the physician. It is important to look for other manifestations such as bruises and burns. The matter is considered in more detail in Chapter 42.

No single lesion is specific for child abuse but certain fracture patterns are suggestive. Fractures before walking age, metaphyseal corner fractures, and multiple fractures at different stages of healing should all alert concern. Spiral fractures of the humerus, femur, and tibia, together with inexplicable rib fractures, should prompt a search for others by skeletal survey. If abuse is suspected the abuse team must be notified. It is, of course, important to rule out other causes of fracture such as fibrous dysplasia, osteogenesis imperfecta.

Inflammatory Synovitis

Transient Synovitis of The Hip

Transient synovitis is the most common cause of hip pain in children [20]. Synonyms include "irritable hip," "observation hip," and "coxalgia fugax." It is a noninfective synovitis characterized by a sudden onset of hip pain and limp in a child who is not systemically ill. Children, more commonly boys, aged 3–8 years are the most vulnerable. The accumulated risk of suffering transient synovitis before 14 years has been shown to be 3% [21]. Repeated episodes occur in 10%, usually within 6 months of the first episode [22].

Etiology

The cause is unknown but trauma, infection, and allergy have been implicated. An infectious etiology is supported by the finding that children have often had a preceding viral upper respiratory tract infection and that the synovitis is seen most often in the autumn, when the incidence of viral infection is high.

Clinical Findings

The child may present with only a limp but may complain of pain in hip, thigh, or knee. Hip movement may vary from slightly to very considerably restricted and some children cannot bear weight.

The patient is usually afebrile but may have a temperature of up to 38–39°C without being systemically ill. The hip joint is typically held in flexion and abduction to accommodate an effusion in the joint. Internal rotation of the hip is limited and painful, the most consistent finding in transient synovitis and is best looked for with the patient prone [23].

The synovitis commonly lasts for only a few days and there is usually complete resolution of the symptoms. The long-term effects of transient synovitis are probably benign [24]. In a long-term follow-up of 23 patients De Valderrama [25] found that up to 50% developed coxa magna, with a slight risk of developing arthritis in the involved hip. However, 67% of his patients spent 3–5 months in hospital, which suggests a more severe disorder than our present concept of "transient synovitis."

It has been postulated that transient synovitis is a precursor of Legg–Calvé–Perthes' disease [26]. Kallio et al. [27], however, found no case of Legg–Calvé–Perthes' disease after 1 year in their study of 119 children with transient synovitis. They suggest that cases described in the literature were examples of early stage Legg–Calvé–Perthes'. While some

recommend a radiograph of the hip 3 months after the synovitis to exclude Legg–Calvé–Perthes', this is not justified in the asymptomatic child.

Investigations

Conventional *radiographs* are normal in typical transient synovitis. Apparent capsular distension and lost fat planes depend on rotation of the leg and are not true indicators of an effusion.

Ultrasound is the method of choice for diagnosing a joint effusion. Intracapsular synovitis and fluid can be directly visualized and measured. The child is positioned supine with the leg in the neutral position. Anterior ultrasonography shows the distance between the femoral neck and the anterior joint capsule (Fig. 25.1). A full blood count, ESR, and CRP may reassure that there is no infection.

Treatment

This is symptomatic, resting in bed with the hip flexed or non-weight-bearing with crutches and anti-inflammatory medication. Unless infection is suspected children should not need hospital admission. When the hip is very irritable, an ultrasound-guided hip aspiration allows the synovial fluid to be analyzed for infection and swiftly relieves discomfort.

Differential Diagnosis

It may be difficult to distinguish transient synovitis from other hip disorders. Early Legg–Calvé–Perthes' disease is clinically similar to transient synovitis. Initial radiographic changes in Legg–Calvé–Perthes' may be subtle. When in doubt a bone scan or MRI may help to distinguish them.

Juvenile idiopathic arthritis, if seronegative, may initially be difficult to diagnose, but the insidious onset and protracted course serve to distinguish it.

Other diagnoses to be considered include osteoid osteoma of the proximal femur with reactive synovitis, slipped capital femoral epiphysis in its early stages, or bone or soft tissue infections in the pelvis. Plain radiographs are rarely diagnostic and MRI or bone scintigraphy may be useful (Fig. 25.4).

The critical differential diagnosis of transient synovitis is *septic arthritis,* which may need urgent drainage and systemic antibiotics. The clinical findings may be similar, but a high temperature is uncommon in transient synovitis. In one study, 97% of children with septic arthritis had an ESR greater than 20 mm/h, a temperature of more than 37.5°C, or both [28]. There is, however, an overlap in the parameters and in the same study 47% of the patients with transient synovitis

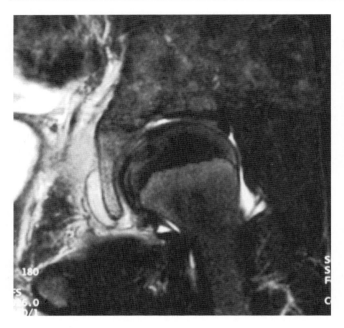

Fig. 25.4 MRI of an 11-year-old with a limp and a temperature of 38°C. There was slight tenderness over the left hip but normal movement. Radiographs and ultrasound images were normal but the MRI shows an *abscess on the inner side of the acetabulum*

Table 25.3 Four-parameter* assessment for septic arthritis [29]

Number of parameters present	Probability for septic arthritis (%)
0	0.2
1	3.0
2	40.0
3	93.1
4	99.6

*Fever >38.5°; non-weight-bearing; ESR > 40 mm/h; white blood count > 12,000 cells/mm³

had similar positive parameters. The C-reactive protein value guides the clinician better but the general rule is that any child with a fever and an increased ESR should be suspected of having septic arthritis.

In one study Kocher et al. [29] considered four independent parameters to distinguish between the two entities (Table 25.3).

The consequences of overlooking septic arthritis can be devastating: patients with two or more positive parameters should have the affected joint aspirated.

Juvenile Idiopathic Arthritis

This generalized systemic arthritis differs from adult rheumatoid arthritis in both course and prognosis. Subgroups are described on the basis of joint involvement and systemic disease. The condition is considered in detail in Chapter 13.

Juvenile idiopathic arthritis often presents with single joint involvement. The onset is usually gradual and less severe than that seen in infection. If the lower extremity is involved, the child may present with an antalgic limp, joint swelling, and slight discomfort. The diagnosis is often made by exclusion and blood tests may help. If the joint is aspirated the cell count is usually 2,000–50,000 cells/mm³ range, whereas in infection the count usually exceeds 50,000.

Reactive Arthritis

This describes a systemic disease not limited to joints alone, despite its name. Reactive arthritis is a response to infection elsewhere in the body, such as the upper airway, gastrointestinal, or urogenital tracts. It is probably autoimmune and results from a crossover reaction between synovial and infectious antigens. The knee, ankle, or hip is usually involved and the patient feels unwell and feverish. The arthritis develops acutely with severe pain and there is often a migratory polyarthritis. If the condition follows a group A streptococcal pharyngitis it can be diagnosed by the presence of an antibody response to group A streptococcus, usually 1–2 weeks after the infection.

The clinical presentation can mimic septic arthritis [30] and may warrant joint aspiration. The joint fluid is sterile but the white blood cell count in the joint fluid is frequently increased.

The reactive arthritis group of diseases merges with others such as Reiter's syndrome and ankylosing spondylitis. In the spondyloarthropathies, the sacroiliac joint is frequently involved and peripheral joint symptoms occur in most children. An enthesopathy, with pain and tenderness at tendon–bone junctions, offers an early diagnostic clue. The inflammation at these sites is often striking and causes a significant limp. The strong association with a positive HLA B27 suggests a genetic factor. Reactive arthritis may also follow acute rheumatic fever and enteric infections from bacteria such as *Shigella, Salmonella*, and *Yersinia*.

Virus infections may also give rise to reactive arthritis or arthralgia. This usually lasts for 1–2 weeks and may be migratory. It may follow rubella infection or immunization, alphavirus infection, or herpes virus infection.

Reactive arthritis is often a diagnosis of exclusion.

Infections

Osteomyelitis

Osteomyelitis occurs at any age in childhood (see Chapter 10) and is caused by the hematological spread of bacteria which usually seed in the metaphyses of long bones, especially those of the femur, the pelvis, and the tibia [31]. Osteomyelitis of the pelvis or upper femur is often adjacent to the hip and can present with hip pain and gait disturbance [32]. Established infections in bone can spread into the adjacent joint, either through the epiphysis in very young children or in the hip, directly from the intracapsular metaphysis. It is important always to examine adjacent joints, as 30% of patients have associated septic joint involvement [33].

Pelvic osteomyelitis presents with fever, pain, and limping. There may be localized tenderness. Most patients have pain and reduced hip movement, which is less marked than in septic arthritis of the hip. If the abscess is located in the obturator internus muscle it can easily be mistaken for septic arthritis of the hip (see Fig. 25.4) [34]. Radiographic changes develop late and ultrasound, MRI, or bone scan allow much earlier diagnosis.

Subacute osteomyelitis is becoming more common. The patient often presents with a painful limp but the diagnosis is frequently delayed as the symptoms develop slowly, the patient is afebrile, and laboratory tests are often normal (Fig. 25.5).

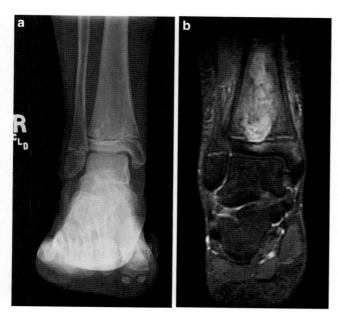

Fig. 25.5 (**a**) Radiograph of a 14-year-old boy's ankle showing a lytic lesion in the distal tibial metaphysis. He gave a 7-week history of a limp and pain but had no fever and only slight tenderness. (**b**) MRI shows the lesion crossing the physis with some edema in the epiphysis. Surgery confirmed *subacute osteomyelitis*

Septic Arthritis

Prompt, accurate diagnosis is essential to allow early treatment and obtain optimal results (see Chapter 10). Septic arthritis of the hip, knee, and ankle account for more than 90% of all cases [1.]

The patient is usually febrile, with a temperature greater than 38°C, and presents with a painful joint that is warm and red with limited, painful movement. In early childhood the fever can be absent or mild. The child who has received antibiotics or is immunodeficient may lack typical symptoms and signs. If the hip joint is involved it is held flexed, abducted, and externally rotated. All movement is restricted and pain may give rise to "pseudoparalysis," especially in infants. Groin or proximal thigh swelling will often be present.

The differential diagnoses include transient synovitis, juvenile idiopathic arthritis, osteomyelitis, Lyme disease, Legg–Calvé–Perthes' disease, and slipped capital femoral epiphysis. Plain radiographs are usually normal in early septic arthritis, although subtle subluxation of the hip occurs early in infants. Even osteomyelitis may be radiologically invisible for many days. The definitive test for septic arthritis of any joint is aspiration, usually guided by ultrasound.

In infection, the joint fluid is usually cloudy with a cell count of more than 50,000 cells/mm³, most being polymorphonuclear cells. In joint infection and acute rheumatoid arthritis, the synovial fluid glucose level is characteristically lowered. Bacteriological culture is positive in only 30–80%. Patients with negative cultures run a clinical course similar to those with positive cultures and should receive the same aggressive treatment [35].

The treatment of septic arthritis in the hip is immediate open drainage and irrigation. It should be regarded as an orthopaedic emergency, because of the possible severe sequelae. These include avascular necrosis of the femoral head, subluxation or dislocation, and growth plate injury. A good outcome depends on prompt decompression. Complications are more frequent in infants under 6 months old, when treatment is delayed for more than 2–3 days and with adjacent osteomyelitis of the proximal femur. The knee and ankle must be treated depending on disease duration and the response to antibiotics, with repeat aspirations, arthroscopic drainage, or arthrotomy.

Discitis

This disc space disease ranges from a benign self-limiting inflammation to a true osteomyelitis involving adjacent bone [36]. It is usually seen in younger children aged 2–6 years (see Chapter 35). The cause of infection is probably bacterial but may, in milder cases, be viral.

The young child usually presents with a limp or refusal to walk or sit, whereas in the older child back or neck pain is more common. If the patient is walking the gait is stiff and guarded.

Physical examination shows a rigid spine with loss of the lumbar lordosis, muscle spasm, and limited straight leg-raising. The ESR and white blood count are usually increased. Plain radiographs are negative in the first 3–6 weeks of the disease but disc space narrowing and erosion of the vertebral bodies may develop later. Bone scintigraphy may help but MRI seems more reliable in establishing an early diagnosis. MRI is probably the best imaging modality for any child with inexplicable back pain.

Pyogenic sacroiliitis may present as back or hip pain and the patient may have a limp [37]. An epidural abscess can, in the early stages, present in a similar fashion [38].

Psoas Abscess

A psoas abscess is uncommon in countries where tuberculosis is no longer endemic but may occur with infections of the spine or abdomen. The child has a painful limp and a hip flexion contracture. Psoas contracture may be seen following an intramuscular bleed in hemophilia or in patients on anticoagulants. Diagnosis is helped by ultrasound and MRI [39].

Lyme Disease

Lyme disease is caused by the spirochete *Borrelia burgdorferi* and is transmitted to humans by the bite of an infected tick.

While presentation varies greatly, the first sign is usually a circular rash—erythema migrans that appears in 75%. It appears from a few days to a month after the tick bite and can expand with a central clear zone giving a "bull's eye" appearance.

Early manifestations include fatigue, fever, cardiac irregularity, and Bell's palsy, with arthritis and polyneuropathy as later signs. Arthritis, however, can be an early sign and the disease should always be considered in areas where it is endemic [40]. Large joints such as the knee, ankle, or hip are usually affected and the symptoms and signs may resemble pauciarticular juvenile arthritis.

If an effusion is present, aspiration for diagnostic purposes is recommended as there is a considerable overlap in the clinical and laboratory presentation of Lyme disease and septic arthritis [41].

There are three types of antibody tests used to diagnose Lyme disease: enzyme-linked immunosorbent assay (ELISA), indirect fluorescent antibody (IFA), and the western blot test. The most commonly used is the ELISA, which is the most sensitive and rapid test; however, the western blot

test is the most specific and used to detect chronic Lyme disease. Most patients with acute Lyme disease can be treated successfully with a short course of oral antibiotics such as doxycycline, amoxicillin, or cefuroxime. Patients with cardiac or neurological involvement or chronic disease may need a longer period of treatment.

Other Causes of a Limp

Many common childhood hip problems present with a limp. A simple but valuable observation is that a healthy child with a limp should, until proven otherwise, be assumed to have hip dysplasia if younger than 4 years, Legg–Calvé–Perthes' disease if 4–9 years old, and a slipped upper femoral epiphysis if older than 9 years. These are discussed in detail in Chapters 26, 27, and 28, respectively.

Many "knee" symptoms are referred from the hip but there are mechanical disorders of the knee that cause a child to limp. These include patellar instability, dislocations, and osteochondrotic lesions (Chapter 29). Because the growth plates around the knee contribute most to growth, they are the most vulnerable to benign and malignant tumors.

At the foot and ankle, limping in an otherwise healthy child may be caused by osteochondritis dissecans, typically of the talar dome. Recurrent sprains, limping, and peroneal spasm with exercise are complications of a tarsal coalition. Osteochondritis of the navicular (Köhler's disease) and osteochondrosis of the head of the second metatarsal (Freiberg's disease) present with a limp and localized pain and tenderness. It is well to remember also that limping is sometimes caused by a foreign body in either the shoe or the soft tissues of the foot. Pseudomonas infection should be suspected if the child was wearing sneakers at the time of a puncture injury to the foot [42].

Köhler's disease is an avascular necrosis of the tarsal navicular, seen mainly in boys 3–8 years. Patients present with a limp and pain over the medial arch of the foot with local tenderness. Radiographs show a small sclerotic navicular. Fragmentation may be seen but in the absence of symptoms this is a normal variant.

Tumors

Fisher and Beattie [2] reported tumors as the cause of a limp in fewer than 1% of children. However, the possibility must be borne in mind as the consequences of a "missed" or late diagnosis can be very serious (see Chapter 14).

It is important to remember that the tumor causing a painful limp may not be in the lower extremity or pelvis: cerebral and spinal cord tumors may present with a limp [43].

Two tumors that often present with a limp are leukemia and osteoid osteoma. Patients with suspected tumors should

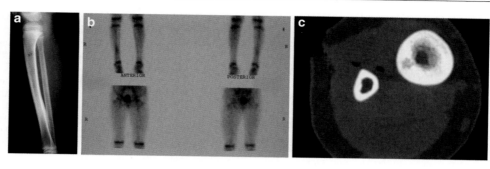

Fig. 25.6 Radiographs of a 7-year-old girl with a limp and right tibial tenderness. (**a**) Plain radiograph shows posterolateral cortical tibial thickening. (**b**) Bone scintigraphy shows increased uptake in the distal tibia. (**c**) CT scan illustrates a typical *osteoid osteoma*

have anteroposterior and lateral radiographs performed. Further studies such as bone scintigraphy, CT, and MRI will usually be necessary both for diagnosis and to stage the tumor.

Leukemia

Leukemia is the commonest childhood malignancy and may present at any age. The orthopaedic surgeon may see the patient first as some will present with a limp [44]. Clinical signs are vague but include fever, lethargy, bruising, and infection. Bone aches and joint pains are frequent and often present asymmetrically in the hips or knees. The symptoms may resemble those of juvenile idiopathic arthritis.

Radiological signs are nonspecific and include osteoporosis, periosteal reaction, sclerosis, or lytic lesions. Metaphyseal lucencies (leukemic lines) are often the first radiological change, commonly around the knee. However, this banding is nonspecific and can be seen also in malnutrition, juvenile idiopathic arthritis, and septicemia. Bone pain is caused by the proliferation of hemopoietic tissue within the medullary canal and may occur without any obvious radiological changes.

The patient will have anemia, thrombocytopenia, and an increased ESR. Surprisingly, about 50% have a low leucocyte count. The diagnosis is confirmed by bone marrow aspiration.

Osteoid Osteoma

This presents as a painful bone lesion in children usually over the age of 5 years. Most lesions are located in the lower limbs but can occur elsewhere (e.g., in the spine); the child presents with pain and a limp. Pain occurs after activity and typically at night, when it is relieved by aspirin.

There may be tenderness, increased warmth, and swelling if the tumor is superficial. The diagnosis can sometimes be made on plain radiographs, where periosteal thickening and endosteal sclerosis are seen. Bone scintigraphy shows increased uptake, but the nidus is best visualized with a CT scan (Fig. 25.6).

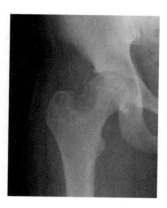

Fig. 25.7 Radiograph of the right hip of a 15-year-old boy who had limped for several months. The large lytic lesion in the femoral neck and greater trochanter was shown at biopsy to be an *aneurysmal bone cyst*

Histiocytosis-X (Langerhans' Cell Histiocytosis [LCH])

Eosinophil granuloma is the commonest of these. If in the lower extremity, it can cause pain and a limp. Spinal involvement may lead to vertebral body collapse (vertebra plana). There may be systemic upset in which case up to 20% may have pulmonary involvement.

Radiograph shows a lytic destructive lesion with a periosteal reaction which may mimic other tumors. CT scans and MRI may help but an unequivocal diagnosis can only be made by biopsy.

Bone Cysts

Unicameral bone cysts or aneurysmal bone cysts may present with a complete fracture or with a limp due to microfracture. The diagnosis is frequently not be made until a fracture occurs (Fig. 25.7).

References

1. Lawrence LL. The limping child. Emerg Med Clin North Am 1998; 16:4:911–929.
2. Fischer SU, Beattie TF. The limping child: Epidemiology, Assessment and Outcome. J Bone Joint Surg 1999; 81B 1029–1034.

3. Hensinger RN. Limp. Pediatr Clin North Am 1986; 33: 6:1355–1362.
4. Sutherland D. The development of mature gait. Gait Posture 1997; 6:163–170.
5. Dabney KW, Lipton G. Evaluation of limp in children. Curr Opinion Pediat 1995; 7:88–94.
6. Phillips WA. The child with a limp. Orthop Clin North Am 1987; 18:4:489–501.
7. Renshaw TS. The child who has a limp. Pediatr Rev 1995; 16: 12:458–465.
8. Huttenlocher A, Newman TB. Evaluation of the erythrocyte sedimentation rate in children presenting with limp, fever or abdominal pain. Clin Pediatr 1997; 339–344.
9. Unkila-Kallio L, Kallio MJT, Eskola J, Peltola, H. Serum C-reactive protein, erythrocyte sedimentation rate and white blood cell count in acute hematogenous osteomyelitis of children. Pediatrics 1994; 93:59–62.
10. Myers MT, Thompson GH. Imaging the child with a limp. Pediatr Clin North Am 1997; 44:3:637–658.
11. Blatt SD, Rosenthal BM, Barnhart, DC. Diagnostic utility of lower extremity radiographs of young children with gait disturbance. Pediatrics 1991; 87:138–140.
12. Connolly LP, Treves ST. Assessing the limping child with skeletal scintigraphy. J Nucl Med. 1998; 39:6:1056–1061.
13. Aronson J, Garvin K, Seibert J, et al. Efficiency of the bone scan for occult limping toddlers. J Pediatr Orthop 1992; 12: 38–44.
14. Pennington WT, Mott MP, Thometz JG, et al. Photopenic bone scan osteomyelitis: a clinical perspective. J Pediatr Orthop 1999; 19:695–698.
15. Terjesen T, Osthus P. Ultrasound in the diagnosis and follow-up of transient synovitis of the hip. J Pediatr Orthop 1991; 11:608–613.
16. Choban S, Killian JT. Evaluation of acute gait abnormalities in preschool children. J Pediatr Orthop 1990; 10:74–78.
17. Ogden JA. Skeletal Injury in a Child. Philadelphia: Lee & Febiger. 1982.
18. Walker RN, Green NE, Spindler KP. Stress fractures in skeletally immature patients. J Pediatr Orthop 1996; 16:578–584.
19. Lombardo SJ, Retting AC, Lerlan RK. Radiographic abnormalities of the iliac apophysis in adolescent athletes. J Bone Joint Surg 1983; 65A:444–455.
20. Bickerstaff DR, Neal LM, Brennan PO. An investigation into the etiology or irritable hip. Clin Pediatr 1991; 30:6:353–356.
21. Landin LA, Danielsson LG, Wattsgard C. Transient synovitis of the hip. J Bone Joint Surg 1987; 69B:238–242.
22. Illingworth CM. Recurrences of transient synovitis. Arch Dis Child 1983; 58:620–623.
23. Haueisen DC, Weiner SD. The characterization of "transient synovitis of the hip" in children. J Pediatr Orthop 1986; 6:11–17.
24. Sharwood PF. The irritable hip syndrome in children. Acta Orthop Scan 1981; 52:633–638.
25. DeValderrama JAP. The "observation hip" syndrome and its late sequelae. J Bone Joint Surg. 1963; 45B:462–470.
26. Winstrand H. Transient synovitis of the hip in the child. Acta Orthop Scand Suppl. 1986; 57:219.
27. Kallio P, Ryoppy S, Kunnamo I. Transient synovitis and Perthes disease. J Bone Joint Surg 1986; 68B:808–811.
28. DelBeccaro MA, Campoux AN, Bockers T, Mendelman, PM. Septic arthritis versus transient synovitis of the hip: the value of screening laboratory tests. Ann Emerg Med 1992; 21:1418–1422.
29. Kocher MS, Zurakowski D, Kasser JR. Differentiating between septic arthritis and transient synovitis of the hip in children: an evidence based clinical prediction algorithm. J Bone Joint Surg 1999; 81A:1662–1670.
30. Birdi N, Allen U, D' Astous J. Poststreptococcal reactive arthritis mimicking acute septic arthritis: a hospital-based study. J Pediatr Orthop 1995; 15:661–665.
31. Scott, RJ, Christofersen, MR, Robertson WW, Davidson RS, Rankin L, Drummond DS. Acute osteomyelitis in children: a review of 116 cases. J Pediatr Orthop 1990; 10:649–652.
32. Mustafa MM, Saez-Llorens X, McCracken GH, Nelson JD. Acute hematogenous pelvic osteomyelitis in infants and children. Pediatr Infect Dis J 1990; 9:6:416–421.
33. Perlman MH, Patzakis MJ, Jumar PI, Holtom P. The incidence of joint involvement with adjacent osteomyelitis in pediatric patients. Pediatr Orthop 2000; 20:40–43.
34. Viani RM, Bromberg K, Bradley JS. Obturator internus muscle abscess in children: report of seven cases and review. Clin Infect Dis 1999; 28:117–122.
35. Lyon RM, Evanich JD. Culture-negative septic arthritis in children. J Pediatr Orthop 1999; 19:655–659.
36. Ring D, Johnson CE, Wenger DR. Pyogenic infectious spondylitis in children: the convergence of discitis and vertebral osteomyelitis. J Pediatr Orthop 1995; 15:652–660.
37. Hollingworth P. Differential diagnosis and management of hip pain in childhood. Br J Rheumatol 1995; 34:78–82.
38. Jacobsen FS, Sullivan B. Spinal epidural abscesses in children. Orthopaedics 1994; 17:1131–1138.
39. Malhotra R, Singh KD, Bhan S, Dave PK. Primary pyogenic abscess of the psoas muscle. J Bone Joint Surg 1992; 74A:278–284.
40. Rose CD, Fawcett PT, Eppes SC, et al. Pediatric Lyme arthritis: clinical spectrum and outcome. J Pediatr Orthop 1994; 14:238–241.
41. Willis A, Widmann R, Flynn J, et al. Lyme arthritis presenting as acute septic arthritis in children. J Pediatr Orthop 2003; 23:114–118.
42. Jacobs RF, McCarthy RE, Elser JM. Pseudomonas Osteochondritis complicating puncture wounds of the foot in children: a ten-year evaluation. J Infect Dis 1989; 160:657–661.
43. Skaggs DL, Roberts JM, Codsi MJ, et al. Mild gait abnormality and leg discomfort in a child secondary to extradural ganglioneuroma. Am J Orthop 2000; 29:111–114.
44. Tuten HR, Gabos PG, Kumar SJ, Harter GD. The limping child: a manifestation of acute leukemia. J Pediatr Orthop 1998; 18:625–629.

Chapter 26

Developmental Dysplasia of the Hip

Michael K.D. Benson and Malcolm F. Macnicol

Introduction

This common disorder, which ranges from mild, spontaneously resolving instability in the newborn to complete dislocation with secondary acetabular and proximal femoral deformity, continues to provoke debate about its assessment and management.

Embryology and Development

An understanding of development of the hip joint allows an insight into the dysplasias and vascular insults to which it is vulnerable.

Three weeks after fertilization primitive limb buds are already beginning to form in the embryo. Strayer demonstrated that these are initially filled with mesenchyme which differentiates in time to form all joint components except for the blood vessels and nerves [1].

The *6-week* embryo is 12-mm long. Areas within the mesenchyme have condensed to outline the ilium, ischium, pubis, and femoral shaft. Rapid differentiation follows. The femoral head appears slightly later than the femoral shaft but by *7 weeks,* when the embryo is 17-mm long, an inter-zone develops between the femoral head and the acetabulum. Three separate layers develop within this inter-zone and come to form the perichondrium of the acetabulum and the femoral head together with the synovial membrane.

By 8 *weeks* the embryo is 30-mm long and blood vessels have grown into the ligamentum teres. There is the beginning of angulation of the femoral neck upon the femoral shaft. The cleft which heralds the true joint cavity begins to develop by apoptosis and the acetabular labrum is identifiable as a separate entity.

At 11 *weeks* the embryo is 50-mm long. The femoral head is spherical and 2 mm in diameter. It is clearly separate from the acetabulum and Watanabe [2] showed that it was possible experimentally to dislocate the hip for the first time at this age. The neck–shaft angle now measures 130–150°; it is already possible to detect femoral anteversion of between 5 and 10°; the vascular supply to the hip is established.

The *16-week* fetus is 120-mm long. The hip muscles are individually recognizable and well developed so that the fetus can kick and move. The femoral shaft shows early ossification within its cartilage anlage but the femoral head and trochanters remain cartilaginous until well after birth (Fig. 26.1). In utero fetal hips lie typically in flexion, abduction, and external rotation, with the left hip usually being the more rotated. The blood supply to the femoral head is predominantly through the epiphyseal and metaphyseal vessels. The vessels in the ligamentum teres are insignificant at this stage but contribute more to the femoral head blood supply later in gestation.

During the *last 20 weeks* of intra-uterine life the hip joint enlarges and matures. In 1912, Le Damany [3] showed neatly that the capacity of the acetabulum relative to the femoral head decreases in the last 3 months of gestation; the studies of Ralis and McKibbin in 1973 [4] confirmed that the acetabular capacity and depth are least at birth and the femoral head therefore most vulnerable to displacement. Neck–shaft angulation, femoral neck anteversion, and acetabular orientation have been interpreted very differently by different authors. The flexed position of the pelvis upon the lumbar spine and the tightly flexed hips contribute to this confusion because the anatomical position is not achieved until the neonatal lumbar kyphosis and the fixed hip flexion present at birth are lost. Most believe that femoral neck anteversion increases during the second half of fetal life reaching an average of 35° at birth. The neck–shaft angle probably changes little: it averages 135–140° at birth.

At birth the femoral shaft has usually ossified to just above the lesser trochanter. The femoral head and greater trochanter combine in a common proximal chondro-epiphysis (Fig. 26.1). The ossific nucleus is occasionally

M.K. Benson (✉)
Nuffield Orthopaedic Centre Oxford, UK

M. Benson et al. (eds.), *Children's Orthopaedics and Fractures,*
DOI 10.1007/978-1-84882-611-3_26, © Springer-Verlag London Limited 2010

Fig. 26.1 Maturation of the
femoral head in the first 5 years

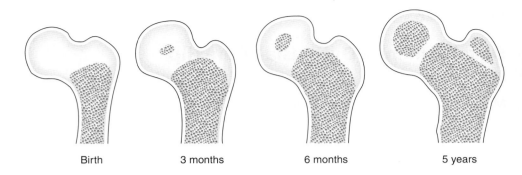

Birth   3 months   6 months   5 years

present within the femoral head at birth but usually does not appear for 3–6 months. In black Africans ossification is often present at birth but this is rare in Caucasians. Ossification of the pelvis is well advanced although the pubis lags behind the ischium and ilium.

Hip Growth After Birth

Acetabular growth is complex: the triradiate cartilage contributes 70%, enlarging both in diameter and depth. At the interface between the pelvic bones and the triradiate cartilage double growth plates allow the circumferential enlargement of the cavity to accommodate the growing femoral head. Growth plates extend also beneath the articular surface of each pelvic bone [5]. The acetabular ring epiphysis which surrounds the acetabular margin contributes nearly 30% to acetabular depth. Small centers of ossification appear in the ring epiphysis between 11 and 14 years. It usually fuses to the acetabular margin in mid-adolescence. Persistent hip instability may lead to failure of fusion and is an indicator of this instability. The triradiate cartilage closes at about 11 years in girls and a year later in boys.

At birth the femoral neck is short and the greater trochanter only slightly distal to the femoral head (Fig. 26.1). Differential growth in the proximal chondro-epiphysis allows the neck to lengthen and the trochanter to lateralize. Although the ossific nucleus in the femoral head should be seen radiologically by 6 months its appearance is often delayed for several months if the hip is dislocated. The greater trochanter starts to ossify by the fourth and the lesser trochanter by the eighth year. The proximal femoral physeal plate contributes about 30% to the eventual length of the femur.

Blood Supply

Despite its rich blood supply, the femoral head is vulnerable to infarction. This is the consequence partly of its deformable cartilaginous structure and partly of its end-arterial blood supply. The two main sources of blood supply to the proximal femur arise from the medial and lateral circumflex vessels, each of which arises typically from the profunda femoris artery (Fig. 26.2). The lateral circumflex artery and its ramifications supply the lateral and anterior part of the chondro-epiphysis, largely the greater trochanter. The postero-superior branch of the medial circumflex artery supplies the bulk of the intracapsular blood supply to the femoral head. At birth the artery of the ligamentum teres supplies only a small area around the fovea. Although each supplying vessel branches extensively in the proximal epiphysis Trueta [6] demonstrated that there is no intercommunication between the systems as each is end arterial. There is then a vascular ring around the hip joint arising predominantly from the medial and lateral circumflex arteries. Additional contributions come from the superior gluteal artery and an ascending branch from the first perforating artery. There is a second, often smaller and incomplete, subsynovial vascular anastomosis. The dominant posterior supply perforates the capsule posteriorly and passes proximally with the synovial reflection to the femoral head. The vessels are bound firmly to the femoral neck by the reflected retinacular portion of the capsule and the periosteum. The epiphyseal and metaphyseal arteries arise directly from these posterior vessels. Chung [7] showed in elegant post-natal perfusion studies that the epiphyseal plate acts as an absolute barrier between the epiphyseal and metaphyseal blood supplies, although there may be a limited and incomplete anastomosis at the periphery.

An extensive cartilage canal vascular network ramifies through the femoral head. These canaliculi may be occluded by pressure. If the hip is forced into extreme flexion and abduction the posterior vessels may be compressed between the short femoral neck and the acetabular margin. Full extension and internal rotation may also "ring out" the retinacular vessels and lead to avascular necrosis.

Displacement and Dysplasia of the Hip

In 1989 Klisic [8] suggested that the umbrella term "developmental dysplasia of the hip" (DDH) should replace "congenital dislocation of the hip" (CDH) as it embraced the concepts of instability and imperfect formation but had the further

Fig. 26.2 The vascular supply of the infant's hip at 6 months. Note that the femoral head is supplied predominantly by the ascending branches of the medial circumflex artery

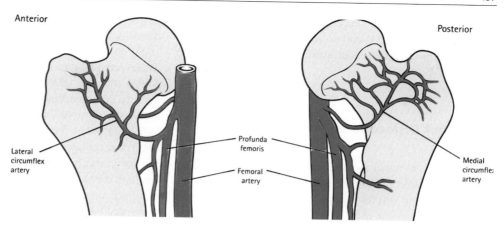

advantage of not specifying *when* the displacement or dysplasia occurred. This may have medico-legal consequences. It is nonetheless accepted that congenital factors contribute to developmental abnormalities.

The hip joint during early infancy is vulnerable to displacement. Although the clinical signs of instability may be subtle, they are usually detectable by careful examination. Early recognition and treatment in the neonatal period may prevent progressive subluxation or dislocation. Early treatment encourages the hip joint to grow normally and makes dysplasia less likely. It limits the otherwise inevitable progression to deformation, lost function, and eventual osteoarthritis.

Etiology

Genetic, gender, environmental, hormonal, and mechanical factors may predispose the hip to displace.

Genetics and Gender

The inheritance of DDH is multifactorial. Hip dysplasia is approximately nine times more common in females than males. If one child is born with hip dysplasia there is a 6% likelihood that a second child will have dysplasia also. In identical twins if one has DDH the second has a 34% chance of having displacement also. It is not clear, however, what the inherited factors are: these may, for example, reflect joint laxity or an abnormality of uterine shape. Ethnic background is important. Congenital dislocation is almost unknown in black Africans but is common in Japan and the Middle East.

Environmental and Mechanical Factors

So-called packaging anomalies in utero are important. In association with oligohydramnios or an eccentric uterine shape, the fetus may be squashed in utero. When cramped, freedom of movement is limited and the fetus cannot move around by kicking. Breech presentation is more common which independently makes displacement of the hip more likely. The infant with packaging abnormality may have an eccentric head shape (plagiocephaly), postural scoliosis, torticollis, eccentric hip movement (with greater abduction at one hip and greater adduction at the other), or calcaneovalgus foot positioning. As first-born children appear more vulnerable to hip displacement presumably uterine and abdominal muscular tone are greatest in a first pregnancy and hence the fetus has less freedom to move.

While club foot had been considered to increase the likelihood of associated DDH, Chan et al. [9] found that it did not predispose to hip displacement. They reviewed 1127 isolated DDH hips and reported that breech presentation, oligohydramnios, female sex, and primiparity were confirmed as major risk factors. There appeared to be an increased risk when a breech-presenting child was delivered vaginally rather than by caesarean section. High birth weight, post-maturity, and older maternal age slightly increased the risk of DDH. Breech presentation led to DDH in 2.7% of girls and 0.8% of boys. The left hip is up to four times more likely to dislocate than the right. This reflects the predominant left occiput anterior position of the fetus in utero in which the left hip is relatively adducted. Knee dislocation, almost invariably associated with breech presentation, was very likely to occur together with DDH.

Hormones

Carter and Wilkinson in 1960 [10] suggested that increased maternal hormone concentrations may cause pathologically lax tissues in some newborn infants. Although other studies failed to demonstrate consistently high levels of maternal hormones it is not possible to measure end organ sensitivity. The hips of girls and boys are anatomically identical at birth and this suggests that girls are more susceptible to female hormones than boys and hence at greater risk of hip displacement. Vogel et al. [11] found no relationship between serum levels of the polypeptide relaxin and hip instability in 21,865 newborns.

Syndromic Dislocations

It is important to remember that neonatal hip anomalies may be part of many syndromes and one abnormality should always prompt a careful search for others. Neuromuscular imbalance may cause the atypical congenital hip displacement seen in association with arthrogryposis and spina bifida, severe joint laxity, major chromosome defects, and a wide variety of other syndromes such as Down's and the thrombocytopenia-absent radius (TAR) syndrome.

When atypical "teratological" dislocations occur they are characterized by being irreducible at birth. Such hips need a different therapeutic approach. Standard neonatal splintage may be both fruitless and dangerous; it is often wise to wait until later in the first year of life before considering surgical treatment.

Patho-anatomy

In the typical hip displacement of the newborn, the only anatomical abnormalities appear to be stretching of the hip capsule and elongation of the ligamentum teres. McKibbin [12] showed the acetabulum and its labrum, the femoral head, and the orientation of femur and acetabulum appear essentially normal. At birth, the tight fit between femoral head and acetabulum is maintained by the surface tension created by the synovial fluid. It is very difficult to dislocate the normal neonatal hip in a postmortem specimen.

If the displaced hip is not reduced it may become permanently subluxated or dislocated. Eccentric pressure upon the head leads to segmental flattening, uneven growth, and increased femoral neck anteversion. The acetabulum, lacking the normal stimulus of a spherical contained femoral head, fails to develop anterosuperiorly, particularly if the rim is directly compressed by the displaced femoral head. This leads to loss of sphericity, a shallow, oval shape, and apparent anteversion. The labrum of the subluxating hip is typically stretched and everted. As the labrum stretches it takes with it part of the pre-osseous cartilage of the acetabular margin. The enveloping hip capsule is invaginated in front and below by the ilio-psoas tendon, adaptively shortening with time. Indentation of the capsule may produce the so-called hourglass capsular deformity. In time a secondary acetabulum develops: with subluxation this forms in the anterosuperior

part of the roof of the true acetabulum; with dislocation it develops in the iliac wing above the true acetabulum.

Subluxation blends almost imperceptibly into dislocation. The everted labrum may become squashed and distorted and folded into the joint, carrying with it part of the acetabular ring epiphysis and a sleeve of capsule. This complex is called the "limbus" and may prevent reduction (Figs. 26.3 and 26.4). When the head is not contained within the acetabulum the acetabular floor thickens and this contributes to the increasingly shallow acetabulum. The fibro-fatty pulvinar and the transverse acetabular ligament hypertrophy may encroach on the entrance to the acetabulum. The superior, elongated hip capsule may adhere to the outer iliac wing. The muscles that span the hip, particularly the ilio-psoas but also the adductors and hamstrings, shorten and contribute to the maintenance of hip displacement (Fig. 26.4).

Avascular necrosis does not occur spontaneously in the subluxated or dislocated hip. When it does occur it is iatrogenic. The growth and shape of the acetabulum are dependent upon the contained femoral head. Experimentally, if a square block is placed in the hip joint the acetabulum will grow square. The capacity for remodeling of the femoral

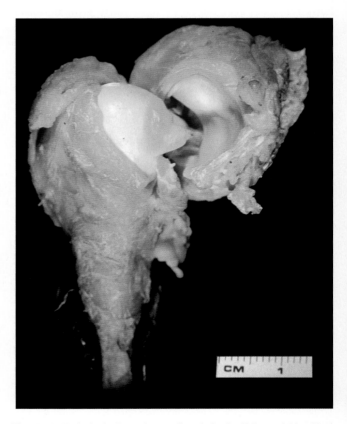

Fig. 26.3 Pathological specimen of an infant's dislocated hip. Note the oval femoral head, the hypertrophic ligamentum teres, the inverted limbus, and the eccentric position the femoral head occupied in the acetabulum

Fig. 26.4 (**a**) Anatomy of the normal hip: the labrum envelops the head and deepens the acetabulum. (**b**) In the subluxating hip the labrum everts; the head lies eccentrically in the acetabulum which deforms. (**c**) In the dislocated hip the cartilaginous acetabular margin deforms and the labrum may invert and obstruct reduction. (**d**) The ilio-psoas tendon may invaginate the capsule anteriorly and inferiorly

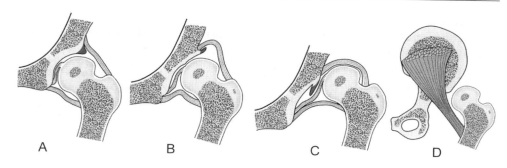

head and acetabulum when correctly relocated is excellent for the first few months but slowly decreases thereafter. From the age of 3 years this spontaneous remodeling capacity decreases relentlessly.

Incidence

There remain problems with assessing hip dysplasia and displacement. Before neonatal clinical screening was implemented the figures represented only late presenters; when clinical screening was introduced widely in the 1950s the incidence appeared to rise and ultrasound screening in the 1980s heralded a further upturn. If we simply consider neonatal instability, Barlow showed in 1962 [13] that 1 in 60 neonates had hip instability demonstrable by clinical examination alone. He noted that the capsular laxity causing instability usually tightened without treatment and that in 80% the instability resolved. With ultrasonographic techniques the neonatal incidence of instability may appear substantially higher with some estimates up to 6%. In the UK, Macnicol's value of 1 in 400 children [14] is probably close to the overall British incidence. In the native North American, instability has been reported to be as high as 1 in 5, but the condition is virtually absent in the black African. The left hip is displaced three times more often than the right at birth and in 20% the displacement is bilateral.

Although most neonatal instability resolves spontaneously, should it fail to do so children may present at walking age with a painless limp and leg shortening. Some, with partially displaced hips, will present as painful dysplasias in adolescence or early adult life. It should be noted that unrecognized or untreated dysplasia is responsible for up to 30% of those adults under the age of 45 years who develop degenerative hip arthritis.

Screening

Roser noted in 1879 [15] that some children's hips could be "dislocated by adduction of the leg and then reduced again by abduction." Little was made of this observation until 1937 when Ortolani [16] described the test named after him and the "snap of entry" of the dislocated hip as it reduced. Von Rosen [17] introduced routine clinical screening of newborns in Sweden in 1957. This dramatically reduced the incidence of late presentation. Palmén's [18] ground-breaking Swedish study led many to believe that the specter of the late-presenting hip dislocation could be avoided.

Preventing late-presenting dislocation remains the goal of neonatal screening programs. When the clinical tests of von Rosen and Barlow (v.i.) were introduced it was believed initially that clinical examination alone would avoid late-presenting DDH. This has proved not to be the case. There seems little doubt that clinical screening is more reliable when performed by experienced and dedicated staff. Without these the likelihood of clinical diagnosis is probably less than 50% [19]. Recognizing that not all dysplastic hips could be clinically diagnosed led to the concept of secondary screening: in the UK statutory guidelines ensured that babies' hips should be re-examined at 6 weeks and at 6–9 months. The guidelines stopped short of specifying the qualifications and experience needed to examine: typically a junior doctor performed the neonatal examination, a general practitioner the 6-week examination, and a nurse or health visitor the last screening. It was a recipe which ensured that children with DDH would continue to be diagnosed late.

Over 25 years ago Graf introduced the technique of ultrasonographic (US) screening of the infant's hip [20]. This radically changed our understanding of hip problems in infancy as the anatomy of the child's hip could be better understood non-invasively. As US screening was refined and developed its use became widespread and in some European countries it became routine for all neonates to have their hips examined by ultrasound. In other countries ultrasonography was reserved for those felt to be at special risk of dysplasia. Analyses of risk and cost–benefit around the world drew different conclusions. In Austria, Germany, and Italy all infants are screened with US. In the United States, Canada, the UK, and Scandinavia only those with at-risk factors or clinical abnormality undergo US examination.

Lehmann et al. [21] were not convinced from their meta-analysis that universal screening could be recommended. Conversely, Clegg [22] believed that cost analysis showed that it should be. He believed that many analyses failed to account fully for the heavy costs associated with late diagnosis, complex treatment, and the premature arthritis that stems from imperfect reduction and persisting dysplasia.

Why should there be doubt? If infants are screened by ultrasound shortly after delivery up to 6% may show instability. If rescreened at 4 weeks most instability has resolved so if routine screening is undertaken it should not be earlier than 3 weeks. Since splintage carries small but finite risks of avascular necrosis it is important that infants should not be over-treated.

Risk Factors for DDH

- Breech presentation either before or during delivery.
- Family history of hip dysplasia in a first-degree relative.
- Evidence of "packaging" anomaly such as torticollis or calcaneovalgus feet.
- Oligohydramnios and/or maternal hypertension.
- Dislocated knees.
- First-born children.
- Girls (who are up to nine times more likely to be affected by hip displacement than boys).
- Syndromes associated with hip anomalies.
- Increased birth weight (over 4.5 kg).

Where selective US screening is performed only some of these risk factors are usually considered. These include a positive family history, breech presentation, associated musculo-skeletal anomaly, and evidence of a cramped intra-uterine position. Clearly if there is any suggestion clinically of hip instability this is the prime reason for ultrasound scanning.

Clinical Examination

Ideally the baby should be relaxed and warm. All clothing, including the nappy, should be removed and the baby placed on a firm surface that allows easy access. General examination of the skull, trunk, arms, and legs should be swift and gentle. Asymmetry or malformation should be looked for. When examining the hip it must be remembered that all newborns have a physiological flexion deformity of 30–40° which may take several months to resolve.

It is important to establish a routine hip examination. The following is recommended:

1. Look for thigh asymmetry. Is one leg shorter? Is one leg more externally rotated than the other? Is there thigh crease asymmetry; in particular is there a deeper groin crease on one side than the other? Does the perineum look too wide? A dislocated hip may look no different from the normal hip, although with the hips flexed one knee may appear lower than the other (Galeazzi's sign).
2. Palpation of bony landmarks may help. Does one trochanter lie higher than the other in relationship to the anterior superior spine? When palpating deep to the femoral artery does one socket feel empty by comparison with the other? When palpating the buttock the greater trochanter may be mistaken for a displaced femoral head.
3. (a) Ortolani's test [16] is key in deciding if the hip is dislocated. With the baby's hip and knee flexed, the thumb in the groin, and the fingers over the greater trochanter, gently abduct the hip (Fig. 26.5a). In the first few weeks of life it should be possible to abduct the hip 90° until the knee is flat on the table. If abduction is restricted gently lift the leg forward and repeat the abduction maneuver. If the hip is dislocated this may allow the femoral head to slide into the acetabulum. Ortolani described the "jerk of entry" or clunk associated with this reduction, which shows that the hip is habitually dislocated at rest but reducible. If abduction is limited and cannot be completed it should be assumed, until proven otherwise, that the hip is dislocated and irreducible.
3. (b) Barlow's test [13] is performed when the Ortolani test is negative. The hip is therefore in joint. It is a provocative test to see if the hip will subluxate or dislocate out of the acetabulum. With the hips and knees flexed and in slight adduction, the thumb on the inner proximal thigh pushes gently backward and laterally (Fig. 26.5b). When capsular laxity or instability is present the femoral head may be felt to jump over the posterior acetabular border and reduce either spontaneously or by Ortolani's maneuver. The test therefore demonstrates whether the normally located hip is unstable.

Asymmetry or limited abduction should alert the examiner as much as the clunk of reduction or displacement. The "click" is usually of little significance and represents a transient vacuum phenomenon or a tendon snap at hip or knee. The tests should therefore be conducted with the knee fully flexed in order to remove this artifact. The pathological clunk is usually not audible but palpable. In any clinical screening program the infant who causes concern should be re-examined, preferably by an experienced examiner with access to US testing.

Fig. 26.5 (**a**) Ortolani's test: when the hip is normally located, full abduction of the flexed hip is possible. Note the reduced abduction of the left hip. (**b**) Barlow's test: with the hip flexed and adducted, posterior and lateral pressure from the thumb on the proximal femur will demonstrate if instability is present

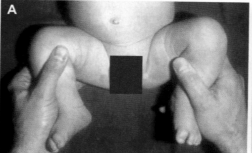
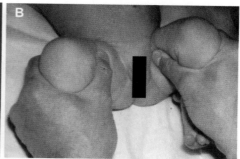

Investigations

Ultrasound

Although careful clinical examination of the infant should detect instability, it is clear that a proportion of children are not diagnosed by the initial clinical screening. This may reflect inexperience of the examiner, an inadequate screening program, or a hip in which the abnormality is not physically detectable at birth.

The neonatal hip is largely cartilaginous and although a pelvic radiograph may help, it is difficult to interpret. In 1984, Graf [19] delineated the different appearances of the infant's hip as "seen" ultrasonographically. The investigation is non-invasive and gives both a static and a potentially dynamic portrayal of the hip joint and any soft tissue distortions. A linear scanner should be used, and the images are produced graphically upon a screen or as hard copies. A variety of different projections and views have been defined.

Graf has shown that a mid-sagittal scan of the hip allows the contour of the femoral head and acetabulum to be gauged. Figure 26.6 illustrates his technique for measuring the bony (α[alpha]) and cartilaginous (β[beta]) angles upon the scan. An analysis of these angles allows quantification of the maturity of the hip and the severity of any dysplasia. Figure 26.7 illustrates a normal and a dislocated hip and Table 26.1 lists Graf's classification. He recognized immaturity and advised splintage for all hips worse than type IIc, with careful review of all but type I normal hips.

Other systems for classifying the US appearances have evolved. The Morin [23] classification assesses acetabular depth relative to head size: this gives a measure of head coverage. It is simpler than Graf's technique. The Suzuki method [24] scans from the front, but the images obtained are more difficult to interpret. Adequate statistical comparison of the systems has not been made.

US has increased considerably our understanding of the morphology of hip development. The natural history of each

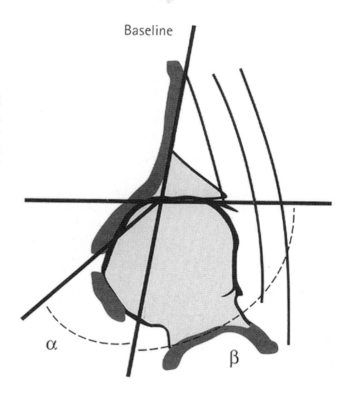

Fig. 26.6 Diagram of the US appearance of a reduced but dysplastic hip. An α [alpha] angle under 60° suggests a poor bony acetabular roof. A large β [beta] angle, as here, shows a poor cartilage roof cover

type of hip appearance is, however, difficult to evaluate. Not surprisingly, investigators have been tempted to treat hips that appear to be morphologically dysplastic. It is not always clear whether treatment or simple maturation has allowed such hips to improve.

US may be used not only statically but also dynamically. If the examiner attempts to displace the hip by Barlow's test, graphic images of the maneuver are easily obtained. Clarke et al. [25] focused attention on this hip instability and Engesaeter et al. [26] suggested that dynamic instability was of greater prognostic significance than morphological appearance.

Fig. 26.7 (**a**) US of normal hip and (**b**) its graphic interpretation. (**c**) US of dislocated hip and (**d**) its graphic interpretation

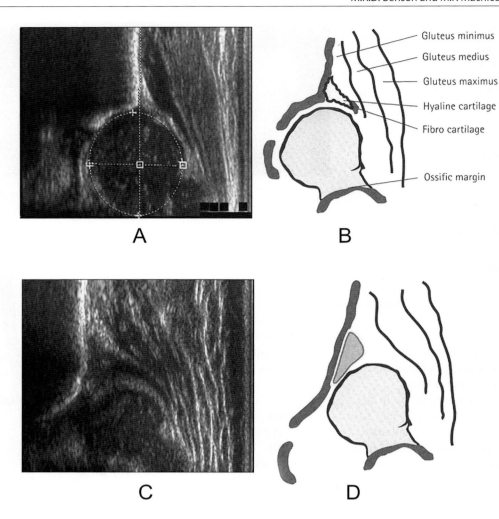

Table 26.1 Graf'S Ultrasonographic Classification of Hip Dysplasia

Hip type	Bony roof	Bony rim	Cartilage rim	α [alpha]: bony roof angle (°)	β [beta]: cartilage roof angle (°)
Ia	Good	Angular	Narrow; covers head	60	<55
Ib	Good	Sl. Rounded	Wide; short; covers head	60	<55
IIa + delay in ossification ≈ age	Adequate	Round	Wide; covers head	50–59	>55
IIa – delay; immature	Deficient	Round	Wide; covers head	50–59	>55
IIb delay ossification > 3 months	Deficient	Round	Wide; covers head	50–59	>55
IIc: critical (any age)	Deficient	Round to flat	Wide; covers head	50–59	70–77
D: decentered (any age)	Deficiency severe	Round to flat	Displaced	43–49	70–77
IIIa	Poor	Flat	Displaced with no structural alteration	<43	>77
IIIb	Poor	Flat	Displaced with structural alternation	<43	>77
IV	Poor	Flat	Displaced infero-medial	<43	>77

In Austria, Italy, and Germany, it has become a national requirement that all babies should undergo US examination after birth. In Britain and the United States, US examination is reserved for those children who are suspected of a clinical anomaly or to be at high risk by virtue of family history or breech presentation. Clegg et al. [22] have shown that universal US screening may prove cheaper than treating late those children with a missed diagnosis of DDH. It remains to be seen whether the routine neonatal use of US will become the norm.

US has established a secure role for monitoring the progress of treatment. In the first few months of life, before the developing ossific nucleus develops in the femoral head, it allows the surgeon to assess the quality of reduction and to monitor acetabular depth. It has the great advantage over other imaging techniques that it is non-invasive and is relatively inexpensive. The danger is that it may lead the unwary to over-treat a condition that often resolves.

Radiography

Where US equipment is not available a standardized antero-posterior pelvic radiograph is of value. Clearly, it is impractical to investigate all babies in this manner, but in suspicious cases, particularly if there is a suggestion of skeletal deformation or asymmetry [27], Bertol and Macnicol highlighted how a carefully taken film adds to the precision of neonatal diagnosis [28].

It should be remembered that the *bony* contours demonstrable radiographically give an imperfect indication of the quality of the *cartilaginous* acetabular roof. Nonetheless, the bony acetabular contour may be assessed by the acetabular index (Fig. 26.8). While this is prone to some measurement error it should be compared, as shown by Tönnis [29], with the angle expected at the child's age. The "medial gap" [27] between ischium and its closest femoral landmark should not

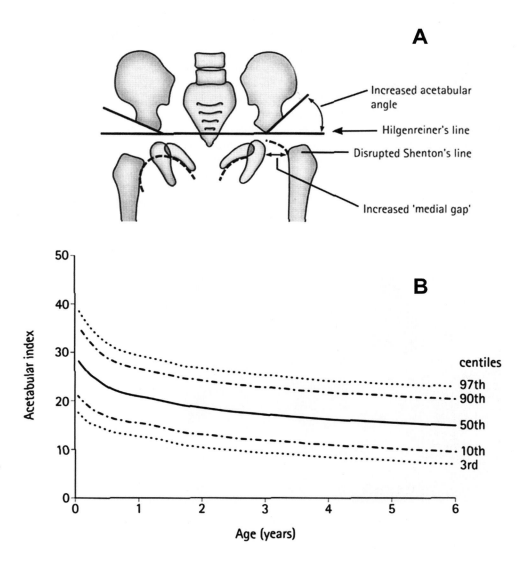

Fig. 26.8 (a) The features of an infant's radiograph that are used to determine the acetabular index. Note also Shenton's line and its disruption; the increased "medial gap" when the hip is displaced. (b) Graph (after Tönnis) demonstrating the change in acetabular angle with time

measure more than 5 mm on a standardized radiograph. A smoothly curved line produced along the lower border of the superior public ramus should follow the curve of the lower border of the medial femoral neck (Shenton's line). Once the ossific nucleus appears in the femoral head (between 3 and 6 months), radiological assessment becomes easier. The ossific nucleus should lie wholly beneath the triradiate cartilage in infancy and early childhood and medial to the perpendicular dropped from the lateral acetabular margin.

After a child has been treated for hip instability, sequential review with serial ultrasonograms and later radiographs is important to ensure that the hip develops normally. When it becomes possible, the child should stand for a weight-bearing film. In the younger child, the acetabular index should be measured at each review and compared with expected development (Fig. 26.8).

Hip displacement causes the ossific nucleus of the femoral head to appear later and smaller than its normal counterpart. Furthermore, the ossific nucleus may be eccentric within the femoral head. As the child grows older and the ossific nucleus enlarges, the center of the femoral head and its sphericity may be estimated by using Mose's concentric rings (Fig. 26.9). Once the center of the femoral head is known, the acetabular cover of the femoral head, the so-called center–edge angle of Wiberg [30], may be measured. In the child this should measure at least 15°; in the adult it should be more than 25°. Severin [31] produced a scheme of classification of later hip dysplasia based upon its radiological appearance and the center–edge angle (Table 26.2). Although imperfectly reproducible, it remains the most widely used system for judging outcomes of treatment.

Table 26.2 Severin's radiographic classification of hip dysplasia

Classification	Radiographic appearance	Center–edge angle (after Wiberg)
Class I	Normal	
Ia		6–13 years: > 19°
		Over 14 years: > 25°
Ib		6–13 years: > 15–19°
		Over 14 years: 20–25°
Class II	Moderate deformity of head, neck, or socket	
IIa		6–13 years: > 19°
		Over 14 years: > 25°
IIb		6–13 years: 15–19°
		Over 14 years: 20–25°
Class III	Dysplasia without subluxation	6–13 years: < 15°
		Over 14 years: < 20°
Class IV		
IVa	Moderate subluxation	>0°
IVb	Severe subluxation	<0°
Class V	Head lies in false socket in upper true acetabulum	
Class VI	Re-dislocation	

When a decision is being taken as to whether additional radiographs of the child's hip should be taken, the risk of irradiation should not be forgotten. Gonadal shields should be used and unnecessary films avoided.

Avascular Necrosis

Idiopathic necrosis is very rare in infancy and young childhood. When it occurs in children with DDH it is almost always iatrogenic. We have seen how the cartilaginous femoral head of infancy is vulnerable to pressure which flattens the canaliculi and obliterates the end-arterial blood supply. The short femoral neck makes compression of the posterior retinacular vessels between acetabular margin and neck all too easy if the hip is held in extreme abduction and flexion. Equally, the vessels may be stretched and wrung out by forced internal rotation. The head is particularly vulnerable if it remains dislocated or subluxed.

If the epiphysis alone is injured, the ossific nucleus may be late in appearing and mottled or fragmented when it does. Salter et al. [32] showed that if the nucleus had not ossified by 1 year it had probably been damaged. The epiphyseal injury may lead to coxa plana or magna and secondary acetabular dysplasia. Occasionally, of course, other disorders such as thyroid deficiency or epiphyseal dysplasia may delay ossification.

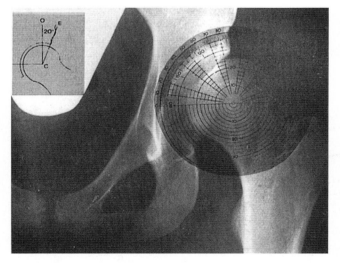

Fig. 26.9 Radiograph with Mose's rings superimposed. The center of the femoral head and the center–edge angle are readily measured. In the insert the angle is 20° and on the radiograph 0°

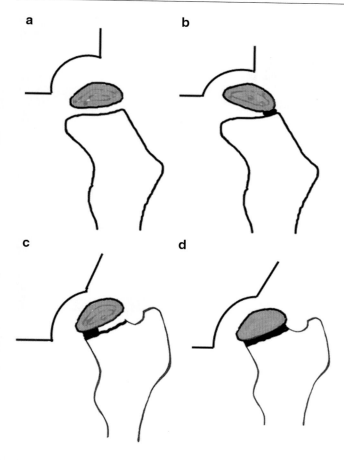

Fig. 26.10 Kalamchi and McEwan's avascular necrosis classification: (**a**) Type I: changes in the ossific nucleus only—mottling or late appearance. (**b**) Type II: ossific nucleus injury and lateral growth plate early closure—valgus tilt. (**c**) Type III: epiphyseal and medial growth plate injury—progressive varus; some trochanteric overgrowth; modest acetabular dysplasia. (**d**) Type IV: epiphyseal and whole growth plate injury—short neck; major trochanteric overgrowth; subluxation with marked dysplasia

The avascular insult may affect not only the epiphysis but also the growth plate. When it does, part or all of the plate may be affected. Kalamchi and MacEwan [33] described lateral, central, and complete injuries to the physis (Fig. 26.10). These produce deformities of the head and neck which become more apparent with growth. The head and neck deformity leads to secondary adaptive acetabular changes, many of which lead in turn to poor head cover and subluxation (Fig. 26.11). Leg length may be severely affected.

The risk of ischemia varies with age, treatment modality, surgical experience, and the form of splintage. It concerns all who treat children and dictates the need for careful splint supervision, avoidance of extreme positions of the leg, and the importance of long-term review.

Treatment

At Birth

We have seen how most neonatally unstable hips resolve spontaneously. Sadly there remains no clear indicator for those that need treatment. The hip that is dislocated rather than dislocatable may be less likely to recover. The hip that is irreducible at birth, the so-called teratological hip, is least likely to reduce.

The dislocatable hip: When the hip is loosely in joint no treatment should be given from birth. The situation should be carefully explained to the family and the infant reviewed in 3–4 weeks for further clinical and US evaluation. If instability persists or there is US evidence of acetabular dysplasia the hips should be splinted in flexion and abduction.

The dislocated but reducible hip: Such hips should have prompt US assessment. Some would observe for 3 weeks to see if spontaneous reduction occurs. Some would splint from birth. The evidence is not there to decide but a clear local policy should be established.

The irreducibly dislocated hip: Early confirmation by US is important to distinguish the irreducible dislocation from the "skew" baby. Marked molding may cause the infant to have one or several findings: plagiocephaly, correctable scoliosis, calcaneovalgus feet, or asymmetry of hip abduction and adduction. It seems sensible to undertake a trial of reduction. Rigid abduction splintage should never be applied but flexible splints such as the Pavlik harness are effective, applied as soon as possible after birth. The infant is monitored carefully both clinically and by US. If the hip reduces within 2 weeks splintage is continued until stability and acetabular maturation develop. If the hip does not reduce progressively within 2 or 3 weeks splintage should be discarded and the child left free until older.

The "at risk" infant: Infants with a recognized risk such as breech presentation or affected family member should be reviewed clinically and with US within 6 weeks of delivery. If they are found to be normal they may safely be discharged from further review. If there is any evidence of instability, displacement, or dysplasia they too should be splinted and serially reviewed. Figure 26.12 outlines the treatment algorithm used in Oxford.

Splintage: It may be asked why all infants are not splinted. Programs have indeed been recommended where all newborns are treated with double nappies or simple abduction splints. There is some evidence that late-presenting problems may be fewer but all splints carry a small but finite risk of avascular necrosis, a complication which imperils the future of the hip. This danger has modified our approach to US. In the early heady days of the new technique subtle immaturity

Fig. 26.11 (**a**) An 8-month-old girl with right DDH. (**b**) Position after 3 months splintage. (**c**) The right ossific nucleus has grown imperfectly, with a fragmented ossific nucleus. (**d**) At 5 years there is loss of epiphyseal height and modest residual dysplasia

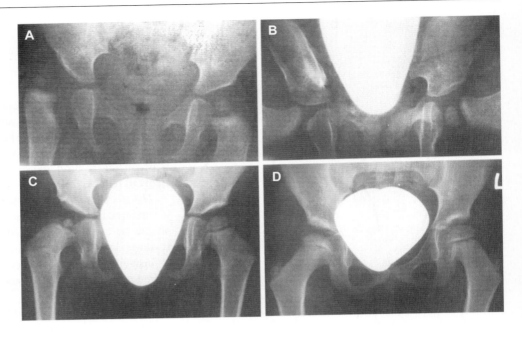

and instability of the neonatal hips led to splintage rates of up to 10%. While the great majority came to no harm a few developed avascular necrosis not only in the affected but also in the contralateral normal hip. Most centers now splint 4–6 infants per 1000. It is difficult to compare splintage rates as DDH incidence varies so widely around the world but each country should have an expected norm. If selection for splintage is not carefully evaluated it will call into question the local screening process.

Types of splint: The principle of any splint is to reduce the hip and maintain reduction safely while the capsule tightens and the acetabulum molds to its proper shape around the femoral head. The Malmö or von Rosen splint was the first widely used. It was pioneered in Sweden and remains in common use. It is H shaped, made of a malleable metal core, padded and encased in a waterproof shell (Fig. 26.13). The splint hooks over the shoulders and under the flexed and abducted thighs. It is essential that some freedom of movement be retained: 30° of flexion and 30° of abduction must be left to avoid compression of the head in the acetabulum and to minimize the risk of avascular necrosis. It is applied next to the skin and should not be removed by the family. Careful, regular supervision is needed to ensure it is used properly and does not tighten as the baby grows.

The Pavlik harness has gained widespread popularity (Fig. 26.13). A simple harness is fitted over the shoulders and around the chest. Front- and back-legging straps are attached to this and hooked under the feet. This ensures the hips are flexed to at least 90°. The straps are so adjusted that, with hips and knees flexed to a right angle, the knees just meet in

the midline. Just as with the von Rosen splint it is essential the harness is not too tight. It was believed at one time that the infant "kicked" the displaced hip into joint. Suzuki et al. [24], however, demonstrated that reduction occurs when the infant relaxes or sleeps.

Both Malmö and Pavlik splints demand some restrictions on bathing and clothing. A variety of other splints are available. Examples include the Craig splint and the Frejka pillow. These are positioned over the nappy and regularly removed. Help from trained support staff, health visitor, or "mothers' club" is essential. We should remember that new mothers are upset when their children need treatment, and care and tact are very important. Fortunately splintage rarely affects bonding between mother and child.

All splints carry the risk of complications: the most serious are avascular necrosis and failure to reduce and stabilize the hip. Bradley et al. [34] noted in addition that skin rashes, temporary femoral nerve palsy, inferior subluxation of the hip, and cavus foot deformity may be occasional complications. Early advice to nurse children prone in splints was set aside when it was recognized that prone lying may increase susceptibility to cot death. It is thought that children are safer lying supine or on their sides.

Splintage does not always succeed. There has been a general trend to prefer Pavlik harnessing to more rigid splintage. The European multicenter trial of 1988 [35] showed a success rate of 92% for those without irreducible dislocation and an avascular necrosis rate of 2.4%. In a small series comparing children splinted with Pavlik harness, von Rosen, and Craig splints the von Rosen was found to be the most reliable [36].

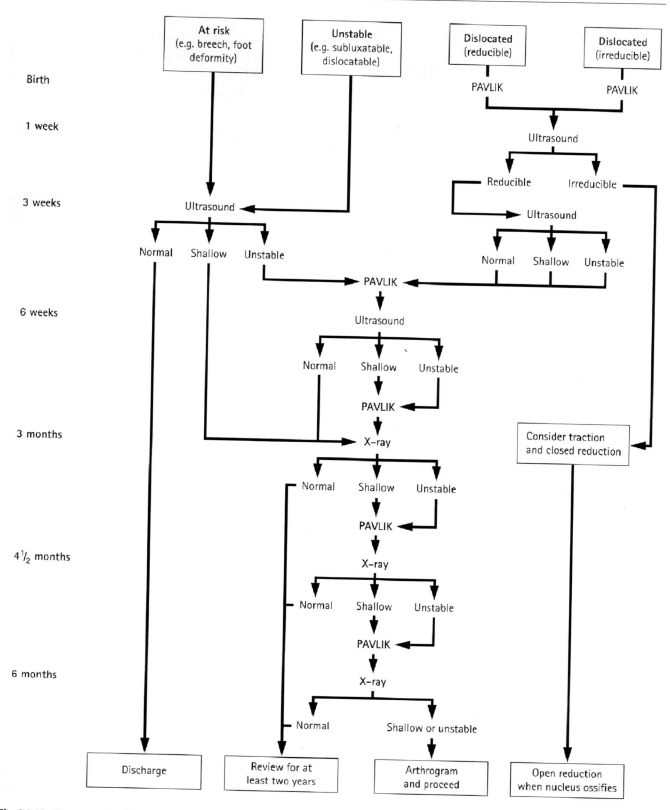

Fig. 26.12 Treatment algorithm for developmental dysplasia of the hip in the first 6 months

Fig. 26.13 Abduction splints in infancy. (**a**) The von Rosen splint. Flexion and abduction are readily obtained but care is needed to avoid extreme abduction. (**b**) The Pavlik harness maintains hip flexion and abduction but allows more freedom of movement

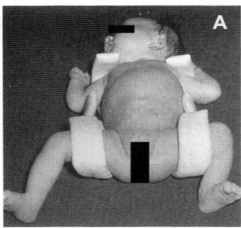 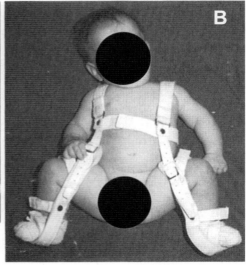

Treatment in the First Few Months

The best time to treat babies with unstable hips is in the first few weeks of life. Failed primary screening, failed primary splintage, and secondary screening still lead to an appreciable number of infants presenting with dislocation later in their first year. In the first few months children with hip subluxation or dislocation may still be treated in simple splintage, and the Pavlik harness is used widely. Nakamura et al. [37], who used the harness for slightly older children (1–12 months: mean 4.8), found it successful in 83% with an avascular necrosis rate of 12%. Once again, careful supervision and repeated US are needed to ensure reduction and compliance. In general, the later the diagnosis, the longer the period of splintage needed. As a rule of thumb children at birth need 6 weeks and those of age 3 months need 3 months. Satisfactory acetabular maturation and stability must be demonstrated before splintage is discontinued. Furthermore, children should be regularly reviewed clinically and radiographically until at least the age of 2 years to ensure their hips develop normally with no evidence of ischemic change.

Treatment Before 12 Months

When the hip has been displacing or displaced for several months the clinical findings change. While in early infancy most unstable hips are readily reducible, this becomes less likely after 3 or 4 months. The abnormal hip tends to become irreducibly subluxated or dislocated. The clinical signs also change. The affected leg may look shorter and lie more clearly in external rotation. Thigh creases, although notoriously unreliable as a diagnostic aid, may show a deep

unmatched groin crease on the affected side posteriorly. Galeazzi's sign of the lower-lying knee when hips and knees are flexed may be more apparent. *The cardinal finding, however, is restricted abduction of the flexed hip.* It is, not surprisingly, more difficult to recognize this lost abduction when both hips are displaced as there is no normal hip for comparison. The loss of abduction may be subtle, only 15–20°. While many surgeons continue to rely on US for diagnosis, many prefer radiographs after the age of 3–4 months.

It may be reasonable to undertake a trial of Pavlik harnessing for infants up to 8 months old with subluxation only but it is fruitless and potentially dangerous for children older than this. If the hip fails to show progressive reduction over the course of the first 2 weeks the harness should be discarded as the postero-superior acetabulum may be flattened by the pressure of an eccentrically lying femoral head. Furthermore, the risk of avascular necrosis of the femoral head increases.

If the hip is reducible in a harness it may need to be used full time for several months to allow the acetabulum to mature properly. There has been argument as to whether splintage should be discarded promptly or weaned. While most surgeons have practiced weaning there is evidence to suggest that, once the hip is stable and the acetabulum well formed, splintage may be discarded without.

Macnicol [38] highlighted the postural asymmetry, "infantile skeletal skew," which may develop when the child lies exclusively on one side. On the habitually dependent side hip abduction is greater and adduction less than the opposite side. By contrast the upper hip, which falls into adduction, has increased adduction but decreased abduction (Fig. 26.14). Radiographically the pelvis seems to be tilted and the appearance of the ossific nucleus on the adducted side may be delayed. Simple stretching and alternate positioning may be

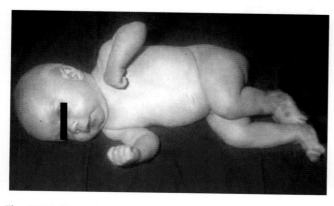

Fig. 26.14 Postural asymmetry in the side-lying child. Note the plagiocephaly, the dependent abdomen encouraging scoliosis and the asymmetric hip position

sufficient to allow such hips to develop normally without formal splintage. If splintage is used the hip must never be abducted forcibly.

It is debatable how the young infant over 3 months old with an irreducible dislocation should be treated. Some suggest treatment should be deferred until ossification begins within the femoral head, believing that this increases stability of the femoral head, making it less vulnerable to pressure and avascular necrosis. Segal et al. [39] showed experimentally in a porcine model that the presence of the ossific nucleus appears to protect the cartilaginous femoral head from compressive ischemic injury. The presence of the ossific nucleus before reduction was statistically significant in avoiding avascular necrosis, which was more frequent when children were treated by open or closed reduction in the first year of life. Luhmann et al. [40], however, found in their series that the ossific nucleus appeared not to be protective against avascular necrosis and believe that the displaced hip should be reduced at diagnosis rather than waiting for nuclear ossification. There is no consensus about this matter.

Closed Hip Reduction

When simple abduction splintage fails alternative treatment is necessary. Children were commonly treated by skin traction for a period ranging from a few days to several weeks. The theoretical aim of such traction was to stretch the soft tissues and to minimize the likelihood of pressure necrosis when the hip was reduced. The Morin School in France continues to use such traction for several weeks and has an excellent record of successful closed reduction with satisfactory long-term outcomes. Their latest results are awaited. This has not always been matched by others. Traction was widely discontinued in the United States, partly because of the cost–benefit aspect and partly because there was some

evidence to suggest that it conferred no benefit either on the reduction itself or on the risk of avascular necrosis. Many centers throughout the world have now abandoned traction as a consequence. Weinstein and Ponseti [41] also suggested that traction may allow the labrum and part of the pre-osseous acetabular rim cartilage (the limbus) to become incarcerated in the hip joint and make subsequent reduction more difficult.

For the 3- to 9-month-old infant whose displaced hip shows no femoral head ossification it is sensible to examine the hip under anesthesia. This also offers the opportunity to carry out an arthrogram.

Arthrography

Injecting contrast medium into the hip joint outlines the femoral head and acetabulum and demonstrates whether the hip will reduce satisfactorily. Any obstacles to reduction can be assessed and a decision taken as to whether closed reduction is possible. Injection into the joint may be made anterolaterally, anteriorly, laterally over the greater trochanter, or infero-medially. The needle should be inserted into the joint under image intensifier control. The joint should not be overdistended with contrast medium as this may obscure the features one hopes to demonstrate. It is best if the contrast medium is diluted 50%. The arthrogram allows the surgeon to examine the hip in a variety of positions, judging the one that allows the best "fit."

In the normal hip the spherical femoral head sits within a spherical acetabulum. The cartilaginous acetabular roof "covers" the femoral head and the labrum extends clearly beyond this. The limbic "thorn," the interval between labrum and capsular reflection, suggests the labrum is correctly located and the acetabular margin not deformed. The so-called zona orbicularis is produced by slight out-pouching of the synovium between the limbs of the Y-shaped ligament of Bigelow. The acetabular fossa and the transverse ligament indentation should be identified. The contrast medium should extend far enough down the neck to delineate the normal capsular attachments and should assess its capacity (Fig. 26.15).

With subluxation a crescent of the contrast may be seen centrally. When, as often happens, subluxation is associated with acetabular insufficiency, this crescent may shift from central to superior when longitudinal traction is applied to the leg and the head centralizes more normally into the acetabulum.

Progressive degrees of subluxation and dislocation may deform and entrap the limbus (the labrum, deformed pre-osseous rim cartilage, and a capsular fold) within the joint. The ligamentum teres is often hypertrophic and may be seen as an obstacle to reduction; the transverse ligament may

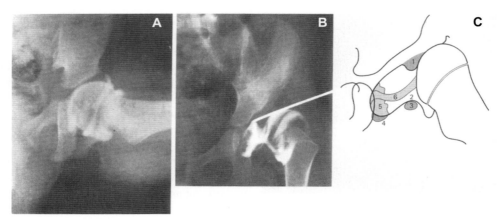

Fig. 26.15 (**a**) Arthrogram of a reduced hip in the frog lateral position. Although the bony acetabulum is deficient, the cartilaginous roof is satisfactory and the labrum normally located. The prognosis is good with simple abduction splinting. (**b**) Arthrogram of dislocated hip in neutral. The injecting needle is superolateral. The infolded labrum and deformed cartilaginous acetabular margin are clearly seen. The deep inferior indentation is made by the ilio-psoas. (**c**) Line diagram of arthrogram findings: (1) deformed acetabular rim and infolded limbus; (2) capsular "waisting" by the invaginating ilio-psoas (3); (4) inferior transverse acetabular ligament; (5) fibro-fatty pulvinar; (6) ligamentum teres

encroach upon the inferior aspect of the hip joint. When the hip is displaced the ilio-psoas tendon may indent the anterior-inferior capsule creating an hourglass constriction.

The arthrogram defines the hip as

- Normal.
- Subluxing with no block to reduction.
- Dislocated or dislocatable but fully reducible.
- Dislocated with an obstacle to reduction.
- Subluxated in a partially dislocated position that cannot be reversed.

Femoral anteversion may be assessed by the amount of rotation needed to align the femur optimally. The acetabulum may show varying severities of dysplasia or delayed ossification.

Management

Closed Reduction

If the child's hip is reducible, closed reduction should be undertaken. Almost invariably the hip needs to be held in flexion and abduction. Care is needed to assess the position of greatest stability and the position in which redisplacement occurs. Too little abduction and the hip dislocates; too much abduction and avascular necrosis follows. The safe zone of Ramsey [42] should be selected. It is a wise precaution to carry out a percutaneous tenotomy of the adductor longus tendon. This is performed simply by holding the flexed hip in abduction, identifying the tendon between finger and thumb, and dividing it with a small tenotome. The maneuver often adds an extra 20° of abduction and increases the safe zone in which a plaster cast may be applied.

Salter highlighted the importance of holding the leg in the right position. He advocated the "human" position in contradistinction to the "frog" position which he believed should be reserved for frogs. The treated hip should be flexed to at least a right angle and abducted to no more than 45–50°, allowing at least 30° of flexion and 30° of abduction beyond the position to be maintained. Unless care is taken there is a tendency for progressive abduction to occur as the hip spica is applied. It is important to not allow the hip to displace backward, careful molding over the greater trochanter restricting this (Fig. 26.16). The spica should extend to the lower thorax but allow the umbilicus to be visible. For hips with mild subluxation it is reasonable to keep the spica above the knee only; for severe subluxation or dislocation in general it is better to incorporate the knee in flexion to minimize hamstring tightness. The ankle and foot may be left free or incorporated in the plaster initially.

When the child wakes it is important to ensure that the hip does not subluxate or dislocate within the plaster cast. A plain radiograph in the plaster is not adequate for assessment: three-dimensional views are needed. While a computed tomography (CT) scan is entirely reasonable it carries the risk of significant gonadal irradiation and where possible a magnetic resonance imaging (MRI) scan is preferable [43]. As the child is incarcerated in plaster, movement artifact is usually not a problem (Fig. 26.17).

Hip spicas need to be changed after 4–6 weeks. The child should then be re-examined under anesthesia with the plaster

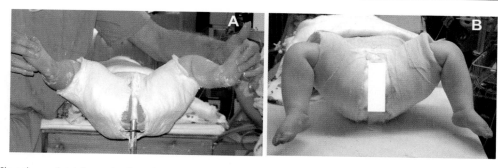

Fig. 26.16 (**a**) Hip spica maintaining reduction. At application care is taken to avoid excess abduction. Molding behind the trochanters makes posterior subluxation unlikely. (**b**) The completed double half hip spica

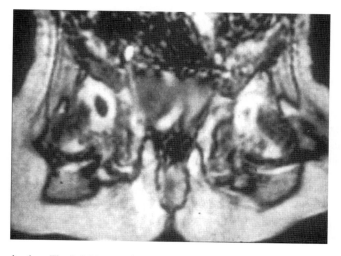

Fig. 26.17 MRI following closed reduction. The left hip acetabular roof is largely cartilaginous; the femoral head has a much smaller ossific nucleus but the head is well applied to the triradiate cartilage

removed and hip stability and alignment checked. At this stage a further 4–6 weeks in a hip spica is usually preferable to a removable abduction splint. After 3 months it is usually safe to remove the plaster cast and continue abduction splintage until satisfactory maturation has been radiologically confirmed. Careful follow-up until skeletal maturity is essential.

Open Reduction

If the arthrogram demonstrates that the hip is not reducible careful decision making is necessary. Some surgeons proceed directly to open reduction under the same anesthetic. Others prefer to wait until the ossific nucleus appears. Where the dislocation is clearly teratological and a well-formed false acetabulum has developed above the true acetabulum, it is advisable to wait for ossification as the risk of avascular necrosis is particularly high.

Open reduction is clearly necessary when closed reduction is not possible. It is also needed when teratological dislocation has delayed treatment until the ossific nucleus

has appeared in the cartilaginous femoral head. When there is a defined obstruction, such as an inverted limbus or an encroaching transverse acetabular ligament, surgical reduction is mandatory. The hip may be approached by the medial, anterolateral, or posterior approaches.

Medial approach: the incision is made parallel to adductor longus or transversely below the groin crease (Fig. 26.18); the transverse scar does not lengthen with growth and is cosmetically satisfactory. The femoral neurovascular bundle is retracted laterally. The lesser trochanter and its attached psoas tendon are approached from in front or behind adductor brevis. Care should be taken to protect the vessels adjacent to it. The psoas tendon is released from its insertion and allowed to retract proximally. This exposes the infero-medial hip capsule. Through a T incision, with its long limb along the femoral neck, the transverse acetabular ligament, the pulvinar, and the ligamentum teres may be inspected; the labrum is rarely seen because it lies posteriorly and superiorly. The approach allows release of the inferior capsule, division of the transverse ligament, and, if needed, excision of the ligamentum teres. This combination usually allows the femoral head to reduce deeply [41, 44].

Fig. 26.18 The medial adductor approach to the hip

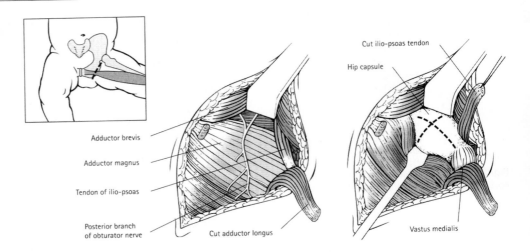

In general, the medial approach is appropriate only for the child under walking age. It is contraindicated when there is a large inverted limbus. A capsulorrhaphy cannot be performed and the medial circumflex artery may be damaged, causing avascular necrosis although its severity depends at least in part upon the preoperative management and the position in plaster. The approach is relatively bloodless, and the recovery of hip movement is usually excellent. Damage to the iliac apophysis is avoided.

Anterolateral approach: this was originally through a Smith-Petersen approach, but this leaves a cosmetically ugly scar. A "bikini" transverse incision below the iliac crest centered upon the anterior superior spine is preferred (Fig. 26.19). The space between sartorius and tensor fasciae latae is developed after identifying, protecting, and retracting the lateral femoral cutaneous nerve. The anterior one-third of the iliac apophysis is split by incising sharply through cartilage to bone. The apophysis with the abductor muscles and periosteum in one sheet are stripped from the outer surface of the ilium. The straight and reflected heads of rectus femoris are divided and reflected distally, exposing the superior and anterior hip capsule. The psoas tendon within the iliacus at the pelvic brim is identified, rolled forward, and divided to provide muscle lengthening without loss of continuity.

A T-shaped incision is made in the hip capsule. The capsulotomy should skirt the capsular attachment to the pelvis, and the long arm of the T should pass along the anterior femoral neck. Hip dislocation is accomplished by adducting, extending, and externally rotating the leg. The femoral head is almost invariably slightly flattened and oval. Inspection of the acetabulum may be difficult. The ligamentum teres is the guide to the acetabular depth. It is usually excised as it is hypertrophic and contributes negligibly to capital epiphyseal blood supply after infancy. The transverse ligament, which blocks reduction inferiorly, should be divided. If a limbus is present and inverted, it should be preserved as it is composed partly of pre-osseous cartilage. It may be made more pliant by making one or two radial cuts, allowing it to be everted over the femoral head.

The acetabulum should be palpated to ensure that no other obstacle prevents reduction, as adhesions and capsular bands

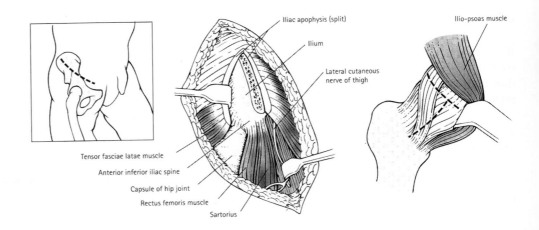

Fig. 26.19 The anterolateral approach to the hip

often extend below the femoral head. Image intensification helps to ensure the head is deeply reduced. Often, a thickened acetabular floor appears to "lateralize" the head. If in doubt, a small pledget soaked in radio-opaque dye may be inserted between head and socket to determine radiographically the adequacy of reduction.

As neither femoral head nor acetabulum is spherical, it is inaccurate to describe the reduction as "concentric" but the position of "best fit" must be estimated. Because of increased femoral anteversion this is usually with the hip flexed, abducted, and internally rotated, each by 30–40°. Capsulorrhaphy is performed by excising the redundant capsule superiorly (removing the superior triangle from the T-shaped incision) or by reefing the capsular margins. Rectus femoris is re-attached and the iliac apophysis is carefully repaired to ensure that it does not become deformed. The hip is maintained in a hip spica in sufficient flexion, abduction, and internal rotation for the head to be fully contained by the acetabulum but avoiding extreme positioning.

In the infant before walking age, it is unlikely that secondary femoral or acetabular procedures will be necessary, and 3 months of plaster immobilization is usually sufficient, followed by a period of abduction bracing if the acetabular response is slow. In the older child, secondary procedures become progressively more likely and it is often advisable to consider them coincidently with open reduction (Fig. 26.20).

Posterior approach: the hip may be approached posteriorly, either through a curved posterolateral or a simple transverse posterior incision. The approach has not gained wide popularity because, although theoretically attractive in giving good access to the limbus, it does not allow an effective capsulorrhaphy, psoas tenotomy has to be performed distally, and there is a significant risk of interfering with the posterior blood supply. Furthermore, if a later pelvic procedure is required, a second incision has to be made.

Treatment of the Toddler

The toddler with a hip dislocation presents typically with an abnormal gait. On average, children with a dislocated hip walk only 1–2 months later than their peers. Children walk with a combined short leg and Trendelenburg limp. The child walks on tiptoe on the affected side, with truncal asymmetry and external rotation of the leg. Clinical signs include elevation of the greater trochanter, flattening of the buttock, and hollowing below the femoral triangle. A groin lump may be palpable with the hip extended, where the femoral lies extruded anterosuperiorly. True shortening is demonstrable when the dislocation is unilateral. It is very rare to be able to reduce the dislocated hip of a child of walking age. Characteristically, abduction in flexion is markedly restricted. When both hips are dislocated, the child walks with a bilateral Trendelenburg lurch and develops hyperlordosis of the lumbar spine.

As in the younger infant, the principles of management in the toddler are straightforward: the hip should be reduced as atraumatically as possible. Reduction should be maintained for the minimum time necessary for stability to be assured.

Treatment of late-presenting congenital hip dislocation was once by forcible manipulation under anesthesia and splintage of the hip in the fully abducted and/or internally

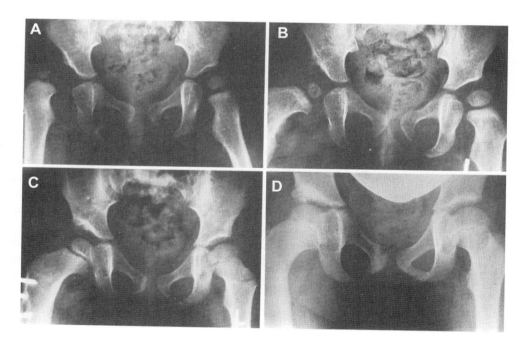

Fig. 26.20 (a) An 18-month-old girl with late-presenting right DDH: note the thick acetabular floor, the steeply sloping acetabular roof, and the smaller ossific femoral head nucleus. (b) Six weeks after open reduction. The lines of temporary growth arrest show symmetrical physeal growth. (c) One year after derotation femoral osteotomy. (d) At age 10 years the hip is stable. The acetabulum has improved and its ring epiphysis ossified but not yet united

rotated position, sometimes for up to 2 years. While many hips were successfully reduced by this technique, avascular necrosis of the femoral head occurred in over 50% of cases. The risk of necrosis remains with current management but the incidence is now much lower.

Twenty years ago, few surgeons would have considered operating on an older child unless the soft tissue contractures associated with dislocation had been at least partly overcome by preliminary traction. Although many continue to advise traction, either at home or in hospital, an increasing number do not, believing that shortened muscles may be lengthened at operation by tenotomy. Inevitably, financial considerations influence the decision. If traction is used it must be carefully supervised: tapes and bandaging must be regularly changed and carefully applied. It may be of simple "gallows" type or progressive abduction in flexion may be achieved if a hoop is placed over the bed. Traction in extension is particularly suitable for the older child, and modified Pugh's traction on a 45° tilted mattress is valuable as the child may lie either prone or supine and is easier to entertain.

For the child older than 2–3 years with a high dislocation, femoral shortening is often necessary to achieve reduction without femoral head compression [45, 46].

Is the Hip Reducible?

Whether or not preliminary traction has been used the child's hip should be examined under general anesthesia. Some surgeons are happy to rely solely on their clinical examination and image intensification but we recommend further evaluation by arthrography. It is essential to decide upon the shape of the femoral head and acetabulum (both of which may be largely cartilaginous). If the head reduces does it do so deeply and congruously? Are there obstacles to reduction and if so what are they? If the hip reduces what is the best position of reduction and how stable is the hip with movement?

The reducible hip: the most satisfactory reduction position should be recorded remembering that extreme positioning is not safe. This may be in 90° of flexion and 45° of abduction (the "human" position) or in modest flexion, abduction and internal rotation (typically 30° of each). It is wise to perform a tenotomy of the adductor longus. Some advise an open psoas tenotomy to further safeguard against undue head pressure. A one-and-a-half or double hip spica is applied in the safe position and changed under anesthesia 4–6 weeks later. It is wise to confirm the initial position postoperatively by MRI or CT scan. After 3 months in a hip spica an abduction brace should be used and retained until adaptive capsular shortening has occurred and the deformed cartilage of the acetabular roof has begun to ossify.

The irreducible hip: the arthrogram may show the hip cannot be reduced and clarifies the obstacles. One French school practices several weeks of traction followed always by closed reduction: where the head stands off from the acetabulum they have found that gradual penetration occurs without incarceration of the limbus. Their long-term results are very good but not yet published. Most centers recommend open reduction when the hip will not reduce under anesthesia. We prefer the anterolateral approach for these older children. The principles of this reduction are no different from those in the younger child, although femoral head deformity may be more pronounced. Femoral anteversion and valgus may be marked, and the acetabulum is shallow and anteverted. If the labrum has been inverted, it becomes more rigid, making it difficult to evert. It is sensible to carry out an intramuscular psoas tenotomy and adductor tenotomy to minimize head pressure following reduction.

In children younger than 18 months, careful reduction of the hip and capsular plication usually promote satisfactory development. In older children, a secondary bony procedure, either to realign the acetabulum or the femur, becomes increasingly advisable. Pelvic osteotomy is not recommended for children under 18 months as the bone graft used tends to crush or displace. After the age of 18 months, however, if the acetabulum is markedly dysplastic, it is wise to consider a pelvic osteotomy to make secondary operation less likely.

If, even after release of the adductors and ilio-psoas, the femoral head appears to reduce too tightly, concurrent femoral shortening should be undertaken. If extending the flexed knee provokes redislocation the hamstrings are too tight and again the femur should be shortened. It is sensible to consider coincident femoral shortening for any child over 2½ years, for the child with a teratological dislocation, and for any child with a neuromuscular disorder such as arthrogryposis. The operation was first described in 1928 by Hey-Groves [45], but was more recently popularized by Klisic [46].

A child immobilized in a hip spica for 3 months is vulnerable to osteoporotic femoral fracture, typically a greenstick supracondylar. Gentle mobilization is important therefore after spica removal and where possible a day or two of supervised in-patient physiotherapy is helpful.

It is important to mobilize the child for a few days in hospital once a hip spica has been removed, because the osteoporotic femur may fracture. A graduated approach to splintage further reduces risks and progression from full-length hip spicas to pantaloon casts and then removable abduction braces are recommended.

While every optimism may be felt for the promptly recognized and treated neonatal unstable hip, the surgeon should be cautious of promising normal outcomes for older children. There is little doubt that the quality of the long-term result is poorer [41, 47] and each child who has been treated for hip dislocation should be reviewed at least until skeletal maturity.

Treatment in Later Childhood

The majority of children over toddler age who present with congenital hip dislocation represent the failures of earlier management. It is rare for the untreated child with congenital hip dysplasia to develop pain before adolescence. Even then, pain is likely to be experienced as discomfort or fatigue after exercise. In contrast, the child who has been treated unsuccessfully is likely to develop pain in early childhood.

Gibson and Benson [47] showed the long-term results of treatment for the older child deteriorate for a variety of reasons: femoral head and acetabular deformity become more marked, femoral anteversion increases, the acetabulum fails to develop anteriorly, and the capacity for remodeling decreases rapidly after the age of 3 years.

Where bilateral dislocation is present, the child stands with a hyperlordotic lumbar spine, which is not present in unilateral dislocation. Shortening becomes more pronounced. Palpation of the groin beneath the inguinal ligament reveals an "empty" acetabulum. The trochanter is high and proximal and may be felt deeply in the buttock, where it is carried by the increasing anteversion of the femoral head and neck.

The principles of treatment for the older child remain exactly the same as before: the hip needs to be reduced atraumatically, preventing abnormal pressure upon the reduced femoral head. To accomplish this many surgeons previously recommended preoperative skin traction but this is now rarely used. Intra-operative femoral shortening reduces the pressure upon the reduced femoral head and is almost always advisable in the child over the age of 2½ years. Such femoral shortening may with profit be combined with derotation sufficient to counteract the excessive anteversion. It is prudent to lengthen the ilio-psoas intra-operatively to minimize further femoral head pressure.

Femoral Osteotomy

Osteotomy of the proximal femur is readily carried out through a lateral thigh incision. An L-shaped incision at its origin allows vastus lateralis to be reflected forward, just below the level of the greater trochanter; the trochanteric growth plate should not be injured. It is sensible to insert wires into the proximal femur so that, after rotation or varus, parallel alignment of the wires confirms that the desired alteration has been achieved. Image intensification should be used if possible. Ideally, the osteotomy should be performed above the level of the lesser trochanter, but this may not be possible if shortening is required. In tiny children the osteotomy is held with a small plate as a "bone suture" (Fig. 26.20). In the older child a blade plate is preferable, and from the age

of 5 or 6 years, compression at the osteotomy site obviates the need for plaster fixation.

Although femoral osteotomy may be necessary, there is a tendency to use it less often than in the past. Typically, the varus introduced at osteotomy resolves within 3 years [48] and the shortening corrects by relative overgrowth within the same period.

It is now uncommon for the child with hip dislocation who is older than 2 years to be treated non-operatively. The surgical approach favored is almost always the anterolateral, which provides the best exposure of the hip joint and its contents. In established dislocation, the superior capsule is usually firmly adherent to the side wall of the ilium above the true acetabulum and needs to be elevated and mobilized superiorly and posteriorly if the labrum is to be everted from the joint. The redundant superior capsule should be excised and a careful capsulorrhaphy performed when the head has been fully reduced.

The femoral head and acetabulum are always deformed in the long-established dislocation, but it is important to ensure that the femoral head is seated as deeply as possible in the true acetabulum. If it is impossible to evert the labrum, radial cuts should make it possible to retain it. It is unnecessary to remove the acetabular fat pad (pulvinar), but the transverse ligament should be divided. The inferior capsule may need careful release to allow the femoral head to descend fully. The posterior capsule should not be divided but in some circumstances, particularly after previous failed surgery, it cannot be avoided; great care should then be taken to divide the capsule at the acetabular margin. The procedure is most likely to be necessary where the hip has dislocated posteriorly as a consequence of excessive internal rotation at previous open reduction.

Pelvic Osteotomy

Careful preoperative analysis and intra-operative assessment should help to decide if pelvic osteotomy is necessary. The capacity of the acetabulum to remodel around the femoral head is maximal in infancy and decreases steadily after the first 3 or 4 years. If, therefore, the acetabulum contains the femoral head poorly, attempts should be made to improve the acetabular cover.

In the typical dislocation, the anterior limb of the triradiate cartilage is inadequately stimulated and the anterior acetabulum fails to develop. This produces a shallow and apparently anteverted acetabulum. If the acetabulum is flat and oval, its shape may be improved by the Pemberton [49] peri-capsular osteotomy. This is described below, but in essence a curvilinear osteotomy is made above the acetabulum and the roof is folded downward to improve acetabular congruity and cover.

If the femoral head and the acetabulum fit well but the acetabulum is too open, the Salter [50] innominate osteotomy, which rotates the whole acetabulum forward and laterally, is to be preferred. Klisic [46] made popular the simultaneous performance of open reduction, femoral shortening, and pelvic osteotomy. Some surgeons, however, prefer to reserve pelvic osteotomy for those children in whom it may be seen that the acetabulum is failing to develop adequately after reduction [51]. The stress to the child and family of multiple hip surgery in childhood and the disadvantages of repetitive plaster immobilization should not be underestimated, and where expertise and facilities allow, the surgeon should attempt both to reduce and stabilize the hip at the time of the first operation. The risk of redislocation should increase only marginally.

Wherever possible, it is best to reshape and realign the acetabulum so that articular cartilage covers the femoral head. In the child older than 4 or 5 years, acetabular and femoral head deformity may be such that this is impracticable. Under these circumstances, when the hip is subluxated and the acetabular volume reduced, a salvage procedure such as the medial displacement osteotomy of Chiari [52] or a shelf procedure may be a better solution.

Although shortening, rotational, and varus osteotomy may be necessary, both to decrease pressure upon the femoral head and to reorientate the proximal femur, it has been shown by Williamson and Benson [53] that femoral osteotomy alone in later childhood is inadequate treatment for the subluxated hip.

Because of the deteriorating results of treatment with age, many surgeons suggest that the child older than 7 years with bilateral hip dislocation should be left untreated because operation has a high chance of increasing the likelihood of adolescent hip pain. Where the dislocation is unilateral, however, most surgeons continue to advocate reduction and reconstruction in older children to preserve leg length and spinal symmetry.

The Innominate Osteotomy

Salter's osteotomy [50] is suitable for the child between the ages of 2 and 6 years with a dislocated hip and may be appropriate for the subluxating hip in the older child and adolescent. Certain criteria are necessary for the osteotomy to be undertaken. The hip should reduce concentrically and preserve a virtually normal range of movement. If open reduction is performed at the same time, hip reduction should be congruous and confirmed radiologically. It should be apparent that subluxation of the hip anterosuperiorly as it is moved from flexion into extension is prevented when the leg is internally rotated and abducted. It is precisely this

maldirectional instability that the innominate osteotomy is designed to correct.

The innominate osteotomy lengthens the leg; avoidance of this lengthening is possible by combining it with a varus rotational osteotomy [53] or by notching the upper pelvic segment in the older child [54]. Overzealous femoral internal rotation or derotational osteotomy may allow the femoral head to displace posteriorly, as the innominate osteotomy achieves improved anterolateral cover at the expense of posterior support. As already noted, in the child older than 3 years, it may be wise to shorten the femur to lessen pressure upon the reduced femoral head. Theoretically, an innominate osteotomy may increase pressure upon the femoral head, but Salter has argued that the pressure increase is trivial.

The innominate osteotomy (Figs. 26.21 and 26.22)is best performed through a transverse incision just below the iliac

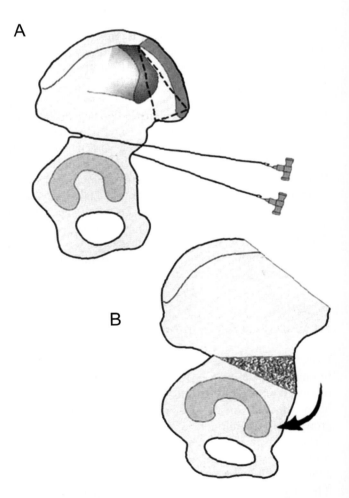

Fig. 26.21 The innominate osteotomy of Salter. (**a**) The Gigli saw transects the ilium at the level of the anterior inferior spine. (**b**) The wedge of bone harvested from the iliac crest is inserted into the osteotomy, allowing the distal pelvic fragment and acetabulum to rotate forward and laterally

Fig. 26.22 (**a**) Previously treated DDH has left this girl with Type II avascular necrosis, dysplasia, and mild subluxation. (**b**) After an arthrogram confirmed sphericity and congruity she was treated by innominate osteotomy and varus femoral osteotomy. (**c**) The appearance 5 years later

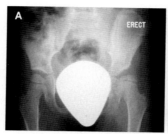
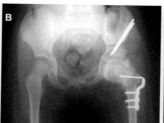
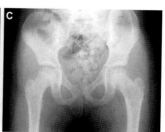

crest. The iliac apophysis is split and the split halves are elevated subperiosteally from the iliac wing, in continuity with the gluteal muscles externally and the iliac muscles medially. Great care should be taken in exposing the sciatic notch, and the retractors placed through this notch should be clearly seen and felt to be subperiosteal. The psoas tendon should be divided intramuscularly by rolling it at the level of the pelvic brim. A curved introducer passed through the sciatic notch allows the Gigli saw to be introduced subperiosteally through the notch.

A transverse pelvic osteotomy is then performed at the level of the anterior inferior iliac spine. Where the hip joint has not been opened the thigh is placed in flexion, abduction, and external rotation. Downward leverage upon the knee allows the distal pelvic fragment to rotate anterolaterally. Its direction may be helped by gentle downward traction using a towel clip placed through the anterior inferior spine or by pulling the posterior edge of the lower fragment forward with a small Lambotte hook. A wedge of bone taken from the anterior superior iliac spine is trimmed and fashioned to fit into the triangular gap so created. It is important to keep the osteotomy closed posteriorly. Once the bone graft is safely placed, two threaded wires should be passed across the osteotomy and screened radiographically to ensure that joint penetration has not occurred. The implants are cut short, but should be left slightly proud of the closed iliac apophysis.

The wound is closed in layers, taking care to re-appose the iliac apophysis carefully. A one-and-a-half hip spica is applied with the hip in 20–30° of flexion and abduction but neutral rotation. The osteotomy unites in 6 weeks. It was once the routine to remove these wires but they are now often retained.

Complications that may occur with this procedure are often the result of faulty technique [55]. The operation should not be performed unless it is possible to reduce the hip satisfactorily. Redislocation may occur if open reduction is performed simultaneously [51]. The bone graft may slip or resorb, wires may penetrate the joint or extrude, the sciatic, femoral, or lateral femoral cutaneous nerves may be injured, and there may be deformity of the ilium consequent upon splitting the iliac apophysis.

Pemberton Acetabuloplasty

Where the femoral head and acetabulum do not "match," and where arthrography has demonstrated a bilocular or "double diameter" acetabulum in association with subluxation, it may be wise to reshape rather than to redirect the acetabulum, in the manner described by Pemberton [49]. Pemberton's procedure allows an incomplete iliac osteotomy to hinge through the triradiate cartilage. This hinge alters the volume of the acetabulum and is therefore applicable for the dysplastic oval socket. The triradiate cartilage must be open and it is therefore most useful for children 3–11 years old. The approach is similar to that described for an innominate osteotomy. Careful preoperative radiographic checking is essential. A series of curved osteotomies is passed above the hip joint, curving medially and posteriorly to the triradiate cartilage, usually at a distance of about 1 cm from the acetabular margin. Care must be taken to ensure that articular penetration does not occur. A curved bone graft is taken from the anterosuperior iliac spine and inserted into the gap created as the acetabular margin is levered down with the osteotome. When the bone graft is tapped into place the position is usually stable so that internal fixation is unnecessary (Figs. 26.23 and 26.24).

The risk of joint penetration is real in this procedure, and there is a slight increase in the risk of avascular necrosis from pressure directed upon the femoral head by the levered-down acetabular roof. The triradiate cartilage may rarely be injured and cease to grow.

The Pemberton acetabuloplasty, just like the innominate osteotomy, may be performed in isolation or as part of a complex open reduction in the older child, in whom it may be combined with femoral shortening and rotation.

Other Procedures

The Dega pelvic osteotomy [56] is similar to the Pemberton, except that the pelvic cut is not curved, but directed obliquely downward and medially to the triradiate cartilage from an anteroposterior axis 2 cm above the acetabular margin. It similarly reduces acetabular size, but increases lateral rather than anterior cover.

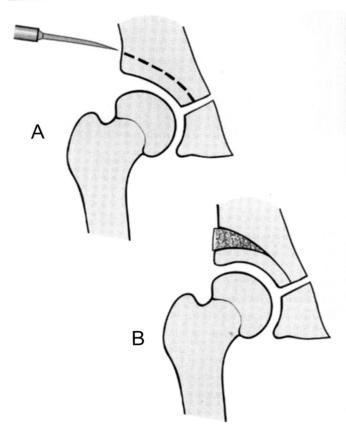

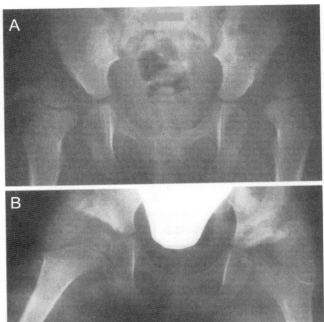

Fig. 26.24 (**a**) Two-and-a-half-year-old girl with right hip subluxation and left hip dislocation. (**b**) Following open reduction of the left hip and bilateral Pemberton osteotomy

Fig. 26.23 The pelvic osteotomy of Pemberton. (**a**) The osteotomy curves 1 cm from the acetabular margin up to the triradiate cartilage. (**b**) Hinging at the triradiate cartilage allows the acetabular roof to be levered down and stabilized with a bone graft

Macnicol [57] has described and illustrated the variety of more complex acetabular osteotomies. As skeletal maturity approaches, the Salter osteotomy in isolation may not allow sufficient rotation about the axis passing from symphysis pubis to greater sciatic notch, unless osteotomies of the superior pubic ramus and ischium are performed coincidentally. This triple innominate osteotomy, as described by Tönnis [29], allows greater rotation and displacement of the acetabulum: the innominate osteotomy element is supplemented by osteotomies of the superior pubic ramus and ischium as close as possible to the acetabulum. This allows much greater rotation of the acetabulum and improved femoral head cover. It must always be remembered that such reorientation decreases posterior cover and care is needed not to over-correct. The triple osteotomy is most useful in children aged 7–14 years whose triradiate cartilage is still open.

Residual dysplasia often merits treatment after maturity. When an adolescent or young adult develops discomfort with exercise and radiographs demonstrate marked uncovering of the femoral head, a periacetabular osteotomy should

be considered. A careful history and examination may suggest the "rim syndrome" described by Klaue et al. [58]. The patient describes sudden sharp groin pain that accompanies twisting movements. There is often a feeling that the leg may "give way." Although the hip may appear to move freely at examination, pain is typically produced when the flexed hip is pressed into adduction and internal rotation. The cause is usually a torn labrum, which may be associated with a ganglionic cyst in the labrum itself or in the bony pelvis. The tear is best demonstrated by gadolinium-enhanced MRI. Increasingly hip arthroscopy is used to assess the hip since labral tears, loose bodies, and articular cartilage flaps are amenable to arthroscopic debridement. It must be remembered that unless the *cause* of the rim syndrome is addressed, further intra-articular injury is almost inevitable, with resultant osteoarthritis.

If a complex, periacetabular osteotomy is considered, careful preoperative planning is essential. A three-dimensional CT scan best allows spatially correct reconstruction of the hip joint. Significant head deformity and arthritis are contra-indications. Ganz [59] has provided clear prerequisites and technical advice for his Bernese osteotomy (Fig. 26.25). Periacetabular osteotomies are complex and risks include neurovascular injury, non-union and mal-union, and over-correction. They are less satisfactory if significant arthritis is present and are not indicated when there is poor congruity between the femoral head and acetabulum.

Fig. 26.25 The complex peri-acetabular osteotomy of Ganz. (**a**) The lines on the hemi-pelvis show the cuts necessary to rotate the acetabular fragment while preserving continuity of the posterior pelvic column. (**b**) Diagrammatic representation of the displacement highlighting that the acetabulum is not displaced laterally

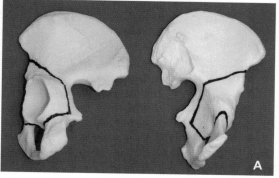
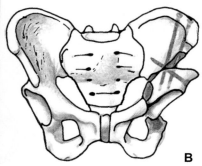

Salvage Procedures

Shelf Arthroplasty

There have been many techniques described to fashion a stabilizing bony shelf above the dysplastic hip. The Staheli technique is widely practiced [60]. Where there is mild or modest subluxation in the child whose hip is not fully containable by a dysplastic acetabulum the shelf is a low-risk procedure to stabilize the femoral head. Whenever possible, it is preferable to realign or reshape the acetabulum to cover the femoral head with true articular cartilage. If this is not possible and the child is developing fatigue discomfort the Staheli shelf arthroplasty is effective.

The superior hip capsule is exposed through a bikini incision and anterior approach. The straight and reflected heads of rectus femoris are defined. Preserving the insertion of the straight head, the reflected head is divided anteriorly and dissected backward off the hip capsule. Its posterior origin is preserved. Taking care not to injure the growth plate at the acetabular margin, a guide wire is inserted slightly cephalad above the capsular insertion. The position should be checked with an image intensifier. A curvilinear slot is made with drill holes and small osteotomes above the capsule and into this slot are inserted coraco-cancellous strips of bone taken from the outer table of the ilium. The reflected head of rectus femoris is laid on top of these bone strips and sutured back to the straight head, so applying the bone graft securely to the superior capsule. Additional cancellous graft is placed above this and the iliac apophysis repaired, holding the graft in place (Fig. 26.26). There is evidence that the graft stimulates growth of the true acetabular margin, increasing articular cartilage cover with time.

The Chiari Osteotomy

Where subluxation is fixed and the femoral head is uncovered, the Chiari medial displacement osteotomy should be considered. Although Chiari [52] first envisaged his procedure as being most applicable to the child 4 or 5 years old, it has become increasingly reserved for the older child, adolescent, and young adult with irreversible and symptomatic acetabular dysplasia. Articulation with the abnormally located false acetabulum may have to be accepted but the femoral head cover is improved to increase stability and decrease harmful shear forces. A shelf procedure affords good support if acetabular insufficiency is mild to moderate, but when the hip joint is lateralized by marked thickening of the acetabular floor, medialization of the femoral head is advisable. These greater degrees of hip deformity benefit from the salvage effect of the Chiari osteotomy, which produces an iliac bone buttress above the superior, uncovered hip capsule.

The procedure reduces loading through the femoral head both by increasing the area of contact and by medializing the fulcrum of the hip. The operation should be carried out using an orthopaedic table and with image intensifier control (Fig. 26.27). A skin-crease bikini incision affords adequate exposure and heals well [61]. The iliac osteotomy should be made just above the hip capsule. The osteotomy level must be checked radiographically as the reflected fibers of the hip capsule are often well above the elected site for osteotomy. Ideally, the osteotomy should be gently curved from front to back, to follow the contour of femoral head and capsule. The angle of the osteotomy should be almost transverse or slightly cephalad. Increasing the upward obliquity of the osteotomy imperils the sacroiliac joint and, by functionally weakening the abductor muscles, makes a persistent Trendelenburg gait more likely.

If 50% displacement at the osteotomy is planned, Benson and Jameson-Evans [62] showed that this allows only up to 2 cm of shift as the ilium is only 3 cm wide at this level. The osteotomy must not be allowed to hinge like a book posteriorly as this causes a false radiographic appearance of good femoral head cover. Anterior femoral head support can be increased by additional bone grafting although this may restrict hip flexion.

Fig. 26.26 (**a**) Diagram of the Staheli shelf arthroplasty: the graft is held on the capsule by the reflected head of rectus femoris. (**b**) A poorly covered hip treated by shelf arthroplasty

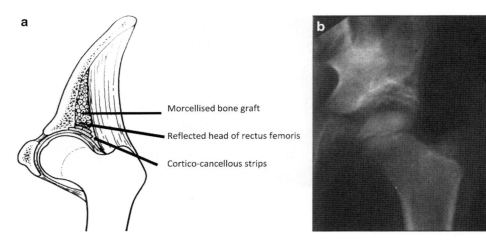

Fig. 26.27 (**a**) Chiari osteotomy. Subluxation is marked; there is incongruity between head and acetabulum and a loose marginal fragment confirming instability. (**b**) After Chiari osteotomy the head is stabilized

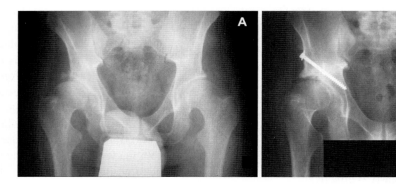

If the osteotomy is fixed with a compression screw, the leg can be moved freely during the recovery period, allowing the patient to return home using crutches a few days postoperatively. Weight bearing is progressively increased over the first 2 months and the limp usually disappears or lessens by 1 year. Because the hip is effectively stabilized, pain relief is significant and lasting. There is a concurrent halt in femoral head migration, and a gratifying degree of pelvic remodeling as Macnicol et al. have shown [63].

Early complications include too low an osteotomy, with breaching of the joint, excessive or inadequate displacement, injury to adjoining nerves and vessels, and problems with wound healing. Late complications are rare, but delayed union has been reported if internal fixation is inadequate, and pelvic ligamentous pain may retard early progress. Damage to the joint produces ankylosis, and numbness in the distribution of the lateral femoral cutaneous nerve may be remarked upon. The osteotomy is contraindicated in the presence of arthritis [64], particularly if there is significant impingement pain and stiffening. Unilateral procedures probably increase the necessity of caesarian section only slightly, bilateral osteotomies rather more. It may be appropriate to carry out a concomitant femoral realignment osteotomy, incorporating varus, valgus, rotation, or extension, depending upon the

resultant congruency of the joint. Windhager et al. [65], in their review of Chiari's own osteotomies after 20–34 years, found the overall result good in 51%, fair in 30%, and poor in 18%. They noted that results were more durable in younger patients. Remodeling of the pelvis occurs around the femoral head. If the osteotomy stabilizes the hip well revision by arthroplasty is avoided in 80% of cases 30 years postoperatively [63].

Capsuloplasty

Femoral head and acetabular deformities may become so pronounced, particularly after failed surgery, that congruous reduction cannot be achieved. If this disparity is pronounced, the Colonna [66] procedure should not be forgotten (Fig. 26.28). A circumferential acetabular capsulotomy is performed and the capsule sutured as an envelope over the femoral head. Using serial reamers, the acetabulum is enlarged to accept the femoral head enveloped in its capsular mantle. Where necessary, the femur may be shortened and rotated appropriately. The Colonna arthroplasty provides a stable articulation, but mobility is clearly less

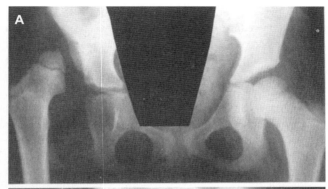

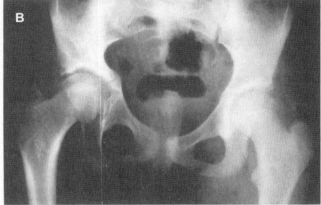

Fig. 26.28 Colonna arthroplasty. (**a**) Late dislocation and severe incongruity. (**b**) Fifteen years after the capsular arthroplasty of Colonna

satisfactory and discomfort more likely than in a more optimally reduced hip. Nonetheless, the restoration of anatomical alignment makes secondary surgery in adult life a great deal more straightforward. Pozo et al. [67] found 70% of 44 hips so treated had good function at a mean follow-up of 20 years.

Trochanteric "Overgrowth"

In children in whom acetabular development is satisfactory but limp and pain are present, the mechanics of the hip may be improved by correcting marked degrees of femoral anteversion, by shortening the femur if there is a "long leg dysplasia," and by distal transfer of the greater trochanter (Fig. 26.29) if the femoral neck is short and the abductor mechanism abnormal [68]. These relatively small surgical adjustments may give considerable improvements in function, endurance, and pain relief if they allow the coaptive relationship between the femoral head and the acetabulum to improve.

Pelvic Support Osteotomies

When the hip is dislocated in later childhood and adolescence both femoral head and acetabulum become so deformed that reduction, even if technically possible, does not provide pain relief and progressive deformity may follow. Fixed flexion, adduction, and external rotation lead to progressive apparent shortening, a deteriorating gait, and secondary back and knee discomfort.

In the adult hip arthrodesis or total joint arthroplasty is a last resort. Recent advances in hip arthroplasty, particularly surface replacement, make this a more attractive option in the young and active adult but the long-term results are still unknown. Furthermore, there is some genetic concern about metal ion release in young women. Revision arthroplasty of the fused hip is also an available but daunting option.

A Schanz sub-trochanteric osteotomy (Fig. 26.30) incorporating valgus, extension, and a little rotation may relieve pain, improve leg alignment and gait, and provide salvage for many years. It may furthermore be combined with distal femoral lengthening [69].

Fig. 26.29 (**a**) Distal transfer of the greater trochanter. Treatment of DDH has caused avascular change in the femoral head and premature growth plate closure. There is relative overgrowth of the greater trochanter. (**b**) More effective abductor power has been achieved by lateral and distal transfer of the greater trochanter, here stabilized by two screws

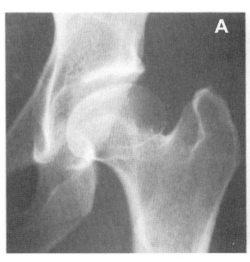

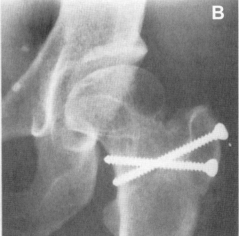

Fig. 26.30 The pelvic support osteotomy of Schanz, 30 years after sub-trochanteric valgus, extension osteotomy. Although severe arthritis has developed the major adduction and flexion deformity has not recurred

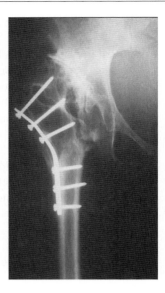

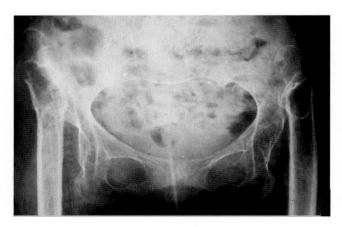

Fig. 26.31 Untreated dislocations in an 88-year-old woman. She has limped throughout her life, has modest back pain but little hip pain

Outcomes

There are few studies of untreated dysplasia. Wedge and Wasylenko [70] contacted 54 adults with 80 affected hips. Although limp was universal many did not develop pain until later adult life. Fifty-nine percent had only fair or poor grading scores. Arthritis developed earlier and was more frequent when a well-formed false acetabulum developed, especially when the hip was subluxated rather than fully dislocated. Unilateral dislocation often led to ipsilateral knee valgus and arthritis. However, the incidence of symptomatic lumbar spondylosis was not increased (Fig. 26.31).

Inevitably we have modified outcomes by treatment. Provided the hip is reducible and avascular necrosis is avoided, neonates and young infants treated promptly should develop a nearly normal hip.

Children with an irreducible hip at birth do less well. Attempts to reduce the hip neonatally may fail and lead to avascular necrosis. Teratological dislocations often present with considerable femoral head deformity so that it is not surprising to find that long-term outcomes are less satisfactory.

Malvitz and Weinstein [71] reviewed 152 young adults after they had been treated by closed reduction at an average age of 21 months. In 60% there was evidence of some proximal femoral growth disturbance; 43% of the treated hips were developing degenerative arthritis, and 36% were still subluxated.

Morcuende et al. [72] then reviewed the Iowa experience with open reduction via a medial approach. A total of 93 hips in 76 children (average age 14 months) were followed up for 4–23 years. Avascular necrotic change was observed in 43%, and 29% had residual dysplasia. The patients were too young at follow-up to assess the incidence of premature arthritis.

Angliss et al. [73] reviewed 147 children with 191 dislocated hips treated surgically for DDH at an average age of 33 years. Thirteen percent showed evidence of some avascular necrosis in the first 5 years. Mild or moderate hip arthritis developed by the mid-thirties in 40% of patients. Arthritis was more likely when the limbus was excised at operation, when residual subluxation was present, and if avascular necrosis developed. Increasing age at presentation also adversely affected the outcome.

Thomas et al. [74] recently reviewed at 45 years postoperatively those children treated by open reduction and innominate osteotomy between the ages of 18 months and 5 years. Of 51 hips with available radiographs, 22 revealed moderate or severe arthritis. Those with bilateral DDH fared worse but the age at operation seemed to make little difference.

Later treatment leads to poorer results because it is more difficult to achieve and maintain a stable reduction. The acetabulum often fails to develop sufficiently and any residual subluxation inevitably worsens with time. Unfortunately, it is not possible to predict outcome accurately for many years after treatment, because the subtle changes of growth disturbance in the proximal femur, especially premature lateral growth arrest, may not appear until adolescence. Therefore, it is imperative that all children treated for developmental dysplasia of the hip be followed by serial radiographs at least until skeletal maturity and that residual instability is recognized and treated as early as possible.

Conclusion

In dealing with displacement and developmental dysplasia of the hip, the overriding principle is to achieve a stable reduction of the femoral head. Treatment is most effective in the neonatal period. With increasing age, there is a greater reliance upon surgery. The surgeon must be constantly alert to the dangers of pressure (avascular) necrosis of the proximal femur and re-displacement. Irrevocable changes occur in the older child, particularly after failed or inadequate surgery, so that the prognosis becomes increasingly poor.

References

1. Strayer LM. The embryology of the human hip. Clin Orthop Rel Res 1971; 74:221–240.
2. Watanabe RS. Embryology of the human hip. Clin Orthop Rel Res 1974; 98:8–26.
3. Le Damany P. Variation en potordeur du cotyle humain aux divers ages. Bulletin Société des Sciences et Medicine d'Ouex 1912; 1974; 12:410.
4. Ralis ZA, McKibbin B. Changes in shape of the human hip in joint during its development and their relationship to its stability. J Bone Joint Surg 1973; 55B:780–785.
5. Portinaro NM, Murray DW, Benson MKD. Microanatomy of the acetabular cavity and its relation to growth. J Bone Joint Surg (Br) 2001; 83:377–383.
6. Trueta J. The normal vascular anatomy of the human femoral head during growth. J Bone Joint Surg 1957; 39B:358–394.
7. Chung SM. The arterial supply of the developing proximal end of the femur. J Bone Joint Surg Am 1976; 58:961–970.
8. Klisic P, Pajic D. Progress in the preventative approach to developmental dysplasia of the hip. J Paediatr Orthop 1993; Part B, 2:108–111.
9. Chan A, McCaul KA, Cundy PJ, et al. Perinatal risk factors for developmental dysplasia of the hip. Arch Dis Child Fetal Neonatal Ed 1997; 76:F94–100.
10. Carter CO, Wilkinson J. Genetic and environmental factors in the aetiology of congenital dislocation of the hip. Clinical Orthop 1960; 33:119–128.
11. Vogel I, Andersson JE, Uldbjerg N. Serum relaxin in the newborn is not a marker of neonatal hip instability J Pediatr Orthop 1998; 18(4):535–537.
12. McKibbin B. Anatomical factors in the stability of the hip in the newborn. J Bone Joint Surg 1970; 52B:148–159.
13. Barlow TG. Early diagnosis and treatment of congenital dislocation of the hip. J Bone Joint Surg 1962; 44B:242–301.
14. Macnicol MF. Results of a 25-year screening programme for neonatal hip instability. J Bone Joint Surg 1990; 72B:1057–1060.
15. Roser W. Ueber angeborene Hueftverrenkung. Langenbeck's Archiv fuer klinische Chirurgie 1879; 24:309–313.
16. Ortolani M. Un segno poco noto e sua importanza par la diagnosi di preluzzione congenitale dell'ance. Pediatria 1937; 45:129.
17. Von Rosen S. Diagnosis and treatment of congenital dislocation of the hip in the new-born. J Bone Joint Surg 1962; 44B:284–291.
18. Palmèn K. Preluxation of the hip joint. Diagnosis and treatment in the newborn and the diagnosis of congenital dislocation of the hip joint in Sweden during the years 1948–60. Acta Paediatr (Suppl 129) 1961;50: 1–71.
19. Godward S, Dezateaux C. Surgery for congenital dislocation of the hip in the UK as a measure of outcome of screening. Lancet 1998; 351(9110):1149–52.
20. Graf R. Classification of hip joint dysplasia by means of sonography. Arch Orthop Trauma Surg 1984; 102:248–255.
21. Lehmann HP, Hinton R, Morello P, Santoli J. Developmental dysplasia of the hip practice guideline: technical report. Committee on Quality Improvement, and Subcommittee on Developmental Dysplasia of the Hip. Pediatrics 2000; Apr. 105(4):E57.
22. Clegg J, Bache CE, Raut W. Financial justification for routine ultrasound screening of the neonatal hip. J Bone Joint Surg 1999; 81B:852–857.
23. Morin C, Harcke HT, MacEwan GD. The infant hip: real-time US assessment of acetabular development. Radiology 1985; 157:673–677.
24. Suzuki S, Kasahara Y, Futami T, et al. Ultrasonography in congenital dislocation of the hip. Simultaneous imaging of both hips from in front. J Bone Joint Surg 1991; 73B:879–83.
25. Clarke NMP, Harcke HT, McHugh P, et al. Real-time ultrasound in the diagnosis of congenital dislocation and dysplasia of the hip. J Bone Joint Surg 1985;67B:406.
26. Engesaeter LB, Wilson DJ, Nag D, Benson MK. Ultrasound and congenital dislocation of the hip. J Bone Joint Surg 1990; 72B:197–200.
27. Dunn PM. Perinatal observations on the aetiology of congenital dislocation of the hip. Clin Orthop 1976; 119:11.
28. Bertol P, Macnicol MF, Mitchell GP. Radiographic features of neonatal congenital dislocation of the hip. J Bone Joint Surg 1982; 64B:176–179.
29. Tönnis D. Congenital Dysplasia and Dislocation of the Hip. Berlin: Springer; 1986.
30. Wiberg C. Studies on dysplastic acetabulae and congenital subluxation of the hip joint. Acta Chirurgica Scandinavica 1939; Suppl 58.
31. Severin E. Contribution to the knowledge of congenital dislocation of the hip joint. Acta Chir Scandinavica 1941; 84: Suppl 63.
32. Salter RB, Kostuik J, Dallas S. Avascular necrosis of the femoral head as a complication of treatment of congenital dislocation in young children: a clinical and experimental study. Can J Surg 1969; 12:44.
33. Kalamchi A, MacEwan GD. Avascular necrosis following treatment of congenital dislocation of the hip. J Bone Joint Surg 1980; 62A:876–888.
34. Bradley J, Weatherill M, Benson MKD. Splintage for congenital dislocation of the hip. Is it safe and reliable? J Bone Joint Surg 1987; 69B:259–263.
35. Grill F, Bensahel H, Canadell J, et al. The Pavlik harness in the treatment of congenital dislocating hip. J Pediatr Orthop 1988; 8(1):1–8.
36. Wilkinson AG, Sherlock DA, Murray GD. The efficacy of the Pavlik harness, the Craig splint and the von Rosen splint in the management of neonatal dysplasia of the hip. J Bone Joint Surg Br 2003; 85:1085–1086.
37. Nakamura J, Kamegaya M, Saisu T, et al. Treatment for developmental dysplasia of the hip using the Pavlik harness. J Bone Joint Surg 2007; 89-B:230–235.
38. Macnicol M F. Congenital dislocation of the hip. In: Bennet GC, ed. Paediatric Hip Disorders. Oxford: Blackwell; 1987: 64–113.
39. Segal LS, Schneider DJ, Berlin JM, et al. The contribution of the ossific nucleus in the structural stiffness of the capital femoral epiphysis: a porcine model for DDH. J Pediatr Orthop 1999; 19:433–437.
40. Luhmann S, Schoenecker PL, Anderson AM, Bassett G. The prognostic significance of the ossific nucleus in the treatment of congenital dysplasia of the hip J Bone Joint Surg 1998; 80-A:1719–1727.
41. Weinstein SL, Ponseti IV. Congenital dislocation of the hip: open reduction through a medial approach. J Bone Joint Surg 1979; 61A:119–124.

42. Ramsey PL, Hensiger RN, MacEwan GD. Congenital dislocation of the hip. Use of the Pavlik harness in the child during the first 6 months of life. J Bone Joint Surg Am 1976; 58:1000–1004.

43. McNally EG, Tasker A, Benson MK. MRI after operative reduction for developmental dysplasia of the hip. J Bone Joint Surg Br 1998; 79:724–726.

44. Ludloff K. The open reduction of congenital hip dislocation by an anterior incision. Am J Orthop Surg 1913; 10:438–454.

45. Hey-Groves E. The treatment of congenital dislocation of the hip. Robert Jones Birthday Volume. Oxford: Oxford University Press; 1928.

46. Klisic P. Combined procedure of open reduction and shortening of the femur in treatment of congenital dislocation of the hip in older children. Clin Orth 1976; 119:60.

47. Gibson PH, Benson MKD. Congenital dislocation of the hip. Review at maturity of 147 hips treated by excision of the limbus and derotation osteotomy. J Bone Joint Surg 1982; 64B:169–175.

48. Sangavi SM, Szoke G, Murray DW, Benson MK. Femoral remodeling after subtrochanteric osteotomy for developmental dysplasia of the hip. J Bone Joint Surg 1996; 8B:917–923.

49. Pemberton PA. Pericapsular osteotomy of the ilium for treatment of congenital subluxation and dislocation of the hip. J Bone Joint Surg 1965; 47A:65–86.

50. Salter RB. Innominate osteotomy in the treatment of congenital dislocation and subluxation of the hip. J Bone Joint Surg 1961; 43B:518–539.

51. Macnicol MF, Bertol P. The Salter innominate osteotomy: should it be combined with concurrent open reduction? J Paediatr Orthop B 2005; 14:415–21.

52. Chiari K. Beckenosteotomie zur Pfannendachplastik. Wiener Medizinische Wochenschrift 1953; 103:707–713.

53. Williamson DM, Benson MKD. Late femoral osteotomy in congenital dislocation of the hip. J Bone Joint Surg 1988; 70B:614–618.

54. Kalamchi A. Modified salter osteotomy. J Bone Joint Surg Am 1982; 64:183–187.

55. Morscher E. Our experience with Salter's innominate osteotomy in the treatment of hip dysplasia. In: Weil UH, ed. Progress in Orthopaedic Surgery. vol 2. Berlin: Springer; 1978.

56. Dega W, Krol J, Polakowski L. Surgical treatment of congenital dislocation of the hip in children; a one step procedure. J Bone Joint Surg Am 1959; 41A(5):920–934.

57. Macnicol MF. Color Atlas and Text: Osteotomy of the Hip. London: Mosby-Wolfe; 1995.

58. Klaue K, Durnin CW, Ganz R. The acetabular rim syndrome. A clinical presentation of dysplasia of the hip. J Bone Joint Surg 1991; 73B:423–429.

59. Ganz R, Klaue K, Vinh TS, Mast JW. A new periacetabular osteotomy for the treatment of hip dysplasias. Technique and preliminary results. Clin Orthop 1988; 232:26–36.

60. Staheli LT, Chew DE. Slotted acetabular augmentation in childhood and adolescence. J Pediatr Orthop 1992; 12(5):569–80.

61. Reynolds DA. Chiari innominate osteotomy in adults: technique, indications and contraindications. J Bone Joint Surg 1986; 68B:45–54.

62. Benson MKD, Jameson-Evans DC. The pelvic osteotomy of Chiari: an anatomical study of the hazards and misleading radiological appearances. J Bone Joint Surg 1976; 58B:164–168.

63. Macnicol MF, Lo HK, Yong KF. Pelvic remodeling after the Chiari osteotomy: a long-term review. J Bone Joint Surg [Br] 2004; 86-B:648–54.

64. Högh J, Macnicol MF. The Chiari pelvic osteotomy. A long-term review of clinical and radiographic results. J Bone Joint Surg 1987; 69B:365–373.

65. Windhager R, Pongracz N, Schonecker W, Kotz R. Chiari osteotomy for congenital dislocation and subluxation of the hip. Results after 20 to 34 years follow-up. J Bone Joint Surg Br 1991; 73(6):890–5.

66. Colonna PC. Capsular arthroplasty for congenital dislocation of the hip: indications and technique. J Bone Joint Surg 1965; 47A:437.

67. Pozo JL, Cannon SR, Catterall A. The Colonna-Hey Groves arthroplasty in the late treatment of the hip. A Long-Term Rev 1987 Mar; 69(2):220–228.

68. Macnicol MF, Makris D. Distal transfer of the greater trochanter. J Bone Joint Surg 1991; 73B:838–841.

69. El-Mowafi H. Outcome of pelvic support osteotomy with the Ilizarov method in the treatment of the unstable hip joint. Acta Orthop Belg 2005; 71:686–691.

70. Wedge JH, Wasylenko MJ. The natural history of congenital disease of the hip. J Bone Joint Surg 1979; 61-B:334–338.

71. Malvitz TA, Weinstein SL. Closed reduction for congenital dysplasia of the hip. Functional and radiographic results after an average of 30 years. J Bone Joint Surg 1994; 76A:1777–1792.

72. Morcuende JA, Meyer MD, Dolan LA, Weinstein SL. Long-term outcome after open reduction through an anteromedial approach for congenital dislocation of the hip. J Bone Joint Surg 1997; 79A:810–817.

73. Angliss R, Fujii G, Pickvance E, et al. Surgical treatment of late developmental displacement of the hips: results after 33 years. J Bone Joint Surg 2005; 87-B:384–394.

74. Thomas S, Wedge J, Salter RB. Outcome at 45 years after open reduction and innominate osteotomy for late-presenting developmental dislocation of the hip. J Bone Joint Surg Am 2007; 89:2341–2350.

Chapter 27

Legg–Calvé–Perthes Disease

Andrew M. Wainwright and Anthony Catterall

Introduction

Legg–Calvé–Perthes disease is caused by infarction of the upper femoral epiphysis complicated by trabecular fracture and associated with a process of repair (Fig. 27.1) [1]. The infarct may be variable in extent and the disorder also varies in its outcome: at best the effects may be limited to a childhood limp which can resolve spontaneously. At worst, if the femoral head segmental collapses and subsequent deformity fails to remodel well, it may lead to shortening, stiffness, and premature hip arthritis.

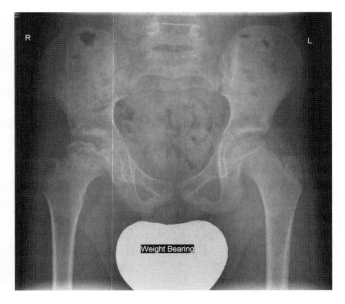

Fig. 27.1 AP view of a hip with Legg–Calvé–Perthes disease on the right side in an eight year old boy

Its Name

The condition has been known variously as coxa plana, osteochondritis deformans juvenilis, Perthes disease, Legg–Perthes disease, and Legg–Calvé–Perthes disease, to which Waldenström's name is sometimes added.

The first description of the condition is generally credited in 1909 to Henning Waldenström [2], Professor of Orthopaedics in Stockholm. He considered it to be a benign form of tuberculosis (then a common cause of hip problems). In fact, the earliest description was published in 1897 by a Czech surgeon Karel Maydl [3], Professor of Surgery in Prague [4].

The term most often used, Legg–Calvé–Perthes disease, is named after the three clinicians who independently recognized that this was a separate problem from tuberculosis of the hip in 1910:

- Arthur Legg [5] (at that time, a junior orthopaedic surgeon at Harvard Medical School, Boston)
- Jacques Calvé [6] (Director of the Institute Calvé, Berck-Plage, France)
- Georg Perthes [7] (Head of Surgery in Tübingen, Germany)

Any condition known by an eponym is intriguing and implies that the condition is not fully understood. Despite several hundred research papers, many of which are contradictory, the underlying etiology remains unknown, the course of the disease difficult to predict, and the best method of treatment not determined.

For brevity in this chapter the condition will be referred to as Perthes disease.

Epidemiology

The incidence of newly diagnosed cases is around 1 in 10,000 children per year [8, 9]. The clinical onset is usually between 4 and 7 years and rarely outside the range of 2–13 years. The

A.M. Wainwright (✉)
Nuffield Orthopaedic Centre, Oxford, UK

M. Benson et al. (eds.), *Children's Orthopaedics and Fractures*,
DOI 10.1007/978-1-84882-611-3_27, © Springer-Verlag London Limited 2010

condition affects boys much more often than girls with a 4:1 ratio [1, 9, 10]. The condition is bilateral in 15% of patients and the disease then runs a more severe course [9, 11].

There is variation between population groups worldwide. There is a marked increased risk in white children compared with black children (10.8 compared to 0.45 per 100,000, respectively in South Africa) [12]. There is also variation regionally within counties; in the UK, the annual incidence is 5.5/100,000 in Wessex and 11.1/100,000 in Liverpool [8]. It is a condition that seems to be associated with social deprivation [9, 10].

There is no evidence that the majority of children with Perthes disease have had a preceding irritable hip. Of the few children with recurrent irritable hip only those with over 2 years delay in bone growth were found to have Perthes disease [13].

Etiology

The cause of the condition is unknown, although there are several theories about its etiology. It is generally agreed that "in a susceptible child the changes are the consequence of ischemia of variable duration, after which the process of repair produces a growth disturbance, which if uncontrolled leads to femoral head deformity with subsequent arthritis" [1].

Inherited Factors

There are some inherited conditions that are similar to Perthes disease, such as the multiple epiphyseal dysplasias. These inherited conditions which mimic Perthes disease need to be excluded when considering the evidence for inheritance in Perthes disease. Also it may be difficult to separate inherited from environmental factors in families. Despite this it is widely believed that there is no clear evidence for a strongly inherited component. This is based on studies of first-degree relatives, twin studies, and the difference in incidence between the sexes, when mimics of Perthes disease, such as the dysplasias, are excluded [14].

There are epidemiological studies that have analyzed the age of onset and associated anomalies [15, 16]. The distributions fit best with models of disease which suggest a single cause acting prenatally. This may be either genetic or environmental. When Perthes disease affects more than one family member this may be caused by environmental factors.

Thrombophilia Theory

It has been proposed that children with Perthes disease may have an underlying coagulation defect which leads to vascular thrombosis—i.e., they are thrombophilic. Reports have shown associations with hypercoagulable conditions such as protein C and protein S deficiency and resistance to activated protein C [17, 18]. Subsequent studies have failed to confirm these findings [19], although others have found a prolonged activated partial thromboplastin time [20–22]. It has been noted that children with Perthes disease with a homozygous Factor V Leiden mutation have more severe disease [23]. Other mutations have been found in the coagulation cascade [24]. The whole of this theory may support the concept of the "susceptible child."

Recurrent Infarction

Several authors have suggested that recurrent infarction is responsible for the disease, although the cause for recurrent infarction has not been established [1, 25]. Experimental work in animals [26, 27] has shown that tying a ligature around the femoral head can cause the pathological changes of ischemic necrosis but not all of those seen in Perthes disease. It is possible that the cause is a tamponade effect—this theory has been examined experimentally in dogs [28].

Growth Arrest Theory

There may be an underlying constitutional problem predisposing children to Perthes disease as it is known to be associated with delayed bone age [29]. The bone age of affected children often lags 2–3 years behind their chronological age. There are abnormalities of levels of growth factors including insulin-like growth factor binding protein 3 [30]. Other studies have shown decreased birth weight [14].

Many of these factors are also associated with social deprivation, such as small stature and delayed bone age [14, 15, 29], dietary deficiency [31], and passive smoking [32].

Course of the Disease

Waldenström described the chronological stages [33] of the disease (Table 27.1).

These stages have been modified based on the radiological appearances (the Elizabethtown classification) [34] and are now recognized as shown in Table 27.2.

Table 27.1 Waldenström's chronological stages

The evolutionary period is divided into two stages
a. *The initial stage*—the epiphysis is dense, with "decalcinated" spots, flattened, and uneven at its margins
b. *The fragmentation stage*—the epiphysis is extremely flattened and divided; it often starts with a few small pieces, progresses to many small granules, and appears atrophied

The healing period—the epiphysis becomes homogenous and there is evidence of recalcification

The growing period—normal growth and ossification of the deformed femoral head

The definite period—the permanent residual features

Table 27.2 The Elizabethtown classification

Stage I	Initial stage
Stage II	Fragmentation stage
Stage III	Healing phase
Stage IV	Definitive stage

Pathological Findings

Histologically, several changes follow sequential infarction of the femoral head [35]. A variable amount of the femoral capital epiphysis may be affected:

- *Synovial tissue* becomes inflamed and causes an effusion.
- *Articular cartilage* is mostly nourished from synovial fluid and continues to grow (even though the underlying bone has lost its source of nutrition). Cartilage becomes thicker on the medial femoral head and the acetabular floor. At its deep surface it may transform to fibrocartilage.
- *Growth plate* cartilage columns become distorted and do not undergo normal ossification. The changes occur maximally under the involved part of the epiphysis, leading to a growth disturbance and tilting of the femoral epiphysis on the neck. On the superior and lateral aspect of the femoral neck there is reactivation of the growth plate with thickened cartilage. This contributes to the formation of a coxa magna.
- *Epiphysis:* in the early phases, the trabeculae and subchondral bone plate become necrotic and fragmented due to crushing of the bony epiphysis. This starts from the anterior margin and proceeds posteriorly to a variable extent. This leads to a subchondral fracture. In the adjacent, unaffected areas of the epiphysis the appearances are normal, with some remodeling. Later in the reparative phase there is new bone deposition on the necrotic trabeculae (creeping substitution) and a callus-like cartilaginous tissue adjacent to the loose necrotic bone.

- *Metaphysis:* the central marrow contains adipose tissue; sclerotic-rimmed osteolytic lesions containing fibrocartilage occur. There is disorganized ossification and extension of the growth plate down into the metaphysis (giving the radiological appearance of metaphyseal "cysts").

In summary, two pathological processes result in the changes seen in established disease leading to a change in shape mainly in the anterior and lateral aspects of the femoral head: infarction in the epiphysis of a variable extent with trabecular fracture and a growth disturbance in cartilage and physis.

Clinical Features

Symptoms

Children present with pain in the hip or, more commonly, the knee [36]. Often the reason for orthopaedic referral is not that the child has symptoms, but that relatives or teachers have noticed a limp. In general the child feels well and has no previous medical history of joint problems.

Signs

As noted previously, the clinical onset is within a narrow age range, i.e., children of junior school age. Affected children may be of short stature and be hyperactive. The limbs may be disproportionately shorter than the trunk.

The first sign of Perthes disease is usually a limp. Waldenström reported that at first the limping may be so slight that it may not be noticeable to the eye, but heard when the child walks across the floor with shoes on [36]. In the later phases the child may develop a Trendelenburg gait because of femoral head deformity, lost abduction, trochanteric overgrowth, and/or abductor dysfunction.

Examination on the couch typically reveals fixed flexion, restricted movement, and variable leg length discrepancy. Depending upon the extent of the disease the following signs are evident:

- In *extension* there is limited abduction and internal rotation. If there is early or established femoral head deformity, the leg abducts and externally rotates as the hip flexes. An adduction contracture is a sign of severe disease with lateral impingement.

- In *flexion* there is usually no adduction or internal rotation and, with head deformity, it may not be possible to adduct to neutral.

Differential Diagnosis

Other conditions may mimic Perthes disease, affecting just one hip or both [37]:

- *Multiple epiphyseal dysplasias* must be excluded if the disease is bilateral—there are similar changes at the hip, but the changes are bilateral, symmetrical, and there may be other epiphyses involved.
- *Spondylo-epiphyseal dysplasias* produce an uninvolved but cup-shaped metaphysis. Clinical examination shows a short trunk and spinal radiographs confirm platyspondyly. Other epiphyses may be affected.
- *Hypothyroidism* leads to delayed epiphyseal maturity, a wide metaphysis and classic clinical signs.
- *Gaucher's disease* (a storage disorder) differs in that the femoral epiphysis fails to remodel and there is associated anemia, thrombocytopenia, and hepatosplenomegaly.
- *Infection*—Sub-acute septic arthritis or osteomyelitis of the femoral neck can mimic these changes; tuberculosis of the hip was the classic differential diagnosis and worldwide this condition remains prevalent.
- *Eosinophilic granuloma* often presents with a high erythrocyte sedimentation rate (ESR) and other lesions may be apparent on a skeletal survey.
- *Lymphoma* deposits in the femoral neck cause complete infarction and the change is progressive.
- *Femoral head osteonecrosis* can be associated with sickle cell disease, steroid treatment, leukemia, and immunosuppression.
- *Hemophiliacs* may develop major femoral head infarction as a consequence of intra-articular bleeds. A positive family history and other signs of the bleeding disorder should clarify.
- *Mucopolysaccharidoses* often have delayed femoral head ossification and fragmentation.

These conditions can usually be differentiated from Perthes disease: ossification of the femoral capital epiphysis is usually delayed, the changes are often bilateral, synchronous, and symmetrical. In addition, the other systemic features of these conditions are apparent. *Bilateral Perthes disease affects each hip at a different time and with different severity.*

Radiographic Features

The radiographic features are best seen on an anteroposterior (AP) view of the pelvis and a frog lateral (Lauenstein view of the hip—i.e., in flexion, abduction, and external rotation). The changes seen depend upon the duration, stage, and severity of the disease. These changes form the basis for the classifications outlined below. One of the earliest signs is medial joint space widening. Some widening of the joint is often present in the opposite hip, compared with controls.

Classification of Severity Based on Radiographs

Radiographs yield information that allows objective assessment. For this reason there have been several classification systems that depend upon radiographic appearances alone. The classifications do offer reliable comparisons for investigators comparing the results of different treatment.

There is probably an overemphasis on radiographic findings, as these do not necessarily help to determine treatment for a particular child; this should be based more upon clinical findings.

Three systems are widely used to classify the radiological severity of Perthes disease. Each is named after its originator.

Catterall Classification

Catterall classification [37] is based on good quality AP and lateral radiographs (Fig. 27.2, Tables 27.3 and 27.4). The four groups are based on increasing proportions of femoral head involvement:

- *Group 1*—only the anterior part of the epiphysis is involved on the lateral view. No collapse of the femoral head is seen and complete absorption of the involved segment is seen without sequestrum formation. This is followed by regeneration. The AP view may show a cystic epiphysis, but there is no loss of height and metaphyseal changes are unusual.
- *Group 2*—more of the anterior epiphysis is involved and this may collapse, leaving a dense sequestrum. On the AP view a dense oval mass may be visible with viable fragments medially and laterally which maintain height. On the lateral view, a V, characteristic of this group, may separate the sequestrum posteriorly from the viable fragments.

Fig. 27.2 The Catterall classification groups I–IV, which are classified according to radiographic features of the epiphysis and metaphysis

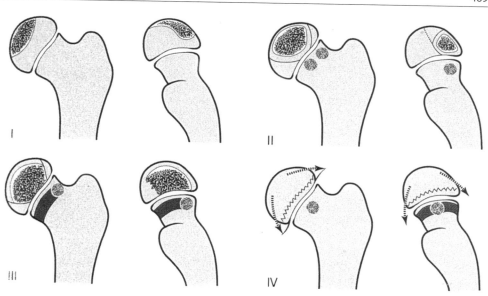

Table 27.3 Epiphyseal signs

Radiological signs	Group			
	I	II	III	IV
Sclerosis	No	Yes	Yes	Yes
Subchondral fracture line	No	Anterior half	Posterior half	Complete
Junction involved	Clear	Clear	Sclerotic	No
Uninvolved segments		Often "V"		
Viable bone at growth	Anterior margin	Anterior half	Posterior half	None
Triangular appearance to medial/lateral aspects	No	No	Occasional	Yes

Table 27.4 Metaphyseal signs

Radiological signs	Group			
	I	II	III	IV
Localized	No	Anterior	Anterior	Anterior or central
Diffuse	No	Yes	Yes	Yes
Posterior remodeling	No	No	No	Yes

- *Group 3*—only a small part of the epiphysis does not sequestrate. The AP view shows the appearance of a "head within a head," with later collapse of the central sequestrum and very small normal segments medially and laterally. The lateral segment is often small and osteoporotic and this becomes laterally displaced with collapse, producing a broadened neck. Metaphyseal changes are more generalized and associated with a broad femoral neck.
- *Group 4*—the whole epiphysis is sequestrated and total collapse of the epiphysis produces a dense line on the AP view. Early loss of height between the physis and the acetabular roof indicates flattening of the head. The epiphysis can "mushroom" anteriorly and laterally and metaphyseal changes can be extensive

Salter and Thompson Classification

Salter and Thompson described a simple two-group classification [38] based on the width of the subchondral fracture (Figs. 27.3 and 27.4), which reflects the extent of femoral head involvement:

- Group A (less than half of the head),
- Group B (more than half of the head)

The authors state that it may be applied early in the disease when the subchondral fracture is detectable. Unfortunately, the subchondral fracture line is seen radiologically in fewer than 50% of affected children.

Herring Classification

Herring et al. described a classification system [39] based upon the extent of involvement of the "lateral pillar" of the femoral head (Fig. 27.5). In the original report the lateral pillar is described as the area in the lateral 15–30% of the femoral head on a true AP film. Subsequently they have

Fig. 27.3 The Salter–Thompson classification

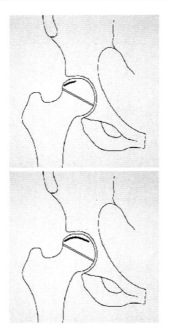

Fig. 27.5 The Herring lateral pillar classification

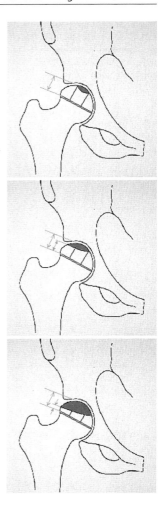

reported that the lateral pillar may be between 5–30% of the femoral head [40] so this makes the classification difficult to apply accurately.

This pillar height is compared with the unaffected hip, ignoring the amount of collapse of the central and medial pillars:

- Group A (no involvement of the lateral pillar)
- Group B (>50% of the lateral pillar height maintained)
- Group C (<50% of the lateral pillar height maintained)

A fourth group, the B/C border, has been added to this classification system by the originators. They noted that it may be difficult to differentiate between Groups B and C [40], hence the addition of this fourth, intermediate group.

Other Systems

Two more recent classification systems have been described since the description of these established systems.

Sugimoto's system assesses combined lateral and posterior pillar involvement [41]. This appears to offer a reasonable association with the amount of deformity at maturity, but needs to be confirmed by others.

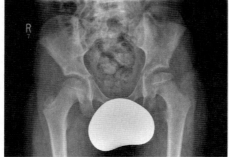
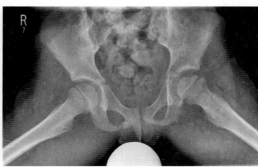

Fig. 27.4 Radiographs of a subchondral fracture

The deformity index, based upon an AP radiographic view only, has been recommended as a simple predictor of eventual radiological outcome (Fig. 27.6) [42]. While this appears to be reliable and valid in the hands of its users, only further application will determine its value. Unlike its predecessors [43, 44], it does not take into account the unseen cartilaginous part of the head seen on an arthrogram, nor does it assess different projections of the deforming femoral head. Loss of sphericity, best demonstrated arthrographically, improves prognostication by helping to differentiate between Herring Groups B and C [44].

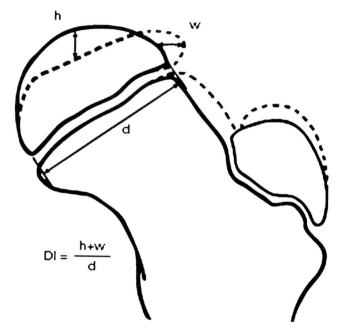

$$DI = \frac{h+w}{d}$$

Fig. 27.6 The deformity index. Reproduced with permission and copyright © of the British Editorial Society of Bone and Joint Surgery [42]

Other Investigations and Their Value

Ultrasound scans can be useful to investigate children with hip pain, as they are safe, inexpensive, and reproducible. When combined with aspiration they help to differentiate Perthes disease from the irritable hip and septic arthritis. Capsular distension that persists for more than 6 weeks suggests Perthes disease rather than hip irritability [45]. Other diagnostic markers shown to be useful in making the diagnosis are articular cartilage thickening and quadriceps atrophy [46].

Radioisotope bone scans have a higher sensitivity and specificity than radiographs and show the onset of revascularization earlier [47]. They have been used to classify

three patterns of disease [48] based on the fact that bone revascularization can occur by the recanalization of existing vessels or by neovascularization. Recanalization occurs rapidly (minutes to weeks), whereas neovascularization is prolonged (months to years). Conway reported [48] that these processes can be differentiated by scintigraphy and proposed three "tracks" that may be followed:

A. "All right track" scintigraphic pattern represents the recanalization process, a process of short duration and good prognosis.
B. "Bad track" scintigraphic pattern represents the process of neovascularization, a process of long duration and poorer prognosis.
C. "Complications" of the healing process (collapse, extrusion), particularly during the resorptive phases of bone reconstitution when the bone is weakened, can cause conversion from track A to track B.

These early tracks appear to correlate well with the radiographic-based classifications that cannot be applied until later [49]; 96% of Conway A hips later showed appearances of Herring A or B (the majority were Catterall type 2), and 82.8% of Conway B hips later showed signs of Herring C (the majority were Catterall type 3 or 4). If more severe (Herring C, Catterall 4) disease can be detected earlier with certainty, then earlier treatment may give better results in this difficult group [50].

Magnetic resonance imaging (MRI) with gadolinium enhancement has revealed Perthes disease changes in younger children which may predate the radiographic changes by up to 3 months [51]. Although MRI can give earlier information on the extent and location of involvement and healing, there is little evidence that it produces information that would alter management [52, 53]. Arthrography is as good as, or better than, MRI in determining the shape of the articular surface and lateral subluxation.

Prognosis at Maturity

There is an association between radiographic features at maturity and subsequent progression to osteoarthritis. Using concentric circular templates (Mose rings), a measure of sphericity is gauged from an AP and lateral view taken at maturity. More than 2 mm deviation between these views indicates lost sphericity and adversely affects outcome [54, 55].

Stulberg et al. assessed the sphericity and congruency of the hip at maturity [56]. From a longitudinal study over three to four decades, the prognosis for arthritis was shown to be related to the congruency between the femoral head

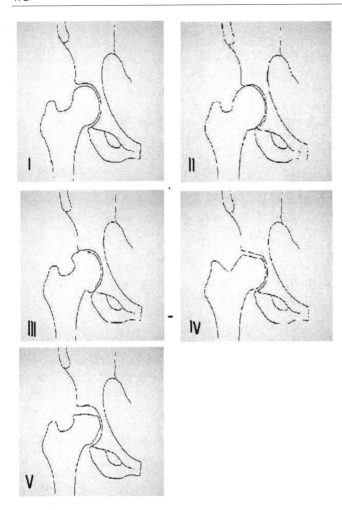

Fig. 27.7 The Stulberg classification

and acetabulum [57]. Five classes of deformity are described (Fig. 27.7 and Table 27.5).

There is considerable interobserver variability using this system. This is because some of the criteria are not clearly defined (e.g., a "flat head," and a "steep acetabulum") [58].

Table 27.5 Stulberg's classes of deformity

Class I Completely normal hip joint

Class II Spherical femoral head but with one or more of the following characteristics:
- A larger than normal (although spherical) femoral head (coxa magna)
- Shorter than normal femoral neck (coxa brevis)
- Abnormally steep acetabulum

Class III Non-spherical (ovoid or mushroom shaped or umbrella shaped), but not flat, femoral head (Class II characteristics are also present)

Class IV Flat femoral head and abnormalities of the femoral head, neck, or acetabulum

Class V Flat femoral head and a normal femoral neck and acetabulum

This system at maturity is often used as a surrogate for long-term prognosis. In the original series, the rate of arthritis at final follow-up (of an average 40 years) was 0, 16, 58, 75, and 78% for each grade (I–V), respectively. The Stulberg classes are often grouped into three types of congruency and sphericity:

1. *Spherical congruency* (class I and II hips)—in hips in this category early arthritis does not develop;
2. *Aspherical congruency* (class III hips)—mild to moderate arthritis develops in late adulthood; and
3. *Aspherical incongruency* (class IV and V hips)—severe arthritis develops before the age of 50 years in these hips

Prognosis and the "Head at Risk"

One of the challenges in Perthes disease is to determine the prognosis for an individual. A proportion of involved hips do well with no intervention but there is a group of children which does poorly with progressive deterioration in femoral head shape. Ideally the prognosis should be made early enough in the disease process to allow an intervention which will modify the natural history.

The most widely accepted prognostic factor is the patient's age at onset. This may reflect the time available for remodeling. There is a better chance of recovery when the onset is before the age of 6 years, and worse after the age of 8. This is not true for every case; although 80% of children with Perthes disease before the age of 6 have a good prognosis, half of those under 6 years with a Herring type B/C or C hip do poorly [59]. However, the older child has a higher ratio of epiphyseal bone to cartilage and consequently a greater potential for collapse of the bony epiphysis.

Girls appear to have a poorer prognosis than boys, possibly because girls reach skeletal maturity at an earlier age with less time for remodeling and also have a higher amount of head involvement (Catterall type 3 or 4).

Catterall described several clinical and radiological "head at risk" signs [60] which define factors contributing to a worse outcome (Table 27.6). Gage originally described a curved rather than straight lateral metaphysis [61] and Schlesinger has suggested that the V-shaped lytic appearance be called Catterall's sign [62].

The advantage of combining clinical with radiological assessment and looking for poor prognostic signs is that it helps to manage the individual child. A child can be managed conservatively if a good range of movement is maintained and radiographs do not show two or more of the radiological "at risk" signs. This is particularly the case in the younger child. Conversely when movement is lost early and

Table 27.6 Catterall's "head at risk" signs

Clinical signs
1 An obese child
2 A decreasing range of movement
3 Adduction contracture in extension
4 Flexion with abduction

Radiological signs
1 Calcification lateral to the epiphysis
2 Diffuse metaphyseal reaction
3 Femoral head lateral subluxation
4 A horizontal growth plate
5 Gage (Catterall) sign

the sign of "flexion with abduction" appears, femoral deformity is occurring and the child may need definitive treatment. This is irrespective of age and the extent of radiological involvement.

It is generally agreed that the four major factors which determine a poor prognosis are

- greater age of the patient at onset,
- greater extent of involvement of the femoral head,
- loss of containment of the femoral head in the acetabulum in the weight-bearing position, and
- loss of motion of the hip.

Treatment Options

Several treatment options have been proposed. A large pan-European study of treatment indications in Perthes disease [63] showed that the indications varied widely between surgeons and appeared to be based more upon personal experience than on scientific data. The different potential forms of treatment are outlined below, followed by a suggested approach to management for a child who presents with Perthes disease.

Conservative Treatment

Bed Rest

Historically, treatment was aimed at preventing weight bearing until the femoral head had re-ossified. This included prolonged strict bed rest, sometimes with months in hospital (Fig. 27.8), often with the use of traction on a frame or in a spica cast. A 17-year review of this treatment in Cardiff showed that this can give good results: 88% children had a good result and only 2% a poor result [64]. Significant problems with these regimens were muscle atrophy, osteoporosis, leg shortening, lost thoracic kyphosis, urinary calculi, social, academic, and emotional problems, and hospital costs.

Physiotherapy

Physiotherapy helps to relieve muscle spasm and regain abduction. Most children can avoid excessive physical activity, limit weight bearing with crutches, and take non-steroid anti-inflammatory drugs if their pain increases. Wherever possible the treatment should encourage children to retain hip flexibility by range of motion exercises, avoid schooling interruption, maintain social integration with their friends but minimize excessive stress through the weakened bone.

Pharmacological Treatment

It has been suggested that femoral head collapse may be reduced by medication such as bisphosphonates in the early stages of the disease. There are studies in animal models of femoral head ischemia which indicate that the use of bisphosphonates improves head sphericity [65, 66]. It will be interesting to see whether children benefit similarly in the medium to long term. Any side effects from the medication will need to be monitored closely.

Containment Treatment

Most methods of interventional treatment are based on the concept of "containment." The concept of containment assumes that the acetabulum will contain and mould the softened femoral head and result in a spherical, congruous joint, and avoid degenerative arthritis. Although containment is not clearly defined, over 80% coverage is commonly accepted to prevent extrusion of the femoral head and lateral compression. It is important that this is done at an early stage in the disease.

If containment treatment is needed, the three methods of containment that have been widely used are the weight-bearing orthosis, femoral osteotomy, and/or acetabular osteotomy.

Weight-Bearing Abduction Braces

Petrie devised an abduction brace which allowed the child to be out of hospital but caused stiff knees, very awkward ambulation, and a cumbersome cast. Devices such as the Atlanta Scottish Rite brace were designed to keep the hips abducted, while permitting mobility at the hip. Arthrography was often

Fig. 27.8 Historical treatment with bed rest

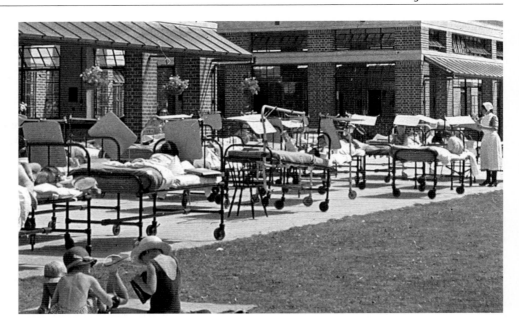

used prior to bracing to assess congruency in different positions to determine the "best-fit" position for containment, with good congruency and the avoidance of hinge abduction. Serial radiographs and clinical assessment of the range of movement were used to guide when weaning from the brace should begin. Some clinicians kept children in a brace until the lateral column re-ossified and sclerotic areas in the epiphysis had resolved.

There are problems with these abduction devices: pain and spasm may result in wide abduction of the *normal* hip and little or no abduction of the abnormal hip; then containment is not achieved. Hinge abduction may occur if the supero-lateral portion of a deformed femoral head impinges on the lateral acetabulum. This impingement damages the acetabular margin which loses its horizontal plane and slopes upward. This further increases the tendency for subluxation. In the older child bracing is difficult due to compliance and psychosocial issues. This form of treatment is not widely used in Europe [63], and in the United States several authors now advise against bracing for severely involved hips [67]. This was confirmed in the long-term follow-up by the Herring Group [68].

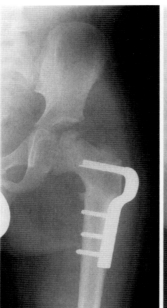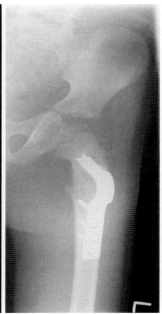

Fig. 27.9 Varus femoral osteotomy

Femoral Varus Osteotomy

Varus osteotomy of the proximal femur (Fig. 27.9) aims to center the femoral head more deeply within the acetabulum and allow weight bearing with the limb in a normal position without the encumbrance of an abduction brace. The goal is to cover the entire ossified femoral epiphysis of a "head at risk" with the ossified acetabulum [69, 70].

The prerequisites for varus derotation osteotomy include a good range of motion, hip congruency, and the ability to contain the femoral head in the acetabulum in abduction (assessed with an arthrogram). The procedure must be performed early in the initial or fragmentation stage of the disease. Many studies report good results with this operation [70–72] and it allows correction of the flexion deformity and rotational profile.

In the older child if the neck–shaft angle postoperatively is less than 115° the varus may not correct with subsequent remodeling. The greater trochanter should be kept distal to the level of the femoral head to prevent an abductor lurch. Sometime this requires distal transfer of the greater trochanter at the same operation or at a later time. Other procedures may later be required to manage limb shortening (of an already short limb), reverse the varus if it persists or remove plates and screws.

Acetabular Osteotomy

Salter described his innominate osteotomy for the subluxated hip (Fig. 27.10). He recommended that the osteotomy should be performed only in hips with a full (or almost full) range of movement, and a round (or almost round) femoral head with reasonable congruency in abduction. The child should be over 6 years old, more than 50% of the femoral head should be affected (Salter–Thompson group B) and the hip be seen to subluxate in the weight-bearing position.

Salter's osteotomy is reported to give good results, particularly in the older child with whole-head involvement [34, 73]. Potentially, it avoids further limb shortening and abductor weakness and leaves a more cosmetic scar.

The innominate osteotomy in isolation may not provide sufficient head cover or stability, particularly in the older child. Sometimes the procedure is performed in combination with a femoral osteotomy [74, 75]. This may be useful to contain a large, deformed femoral head, avoid an extreme varus neck–shaft angle, maintain leg length equality, and decrease intra-articular pressure. In the older child a triple pelvic osteotomy may be needed to rotate the acetabulum sufficiently to offer adequate head cover.

Valgus, Extension Femoral Osteotomy

This operation may be an effective salvage procedure in late-presenting cases where decreasing abduction is associated with femoral head overgrowth and mushroom deformity. When an arthrogram demonstrates femoral head deformity with unstable movement and hinge abduction in neutral but better stability in adduction and flexion, a valgus, extension upper femoral osteotomy will improve stability as the child stands and walks. It will also improve leg length and provide a more normal abductor lever arm. The rotational and sagittal correction can improve symptoms, function, and remodeling of the hip in patients with Perthes disease [76, 77] (Fig. 27.11). Care must be taken to lateralize the femoral shaft as the osteotomy is closed. Failure to do this can lead to proximal femoral deformity making potential arthroplasty more difficult. The procedure should not be undertaken before reconstitution of the femoral head nears completion.

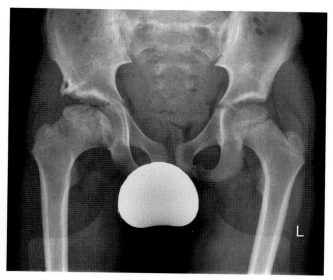

Fig. 27.11 Radiograph of shelf osteotomy

Shelf Procedures

Lateral shelf arthroplasty (Fig. 27.11) or the Chiari osteotomy may add cover to the femoral head although both rely upon capsular conversion to fibrocartilage for this improvement. The shelf arthroplasty [78, 79] is the ideal procedure for the child presenting over the age of 8 years. It increases coverage and stability of the femoral head while decreasing subluxation. If hip stability is achieved, the

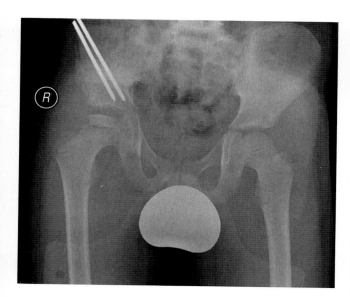

Fig. 27.10 Radiograph of Salter innominate osteotomy

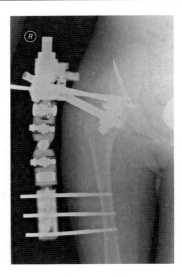

Fig. 27.12 Radiograph of distraction with external fixator

longevity of the hip improves [80]. Lateral support is helpful when there is inadequate acetabular coverage or when hinge abduction is developing. It was found to be less effective for children over the age of 11 years, especially girls [78], but offers pain relief and the maintenance of a stable, congruent hip [81]. Some suggest that shelf arthroplasty may help in the late fragmentation stage when hinging is more marked, improving moulding of the deformed femoral head.

Hip Distraction

Arthrodiastasis, distraction of the joint (Fig. 27.13), has been proposed as early treatment in the disease, before any significant collapse of the femoral head had occurred. The aim

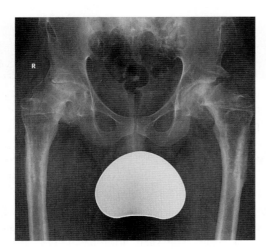

Fig. 27.13 Radiograph of a twenty year old man. He had been diagnosed with bilateral Perthes disease at age ten and had a corrective ostcotomy on both sides. Since this he experienced a reduced ROM and painful hips

is to halt further fragmentation and collapse [82]. Typically, this requires 4 months in an articulated fixator. Although the early results seemed promising, the longer term benefits have not been demonstrated (Fig. 27.12).

Other Procedures

After reossification of the femoral head there is a potential for late remodeling of the hip joint. There are circumstances when intervention is required to salvage a deformed head that is causing incongruity.

Cheilectomy

If there is femoro-acetabular impingement, excision of the extruded part of femoral head (cheilectomy) has been attempted. Ganz has shown that the hip may be dislocated with only small risk of avascular necrosis provided great care is taken to protect the posterior vessels [83, 84]. This may allow better re-shaping of the head and improve on the previously reported results of cheilectomy which often caused stiffness and pain and yielded poor long-term outcomes [85].

Arthrodesis

Surgical fusion of the hip may be indicated in young men at maturity with unilateral disease, severe functional impairment, and hip deformity.

Arthroplasty

This may be necessary after skeletal maturity if there is severe deformity and arthritis. Surface replacement may be possible and gives results equivalent to conventional replacement in Perthes disease [86].

Published Results of Treatment Regimens

It is difficult to compare previous studies. Most research has been published as case series and there are many conflicting findings following the same treatment modality. The age at onset, the stage and severity of the disease, the treatment regimens, the length of follow-up, and the outcome measures yield too many variables for easy analysis. Furthermore our measures of sphericity and head shape lack inter-observer precision. Finally, there is a long lag period of three or four decades between the onset of the disease and its degenerative effects on the hip.

There has been one proposal for a Cochrane systematic review to be published; however, the results of this review are not yet available [87].

The large prospective, multicenter study published from the Legg–Calvé Perthes Study Group in North America [68] compared the results of various interventions as determined by the treating surgeon in each center. In essence their findings by Herring type is summarized as

- *Group A hips* have an excellent prognosis and require no specific treatment.
- *Group B hips* in children whose disease started before 8 years of age have a good prognosis and require only symptomatic treatment.
- *Group B/C border hip* in children with Perthes disease starting before 8 years of age have a poorer prognosis but do not appear to benefit from surgical treatment.
- *Group B and B/C border hips* in children with Perthes disease starting after 8 years (or bone age over 6 years) have a significantly better outcome if treated with an innominate or a varus femoral osteotomy.
- *Group C hips* have an unfavorable prognosis in children regardless of age or surgical treatment (Fig. 27.13).

The other large prospective review with medium-term follow-up yielded similar findings [88]. In this series, although the lateral pillar classification was related to outcome, the strongest predictor of outcome was the percentage of femoral head involvement and age at diagnosis. The recommendation from this study was that a child aged 6 and over, with more than 50% femoral head involvement (Catterall groups 3 and 4) had a better outcome if treated with a femoral varus osteotomy.

Suggested Management of a Child with Perthes Disease

Many treatment protocols rely upon the radiographic appearances, despite the difficulties in applying classification systems early in the disease process. Although radiographs provide information that is measurable, they are not so helpful in making treatment decisions.

After making the diagnosis, management depends upon the clinical findings and the child's age at disease onset. The clinical examination gives the best assessment of the deformity of the femoral head. If there are clinical signs of deformity, the containment and congruity of the femoral head in the acetabulum in the weight-bearing position should be assessed further under anesthesia with an arthrogram.

Children who likely have a poor prognosis have clear clinical signs early in the disease, including

- poor ranges of movement
- decreased abduction in extension
- flexion into abduction
- fixed flexion deformity of over 20°
- inability to adduct or internally rotate the flexed hip to neutral
- leg length discrepancy

A suggested protocol for treatment follows based upon age and clinical findings. Under 6 years—the outlook is generally good:

- maintain range of movement, with physiotherapy and swimming
- restrict impact activities such as jumping during early phases
- crutches may be needed to help off-load the hip and relieve pain
- simple analgesia

The exception to a conservative approach is the child with whole-head involvement (Catterall group 4) when the prognosis can be improved by femoral or innominate osteotomy.

For children 6–8 years:

- as above
- monitor closely for clinical signs of a head at risk but, if clinical signs of head at risk are found, perform an examination under anesthesia and a dynamic arthrogram. This will demonstrate whether

1. the head is contained and stable. Plan monitoring and maintain hip motion and regular review for signs that would indicate the need for surgery (head at risk)
2. the head can be contained in abduction (+/–flexion). This is the indication for a femoral or pelvic osteotomy
3. the head cannot be contained but is uncovered and hinges. A lateral shelf acetabuloplasty will give support

Over 8 years as the prognosis is poorer an early examination under anesthesia and arthrogram to ascertain that

- the head is contained and stable (unusual). Any further loss of movement is an indication for definitive treatment
- the head can be contained in abduction. This is the best indication for a pelvic osteotomy or possibly a shelf procedure, before there is loss of epiphyseal height and deformity

- the head cannot be contained but is uncovered and has unstable movement with hinging. In the fragmentation or early healing stages a shelf arthroplasty is appropriate

The child at any age with late femoral head deformity:

- If the child has a painful limp with shortening and an arthrogram which shows femoral head deformity, unstable movement, and hinge abduction but stability in adduction and flexion. A valgus, extension upper femoral osteotomy, will produce stable movement, improve leg length, and produce a more normal abductor lever arm

Summary

There is still much to be learned about Legg–Calvé–Perthes disease. If the cause can be determined, then prevention or disease limitation may be possible in the future. It is apparent that a group of children need only symptomatic treatment: these tend to be younger and have a good range of movement. There is another group in which the hip progresses to a symptomatic arthropathy at an early age. One of the challenges is to improve upon the natural history by surgical intervention as soon as the clinical signs are detected.

References

1. Catterall A. Legg-Calvé-Perthes Disease. Edinburgh: Churchill Livingstone; 1982.
2. Waldenström H. Der obere tuberkulöse Cullumherd. Zeitschrift für Orthopädische Chirurgie 1909; 24: 487–512.
3. Maydl K. Coxa vara und Arthritis deformans coxae. Wiener klinische Rundschau 1897; 11:153.
4. Enersen, OD. Legg-Calvé-Perthes disease. At: http://www.whonamedit.com/synd.cfm/908.html. Accessed 7 October 2008.
5. Legg AT. An obscure affection of the hip-joint. Boston Med Surg J 1910; 162: 202–204.
6. Calvé J. Sur une forme particulière de pseudo-coxalgie greffée sur des déformations caractéristiques de l'extrémité supérieure du fémur. Revue de chirurgie 1910; 42: 54–84.
7. Perthes G. Über Arthritis deformans juvenilis. Deutsche Zeitschrift für Chirurgie 1910; 107: 111–159.
8. Barker DJP, Dixon E, Taylor JF. Perthes disease of the hip in three regions of England. J Bone Joint Surg [Br] 1978; 60-B: 478–480.
9. Kealey WDC, Moore AJ, Cook S, Cosgrove AP. Deprivation, urbanisation and Perthes disease in Northern Ireland. J Bone Joint Surg 2000; 82B: 167–171.
10. Margetts BM, Perry CA, Taylor JF, Dangerfield PH. The incidence and distribution of Legg-Calve-Perthes disease in Liverpool, 1982–1995. Ach Dis Child 2001; 84: 351–354.
11. Van de Bogaert G, de Rosa E, Moens P, et al. Bilateral Legg-Calvé-Perthes disease: different from unilateral disease? J Paediatr Orthop 1999; part B 8: 165–168.
12. Purry NA. The incidence of Perthes disease in three population groups in the Eastern cape region of South Africa. J Bone Jt Surg [Br] 1982; 64-B:286–288.
13. Keenan WNW, Clegg J. Perthes disease after "irritable hip": delayed bone age shows the hip is a "marked man." J Pediatr Orthop 1996; 16: 20–23.
14. Wynne-Davies R, Gormley J. The etiology of Perthes disease: genetic, epidemiological and growth factors in 310 Edinburgh and Glasgow patients. J Bone Joint Surg [Br] 1978; 60-B: 6–14.
15. Hall AJ, Barker DJ, Dangerfield PH, et al. Small feet and Perthes disease: a survey in Liverpool. J Bone Joint Surg [Br] 1988; 70-B: 611–13.
16. Wiig O, Terjesen T, Svenningsen S, Lie SA. The epidemiology and etiology of Perthes disease in Norway. J Bone Joint Surg [Br] 2006; 88-B: 1217—1223.
17. Glueck CJ, Glueck HI, Greenfield D, et al. Protein C and S deficiency and hypofibrinolysis: pathophysiologic causes of Legg Perthes disease. Pediatr Res 1994; 35: 383–388.
18. Glueck CJ, Brandt G, Gruppo R, et al. Resistance to activated protein C and Legg-Perthes disease. Clin Orthop 1997; 338: 139–152.
19. Hayek S, Kenet G, Lubetsky A, et al. Does thrombophilia play an aetiological role in Legg-Calvé-Perthes disease? J Bone Joint Surg [Br] 1999; 81-B: 686—690.
20. Gallistl S, Reitinger T, Linhart W, Muntean W. The role of inherited thrombotic disorders in the etiology of Legg-Calvé-Perthes disease. J Paediatr Orthop 1999; 19: 82–83.
21. Sirvent N, Fisher F, El Hayek T, et al. Absence of congenital prethrombotic disorders in children with Legg-Perthes disease. J Pediatr Orthop 2000; part B 9: 24–27.
22. Thomas DP, Morgan G, Tayton K. Perthes disease and the relevance of thrombophilia. J Bone Joint Surg 1999; 81B: 691–695.
23. Kealey WDC, Mayne EE, McDonald W, et al. The role of coagulation abnormalities in the development of Perthes disease. J Bone Joint Surg [Br] 2000; 82B, 744–746.
24. Dilley A, Hooper WC, Austin H, et al. The beta fibrinogen gene G-455-A polymorphisms a risk factor for Legg-Perthes disease. J Thromb Haemost 2003; 1: 2317–2321.
25. McKibbin B, Rális Z. Pathological changes in a case of Perthes disease J Bone Joint Surg [Br] 1974; 56-B (3): 438.
26. Salter RB, Bell M. The pathogenesis of deformity in Legg- Perthes disease—an experimental investigation. J Bone Joint Surg 1968; 50B: 436.
27. Kim H, Su P-H. Development of flattening and apparent fragmentation following ischemic necrosis of the capital femoral epiphysis in a piglet model. J Bone Joint Surg [Am] 2002; 84(8): 1329–1334.
28. Kemp HB. Perthes disease: an experimental and clinical study. Ann R Coll Surg Engl 1973; 52(1): 18–35.
29. Burwell RG, Dangerfield PH, Hall DJ, et al. Perthes disease. An anthropometric study revealing impaired and disproportionate growth. J Bone Joint Surg [Br] 1978; 60B: 461–477.
30. Matsumoto T, Enomoto H, Takahashi K, et al. Decreased levels of IGF binding protein 3 in serum from children with Legg Calvé Perthes disease. Acta Orthop Scand 1998; 69: 125.
31. Hall AJ, Margetts BM, Barker DJ, et al. Low blood manganese levels in Liverpool children with Perthes disease. Paediatr Perinat Epidemiol 1989; 3: 131–135.
32. Mata SG, Aicua EA, Ovejero AH, Grande MM. Legg-Calvé-Perthes disease and passive smoking. J Pediatr Orthop 2000; 20: 326–330.
33. Waldenström H. The first stages of coxa plana. J Bone Joint Surg 1938; 20: 559–566.
34. Canale ST, D'Anca AF, Cottler JM, Snedden HE. Innominate osteotomy in Legg Calvé Perthes disease J Bone Joint Surg 1972; 54-A: 25–40.

35. Catterall A, Pringle J, Byers PD. A review of the morphology of Perthes disease. J Bone Joint Surg [Br] 1982; 64B: 269–275.

36. Waldenström H. The definite form of the coxa plana. Acta Radiol 1922; 1: 384–394.

37. Catterall A. The natural history of Perthes disease. J Bone Joint Surg [Br] 1971; 53B: 37–53.

38. Salter RB, Thompson GH. Legg-Calvé-Perthes disease. The prognostic significance of the subchondral fracture and a two-group classification of the femoral head involvement. J Bone Joint Surg 1984; 66A: 479–489.

39. Herring JA, Neustadt JB, Williams JJ, et al. The lateral pillar classification of Legg-Calvé-Perthes disease. J Pediatr Orthop 1992; 12: 143–150.

40. Herring JA, Kim HT, Browne R. Legg-Calvé-Perthes Disease. Part I: classification of radiographs with use of the modified lateral pillar and Stulberg classifications. J Bone Joint Surg 2004; 86-A: 10–12.

41. Sugimoto Y, Akazawa H, Miyake Y, et al. A new scoring system for Perthes disease based on combined lateral and posterior pillar classifications. J Bone Joint Surg [Br] 2004; 86-B: 887–891.

42. Nelson D, Zenios M, Ward K, et al. The deformity index as a predictor of final radiological outcome in Perthes disease J Bone Joint Surg [Br] 2007; 89-B: 1369–1373.

43. Shigeno Y, Evans G. Revised arthrographic index of deformity for Perthes disease. J Ped Orthop 1996; 5: 44–47.

44. Ismail M, Macnicol MF. Prognosis in Perthes disease: a comparison of radiographic predictors. J Bone Joint Surg [Br] 1998; 88-B: 310–314.

45. Eggl H, Drekonja T, Kaiser B, Dorn U. Ultrasonography in the diagnosis of transient synovitis of the hip and Legg-Calvé-Perthes disease. J Pediatr Orthop 1999; part B 8: 177–180.

46. Robben SGF, Meradji M, Diepstraten AFM, Hop WCJ. US of the painful hip in childhood: The diagnostic value of cartilage thickening and muscle atrophy in the detection of Perthes disease. Radiol 1998; 208: 35–42.

47. Sutherland AD, Savage JP, Paterson DC, Foster BK. The nuclide bone-scan in the diagnosis and management of Perthes disease. J Bone Joint Surg [Br] 1980; 62B: 300–306.

48. Conway JJ. Scintigraphic classification of Legg-Calvé-Perthes disease. Semin Nucl Med 1993; 23(4): 274–295.

49. Van Campenhout A, Moens P, Fabry G. Serial bone scintigraphy in Legg-Calvé-Perthes disease: correlation with the Catterall and Herring classification. J Pediatr Orthop B 2006; 15(1): 6–10.

50. Diméglio A, Canavase F, Ali M, Kelly P. Surgical treatment of Legg-Calvé-Perthes disease; improved results for severe forms Catterall IV/Herring C. J Child Orthop 2008; 2 (Suppl 1): S27#.

51. Gent E, Antapur P, Fairhurst J, et al. Perthes disease in the very young child. J Pediatr Orthop B 2006; 15:16–22.

52. Kaniklides C, Lönnerholm T, Moberg A, et al. Legg-Calvé-Perthes disease. Comparison of conventional radiography, MR imaging, bone scintigraphy and arthrography. Acta Radiol 1995; 36: 434–439.

53. Jaramillo D, Galen TA, Winalski CS, et al. Legg-Calvé-Perthes disease. MR imaging evaluation during manual positioning of the hip—comparison with conventional arthrography. Radiol 1999; 212: 519–525.

54. Mose K. Methods of measuring in Legg-Calvé-Perthes disease with special regard to the prognosis. Clin Orthop Relat Res. 1980; 150: 103–109.

55. Mose K, Hjorth L, Ulfeldt M, et al. Legg Calvé Perthes disease. The late occurrence of coxarthrosis. Acta Orthop Scand Suppl 1977; 169: 1–39.

56. Stulberg SD, Salter RB. The natural course of Legg-Perthes disease and its relationship to degenerative arthritis of the hip. A long-term follow-up study. Orthop Trans 1977; 1: 105–106.

57. Stulberg SD, Cooperman DR, Wallensten R. The natural history of Legg-Calvé-Perthes disease. J Bone Joint Surg 1981; 63A: 1095–1108.

58. Neyt JG, Weinstein SL, Spratt K. Stulberg classification system for evaluation of Legg-Calvé-Perthes disease: Intra-rater and inter-rater reliability. J Bone Joint Surg 1999; 81: 1209–1216.

59. Rosenfeld SB, Herring JA, Chao JC. Legg-Calvé-Perthes disease: A review of cases with onset before 6 years of age. J Bone Joint Surg Am 2007; 89: 2712–2722.

60. Catterall A. Legg-Calvé-Perthes disease. Clin Orthop and Rel Res 1981; 158: 41–51.

61. Gage HC. A possible early sign of Perthes disease. Br J Radiol 1933; 6: 295–297.

62. Schlesinger I, Crider RJ. Gage's sign—revisited! J Paediatr Orthop 1988; 8: 201–202.

63. Hefti F, Clarke NMP. The management of Legg-Calvé-Perthes disease: is there a consensus? J Child Orthop 2007; 1:19–25.

64. Brotherton BJ, McKibbin B. Perthes disease treated by prolonged recumbency and femoral head containment. J Bone Joint Surg [Br] 1975; 57-B:620.

65. Little DG, McDonald M, Sharpe IT, et al. Zoledronic acid improves femoral head sphericity in a rat model of Perthes disease. J Orthop Res 2005; 23: 862–868.

66. Kim HKW, Randall TS, Bian H, et al. Ibandronate for prevention of femoral head deformity after ischemic necrosis of the capital femoral epiphysis in immature pigs. J Bone Joint Surg Am 2005; 87: 550–557.

67. Martinez AG, Weinstein SG, Dietz FR. The weight-bearing abduction brace for the treatment of Legg-Calvé-Perthes disease. J Bone Joint Surg Am 1992; 74: 12–21.

68. Herring JA, Kim HT, Browne R. Legg-Calvé-Perthes Disease. Part II: Prospective Multicenter Study of the Effect of Treatment on Outcome. J Bone Joint Surg Am 2004; 86: 2121—2134

69. Somerville EW. Perthes disease of the hip. J Bone Joint Surg Br 1971; 53-B: 639–649.

70. Lloyd-Roberts G, Catterall A, Salamon P. A controlled study of the indications for and the results of femoral osteotomy in Perthes disease J Bone Joint Surg 1976; 58-B: 31–36.

71. Fulford GE, Lunn PG, Macnicol MF. A prospective study of non-operative and operative management for Perthes disease. J Pediatr Orthop 1993; 13: 281–285.

72. Coates CJ, Paterson JMH, Woods KR, et al. Femoral osteotomy in Perthes disease: results at maturity. J Bone Joint Surg [Br] 1990; 72-B:581–585.

73. Paterson DC, Leitch JM, Foster BK. Results of innominate osteotomy in the treatment of Legg-Calvé-Perthes disease. Clin Orthop 1991; 266: 96–103.

74. Crutcher JP, Staheli LT. Combined osteotomy as a salvage procedure for severe Legg-Calvé-Perthes disease. J Pediatr Orthop 1992; 12: 151–156.

75. Olney BW, Asher MA. Combined innominate and femoral osteotomy for the treatment of severe Legg-Calvé-Perthes disease. J Pediatr Orthop 1985; 5: 645–651.

76. Bankes MJK, Catterall A, Hashemi-Nejad A. Valgus extension osteotomy for 'hinge abduction' in Perthes disease: results at maturity and factors influencing the radiological outcome. J Bone Joint Surg [Br] 2000; 82-B:548–554.

77. Yoo WJ, Choi IH, Chung CY, et al. Valgus femoral osteotomy for hinge abduction in Perthes disease. Decision-making and outcomes. J Bone Joint Surg [Br] 2004; 86; 726–730.

78. Daly K, Bruce C, Catterall A. Lateral shelf acetabuloplasty in Perthes disease: a review at the end of growth. J Bone Joint Surg [Br] 1999; 81-B: 380–384.

79. Willett K, Hudson A, Catterall A. Lateral shelf acetabuloplasty: an operation for older children with Perthes disease. J Pediatr Orthop Surg 1992; 12:563–568.

80. Kruse RW, Guille JT, Bowen JR. Shelf arthroplasty in patients who have had Legg-Calvé Perthes disease: a study of long-term results. J Bone Joint Surg [Am] 1991; 73-A:1338–1347.

81. Freeman R, Kandil Y, Wainwright A, et al. The outcome of patients with hinge abduction in severe Perthes disease treated by shelf acetabuloplasty. J Children Orthop 2007; 1 (Suppl 1): S35.

82. Maxwell SL, Lappin KJ, Kealey WD, et al. Arthrodiastasis in Perthes disease. Preliminary results. J Bone Joint Surg [Br] 2004; 86(2):244–250.

83. Ganz R, Gill TJ, Gautier E, et al. Surgical dislocation of the adult hip a technique with full access to the femoral head and acetabulum without the risk of avascular necrosis. J Bone Joint Surg Br 2001; 83: 1119–1124.

84. Lavigne M, Parvizi J, Beck M, et al. Anterior femoroacetabular impingement: part I. Techniques of joint preserving surgery. Clin Orthop Relat Res 2004; 418:61–66.

85. Rowe SM, Jung ST, Cheon SY, et al. Outcome of Cheilectomy in Legg-Calve-Perthes disease; Minimum 25-year follow-up. J Pediatr Orthop 2006; 26: 204–210.

86. Boyd HS, Ulrich SD, Seyler TM, et al. Resurfacing for Perthes disease: an alternative to standard hip arthroplasty. Clin Orthop Relat Res 2007; 465: 80–85.

87. Maxwell L, Kealey D. Surgical management of Perthes disease (Protocol). Cochrane Database of Systematic Reviews 2002; 2: CD003829.

88. Wiig O, Terjesen T, Svenningsen S. Prognostic factors and outcomes of treatment in Perthes disease: a prospective study of 368 patients with five-year follow-up. J Bone Joint Surg [Br] 2008; 90-B: 1364–1371.

Chapter 28

Slipped Capital Femoral Epiphysis

Malcolm F. Macnicol and Michael K. D. Benson

Introduction

Posterior slipping of the upper (capital) femoral epiphysis (SUFE) is the most common cause of hip disability in early adolescence, until the growth plate closes. A number of factors contribute to a relative weakening of the growth plate and its surrounding fibrocartilaginous perichondrial ring, culminating in a shearing displacement through the zone of hypertrophic cartilage. The resultant symptoms and loss of function may be trivial or profound. Treatment is directed at preventing progressive slippage, minimizing deformity, and avoiding the major complications of avascular necrosis (AVN) and chondrolysis. Incidence: The incidence of SUFE is 2–3 per 100,000 children and adolescents [1] and is dependent upon race, gender, and geographical region. Minor slips which stabilize are often missed and the incidence also seems to be rising as a result of increasing obesity in youngsters [2]. The male predominance is now less marked, a ratio of 2:1 being recorded [3]. Boys usually present between the ages of 14 and 16 years whereas girls are afflicted between 11 and 13 years; after menarche girls are almost immune to the condition. The left hip is affected in 60% of cases initially but in 20–25% of cases the contralateral epiphysis may slip at a later date [4]. Subtle changes of pre-slipping in the opposite hip are evident in a further 40%. Rarely, both epiphyses may displace simultaneously but usually there is a delay of 6–18 months [5–7] between the sides, sometimes as long as 4–5 years. Younger boys are particularly at risk of a contralateral slip. Stasikelis et al. [8] found the Oxford pelvic bone age score [9] to be predictive: all their male patients under 11 years and 7 months developed a contralateral slip whereas only 9 of 22 did so between the ages of 11 years 8 months and 14 years 11 months. No cases presented secondarily over the age of 15 years, in accordance with the finding that closure of the triradiate cartilage is protective [10].

Racial variations are recognized, SUFE being relatively rare in southern Asia, Japan, China, and Africa but 4–5 times as common in Polynesians and 2.2 times in African-Americans compared to whites [1]. Obesity and variable radiographic surveillance may account for some of the differences in prevalence but neither Loder et al. [11] nor Kordelle et al. [12] have been able to establish acetabular morphological changes as contributory. Bilaterality is twice as common in African-Americans (34%) than in whites, Hispanics, and Asians. Hansson et al. [13] noted increased rates of SUFE during summer and autumn and in rural versus urban populations living above the 40° northern latitude, perhaps implicating physical activity as a precipitant. According to Rennie [14] the disorder appears to be autosomal dominant with variable penetrance, causing a 7% risk of a second family member being affected.

Etiology

The interplay of factors that contributes to SUFE is intriguing, mechanical stress, repetitive trauma, anatomical factors, endocrinopathies, and immunological abnormalities being considered separately and together as etiologically important.

Biomechanical Factors

Chung et al. [15] showed that the perichondrial fibrocartilaginous ring surrounding the growth plate contributes significantly to the ability of the epiphysis to withstand shear

M.F. Macnicol (✉)
University of Edinburgh, Edinburgh, UK; Royal Hospital for Sick Children, Edinburgh, UK; Murrayfield Hospital, Edinburgh, UK; Royal Infirmary; Edinburgh, UK

M. Benson et al. (eds.), *Children's Orthopaedics and Fractures*,
DOI 10.1007/978-1-84882-611-3_28, © Springer-Verlag London Limited 2010

forces. It is firmly bound to neighboring subperiosteal meta-physeal bone and is the strongest during infancy. The ring decreases in volume and strength progressively and coinci-dentally the physeal plate widens during the growth spurt in early adolescence. At this stage the mammillary processes at the epiphyseal–metaphyseal junction offer more intrinsic resistance to shearing forces than the perichondrial ring.

Shear stress across the growth plate is minimized by a hor-izontal physis and anteverted femoral neck. Gelberman et al. [16] found SUFE to correlate with neck retroversion and it is highly unusual to encounter the condition in a patient with femoral anteversion. Whereas anteversion averages 10.6° in adolescents of normal physique the figure also decreases to 0.4° in the obese [17]. Mirkopoulos et al. [18] found that patients with a slip had a more vertical proximal femoral physis, the effective decrease in neck–shaft angle also con-tributing to increased shear forces. Rarely, the epiphysis may slip into a valgus position although it is not known if this occurs when the growth plate is more horizontal. Because 5–6 times of body weight is applied to the femoral head during running and jumping it is also established that body weight and repetitive trauma contribute to the risk of SUFE.

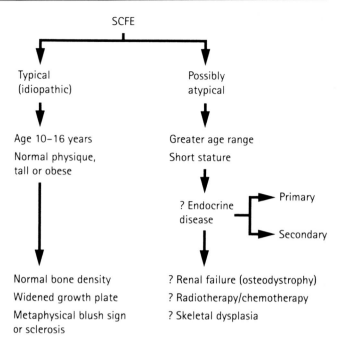

Fig. 28.1 Clinical differences between typical and atypical cases of slipped epiphysis

Endocrine Factors

Short stature, extremes of physique, and hypogonadism may predispose to SUFE, especially at an earlier stage in childhood when bilateral slips may develop. Appreciation of this atypical slip is important (Fig. 28.1) and these children should be referred for review by a paediatri-cian. Blethen and Rundle [19] found that growth hormone (GH) treatment for established GH deficiency, Turner's syn-drome, or chronic renal failure enhances the risk of SUFE. Estrogen is known to increase the strength of the growth plate by causing it to narrow so that girls after menar-che are protected from SUFE. When children with pan-hypothyroidism are treated with growth hormone, there is a significant risk of slip, particularly if sex hormones are not given concurrently. A deficiency of sex hormones will delay epiphyseal closure, thus increasing the time span when slipping may occur. This hormonal imbalance may also result in obesity, adding to the adverse mechanical factors.

Other endocrinopathies have been implicated, includ-ing hypothyroidism, primary and secondary hyperparathy-roidism (where epiphyseal slips may also occur at the wrist), hypogonadism, and an association with craniopharyngioma and optic glioma. Previous irradiation therapy may also increase the risk of SUFE in a dose-related manner [20].

Immunological Factors

Eisenstein and Rothschild [21] reported an association between SUFE and increased serum immunoglobulins, par-ticularly IgA. Patients with chondrolysis showed a greater increase in IgM. It was proposed that epiphyseal slipping was either a localized manifestation of a generalized inflam-matory disorder or, more probably, that the slip exposes a tissue proteoglycan that acts as an antigenic stimulus for immunoglobulin and complement (C3) production.

Synovial fluid assays in SUFE sometimes reveal elevated immune complexes compared to normal joints, at a time when serum levels are normal. Cell death and the local inflammatory response could therefore increase the risk of further slippage and chondrolysis. As yet, the evidence for these associations is unconvincing.

Pathophysiology

The growth plate structural changes in SUFE have been assessed mainly by core biopsies. Apart from hyperpara-thyroidism, when the displacement may occur in the metaphy-sis, the slip develops through the zone of hypertrophic cartilage where the enlarging chondrocytes lie in irregular clusters [22] within a matrix which is weakened by a lack of col-lagen fibrils. Abnormal accumulation and distribution of glycoproteins and proteoglycans may inhibit the process of chondrocyte apoptosis [23, 24].

In the pre-slip stage the synovium is edematous and hyperemic while the growth plate appears widened [25]. Softening and decalcification of the metaphysis produce juxta-epiphyseal osteopenia radiographically. In the second stage of true displacement the slip progresses incrementally, although a sudden shearing force may lead to the so-called acute-on-chronic slip. In reality, displacement results from pathological movement not of the epiphysis but of the femoral neck which adducts, externally rotates, and shifts proximally like the fractured neck of femur in the elderly.

The capital epiphysis remains within the acetabulum, constrained by the ligamentum teres, the labrum, and surface tension. Griffiths [26] confirmed that the epiphysis comes to lie posterior to the femoral neck but that an anterior radiographic projection of the hip gives a misleading appearance of medial displacement. It is therefore helpful to rotate the femur during surgery to fix the epiphysis as this identifies the precise position of the epiphysis and screw tip under image intensifier. In rare cases the slip is acute, catastrophic, and unstable [27], so that imaging of a true lateral of the hip proves almost impossible.

The periosteum is torn through anteriorly as the slip progresses while posteroinferiorly, where it is lifted up from the neck of the femur, the callus forms. In the chronic slip with a history of over 3 weeks re-modeling of the callus stabilizes the displaced epiphysis, as with any fracture. The posterior retinacular vessels are stripped up with the periosteum and eventually shorten. Manipulation may therefore stretch the arterial supply and produce epiphyseal ischemia. The uncovered, anterior portion of the residual proximal femoral growth plate appears bluish-grey with islands of bone and cartilage. Impingement may later develop anteriorly between this metaphyseal "bump" and the acetabular rim although re-modeling in lesser slips eventually reduces this.

The synovial membrane and periosteum remain hyperemic and edematous throughout the slipping phase. Eventually, the inflammatory process subsides and the growth plate closes prematurely, on average 19 months after the onset of symptoms in the untreated case.

Clinical Features

Pain in the groin or knee, limp, and restricted hip movements characterize SUFE. Despite a limp, which may be painless, and an externally rotated leg (Fig. 28.2), diagnosis may be delayed by weeks or months. The knee may be the only symptomatic site [28] and radiographs are mistakenly confined to that joint. It is therefore essential to examine and possibly image the hips in any child or adolescence with a limp

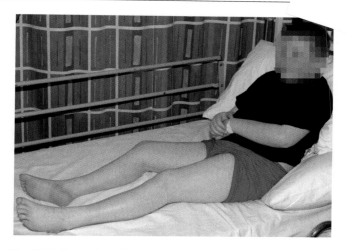

Fig. 28.2 External rotation and shortening of the right leg as a result of slipped epiphysis

and knee pain, particularly if knee examination is normal. An antalgic or Trendelenburg gait should also be tested for.

Classification

The condition is graded by the length of history, the extent of the slip, and by the disability in regard to weight bearing. Loder et al. [27] proposed that an unstable acute slip prevents the patient from weight bearing due to pain, even when crutches are being used. Active straight leg raising is also impossible with an unstable SUFE.

The involved limb lies in external rotation and adduction when displacement is severe. With a mild slip internal rotation and adduction of the flexed hip are painful and possibly limited. In more marked slipping abduction, flexion and internal rotation are decreased. As the examiner flexes the affected hip the thigh rolls typically into external rotation, producing the "figure 4" position. Flexion may be more limited than extension. Movement is more restricted in the acute slip, probably because the hemarthrosis or tense effusion causes pronounced muscle spasm. Shortening of the leg is rarely more than 2 cm, a combination of real and apparent loss of length.

Acute Slip

The history is less than 2–3 weeks by definition and the symptoms are usually marked. Approximately 20% of cases present acutely and AVN may complicate the condition in up to 50% of cases. A type I (Salter–Harris) fracture is a different entity, occurring in a normal patient with no prodromal symptoms who has been injured by a severe traumatic event. In both conditions reactive bone changes are yet to be seen on radiographs or scans.

Chronic Slip

The history is more than 3 weeks' duration with no defined trauma or sudden pain. Limp may be painless and unnoticed by the patient or family. Radiographs reveal posterior tilting of one or both capital epiphyses with associated metaphyseal re-modeling.

Acute-on-Chronic Slip

Although the patient has been symptomatic for more than 3 weeks, a sudden increase in pain and disability suggests a rapid further displacement of the epiphysis. This presentation accounts for about half of all treated cases.

It is not entirely clear why some epiphyses slip minimally and then stabilize, and why others displace progressively or in one, catastrophic shift. Knight et al. [29] found that of the 30% who present with a chronic slip, 50% have displaced less than 30°. Acute episodes of slipping superimposed upon chronic mild displacement result in periods of hip irritability and variable deformity.

Measuring the Slip

Although radiographic alterations are evident on the anteroposterior radiographs in SUFE the classic lateral projection method was proposed by Southwick [30] (Fig. 28.3) when describing his corrective proximal femoral osteotomy. If pain and spasm allow, a frog lateral view is attempted. Forcible positioning is both uncomfortable and risky so it may be wiser to obtain a "cross-table" lateral.

Radiographic imaging of the slip at operation is difficult and may be misleading. When the leg is externally rotated the epiphysis appears to be tilted medially; when the hip is internally rotated the tilt appears to be posterolateral. To demonstrate the displacement best the hip should be flexed 20–30°, the knee flexed to 90° and the thigh supported in 30° of external rotation. This reduces the parallax effect [26, 31] which can also be reduced by screening the hip while rotating the leg until the epiphysis is best visualized.

The degree of posterior slip is defined as follows:

Mild – the head–shaftangle is less than 30° (Fig. 28.3)
Moderate – the angle is 30–60°
Severe – the angle is more than 60°

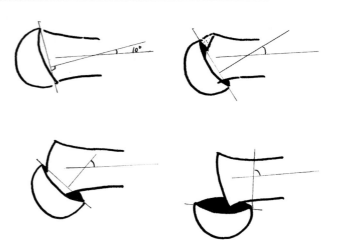

Fig. 28.3 The lateral projection of the affected hip shows neck retroversion and the extent of epiphyseal displacement in degrees

The tilt is compared to the contralateral hip which is often retroverted or may also be affected by a mild slip. Southwick also noted that the anteroposterior (AP) view offered a measure of the axis of the femoral neck versus the base of the capital epiphysis, considering the normal angle to be 145°.

Wilson [32] quantified displacement on the lateral view using the ratio of slip distance to the diameter of the femoral neck proximally. A mild slip is less than 33%, a moderate is 33–50%, and severe is more than 50% displacement. Complete displacement (100%) is a 90° Southwick angle.

Figure 28.4 shows some of the changes seen on an AP radiograph of a slip:

1 Klein's line [33] intersects the lateral segment of the epiphysis but this intersection is reduced or absent on the abnormal side (Trethowan's sign).
2 A break in Shenton's arc develops progressively.
3 Scham's sign [34] describes the absence of the normal overlap between the proximal, medial metaphysis, and the acetabular wall (pubic component).
4 Steel's metaphyseal blanch sign [35] develops as the posteriorly slipping epiphysis overlaps the proximal femoral neck.
5 Concurrently, the height of the epiphysis reduces as it tilts.
6 Relative osteopenia occurs in the femur and hemipelvis on the abnormal side as weight bearing is reduced.

It is particularly important to look for these subtle signs and to augment this with a frog lateral view. Computed tomography (CT) scans or magnetic resonance (MR) imaging depict the anatomy accurately and are therefore of value, principally in the established or healed case when corrective osteotomy is being planned.

Fig. 28.4 The anteroposterior radiographic projection shows a number of signs. See text for the six alterations

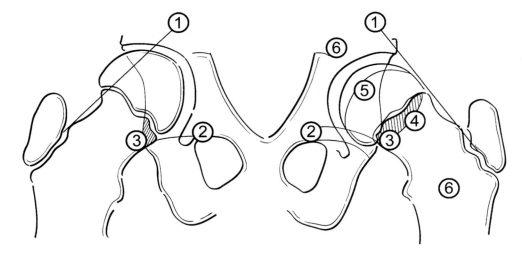

Alternative Imaging (Early)

Imaging of the hips by radiography can be augmented by ultrasound [36] which demonstrates the effusion and possibly the shift of the epiphysis on the metaphysis. Similarly, MR scanning may be appropriate in the acute situation, allowing some definition of the abnormal anatomy and possible changes in the "pre-slipping" phase, although the value of this over radiographs has been disputed [37]. Images are degraded by the presence of metallic implants in the proximal femur postoperatively.

Alternative Imaging (Late)

Bone scanning with technetium (Tc-99m) was assessed prior to treatment by Rhoad et al. [38]. Since ischemia was identified in 6 of the 10 unstable but none of the stable hips the scan was a useful predictor of outcome prior to surgical treatment. None of the unstable hips with normal isotope uptake subsequently developed AVN. Owing to restrictions in the acute availability of this investigation in many health care systems, bone scanning cannot yet be considered a standard investigation in the urgent management of SUFE.

Bone scans are more commonly used to assess the presence of AVN or chondrolysis postoperatively, particularly in the severe slips or after corrective osteotomy at the femoral neck. These two complications invariably lead to stiffness and discomfort but whereas AVN leads to reduced epiphyseal isotope uptake, chondrolysis produces increased uptake in the acetabulum as well as the epiphysis.

CT scans are of value postoperatively, first to assess the position of the screw if there is concern about implant position or joint penetration, and second to improve later realignment surgery (Fig. 28.5). Axial CT scans allow detailed

measurement of the slip angle between the axis of the femoral neck and the tangent across the base of the epiphysis [39]. Bone stock and femoral dimensions can also be gauged with 3D CT scanning (Fig. 28.6).

Surgical Treatment

The objectives of orthopaedic management are as follows:

1 Early diagnosis and definition of the slip
2 Avoidance of forced manipulation (Fig. 28.7)
3 Stable fixation of the slipped epiphysis
4 Consideration of the risks of contralateral slippage
5 Monitoring for AVN or chondrolysis
6 Timed contralateral distal femoral epiphysis for leg length discrepancy
7 Later corrective osteotomy if appropriate.

In Situ Fixation

Conservative treatment with a hip spica cast is no longer appropriate and carried a high rate of complications. Percutaneous fixation (Fig. 28.8) is effective for mild to moderate chronic and acute-on-chronic slips, using a single cannulated, full-threaded screw placed as centrally in the epiphysis as possible [40]. For greater degrees of slip the guide wire and subsequent screw need to be placed through a more anterior site in the femoral neck. Even if the line of the insertion is marked out on the skin of the proximal thigh using anterior and lateral projections on the image intensifier it is often necessary to expose the femur more formally.

Fig. 28.5 CT scans reveal the posterior epiphyseal slip and three artifacts from previous pinning

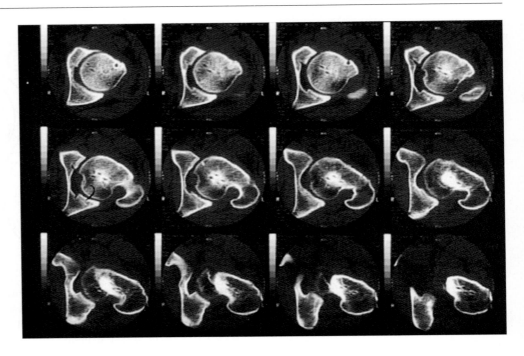

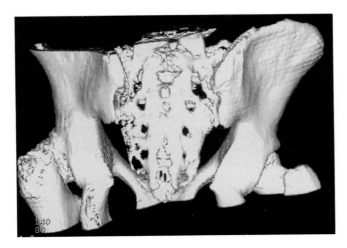

Fig. 28.6 Imaging with 3D CT shows posterior shift of the epiphysis and external rotation of the femur

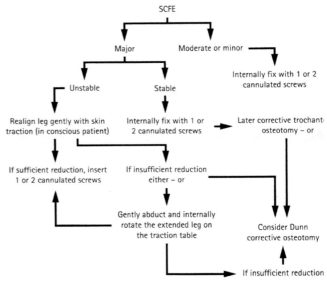

Fig. 28.7 Flow diagram to outline the surgical approach for slipped epiphysis

The epiphysis must be clearly visualized throughout the procedure to ensure that the guide wire or screw do not penetrate the joint. Greenhough et al. [41] reported a high complication rate with multiple pins but a single cannulated screw applied with compression and five threads in the epiphysis [42] should offer good stability. An arthrogram has been recommended after pinning [43] or cannulated screw insertion [44], while the patient is still anesthetized, although this does not rule out joint penetration completely [45]. The hip should also be assessed through a full range of movement to check for crepitus or obstruction and definitive AP and lateral radiographs obtained at the end of the procedure.

With slips of greater than 30° the medullary aperture begins to close (Fig. 28.9) and an anterior neck insertion is inevitable (Figs. 28.10 and 28.11). This helps to avoid the crucial lateral epiphyseal vessels which enter the epiphysis at its posteroinferior quadrant [46] and anastomose with vessels from the ligamentum teres and other retinacular vessels.

Fig. 28.8 The stages in percutaneous pinning

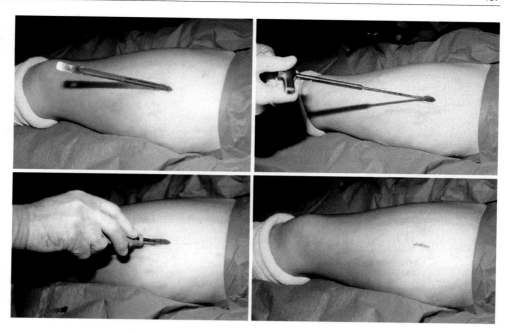

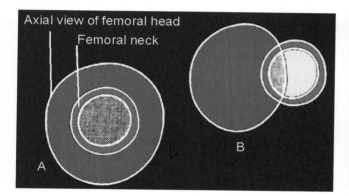

Fig. 28.9 The aperture shared by the femoral neck and epiphysis (**a**) gradually closes off as the slip increases (**b**)

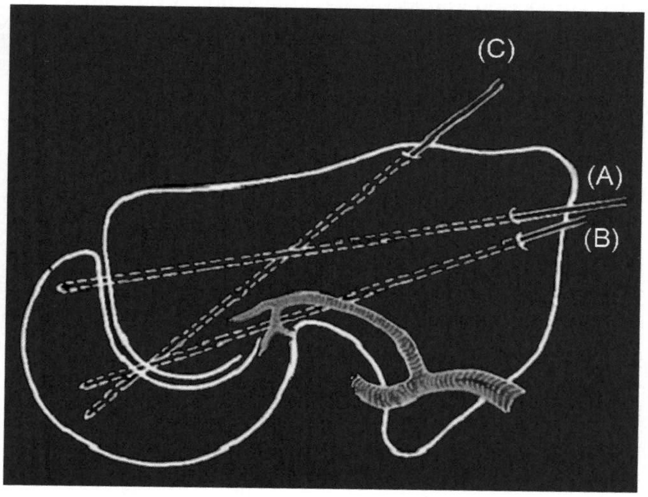

Fig. 28.10 The trajectory of the guide wire is important. A conventional insertion may either result in a poor fixation in the anterior epiphysis (**a**) or, if directed more posteriorly, may breach the posterior cortex of the neck and thus injure the vital retinacular vessels (**b**). A more anterior starting point with the guidewire will allow the neck to be traversed within the neck and the center of the epiphysis to be reached (**c**)

The Unstable Slip

Management of the major acute slip is controversial and beset with concerns. The risk of stretching the posterior retinacular vessels is considerable when the leg is manipulated under general anesthesia to reduce the slip. Gently rolling the extended leg internally with the thigh supported and slightly abducted may lessen the slip angle, making in situ fixation possible [47]. In the heavier child double guide wire fixation may be indicated to achieve epiphyseal stability, while maintaining internal rotation and some abduction of the hip. This permits double screw fixation [48] thus increasing implant strength by 33% [49], although complications may be increased. De Sanctis et al. [50] found that single cannulation screw fixation was effective for both stable and unstable slip if the implant was properly positioned in the epiphysis.

Timing the surgery may be important in the management of the unstable hip. Kalogriantis et al. [51] have suggested treatment within 24 h if possible, when the risk of stretching the retinacular vessels with gentle manipulation may be less (Fig. 28.7). AVN complicated those hips treated between 24 and 72 h. In view of the isotope bone scan results of Rhoad

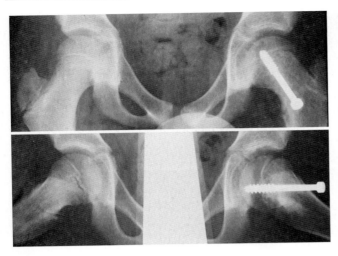

Fig. 28.11 Radiographs to show cannulated screw fixation of a moderate slip

et al. [38] it still remains a concern as to whether there is any truly safe period to operate upon the acute, severe slip [52].

The etiology of this chondrolysis is unclear although pin penetration and the obsolete use of a spica cast produce high rates. It may complicate subcapital, basal neck (cuneiform) [53, 54], and even later corrective trochanteric osteotomy. An increased risk in African-American and Hawaiian children has been reported [55].

The joint space narrows due to softening and thinning of articular cartilage on both sides of the joint. A villous synovitis develops with the eventual formation of adhesions. As cartilage is lost the subchondral bone is exposed, leading to pain and progressive osteoarthritis.

Treatment comprises physiotherapy to maintain as much hip movement as possible. If symptoms are severe, weight bearing is reduced for a variable period and non-steroidal anti-inflammatory drugs may be appropriate. Infection should be ruled out by joint aspiration and a CT scan will visualize whether the screw or pin has penetrated the joint. Arthrodesis or hip resurfacing arthroplasty is a later option, but realignment, sometimes useful in cases of segmental AVN, is not effective. Standard bone grafting and vascularized fibular grafts are ineffectual.

Later Proximal Femoral Osteotomies

In cases where the growth plate has closed following in situ fixation, with an established slip angle of 30–60°, a later corrective intertrochanteric osteotomy is indicated. For lesser slips re-modeling may improve alignment in the younger

patient, but this phenomenon ceases with skeletal maturity. Osteoplasty by removal of the prominent neck bump anteriorly [56] may be indicated when there is evidence of femoro-acetabular impingement.

Urgent Subcapital Osteotomy

There is a limited place for these procedures, provided that the surgeon is experienced in this demanding technique. When the epiphysis proves to be irreducibly displaced through 70–90°, the Dunn procedure [57, 58] allows the slip to be fully corrected. It is imperative to obtain full surgical access through an anterolateral or anterior approach. The plane of dissection is between the abductors and tensor fasciae latae, with or without greater trochanteric osteotomy, exposing the femoral neck superiorly and anteriorly (Fig. 28.12). The operation may be undertaken with the patient lying supine [59] or lying on the unaffected side with the image intensifier positioned appropriately.

The posterior retinacular vessels of the femoral neck must not be damaged and this is ensured by

1 leaving the soft tissues over the posterior neck undissected
2 shortening the femoral neck 1–2 cm to allow gradual repositioning of the epiphysis without tensioning the vessels
3 gentle positioning of the thigh in abduction and slight internal rotation while inserting a central, cannulated screw with compression

The curved line of the femoral neck and the saucer-shaped inferior epiphyseal surface (Figs. 28.13 and 28.14) should fit together snugly and the hip carefully screened to assess stability of fixation and possible pin penetration. Postoperative mobilization depends upon the security of fixation and whether a greater trochanteric osteotomy has been used. If hip movements comparable to the normal side are regained rapidly over the first few days the likelihood of AVN is low. Partial weight bearing can be permitted with crutches within the first week postoperatively, with full weight bearing by 6 weeks.

AVN is reported in 20–25% of patients [60] (Fig. 28.15), with varying rates of chondrolysis in different series [59]. Shortening of the affected leg is approximately 1.5 cm and since the growth plate has been ablated the discrepancy may increase unless contralateral prophylactic fixation of the proximal epiphysis has been deemed advisable. If this is not the case, particularly with the younger patient, a distal femoral epiphysiodesis should be undertaken at the appropriate time [61].

Fig. 28.12 Stages in the Dunn osteotomy

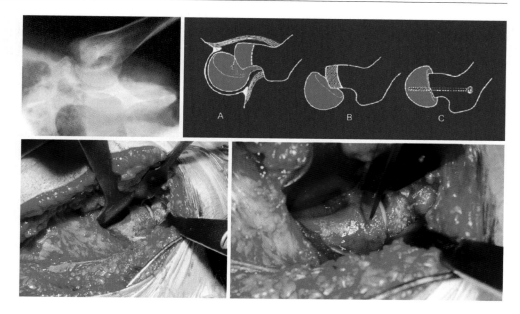

Fig. 28.13 The femoral neck must be shortened so that repositioning the epiphysis does not stretch or damage the posterior retinacular vessels

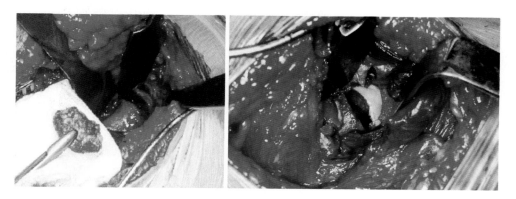

The Fish osteotomy [62, 63] is a similar procedure undertaken less acutely. Provided that the growth plate is still open, best confirmed by axial CT scanning, correction is possible by removing callus and an appropriate wedge of proximal metaphyseal bone. The anterolateral approach is used and the growth plate defined with a needle. The AVN and chondrolysis rates remain as complications.

Contralateral Prophylactic Fixation

Bilateral epiphyseal slips occur in 95% of patients with chronic renal osteodystrophy [64] and in 61% of endocrinopathies [65]. These slips are usually severe and therefore merit bilateral fixation unlike the often asymptomatic minor slips seen in athletic individuals [66] which may still predispose to later osteoarthritis due to femoro-acetabular impingement (Fig. 28.16)

The risk of severe contralateral slip is greater in younger children who have already suffered from an unstable slip, so there is a case for bilateral fixation, particularly if social circumstances cause concern. Jerre et al. [4] reported a contralateral slip rate of 20–25% and since only one in ten of these will be unstable, the risk of developing an unstable contralateral slip is in the order of 1–2%. Nevertheless, the risks of a later, major contralateral slip is such that careful monitoring every 3–6 months is warranted [67].

The complications from contralateral fixation are low [68], particularly as operative techniques have improved. It is therefore prudent to fix the contralateral hip in prepubertal children, particularly if the triradiate cartilage is open or when the Oxford pelvic bone age score, as modified by Stasikelis et al. [69], confirms that the patient is relatively immature. Vigilant follow-up in the orthopaedic outpatient clinic is mandatory until the proximal femoral growth plates fuse. It is a calamity if a patient with a poor result from one unstable slip sustains a contralateral unstable slip with subsequent complications.

Fig. 28.14 Dunn procedure
a) the right hip treated by Dunn
procedure with b) right hip of the
same patient three years later
after metal removal c) acute slip
of the left hip in 13 year old boy
d) after Dunn procedure without
trochanteric osteotomy

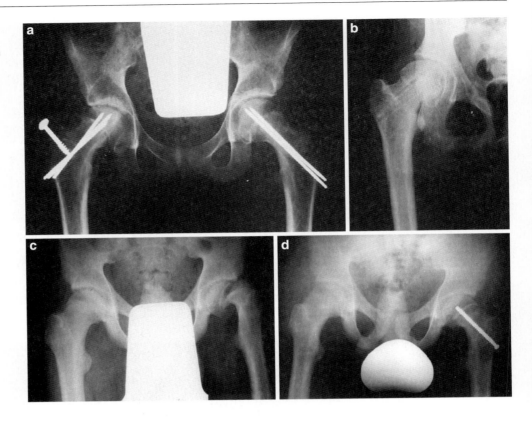

Fig. 28.15 The radiographic
appearances 20 years after a right
Dunn osteotomy complicated by
segmental avascular necrosis and
subsequent osteoarthritis

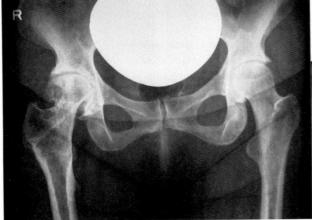
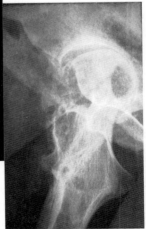

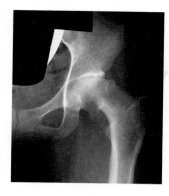

Fig. 28.16 Pistol grip deformity of the left hip in a 20 year old girl, who had an acute-on-chronic slip on the left side at age 14 years

Complications

Operative

Difficulties in imaging the true lateral view of the hip, both preoperatively and during the surgical procedure, may result in the pins or cannulated screw being inserted inaccurately leading to later loss of reduction, implant breakage or penetration into the joint. The guide wire may fracture if it bends during positioning of the leg to maintain slip reduction thus snaring against the cannulated reamer. The surgeon should therefore be prepared to enlarge the wound if these technical difficulties arise. Migration of pins may occur and clustering their tips may produce segmental necrosis [46]. A fracture may develop at the stress riser where the implant has been inserted. Lastly, the standard surgical complications of nerve and vessel injury, infection, and hypertrophic scar may occur.

Avascular Necrosis

As previously discussed the most common cause of AVN is manipulative reduction of the slipped epiphysis (Fig. 28.17) although it can occur rarely in the untreated, unstable hip. The rate of AVN increases if the partial or complete reduction has been for a mild slip (12.5%), a moderate slip (70%), or a severe slip (75%) [70].

Postoperative stiffness is the first sign that necrosis may be present, cell death producing a continuing reactive effusion and muscle spasm. The radiographic changes are evident by 6–12 months (Fig. 28.17) [71], although minor changes and loss of femoral head sphericity may not appear until a few years later, with the inevitable hastening of osteoarthritis. MR and isotope bone scanning confirm AVN,

which may be partial (segmental) or total, at an early stage postoperatively.

Chondrolysis

This complication has been discussed in relation to the unstable slip. An autoimmune reaction has been proposed [21], resulting in a lack of synovial fluid production. There is no clear-cut association with intra-articular pin penetration [41, 72].

Later Surgical Procedures

Corrective Femoral Osteotomy

Southwick described his triplane valgus, extension, and internal rotation distal segment correction in 1967 [30]. With the removal of carefully executed bone wedges at the level of the lesser trochanter (Fig. 28.18) following preoperative planning, the principal components of the deformity can be corrected. Fixation with fixed angle blade plates and screws (Fig. 28.19) avoids the need for postoperative immobilization and achieves excellent or good results in 87% of patients at 18 years.

Imhauser [73, 74] and Griffiths [26] corrected the extension and external rotational deformities, satisfactory results being reported for moderate and severe SUFE [75]. These intertrochanteric osteotomies are distal to the site of deformity and correction is limited but usually sufficient to improve gait. AVN is not a risk although loss of fixation (with re-operation needed), delayed union, fracture, and occasionally chondrolysis have been reported. Later osteoarthritis still develops in many cases. In patients where the growth plate was open Southwick found that closure of the physis was probably hastened by the realignment which increased axial compression when weight bearing.

Implant Removal

As many of these patients will require a later hip arthroplasty, removal of blade plates and screws is advisable once the growth plate and osteotomy have united. Apart from requiring a second anesthetic the removal of implants is often difficult, so an asymptomatic single cannulated screw should be left in situ.

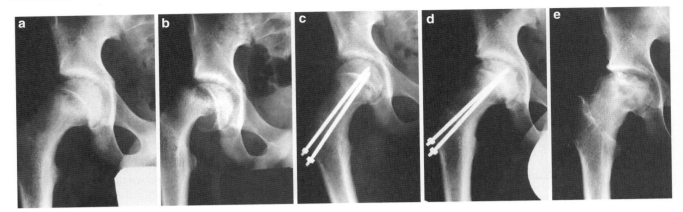

Fig. 28.17 A minor slip of the right upper femoral epiphysis was not appreciated although many of the pathological signs detailed in Fig. 28.4 are present (**a**). The epiphysis slipped significantly a few days later (**b**) and was reduced anatomically by manipulation under anesthesia (**c**). Avascular necrosis and loss of joint space became progressively more obvious (**d**, **e**)

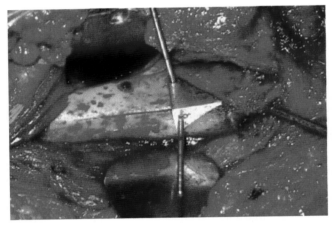

Fig. 28.18 Metal templates allow the excision of precisely measured bone wedges as part of a Southwick, triplane osteotomy

Conclusion

Failure to diagnose the slipped capital femoral epiphysis remains the main concern in this condition. As a cause of limp in childhood, it accounts for only 0.5% of the total number of hip conditions that are encountered. It is this relative rarity that makes slipped epiphysis difficult to diagnose, coupled with its insidious onset in some children and adolescents, and the fact that pain is commonly referred to the ipsilateral knee. In any child who is abnormally short, or in whom the medical history is complex, and particularly in the later stages of childhood and in adolescence, the possibility of slipped upper femoral epiphysis must be entertained.

Fig. 28.19 A valgus, derotation (biplanar) proximal femoral osteotomy corrects leg alignment although some head–neck deformity has to be accepted

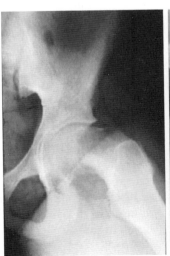
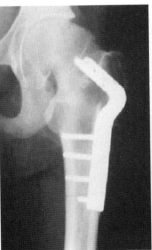
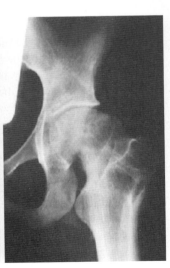

References

1 Loder RT. The demographics of slipped capital femoral epiphysis. An international multicentre study. Clin Orthop 1996; 322:8–27.

2 Kelsey JL, Acheson RM, Keggi KJ. The body build of patients with slipped capital epiphysis. Am J Dis Child 1972; 124:276–81.

3 Hansson LI, Hagglund G, Ordeberg G. Slipped capital femoral epiphysis in Southern Sweden 1910–1982. Acta Orthop Scand Suppl 1987; 226:1–67.

4 Jerre R, Billing L, Hansson G, et al. The contralateral hip in patients treated for unilateral slipped upper femoral epiphysis: long term follow up of 61 hips. J Bone Joint Surg [Br] 1994; 76B:563–7.

5 Sorensen KH. Slipped upper femoral epiphysis. Clinical study on etiology. Acta Orthop Scand 1968; 39:499–517.

6 Hagglund G, Hansson LI, Ordeberg G. Bilaterality in slipped upper femoral epiphysis. J Bone Joint Surg [Br] 1988; 70B:179–81.

7 Loder RT, Aronson DD, Greenfield ML. The epidemiology of bilateral slipped capital femoral epiphysis: a study of children in Michigan. J Bone Joint Surg [Am] 1993; 75A:1141–9.

8 Stasikelis P, Sullivan C, Phillips W, et al. Slipped capital femoral epiphysis: prediction of contralateral involvement. J Bone Joint Surg [Am] 1996; 78A:1149–55.

9 Acheson R. The Oxford method of assessing skeletal maturity. Clin Orthop 1957; 10:19–26.

10 Puylaert D, Dimeglio A, Bentahar T. Staging puberty in slipped capital femoral epiphysis: importance of the triradiate cartilage. J Pediatr Orthop 2004; 24:144–7.

11 Loder RT, Mehbod AA, Meyer C, et al. Acetabular depth and race in young adults, a potential explanation of the differences in the prevalence of slipped capital femoral epiphysis between different racial groups. J Pediatr Orthop 2003; 23:699–702.

12 Kordelle J, Richolt JA, Millis MB, et al. Development of the acetabulum in patients with slipped capital femoral epiphysis: a three-dimensional analysis based on computed tomography. J Pediatr Orthop 2001; 21:174–8.

13 Hansson LI, Hagglund G, Ordeberg G. Epidemiology of slipped capital epiphysis in Southern Sweden. Clin Orthop 1984; 191: 82–94.

14 Rennie AM. The inheritance of slipped upper femoral epiphysis. J Bone Joint Surg [Br] 1982; 64B:180–4.

15 Chung SMK, Batterman SC, Brighton CT. Shear strength of the human capital epiphyseal plate. J Bone Joint Surg [Am] 1976; 58A:99–103.

16 Gelberman RH, Cohen MS, Shaw BA, et al. The association of femoral retroversion with slipped capital femoral epiphysis. J Bone Joint Surg [Am] 1986; 68A:1000–7.

17 Galbraith RT, Gelberman RH, Hajek PG, et al. Obesity and decreased femoral anteversion in adolescence. J Orthop Res 1987; 5:523–8.

18 Mirkopulos N, Weiner DS, Askew M. The evolving slope of the proximal femoral growth plate relationship to slipped capital femoral epiphysis. J Pediatr Orthop 1988; 8:268–73.

19 Blethen SL, Rundle AC. Slipped capital femoral epiphysis in children treated with growth hormone: a summary of the national cooperative growth study experience. Horm Res 1996; 46:113–6.

20 Loder RT, Hensinger RN, Alburger PD, et al. Slipped capital epiphysis associated with radiation therapy. J Pediatr Orthop 1998; 18:630–6.

21 Eisenstein A, Rothschild S. Biochemical abnormalities in patients with slipped capital femoral epiphysis and chondrolysis. J Bone Joint Surg [Am] 1976; 58A:459–67.

22 Mickelson MR, Ponseti IV, Cooper RR, et al. The ultrastructure of the growth plate in slipped capital femoral epiphysis. J Bone Joint Surg [Am] 1977; 59A:1076–81.

23 Kerr JFR, Wyllie AH, Currie AR. Apoptosis—basic biological phenomenon with wide-ranging implications in tissue kinetics. Brit J Cancer 1972; 26:234–42.

24 Roach HI, Aigner T, Kouri JB. Chondroptosis: a variant of apoptotic cell death in chondrocytes? Apoptosis 2004; 9:265–79.

25 Howorth B. Slipping of the capital femoral epiphysis: pathology. Clin Orthop 1966; 48:33–9.

26 Griffiths MJ. Slipping of the upper femoral epiphysis. Ann Roy Coll Surg 1976; 58:34–42.

27 Loder RT, Richards BS, Shapiro PS, et al. Acute slipped capital femoral epiphysis: the importance of physeal stability. J Bone Joint Surg [Am] 1993; 75A:1134–40.

28 Matava MJ, Patton RM, Luhmann S, et al. Knee pain as the initial symptom of slipped capital femoral epiphysis: an analysis of initial presentation and treatment. J Pediatr Orthop 1999; 19:455–60.

29 Knight DJ, Dreghorn C, Main SG. Slipped capital femoral epiphysis in Glasgow. J Pediatr Orthop 1987; 7:283–7.

30 Southwick WO. Osteotomy through the lesser trochanter for slipped capital femoral epiphysis. J Bone Joint Surg [Am] 1967; 49A:807–34.

31 Billing I, Severin E. Slipping epiphysis of the hip; a roentgenological and clinical study based on a new roentgen technique. Acta Radiol 1959; 51:1–76.

32 Wilson PD. The treatment of slipping of the upper femoral epiphysis with minimal displacement. J Bone Joint Surg [Am] 1938; 20A:379–99.

33 Klein A, Joplin RJ, Reidy JA, et al. Roentgenographic features of slipped capital epiphysis. Am J Roentgenol 1951; 66:361–74.

34 Scham SM. The triangular sign in the early diagnosis of slipped capital femoral epiphysis. Clin Orthop 1974; 103:16–7.

35 Steel HH. The metaphyseal blanch sign of slipped capital femoral epiphysis. J Bone Joint Surg [Am] 1986; 68A:920–2.

36 Kallio PE, Mah ET, Paterson DC, et al. Ultrasound in slipped capital femoral epiphysis. Diagnosis and assessment of severity. J Bone Joint Surg [Br] 1991; 738:884–9.

37 Tins BJ, Cassar-Pullicino VN. Slipped upper femoral epiphysis. In: Davis AM, Johnson K eds. Imaging of the hip and bony pelvis. Techniques and applications. Springer, Berlin 2005; pp 173–94.

38 Rhoad RC, Davidson RS, Heyman S, et al. Pre-treatment bone scan in SCFE: a predictor of ischemia and avascular necrosis. J Pediatr Orthop 1999; 19:164–8.

39 Cohen MS, Gelberman RH, Griffin PP, et al. Slipped capital femoral epiphysis: assessment of epiphyseal displacement and angulation. J Pediatr Orthop 1986; 6:259–64.

40 Morrissy RT. Slipped capital femoral epiphysis: technique of percutaneous in situ fixation. J Pediatr Orthop 1990; 10:347–50.

41 Greenhough CG, Bromage JD, Jackson AM. Pinning of the slipped upper epiphysis—a trouble-free procedure? J Pediatr Orthop 1985; 5:657–60.

42 Carney BT, Birnbaum P, Minter C. Slip progression after in situ single screw fixation for stable slipped capital femoral epiphysis. J Pediatr Orthop 2003; 23:584–9.

43 Bennet GC, Koreska J, Rang M. Pin placement in slipped capital femoral epiphysis. J Pediatr Orthop 1984; 4:574–8.

44 Lehman WB, Minche D, Grant A, et al. The problem of evaluating in situ pinning of slipped capital femoral epiphysis. An experimental model and review of 63 consecutive cases. J Pediatr Orthop 1984; 4:297–303.

45 Shaw JA. Preventing unrecognised pin penetration into the hip joint. Orth Rev 1984; 13:142–52.

46 Brodetti A. The blood supply of the femoral neck and head in relation to the damaging effects of nails and screws. J Bone Joint Surg [Br] 1960; 428:794–801.

47 Aronsson DD, Loder RT. Treatment of the unstable (acute) slipped capital femoral epiphysis. Clin Orthop 1996; 322:99–110.

48 Macnicol MF, Macindoe N. Management of severe slippage of the capital femoral epiphysis. Curr Orth 1996; 10:180–4.

49 Karol LA, Doane RM, Cornicelli SF, et al. Single versus double screw fixation for treatment of slipped capital femoral epiphysis: a biochemical analysis. J Pediatr Orthop 1992; 12:741–6.

50 De Sanctis N, DiGennaro G, Pempinello C, et al. Is gentle manipulative reduction and percutaneous fixation with a single screw the best management of acute and acute on chronic slipped capital epiphysis. A report of 70 patients. J Pediatr Orthop B 1996; 5:90–5.

51 Kalogriantis S, Khoon Tan C, Kemp GJ, et al. Does unstable slipped capital femoral epiphysis require urgent stabilisation? J Pediatr Orthop B 2007; 16:6–9.

52 Weinstein S. Natural history and treatment outcomes of childhood hip disorders. Clin Orthop 1997; 344:227–34.

53 Kramer WG, Craig WA, Noel S. Compensating osteotomy at the base of the femoral neck for slipped capital femoral epiphysis. J Bone Joint Surg [Am] 1976; 58A:796–800.

54 Barmada R, Bruch RF, Gimbel JS, Ray RD. Base of the neck extracapsular osteotomy for correction of deformity in slipped capital femoral epiphysis. Clin Orthop 1978; 132:98–101.

55 Carney BT, Weinstein SL, Noble J. Long-term follow-up of slipped capital femoral epiphysis. J Bone Joint Surg [Am] 1991; 73A: 667–74.

56 Heyman S, Herndon C, Strong J. Slipped femoral epiphysis with severe displacement: a conservative operative technique. J Bone Joint Surg [Am] 1957; 39A:293–303.

57 Dunn DM. The treatment of adolescent slipping of the upper femoral epiphysis. J Bone Joint Surg [Br] 1964; 46B:621–9.

58 Dunn DM, Angel JC. Replacement of the femoral head by open operation in severe adolescent slipping of the upper femoral epiphysis. J Bone Joint Surg [Br] 1978; 60B:394–403.

59 Macnicol MF, ed. Color Atlas and Text of Osteotomy of the Hip. London: Mosby-Wolfe; 1996:139–44.

60 Szypryt EP, Clement DA, Colton CL. Open reduction or epiphysiodesis for slipped upper femoral epiphysis. J Bone Joint Surg [Br] 1987; 64B:737–42.

61 Macnicol MF, Gupta M. Epiphysioidesis using a cannulated tube saw. J Bone Joint Surg [Br] 1997; 97B:307–9.

62 Fish J. Cuneiform osteotomy of the femoral neck in the treatment of slipped capital femoral epiphysis. J Bone Joint Surg [Am] 1984; 66A:1153–68.

63 Fish J. Cuneiform osteotomy of the femoral neck in the treatment of slipped capital femoral epiphysis. J Bone Joint Surg [Am] 1994; 76A:46–59.

64 Loder RT, Hensinger RN. Slipped capital femoral epiphysis associated with renal failure osteodystrophy. J Pediatr Orthop 1997; 17:205–11.

65 Loder RT, Wittenberg B, DeSilva G. Slipped capital femoral epiphysis associated with endocrine disorder. J Pediatr Orthop 1995; 15:349–56.

66 Murray RO, Duncan C. Athletic activity in adolescence as an aetiological factor in degenerative hip disease. J Bone Joint Surg [Br] 1971; 53B:406–19.

67 Maclean JGB, Reddy SK. The contralateral slip. An avoidable complication and indication for prophylactic pinning in slipped upper femoral epiphysis. J Bone Joint Surg [Br] 2006; 88B:1497–501.

68 Seller K, Raab P, Wild A, et al. Risk benefit analysis of prophylactic pinning in slipped capital femoral epiphysis. J Pediatr Orthop 2001; 10:192–6.

69 Robb JE, Annan IH, Macnicol MF. Guidewire damage during cannulated screw fixation for slipped capital femoral epiphysis. J Pediatr Orthop B 2003; 12:219–22.

70 Tokmakova KP, Stanton RP, Mason DE. Factors influencing the development of osteonecrosis in patients treated for slipped capital femoral epiphysis. J Bone Joint Surg [Am] 2003; 85A:798–801.

71 Krahn TH, Canale ST, Beaty JH, et al. Long term follow up of patients with avascular necrosis after treatment of slipped capital femoral epiphysis. J Pediatr Orthop 1993; 13:154–8.

72 Vrettos B, Hoffman EB. Chondrolysis in slipped upper femoral epiphysis: long-term study of the etiology and natural history. J Bone Joint Surg [Br] 1993; 75B:456–61.

73 Imhauser G. Zur Pathogenese und Therapie der jugendlichen Huftkopflosung. Orthop 1957; 88:3–41.

74 Imhauser G. Spaetergebnisse der sog Imhauser Osteotomie bei der Epiphysen loesung. Z Orthop 1977; 115:716–25.

75 Parsch K, Zehender H, Buehl T, Walker S. Intertrochanteric corrective osteotomy for moderate and severe chronic slipped capital femoral epiphysis. J Pediatr Orthop B 1999; 8:223–30.

Chapter 29

The Knee

David M. Hunt and Malcolm F. Macnicol

Introduction

The child's knee is vulnerable to mechanical problems, although the relative frequency of complaints varies with age. For example, instability of the knee in a child is more likely to result from a patellofemoral problem than from a torn meniscus. Isolated congenital abnormalities are often of minor degree, whereas more severe problems are usually found in association with lower limb dysplasias and syndromes. The stiff, congenital knee dislocation that is seen in Larsen's syndrome is an example. Because the growth plates above and below the knee make such a major contribution to longitudinal growth, trauma and infection at these sites in early life can have disastrous consequences, causing leg length discrepancy and deformity. Primary tumors found in the region of the knee, both benign and malignant, are specific for age (see Chapter 14).

Referred pain from the hip and lumbar spine can sometimes be confusing: in such conditions as slipped capital femoral epiphysis, the first radiograph in the patient's file is invariably one of the knee. Further difficulty and confusion become apparent when a psychological cause for knee pain or bizarre gait is suspected. It is a mistake to focus so much on the knee as to forget the child and the parents. Great caution and diplomacy should be exercised in this area.

The classic presentation of knee malfunction includes pain (particularly in the older child), clicking and/or giving way, effusion, and locking which is most likely to be the pseudo-locking of patellar instability or tibiofemoral subluxation than meniscal (discoid lateral meniscus or an unstable tear). Yet in many cases the younger child will have no complaint to make; it is parental concern about deformity, whether resolving and benign or structural and progressive, which promotes orthopaedic review. As detailed in Chapter 2, gait, knee alignment, patellar tracking, and increases or decreases in the four arcs of movement (flexion/extension, coronal laxity, rotation, and anteroposterior glide) should be recorded and compared to the opposite knee. Testing should quantify mild, moderate, and major effusions [1], areas of diagnostic tenderness, and maltracking of the patella both passively and under load with the patient sitting at the edge of the examining couch.

Knee Deformity

Genu Recurvatum

Familial joint laxity is a common cause of symmetrical physiological genu recurvatum, usually seen in girls. Such laxity may predispose the child to ligament sprains and may be associated with patellar instability. When unilateral or severe, recurvatum is more likely to be pathological. One must distinguish between congruous hyperextension, anterior subluxation of the tibia, and complete anterior dislocation of the tibia on the femur.

Congenital Dislocation of the Knee

Congenital dislocation of the knee is rare [2], about 1% of the frequency of developmental dysplasia of the hip (DDH), which is detected in 1–2 per 1000 live births. It is clinically obvious and therefore unlikely to be missed although varying degrees of knee hyperextension may be erroneously included. Curtis and Fisher [3] represented the increasing severity of the deformity (Fig. 29.1a), the joint appearing "back to front" with an obvious transverse anterior skin crease (Fig. 29.1b) and the femoral condyles prominent posteriorly because the tibia is displaced. The hamstring tendons subluxate anteriorly, potentiating the deformity.

D.M. Hunt (✉)
Department of Orthopaedics, St. Mary's Hospital, London, UK

M. Benson et al. (eds.), *Children's Orthopaedics and Fractures*,
DOI 10.1007/978-1-84882-611-3_29, © Springer-Verlag London Limited 2010

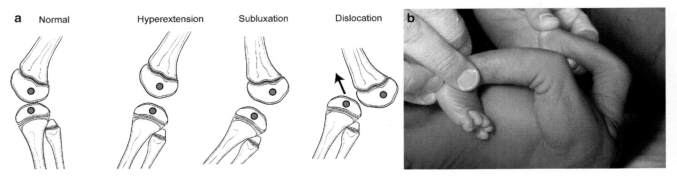

Fig. 29.1 (**a**) Congenital dislocation of the knee is a continuum of deformity although a grading of severity has been proposed [3]. (**b**) The knee is clearly abnormal with a transverse anterior skin crease

Hyperextension with slight subluxation is probably an intrauterine moulding deformity, analogous to neonatal hip instability. In normal infants the knee often reduces with a clunk as it is flexed, the hamstrings and iliotibial band shifting to the flexor side of the knee axis. If the knee can be flexed to 30–40°, splintage with increasingly flexed anterior casts and physiotherapy produces a satisfactory result. Splintage can be discontinued at 6–8 weeks, the knee returning to a normal shape, with minimal residual hyperextension and slight loss of flexion.

More severe knee dislocation is recalcitrant to conservative measures. Other abnormalities are usually present including a dysplastic patella tethered proximally by a shortened, fibrotic quadriceps tendon, and obliteration of the suprapatellar pouch. Ultrasound scanning can be helpful in identifying the patella (Fig. 29.2) [4]. Abnormalities or absence of the cruciate ligaments are present [5] and associated anomalies include DDH, clubfoot, calcaneovalgus, dislocation of the elbow, and syndromes such as arthrogryposis.

Skeletal traction is contraindicated so a sequential release is undertaken, involving the fascia lata and vastus lateralis, a V–Y lengthening of the distal quadriceps and any tethering adhesions. The surgery is best undertaken by 6 months of age so that secondary changes are avoided. Delay may lead to a progressive, sloping deformity where the posterior tibia abuts against the distal, anterior femur, a deformity that makes stable open reduction difficult. Failure to elongate the lateral tethers leads to a valgus deformity, again difficult to correct.

An extremely rare form of congenital snapping knee has been described [6,7]. The tibia subluxates anteriorly in extension and reduces with a pronounced clunk at 30° of flexion. The condition is often part of a syndrome (Larsen's, Catel-Manzke, or congenital short tibia) and the dysmorphic nature of the joints becomes obvious as the child grows. Division and possibly re-routing of the iliotibial band together with suturing of the biceps tendon to the vastus lateralis control the subluxation.

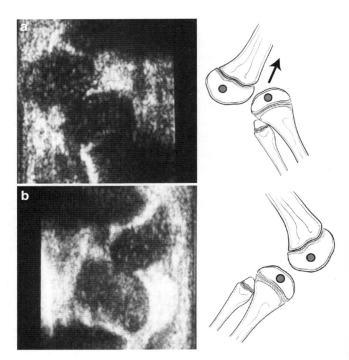

Fig. 29.2 Ultrasound of congenital dislocation of the knee. (**a**) At birth. (**b**) Reduced

Neurological Hyperextension

Secondary Genu Recurvatum

The hyperextended knee is a common feature of several neurological conditions. The usual mechanism is muscle imbalance, in which a strong or spastic quadriceps group overcomes the action of weak hamstrings. Very occasionally, the hamstring deficit may be due to excessive and inappropriate release in patients with cerebral palsy.

In poliomyelitis, hamstring paralysis in the presence of active quadriceps can produce stretching of the posterior soft tissues of the knee, and eventually a gross recurvatum that is extremely difficult to control without a caliper. Posterior soft tissue reefing procedures are not successful, and probably the best surgical option at maturity is the anterior patellar bone block, fixing the patella to the upper tibia so that it acts as a "doorstop" in extension.

In the totally flail knee, it is well to remember that slight hyperextension enables the patient to lock out and therefore stabilize the knee when walking.

A second cause of neurological recurvatum arises when the knee is forced into hyperextension by an equinus foot; this is seen in cerebral palsy and sometimes after head injury. Early lengthening of the tendo-Achilles will prevent progression of knee deformity and improve gait.

Post-traumatic Tibial Recurvatum

Injury to the anterior half of the proximal tibial growth plate and the apophysis of the tibial tuberosity may produce a progressive recurvatum of the knee if there is sufficient skeletal growth remaining (Fig. 29.3a) [8]. The Salter–Harris type V fracture, with or without a splitting of the physis, results from compression if the knee is hyperextended and may be associated with cruciate ligaments tears.

Moroni et al. [9] described the role of proximal tibial osteotomy at skeletal maturity. If the injury is recognized earlier than this, an epiphysiodesis or posterior stapling will prevent the inexorable increase in angulation and a contralateral proximal tibial epiphysiodesis should be considered to prevent leg length discrepancy.

The osteotomy should be supratubercular (Fig. 29.3b), as close to the deformity as possible. An anterior opening wedge using bank bone is effective, without osteotomy of the fibula. A posterior closing wedge osteotomy [10] may

be more risky and further shortens the tibia. Choi et al. [11] have described the successful use of the Taylor spatial frame to produce graded correction of the proximal tibial slope. The osteotomy should start below the tibial tuberosity if patellar positioning is acceptable although in most cases the lack of anterior tibial growth produces a relative patella alta.

Tibial recurvatum also develops in certain skeletal dysplasias. Associated ligament laxity may prevent successful correction and the subchondral plate is characteristically softened and unreliable. Iatrogenic recurvatum is now rare but used to complicate prolonged traction with the knee in extension (frame knee), cast immobilization, proximal tibial traction wire or pin fixation, and tibial tuberosity transfer before skeletal maturity.

Flexion Deformity

During the first few days of life, a mild physiological flexion deformity of the knee is commonplace and rapidly resolves. More obvious and permanent fixed flexion may be seen at birth in arthrogryposis and spina bifida, whereas in cerebral palsy, myopathic and infective conditions, and juvenile idiopathic arthritis the deformity appears later. Serial plaster splints or slabs applied during the first few weeks of life can be effective, but attention needs to be paid to the skin, especially in children who have impaired sensation. The chief shortcoming of serial splintage is that, although the knee may indeed straighten, the correction is often spurious, with the knee hinging open at the back and the tibia impacting against the femoral condyles and failing to glide forward in a normal and congruous fashion. To overcome this problem, reverse dynamic slings [12] have been used in hemophilia and are certainly applicable in the older child.

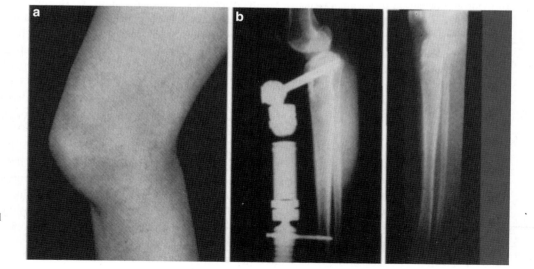

Fig. 29.3 (a) Recurvatum after proximal tibial growth plate injury: Note the prominence of the posterior femoral condyles (b) Pre- and postoperative lateral radiographs after correction of genu recurvatum using a distraction frame

Fig. 29.4 Supracondylar
extension osteotomy of the femur
for fixed flexion deformity.
Recurrence of the knee flexion
deformity with growth and later
reversal of some of the correction

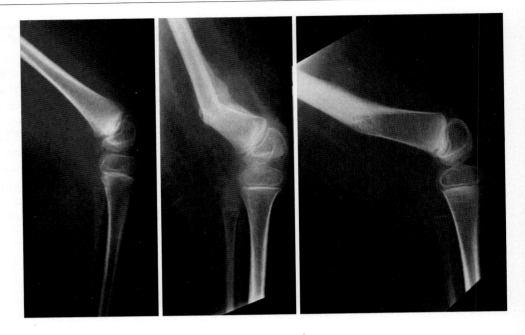

The surgical correction of paediatric deformity includes an extensive soft tissue release since the effects of supracondylar extension osteotomy alone will reverse with further skeletal growth (Fig. 29.4). The posterior exposure is achieved by medial and lateral longitudinal incisions or a transverse lazy "S" incision provided that skin is allowed to heal postoperatively before stretching casts are applied. The hamstring tendons and posterior cruciate ligament are divided after careful identification of the popliteal vessels and the common peroneal and posterior tibial nerves. The posterior capsule should be released fully after opening the joint space posteriorly.

Nerves and vessels must be protected from the deleterious efforts of rapid extension of the knee, the same principle applying to correction of severe valgus. In younger patients serial casts work well but they lose their effectiveness after puberty. Arthrogrypotic deformity corrects reasonably well with soft tissue release and possibly osteotomy [13, 14] (see Chapter 20) or by circular frame distraction [15].

Valgus Deformity

Physiological valgus of the knee ceases to be a functional or cosmetic problem in most children by the age of 6 years, the tibiofemoral angle spontaneously decreasing [16]. An intermalleolar distance of greater than 5 cm when standing may merit review in mid-childhood but there is no evidence that osteoarthritis will develop prematurely in the valgus knee.

It is invidious to state that a definite intermalleolar distance at the age of 12 years should be surgically corrected but concern about function is legitimate if the distance exceeds 15 cm, allied to a valgus angulation of 15°. Medial ligament pain, limp, and the onset of patellar subluxation reinforce the decision to operate, although physiotherapy, weight reduction when appropriate and medial shoe wedges may prove effective.

When valgus appears to be increasing medial stapling [17, 18] or epiphysiodesis [19, 20] are effective. A standing radiograph film will demonstrate any obliquity of the knee joint and confirm whether staples should be placed above rather than below the knee. Strong implants are required and experience has shown that a 10-cm intermalleolar gap will close in approximately 1 year. Obviously, there must be sufficient potential growth to effect the correction and the staples must be removed as soon as physiological alignment is achieved. Failure to time staple removal accurately will convert a knock-knee to a bow leg deformity, causing immense dissatisfaction. Staples should be inserted extraperiosteally, as should any form of plate and screw anchorage. Even with correctly timed removal the effects of the stapling may persist causing over-correction [21] (Fig. 29.5), so careful clinical and radiographic monitoring is essential until skeletal maturity.

Distal femoral osteotomy is the only option at the end of growth [22, 23]. Valgus deformity may be secondary to loss of abduction due to stiffness in the ipsilateral hip or may present as a complex deformity in skeletal dysplasia, requiring an abduction (valgus) osteotomy of the proximal femur as well as corrective osteotomies above and below the knee (Fig. 29.6).

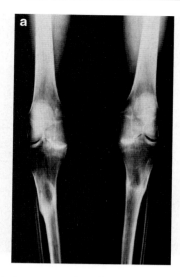

Fig. 29.5 Surgical over-correction of genu valgum in adolescence led to genu varum and later osteoarthritis in adult life

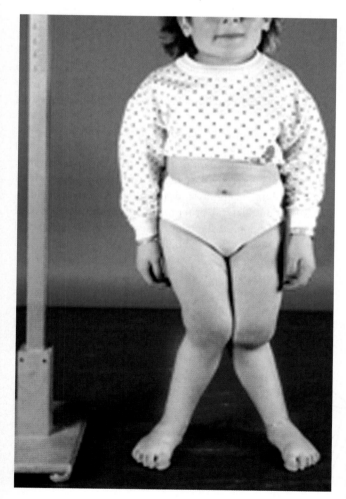

Fig. 29.6 Complex deformity with hip adduction and genu valgum requiring multi-level osteotomies

Post-fracture Genu Valgum

Unilateral and initially progressive genu valgum may follow a proximal, metaphyseal tibial fracture [24], particularly if there is tibial comminution and associated fibular fracturing (Fig. 29.7). Many theories have been advanced to explain the asymmetrical physeal growth, including inadequate primary reduction or splintage, differential vascular stimulation of the growth plate, unusual loading through the proximal tibia, interposition of soft tissues in the fracture site medially (pes anserinus, periosteum, tibial collateral ligament), and tethering by the shortened (united) fibula. It is wise to await the spontaneous correction of the deformity although this is not always assured.

Genu Varum

Babies are usually born with bow legs which persist through the toddler stage. The appearance may be accentuated by internal tibial torsion and these "late correctors" may be a cause of great anxiety for parents. Resolution or progression of the deformity can be monitored photographically and the diagnosis of a possibly pathological deformity is made by asking five questions:

1. Is the child short or disproportioned as may occur in skeletal dysplasia or endocrine disorders?
2. Is the deformity unilateral or asymmetrical, perhaps following trauma or infection?
3. Is there a family history of a syndrome such as familial hypophosphatemic rickets?
4. Is the deformity excessive for the child's age? (progressive varus after the age of 3 years)
5. Is the angulation within the physiological pattern for age (Fig. 29.8)?

Tibia vara or Blount's disease [25] was first recognized by Erlacher in 1922 [26], before an extensive review of the condition by Blount. Repetitive, compressive injury of the proximal tibial growth plate medially leads to progressive varus. There is later overgrowth of the lateral tibial physis and of the distal, medial femoral epiphysis.

Langenskiold [27] classified infantile tibia vara into grades of severity that worsened with increasing age (Fig. 29.9). Stages I and II can be expected to resolve fully but surgical realignment by osteotomy becomes increasingly likely thereafter. The radiographic tibiofemoral [15] and metaphyseal–diaphyseal [28] (Fig. 29.10) angles are monitored, the latter being pathological when it exceeds 15°.

Fig. 29.7 Post-proximal tibial metaphyseal fracture valgus correcting spontaneously with growth

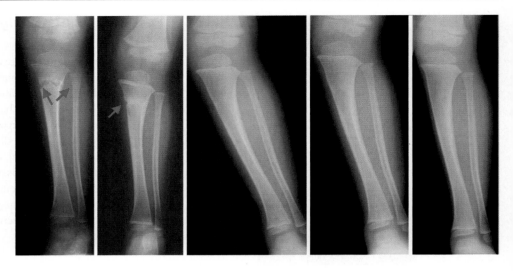

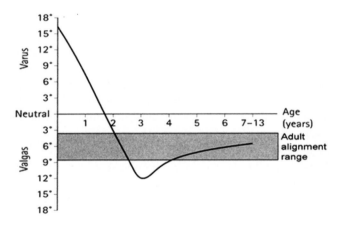

Fig. 29.8 Graph showing normal progression from varus to valgus with age

The etiology of Blount's disease includes increased body weight, level of activity, and angular deformity. The postero-medial corner of the proximal tibial growth plate fails under load and in severe cases the femur may develop a lateral bow. The incidence is estimated at 0.05 per 1000 live births with variations between populations dependent upon age of walking [29], body mass, and the stage at which surgical correction is undertaken. Satisfactory correction from a single tibial osteotomy is more certain if undertaken by the age of 4 years [30] although the Scandinavian experience is of a more benign condition that can be surgically treated effectively up to the age of 8 years [31]. The internal rotation deformity should also be corrected. Recurrence is likely if a bone bar is missed.

The bone bar or tether can be mapped by magnetic resonance (MR) scanning (see Chapter 41) and should be excised in patients under 10 years of age at the time of osteotomy. After this age corrective osteotomy can be combined with a lateral or complete epiphysiodesis, and in unilateral Blount's disease a contralateral proximal tibial epiphysiodesis will prevent a leg length discrepancy. In severe or late, neglected cases elevation of the medial tibial plateau [32, 33] is achieved with an elevating osteotomy (Fig. 29.11) or using a distraction frame.

Adolescent Blount's disease is usually unilateral and less severe than the infantile form. Pain may precede the deformity and shortening of up to 2 cm develops. Internal tibial

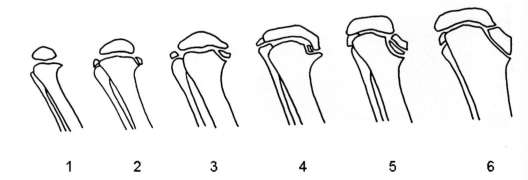

Fig. 29.9 Grades of severity in Blount's disease [26]

1   2   3   4   5   6

Fig. 29.10 The metaphyseal–diaphyseal angle of Levine and Drennan [27] (**a**) Clinical photograph. (**b**) Radiological metaphyseal–diaphyseal angle

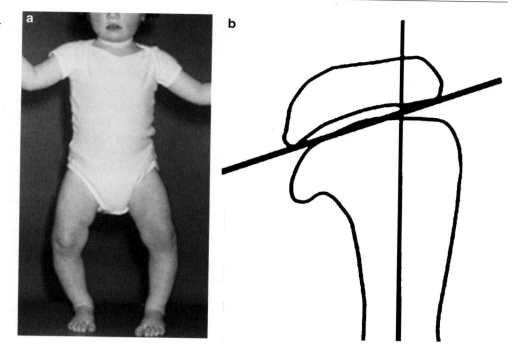

Fig. 29.11 (**a**) MRI showing the unossified medial tibial condyle. (**b**) Pre- and postoperative radiographs of elevation of the medial tibial plateau which is occasionally required in the neglected or recurrent case

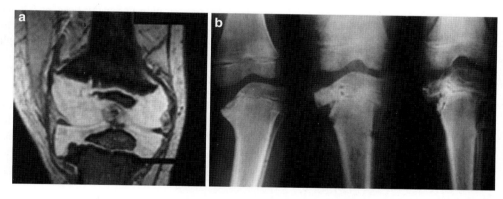

torsion is less obvious and the shape of the tibial epiphysis is relatively normal with no beaking of the medial tibial metaphysis. The proximal tibial and lateral, distal femoral growth plates are widened.

Corrective osteotomy with lateral proximal tibial epiphysiodesis is a reliable means of improving alignment. Leg length discrepancy is prevented by appropriately timed epiphysiodesis above and below the opposite, normal knee joint. Distraction osteogenesis offers an alternative approach [34] with further refinements described by Coogan et al. [35].

A variety of osteotomies have been described (Fig. 29.12):

- Transverse opening or closing wedge [36]
- Inverted arcuate [37]
- Dome or arcuate [38]
- Oblique coronal [39]
- Serrated W–M [40]
- Oblique sagittal [41]
- Spike [42]

Traditionally the dome osteotomy has been popular and is relatively easy to perform [43]. Correction of coronal, sagittal, and axial (rotational) deformities is not possible with the transverse, spike, oblique, and serrated osteotomies. Conventional fixation with Steinmann pins, screws, or plates requires precision, so external fixation may be preferred, allowing alignment to be adjusted postoperatively.

Complications of proximal tibial osteotomy [44] include common peroneal and other nerve deficits, compartment syndrome, laceration of the anterior tibial artery, inaccurate correction, failure of fixation with recurrent deformity, pin site and wound infections, and limb length inequality. The correction of the internal rotation of Blount's disease may

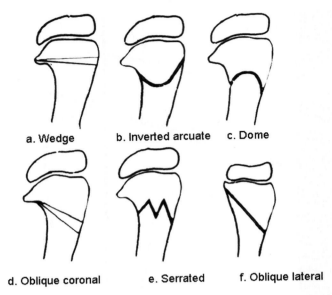

a. Wedge   b. Inverted arcuate   c. Dome

d. Oblique coronal   e. Serrated   f. Oblique lateral

Fig. 29.12 Proximal tibial corrective osteotomies described in the literature

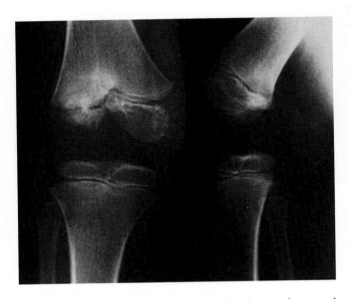

Fig. 29.13 Post-infective knee deformity following meningococcal septicemia

imperil arterial supply at the level of the proximal tibial diaphysis.

Coronal deformity may follow infection (Fig. 29.13) or trauma, nutritional and renal rickets, or skeletal dysplasia, including focal fibrocartilaginous dysplasia which affects the tibia or, very rarely, the femur [45]. Leg lengthening may also increase or produce angulation at the knee.

Anterior Knee Pain

Many of the diagnoses associated with anterior knee pain produce similar symptoms which accounts for the confusion about this condition. Aglietti, Buzzi, and Insall [46] have stressed that there is no single symptom or sign that is in itself diagnostic of patellar pain. There is, however, a pattern of symptoms which are specific for patellar pain and the patella is the usual cause of true "anterior knee pain." The importance of taking a thorough and careful history regarding, for example, the onset and the site of the pain and aggravating factors cannot be over-emphasized. The aim is to make a specific diagnosis in each case and not to lump these patients together as "just anterior knee pain" and untreatable. The onset of symptoms may follow an acute event such as a direct blow on the knee or a twisting injury with minor subluxation of the patella, both resulting in chondral damage and subsequent pain. Often the onset is slow, as a result of over-use such as excessive running. Careful examination will indicate the site of the pain and whether or the lesion is in bone, cartilage, or soft tissue.

It is then helpful to consider the causes of anterior knee pain under the headings "Distinct diagnoses" and "Obscure diagnoses" (see Table 29.1)[47]. The first group is made up of mainly focal pathological lesions, for which logical treatment can be applied and outcome predicted. The second is a spectrum of conditions ranging from anterior knee pain of unknown cause through chondromalacia to dynamic problems of maltracking, subluxation, and excessive lateral pressure. It includes pain referred either from the spine or the hip which must be considered when the examination of the knee is normal.

Table 29.1 Causes of anterior knee pain

Distinct diagnoses	Obscure diagnoses
Overuse	
Osgood–Schlatter's condition	Idiopathic knee pain
Sinding–Larsen–Johansson syndrome	Chondromalacia patellae
Bipartite patella	Maltracking and malalignment
Stress fracture, tendinitis	Shift/tilt and instability
Trauma	Excessive lateral pressure syndrome
Osteochondritis dissecans	Neurogenic pain
Bone bruising	Regional pain syndrome
Meniscal and ligament tears	Referred pain
Syndromes and dysplasias	Psychogenic
Tumors	
Plicae and bursae	
Iatrogenic	
Infrapatellar contracture, e.g., post-ACL reconstruction or patellar realignment	
Scar neuroma	

Distinct Causes of Anterior Knee Pain

Osgood–Schlatter's Condition

This is a condition affecting the young athlete. Pain is situated very precisely over the tibial tuberosity so diagnosis is rarely a problem as patients point exactly to where the pain is. It has been estimated to occur in 21% of athletic children but only in 4% of non-athletes [48]. Boys are more commonly affected between the ages of 13 and 14. In girls the onset is earlier (10–11 years). The cause is repetitive microtrauma at the insertion of the patella tendon into the tibial tuberosity apophysis which, being softer and thus weaker than the normal attachment of tendon to bone (Fig. 29.14), stretches or microfractures the tuberosity, giving rise to the pain. The bone is growing faster than soft tissue and therefore in this condition, tightness of the quadriceps and hamstrings is a feature. The tuberosity will increase in size, resulting in a large bump over the front of the tibia. This can develop into a separate ossicle which may cause persistent pain after skeletal growth ceases, interfering with kneeling and requiring surgical removal at maturity. The most important feature of the pain is that it rapidly settles with rest and never occurs at night. The condition resolves spontaneously when soft tissue growth catches up, usually in 1–2 years. There is really no differential diagnosis but sometimes there is alarm about a possible tumor. A radiograph is a definitive but unnecessary investigation. Ultrasound scanning can relieve anxiety about malignancy.

Treatment consists of reassurance and a policy of allowing activity but letting the child stop when the pain starts. The problem is that these children are often athletically gifted and are under pressure to perform. The importance of a good warm-up and stretching program has recently been appreciated and is very helpful in overcoming muscle tightness, thus reducing symptoms.

Appreciation of the value of a stretching program has rendered the use of casts or bracing obsolete. The application of

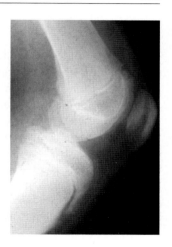

Fig. 29.14   A lateral radiograph of Osgood–Schlatter's condition

an anti-inflammatory, non-steroid gel may relieve local tenderness but is little more than a placebo. Occasionally, an acute flexion injury will avulse part of the tibial tuberosity which must not be confused with Osgood–Schlatter's condition (see Chapter 32).

Sinding–Larsen–Johansson

This occurs in the same age group of children but the point of tenderness and pathology are located at the lower pole of the patella. The lateral radiograph of the patella may be normal or there may be speckled calcification or a small ossicle at the lower pole. It occurs in the same age group and patient population as Osgood–Sclatter's condition and treatment is the same. Acute pain and tenderness following a sudden flexion injury should raise the possibility of a sleeve fracture of the patella when ultrasound is more revealing than a plain radiograph [49] (Fig. 29.15). Both Osgood–Schlatter's and Sinding–Larsen–Johansson conditions are more likely with patella alta.

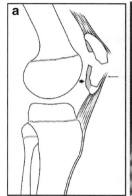
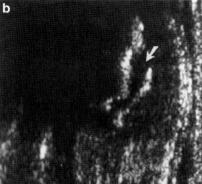
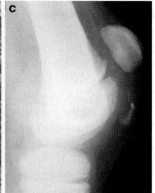

Fig. 29.15 (**a**) Line drawing of a patellar sleeve fracture. (**b**) Ultrasound showing the periosteal sleeve. (**c**) Later radiograph of a missed case showing new bone formation in the sleeve, giving the appearance of a double patella

Bipartite Patella

The patella ossifies from multiple centers. Any of these may persist, failing to fuse. Occasionally they can be painful, probably a form of traction apophysitis in the immature skeleton. By far the most common is the supero-lateral center and traction is from the vastus lateralis. The pain is made worse by squatting. Treatment is as for other traction conditions such as Osgood–Schlatter's disease, employing an effective thigh muscle stretching program until symptoms settle. Very occasionally, a sudden flexion injury can cause avulsion of the fragment in which case reattachment is required to preserve the integrity of the extensor mechanism.

Sleeve Fracture of the Patella

This is a diagnosis which is often missed. It presents as an acutely painful knee after a fall or landing heavily, forcing the knee into flexion. The swelling may be minimal and the only finding is a variable degree of patellar alta and tenderness at the lower pole. Active knee extension is restricted or impossible. The avulsed periosteal sleeve, usually from the lower pole of the patella, is not visible radiographically. Ultrasound is very helpful but an awareness of the possibility of this injury is the most important factor (Fig. 29.15). Open reduction and reattachment of the sleeve is necessary to avoid an extensor lag and the embarrassment of a large bony lump appearing at the lower end of the patella [49].

Stress Fractures of the Patella

Stress fractures of the lower pole of the patella occur in spastic children with flexed knee gait and are a cause of pain and further deterioration in walking [50]. These fractures cannot heal unless steps are taking to correct the fixed flexion deformities of the knees.

Osteochondritis Dissecans

Osteochondritis dissecans is one of the causes of anterior knee pain. The symptoms are initially non-specific and related to activity, not necessarily to the site of the lesion. Rarely, the lesion is on the patella or in the trochlear groove, in which case the pain will be truly anterior.

Males are affected twice as commonly as females. Two distinct types are recognized: the juvenile type which starts before the growth plates fuse, commonly before the age of 12 years, and the adult type starting after the growth plates have fused.

The cause of the lesion is not known. Repetitive trauma is unlikely as the condition is often bilateral and symmetrical. It usually occurs on the lateral side of the medial femoral condyle which is not a site subjected to trauma except perhaps in those with excessive recurvatum which allows the tibial spine to impinge against the femoral condyle more easily (Fig. 29.16).

Transient ischemia of the affected part is another possibility, resulting in an ossification defect which fails to heal [51]. The lesion starts in the subchondral bone and may lead to separation and fragmentation, causing the overlying articular cartilage to split and the fragment to hinge and eventually displace.

The child often walks with an antalgic gait, resisting full extension. In addition to a sensation of catching or of giving way and, later, locking, there may be an effusion and Wilson's sign can be helpful if positive: the knee is flexed to 90°, the tibia is internally rotated and the knee extended. A positive sign is pain felt at the 30° mark when the medial tibial spine impinges against the medial femoral condyle at the classic site. It is relieved by external rotation of the tibia and reproduced again on internal rotation. Often with careful examination, a tender spot at the site of the lesion can be found.

The first investigation should be the four standard radiographic views of the knee, of which the notch or tunnel view is usually the most helpful. A technetium bone scan will assess the presence or absence of hyperemia at the site of the lesion and this has been linked to the likelihood of healing [52].

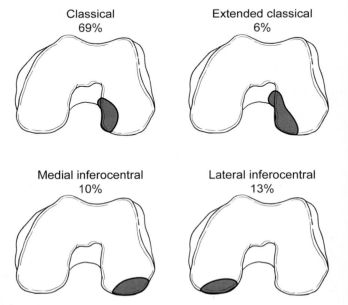

Fig. 29.16 The incidence of osteochondritis dissecans in different positions in the knee [56]

Table 29.2 MRI signs of osteochondritis dissecans (De Smet 1997)

1. A line of high signal intensity > 5 mm long deep to the OCD lesion (T2)
2. An area of homogeneous signal >5 mm in diameter deep to the lesion (T2)
3. A focal defect > 5 mm in the articular surface (T1)
4. A line of high signal crossing the subchondral plate into the lesion (T2)

The biggest advance in the management of this condition has been magnetic resonance imaging (MRI) which has largely replaced isotope bone scanning, especially when combined with arthrography in the form of gadolinium enhancement. De Smet [53] identified four MRI signs, observing that the volume of the area of high signal behind the lesion was the most valuable for predicting outcome (Table 29.2).

The high signal line on T2 and the articular cartilage breach on T1 are the most relevant for predicting healing. The advantage of MRI is that surgical intervention in the form of arthroscopy may be avoided and repeat scans can be used to monitor progress (Fig. 29.17).

The aim of treatment is to promote healing. In the juvenile type, where the growth plates are open, the chances of spontaneous healing are high. Treatment is non-operative with a program of rest followed by graduated activity. This extends for a minimum of 3 months. The initial treatment is rest from all activity using crutches and a brace. Protected weight bearing is allowed. After 6 weeks, if the knee is pain-free and not swollen, the brace is discontinued but protected weight bearing is continued for a further 6 weeks. Physiotherapy can start with a supervised, progressive program of mobilizing exercises and low-impact quadriceps and hamstring strengthening. The child should do this for at least 3 months before adding running, jumping, or side-stepping movements. An MRI showing healing is helpful at this stage.

Arthroscopy is indicated in the older child, or the occasional younger one when symptoms persist for more than 6 months, particularly if there are episodes of locking, sharp pain, and an effusion. Characteristically, there is progression and separation of the lesion with a breach in the articular cartilage.

The lesion is inspected and probed. If stable, drilling with a Kirschner wire often stimulates healing. This can be done retrograde under image intensifier control from a point on the femoral condyle just distal to the growth plate. The arthroscopic guides used for the placement of tunnels in cruciate ligament reconstruction are helpful for accurately drilling into the lesion from the deep surface. Alternatively, transarticular drilling, either open or arthroscopically, is acceptable. If the lesion is unstable but not displaced, it can be held with bone pegs taken from the proximal tibia, with biodegradable pins or using variable thread headless screws (Fig. 29.18).

Debate surrounds the management of the bone fragment when it is almost totally detached or has become loose in the joint. Nearly all affected patients are skeletally mature. Small fragments, less than 1.5 cm in diameter, are probably best removed and the base curetted. Drilling or microfracture with chondral picks stimulates the influx of pluripotential cells into the defect to produce fibrocartilage [54].

Lesions greater than 1.5 cm should be replaced if possible. The base of the defect should again be curetted, drilled, or microfractured (Fig. 29.19). The fragment may need to be trimmed to fit the defect and then fixed as for the stable lesion. The end result must leave a smooth, congruous, or even slightly depressed surface. If an accurate fit is not possible the fragment should be discarded. Treatment of these defects by chondrocyte transplantation is an area where this newer technique may be successful [55].

Rehabilitation must be taken slowly after any of these procedures, with protected weight bearing for at least 9 months.

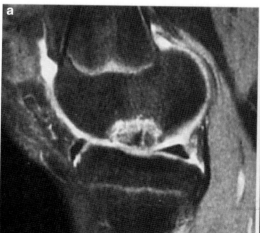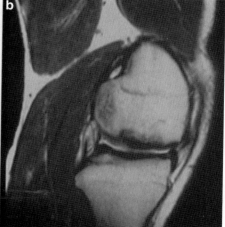

Fig. 29.17 (**a**) T2-weighted MRI showing osteochondritis dissecans of the medial femoral condyle with a line of high signal deep to the lesion. (**b**) T1-weighted MRI of an osteochondritis dissecans lesion in the lateral femoral condyle showing a breach in the articular cartilage

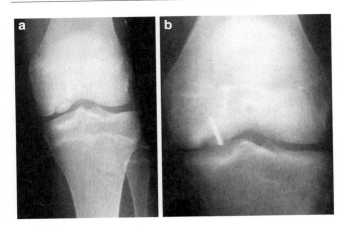

Fig. 29.18 (**a**) An osteochondritis dissecans lesion in the extended classical position in the medial femoral condyle. (**b**) Fixation with a variable thread screw

In summary, the natural history of osteochondritis dissecans depends upon the age of the child at the onset of symptoms. The juvenile type, before skeletal maturity, heals with minimal risk of developing osteoarthritis at 30 years if it is in the classical position. In any other position, osteoarthritis is likely particularly if it involves a weight-bearing surface. Lesions of the lateral femoral condyle appear to do worst but these comprise only 15% of all cases [56]. The adult type does less well and the fragment may not heal, predisposing to osteoarthritis [57]. It is a reasonable estimate to say that the onset of osteoarthritis is accelerated by 10 years.

Bone Bruises

The entity of the bone bruise or contusion was largely theoretical until the advent of MRI which shows bruising very clearly. Following a direct blow or a high-velocity fall, often in association with anterior cruciate and medial collateral ligament injury, the lateral femoral condyle impacts on the posterior tibial plateau as the knee twists. Similarly, acute varus angulation can produce a lateral ligament tear and medial bruising. They are self limiting and no treatment is required apart from protection from similar injuries until the symptoms of pain and possibly swelling have settled.

Reassurance, backed up by a positive MRI, is enough to convince the child and parents of the need to modify activity, usually for about 6 weeks.

Plicae and Bursae

Popliteal Cysts

Popliteal cysts are twice as common in boys and usually present before the child has reached the age of 10 years as an asymptomatic fluctuant swelling just to the medial side of the popliteal fossa. If there is doubt about the cystic nature of the lesion, trans-illumination will settle the issue. This technique is a great deal, less expensive than ultrasound or MRI scanning which is unnecessary. If there is concern about enlargement or a possible diagnosis of villonodular synovitis or chondromatosis, an ultrasound is all that is required. The most common cause is a semi-membranosus bursa which is better felt in extension than in flexion; the knee is otherwise normal. Dinham [58] drew attention to the very high recurrence rate after surgical removal, and the natural tendency of these cysts to disappear spontaneously. Operation without a very good reason is unjustified and reassurance is all that is required.

Plicae

Much has been made of the importance of plicae in knee surgery. The common sites of plicae are well known (Fig. 29.20) and they are very rarely of significance in children. They can cause pain over the medial femoral condyle on squatting especially when thickened in some skeletal dysplasias or inflammatory conditions. They do not cause "snapping" of the knee which in children is due to a discoid meniscus or rarely to the semi-membranosus during flexion.

Ganglion Cysts

Ganglia occur at many sites in the knee. They are found in the substance of the anterior or posterior cruciate ligaments

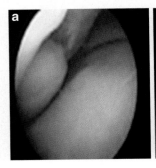
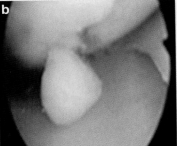
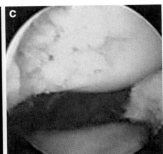

Fig. 29.19 (**a–c**) An osteochondral fragment detached and with an irregular fit; it was removed and the defect treated by microfracturing

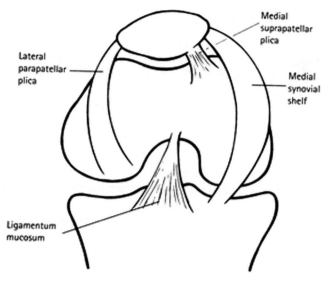

Fig. 29.20 The sites of synovial plicae

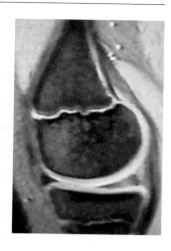

Fig. 29.21 MRI showing a normal bright signal within the posterior horn of the paediatric medial meniscus, potentially mistaken for degeneration or a tear

where they are usually an incidental finding but can cause a deep ache, often confused with anterior knee pain. The most common site is in association with a lateral meniscal radial tear which allows synovial fluid to leak out into the subcutaneous layer. These do occur in adolescence and even younger children and pathologically they are indistinguishable from a ganglion. They are easily palpable, typically when the knee is in extension, and they disappear when the knee is flexed. Treatment is by excising the tear and decompressing the cyst arthroscopically from inside the knee [59].

The real concern is that the diagnosis is correct. Occasionally, the cause of a lump in or around the knee will be pigmented villonodular synovitis, synovial chondromatosis, or even a hemangioma. MRI is then essential before exploring these lesions.

Meniscal Lesions

Meniscal Tears

Meniscal tears in childhood are rare, accounting for 2% of all meniscal tears [60]. The paediatric incidence does appear to be increasing with more participation in contact sports, often combined with anterior cruciate ligament (ACL) rupture [61]. Careful clinical examination will establish the diagnosis but can be difficult if the knee is swollen. MRI has greatly improved the diagnosis but a high signal associated with increased vascularity seen within the substance of the meniscus can resemble mucoid degeneration (Fig. 29.21). It should not be mistaken for a tear, especially at the menisco-synovial junction, or for a hypermobile lateral meniscus.

Arthroscopy still has a place in the diagnosis if the symptoms cannot be accounted for or if the knee is swollen and locked. Meniscal tears in childhood should be treated very conservatively. Minor tears, less than 1 cm long, and partial thickness tears, heal. More extensive tears should be repaired. The increased vascularity and cell population of the meniscus will facilitate healing but the idea that the meniscus can regenerate in childhood is a myth.

McNicholas et al. [62] reviewed clinically 63 adolescents 30 years after open meniscectomy. While 71% said they were satisfied with their knees, 36% had significant joint narrowing. These findings reinforce the earlier views of King [63] and Fairbank [64] who were the first to recognize the importance of the menisci and the relationship between meniscectomy and later osteoarthritis.

Meniscal repair is now an accepted procedure for the appropriate tear. The indications can be extended in children where the increased vascularity, biochemical factors, and histological structure of the meniscus give greater scope for healing. The blood supply of the outer one-third of the meniscus and the concept of red and white zones is attributed to Arnoczky and Warren [65]. They showed that the vascularity of the adult meniscus does not extend more than 5 mm from the menisco-capsular junction. This is the white–white zone and repair will not succeed. Less than 3 mm from the junction is the red–red zone and repair is very likely to succeed. Between 3 and 5 mm is the red–white zone where repairs have a reasonable chance of healing, especially in younger patients [66].

The prime indications for meniscal repair are as follows:

- an unstable longitudinal tear in the red/white zone within 3–5 mm of the rim (tears less than 1 cm long can be expected to heal without suturing)
- an injury less than 8 weeks old
- a patient aged less than 20 years old

- a stable knee (an associated ruptured ACL is an absolute indication for ligament reconstruction)

A variety of techniques for repair are recognized. Open repair was popularized by De Haven and Hales [67]. An arthroscopic inside-out technique was the next to be developed and is still the best tried and most successful (Fig. 29.22). Recently, all-inside techniques using toggle devices and self-tying sutures have been advocated. The results of meniscal repair are still not established although healing rates as high as 75% for the standard inside-out suture repair can be expected [68].

In general terms, preservation of meniscal tissue is the main priority. The place of meniscal allograft in the skeletally immature is not established. It is as yet an unproven procedure [69].

The hypoplastic, hypermobile medial meniscus is an occasional cause of pain with activity, caused by the femoral condyle contacting the tibial plateau in extension. Modification of activity is all that is required.

Discoid Meniscus

The discoid meniscus is a true congenital malformation that occurs in 0.4–5% of the population although the incidence may be as high as 16.6% in the Japanese [70, 71]. It is often bilateral and almost always involves the lateral meniscus although it has been reported, very rarely, in the medial meniscus. Three types have been described by Watanabe [72] and this classification largely determines the treatment:

- Type I Complete: the meniscus is a round disc completely covering the tibial plateau. It has normal attachments and so is stable.
- Type II Incomplete: this is simply a thicker and wider than normal meniscus but leaves some of the tibial plateau uncovered. It also has normal attachments and is stable.
- Type III Wrisberg type: this often causes confusion. It may be complete or incomplete and is distinguishable at arthroscopy by its thickened posterior edge. Its main feature is that it is only attached posteriorly by the Wrisberg ligament and has no attachment to the posterior capsule. So during flexion, the meniscus can move forward and laterally [73] (Fig. 29.23).

The cause is not known. It is a myth that all menisci start as discs and develop into the normal crescent shape [74]. Histologically, there is always some mucoid degeneration which will develop into a horizontal tear making preservation of meniscal tissue, when treated, difficult.

The first indication that a child has a discoid meniscus may come as young as 3 years old. Classically, the knee starts to "clunk" on flexing and extending. It can be dramatic and cause distress although it is not particularly painful. This tends to stop happening as the physiological valgus of the knee decreases, and the child is symptom-free until a tear

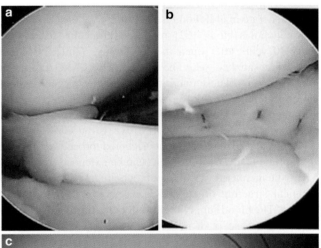

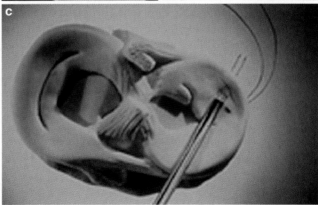

Fig. 29.22 (**a**) A displaced bucket handle tear of the medial meniscus. (**b**) Tear reduced and held with three inside-out sutures. (**c**) The technique of inside-out meniscal repair (courtesy Smith and Nephew)

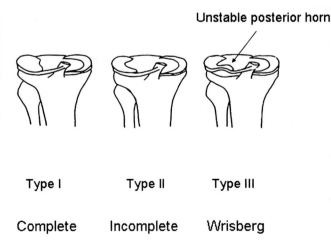

Fig. 29.23 The Watanabe classification of discoid lateral menisci

Fig. 29.24 (**a**) MRI appearances and (**b**) specimen of a discoid torn meniscus

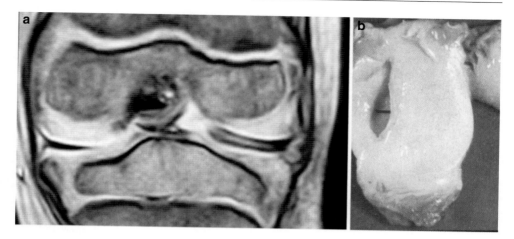

develops or the knee locks due to an unstable meniscus later in childhood or more usually in adolescence.

MRI scan is often diagnostic although a discoid meniscus can be missed (Fig. 29.24). The radiographic appearance is unreliable; widening of the lateral joint space, flattening of the lateral femoral condyle, and cupping of the lateral tibial plateau are not specific.

Management depends upon the type and the degree of symptoms. Treatment of discoid menisci found incidentally on MRI is not justified unless the symptoms are appropriate. At arthroscopy, visualization of the meniscus can be difficult as the lateral compartment is filled with tissue. Probing will reveal a tear but it is the posterior rim which needs to be carefully inspected and probed to test for stability. This will be easier after a tear has been excised. The rim is usually thickened and very mobile, easily pulled into the intercondylar notch or under the femoral condyle. It is then clear there are no posterior capsular attachments. If this is the case a subtotal meniscectomy is still recommended. Attempting to stabilize an unstable posterior horn is hazardous and success is most unlikely. If the meniscus is stable, the tear is excised arthroscopically and the rim saucerized.

While preservation of meniscal tissue is the ideal, the tears are often horizontal and the remaining meniscus is of poor quality. Relatively short-term outcomes at about 5 years are good following total meniscectomy whereas at 20 years most have symptoms and radiographic signs of osteoarthritis [75]. It remains to be seen if partial meniscectomy and repair of the unstable and abnormal meniscal tissue will achieve healing, thus providing some protection and possibly improving this outcome.

Ligament Problems

Congenital absence of the ACL is rare and usually seen only in association with congenital dislocation of the patella or lower limb dysplasias such as congenital short femur or tibia with a hypoplastic fibula and absent lateral rays of the foot [76]. Patients tolerate the instability surprisingly well, but if a leg-lengthening procedure is undertaken deformity and laxity are likely to become worse. Modern bracing techniques can provide an acceptable alternative to reconstruction.

Ligament injury is rare in childhood because the ligaments are stronger than the bones and their attachments blend directly with epiphyseal cartilage or periosteum. The proximal tibial epiphysis is relatively protected by the collateral ligaments which cross the growth plate, whereas at the femur the attachment is to the epiphysis (Fig. 29.25). A severe injury will cause a fracture separation through the lower femoral or, rarely, the upper tibial growth plate in childhood.

A typical injury likely to rupture a ligament in an adult will then result in just a sprain or avulsion of a fragment of cartilage and bone in childhood, for example, avulsion of the tibial spine or a fracture of the tibial tuberosity (Fig. 29.26). Meyers and McKeever [77] classified tibial spine avulsions according to the degree of displacement, stressing the importance of accurate reduction to preserve stability (Table 29.3) (see Chapter 38).

Ligament injuries, including mid-substance rupture of the ACL rather than the more common avulsion of the tibial spine, are increasing in frequency in juveniles [78]. This reflects increased involvement in intense sporting activities. The results of conservative treatment of ACL injuries have the same poor outlook as in adults [79]. Fear of damaging the physis, producing deformity or even growth arrest, is the reason for reluctance to reconstruct ligaments in the immature although increasingly reconstruction is undertaken, particularly if there is a meniscal tear which has been repaired. Extra-articular and non-anatomical reconstructive operations are generally unsatisfactory. A standard hamstring reconstruction drilling across both the tibial and femoral physes, using fixation placed well away

Fig. 29.25 (**a**) The collateral ligaments showing the attachments in relation to the epiphyses. (**b**) The incidence of fracture types and ligament injuries in relation to age

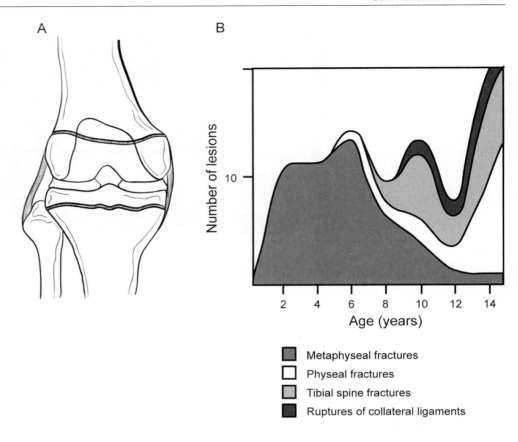

Fig. 29.26 (**a**) Tibial spine avulsion fracture. (**b**) Fragment fixed back with a small cannulated screw

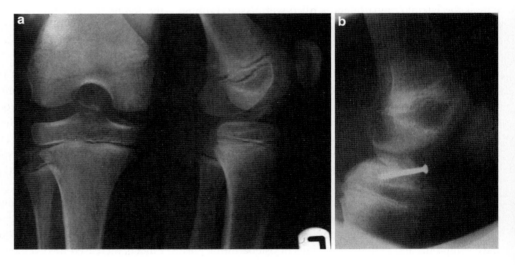

from the growth plate, does seem to be effective and carries a minimal risk of growth disturbance. Reconstruction should only be recommended when there is an appreciable risk of the child sustaining further damage such as a meniscal tear.

A standard four-strand hamstring graft is taken and should fill the tunnel as fully as possible. At arthroscopy, the remnant of the ACL is removed and if the notch is considered narrow, a notchplasty performed. Reconstruction is performed by a standard arthroscopic technique using the same guides as in the adult. The drill holes are made slowly to minimize heating and destruction of tissue at the physis. The holes are cleared of loose bone. A closed loop endobutton is used proximally. The graft is inserted and the button flipped. Distally, a screw placed alongside the graft should not be used as there is a small risk of it crossing the growth plate. A washer and screw placed transversely across the tibia

Table 29.3 Classification of tibial spine avulsion injuries. Meyers and Mckeever [77]

Grade 1. Undisplaced
Grade 2. Partially displaced (up to 50%)
Grade 3. Completely displaced + rotation
Grade 4. Comminuted

is recommended (Fig. 29.27). Postoperatively, a brace may be used but is not essential although it does emphasize the need for gradual rehabilitation. Children will tend to progress too rapidly if the knee feels comfortable.

The complications of this procedure are no different from those of the same procedure in adults. The real concerns are growth disturbance with leg length discrepancy or a valgus deformity caused by tethering. The grafts grow with the child (Fig. 29.28) and reports of growth disturbance are largely anecdotal, usually associated with injudicious placement of a fixation device [80]. If possible, sporting activity should be modified until maturity because of the risk and the consequences of re-rupture. The results are comparable to those in adults but with a slightly higher rate of re-rupture and meniscal tears [81].

Posterior cruciate ligament injuries in childhood are very rare and more likely to be the pull-off or avulsion type accompanied by a bony fragment. This should be reattached back if displaced more than 5 mm or if the tibia drops back markedly. With the increased use of domestic trampolines and participation in extreme sports, mid-substance ruptures are being seen more often. The principle is to delay reconstruction until skeletal maturity and it is unusual for an immature patient to require reconstruction. The drill hole through the tibia is necessarily very close to the back of the tibia at the level of the physis and damage will be more extensive than the more direct tunnel for anterior cruciate reconstruction. The risk of growth disturbance is therefore much greater and not justified in most cases [82].

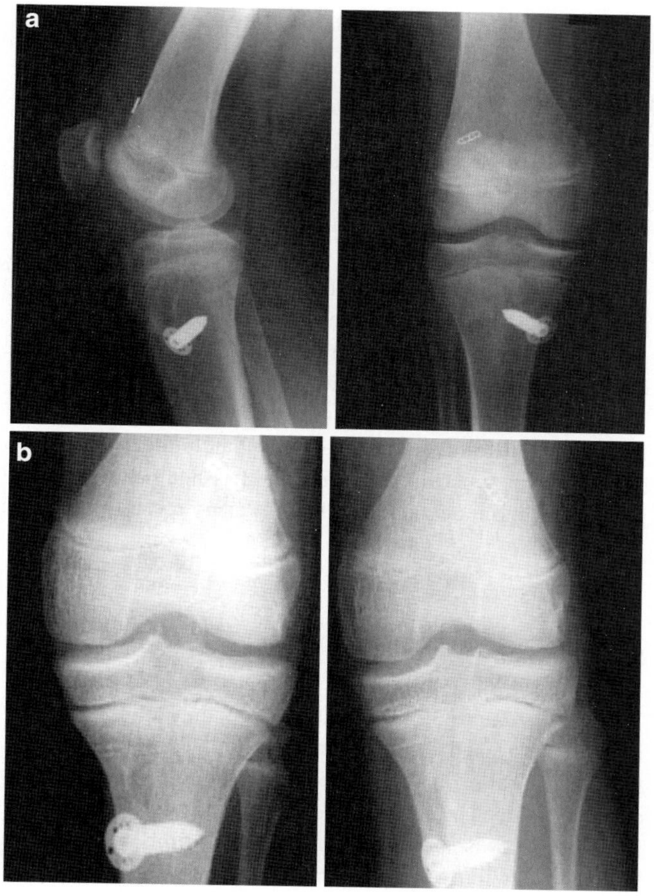

Fig. 29.28 (a) Immediate postoperative radiograph. (b) The same view, 2 years later, showing considerable growth of the whole graft length

Multiple ligament injury associated with a dislocated knee is fortunately very rare in children. A conservative approach should be adopted with good results being obtained using simple plaster cast immobilization following reduction.

Other Distinct Causes

There are a number of other diagnoses which cause knee pain which are rare in children and so not appropriate for inclusion in this chapter. These are patellar tendinitis (jumper's knee), quadriceps tendinitis, and Hoffa's fat pad syndrome. A foreign body such as glass or a needle, or a neuroma, causes knee pain, which is usually, but not always, obvious from the history. Other causes of pain which are covered elsewhere in this book include bone tumors which have a predilection for the region of the knee (Chapter 14) and skeletal dysplasias (Chapter 7 and Chapter 8). Bone and joint infection and inflammatory arthritis are also common in the knee and are covered in Chapter 10 and 13, respectively.

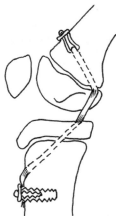

Fig. 29.27 Line drawing of transphyseal anterior cruciate ligament reconstruction in a child

Obscure Causes of Anterior Knee Pain

Idiopathic Knee Pain

This is knee pain for which no distinct cause can be found. It is most commonly associated with malalignment with or without chondral damage and is known as chondromalacia. The two conditions are often related. Anterior knee pain is specific. It is an aching pain, felt over the medial side of the patella, which is made worse by loading the joint such as going up stairs or after prolonged sitting. It causes catching, crepitus, or even locking in extension.

In a deep squat, up to 17 times the body weight is loaded through the patella. Additionally, the patella bears the brunt of overuse or repetitive stressing so it is not surprising that pain is common, occurring in 15% of army recruits [83].

Malalignment

The terms malalignment, maltracking, and patella instability are often used loosely and interchangeably to describe patellofemoral problems with or without pain. This leads to confusion. Each needs to be defined and used specifically. Malalignment is a description of lower limb morphology which results in excessive compression of the patella in the trochlea groove. It occurs with varus or valgus knees, recurvatum, persistent femoral anteversion, compensatory external tibial torsion, and patella alta. A feature is an increased Q angle, a consequence of internal torsion of the femur compensated for by external torsion of the tibia as the child grows. It is measured by dropping a line from the anterior superior iliac spine to the center of the patella and then from the center of the patella to the tibial tuberosity (Fig. 29.29). Although normally less than 10°, it is not an indicator of maltracking which can occur with or without malalignment. It is also a poor indicator of patellar instability. An unstable patella can occur in the presence of malalignment, maltracking, or both. It can also occur in the absence of both. It is perfectly possible for a normally aligned, normally tracking patella to dislocate although this is usually a significantly traumatic event. It is of no surprise that there is confusion about the terminology used in this condition.

Recurvatum, genu valgum, femoral anteversion, and increased Q angle are as common in patients without symptoms as they are in those with pain. Malalignment is, however, a cause of anterior knee pain when there is tightness of the quadriceps and hamstrings and when femoral anteversion and an increased Q angle are combined [84]. There has been no proven connection between forefoot pronation or valgus flat foot and anterior knee pain.

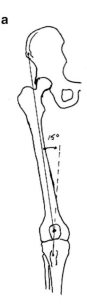
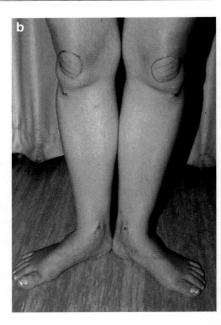

Fig. 29.29 (a) The Q angle. The angle between line from the superior iliac spine to the center of the patella and from the center of the patella to the tibial tuberosity. (b) An increased Q angle as a result of compensatory lateral tibial torsion for persistent femoral anteversion causing intoeing in childhood

Maltracking

This refers, again specifically, to a patella that fails to track symmetrically in the femoral trochlear groove during flexion and extension. This phenomenon has been extensively studied by Fulkerson [85]. He introduced the concept of "subluxation" and "tilt" of the patella (Figs. 29.30 and 29.31). This is measured on a simple sky-line patellar radiograph in 30° of flexion or in extension on a computed tomography (CT) cut. Shift alone, tilt alone, and a combination of both occur and treatment should be directed specifically to treating which of these is present.

Maltracking in extension is almost always lateral and can be demonstrated on clinical examination. The patient, sitting on the edge of a couch, extends the knee against gravity and, as the patella disengages from a position of stability in the trochlear groove, it shifts laterally. This physical sign is usually seen as the knee extends from 20° of flexion to full extension, and may be associated with and inhibited by pain. It may also be seen by simply asking the patient to contract the quadriceps with the knee extended when the patella will jump laterally, sometimes known as the "inverted J" sign. The confusion with this pattern of maltracking is that when mild it may be a cause of anterior knee pain and the skyline view will be normal; when more severe it can cause recurrent dislocation of the patella, especially in childhood and

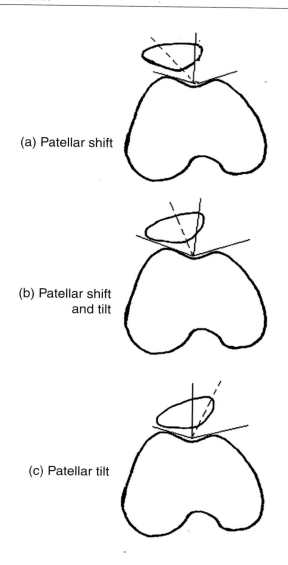

(a) Patellar shift

(b) Patellar shift
and tilt

(c) Patellar tilt

Fig. 29.30   Patellar shift and tilt

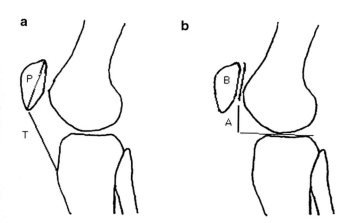

Fig. 29.31   (**a**, **b**) Measurements of patellar height

adolescence. At its most extreme, the patella dislocates laterally in extension, relocating on flexing the knee. It is caused by quadriceps tightness. The lateral retinaculum may or may not be tight. Again, the skyline view may be normal but there is likely to be some evidence of either tilt or subluxation or even both. There will often be patella alta on a lateral view. Associated femoral anteversion and an increased Q angle are incidental and not diagnostic.

Maltracking in flexion is difficult to see clinically but, by definition, present on the skyline view. The usual finding is lateral tilt, due to a tight lateral retinaculum. It is often a cause of lateral patellar pain but if severe and in the hypermobile, it can cause dislocation in flexion.

Patellar Dislocation and Instability

The anatomical relationship of the patella to the femoral sulcus or trochlea is complex, extension producing contact between the lower pole of the patella and the trochlea, and flexion a deeper engagement with the upper pole. Static soft tissue restraints include the medial patellofemoral ligament which contributes 60% of medial stability [86], the lateral fascial superficial oblique and deep transverse (lateral patellar ligament) components of the retinaculum, and the patellar inferior pull which may be compromised by patella alta and lateral condylar "conflict" or abnormal impingement. Medial patellomeniscal and lateral patellotibial ligaments are also recognized.

Dynamic control is achieved by the vastus medialis oblique muscle which works in tandem with the medial patellofemoral ligament and further contributions from the remaining components of the quadriceps mechanism. With a history of patellar subluxation or dislocation there is a 50% likelihood of further episodes of instability; after acute dislocation the risk of further maltracking is approximately one in five. The presence of ligament laxity, lower limb torsional abnormalities (Chapter 2), increased Q angle, and patella alta worsen the prognosis, as do overt maltracking, patellar tilt, and apprehension (Figs. 29.29, 29.30, and 29.31).

Imaging of the knee in the older adolescent includes:

1. Radiographic views:

   a. anteroposterior (osteochondral lesions/ loose bodies and lateral femoral condylar lesions)
   b. lateral (patella alta, trochlea dysplasia) (Fig. 29.31).
   c. skyline (taken in 30–40° of flexion, with or without weight-bearing stress, to show subluxation or tilting of the patella and the congruence angle, trochlear dysplasia, and other patellofemoral relationships in largely static positions) (Fig. 29.30).

2. MR scans (bone bruising, chondral defects, avulsed osteo-chondral fragments, the medial patellofemoral ligament, and further morphological details of the patellofemoral joint).
3. CT scans (axial views are preferred to potentially misleading sagittal images and depict the tibial tubercle–trochlear groove offset [87] (Fig. 29.32) and the rotational profile of the lower limb).

Soft tissues procedures include percutaneous or open, extra-articular lateral release, medial retinacular imbrication or medial patellofemoral ligament reconstruction, and V–Y quadricepsplasty for severe patella alta with habitual dislocation or congenital knee dislocation. Habitual or obligatory lateral dislocation occurs every time the knee flexes. The condition is a manifestation of a shortened quadriceps mechanism, often in association with genu valgum. Tension along the anterior structures causes the patella to sublux or dislocate laterally repeatedly. With time the intrinsic stability of the patella is lost as it becomes increasingly dysplastic and the sulcus flattens laterally. The pathological anatomical changes are comparable to the progressive deformity of untreated developmental dysplasia of the hip.

Arthroscopic lateral release may prove sufficient although other augmentation procedures are usually indicated. Distally, a patellar tendon medialization by the Roux–Goldthwaite procedure or alternative soft tissue realignment is effective for lateral dislocation in extension (Fig. 29.33). Very occasionally, proximal or distal femoral rotational osteotomy is necessary but skeletal procedures such as

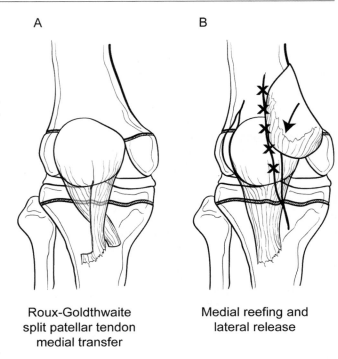

A

B

Roux-Goldthwaite
split patellar tendon
medial transfer

Medial reefing and
lateral release

Fig. 29.33 (**a**) The Roux–Goldthwaite procedure is safe and generally effective in the older child or adolescent. (**b**) Lateral release and medial reefing for post-traumatic recurrent dislocation. Note cutting off of top of Roux-Goldthwaite

trochleoplasty or tibial tubercle transfer should not be undertaken until the end of growth.

Unfortunately, most interventions do not retard the degenerative changes which follow chronic patellofemoral instability. Osteoarthritis may take more than 5 years to develop but the condition tends to progress, perhaps offering some patellar stability with time. Microfracturing or drilling of cartilage defects and chondral grafting do not have a role in patellofemoral instability syndromes during childhood. In osteochondritis dissecans, however (see above), there is a place for these techniques.

Excessive Lateral Pressure Syndrome

This is a consequence of maltracking and a tight lateral retinaculum, causing excessive wear on the lateral facet of the patella. It is a very specific and identifiable cause of anterior knee pain.

Chondromalacia Patellae

Chondromalacia patellae remain a difficult subject. It is helpful to remember that it is a physical sign and not a symptom or a diagnosis in itself although it is commonly used as

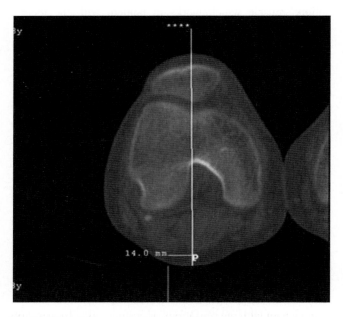

Fig. 29.32 A CT scan showing the tibial tubercle-trochlear groove "offset," a predisposing factor for patellar instability if greater than 15 mm

such. It describes softening of the articular cartilage, recognized by crepitus on compression of the patella against the femur or pain when the quadriceps are contracted while the examiner's index finger is held across the insertion into the upper pole of the patella as in Clarke's test. The confusion is because it has multiple causes which may be idiopathic, post-traumatic, or secondary to maltracking or malalignment. The term describes a pathological lesion of articular cartilage, which when mild may be reversible, but when severe merges with osteoarthritis. As chondromalacia is most often seen in the medial facet of the patella and osteoarthritis on the lateral it is concluded that the one does not necessarily lead to the other. As with osteoarthritis the symptoms are not always proportional to the macroscopic appearance. Standard radiographs may appear normal but MRI scanning is the most useful test and can show the changes well.

Management

Treatment of all the conditions giving rise to obscure anterior knee pain should be conservative. This means physiotherapy and, where there is overuse, activity modification. Physiotherapy consists initially of a comprehensive stretching program for the quadriceps, hamstrings, iliotibial band, and lateral retinaculum. This will include patellar mobilizations. Then isometric and inner range strengthening exercises are added, concentrating on the inner quadriceps and vastus medialis obliquus. Taping, the use of a patellar brace and foot orthoses can all be tried for symptomatic relief but the results are variable. This regimen will be successful in 80% [88]. In the remaining 20%, arthroscopic irrigation may prove beneficial. The patella is inspected and tracking can be further assessed by flexing and extending the knee while examining the patella. Tracking is best seen from a lateral suprapatellar portal.

The modified Outerbridge classification is used to record the damage to the articular surface of the patella [89]:

- Grade I: "closed disease": the articular surface is intact. There may be a slightly blistered appearance or a soft bulky feel when the area is probed with a hook.
- Grade II: "open disease": the probe will now reveal fibrillation and fissures that may or may not be obvious at first sight.
- Grade III: wide spread fibrillation or "cauliflower" appearance.
- Grade IV: the fibrillation is full thickness and erosive changes extend down to the bone which may be exposed.

The size of the lesion should also be recorded using the hook of the probe as a measure.

When there is a definite diagnosis such as excessive lateral pressure syndrome, surgery directed toward correction of this is indicated if physiotherapy has failed. In this instance, there will always be tilt, with or without subluxation. The lateral retinaculum is tight and lateral release may be effective. It should be stressed that the indications for lateral release are very few and it must only be undertaken when there is tilt. It can be done open or arthroscopically but an adequate release must be performed to allow the lateral border of the patella to be elevated perpendicular to the trochlea by the end of the procedure.

Neuropathic Pain

Children with chronic or recurrent pain often locate their symptoms to the knee [90]. The commonest conditions causing pain are post-traumatic or post-surgical peripheral neuropathic pain such as a scar neuroma, complex regional pain syndromes types 1 and 2, and neuropathic pain due to a nerve tumor.

The diagnosis of a scar neuroma is usually straightforward. It is then strictly a "distinct diagnosis" but it is not a cause of knee pain, hence its inclusion as an "obscure diagnosis." Scars around the knee are often complicated by areas of numbness as cutaneous nerves are difficult to avoid and so neuromas in the scars also occur. The management is the same as for any neuroma with the use of local anesthetic patches to confirm the diagnosis and excision if troublesome (see Chapter 23: Part II).

Similarly, nerve tumors are a distinct diagnosis but are included as they may present as knee pain. There may be a palpable tumor which can be confused with a popliteal cyst or ganglion. Very occasionally a glomus tumor is responsible so this emphasizes the importance of a neurological examination in the assessment of knee pain. These unusual causes of knee pain need to be considered before a generic diagnosis of anterior knee pain is made and no treatment offered.

Complex Regional Pain Syndrome

Complex regional pain syndrome (CRPS) incorporates the previous name of reflex sympathetic dystrophy (RSD) and causalgia or neurogenic pain. CRPS type I is RSD and type II is causalgia [91]. Type I comprises a characteristic, spontaneous pain with the sensations of burning, hypersensitivity, and paresthesia. The limb is cold, mottled, and swollen with waxy skin. There is muscle wasting and stiffness. In type

II, all the above are present but there is also evidence of peripheral nerve damage.

CRPS does occur in children. Recent awareness of this has led to earlier diagnosis and more successful treatment [92]. It is very rare under the age of 6 years, commonly affects the lower limb, and is six times more frequent in girls. This is different from adults where the ratio is more equal.

The usual treatment of antidepressants, sympathetic blockade or local anesthetic, and corticosteroid injections are unpredictable in children. The potential for recovery is much better than in adults and a rehabilitation program of physiotherapy combined with cognitive behavioral therapy can be very successful.

The Swollen Knee

The acutely swollen knee may be a manifestation of a range of conditions, foremost of which will be infection. This raises the question of aspiration and even exploration as an emergency. Children are prone to fall on their knees and whereas metallic foreign bodies such as needles or glass are obvious on radiograph, penetrating pieces of wood and other radiographically less obvious material may be present. In the acute stage, air may be seen within the joint, and this can give a clue to the depth of the injury. An acute and transient synovitis is quite common in the juvenile knee as a response to trauma, especially if there is joint laxity. The possibility of a missed patellar dislocation with spontaneous relocation should always be remembered.

Synovial chondromatosis in childhood is extremely rare and when it does occur there may be hundreds of tiny cartilaginous "rice particles" within the knee [93]. As these loose bodies are not ossified, the diagnosis will not be made radiologically but by MRI. The multiple, tiny loose bodies must all be washed out; repeat arthroscopy is sometimes required.

Pigmented villo-nodular synovitis is an inflammatory process of unknown cause, although an auto-immune reaction seems likely. The knee is painful, swollen, and stiff. Locking and crepitus may be present if the synovial proliferation is exuberant. The synovium is brown, thickened, and nodular. Subchondral erosions develop secondary to the release of proteolytic enzymes, and these erosions are seen on both sides of the joint. Histological examination reveals multinucleate giant cells and deposits of hemosiderin, which gives the tissue its color. The treatment is arthroscopic synovectomy.

Septic arthritis, an important cause of a swollen knee, must be recognized and drained early if permanent damage and stiffness are to be minimized. The diagnosis depends upon the history, the appearance of the child who is pyrexial and unwell, and a swollen and tender knee that is too painful to move. Immuno-deficiency and sickle cell disease should not be forgotten, and the vaccination history should be checked. The initial radiograph is usually unhelpful, but may show a pre-existing osteomyelitic focus. Late in the disease, articular changes may become apparent.

Arthroscopy offers a most effective method of obtaining synovial fluid and tissue for bacteriological culture and histological review. The joint can be thoroughly inspected and irrigated, and the procedure avoids the greater morbidity of arthrotomy. Arthroscopy should be repeated every 2 days until the knee is no longer swollen and the serum markers of infection are normal. Although at first the knee should be splinted and the child rested in bed, gentle movement of the knee and protected weight bearing should then be encouraged. Systemic antibiotics remain the mainstay of early treatment, depending upon the culture and the sensitivity of the organisms identified. *Staphylococcus aureus* remains the most common organism. Effective initial cover for both staphylococci and streptococci would be flucloxacillin 200 mg/kg per day (given as four equal doses) and ceftriaxone 80 mg/kg per day (see Chapter 10).

Chronic swelling of the knee suggests low-grade inflammation, such as tuberculosis or juvenile arthritis. When faced with a knee that is warm, boggy, and intermittently swollen in a child, it is important to obtain a family history and to examine the child completely. All other joints should be assessed for reduced range of movement and synovitis. A paediatric rheumatology opinion is essential. Surgical intervention, even in the form of arthroscopy, should be resisted as it is likely to make the joint stiffer. This can cause difficulty if there is a question of infection but the chronic nature of the swelling, the thickening of the synovium, and a very high C-reactive protein (CRP) in the absence of fever are against the diagnosis of infection.

The acute, traumatic, swollen knee in children is as likely to be associated with pathology as it is in the adult (Fig. 29.34). A hemarthrosis may be due to an avulsion or shear fracture of articular cartilage with or without a bony fragment attached. Mid-substance rupture of the anterior cruciate and, rarely, the posterior cruciate ligament are being increasingly diagnosed [63].

Psychogenic Pain

A sensitive knee, in the absence of the signs of chronic regional pain syndrome, swelling, or appropriate trauma, can be the site of pain of psychological origin. It tends to occur in early adolescence and the symptoms are out of proportion to the history which may not even include trauma. The child limps badly or may even be in a wheelchair. School avoidance, depression, anxiety, and family dysfunction are

Fig. 29.34 The causes of hemarthrosis in a child

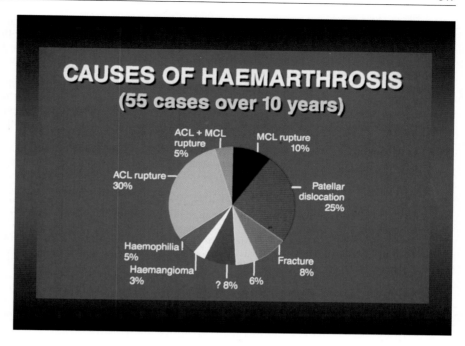

all causes. There may be excessive pressure on a child to perform. A thorough history and examination are vital to be absolutely sure there is no physical cause. Examination may yield important clues. There may be a different range of movement of joints when examined lying down rather than standing up. The limp may disappear when the child walks backward or the child may not be able to do so. The child may stand on the leg when still but avoid taking weight when walking and will resist all attempts to examine the joint although it may appear normal to inspection. There may, rarely, be artifactual marks of self abuse. Once a physical cause is excluded physiotherapists, paediatricians, and psychologists with an interest in this range of conditions can be very successful in treating these children with a combination of physiotherapy, cognitive behavioral therapy, and video feedback.

Tumors

Tumors in childhood (see Chapter 14) show a predilection for the knee, perhaps because the knee is frequently injured. One should therefore have a low threshold for requesting radiographs, especially when the history is short and there is no clear precipitant of the symptoms. As cancer is the second most common cause of death in childhood, bone and soft tissue tumors are of considerable concern particularly as their presentation may be mistaken for other conditions.

Gebhardt et al. reviewed 1999 cases of tumors affecting the knee in childhood and found that knee neoplasia was more common the older the child [94]. Benign bone tumors

comprise 50% of referrals and the most common lesion is the osteochondroma, which can cause a variety of problems. A large posterior swelling will limit knee flexion, whereas medial and lateral excrescences can be the cause of snapping knee and attrition of the hamstring tendons. Multiple lesions may be associated with a growth disturbance and consequent knee deformity of a degree that requires correction. Large lesions may be painful because they are always being knocked during games.

The risk of limb angulation secondary to the osteochondroma is probably not more than 1% and not in itself is considered a reason for excision. Other lesions in decreasing order of frequency are non-ossifying fibroma, chondroblastoma, osteoid osteoma, aneurysmal bone cyst, giant cell tumor, chondromyxoid fibroma, simple bone cyst, and fibrous dysplasia. Osteosarcoma and Ewing's tumor are the principal malignant tumors, and infiltrative conditions such as leukemia and histiocytosis X can occasionally affect the knee. Soft tissue tumors should always be considered as potentially malignant but, fortunately, they are rare and easy to distinguish from popliteal and meniscal cysts.

References

1. Macnicol MF. The Problem Knee, 2nd edition. Oxford: Butterworth Heineman; 1995:8–13.
2. Jacobsen K, Vopalecky F. Congenital dislocation of the knee. Acta Orthop 1985; 7:194–9.
3. Curtis BH, Fisher RL. Congenital hyperextension with anterior subluxation of the knee: surgical treatment and long-term observations. J Bone Joint Surg [Am] 1969; 51A:255–8.

4. Parsch K, Ultrasound diagnosis of congenital knee dislocation. Orthopade. 2002 Mar, 31(3):306–7

5. Katz MP, Grogono BJS, Soper KC. The etiology and treatment of congenital dislocation of the knee. J Bone Joint Surg [Br] 1967; 49B:112–20.

6. Curtis BH, Fisher RL. Heritable congenital tibiofemoral subluxation: clinical features and surgical treatment. J Bone Joint Surg [Am] 1970; 52A:1104–14.

7. Ferris BD, Jackson AM. Congenital snapping knee (habitual anterior subluxation of the tibia in extension) J Bone Joint Surg [Br] 1990; 72B:453–6.

8. Pappas AM, Anas P, Toczylowski HM. Asymmetrical arrest of the proximal tibial physis and genu recurvatum deformity. J Bone Joint Surg [Am] 1984; 66A:575–81.

9. Moroni A, Pezzuto V, Pompili M, Zinghi G. Proximal osteotomy of the tibia for the treatment of genu recurvatum in adults. J Bone Joint Surg [Am] 1992; 74A: 577–86.

10. Bowen JR, Morley DC, McInverny V, MacEwen GD. Treatment of genu recurvatum by proximal tibial closing-wedge anterior displacement osteotomy. Clin Orthop 1983; 179:194–9.

11. Choi JH, Chung CY, Cho TJ, Park SS. Correction of genu recurvatum by the Ilizarov method. J Bone Joint Surg [Br] 1999; 81B:769–74.

12. Stein H, Dickson RA. Reversed dynamic slings for knee flexion contractures in the haemophiliac. J Bone Joint Surg [Br] 1975; 57B:282–3.

13. Del Bello DA, Watts HG. Distal femoral extension osteotomy for knee flexion contracture in patients with arthrogryposis. J Pediatr Orthop 1996; 16:122–6.

14. Murray C, Fixsen JA. Management of knee deformity in clinical arthrogryposis multiplex congenita (amyoplasia congenita). J Pediatr Orthop B 1997; 6:186–91.

15. Brunner R, Hefti F, Tgetgel JD. Arthrogrypotic joint contracture at the knee and foot: correction with a circular frame. J Pediatr Orthop B 1997; 6:192–7.

16. Salenius P, Vankka E. The development of the tibiofemoral angle in children. J Bone Joint Surg [Am] 1975; 57A:259–61.

17. Fraser RK, Dickens DR, Cole WG. Medial physeal stapling for primary and secondary genu valgum in late childhood and adolescence. J Bone Joint Surg [Br] 1995; 77B:733–5.

18. Stevens PM, Maguire M, Dales MD, Robins AJ. Physeal stapling for idiopathic genu valgum. J Pediatr Orthop 1999; 19:645–9.

19. Bowen JR, Leahy JL, Zheng Z, MacEwen GD. Partial epiphysiodesis at the knee to correct angular deformity. Clin Orthop 1985; 198:184–9.

20. Volpon JB. Idiopathic genu valgum treated by epiphysiodesis in adolescence. Int Orthop 1997; 21:228–31.

21. Macnicol MF. The correction of lesser leg length inequalities. Curr Orthop 1999; 13:212–7.

22. Edgerton BC, Mariani EM, Morrey BF. Distal femoral varus osteotomy for painful genu valgum. A 5–11 year follow-up study. Clin Orthop 1993; 288:263–9.

23. Healy WL, Anglen JO, Wasilewski SA, Krackow KA. Distal femoral varus osteotomy. J Bone Joint Surg [Am] 1983; 70A:102–9.

24. Ogden JA, Ogden RN, Pugh L, et al. Tibia valga after proximal metaphyseal fractures in childhood: a normal biologic response. J Pediatr Orthop 1995; 15:489–93.

25. Blount WP. Tibia vara. Osteochondrosis deformans tibiae. J Bone Joint Surg [Am] 1937; 19A:1–10.

26. Erlacher P. Deformierende Prozesse de Epiphysengenend bei Kindern. Arch Orthop Unfallchir 1922; 20:81–4.

27. Langenskiold A. Tibia vara. Acta Chir 1952; 103:9–14.

28. Levine AM, Drennan JC. Physiological bowing and tibia vara: the metaphyseal-diaphyseal angle in the measurement of bow-leg deformities. J Bone Joint Surg [Am] 1982; 64A:1158–63.

29. Bateson EM. The relationship between Blount's disease and bow legs. Brit J Radiol 1968; 41:107–14.

30. Ferriter P, Shapiro F. Infantile tibia vara: factors affecting outcome following proximal tibial ostetomy. J Pediatr Orthop 1987; 7: 1–7.

31. Langenskiold A. Tibia vara: osteochondrosis deformans tibiae. Blount's disease. Clin Orthop 1981; 158:77–81.

32. Siffert RS. Intra-epiphyseal osteotomy for progressive tibia vara: a case report and rationale of management. J Pediatr Orthop 1982; 2:81–3.

33. van Huyssteen AL, Hastings CJ, Olesak M, Hoffman EB. Double-elevating osteotomy for late-presenting infantile Blount's disease: the importance of concomitant lateral epiphysiodesis. J Bone Joint Surg [Br] 2005; 87B:710–5.

34. Monticelli G, Spinelli R. A new method of treating the advanced stages of tibia vara (Blount's disease). Ital J Orthop Traumatol 1984; 10:245–303.

35. Coogan PG, Fox JA, Fitch RD. Treatment of adolescent Blount's disease with the circular external fixation device and distraction osteogenesis. J Pediatr Orthop 1996; 16:450–4.

36. Morrissy RT. Atlas of Pediatric Orthopaedic Surgery. Philadelphia: JB Lippincott; 1992:455–64.

37. Miller S, Radomisli T, Ulin R. Inverted arcuate osteotomy and external fixation for adolescent tibia vara. J Pediatr Orthop 2000; 20:450–4.

38. Van Olm JMJ, Gillespie R. Proximal tibial osteotomy for angular knee deformity in children. J Bone Joint Surg [Br] 1984; 66B:301–6.

39. Rab GT. Oblique tibial osteotomy for Blount's disease (tibia vara). J Pediatr Orthop 1988; 8:715–20.

40. Hayek S, Segev E, Ezra E, et al. Serrated W/M osteotomy. Results using a new technique for the correction of infantile tibia vara. J Bone Joint Surg [Br] 2000; 82B:1026–9.

41. Laurencin CT, Ferriter PJ, Millis MB. Oblique proximal tibial osteotomy for the correction of tibia vara in the young. Clin Orthop 1996; 327:218–24.

42. Dietz FR, Weinstein SL. Spike osteotomy for angular deformities of the long bones in children. J Bone Joint Surg [Am] 1988; 70-A:848–52.

43. Macnicol MF. Realignment osteotomy for knee deformity in childhood. Knee 2002; 4:113–20.

44. Steel HH, Sandrow RE, Sullivan PD. Complications of tibial osteotomy in children for genu varum or valgum. J Bone Joint Surg [Am] 1971; 53A:1629–35.

45. Macnicol MF. Focal fibrocartilaginous dysplasia of the femur. J Pediatr Orthop B 1997; 8:661–3.

46. Aglietti P, Buzzi R, Insall JN. Disorders of the patellofemoral joint. In: Insall JN, Scott WN, eds. Surgery of the Knee, 3rd ed. Philadelphia: Churchill Livingstone; 2001:929.

47. Jackson AM. Anterior knee pain. J. Bone Jt. Surg [Br] 2001; 83-B:937–948.

48. Ogden JA. Radiology of postnatal skeletal development. Patella and tibial tuberosity. Skeletal Radiol 1984; 1:246–57.

49. Hunt DM, Somashaker N. A review of sleeve fractures of the patella in children. Knee 2005; 12:3–7.

50. Lloyd Roberts GC, Jackson AM, Albert JS. Avulsion of the distal pole of the patella in cerebral palsy. J Bone Joint Surg [Br] 1985; 67-B:252–4.

51. Enneking WF. Clinical Musculoskeletal Pathology, 3rd ed. Gainesville FL: University of Florida Press; 1990:166.

52. Cahill BR, Berg BC. 99 m-Technetium phosphate compound joint scintigraphy in the management of juvenile osteochondritis dissecans of the femoral condyles. Am J Sports Med 1983; 11:329–35.

53. De Smet AA, Ilahi OA, Graf BK. Untreated osteochondritis of the femoral condyles: prediction of patient outcome using

radiographic and MR findings. Skeletal Radiol 1997; 26(8): 463–7.

54. Ramappa AJ, Gill TJ, Bradford CH, et al. MRI to assess knee cartilage repair tissue after microfracture of chondral defects. J Knee Surg 2007; 20:228–34.

55. Petersen L, Minas T, Brittberg M, Lindahl A. Treatment of osteochondritis dissecans of the knee with autologous chondrocyte transplantation: results at two to ten years. J Bone Joint Surg [Am] 2007; 85-A (Suppl 2):17–24.

56. Twyman RS, Desai K, Aichroth PM. Osteochondritis dissecans of the knee. A long term study. J Bone Joint Surg [Br] 1991; 73-B:461–4.

57. Linden B. Osteochondritis dissecans of the femoral condyles: a long term follow -up study. J Bone Joint Surg [Am] 1997; 53:769–76.

58. Dinham JM. Popliteal cysts in children. J Bone Joint Surg [Br] 1975; 57:69–71.

59. Glasgow MMS, Allen PW, Blakeway C. Arthroscopic treatment of cysts of the lateral meniscus. J Bone Joint Surg [Br] 1993; 75-B:299–302.

60. Henry JH, Craven PR Jr. Traumatic meniscal lesions in children. South Med J 1981; 74:1336–7.

61. Stanitski CL, Harvell JC, Fu F. Observations on acute knee hemarthrosis in children and adolescents. J Paed Orthop 1993; 13:506–10.

62. McNicholas MJ, Rowley DI, McGurty D, et al. Total meniscectomy in adolescence. A 30-year follow-up. J Bone Joint Surg [Br] 2000; 82-B:217–21.

63. King D. The healing of semilunar cartilages. J Bone Joint Surg [Br] 1936; 18-B:333–42.

64. Fairbank HA. Knee joint changes after meniscectomy. J Bone Joint Surg [Br] 1948; 30-B:664–70.

65. Arnoczky SP, Warren RF. Microvasculature of the human meniscus. Am J Sports Med 1982; 10:90–5.

66. Noyes FR, Barber-Westin SD. Arthroscopic repair of meniscal tears extending into the avascular zone in patients younger than twenty years of age. Am J Sports Med 2002; 30: 589–600.

67. De Haven KE, Hales W. Peripheral meniscal repair; an alternative to meniscectomy. Orthop Transact 1981; 5:399–400.

68. Steenbrugge F, Verdonk R, Verstraete K. Long-term assessment of arthroscopic meniscal repair: a 13 year follow-up study. Knee 2002; 9:181–7.

69. Peters G, Wirth CJ. The current status of meniscal allograft transplantation and replacement. Knee 2003; 10:19–31.

70. Noble J, Hamblen DL. The pathology of the degenerate meniscus. J Bone Joint Surg [Br] 1975; 57-B:180–6.

71. Ikeuchi H. Arthroscopic treatment of discoid lateral meniscus; technique and long term results. Clin Orth Rel Res 1982; 167:19–28.

72. Watanabe M, Takeda S, Ikeuchi H. Atlas of Arthroscopy. Tokyo: Igakushan; 1979.

73. Kaplan EB. Discoid lateral meniscus of the knee joint: nature, mechanism and operative treatment. J Bone Joint Surg [Am] 1957; 39A:77–87.

74. Clark CR, Ogden JA. Development of the menisci of the human knee joint. J Bone Joint Surg [Am] 1983; 65-A:538–47.

75. Räber DA, Friederich NF, Hefti F. Discoid lateral meniscus in children. J Bone Joint Surg [Am] 1998; 80-A:1579–86.

76. Thomas NP, Jackson AM, Aichroth PM. Congenital absence of the anterior cruciate ligament. J Bone Joint Surg [Br] 1985; 67-B:572–5.

77. Meyers MH, McKeever FM. Fractures of the intercondylar eminence of the tibia. J Bone Joint Surg [Am] 1970; 52-A:1677–84.

78. Dorizas JA, Stanitski CL. Anterior cruciate ligament injury in the skeletally immature. Orthop Clin North Am 2003; 34:355–63.

79. Aichroth PM, Patel DV, Zorilla P. The natural history and treatment of rupture of the anterior cruciate ligament in children and adolescents. J Bone Joint Surg (Br) 2002; 84-B:38–41.

80. Kocher MS, Saxon HS, Hovis WD, Hawkins RJ. Management and complications of anterior cruciate ligament injuries in skeletally immature patients: Survey of the Herodicus Society and the ACL Study Group. J Paediatr Orthop 2002; 22:452–57.

81. Kocher MS, Smith JT, Zoric BJ, et al. Transphyseal anterior cruciate ligament reconstruction in the skeletally immature pubescent adolescents. J Bone Joint Surg [Am] 2007; 89-A:2632–9.

82. Harner CD. Posterior Cruciate ligament repair and reconstruction. In Micheli LJ, Kocher MS, eds. The Pediatric Knee. Philadelphia: Saunders Elsevier; 2006:389.

83. Milstrom C, Finestone A, Shlamkovitch N, et al. Anterior knee pain caused by overactivity: a long term prospective follow up. Clin Orth Rel Res. 1996; 331:256–60.

84. Hvid I, Anderson LI. The quadriceps and its relation to femoral torsion. Acta Orthop Scand 1982; 53:577–9.

85. Fulkerson JP, Shea KP. Disorders of patello-femoral alignment. J Bone Joint Surg [Am] 1990; 72-A:1424–29.

86. Amis AA, Firer P, Mountney J, et al. Anatomy and biomechanics of the medial patellofemoral ligament. Knee 2003; 10:215–20.

87. Mulford JS. Assessment and management of chronic patellofemoral instability. J Bone Joint Surg [Br] 2007; 89B:709–16.

88. Kannus P, Natri A, Paakklala T, Järvinnen M. An outcome study of chronic patellofemoral pain syndrome. 7-year follow-up of patients in a randomised, controlled trial. J Bone Joint Surg [Am] 1999; 81-A:355–63.

89. Outerbridge RE. The etiology of chondromalacia patellae. J Bone Joint Surg [Br] 1961; 43-B:752–7

90. McGrath P. Chronic pain in children. In Crombie IK, Croft PR, Linton SJ, eds. Epidemiology of Pain. Seattle WA: IASP Press; 1999:81–82.

91. Stanton-Hicks M, Janig W, Hassenbuch S, et al. Reflex sympathetic dystrophy: changing concepts and taxonomy. Pain 1995; 63:127–33.

92. Wilder RT, Berde CB, Wolohan M, et al. Reflex sympathetic dystrophy in children. Characteristics and follow up of 70 patients. J Bone Joint Surg [A] 1992; 74:910–19.

93. Carey RPL. Synovial chondromatosis of the knee in childhood. J Bone Joint Surg [B] 1983; 65:444–7.

94. Gebhardt MC, Ready JE, Mankin HJ. Tumors about the knee in children. Clin Orth Rel Res 1990; 255:86–110.

Chapter 30

The Foot

John A. Fixsen

Introduction

Foot deformities such as in-toeing, curly toes, and flat feet are common causes of parental anxiety. As a result, they make up a large part of the routine referrals to a children's orthopaedic clinic. The orthopaedic surgeon must not only understand the condition and its natural history but also be able to explain it to the parents and allay their anxiety. A careful history including details of pregnancy, birth, and development, together with examination of the child, both statically on the couch and actively—walking and running—is essential. Time spent explaining the position carefully at the first interview is well spent, particularly if it saves unnecessary follow-up appointments, which tend to reinforce the parents' anxiety that something is wrong as the doctor continues to want to see their child. Clearly, if the parents remain unconvinced or the surgeon unsure as to the outcome or nature of the condition, then continued follow-up is necessary.

The surgeon should remember that there are very few foot deformities that actually prevent walking. If a child's motor development is delayed, parents will nearly always blame the obvious in-toeing gait or flat foot that they can see. The surgeon must look beyond the obvious for the real cause of the problem, such as cerebral palsy, spina bifida occulta, or Down syndrome. It is often a difficult and delicate task to persuade parents that the obvious foot deformity is not the root cause of the problem. Treatment of the foot may not only be unnecessary but will not solve the child's developmental or coordination problems.

In-Toe Gait

In-toeing is probably the single most common cause of referral of a child to a children's orthopaedic clinic. It may arise in the foot itself, in the lower leg, at the hip, or be secondary to a central problem or a combination of some or all of these.

Metatarsus Varus, Adductus, or Adductovarus

In the foot itself, metatarsus varus, adductus, or adductovarus comprise the most common entity producing an in-toe gait. It is essential to differentiate this benign, largely self-resolving condition from congenital talipes equinovarus [1]. In club foot, both the forefoot and the hindfoot are in equinus and varus, whereas in metatarsus varus the forefoot is in varus but the hindfoot is in neutral or valgus, with normal posterior skin creases (Fig. 30.1).

The condition is rarely noted at birth but usually becomes obvious in the first few months of life or when the child starts to walk. The forefoot is in varus or adduction, very often with some supination but no equinus. The hindfoot is in neutral or valgus. The deformity is often best seen from the sole of the foot, and in mild and moderate cases is easily correctable by simple finger pressure on the first ray. It is essential to examine the whole child carefully because metatarsus varus can be associated with neurological conditions such as spina bifida occulta or spinal muscular atrophy, in which case there is usually evidence of muscle wasting and lack of normal movements in the lower limb. There is a very rare rigid form of the condition called serpentine, skew, or "Z-foot" (see below), in which the forefoot is in fixed valgus (Fig. 30.2).

The etiology of metatarsus varus is unknown, although Harris [2] suggested that it could be associated with a persistent prone-lying sleeping position. Recently, prone lying for infants has been associated with the "cot death" syndrome; as a result supine lying has been encouraged, and the incidence of metatarsus varus appears to have reduced considerably.

J.A. Fixsen (✉)
Orthopaedic Department, Great Ormond Street Hospital for Sick Children, London, UK

M. Benson et al. (eds.), *Children's Orthopaedics and Fractures*,
DOI 10.1007/978-1-84882-611-3_30, © Springer-Verlag London Limited 2010

Fig. 30.1 Clinical photographs showing (**a**) anterior and (**b**) posterior views of a patient with metatarsus varus aged 18 months. Note the forefoot and hallux varus but both heels are in slight valgus. There is no equinus and the posterior creases are normal

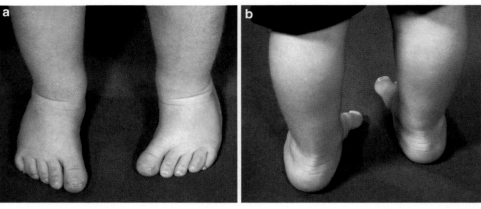

Fig. 30.2 Clinical photographs showing (**a**) anterior and (**b**) posterior views of serpentine, skew, or "Z-feet" in a child aged 4 years

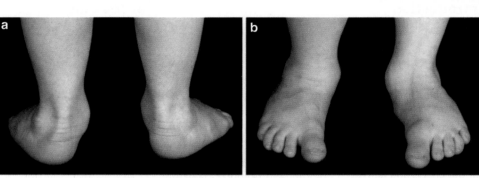

Radiographs show that the metatarsals are adducted relative to the mid- and hindfoot and the talocalcaneal angles are normal or increased in the anteroposterior view (Fig. 30.3). In the rare serpentine, Z, or "skew" foot, the navicular and cuboid are laterally displaced on the talus and the calcaneum (Fig. 30.4).

Treatment

There is considerable argument about the treatment of this common condition. The natural history has been reported by Ponseti and Becker [3] and Rushforth [4], both of whom found that in the majority of patients the condition corrected spontaneously with or without treatment. The former reported that approximately one in nine patients needed treatment. They used plasters, which they pointed out were difficult to apply, and because they worked in a special center for children's orthopaedics they probably had a greater number of difficult cases than average. In Rushforth's series of 130 feet which received no treatment and were followed up for 7 years, 86% corrected completely, 10% showed mild persistence of the deformity, which did not worry the patient or their parents in any way, and only 4% showed persistence of the deformity. Rushforth was unable to predict, until the child reached the age of 3–4 years, which feet were not going to correct. This puts the orthopaedic surgeon in

a considerable dilemma: at least four in five feet will correct spontaneously without any treatment, and it is very difficult to identify those patients requiring treatment. In general, any patient in whom the foot corrects easily to neutral or beyond will probably correct spontaneously. The child with a very rigid deformity and a deep medial crease should be treated initially with stretching by the mother (Fig. 30.5). Ponseti and Becker [3] advised that plastering above the knee was necessary to control the whole leg. They emphasized the difficulty of applying these plasters. They advised that the plasters were changed every 2–3 weeks and that correction was usually obtained within 8–10 weeks, but in some patients relapse occurred after the plasters were removed. Farsetti et al. [5] published a long-term follow-up of untreated and non-surgically treated metatarsus adductus and reported good results in all 16 untreated feet and in 90% of those treated with long leg plasters. Recently, Katz el al. [6] reported treating 85 inflexible feet with below-knee plasters, achieving satisfactory results.

In order to avoid excessive overtreatment of this generally benign condition, the vast majority of these feet should be left alone or, if inflexible, treated with plasters. If, at the age of 3–4 years, there is a persistent deformity, operative correction can be considered. Browne and Paton [7] described an anomalous insertion of the tibialis posterior and noted that the main bulk of the tendon did not attach to the navicular bone, but extended into the forefoot. This was released

Fig. 30.3 Anteroposterior radiographs of both feet in a patient with metatarsus varus (**a**) at 9 months and (**b**) at 3 years 3 months. No treatment was given

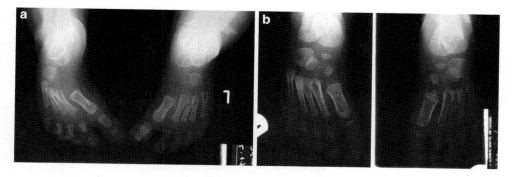

Fig. 30.4 (**a**) Anteroposterior and (**b**) lateral radiographs of true serpentine feet in a boy aged 5 years 4 months. Note the lateral shift of the mid-tarsus on the hindfoot and supination of the forefoot

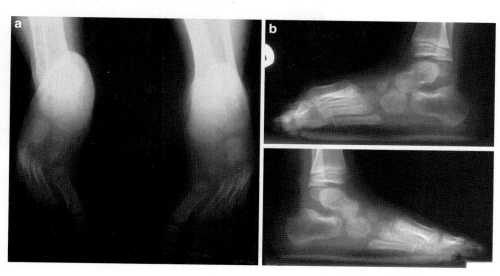

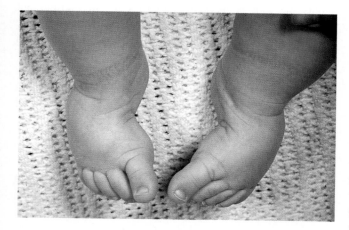

Fig. 30.5 Clinical photograph of a child aged 9 months with severe metatarsus varus showing a marked medial crease. The deformity was rigid and not passively correctable

together with the abductor hallucis and the deformity corrected by plaster. Heyman et al. [8] recommended the more extensive procedure of tarsometatarsal capsulotomies. Stark et al. [9] reported a 41% overall failure rate and a 50% incidence of a painful dorsal prominence at the site of the surgical scar, in a review of this procedure performed over an 18-year period. The author's own limited experience of this operation is similar to that described by Stark et al. [9]. After the child has reached the age of 6 years, multiple metatarsal osteotomies as described by Berman and Gartland [10] can be used. Again, there are significant complications associated with this operation, with failure of correction and damage to the growth plate (physis) of the first metatarsal causing shortening and progressive deformity indicating that this operation should be used with great care. It is extremely rare to see an adult with persistent symptomatic metatarsus varus. On this basis, and the evidence that the majority of these feet correct with time, it is important not to overtreat this condition. In particular, surgery should be avoided unless it is absolutely necessary because it is quite clear that operation can produce symptoms and deformity of greater severity than the condition itself.

Bleck [11] advocated a more radical early approach to conservative treatment with serial plasters. However, he accepted that the results of his study did not make it possible to predict with certainty which feet must be treated and acknowledged the influence of "the public attitude toward deformity" among his treatment population.

Fig. 30.6 (a) Clinical photograph of the feet and lower legs of a patient with Larsen's syndrome. Note the serpentine feet and dislocated knees. (b) AP radiograph of the left foot showing the severe Z-shaped deformity

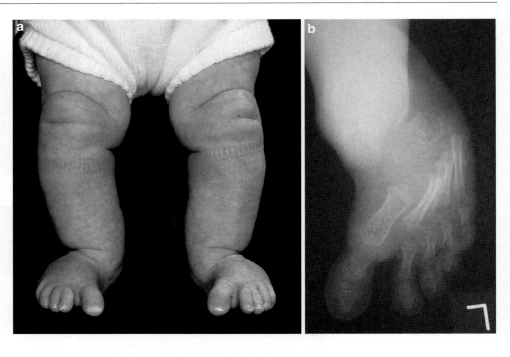

Serpentine, Skew, or "Z-Foot"

A true serpentine, skew, or "Z-foot" is a very rare entity. Kite [12] described 12 examples among a total of 2818 cases of metatarsus varus, an incidence of 0.43%. In this condition the forefoot varus and adduction is fixed and the hindfoot is in fixed valgus. The radiographs show that the navicular and cuboid bones are laterally displaced on the talus and calcaneum with the metatarsals in varus, giving rise to the classical "Z- or S-shaped" foot (Fig. 30.4). This is extremely difficult to treat because all three components of the deformity require correction. Lloyd-Roberts and Clark [13] pointed out that this rare condition may be associated with a ball-and-socket ankle joint, so that fusing the subtalar joint may not correct the valgus. It is important to look at the whole patient, as this condition may be associated with other anomalies such as Larsen's syndrome (Fig. 30.6). Mosca [14], in an important review of skew foot, suggested that, in infants and young children, management should follow that of metatarsus adductus: in older children and adults, only those with symptoms should be treated. In 1995, he described satisfactory short-term results in 10 symptomatic skew feet operated on to correct all three components of the deformity. The operation was performed at an average age of 10 years. The operation combined a reversed Evans [15] type of calcaneal lengthening procedure to correct the hindfoot and midfoot and a medial cuneiform opening wedge osteotomy, as described by Fowler et al. [16], to correct the forefoot. The tendo-Achilles, which was always short, was also lengthened.

Congenital Talipes Calcaneo-Valgus

Postural calcaneo-valgus is the most common position of the foot in the newborn (Fig. 30.7). It is normal to be able to dorsiflex the foot of the neonate so that the dorsum touches the anterior aspect of the tibia; however, there should be a full range of plantar flexion. In congenital talipes calcaneo-valgus the foot is markedly dorsiflexed and everted, but plantar flexion is limited, often to only the neutral position. The condition is more common in firstborn children. It is associated with oligohydramnios and the "molded baby syndrome" described by Lloyd-Roberts and Pilcher [17]. It is said to be associated with congenital dislocation of the hip in 5% of cases, and instability of the hip must be looked for in patients with this deformity. It is very important to look for any suggestion of neuromuscular abnormality, both

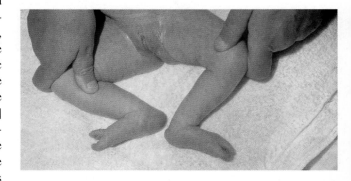

Fig. 30.7 Clinical photograph of typical calcaneo-valgus feet in a newborn infant

in the spine and in the leg, typically wasting or a difference in size between the two legs. The condition must be distinguished from congenital vertical talus (congenital convex pes valgus), in which the forefoot is dorsiflexed and valgus, but the hindfoot is in fixed equinus (see Chapter 33).

If there is no evidence of an underlying abnormality, this condition nearly always responds to simple stretching into plantar flexion and inversion by the mother under instruction from the physiotherapist. This should be done regularly several times a day, probably when the baby is being fed and the nappy changed. In the vast majority of patients, the condition will correct by the age of 3 months. If there is failure to correct by this age, the patient should be looked at very carefully for evidence of any underlying neuromuscular abnormality or generalized condition. It is probably wise to follow-up the child until walking is established.

Parents are often very worried by this condition and believe that their child will have an abnormal foot or difficulty with walking. Some orthopaedic surgeons such as Giannestras [18] advocate a more aggressive policy, with serial plasters followed by modifications to shoe wear. In the author's experience, this type of treatment has not been necessary unless the deformity has been associated with an underlying neuromuscular or skeletal deformity.

Tip-Toe Walking

Persistent Tip-Toe Walking or Persistent Equinus

The mature heel–toe pattern of gait should normally be adopted by the age of 2 years [19]. One of the most important things for an orthopaedic surgeon to recognize is the child who had developed a mature heel–toe pattern of gait but then reverted to a toe–heel or toe–toe gait. This is nearly always pathological, and conditions such as muscular dystrophy, spinal dysraphism, peroneal muscular atrophy (hereditary motor and sensory neuropathy), and spinal tumor must be looked for.

Idiopathic Tip-Toe Walking

In this situation the child persistently walks up on the toes, although when standing may bring the heels to the ground. There may be a degree of hyperextension of the knee and also external rotation of the feet in order to bring the heels to the ground more easily. Typically, the tip-toe gait is more noticeable in bare feet than when wearing shoes. On the couch, dorsiflexion of the foot with the knee extended is sometimes limited, but can be normal with no evidence of

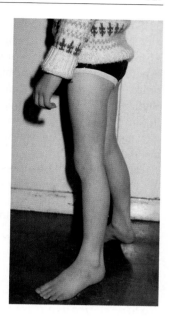

Fig. 30.8 Clinical photograph of a persistent tip-toe walker aged 7 years. Note the heels are well off the ground, the knees extended, and the legs externally rotated

tendo-Achilles shortening. Occasionally true shortening of the tendo-Achilles with fixed equinus is present. Hall et al. [20] described this as idiopathic shortening of the tendo-Achilles. They pointed out that this condition was often not recognized until the child was at school, as it had been accepted that the child habitually walked like this, and that it would correct with time (Fig. 30.8). They advised surgical lengthening of the tendo-Achilles.

Idiopathic tip-toe walking is a diagnosis of exclusion. Neuromuscular disorders such as spastic diplegia and other forms of cerebral palsy should be considered. For a period all patients referred to the orthopaedic department at The Hospital for Sick Children, London, were referred to a paediatric neurologist to determine if it was possible to make a neurological diagnosis in every case of tip-toe walking. A skilled paediatric neurologist was able to find some underlying neurological cause in approximately 50% of tip-toe walkers. This gait is also associated with hyperactive children, learning disorders, autism, and schizophrenia.

In the past, physiotherapy in the form of stretching by the mother or under the supervision of the physiotherapist, plaster casting, and braces have been advised for the treatment of persistent idiopathic tip-toe walking. However, Eastwood et al. [21] showed that tendo-Achilles lengthening (TAL) was significantly better than conservative forms of treatment. In their series of patients, 16% had a positive family history of tip-toe walking and 50% had suffered significant neonatal jaundice. In 20%, muscle biopsies were performed and these showed features suggestive of a neuropathic process, including a predominance of type I muscle fibers. In 1998 Stricker and Angulo [22] also showed that casts and bracing were really no better than no treatment and that surgery gave better results. It was interesting that

32% of their 80 patients had a family history of toe walk-ing, 28% were born prematurely, 16% reported delay in psychomotor development or speech, and 31% had perinatal hyperbilirubinemia. Muscle biopsy was not performed in this series. The investigators concluded that the origin of idio-pathic tip-toe walking was unclear in the majority of cases. In those children who showed persistent heel cord contrac-ture, surgical treatment was more effective than conservative methods.

In a maturity follow-up using gait analysis of idiopathic toe walkers treated either by plasters or by TAL, there were still changes in ankle kinematics and kinetics but this was not detectable visually in most subjects [23].

The Painful Heel

Kohler's Disease (Osteochondritis of the Navicular)

Kohler [24] described a painful self-limiting disease of the tarsal navicular that showed flattening, sclerosis, and frag-mentation of the navicular on radiograph (Fig. 30.9). The tarsal navicular ossifies between the ages of 2.5 and 3.5 years. There are considerable variations in the development and pattern of its ossification, so the radiographic appearances may be irrelevant unless the child also has symptoms and local signs. The condition commonly occurs between the age of 4 and 7 years and, in up to 33% of patients, both feet may be involved. The patient presents with pain, limp, and tenderness over the tarsal navicular. Sometimes there is suf-ficient local swelling redness and warmth for the diagnosis of infection to be considered. Waugh [25], in a careful study of 52 feet, showed the ossification of the tarsal navicular occurred later in boys than in girls. Abnormalities of ossi-fication were more frequent in boys. He was of the opinion that abnormal ossification resulted from compression of the bony nucleus at the critical phase of growth of the navicular bone. Biopsy performed when the question of infection or tumor had been raised showed areas of necrosis and resorp-tion of dead bone, with the formation of new bone similar to that seen in Perthes' disease. Waugh also showed that, within 2–3 years, the appearances of the navicular had returned to normal. Cox [26], in a long-term review of 55 patients, found no evidence of permanent deformity or disability after this disease.

Treatment depends upon the severity of the symptoms. Often, no treatment is necessary and the child will recover spontaneously. Occasionally pain is sufficiently severe to require immobilization of the foot in a below-knee walking plaster or the use of an orthosis for 6 weeks.

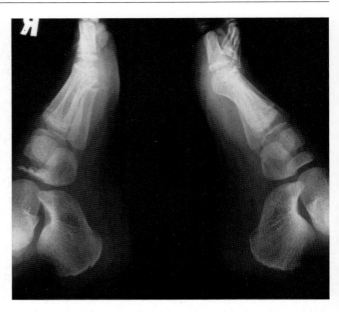

Fig. 30.9 Lateral radiographs of the feet in a 5-year-old child. (Left) Kohler's disease (osteochondritis of the tarsal navicular) in the right foot with flattening, fragmentation, and sclerosis. (Right) The normal left foot for comparison

Calcaneal Apophysitis (Sever's Disease)

Sever described this condition in 1912 [27]. He believed it to be a form of osteochondritis of the calcaneal apophysis. However, the appearance of increased density and fragmen-tation of the calcaneal apophysis is now known to be a normal radiographic finding in the age group concerned (Fig. 30.10).

The child, usually between the ages of 7 and 12 years and more commonly a boy than a girl, presents with pain and tenderness over the insertion of the tendo-Achilles into the calcaneus. The patient commonly finds it more comfortable to wear a shoe with a heel than to walk barefoot. The child is often a keen footballer or gymnast, and the tenderness is accurately localized to the insertion of the tendo-Achilles. This condition is now believed to be a strain of the inser-tion of the tendo-Achilles. It must be distinguished from Achilles tendonitis, which can also occur in children, particu-larly keen sportsmen, but is associated with pain and swelling over the tendo-Achilles above the calcaneus. It is also possi-ble to develop a bursitis in which the small bursa between the posterosuperior corner of the calcaneus and the tendo-Achilles becomes inflamed. The rare subacute osteomyelitis of the calcaneus should also be considered (see below: under *Other Cause of Pain in the Heel*).

Treatment usually consists of temporarily fitting a lift under the heel of the shoe, gentle calf stretching, and reduced activity. If this is not sufficient, a short period in plaster may be necessary, although this is rarely necessary. However, it

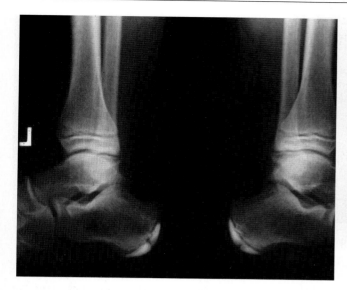

Fig. 30.10 Lateral radiograph of both hindfeet of a child aged 11 years with so-called Sever's disease. The sclerosis and fragmentation of the calcaneal apophysis are normal radiographic appearances at this age. The patient was complaining of pain over the insertion of the tendo-Achilles on the right side only

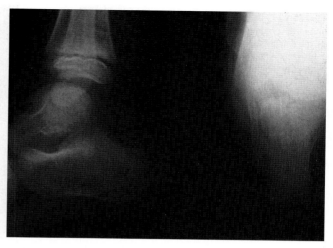

Fig. 30.11 Lateral (*left*) and axial (*right*) radiographs of a child with a fracture of the calcaneus causing a limp. The fracture is only visible on the axial view

is important to regulate activity carefully when the plaster is removed, otherwise the symptoms will recur. This condition can be a considerable nuisance in children who are keen on sport, particularly football and gymnastics.

Calcaneal Boss

This condition is almost entirely confined to adolescent girls, who develop a painful bony swelling over the superolateral corner of the calcaneus. This is almost always associated with wearing a high-heeled court shoe, which causes pressure over this area, resulting in a bursa over the normal prominence of the calcaneus at this site. With time, the feet become accustomed to the pressure of the shoes and the condition settles. Sometimes there is sufficient anxiety and pressure to do something about it that the surgeon may be persuaded to operate. However, it is much better to change the design of shoe and take the pressure off the heel or pad the heel and wait for the condition to subside. If the surgeon is persuaded to remove the bony lump that underlies the swelling, this involves removing a substantial portion of the posterosuperior corner of the calcaneus. Great care must be taken not to damage the terminal branches of the sural nerve and to avoid a painful neuroma which can cause more troublesome symptoms than the original lump. Almost all these patients will respond to modification of footwear and time.

Other Cause of Pain in the Heel

There are a number of other interesting causes of pain in the heel. A child may traumatize the heel by jumping from a height. Fractures of the calcaneus are notoriously difficult to see on radiographs unless an axial view of the os calcis is taken in addition to the conventional anteroposterior (AP) and lateral views (Fig. 30.11).

Infection in the calcaneus often runs an unusual subacute course (see Chapter 10) and has been misdiagnosed as a sprain, ligamentous injury, or Sever's disease [28] (Fig. 30.12).

Generalized bony conditions such as fibrous dysplasia and neurofibromatosis can also present with pain in the heel, as can bone tumors such as bone cysts and osteoid osteoma (Fig. 30.13). The latter may be very difficult to see, and a bone scan can be very useful in the investigation of obscure pain in the heel region.

Flat Feet

Flat Foot (Pes Planus)

In the past there has been great concern among parents and doctors about flat feet. However, a knowledge of the natural history of foot development in the child and the awareness that the ordinary flexible flat foot associated with joint laxity should be considered a normal variant and not a disability have led to a much more rational attitude to this very common condition.

Fig. 30.12 Lateral radiographs showing subacute osteomyelitis of the calcaneus. (*Left*) The initial radiograph was taken 2 months before the second (*right*). Note the development of the lytic lesion (abscess) with time. The patient was initially treated for a strain of the tendo-Achilles at the time of the first radiograph

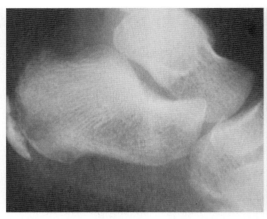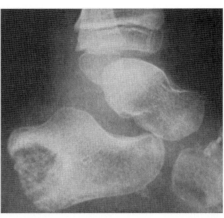

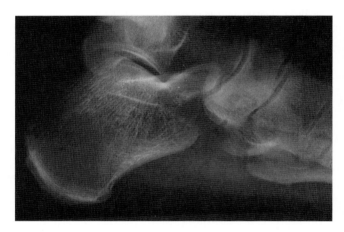

Fig. 30.13 Lateral radiograph of a child with pain in the hindfoot showing a lytic lesion with a central nidus in the tarsal navicular which proved to be an osteoid osteoma

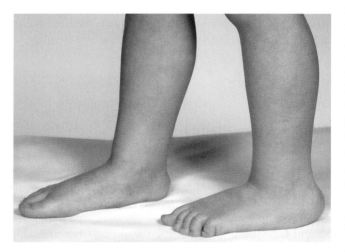

Fig. 30.14 Clinical photograph of a child aged 18 months showing the normal weight-bearing appearance of the feet at this age with flattening of the medial arch

Natural History

Staheli et al. [29] made an important contribution to our understanding of the natural history of foot development in the child.

At birth, the most common position for the foot is in slight dorsiflexion and eversion, a mild calcaneo-valgus. At the end of the first year, when the child begins to stand, the foot nearly always looks flat, particularly because there is a large pad of fat on the medial side of the foot beneath the navicular. This is a normal fat pad, although it can look quite large and sometimes has a considerable vascular element. Between the ages of 1 and 2 years, walking becomes established and the child characteristically stands with the feet everted and externally rotated. As a result the feet look very flat, but this should not be considered an abnormality (Fig. 30.14). Between the ages of 2 and 3 years, the medial arch starts to appear. If, at this stage, a child's feet remain significantly flat, with the medial arch resting near or on the ground, it is most important to test for the presence of joint laxity. The majority of these feet will be so-called flexible flat feet, which are asymptomatic and require no treatment. The assessment of join laxity can be difficult, particularly as it varies considerably between races. Carter and Wilkinson [30] described five tests for joint laxity in the upper and lower limbs that have become accepted as evidence of familial joint laxity (Fig. 30.15), but these do not take into account considerable racial variations. Cheng et al. [31] have shown that among Chinese children, the tests of Carter and Wilkinson are not sufficiently sensitive for children in Hong Kong because they are generally far more flexible than the European children tested by Carter and Wilkinson.

Diagnosis

In the diagnosis of flat foot, the problem is to distinguish the normal variant, usually associated with joint laxity, for which no treatment is necessary, from patients who have a

Fig. 30.15 Line drawings from Carter and Wilkinson of the five tests for joint laxity. (**a**) Hyperextension of the elbows. (**b**) Thumb can be placed on the flexor surface of the forearm. (**c**) Fingers extend parallel to the dorsum of the forearm. (**d**) Feet dorsiflex above 30°. (**e**) Knees hyperextend. Adapted with permission and copyright of the British Editorial Society of Bone and Joint Surgery [30]

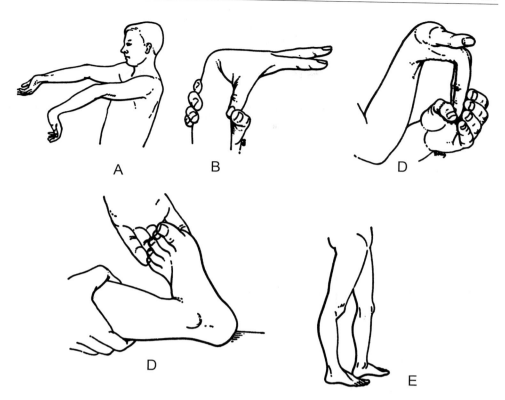

A   B   D

D   E

significant abnormality causing symptoms for which treatment is necessary and which are often due to some underlying cause not arising in the foot. Morley [32], in an unselected series of patients attending routine health clinics, showed that 97% of children younger than 18 months had apparent flat feet. By the age of 10 years, only 4% of children had any evidence of flat feet. In this series, there was no evidence that any treatment such as shoe modifications, insoles, or exercises made any difference to the natural evolution of the feet. Rose et al. in 1986 [33] published the results of an important 25-year study designed to distinguish normal anatomical variants from pathological conditions. They stated that tests for flat foot should relate to function and should be dynamic rather than static. They accepted that all except markedly valgus, everted feet in young children were normal and showed that children progressively developed an arch with time, so that initially broad feet in pre-school children became normal with time, irrespective of whether they had any treatment or not.

Rose et al. [33] pointed out that the great toe extension test is the most useful test for dynamic function of the medial arch. In this test, when the big toe is actively dorsiflexed the medial arch should rise and the tibia externally rotate (Fig. 30.16). The simplest way of testing whether a child has normal flexible flat feet that require no treatment is to get the child to stand on tip-toe. If the arches are restored by this action, the tibia rotates laterally and the heel goes into varus, the feet are normal. Wenger et al. [34], in a most important

prospective study, asked the question: "Can flexible flat feet in children be influenced by treatment?" The conclusion of this study was that flexible flat feet in young children improve with growth. Treatment with corrective shoes, inserts, or specially designed insoles did not alter the natural history of the condition. Rao and Joseph [35] in an interesting study of shod and un-shod children in India suggested that shoe wear in early childhood was detrimental to the development of a normal longitudinal arch, particularly in children with marked joint laxity. However, Echam and Forriol [36] in a similar study of shod and un-shod children in the Congo concluded that footwear made little difference.

Management

In light of the above, as far as management is concerned, there are two types of flat feet:

a. *The common flexible flat foot* is pain-free, associated with normal muscle power and mobility, and has a normal great toe extension test. This type of foot should be considered a normal variant. Frequently it is familial and associated with joint laxity. These feet require no treatment, and there is no evidence that conservative treatment of any sort alters the natural history of the condition.

b. *The pathological type of flat foot.* This is often painful. It may have abnormal muscle power being either weak

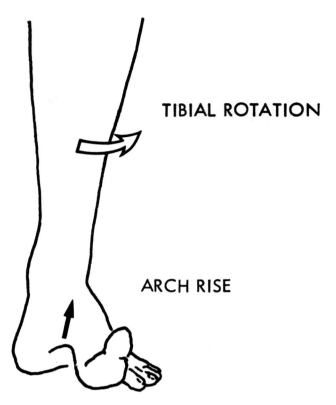

TIBIAL ROTATION

ARCH RISE

The great toe extension test.

Fig. 30.16 Line drawing from showing the great toe extension test. Reproduced with permission and copyright © of the British Editorial Society of Bone and Joint Surgery [33]

or hypertonic and may be associated with abnormal mobility, i.e., excessive movement or rigidity. These feet require careful investigation before treatment. Frequently the problem is due to a generalized condition, often neuromuscular in origin, or to some local condition arising in the foot. Treatment with insoles, shoe modifications, or exercises may be helpful in this type of foot problem, but it is essential to diagnose the underlying cause if possible.

In the rare severe idiopathic flat foot without any underlying cause, but which is developing symptoms, orthopaedic treatment may be necessary. Supporting the foot with insoles, surgical footwear, or an orthosis may relieve both symptoms and excessive shoe wear. In the older child with severe talocalcaneal hypermobility, the Grice type of subtalar arthrodesis will stabilize the subtalar joint very satisfactorily, but at the expense of permanent stiffening of the joint and possible later problems in the ankle. Localized naviculocuneiform fusion to restore the medial arch has not been successful in the long term [37]. The so-called reverse Evans

operation, described by Evans in 1975 [15] and recently popularized by Mosca [14], in which the lateral border of the foot is lengthened by inserting a wedge of bone in the anterior end of the calcaneus, has produced good results. Finally, medial displacement osteotomy of the calcaneus, described by Koutsogiannis [38], was successful in the short term in some cases.

Tarsal Coalition (Peroneal Spastic Flat Foot)

Sir Robert Jones in 1897 [39] drew attention to a form of rigid valgus everted foot in which the peroneal muscles were in spasm. This condition became known as "peroneal spastic flat foot." The association of this clinical syndrome with tarsal coalition was first described by Slomann in 1921 [40] and Badgely in 1927 [41], who reported the presence of a partial or complete calcaneo-navicular bar in association with peroneal spastic flat foot. In 1948 Harris and Beath [42] described talocalcaneal coalition, and a wide variety of forms of tarsal coalition have been described since then. The patient, who is usually in the second decade, presents with characteristic clinical signs, often after minor trauma to the foot or ankle, which are initially diagnosed as a simple twist or sprain. However, the symptoms persist. The patient continues to complain of disability, difficulty with walking and running, and, if the peroneal spasm is not recognized, may be accused of exaggerating the symptoms and a functional overlay. There are usually clear-cut clinical signs: the foot is held flat and in valgus (Fig. 30.17); the medial arch is not restored when the patient attempts to stand on tip-toe; any attempt to invert the foot at the subtalar joint causes pain, usually over the lateral side of the foot, with spasm of the peronei. Rarely, spasm of the tibialis posterior may occur with an inversion deformity [43]. Plain AP and lateral radiographs

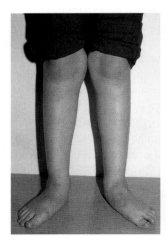

Fig. 30.17 Clinical photograph of a patient with bilateral peroneal spastic flat feet due to bilateral calcaneo-navicular bars

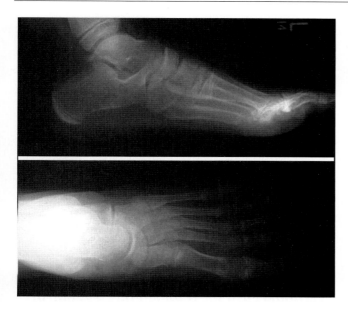

Fig. 30.18 (*Upper*) Lateral radiograph of the foot showing a partial calcaneo-navicular bar and the "anteater's nose" sign. (*Lower*) AP radiograph. Note that the calcaneo-navicular bar is very difficult to see on this view

demonstrate the valgus deformity of the foot. A useful sign of calcaneo-navicular coalition, "The anteater's nose," was reported in 1987 by Oestreich et al. [44]. A 45° oblique radiograph is also very useful when looking for a talonavicular bar. Harris and Beath [42] recommended a 45° axial view for talocalcaneal coalition. A computed tomography (CT) scan is very helpful in the assessment of all forms of tarsal coalition, and particularly talocalcaneal bars (Fig. 30.18).

The inheritance of this condition is interesting. Leonard [45] reported that, among 98 first-degree relatives of 31 patients, 39% had totally asymptomatic tarsal coalition on radiographic examination. The incidence of tarsal coalition in the population is therefore unknown as it is frequently entirely asymptomatic. Leonard postulated an autosomal dominant inheritance of almost full penetrance.

Treatment

The management of this condition can be very difficult. If a patient presents with minor symptoms, a medial arch support or medial wedge on the heel may be sufficient to support the medial arch of the foot and relieve the spasm. Frequently, however, the spasm persists. A manipulation under anesthesia, with or without local injection of hydrocortisone and local anesthetic into the subtalar region, followed by a below-knee plaster with the foot held in neutral for a period of 6–8

weeks, may be necessary. This often relieves the pain while the patient is in plaster, but it commonly relapses when the plaster is removed. Some surgeons, therefore, recommend prolonged splintage for up to 6 months using a carefully molded plastic ankle–foot orthosis. Braddock [46] published the results of conservative treatment in 56 feet followed up for 21 years. This important review showed that about 50% of the patients had suffered minor symptoms, which did not bother them significantly. Only 10% had had persistent symptoms requiring triple arthrodesis. The prognosis for the foot and the response to treatment bore no relation to the radiographic appearances, and symptomatic tarsal arthritis was rare in the long term.

From the surgical point of view, Mitchell and Gibson [47] recommended excision of the calcaneo-navicular bar in patients aged between 10 and 14 years who did not show any secondary changes in other tarsal joints. Macnicol et al. [48] reviewed 16 feet in 11 patients at an average of 23 years after excision of their calcaneo-navicular bars; 67% had had a good or excellent result. Five feet had poor results that responded well to triple arthrodesis. The so-called beaking of the talus on the preoperative radiograph correlated with a poor result from excision of the calcaneo-navicular bar. Dwyer [49] suggested calcaneal osteotomy to treat the valgus hindfoot. Cain and Hyman [50] reported the results of a closing medial wedge osteotomy of the calcaneus with satisfactory relief of pain and improved movement in the majority of the 40 feet operated upon in their series.

CT scanning has made talocalcaneal bars much easier to diagnose and assess. Olney and Asher [51] published an early report recommending resection of the persistently symptomatic talocalcaneal middle facet coalition, even in the present of talar beaking. In 1997 McCormack et al. [52] reported a 10-year follow-up of eight of these patients who had operations in nine feet. Eight of the nine feet had done well, particularly those with smaller coalitions, and none had required further surgery. The authors pointed out that this technique allows the option of a later arthrodesis if the resection does not relieve symptoms.

It is important to remember that a tarsal coalition is not always the cause of a painful peroneal spastic flat foot. It can occur after previous surgery, in particular, overcorrection of the foot in club foot, and in association with juvenile idiopathic arthritis, which frequently affects the subtalar joint in children. It may also be seen in association with infection in the hindfoot and tumors such as an osteoid osteoma. Blockey [53] drew attention to the fact that peroneal spasm can occur without a tarsal anomaly and that the presence of a tarsal anomaly does not mean that the foot is inevitably stiff. He postulated that a tarsal coalition makes the foot more liable to break down under stress and that a minor injury may precipitate peroneal spasm. It is important for the orthopaedic surgeon to recognize this condition and treat it energetically, before the spasm becomes established.

The Toes

Curly Toes

The majority of babies at birth show significant flexion of the toes, particularly the lateral three toes which may also adopt a varus alignment (Fig. 30.19). This often causes anxiety among parents, even before the child starts to walk, particularly if one of the adults in the family or a close relative has recently had problems from toe deformities. In general, if the toe can be passively straightened and there is no fixed deformity, it is most unlikely to cause any symptoms. However, if there is a fixed deformity this may require treatment once the child is established in walking. Many years ago, Trethowan [54] recommended over- and understrapping. Sweetnam [55] was unable to find any evidence that this type of conservative treatment influenced the natural history of the disorder. Most parents found it extremely difficult to persist with this treatment for more than a few months. In the majority of patients curly toes do not cause any symptoms and should be left alone. In the few cases in which there is persistent deformity causing symptoms, surgical correction by simple tenotomy of the flexor tendon, as reported by Menelaus and Ross [56], has given good results from a simple procedure that can be performed on a day-case basis and allows the patient to walk within 24 hours of the operation. Some surgeons recommend the insertion of an axial K wire to hold the digit straight while the tenotomized tendon heals in a lengthened position. This is much simpler than formal transfer of the long-toe flexor into the extensor as described by Taylor [57], which is probably best reserved for patients with severe clawing of the toes associated with neuromuscular imbalance.

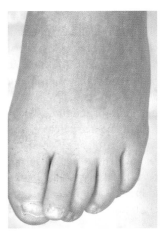

Fig. 30.19 Clinical photograph of an infant showing typical, curly lateral three toes

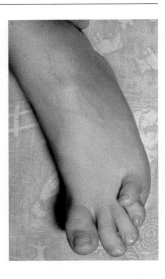

Fig. 30.20 Clinical photograph showing an overlapping fifth toe (congenital elevation of the fifth toe)

Overriding Fifth Toe (Congenital Elevation of the Fifth Toe)

This is a true congenital deformity of the fifth toe which is hypoplastic, elevated, and rotated medially. It overlies the fourth toe (Fig. 30.20). The deformity is fixed and does not correct spontaneously with time. Treatment is required if problems with shoe wear and pressure from the shoes on the toe become troublesome. Conservative measures are rarely successful, and a number of surgical procedures have been described. A simple V-Y plasty, described by Wilson [58], releases the dorsal contracture, but often the toe will not remain corrected after this procedure and the deformity recurs. The double V-Y plasty, described by Butler and reported by Cockin [59], combines a V-Y plasty on the dorsum of the foot and a Y-V plasty on the sole of the foot, connecting the two so that the toe is not only released dorsally but also pulled down into the plantigrade position by the Y-V plasty on the sole. This can provide good correction but must be performed with care to avoid damage to the neuromuscular bundles. Unfortunately, the new, lateralized position of the fifth toe may increase shoe pressure from the side, with resurgence of the deformity. More radical bony procedures such as proximal phalangectomy or even amputation of the fifth toe should be reserved for patients who have failed previous soft tissue surgery.

Hallux Valgus

Hallux valgus in the young child is rare unless it is associated with other major congenital anomalies affecting the foot, such as Apert's syndrome (acrocephalosyndactyly). However, it becomes increasingly common in teenagers. In

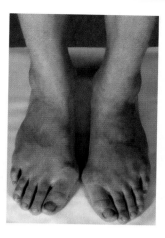

Fig. 30.21 Clinical photograph of bilateral hallux valgus in an adolescent. Note the broad forefoot, prominent medial bunion, and fifth metatarsal bunionette

Corrective Procedures

More than 100 procedures have been described for the correction of hallux valgus. Bony procedures performed before the end of growth in the foot, at 13–14 years of age, are likely to fail because of recurrent deformity. Therefore, in the very rare case in which it is necessary to consider surgery before skeletal maturity, McBride's [61] so-called conservative operation is indicated. If at all possible, the surgeon should try to delay operation until skeletal maturity. Unfortunately, splints, insoles, and physiotherapy have little effect upon hallux valgus, and the only reasonable conservative treatment is to ensure that adequately fitting shoes are worn that do not press on the toes or the bunion.

Once skeletal maturity is reached, there is a bewildering array of osteotomies. Helal et al. [62] reviewed the results of a number of procedures and came to the conclusion that the oblique or Wilson osteotomy gave the most consistent results. The problem with this oblique osteotomy is that it can shorten the first metatarsal and so it is unsuitable if the second toe is particularly long. As in all metatarsal osteotomies, it is absolutely essential that the metatarsal head is not allowed to displace dorsally, thus reducing weight bearing on the first metatarsal head and increasing the pressure on the second metatarsal head, leading to metatarsalgia and, occasionally, stress fracture. The Chevron osteotomy, described by Johnson et al. in 1979 [63], is aimed at reducing the amount of shortening and holding the metatarsal head more firmly. This operation undoubtedly controls the metatarsal head well, but it is important not to damage the blood supply to the metatarsal head and to avoid avascular necrosis, which leads to pain and joint degeneration. Other popular forms of metatarsal osteotomy are the Homann-Thomason, described by Mygind [64] in which a peg is used to hold the head in position, the Mitchell [65], and more recently the scarf osteotomy [66]. Most surgeons will try a variety of these distal osteotomies and then settle on the one which they find works best for them.

In many ways proximal osteotomy at the base of the first metatarsal seems more logical. Clearly, this should be used with great care before skeletal maturity, because the growth plate is proximal and not distal, and must not be damaged. However, although good results have been reported by Simmonds and Menelaus [67], it is a more difficult procedure. It is harder to correct the metatarsal alignment and obtain long-term satisfactory results. It may be necessary, in severe cases, to combine the McBride procedure with a basal osteotomy to obtain full control of the deformity. Mann et al. [68] reported satisfactory results in 93% of patients in whom the combination of a basal crescentic first metatarsal osteotomy was combined with a modified McBride procedure. However, only 7 of 75 patients were younger than 20

the past, it was frequently assumed that this condition was caused by poorly fitting shoes, and parents were blamed for their child's hallux valgus. However, the condition is much more likely to be familial rather than acquired. Patients with this type of foot have a characteristically supple, broad forefoot with hallux valgus and a bunion on the medial side and often a bunionette or fifth metatarsal bunion on the lateral side (Fig. 30.21). Ill-fitting shoes do not cause the deformity, but they can cause symptoms by pressure over the medial side of the metatarsal head, leading to development of a bunion and crowding of the toes.

Medial deviation of the first metatarsal (metatarsus primus varus) is common and may be associated with a lateral deviation of the fifth metatarsal and a bunionette. Metatarsus varus is very common in young children and it is tempting to suggest that hallux valgus is the long-term result; however, there is no good evidence for this. Farsetti et al. [5], in their long-term review of metatarsus varus, found only one case of mild hallux valgus in one foot. In 1960, Piggot [60] in a very useful review showed that up to 20° of valgus at the first metatarsophalangeal joint is within normal limits. Between 20 and 25° of valgus, the big toe is deviated but does not necessarily progress to hallux valgus. Adolescents and young adults with this degree of valgus should be watched. However, once the valgus angle is greater than 25° progressive deformity is almost inevitable. Similarly, lateral subluxation of the proximal phalanx of the big toe on the first metatarsal head leads to inevitable progression of the deformity and, ultimately, degenerative change. The paper by Piggott [60] provides a rational basis for advising surgical correction: up to 20° there is no indication for surgery on account of the deformity itself; between 20 and 25° the situation should be watched; when there is more than 25° of deformity or lateral subluxation of the proximal phalanx on the metatarsal head, it is reasonable to offer surgical correction to prevent further progression and ultimately osteoarthritis in the joint.

Fig. 30.22 Clinical photograph of an overriding second toe. Note inward curling of the third, fourth, and fifth toes

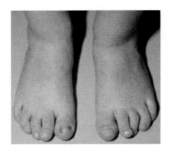

Fig. 30.23 Clinical photograph of severe hallux varus in association with a localized fibrous band

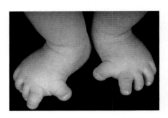

years, and the authors have made no special mention, in the description of the operative technique, of the care necessary to avoid damage to the epiphyseal plate at the base of the first metatarsal in patients in whom it is still open. Recently Davids et al. [69] have reported lateral hemiepiphysiodesis of the great toe for juvenile hallux valgus, with encouraging early results.

Overriding Second Toe

This condition is commonly seen in children's feet, particularly in association with curly third, fourth, and fifth toes (Fig. 30.22). The hallux is in mild valgus and the lateral three toes curl medially, so that the second toe is displaced dorsally and lies at a higher level than the first metatarsal and other toes. The condition is nearly always fully correctable passively and corrects spontaneously when the child starts to walk. Provided there is no fixed deformity, no treatment is indicated and parents can be reassured that, if shoes of adequate width are fitted, once the child starts to walk the condition should not cause any further problems. Very occasionally there is a persistent fixed contracture and tenotomy of the extensor tendon is indicated. Fixed flexion deformity of the third toe can also occur. If this does not correct with passive stretching by the mother, then a fixed hammer toe deformity can develop, causing problems with shoe wear and the development of the toenail. Simple flexor tenotomy or, occasionally, flexor-to-extensor transfer may be necessary if the deformity is symptomatic.

Hallux Varus

Minor forms of this condition are very common in association with metatarsus varus. Provided the deformity is fully correctable passively, the hallux varus should correct as the forefoot varus corrects, without any specific treatment. It can also occur as an isolated phenomenon in association with a localized fibrous band on the medial side of the foot (Fig. 30.23). If this fails to respond to passive stretching, the contracted fibrous band on the medial side of the

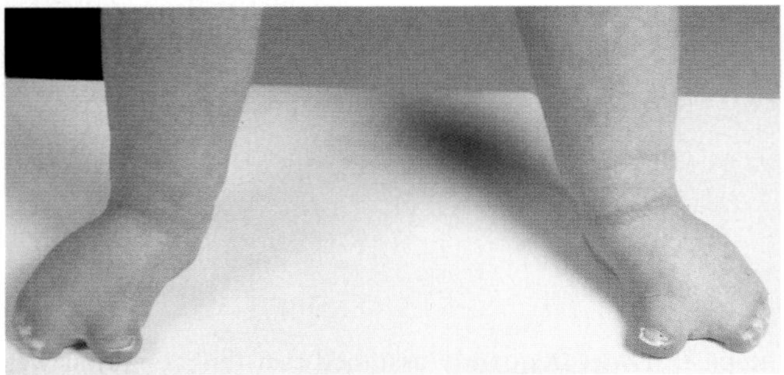

Fig. 30.24 Clinical photograph of the feet of a child with Apert's syndrome and hallux varus. Note syndactyly of the other toes

great toe, the tight abductor hallucis, and shortened medial capsule of the metatarsophalangeal joint of the big toe can be released. Finally, hallux varus may be associated with localized bony anomalies such as abnormal phalanges, duplication and accessory toes, congenital short first metatarsal, and with generalized conditions such as Apert's syndrome (acrocephalosyndactyly) (Fig. 30.24), diastrophic dwarfism, and myositis ossificans progressiva. Quite extensive and complex soft tissue and bony surgery may be necessary to correct hallux varus in these patients. [70, 71].

Hallux Rigidus

Hallux rigidus occurs in children and adolescents. Unlike the condition in adults, it is more common in girls than in boys. McMaster [72] has suggested an acute pathogenesis, or that chronic trauma associated with stubbing or stress on the big toe may cause a chondral or osteochondral injury to the head of the first metatarsal. Radiographically this is often not seen because it is largely or entirely a chondral lesion. As a result of the injury, the patient develops so-called metatarsus primus elevatus from spasm of the flexor of the big toe, with loss of dorsiflexion of the big toe and tenderness over the dorsum of the metatarsophalangeal joint. The patient walks awkwardly on the outer side of the foot as a result of loss of the normal "rock-over" at the first metatarsophalangeal joint. Protection of the joint by a rocker bar may relieve the symptoms, as may a short period of rest in a plaster. If, however, this fails, a dorsal closing wedge osteotomy of the proximal phalanx of the big toe as described by Bonney and MacNab

[73] can produce good results, provided the patient has 30° of plantar flexion before surgery. Citron and Neil [74] reported good long-term results at an average follow-up of 22 years in nine of ten toes treated with dorsal wedge osteotomy of the proximal phalanx. Radiographically the usual changes of degenerative arthritis are not seen in children, but sometimes a defect similar to that of osteochondritis of the knee may be seen on the metatarsal head, as has been reported by Kessel and Bonney [75].

Metatarsus Primus Elevatus

This condition was believed by Lambrinudi [76] to be a primary developmental abnormality. Nowadays, most surgeons would consider this to be secondary to plantar flexor spasm of the big toe. This may be seen in association with hallux rigidus and after surgical procedures on the mid- or hindfoot that cause supination of the foot so that the first metatarsal is elevated and the big toe has to be held in flexion in order to reach the ground. This is seen after surgery for congenital talipes equinovarus and also in neuromuscular conditions such as poliomyelitis and spina bifida. The patient develops pain over the dorsal bunion and also from the flexion of the big toe. It can be a difficult condition to treat unless muscle balance can be restored. This imbalance is commonly associated with a strong tibialis anterior, elevating the first metatarsal, and weakness of the peroneus longus. Lapidus [77] described transfer of flexor hallucis longus through a tunnel in the first metatarsal into the dorsum of the proximal phalanx, with a basal osteotomy of the first metatarsal, for this deformity.

Interphalangeal Valgus of the Big Toe

Sometimes valgus of the big toe occurs, not at the metatarsophalangeal joint but at the interphalangeal joint, usually associated with a congenital anomaly of the distal phalanx. This can cause problems with the distal phalanx pressing on the second toe, or even lying underneath it. Radiographs may show a malformation of the interphalangeal joint, the epiphysis of the distal phalanx often appearing wedge shaped, the base of the wedge being on the medial side. If symptoms are sufficient, the deformity can be corrected either by osteotomy of the proximal phalanx, removing a medially based wedge, or after growth has finished by fusion of the interphalangeal joint, provided there is a full range of pain-free movement at the first metatarsophalangeal joint.

Duplication, Syndactyly, and Accessory Toes

Minor anomalies such as duplication, syndactyly, and accessory toes are quite common. They may occur on their own or in association with generalized conditions such as chondroectodermal dysplasia (Ellis–Van Creveld syndrome) and Apert's syndrome (Fig. 30.24) and also with local abnormalities such as tibial dysplasia. Congenital shortening of the first metatarsal is seen in fibrodysplasia (myositis) ossificans progressiva (Chapter 7) and dysplastic nails in the nail-patella syndrome (onycho-osteodystrophy). It is very important to look at the entire patient in addition to the feet.

Syndactyly frequently needs no treatment. Duplications and accessory toes can sometimes be simply reduced or removed, but occasionally the skeletal architecture is very complex and careful planning and meticulous surgery are necessary. Both Phelps and Grogan [78] and Turra et al. [79] in important reviews of surgery for polydactyly reported good long-term results in the majority of post-axial polydactyly patients but more problems in pre-axial polydactyly due to recurrent hallux varus. Parents may frequently ask for the surgery to be performed early, before the child starts to walk, but often it is better to wait until the child has reached at least the age of 1 year, so that the bony architecture of the foot can be more accurately assessed before surgery is decided upon.

The Accessory Navicular

The accessory navicular (prehallux; os tibiale externum) is one of many benign ossicles which may be detected radiographically in relation to the midfoot and hindfoot. It is the most likely to become symptomatic, particularly in later childhood, and may be familial [80]. The type 1 ossicle is very small, residing within the tibialis posterior tendon; it rarely requires excision. The type 2 is larger (approximately 1 cm in diameter) and is joined to the main navicular through cartilage. The lump is analogous with a bipartite patellar ossicle. Stress, trauma, skeletal growth, and pressure from the inner border of the shoes have all been implicated in the onset of symptoms.

Kidner [81] considered that the accessory navicular was associated with, or even causative of, flat foot. This is now disproved and his relatively complex and potentially hazardous rerouting of the tibialis posterior tendon was shown by Macnicol and Voutsinas [80] to be no better than simple excision of the accessory bone and careful contouring of the residual navicular medially.

The majority of symptomatic feet can be managed conservatively, with reassurance of the child and parents and minor adjustment of the shoes. A magnetic resonance (MR) scan reveals marrow edema [82] and helps to define the extent of the skeletal reaction. If symptoms and scan changes persist, excision of the lesion is achieved through a curved, skin crease incision and longitudinal splitting of the tendon, leaving intact the various attachments of the tibialis tendon to the tarsal bones. Unlike the postoperative splintage advised following the Kidner procedure, the lesser procedure of excision allows partial weight bearing with crutches for a few weeks and a relatively rapid resumption of normal activity.

Symptoms may recur to some extent as the child completes the adolescent growth spurt. It is therefore important to ensure that supportive and comfortable shoes do not give way to fashionable but symptom-provoking footwear.

Congenital Split or Cleft Foot (Lobster Claw Foot)

This is a rare congenital anomaly characterized by failure of development of the central two or three rays of the foot (Fig. 30.25). The first metatarsal may be normal or enlarged and the hallux is usually in valgus. There is then a large cleft and the remainder of the foot is made up of the lateral fourth or fifth rays, with the phalanges deviating medially. The hindfoot is usually normal. The common form is bilateral and inherited as an autosomal dominant with incomplete penetrance. There is a more rare unilateral form, in which there is usually no family history. The condition can occur on its own or in association with clefts of the hands. It can also be associated with cleft lip and cleft palate and deafness.

Surgery may be considered to improve footwear and cosmesis. Abraham et al. [83], in a useful review, classified the deformity into three groups according to severity: type I in which a central partial forefoot cleft is present and can be treated by a soft tissue syndactylism with correction of the hallux valgus if necessary; type II, a complete forefoot cleft involving the tarsus, can be treated by a soft tissue syndactylism with osteotomy of the first ray to aid the soft tissue

closure; and type III in which there is complete absence of the first to the fourth rays, so the patients did not require surgery and managed well in normal shoes with a shoe filler or "false foot."

References

1. Bankart ASB. Metatarsus varus. Brit Med J 1921; 2: 685.
2. Harris NH. Rotational deformities and their secondary effects in the lower extremities in children. J Bone Joint Surg 1972; 54B: 172
3. Ponseti IV, Becker JR. Congenital metatarsus varus. The results of treatment. J Bone Joint Surg 1966; 48A: 702–711.
4. Rushforth GF. The natural history of hooked forefoot. J Bone Joint Surg 1978; 60B: 530–542.
5. Farsetti P, Weinstein L, Ponseti IV. The long term functional and radiographic outcomes of untreated and non-operatively treated metatarsus adductus. J Bone Joint Surg 1994; 76A: 257–265.
6. Katz K, David R, Soudry M. Below knee plaster cast for the treatment of metatarsus adductus. J Paediatr Orthop 1999; 19: 49–50.
7. Browne RS, Paton DF. Anomalous insertion of the tibialis posterior in congenital metatarsus varus. J Bone Joint Surg 1979; 61B: 74–76.
8. Heyman CH, Herndon CH, Strong JM. Mobilisation of the tarso-metatarsal and intermetatarsal joints for the correction of resistant adduction of the forepart of the foot in congenital club foot or congenital metatarsus varus. J Bone Joint Surg 1986; 40A: 299–310.
9. Stark KG, Johanson JE, Winter RB. The Heyman-Hendon tarsometatarsal capsulotomy for metatarsus adductus; results in 48 feet. J Paediatr Orthop 1987; 7: 305–310.
10. Berman A, Gartland J. Metatarsal osteotomy for the correction of adduction of the forepart of the foot in children. J Bone Joint Surg 1971; 53A: 498–506.
11. Bleck EE. Metatarsus adductus: classification and relationship to outcomes of treatment. J Paediatr Orthop 1983; 3: 2–9.
12. Kite JH. Congenital metatarsus varus. J Bone Joint Surg 1967; 46A: 388–397.
13. Lloyd-Roberts GC, Clark RC. Ball and socket ankle joint in metatarsus adductus varus. J Bone Joint Surg 1973; 55B: 193–196.
14. Mosca VA. Flexible flat foot and skew foot. J Bone Joint Surg 1995; 77A: 1937–1945.
15. Evans D. Calcaneovalgus deformity. J Bone Joint Surg 1975; 57B: 170–278.
16. Fowler SB, Banks AL, Parrish TF. The cavovarus foot. J Bone Joint Surg 1959; 41A: 757.
17. Lloyd-Roberts GC, Pilcher MF. Structural idiopathic scoliosis in infancy. J Bone Joint Surg 1965; 47B: 520–523.
18. Giannestras J. Foot Disorders, Medical and Surgical Management, 2nd ed. London: Henry Kimpton; 1973.
19. Sutherland DM, Olsehn R, Cooper L, Woo SLY. The development of mature gait. J Bone Joint Surg 1980; 62A: 336–353.
20. Hall JE, Salter RB, Bhalla SK. Congenital short tendo calcaneus. J Bone Joint Surg 1967; 49B: 695–697.
21. Eastwood DM, Cole G, Dickens DRD. Idiopathic toe walking: is this a neurological problem "solved" by surgery? Proceedings of the British Society of Children's Orthopaedic Surgery. J Bone Join Surg 1996; 78B:(Suppl 1) 11.
22. Stricker SJ, Angulo JC. Idiopathic toe-walking: a comparison of treatment methods. J Paediatr Orthop 1998; 18: 289–293.
23. Stott NS, Walt SE, Lobb GA, et al. Treatment for idiopathic toe-walking: results at skeletal maturity. J Pediatr Orthop 2004; 24: 63–69.

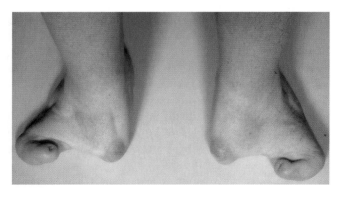

Fig. 30.25 Clinical photograph of the severe form of cleft (lobster claw) foot (Abrahams et al. [78] type III)

24. Kohler A. Uber einer haufige bisher ansheinend uberkannte Erkrankung einzeiner kindlicher Knocken Munchen. Medizinische Wochtenschrift 1908; 55: 1923.

25. Waugh W. The ossification and vascularisation of the tarsal navicular and their relation to Kohler's disease. J Bone Joint Surg 1958; 40B: 765–777.

26. Cox MJ. Kohler's disease. Postgrad Med J 1958; 34: 58–59.

27. Sever JW. Apophysitis of the os calcis. NY Med J 1912; 95: 1025–1029.

28. Antoniou D, Connor AM. Osteomyelitis of the calcaneus and talus. J Bone Joint Surg 1974; 56A: 338–345.

29. Staheli LT, Chew BE, Corbett M. The longitudinal arch. A survey of 882 feet in normal children. J Bone Joint Surg 1987; 69A: 426–428.

30. Carter C, Wilkinson J. Persistent joint laxity and congenital dislocation of the hip. J Bone Joint Surg 1964; 46B: 40–45.

31. Cheng JCY, Chan PS, Hui PW. Joint laxity in children. J Paediatr Orthop 1991; 11: 752–756.

32. Morley AJM. Knock knee in children. Brit Med J 1957; 2: 976–979.

33. Rose GK, Welton CA, Marshal T. The diagnosis of flat foot in the child. J Bone Joint Surg 1986; 67B: 71–78.

34. Wenger DR, Maudlin D, Speck G, et al. Corrective shoes and inserts as treatment for flexible flat foot in infants and children J Bone Joint Surg 1989; 71A: 800–810.

35. Rao UB, Joseph B. The influence of footwear on the prevalence of flat foot. J Bone Joint Surg 1992; 74B: 525–527.

36. Echam JJ, Forriol F. The development in foot print morphology in 1851 Congolese children from urban and rural areas and the relationship between this and wearing shoes. J Pediatr Orthop B 2003; 12: 141–146.

37. Seymour N. The late results of naviculo-cuneiform fusion. J Bone Joint Surg 1967; 49B: 558–559.

38. Koutsogiannis E. Treatment of mobile flat feet by displacement osteotomy of the calcaneus. J Bone Joint Surg 1971; 53B: 96–100.

39. Jones Sir R. Peroneal spasm and its treatment. Report on a meeting of the Liverpool Medical Institution Journal 1897; 17: 442.

40. Slomann MC. Coalition calcaneo navicularis. J Orthop Surg 1921; 3: 586–602.

41. Badgely CE. Coalition of the calcaneus and the navicular. Arch Surg 1927; 15: 75–88.

42. Harris RI, Beath T. Etiology of peroneal spastic flat foot. J Bone Joint Surg 1948; 30B: 624–634.

43. Simmons EH. Tibialis posterior varus foot with tarsal coalition. J Bone Joint Surg 1965; 47B: 533–536.

44. Oestreich E, Mize WA, Crawford AH, Morgan RB. The "anteater's nose." A direct sign of calcaneo navicular coalition on the lateral radiograph. J Paediatr Orthop 1987; 7: 709–711.

45. Leonard MA. The inheritance of tarsal coalition and its relationship to spastic flat foot. J Bone Joint Surg 1974; 56B: 520–525.

46. Braddock GTF. A prolonged follow up of peroneal spastic flat foot. J Bone Joint Surg 1961; 43B: 734–737.

47. Mitchell GP, Gibson JMC. Excision of calcaneonavicular bar for painful spasmodic flat foot. J Bone Joint Surg 1967; 49B: 281–287.

48. Macnicol MF, Inglis G, Buxton RA. Symptomatic calcaneonavicular bars. J Bone Joint Surg 1986; 68B: 128–131.

49. Dwyer FC. Causes, significance and treatment of stiffness of the subtaloid joint. Proc Royal Soc Med 1976; 69: 97–102.

50. Cain TJ, Hyman S. Peroneal spastic flat foot. J Bone Joint Surg 1978; 60B: 527–529.

51. Olney BW, Asher MA. Excision of symptomatic coalition of the middle facet of the talo-calcaneal joint. J Bone Joint Surg 1987; 69A: 539–544.

52. McCormack J, Olney B, Asher M. Talo-calcaneal coalition resection: a 10-year follow up. J Paediatr Orthop 1997; 17: 13–15.

53. Blockey NJ. Peroneal spastic flat foot. J Bone Joint Surg 1959; 37B: 191–202.

54. Trethowan WH. Treatment of hammer toes. Lancet 1925; 1: 1257–1258.

55. Sweetnam DR. Congenital curly toes. An investigation into the value of treatment. Lancet 1958; 2: 398–400.

56. Meneiaus MB, Ross ERS. Open flexor tenotomy for hammer toes and curly toes in childhood. J Bone Joint Surg 1984; 66B: 770–771.

57. Taylor RG. The treatment of claw toes by multiple transfers and flexor to extensor tendons. J Bone Joint Surg 1951; 35B: 539–542.

58. Wilson JN. V-Y correction for varus deformity of the 5th toe. Br J Surg 1953; 41: 133–135.

59. Cockin J. Butler's operation for overriding 5th toe. J Bone Joint Surg 1968; 60B: 78–81.

60. Piggot H. The natural history of hallux valgus in adolescents and early adult life. J Bone Joint Surg 1960; 42B: 749–760.

61. McBride ED. A conservative operation for bunions. J Bone Joint Surg 1928; 10B: 735–739.

62. Helal B, Gupta SK, Gojaseni P. Surgery for adolescent hallux valgus. Acta Orthop Scand 1974; 45: 271–295.

63. Johnson KA, Cofield RH, Morrey BF. Chevron osteotomy for hallux valgus. Clin Orthop Rel Res 1979; 142: 44–47.

64. Mygind H. Operations for hallux valgus. Report of Danish Orthopaedic Association. J Bone Joint Surg 1952; 34B: 529.

65. Mitchell CL, Fleming JL, Allen R, et al. Osteotomy bunionectomy for hallux valgus. J Bone Joint Surg 1958; 40A: 41–49.

66. Crevoisier X, Mouhsine E, Ortolano V, et al. The scarf osteotomy for the treatment of hallux valgus deformity: a review of 84 cases. Foot Ankle Int 2001; 22: 970–976.

67. Simmonds FA, Menelaus MB. Hallux valgus in adolescence. J Bone Joint Surg 1960; 42B: 761–768.

68. Mann RA, Rudicel S, Grabes SC. Repair of hallux valgus with a distal soft tissue procedure and proximal metatarsal osteotomy. J Bone Joint Surg 1992; 74A: 124–129.

69. Davids JR, McBrayer D, Blackhurst DW. Juvenile Hallux Valgus Deformity, Surgical Manager by lateral hemiepiphyseodesis of the great toe metatarsal. J Pediatr Orthop 2007; 27: 826–70.

70. Mubarak SJ, O'Brien J, Davids JR. Metatarsal epiphyseal bracket: treatment by central physiolysis. J Paediatr Orthop 1993; 13: 5–8.

71. Anderson PJ, Hall CM, Evans RD, et al. The feet in Apert's syndrome. J Paediatr Orthop 1999; 19: 504–507.

72. McMaster MJ. The pathogenesis of hallux rigidus. J Bone Joint Surg 1978; 60B: 82–87.

73. Bonney G, MacNab I. Hallux valgus and hallux rigidus. A critical survey of operative results. J Bone Joint Surg 1952; 34B: 366–385.

74. Citron N, Neil M. Dorsal wedge osteotomy of the proximal phalanx for hallux rigidus. J Bone Joint Surg 1987; 69B: 835–837.

75. Kessel I, Bonney G. Hallux rigidus in the adolescent. J Bone Joint Surg 1958; 40B: 668–673.

76. Lambrinudi C. Metatarsus primus elevatus. Proc Royal Soc Med 1938; 31: 1273.

77. Lapidus PW. "Dorsal Bunion": its mechanics and operative correction. J Bone Joint Surg 1940; 22: 627–637.

78. Phelps DA , Grogan DP. Polydactyly of the foot. J Pediatr Orthop 1985; 5: 448–451.

79. Turra S, Gigante C, Businella G. Polydactyly of the foot. J Pediatr Orthop 2007; B 16: 216–220.

80. Macnicol MF, Voutsinas S. Surgical treatment of the symptomatic accessory navicular. J Bone Joint Surg 1984; 66B: 218–222.

81. Kidner FC. The prehallux (accessory scaphoid) in its relation to flat foot. J Bone Joint Surg 1929; 11: 831–834.

82. Miller TT, Staron RB, Feldman F, et al. The symptomatic accessory tarsal navicular bone: assessment with MR imaging. Radiology 1995; 195: 849–53.

83. Abraham E, Waxman B, Shirali S, Durkin M. Congenital cleft foot deformity treatment. J Paediatr Orthop 1999; 19: 404–430.

Chapter 31

The Clubfoot: Congenital Talipes Equinovarus

Deborah M. Eastwood

The clubfoot is a common, classic, paediatric orthopaedic problem. Every orthopaedic surgeon knows what the deformity looks like but most find it more difficult to describe or to define. The etiology is still largely unknown but ideas about treatment have changed considerably over the last few years.

The overall picture of a talipes equinovarus deformity is one of ankle equinus, hindfoot varus, and forefoot adduction with pronation of the first ray giving the appearance of cavus (Fig. 31.1a). The typical, isolated clubfoot is congenital and idiopathic in origin. Some cases are positional or postural in which case the deformity, by definition, resolves completely by 3 months with minimal treatment. At the other end of the spectrum some examples of rigid clubfoot are associated with syndromic conditions and more generalized musculoskeletal problems (Fig. 31.1b). A further subgroup of foot problems are seen in neuromuscular disorders such as spina bifida where the deformity may worsen with time as the neuromuscular imbalance develops (Table 31.1).

Incidence

The incidence of isolated clubfoot varies between racial groups: in Caucasians the rate of idiopathic cases is approximately 1:1000 live births; in Asians, slightly lower at 0.7:1000; and in Aboriginals, Polynesians, Maoris, and native Hawaiians, the rate of 4–6:1000 is significantly higher. All studies agree that boys are more commonly affected than girls: the ratio is usually quoted as 2:1 but rising to 4:1 in the Aboriginal groups. Among live births, approximately 50% of cases are bilateral.

A familial tendency is apparent among first-degree relatives but inheritance is considered by most to be multifactorial (Table 31.2) [1–3].

The complex clubfoot, one that is associated with other congenital anomalies, has an incidence of 0.7–0.9:1000 births and is significantly more likely to be bilateral.

Other factors associated with an increased incidence are first-trimester amniocentesis [4], maternal smoking [5, 6], hyperemesis, and maternal anemia [3].

Antenatal Diagnosis

In developed countries, antenatal ultrasound scans are now used almost universally in the management of the mother and child during pregnancy. Increasingly, ultrasonography is also being used to detect fetal anomalies such as a clubfoot but the false-positive rates can be high, depending upon the timing of the scan, the skill of the operator, and whether or not the scan is primarily assessing the pregnancy or the fetus. The detection of these anomalies has obvious implications for the parents and the medical staff as both groups require accurate information regarding the condition and its prognosis in order to plan management. In certain cases, termination of the pregnancy may be an option.

The overall detection rate of talipes equinovarus foot deformities in utero has improved with time and, currently, in a large non-selected Norwegian population, 77% of cases were identified antenatally [7]. The earliest such cases that can be identified is at 12 weeks but "new" cases can be seen as late as the third trimester [8]. Bar-Hava et al. [9] have noted that the clubfoot deformity can appear as a transient phenomenon and others have noted that the diagnosis, or the complexity of the case, can change during pregnancy in up to 25% of cases [10]. Many authors have stressed the need for sequential and detailed fetal anomaly scans (DFAS) in order to reduce the false-positive rate. Bar-On et al. report a positive predictive value of 83% (a false-positive rate of 17%) [10]. Generally, it is easier to detect bilateral cases

D.M. Eastwood (✉)
Department of Paediatric Orthopaedics, Great Ormond Street Hospital, London, UK

M. Benson et al. (eds.), *Children's Orthopaedics and Fractures,*
DOI 10.1007/978-1-84882-611-3_31, © Springer-Verlag London Limited 2010

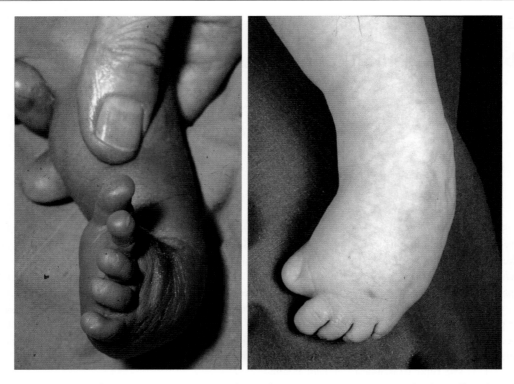

Fig. 31.1 (**a**) Clinical photograph of a unilateral idiopathic clubfoot deformity. (**b**) Clinical photograph of a unilateral syndromic clubfoot deformity

Table 31.1 Types of clubfoot

Type	Characteristic	Other features	Example
Idiopathic	Rigid foot	Isolated finding	
Postural	More supple	Associated with other "moulding" affects, e.g., plagiocephaly	
Neuromuscular	Often rigid but not necessarily so	Altered muscle tone and reflexes. Sensory changes and muscle imbalance	Spina bifida or myelomeningocele
Syndromic	Very rigid	Associated with widespread musculoskeletal abnormalities and often anomalies affecting other systems	Constriction bands; Arthrogryposis; Tibial dysplasia; Larsen syndrome; Pierre Robin; syndrome; diastrophic dwarfism

and these are more likely to be the complex cases [7]. Thus, correspondingly, the false-positive rate is higher in the isolated cases [11]. It is therefore important not only to detect cases but also to classify them accurately. Bar-On et al. [10] reported an accuracy of 73% in obtaining a specific diagnosis of an isolated versus a complex deformity and they noted that all errors were ones of overdiagnosis.

It is important to recognize that the in utero diagnosis of a clubfoot deformity does not correlate with the severity of the condition at birth. Indeed, in some studies a postural clubfoot at birth is considered as a positive finding, while in others such a case is labeled as a false positive: perhaps, the term *functional false positive* should be used for

these cases [12]. Certainly, when counseling parents antenatally, it is important to recognize that some apparently severe foot deformities may require minimal or indeed no postnatal treatment [12, 13]. The rates of surgical intervention quoted almost all predate the widespread use of the Ponseti technique and in terms of contemporary management are probably meaningless. While it is likely that more detailed scans and advancing technology will improve our understanding of the prenatal foot deformity, there is no suggestion as yet that fetal surgery in utero would be helpful.

At present, there is no indication for amniocentesis and karyotyping when an isolated clubfoot is diagnosed by DFAS [14].

Table 31.2 Familial influences on the presentation of clubfoot

Parent(s)	Affected child	% Chance of sibling CTEV
Normal	Male	2.5
	Female	6.5 if male 2.5 if female
Affected	Male or Female	10–25
	Monozygotic twins	Concordance rate 32.5
	Dizygotic twins	Concordance rate 3

Pathoanatomy

The primary pathology in the clubfoot is subluxation of the talonavicular joint. There are associated, similar abnormalities of the calcaneocuboid and talocalcaneal joints. The talar head is readily palpable on the dorsolateral aspect of the foot. Anatomical dissections and radiographic studies [15–17] have shown that the talus is plantarflexed and, with respect to the ankle mortise, the anterior end of the long axis of the talus has rotated laterally even though the actual talar head and neck are tilted medially and plantarward. The calcaneus is also plantarflexed and its long axis is rotated through the subtalar joint but in the opposite direction to that of the talus. This medial spin means that the anterior end of the calcaneus lies medially, while the posterior part lies adjacent to the lateral malleolus. (Fig. 31.2). Both the navicular and cuboid lie medially. All these joint subluxations are held by capsular, ligamentous, or musculotendinous contractures. The structures most commonly identified as being tight are the sheaths of the tibialis posterior tendon and the peroneal tendons, the plantar-based talocalcaneonavicular (or spring) ligament, and the calcaneofibular ligament. These ligaments contain more collagen fibers and increased cellularity on histological examination [18, 19]. Several authors [20, 21] have identified cells with myofibroblastic characteristics on electron microscopy of the medial structures of the clubfoot and consider that these may contribute to the deformities. However, a more recent paper [22] suggested that collagen crosslinking was normal and failed to identify myofibroblasts. Recently, Hattori et al. [23] have shown reduced elasticity in the lateral ligaments and capsule compared to the medial structures, adding weight to the concept of the posterolateral tether.

Abnormalities of muscle infrastructure and insertion have also been identified. There is evidence of intramuscular fibrosis and limited muscle excursion with a predominance of type 1 muscle fibers in the posteromedial muscle groups, noted along with other histological features that suggest a local or regional neurological abnormality [24–26].

The dorsalis pedis artery may be absent or its supply to the foot altered in patients with clubfoot [27, 28]. Recently, Katz et al. [29] have shown a deficient blood flow in this vessel in almost half of clubfoot cases compared with only 8% of

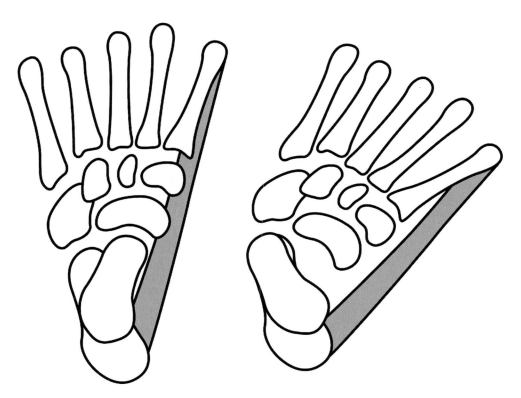

Fig. 31.2 Line diagram of the relationships between the talus and the calcaneus (and the associated tarsal bones) in the normal and the club foot

normal feet. They suggest that the severity of the deformity relates to this.

While, overall, there is agreement regarding these descriptions of the pathological changes associated with a clubfoot deformity, there is still considerable disagreement about their etiology and whether any individual anomaly is a cause or an effect. Many of the histological studies are small and have not been repeated and in the case of fetal dissections, the data may not be representative of the more general example of a clubfoot.

Etiological Theories

Genetic Influences

Many papers [30, 31] have studied the familial incidence of idiopathic talipes equinovarus and noted the different incidence in first-degree versus second- and third-degree relatives and the lack of complete concordance in monozygotic twins. They have concluded that inheritance must be multifactorial. Twin studies have characterized the increased incidence and suggested that the risk for the second monozygotic twin is 1:3 [32, 33]. Recent genetic studies are beginning to identify possible candidate genes. Ester et al. [34] noted that certain chromosomal deletions (on the long arm of chromosome 2) were associated with the clubfoot phenotype. Previous linkage studies have also implicated this region and it may harbor genes that contribute to the development of clubfoot. Single nucleotide polymorphisms (SNPs) in three apoptotic genes were investigated. Programmed cell death that is regulated by these genes is important during growth and development, and the study suggests that apoptotic genetic variation may play a role in clubfoot etiology. The same group of researchers [35] also noted the association of clubfoot with maternal smoking and investigated the biotransformation of environmental exogenous substances such as tobacco smoke which can be modulated by genes such as the N-acetylation genes (NAT1 & 2). Slow NAT2 acetylation may be a risk factor for idiopathic clubfoot with NAT2 being a possible biotransformation candidate gene.

Other Theories

Some long-standing theories on the etiology are now becoming discredited. The increased use of antenatal ultrasound scans has shown that intrauterine fetal *molding* is not a common cause of idiopathic clubfoot deformity although it may account for some of the "late" cases that develop in previously normal fetuses when the relative lack of amniotic fluid in late pregnancy may contribute to a postural clubfoot deformity. Early amniocentesis is associated with an increased incidence of clubfoot, particularly when accompanied by an amniotic fluid leak. Molding at this early stage may have a role in some cases [4].

There is an obvious association between clubfoot deformities and certain *neuromuscular* conditions such as spina bifida, and in these feet, neuromuscular imbalance must be an important factor. Much more subtle or more short-lived episodes of imbalance may be a factor in other idiopathic cases and some of the pathological muscle changes identified would support a resolving neuropathic process [25]. It is difficult to know whether the changes seen are primary or adaptive and more recent studies have failed to substantiate these theories [36].

The primary abnormality may be with the initial formation of the cartilage anlage or a *failure of the normal maturation process* during fetal development. The fetal foot position changes from one of equinovarus to one of calcaneovalgus at about the same time as changes in blood supply to the fetal limb occur. Problems with this maturation process may account for those cases in which the dorsalis pedis pulse is absent and the deformity severe [29].

It is well recognized that the clubfoot is often small and the calf thin and possibly short. Shimode et al. [37] confirmed these findings and quantified the field change that affects growth of the whole lower limb including the femur and thigh. Changes in limb length and girth were more obvious distally than proximally and were significantly more obvious in the operatively treated cases compared to those treated conservatively.

It is unlikely that one single etiological agent or theory can account for all cases of clubfoot deformity. The etiology is probably multifactorial, different influences affecting foot development at different stages with potentially a summative effect on the severity of the deformity. Thus a genetic tendency allied to a mild, temporary neuromuscular imbalance may lead to a foot deformity that could be significantly exacerbated in the later stages of pregnancy by a period of intrauterine molding.

If the relevant influences producing any individual deformity could be identified, this might help to establish a better individual prognosis and affect the choice of treatment.

Clinical Assessment

The diagnosis of a clubfoot deformity is clinical. A full assessment of the child will help to distinguish the idiopathic foot from the "syndromic" foot (Table 31.1) and identify any obvious underlying neuromuscular imbalance. Careful note should be made of skin or soft tissue dimples or signs of an amniotic band as these features are indicative of a "syndromic" foot and are associated with a poorer response to treatment.

The flexibility of the foot is an important feature and the fixed deformities at each level should be identified and quantified as this helps the clinician to understand which tight structures are limiting joint movement and may influence treatment. Deep posterior and medial skin creases are universal in the idiopathic clubfoot and may distinguish this foot from a simple postural deformity.

Classification Systems

Although several systems exist it is becoming apparent that only two are useful in terms of ease of application and communication, reliability, and as a guide to prognosis.

Both of the commonly used systems of Dimeglio [38] (Fig. 31.3) and Pirani [39] (Table 31.3) apply a point score to various physical findings which when summated differentiate between mildly affected feet that require little or no treatment and the more severely affected foot that is likely to require treatment. Flynn et al. [40] showed good inter- and intra-observer correlation with both systems and noted that there was a significant improvement in correlation once the learning curve had been "completed." The Pirani score has been modified, but not revalidated, since this study. Wainwright et al. [41] looked at four commonly used classification systems in the United Kingdom and found the Dimeglio system to be the most reliable.

It is hoped that such systems will be used increasingly to quantify the severity of the clubfoot being treated in order to allow a more valid comparison of treatment methods.

Imaging

Traditionally, plain radiographs have formed part of the baseline evaluation of the clubfoot deformity but often the information obtained was of limited value. Standard radiographic views are difficult to obtain so this tends to invalidate attempts at radiographic measurement, as does the observation that the ossific nuclei may be more eccentrically placed within the cartilage anlage in the clubfoot than in the normal infantile foot. Stress radiographs that theoretically might quantify the flexibility of the infant foot are also difficult to obtain. Radiographs may be useful in simple terms to exclude any obvious bony abnormality such as a tibial dysplasia masquerading as a clubfoot deformity (Fig. 31.4). The lateral and

anteroposterior (AP) talocalcaneal angles should diverge: parallelism in one or both views, particularly on simulated weight bearing, suggests persistent deformity. Radiographs can also identify "false correction" when dorsiflexion is occurring as a result of a midfoot breech.

Computed tomography (CT) and magnetic resonance (MR) scans define the pathoanatomy of the deformity and have been used to document the effects of treatment on the foot, but neither technique is used for primary assessment of the infant clubfoot.

Ultrasound does show promise in evaluating the clubfoot. Several studies have identified ultrasonographic features that are reliably different in the clubfoot and the normal foot and these can be used to assess the foot and monitor the effect of treatment. The most commonly used measurement is the medial malleolar to navicular (MMN) distance which is significantly lower in clubfeet than in normal feet and although the distance increases in both feet with age, the rate of change is significantly less in the clubfoot [42].

Management of the Idiopathic Foot

Over recent years, there has been a reversal in philosophy concerning the most effective treatment of the infant clubfoot deformity with a complete swing away from the extensive surgical approach that all too often seemed to follow "traditional" conservative regimes [43]. Manipulative techniques have been in use for several centuries, the Thomas wrench being an early, extreme example of this, and Kite's method, a more acceptable and popular method in the mid-20th century. Dissatisfaction with the results of these relatively lengthy treatment protocols led to a swing toward surgical releases but the long-term results of such surgery have been disappointing [44]. Not surprisingly, this encouraged a trend back to conservative methods just at the time when one particular technique was reporting improved long-term results. This happened simultaneously with the development of the simple, effective scoring systems mentioned above that allowed practitioners to document the type of foot they were seeing and, to a certain extent, the influence of treatment upon it.

Ponseti Method

The Ponseti [45] method of treatment corrects the clubfoot by a process of serial manipulations and cast applications that sequentially correct the three essential deformities of the foot namely the cavus, the adduction, and the equinovarus. Several minutes of manipulation are required at every cast

Classification			Assessment of Clubfoot by Severity Scale			
Classification grade	Type	Score	Characteristics: Deformity	Points (pts)	Characteristics: Other parameters	Points (pts)
I	Benign	(<5)	90–45°	4	Posterior crease	1
II	Moderate	(=5<10)	45–20°	3	Medial crease	1
III	Severe	(=10<15)	20–0°	2	Cavus	1
IV	Very severe	(=15<20)	<20 to –20°	1	Poor muscle condition	1

Sagittal plane evaluation of equinus

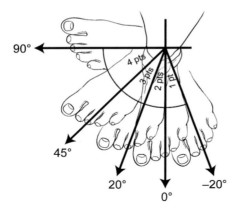

Frontal plane evaluation of varus

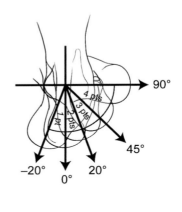

Horizontal plane evaluation of derotation of the calcaneopedal block

Horizontal plane evaluation of forefoot relative to hindfoot

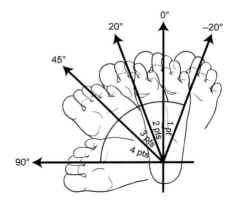

Fig. 31.3 The Dimeglio classification system. Four aspects of the deformity (the equinus, varus, rotation of the foot, and forefoot medial deviation) are scored on a scale of 1 (good) to 4 (bad) with four other categories (depth of posterior crease, medial crease, cavus, and muscle power) being assigned a present/absent score of 0 or 1 to give a total maximum score of 20

change in order to stretch tight structures and allow improved bone and joint alignment prior to the improved position being held with a further cast. The classic casts as advocated by Ponseti and his group involve a small amount of padding and a well-applied above-knee plaster cast. Others have experimented with different casting materials and with shorter casts and feel these modifications work well in their hands.

The standard protocol involves weekly cast changes and an extensive surgical procedure can be avoided in around 95% of cases. Treatment is usually started within a few days of birth.

The cavus deformity in clubfoot is principally a problem of the first ray. In order to correct this, the first ray must be dorsiflexed, effectively supinating the forefoot further. Correction of the cavus realigns the metatarsals, navicular, cuboid, and cuneiforms into the same plane. With the initial cast application, the forefoot is also abducted with laterally based, counterpressure applied over the talar head.

Table 31.3 The Pirani classification

HFCS Hindfoot contracture score	PC	**The severity of the posterior crease** Foot held in maximal correction	0 0.5 1	multiple fine creases one or two deep creases deep creases change the contour of the arch
	EH	**The emptiness of the heel** Foot held in maximal correction	0 0.5 1	tuberosity of calcaneus easily palpable tuberosity of calcaneus more difficult to palpate tuberosity of calcaneus not palpable
	RE	**Rigidity of equinus** Knee extended, ankle maximally corrected	0 0.5 1	ankle dorsiflexes fully ankle dorsiflexes to 'neutral' angle between lateral border of foot and leg $\leq 90°$ ankle dorsiflexion severely limited – fixed equinus. angle between lateral border of foot and leg $>90°$
MFCS Midfoot contracture score	MC	**Severity of the medial crease** Foot held in maximal correction	0 0.5 1	multiple fine creases one or two deep creases deep creases change the contour of the arch
	LHT	**Palpation of the lateral part of the head of the talus** Forefoot held fully abducted	0 0.5 1	navicular completely reduces, lateral talar head cannot be felt navicular partially reduces, lateral talar head less palpable navicular does not reduce, lateral talar head easily felt
	CLB	**The curvature of the lateral border**	0 0.5 1	straight border mild curve of lateral border distally lateral border curves at calcaneo-cuboid joint

Adapted from generally available score sheets

Successive casts continue to correct the talonavicular alignment and simultaneously the calcaneus rotates under the talus with the posterior aspect rotating away from the fibula as the calcaneofibular ligament stretches. At this stage, care must be taken to maintain the forefoot in a neutral position with respect to supination/pronation. Simultaneously, the foot, under the talus, is externally rotated with respect to the leg and the correction continued until abduction/external rotation reaches 70°. Once the midfoot and forefoot deformity has been corrected fully, the equinus deformity can be addressed.

This correction is achieved by pulling down on the heel and applying upward pressure on the entire foot (to avoid a breech or rocker bottomed foot). If 15° of dorsiflexion with 70° of abduction/external rotation cannot be achieved easily, then a percutaneous tenotomy of the Achilles tendon is required. The tenotomy can be performed safely, comfortably, and easily using local anesthetic cream in the clinic, particularly in the young infant, although some practitioners

prefer a general anesthetic procedure, especially in the older child. Following tenotomy, dorsiflexion is achieved and the corrected position is held in the final cast for a period of 2–3 weeks, by which time both clinically and by ultrasound assessment [46] the tendon has reconstituted (Fig. 31.5). The older the child, the longer it takes for the tendon to reconstitute. This may necessitate adjustment of the post-tenotomy casting and splinting regime.

Following removal of the final cast, a foot abduction orthosis (FAO) is applied. The size of the foot is measured at the time of the tenotomy so that the appropriate size of boot is ordered. Comfortable, well-fitting boots are essential. The bar connecting the boots has a slight bend in it which allows the foot to be maintained in some dorsiflexion (Fig. 31.6). The boots are positioned at shoulder distance apart and the feet externally rotated by 70°. Full time use of the FAO is advocated for the first 3 months following cast treatment, then "nap time and night time" use up to walking age. Night time use should be continued for at least a

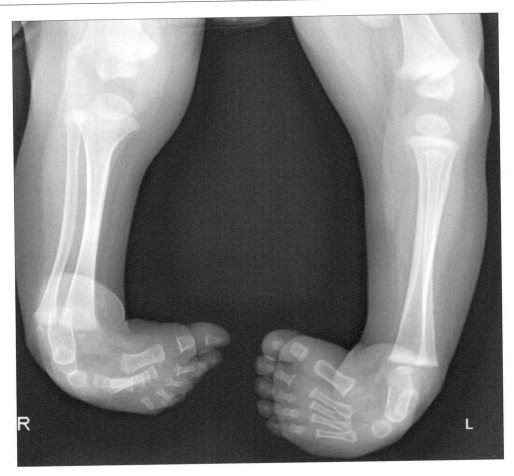

Fig. 31.4 AP radiograph of the distal lower limbs and feet of a child with bilateral clubfoot deformities. The radiograph effectively excludes a tibial dysplasia. Lines drawn through the long axes of the talus and the calcaneus would show a degree of parallelism which would not be seen in the normal foot when these lines should diverge (see also Fig. 31.2)

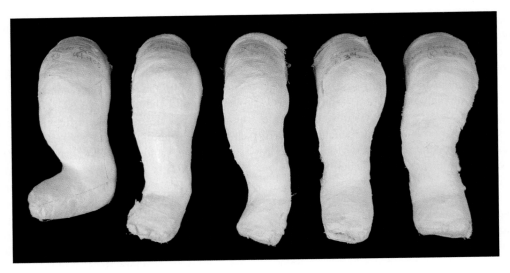

Fig. 31.5 A series of plaster casts demonstrating correction of the clubfoot deformity following treatment with the Ponseti regime. From Eastwood DM. Paediatric orthopaedics. In: Williams NS, Bulstrode CJK, O'Connell PR, eds. Bailey and Love's Short Practice of Surgery, 25th ed. London: Hodder Arnold; 2008. Used with permission

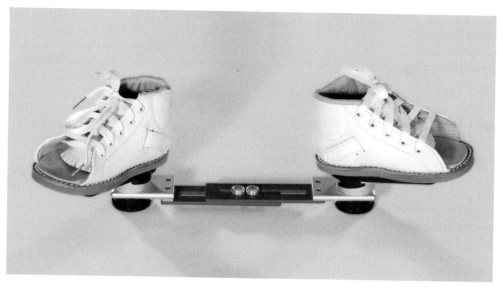

Fig. 31.6 An example of the "boots and bars" foot abduction orthoses used as part of the Ponseti management program

further 12 months with some exponents of the technique, including Ponseti, believing that splint usage until the age of 4 years is essential if full correction of the deformity is to be maintained with a minimal risk of recurrence.

Relative muscle imbalance may be a problem and once the foot is in the corrected position, it is important to stimulate activity particularly in the anterior tibial muscles and the peroneal muscle groups in order to shorten the relative over-lengthening of these muscle-tendon units.

Several different types of FAOs are available and it is certainly true that one splint does not fit all feet. The "short, fat foot" is recognized as a particular problem by many practitioners. However, with all splints, compliance can be a problem and as compliance with treatment is predictive of a successful long-term outcome it is essential that the parents cooperate with the treatment program. Continuity of care and a holistic approach to the family and the child are essential.

Many authors have been able to duplicate Ponseti's results, and in the idiopathic foot, full correction should be achievable in around 95% of cases following a mean of 5–8 casts depending upon the age at which treatment started. A percutaneous tenotomy will be needed in between 65 and 85% of cases depending upon the severity of the foot deformity at the start of treatment. A Pirani score of 5 or more at presentation or a Dimeglio grade IV foot is highly predictive of the need for tenotomy [47]. The pathoanatomy of the clubfoot, including both the abnormal shape of the cartilage anlagen and the abnormal relationships between them, resolves promptly with the Ponseti treatment as confirmed on MR imaging [48]. The changes in mechanical loading result in altered growth in these fast-growing tissues with the interesting observation that with the Ponseti method static

stresses rather than dynamic loading may be influencing tissue adaptation [49].

The manipulation and the casting can be performed by a variety of practitioners as long as they are confident and competent in applying the technique [50, 51]. In developed countries, the tenotomy is performed by surgically trained practitioners but elsewhere clinical medical officers have been trained in this technique [51]. Occasional, significant bleeding complications have been noted. It has been suggested that the tenotomy could be performed using a needle as has been used effectively for the release of the A1 pulley in trigger fingers in the outpatient clinic [52].

Recently, Morcuende et al. [53] have shown that an accelerated treatment protocol, changing casts every 5 days rather than 7, results in a more rapid correction of deformity while allowing the parents to remove the cast the night before their clinic attendance. Leaving the child's foot free to return to its position of deformity from its position of correction results in a longer treatment time compared to those patients in whom the cast is removed in the clinic just prior to the next manipulation and casting session [54].

Radiographic evaluation has confirmed that the Achilles tenotomy is followed by an increase in the lateral tibiocalcaneal angle, indicating that dorsiflexion is occurring at the ankle and not at the midfoot [55]. Koureas et al. [56] have emphasized that the use of a lateral radiograph can identify a rocker bottom deformity or midfoot breech which would prompt an early tenotomy.

Ultrasound monitoring during treatment can demonstrate that correction is occurring although this is usually visible clinically. In appropriately trained hands, scans may be better than radiographs in identifying false correction earlier than would be apparent clinically, and this may prompt changes to the manipulation technique [57].

Recurrent deformity (see below) may be treated by repeated manipulation and casting followed again by FAOs.

Other Methods of Conservative Treatment

Over the years many methods of conservative treatment have been tried using a variety of "stretching and strapping" or "manipulating and plastering" techniques but few methods have been described in great detail. The *Kite method* was popular but has now been shown to be less successful than the Ponseti technique in a randomized study [58]. Kite recommended forefoot correction by abducting the forefoot against pressure applied laterally at the calcaneocuboid joint. This was termed "Kite's error" by Ponseti who believes that the point of counter pressure should be the talar head [45].

The *French or functional method* of clubfoot correction, developed and popularized by Bensahel [59] and Dimeglio [38], is an intensive, dynamic program that emphasizes stretching of the tight medial structures, strengthening of the peroneal muscles, and strapping of the improved foot position. Treatment takes place on a daily basis for the first 2–3 months. The frequency of treatment then drops to 2–3 times per week until 6 months of age with physiotherapy and night splinting continuing until the age of 2–3 years. The addition of continuous passive motion has been found to be beneficial during the first 3 months of treatment. With this program, most authors have found a reduction in the number and the extent of surgical procedures required to obtain a good foot position [60, 61]. Several of these authors feel that the chances of success are higher with the moderately deformed feet scoring less than 10 on the Dimeglio scale. As with the Ponseti method, MR imaging evaluation pre- and post-treatment with the French method has shown improved anatomical relationships in all areas other than hindfoot equinus [62].

Surgical Management

Conservative methods of management of the clubfoot are not applicable to all feet or for all families and an individual approach to the management of the deformity must be defined particularly in the child with a complex foot. For some severe deformities (Dimeglio grades 3 and 4) and for some of those associated with syndromes or neuromuscular conditions, surgical treatment is still the most appropriate choice and surgically treated clubfeet can and do function well at long-term follow-up despite some persistent

abnormalities evident on clinical or radiographic assessment [63, 64] (Fig. 31.7). The most common residual problems are probably stiffness, poor push-off during gait secondary to calf weakness, and a tendency for compensatory external rotation at the hip level to counteract the persistent internal rotation at foot or tibial level.

A large number of surgical approaches and procedures have been described but it is difficult to compare their outcomes due to the lack of a common classification system at the start of surgery. On the whole with all techniques most feet do well, some have a fair result and about 10% do badly.

The indication for surgery is an inability to obtain and maintain reduction of the joint subluxations by conservative means. Surgical intervention must release the tight structures causing these deformities and allow joint realignment to occur. Some feet require little more than a tendo Achilles lengthening, while others require a full peri-talar release. Several authors believe that specific structures are the key to obtaining a good foot position so, for example, the importance of the posterolateral corner with a limited release medially was emphasized by Catterall [65], whereas Simons [66] emphasized correction of the calcaneocuboid joint and felt that division of the talocalcaneal interosseous ligament should be part of the peri-talar release. Others felt that such extensive surgery led to an unacceptably high rate of overcorrection.

Most experienced surgeons have probably developed their own variation of the "a la carte" method popularized by Bensahel et al. [67]. In this pragmatic approach to the surgical treatment of clubfoot, pathologically tight structures are released in sequence until the foot is well aligned. Fractional lengthenings of muscle-tendon units are preferred when possible, and tendons are repaired under some tension to try and prevent postoperative weakness. Once reduction of the joints has been obtained, the position is often maintained by one or more K-wires, ensuring joint reduction during the healing phase. The talonavicular relationship is key and hence one wire crosses this joint. The importance of the calcaneocuboid relationship is emphasized by some authors and a wire across this joint may be required. In those cases where release of the interosseous ligament has been necessary, a talocalcaneal wire will guard against heel valgus. While early movement might be ideal, traditionally immobilization with an above-knee plaster cast has been recommended for 6–8 weeks depending upon the extent of the surgery and the age of the child. Further splinting may be recommended on an individual basis and can be influenced by the etiology of the deformity. Idiopathic clubfeet may require no further orthotic use whereas neuromuscular feet usually do.

The choice of incision(s) must be appropriate to the amount and type of surgery planned. The Cincinnati circumferential incision [68] certainly provides a good exposure to all aspects of the deformity and even though it may not

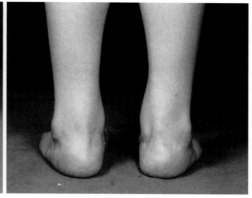

Fig. 31.7 (**a**) Front and (**b**) back-standing clinical photographs of a child whose clubfoot deformity was corrected surgically as an infant

close primarily, several papers have confirmed that healing takes place while the foot is in plaster, without the need for plastic surgical intervention and without compromising the functional outcome. One advantage of the Cincinnati incision is that the scar is cosmetically acceptable, usually lying below the line of a shoe and sock. It does not extend up the leg as the child grows as longitudinal incisions tend to do.

The timing of surgical intervention is not crucial but despite the popularity of an early tenotomy with the Ponseti program, most people feel that early major surgical intervention risks increased scarring and it is still difficult to hold the foot in the plantigrade position until the child is old enough to bear weight. Surgical intervention is often timed for around 9–10 months of age so that removal of the postoperative casts occurs at the time the child is likely to start walking.

Muscle Rebalancing

Even in the idiopathic foot, relative muscle imbalance with poor evertor muscle function can be noted from an early stage. If this persists, despite correction of the foot deformity and despite a strengthening program, then the foot develops a supination deformity that is often dynamic. The standing foot posture may be good but the supination deformity becomes obvious as the child walks. For this type of problem, a split (or total) tibialis anterior tendon transfer to the cuboid or the intermediate cuneiform is considered the procedure of choice. It is important to suture the transferred tendon under sufficient tension and a slightly everted resting foot position at the end of the procedure is ideal. Many clinicians feel this procedure will be required in a significant number of cases treated with the Ponseti technique and the families can be warned about this as treatment commences [45].

Management of the Complex Case

Primary management of the complex clubfoot deformity is essentially similar to that of the idiopathic foot but treatment must take into account associated problems. Neurological conditions may be accompanied by sensory deficits and thus manipulation and casting risks causing pressure sores. Similarly, arthrogrypotic foot deformities may be difficult to treat due to more proximal limb contractures. Associated non-orthopaedic problems may mean that early treatment or cast treatment is not appropriate. While a surgical procedure is more likely in this group of patients than in the idiopathic foot, some success is being achieved in these feet with a modified Ponseti program. In such complex feet an early tenotomy may be justified before full forefoot abduction has been achieved and the postoperative splinting program may require significant adaptation to accommodate other joint deformities [69].

Assessment of Outcome

This is an essential part of long-term management to allow comparison between one method of treatment and another. Unfortunately there are few studies with long-term follow-up to skeletal maturity or beyond but Cooper and Dietz [70] noted good or excellent function in 78% of their patients in a 30-year follow-up. They also reported that radiographic measurements do not correlate with function. The value of many studies has been hampered by poor documentation of the initial deformity both clinically and radiographically. The Pirani [39] and Dimeglio [38] classification systems are being used increasingly pre-treatment and their continued use post-treatment may help to distinguish between subgroups of patients who do well and those who do not. However, neither of these two systems assesses function and objective scores which together with subjective patient-based outcomes need to be developed and studied, with a distinction between the idiopathic foot and the complex foot [71]. A study of 204 children designed to compare subjective and objective outcome measures found a correlation between certain anthropometric measurements and patient satisfaction. A grading system based on foot length, maximal calf circumference, and ankle movement would be relevant and easily applicable to all patients [72]. Andriesse et al. [73] have presented their initial evaluation of a clubfoot assessment protocol (CAP) that has shown good validity and responsiveness, particularly in the moderate to severe feet, when compared to the Dimeglio system. It also has a greater ability to discriminate between different degrees of mobility in the left and right feet in bilateral cases. This assessment protocol concentrates on determining change over time and thus aims to be an instrument that would be valuable for longitudinal follow-up. Further studies are required.

Table 31.4 Questions to consider when faced with a late foot deformity following initial treatment of CTEV

What treatment did the foot have initially?	A failure of Ponseti treatment is likely to present different problems from a failure of surgical treatment.
Was the foot ever fully corrected?	*If so,* why has the foot deformity recurred? (a) Is this a failure of post-operative management? (b) Are there other neuromuscular or syndromic conditions that should be considered? For example, tethering of the cord. (c) Has the previous surgery damaged the developing foot—i.e., are there soft tissue contractures or physeal tethers that are contributing to the progressive deformity? *If not,* why is there residual deformity? (a) Was the initial treatment appropriate? (b) Was the original diagnosis correct?
What is the essence of the deformity?	*Is it:* dynamic or fixed? overcorrection? continuing/recurrent equinovarus?

The Management of Residual or Recurrent Deformity

The assessment and management of foot deformity secondary to the surgical treatment of a clubfoot has been a difficult area for many surgeons over the last few decades. (Fig. 31.8) With the decline of primary surgical management it is possible that these difficult cases will become less common.

When presented with a residual or relapsed foot deformity, it is important that the clinician takes time to review the whole history and conducts a full examination of the foot and lower limb including a neurological assessment of the child. Suitable investigations must be undertaken which may include spinal cord imaging and/or nerve conduction studies to exclude a neurological cause.

The most common problems which cause parental anxiety are the following:

1. foot shape and size (a measure of deformity);
2. walking pattern (although function is usually good);
3. discomfort (which may be more perceived than real as assessed by the child's continuing participation in physical activities).

The clinician should try to identify whether or not the deformity is a residual deformity or a recurrent deformity perhaps by considering the questions in Table 31.4.

It is essential that standing posture and gait pattern are assessed and the clinical examination of the foot and hindfoot should identify what deformity is present at each level

and whether or not it is supple. All too often a combination of deformities exists. The Coleman block test [74] is helpful in determining whether the hindfoot deformity is fixed in relation to a supple forefoot (see Chapter 32).

In cases of complex three-dimensional foot deformities, plain two-dimensional radiographs may be difficult to interpret. It is impossible for the radiographers to obtain a true lateral view of the foot when there is significant forefoot adduction, for example, and thus in order to achieve the "required" position, the patient rotates the foot externally at ankle level. This gives the appearance of a posteriorly placed lateral malleolus and often a "flat-topped talus." However, the flat-topped talus may be a true appearance in cases where an extensive soft tissue release has resulted in compression or avascular change within the talus.

Equinus

A pure equinus deformity is common. Following Ponseti treatment, further casting and a repeat tenotomy of the Achilles tendon should be considered. If the deformity is secondary to post-surgical treatment a repeat tenotomy alone is invariably disappointing and the surgeon should be prepared to perform a posterior release of the ankle and subtalar joint. If there is a flat-topped talus, a repeat release will not be successful as the talus can no longer rotate into dorsiflexion although dome subtalar motion may be regained.

Often there is a concomitant *cavus* deformity which may merit a plantar fascia release.

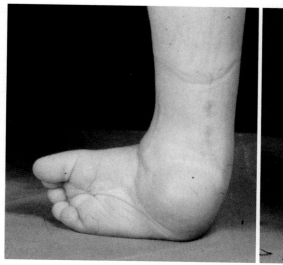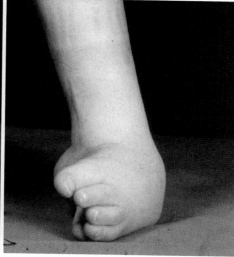

Fig. 31.8 Clinical photographs of a child whose clubfoot deformity was treated surgically as an infant but who still has considerable recurrent or residual deformity

Hindfoot Varus

Hindfoot varus is often associated with under-correction of the original deformity. The deformity is usually rigid and management depends upon the age of the child and on the extent of other deformities. Ponseti casting or a surgical release may be considered, but in a child over the age of 4 years it is likely that a calcaneal osteotomy should be considered. A lateral closing wedge (incorporating some lateral translation) is probably the best method of correcting deformity and maintaining heel height.

Hindfoot Valgus

This is most commonly seen following a major surgical release and a failure to maintain a neutral correction in the postoperative period. Instability of the subtalar joint secondary to division of the talocalcaneal interosseous ligament and/or insufficiency of the tibialis posterior musculature will lead to valgus. If the surgical procedure has left the foot with ineffective plantar ligaments (such as the spring ligament and the calcaneonavicular ligament) the deformity may be more planovalgus than valgus. Other authors [45, 65] have emphasized the importance of the pathological calcaneofibular ligament or "tether." If this is not divided during the initial surgical release, the talus cannot dorsiflex into the ankle mortice and the tether pulls the calcaneus toward the fibula. The hindfoot valgus may be driven by a rigid forefoot supination deformity.

Hindfoot valgus is associated with weakness of push-off and may be painful due to calcaneofibular impingement laterally. Deformity is often progressive as the midfoot collapses.

As with all deformities, management may be conservative or surgical. The surgical options concentrate upon correcting the hindfoot valgus via either a translational or a lengthening calcaneal osteotomy. Concomitant forefoot surgery may also be required if correction of the hindfoot valgus reveals some forefoot supination. Currently, the calcaneal lengthening osteotomy is the procedure of choice for the foot as it maintains some flexibility and is therefore capable of producing some correction when the osteotomy is distracted [75]. In the more rigid foot, other osteotomies should be considered or a subtalar arthrodesis. If the hindfoot deformity is associated with other significant deformity a triple arthrodesis (see below) may be the best option.

Calcaneus

This deformity is unusual and is probably related to over-lengthening of the gastrocsoleus complex. The clinical appearance is similar to that seen in some feet after poliomyelitis and it raises the suspicion of an underlying neurological condition (Fig. 31.9). Treatment is difficult: a calcaneal osteotomy that displaces the tuberosity posteriorly may be effective in improving the cosmetic appearance of the foot and the ability to wear shoes [76]. It does alter the lever arm for the gastrocsoleus but whether this translates into improved function is debatable. Not infrequently, a dorsal soft tissue release is also required to improve the forefoot position.

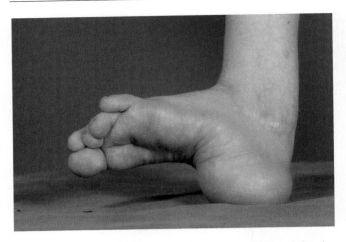

Fig. 31.9 Clinical photograph of a child with a calcaneus deformity secondary to early surgical treatment of a clubfoot deformity

Dorsal Bunion (with Forefoot Supination)

A dorsal bunion with plantar flexion of the first metatarsophalangeal (MTP) joint is a common problem following extensive surgical release of the idiopathic clubfoot when the underlying etiology is probably a persistent muscle imbalance. The weak gastrocsoleus complex means that flexor hallucis longus is relatively overactive when contributing to the push-off phase of gait. The first MTP joint is frequently stiff and physiotherapy designed at regaining and maintaining movement is important. Yong et al. [77] have recently reported good results with a reverse Jones tendon transfer.

A supination deformity of the forefoot often accompanies a dorsal bunion. Again muscle imbalance is a contributory factor with a strong tibialis anterior muscle pull overcoming that of the weak peroneal muscles. The supination deformity may be the root cause of the dorsal bunion.

As mentioned previously, a split or complete tibialis anterior tendon transfer to either the cuboid or the intermediate cuneiform rebalances the foot but the tension in the tendon transfer must be correct and the foot should lie in slight eversion at the end of the procedure [78]. The usual indication for this tendon transfer is a dynamic supination deformity in the presence of a supple forefoot although some report its value in a fixed foot with the transfer simply halting progression of the deformity.

Metatarsus Adductus (the Curved Forefoot)

This deformity, like the others already mentioned, tends not to occur in isolation. Hindfoot varus or indeed valgus (the skew foot) may also be present. Ponseti-type stretching and casting may be helpful but in the more rigid foot, surgery may be necessary. In simple terms, the medial column of the foot is too short and the lateral column too long causing the forefoot to curve inward. Assuming that the hindfoot is relatively well aligned, surgery is first directed toward a release of the tight medial soft tissues which may include scar tissue from previous incisions, the abductor hallucis, and the capsules of the midtarsal and tarsometatarsal joints. A shortening of the lateral column of the foot may then be performed via a closing wedge osteotomy of the cuboid or a calcaneocuboid joint fusion as described by Evans [79]. The wedge that is removed from the lateral side can be inserted in the medial side as a graft in an opening wedge osteotomy of the medial cuneiform [80].

Recurrent Clubfoot Deformity

If all aspects of the deformity have recurred then it may be necessary to repeat the original treatment especially if this was the Ponseti approach. If the recurrence is secondary to a surgical procedure, then clinical judgment is required to decide whether or not the risks of further surgery and subsequent scarring with stiffness are worth the possible benefits.

Intoeing Gait

An intoeing gait is very common in patients with clubfoot. It is possible that the prolonged use of foot abduction orthoses as part of the Ponseti program may reduce the incidence of internal tibial rotation which is often the cause of the intoeing gait. Other factors such as persistent foot deformity and weak peroneal muscles must also be considered. A supramalleolar osteotomy of the tibia with/without fibular osteotomy will significantly improve foot progression.

Leg Length Discrepancy

In severe clubfoot deformity leg length discrepancy may develop with time and some prediction of what the discrepancy is likely to be at skeletal maturity should be made. If the predicted discrepancy is more than 2 cm an epiphysiodesis of the contralateral proximal tibia (or distal femur) at the appropriate time should be considered. Often severe clubfoot deformities following surgical treatment have some residual equinus deformity which can compensate, at least in part, for the discrepancy.

The Ilizarov Method

The use of the Ilizarov principle of gradual distraction of soft tissues and bone to correct residual or recurrent clubfoot deformity by means of the law of tension–stress and the application of an external fixator was first popularized by Grill and Franke in 1987 [81]. They achieved a plantigrade foot in all 10 feet. Since then there have been mixed reports on its use and value. Comparison between these papers is difficult due to a lack of objective assessment of the etiology and the severity of the initial deformity and the use of various methods to achieve deformity correction. Some surgeons use purely soft tissue distraction techniques, while others perform limited soft tissue release in addition, sometimes combined with a midfoot or hindfoot osteotomy. Despite initial optimism, such surgery often leads to stiffening of the affected and neighboring joints, particularly the ankle, which has a detrimental effect on the results. Bradish and Noor [82] reported 76% good/excellent results at a mean of 3 years and noted that in supple feet the addition of a tendon transfer to prevent recurrent deformity was always associated with an excellent outcome. Similar results have been reported by others with slightly longer follow-up [83, 84] although a relatively high rate of secondary surgery was noted [83]. Recently, Freedman et al. [85] reported disappointing results at a mean follow-up of 6.6 years with only 3 out of 21 (15%) good/excellent results and almost 50% of feet requiring revision surgery. Utukuri et al. [86] also showed recurrent deformity in 14 of 23 (61%) patients but patient-based outcomes were good/excellent in around 50% of patients.

The use of this technique does allow for correction of any tibial deformity or shortening at the same time should this be required.

Triple Arthrodesis

A triple arthrodesis should be reserved for the symptomatic, rigid foot with significant deformity. Improvement in symptoms will be achieved only if a stiff, plantigrade foot is achieved and if there is some useful ankle movement. The procedure is never indicated in a patient less than 10–12 years of age because it would have a major effect on the growth of the foot. While it is generally felt that patient satisfaction following this procedure is good, there is little objective information to support this belief. Ramseier et al. [87] reviewed seven patients who had undergone a triple arthrodesis as adults and reported improved outcome according to American Orthopaedic Foot and Ankle Society scores,

with six out of seven patients being satisfied despite residual symptoms and degenerative changes at the ankle. Bennet et al. [88] similarly reported improvement in deformity and hindfoot pain but there was little evidence to suggest that function was improved. It is perceived that triple arthrodesis is more successful in the treatment of a varus deformity than a valgus deformity.

Talectomy

Talectomy remains a radical solution for significant equinovarus deformity in the foot that has undergone multiple previous operative procedures or that has an arthrogrypotic or neuromuscular etiology, particularly if the patient is young. The aim of the procedure is to obtain a stable and pain-free plantigrade foot. On its own, talectomy does not necessarily correct mid- and forefoot deformity and additional procedures may be necessary. In an essentially arthrogrypotic group of patients, Legaspi et al. [89] reported 75% good or fair results at a mean follow-up of 20 years when the initial procedure took place at a mean age of 5 years. Good results have also been reported in bilateral cases [90].

Decision Making in Recurrent/Relapsed Feet

In recurrent clubfoot deformities as in many other areas of paediatric orthopaedics it is important to remember a few important rules (Table. 31.5).

Ponseti and others believe that early treatment is associated with a better outcome because the shape of the cartilaginous bones of the infant foot can be preserved [45]. Congruous joints can develop provided compression is not excessive. If treatment is delayed and later correction is performed surgically with release of contracted joints and ligaments, then all too often the corrected position is unstable perhaps because of articular incongruency. To stabilize

Table 31.5 Points to remember when decision-making in recurrent/relapsed deformities

1	Every operation on the foot will increase stiffness in adjacent joints
2	A supple foot with some deformity may be better than a stiff foot with no deformity
3	The stiff, deformed foot often has the worst outcome
4	The longer the foot has been in a position of deformity, the less likely it is that a normal foot will be obtained with treatment. Due to the abnormal configuration of the bones, it is likely that joint function will also be poor

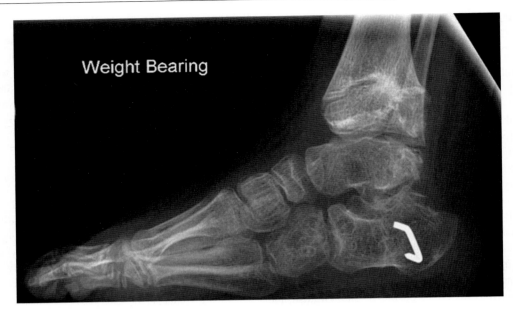

Fig. 31.10 Lateral radiograph of a foot that has had two surgical procedures performed. A growth arrest of the distal tibial physis is noted

the foot, K-wire fixation is advocated and the foot heals with the formation of scar tissue so that the joint may become stiff. This partly accounts for the disappointing relapse rates following late surgical intervention for the primary or recurrent clubfoot deformity [44]. All too often, on talking to parents of children with "difficult" feet, it is apparent that the previous surgical procedure was disappointing in terms of deformity correction. In such cases, it is important to remember that the foot may be deformed but the foot may be comfortable and functional. The asymptomatic foot may benefit from being left alone until such time as pain or change in functional level leads the patient to ask for help. A more extensive surgical procedure may be necessary at that stage but the overall outcome may be better.

Recurrence or relapse is quite common in the first few years following Ponseti treatment. Both problems usually relate to a failure to comply with the FAO and the prolonged period of treatment [91]. Recurrent deformity can be treated with further manipulation and casting and the addition of a tenotomy or tendon transfer as discussed previously. However, if compliance was a problem initially, it may be so again and the clinician must decide whether it is sensible to persevere with one particular type of treatment or obtain and then maintain correction by some other method [92]. While the Achilles tendon can be lengthened once and probably twice, repeated procedures are associated with increasing weakness leading to disability and calcaneus deformity. Following the use of the Ponseti regimen recurrence after the age of 7 years is unlikely. Should a recurrence occur, a neurological cause should be considered [93].

Foot deformity may be secondary to long-standing abnormal mechanics through the deformed joints or to surgical damage to the developing foot. Growth arrest, muscle imbalance, and incongruent joints will all play a role (Fig. 31.10).

Summary

Although much has been learnt about the nature and management of idiopathic clubfoot over the years, much remains to be understood. Further research into the etiology and pathology of the condition is necessary and long-term outcome studies of current methods of treatment will be required.

References

1. Siapkara A, Duncan R. Congenital talipes equinovarus: A review of current management. J Bone Joint Surg 2007; 89-B:995–1000.
2. Carey M, Bower C, Mylvaganam A, Rouse I. Talipes equinovarus in Western Australia. Paediatr Perinat Epidemiol 2003; 17: 87–194.
3. Byron-Scott R, Sharpe P, Hasler C, et al. A South Australian population-based study of congenital talipes equinovarus. Paediatr Perinat Epidemiol 2005; 19:227–237.
4. Cederholm M, Haglund B, Axelsson O. Infant morbidity following amniocentesis and chorionic villus sampling for prenatal karyotyping. BJOG 2005; 112:394–402.
5. Dickenson KC, Meyer RE, Kotch J. Maternal smoking and the risk for clubfoot in infants. Birth Defects Res A Clin Mol Teratol 2008; 82:86–91.

6. Alderman BW, Takahashi ER, LeMier MK. Risk indicators for talipes equinovarus in Washington State 1987–1989. Epidemiology 1991; 2:289–292.

7. Offerdal K, Jebens N, Blaas HG, Eik-Nes SH. Prenatal ultrasound detection of talipes equinovarus in a non-selected population of 49314 deliveries in Norway. Ultrasound Obstet Gynecol 2007; 30:838–844.

8. Keret D, Ezra E, Lokiec F, et al. Efficacy of prenatal ultrasonography in confirmed club foot. J Bone Joint Surg 2002; 84-B:1015–1019.

9. Bar-Hava I, Bronshtein M, Orvieto R, et al. Caution: prenatal clubfoot can be both a transient and a late-onset phenomenon. Prenat Diagn 1997; 17:457–460.

10. Bar-On E, Mashiach R, Inbar O, et al. Prenatal ultrasound diagnosis of club foot: Outcome and recommendations for counseling and follow-up. J Bone Joint Surg 2005; 87-B:990–993.

11. Mammen L, Benson CB. Outcome of fetuses with clubfeet diagnosed by prenatal sonography. J Ultrasound Med 2004; 23:497–500.

12. Tillett RL, Fisk NM, Murphy K, Hunt DM. Clinical outcome of congenital talipes equinovarus diagnosed antenatally by ultrasound. J Bone Joint Surg 2000; 82-B:876–880.

13. Woodrow N, Tran T, Umstad M, et al. Mid-trimester ultrasound diagnosis of isolated talipes equinovarus: accuracy and outcome for infants. Aust NZ J Obstet Gynaecol 1998; 38:301–305.

14. Malone FD, Marino T, Bianchi DW, et al. Isolated clubfoot diagnosed prenatally: is karyotyping indicated? Obstet Gynecol 2000; 95:437–440.

15. Herzenberg JE, Carroll NC, Christofersen MR, et al. Clubfoot analysis with three-dimensional computer modelling. J Paediatr Orthop 1988; 8:257–262.

16. Windisch G, Salaberger D, Rosmarin W, et al. A model for clubfoot based on micro-CT data. J Anat 2007; 210:761–766.

17. Itohara T, Sugamoto K, Shimizu N, et al. Assessment of talus deformity by three-dimensional MRI in congenital clubfoot. Eur J Radiol 2005; 53:78–83.

18. Ippolito E, Ponseti IV. Congenital clubfoot in the human fetus. A histological study. J Bone Joint Surg Am 1980; 62:8–22.

19. Zimny ML, Willig SJ, Roberts JM, D'Ambrosia RD. An electron microscopic study of the fascia and lateral sides of the clubfoot. J Pediatr Orthop 1985; 5:577–581.

20. Fukuhara K, Schollmeier G, Uhthoff HK. The pathogenesis of club foot. A histomorphometric and immunohistological study of fetuses. J Bone Joint Surg Br 1994; 76-B:450–457.

21. Sano H, Uhthoff HK, Jarvis JG, et al. Pathogenesis of soft-tissue contracture in clubfoot. J Bone Joint Surg 1998; 80-B:641–644.

22. Van der Sluijs JA, Pruys JE. Normal collagen structure in the posterior ankle capsule in different types of clubfeet. J Pediatr Orthop B 1999; 8:261–263.

23. Hattori K, Sano H, Saijo Y, et al. Measurement of soft tissue elasticity in the congenital clubfoot using scanning acoustic microscope. J Pediatr Ortho B 2007; 16:357–362.

24. Handelsman JE, Badalamente MA. The club foot: a neuromuscular disease. Develop Med Child Neurol 1982; 24:3–12.

25. Isaacs H, Handelsman JE, Badenhorst M, Pickering A. The muscles in clubfoot—a histological, histochemical and electron microscopy study. J Bone Joint Surg 1977; 59-B:465–472.

26. Macnicol MF, Nadeem RD, Maffuli N, et al. Histochemistry of the triceps surae muscle in idiopathic congenital clubfoot. J Foot Ankle Surg 1992; 13:80–84.

27. Muir L, Laliotis N, Kutty S, Klenerman L. Absence of the dorsalis pedis pulse in the parents of children with club foot. J Bone Joint Surg 1995; 77-B:114–116.

28. Sodre H, Bruschini S, Mestriner LA, et al. Arterial abnormalities in talipes equinovarus as assessed by angiography and the Doppler technique. J Pediatr Orthop 1990; 10:101–104.

29. Katz DA, Albanese EL, Levinsohn EM, et al. Pulsed color-flow Doppler analysis of arterial deficiency in idiopathic clubfoot. J Pediatr Orthop 2003; 23:84–87.

30. Wynne-Davis R. Family studies and the case of congenital talipes equinovarus, talipes calcaneovalgus and metatarsus varus. J Bone Joint Surg 1964; 46-B:445–463.

31. Cowell HR, Wein BK. Genetic aspects of club foot. J Bone Joint Surg Am 1980; 62-A:1381–1384.

32. Lochmiller C, Johnston C, Scott A, et al. Genetic epidemiology study of idiopathic talipes equinovarus. Am J Med Genet 1998; 79:90–96.

33. Engell V, Dambiorg F, Andersen M, et al. Club foot: a twin study. J Bone Joint Surg 2006; 88-B:374–376.

34. Ester AR, Tyerman G, Wise CA, et al. Apoptotic gene analysis in idiopathic talipes equinovarus. Clin Orthop Relat Res 2007; 462: 32–37.

35. Hecht JT, Ester A, Scott A, et al. NAT2 variation and idiopathic talipes equinovarus. Am J Med Genet A 2007; 143:2285–2291.

36. Herceq MB, Weiner DS, Aqamanolis DP, Hawk D. Histologic and histochemical analysis of muscle specimens in idiopathic talipes equinovarus. J Pediatr Orthop 2006; 26:91–99.

37. Shimode K, Myagi N, MajimaT, et al. Limb length and girth discrepancy of unilateral congenital clubfoot. J Pediatr Orthop B 2005; 14:280–284.

38. Dimeglio A, Bensahel H, Souchet P, et al. Classification of clubfoot. J Pediatr Orthop B 1995; 4:129–136.

39. Pirani S. A reliable and valid method of assessing the amount of deformity in the congenital clubfoot. St Louis MO: Pediatric Orthopaedic Society of North America; 2004.

40. Flynn JM, Donohoe M, Mackenzie WG. An independent assessment of two clubfoot-classification systems. J Pediatr Orthop 1998; 18:323–327.

41. Wainwright AM, Auld T, Benson MK, Theologis TN. The classification of congenital talipes equinovarus. J Bone Joint Surg 2002; 84-B:1020–1024.

42. Coley B, Sheils WE 2nd, Kean J, Adler BH. Age-dependent dynamic sonographic measurement of pediatric clubfoot. Pediatr Radiol 2007; 37: 1125–1129.

43. Turco VJ. Resistant congenital clubfoot. One stage posteromedial release with internal fixation. J Bone Joint Surg 1979; 61A: 805–814.

44. Tarraf YN, Carroll NC. Analysis of the components of residual in clubfeet presenting for reoperation. J Pediatr Orthop 1992; 12:207–216.

45. Ponseti IV. Current Concepts Review: Treatment of congenital club foot. J Bone Joint Surg 1992; 74-A:448–454.

46. Barker SL, Lavy CB. Correlation of clinical and ultrasonographic findings after Achilles tenotomy in idiopathic clubfoot. J Bone Joint Surg 2006; 88-B:377–379.

47. Scher DM, Feldman DS, van Bosse HJ, et al. Predicting the need for tenotomy in the Ponseti method for correction of clubfeet. J Pediatr Orthop 2004; 24:349–352.

48. Pirani S, Zesnik L, Hodges D. Magnetic resonance imaging study of the congenital clubfoot treated with the Ponseti method. J Pediatr Orthop 2001; 21:719–726.

49. Brand RA, Siegler S, Pirani S, et al. Cartilage anlagen adapt in response to static deformation. Med Hypotheses 2006; 66:653–659.

50. Shack N, Eastwood DM. Early results of a physiotherapist delivered Ponseti service for the management of idiopathic congenital talipes equinovarus foot deformity. J Bone Joint Surg 2006; 88-B:1085–1089.

51. Tindall AJ, Steinlechner CW, Lay CB, et al. Results of manipulation of idiopathic clubfoot deformity in Malawi by orthopaedic clinical officers using the Ponseti method: a realistic alternative for the developing world? J Pediatr Orthop 2005; 25:627–629.

52. Minkowitz B, Finkelstein BL, Bleicher M. Percutaneous tendo-Achilles lengthening with a large-gauge needle: a modification of the Ponseti technique for the correction of idiopathic club foot. J Foot Ankle Surg 2004; 43:263–265.

53. Morcuende JA, Abbasi D, Dolan LA, Ponseti IV. Results of an accelerated Ponseti protocol for clubfoot. J Pediatr Orthop 2005; 25:623–626.

54. Terrazas-Lafargue G, Morcuende JA. Effect of cast removal timing in the correction of idiopathic clubfoot by the Ponseti method. Iowa Orthop J 2007; 27:24–27.

55. Radler C, Manner HM, Suda R, et al. Radiographic evaluation of idiopathic clubfeet undergoing Ponseti treatment. J Bone Joint Surg 2007; 89-A:1177–1183.

56. Koureas G, Rampal V, Mascard E, et al. The incidence and treatment of rocker bottom deformity as a complication of the conservative treatment of idiopathic congenital clubfoot. J Bone Joint Surg 2008; 90-B:57–60.

57. Desai S, Aroojis A, Mehta R. Ultrasound evaluation of clubfoot correction during Ponseti treatment: a preliminary report. J Pediatr Orthop 2008; 28:53–59.

58. Sud A, Tiwari A, Sharma D, Kapoor S. Ponseti's vs Kite's method in the treatment of clubfoot—a prospective randomized study. Int Orthop 2008; 32:409–413.

59. Souchet P, Bensahel H, Themar-Noel C, et al. Functional treatment of clubfoot: a new series of 350 idiopathic clubfeet with long-term follow-up. J Pediatr Orthop B 2004; 13:189–196.

60. Richards BS, Johnston CE, Wilson H. Nonoperative clubfoot treatment using the French physical therapy method. J Pediatr Orthop 2005; 25:98–102.

61. Van Campenhout A, Molenaers G, Moens P, Fabry G. Does functional treatment of idiopathic clubfoot reduce the indication for surgery? Call for a widely accepted rating system. J Pediatr Orthop B 2001; 10:315–318.

62. Richards BS, Dempsey M. Magnetic resonance imaging of the congenital clubfoot treated with the French functional (physical therapy) method. J Pediatr Orthop 2007; 27:214–219.

63. Turco VJ. Resistant congenital clubfoot. One stage posteromedial release with internal fixation. A follow up report of a fifteen year experience. J Bone Joint Surg Am 1979; 61-A:805–814.

64. McKay DW. New concept of and approach to clubfoot treatment: Section II—correction of the clubfoot. J Pediatr Orthop 1982; 2:347–356.

65. Hudson I, Catterall A. Posterolateral release for resistant clubfoot. J Bone Joint Surg 1994; 76-B:281–284.

66. Simons GW. Complete subtalar release in club feet. Part 1—A preliminary report. J Bone Joint Surg Am 1985; 67-A:1044–1055.

67. Bensahel H, Csukonyi Z, Desgrippes Y, Chaumien JP. Surgery in residual clubfoot: one stage medioposterior release 'a la carte.' J Pediatr Orthop 1987; 7:145–148.

68. Crawford AH, Marxen JL, Osterfeld DL. A comprehensive approach for surgical procedures of the foot and ankle in childhood. J Bone Joint Surg 1982; 64A: 1355–1358.

69. Ponseti IV, Zhivkov M, Davis N, et al. Treatment of the complex idiopathic clubfoot. Clin Orthop Relat Res 2006; 451:171–176.

70. Cooper DM, Dietz FR. Treatment of idiopathic clubfoot. A thirty-year follow-up note. J Bone Joint Surg 1995; 77-A:1477–1489.

71. Vitale MG, Choe JC, Vitale MA, et al. Patient-based outcomes following clubfoot surgery: a 16 year follow-up study. J Pediatr Orthop 2005; 25:533–538.

72. Chesney D, Barker S, Maffulli N. Subjective and objective outcome in congenital clubfoot; a comparative study of 204 children. BMC Musculoskelet Disord 2007; 8:53.

73. Andriesse H, Roos EM, Hagglund G, Jarnlo G-B. Validity and responsiveness of the Clubfoot Assessment Protocol (CAP). A methodological study. BMC Musculoskelet Disord 2006; 7:28.

74. Coleman SS, Chestnut WJ. A simple test for hindfoot flexibility in the cavovarus foot. Clin Orthop Rel Res 1977; 123:60–62.

75. Evans D. Calcaneovalgus deformity. J Bone Joint Surg 1975; 57B:270–278.

76. Mitchell GT. Posterior displacement osteotomy of the calcaneus. J Bone Joint Surg 1977; 59B:233–235.

77. Yong SM, Smith PA, Kuo KN. Dorsal bunion after clubfoot surgery: outcome of reverse Jones procedure. J Pediatr Orthop 2007; 27:814–820.

78. Ezra E, Hayek S, Gilai AN, et al. Tibialis anterior tendon transfer for residual dynamic supination deformity in treated club foot. J Pediatr Orthop B 2000; 9:207–211.

79. Evans D. Relapsed club foot. J Bone Joint Surg 1961; 43-B:722–733.

80. Schaefer D, Hefti F. Combined cuboid/cuneiform osteotomy for correction of residual adductus deformity in idiopathic and secondary clubfeet. J Bone Joint Surg 2000; 82B:881–884.

81. Grill F, Franke J. The Ilizarov distractor for the correction of relapsed and neglected clubfoot. J Bone Joint Surg 1987; 69-B:593–597.

82. Bradish CF, Noor S. The Ilizarov method in the management of relapsed club feet. J Bone Joint Surg 2000; 82-B:387–391.

83. Ferreira RC, Costa MT, Frizzo GG, Santin RA. Correction of severe recurrent clubfoot using a simplified setting of the Ilizarov device. Foot Ankle Int 2007; 28:557–568.

84. Prem H, Zenios M, Farrell R, Day JB. Soft tissue Ilizarov correction of congenital talipes equinovarus—5–10 years post surgery. J Pediatr Orthop 2007; 27:220–224.

85. Freedman JA, Watts H, Otsuka NY. The Ilizarov method for the treatment of resistant clubfoot: Is it an effective solution? J Pediatr Orthop 2006; 26:432–437.

86. Utukuri MM, Ramachandran M, Hartley J, Hill RA. Patient-based outcomes after Ilizarov surgery in resistant clubfeet. J Pediatr Orthop B 2006; 15:278–284.

87. Ramseier LE, Schoeniger R, Vienne P, Espinosa N. Treatment of late recurring idiopathic clubfoot deformity in adults. Acta Orthop Belg 2007; 73:641–647.

88. Bennett GL, Graham CE, Mauldin DM. Triple arthrodesis in adults. Foot Ankle 1991; 12:138–143.

89. Legaspi J, Li YH, Chow W, Leong JC. Talectomy in patients with recurrent deformity in club foot. A long-term follow-up study. J Bone Joint Surg 2001; 83-B:384–387.

90. Letts M, Davidson D. The role of bilateral talectomy in the management of bilateral rigid clubfeet. Am J Orthop 1999; 28:106–110.

91. Ponseti IV. Congenital Clubfoot: Fundamentals of Treatment. Oxford: Oxford University Press; 1996.

92. Haft GF, Walker CG, Crawford HA. Early clubfoot recurrence after use of the Ponseti method in a New Zealand population. J Bone Joint Surg 2007; 89-A:487–493.

93. Lovell ME, Morcuende JA. Neuromuscular disease as the cause of late clubfoot relapses: report of 4 cases. Iowa Orthop J 2007; 27:82–84.

Chapter 32

Pes Cavus

John A. Fixsen

Introduction

Pes cavus, or a high arched foot, is rarely seen at birth or in the first year of life unless it is part of a severe congenital talipes equinovarus. There is a rare, benign form of high arched foot called pes arcuatus; this is occasionally seen as an isolated abnormality in the first year of life and resolves spontaneously. Cavus deformity of the foot develops in the majority of cases in the first or second decade of life.

It is essential that the orthopaedic surgeon distinguishes between a cavovarus foot and a calcaneocavus foot. In the cavovarus foot the heel is in varus and the forefoot in equinus with pronation of the first and sometimes the second ray (Fig. 32.1). This is the basis of the so-called block test described by Coleman and Chesnut in 1977 [1] to distinguish whether the hindfoot varus is secondary to the pronation of the forefoot and the subtalar joint is mobile, or whether the hindfoot varus is fixed. In the calcaneocavus foot (Fig. 32.2), the calf is weak and the heel is in calcaneus and often valgus. The subtalar joint is usually stiff. The forefoot is in equinus or "plantaris," as it is often called. In this type of cavus foot, both the medial and the lateral longitudinal arches are off the ground, and the so-called coin test can be used, in which a small coin can be pushed across underneath both arches of the foot, from medial to lateral. Unlike the cavovarus foot, the lateral arch is raised from the ground in calcaneocavus. Sometimes an elevation of the central metatarsal heads of the forefoot arch develops, causing a tripod foot and increasing pressure over the first and fifth metatarsal heads.

The orthopaedic surgeon should always look for an underlying cause when assessing a cavus foot. The most common cause is a neurological imbalance of the foot and calf muscles. Price et al. [2] showed that the earliest and most severe involvement was in the intrinsic muscles of the foot in patients suffering from a peripheral neuropathy, and this occurred before involvement of the extrinsic muscles of the calf. Deluca and Banta [3] reported a progressive cavovarus deformity of the foot after laceration of the peroneus longus. If a neurological disorder, of either the central or the peripheral nervous system, is suspected, the help of an expert neurologist should be sought. It is also important to investigate the family background, as there is frequently a genetic basis to the deformity. Brewerton et al. [4] published an important paper on the etiology of pes cavus and found that, in 67% of patients, a neurological cause could be found. The commonest neurological condition in their series was peroneal muscular atrophy or Charcot–Marie–Tooth disease, which is now included under the hereditary motor and sensory neuropathies. In a recent study of patients with bilateral cavovarus feet, 78% were found to have Charcot–Marie–Tooth disease [5]. The other conditions that should be considered are cerebral palsy, poliomyelitis, spina bifida and spinal dysraphism, benign spinal cord tumors, and syrinx of the spinal cord. Sometimes the neurological cause can be treated, as in the case of diastematomyelia, a spinal cord tumor, or a syrinx. Talipes equinovarus, particularly in its more severe forms, often has a cavus component. Similarly, cavus may develop after treatment of club foot. If no underlying cause can be found, then the term idiopathic can be accepted.

Pes Cavovarus

This type of foot may be associated with congenital talipes equinovarus or it may be the sequel of its treatment. It is also commonly seen in association with the peripheral neuropathies. In the past, the terms Charcot–Marie–Tooth disease and peroneal muscular atrophy were commonly used. However, the modern term is hereditary motor and sensory neuropathy (HMSN), as this emphasizes not only the motor problems but also the sensory aspect of these disorders. These tend to affect deep pain, temperature sensation, and

J.A. Fixsen (✉)
Orthopaedic Department, Great Ormond Street Hospital for Sick Children, London, UK

M. Benson et al. (eds.), *Children's Orthopaedics and Fractures*,
DOI 10.1007/978-1-84882-611-3_32, © Springer-Verlag London Limited 2010

Fig. 32.1 Clinical photographs of bilateral cavovarus feet. (**a**) Posterior view showing bilateral heel varus. (**b**) Lateral view showing cavus and forefoot equinus with pronation of the first and second rays. Note that the lateral longitudinal arch rests upon the ground

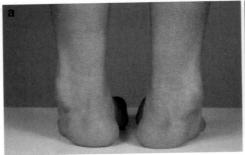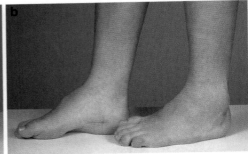

proprioception, rather than superficial sensations. As a result, these patients may present with "giving way" of the ankle or the knee, and with penetrating ulcers over the toes. HMSN was described by Harding and Thomas in 1980 [6]. Initially, two types were described; subsequently, further types were added (see Chapter 15).

Type I HMSN, sometimes called Charcot–Marie–Tooth type I, is the so-called hypertrophic type. This is dominantly inherited and usually appears in the first decade of life. Seventy percent of those affected are likely to develop pes cavus. The upper limbs below the elbow may be involved and 10–12% of patients are likely to develop significant scoliosis. On examination, hypertrophy of the peripheral nerves can be palpated, best seen in the subcutaneous nerves of the neck. Nerve conduction is significantly reduced, at 20–30 m/s, and is most easily recorded in the median nerve of the forearm. Other family members are often unaware that they suffer from the same condition because the phenotype is very variable. It is important to examine them, and often they will show minor abnormalities in the feet and of their median nerve conduction time.

Type II HMSN is called the axonal type (Charcot–Marie–Tooth type II). It is less commonly seen in children and tends to develop from the second to the sixth decades of life. The nerve conduction time is normal in these patients, and pes cavus and scoliosis are less common. Affected individuals present to orthopaedic surgeons with problems of balance and calf weakness, such as recurrent and unexplained ankle sprains, giving way of the knee and subluxation of the patella, or generalized clumsiness and weakness. In this form, inheritance may be dominant, recessive, or X-linked.

Type III HMSN is the so-called Dejerine–Sotta type. These patients tend to present to the paediatrician or neurologist with severe problems of abnormal motor development. They have a very slow conduction time of less than 5 m/s. The other types have complex neurological problems, with pyramidal signs, optic problems, and deafness, and are unlikely to present to the orthopaedic surgeon.

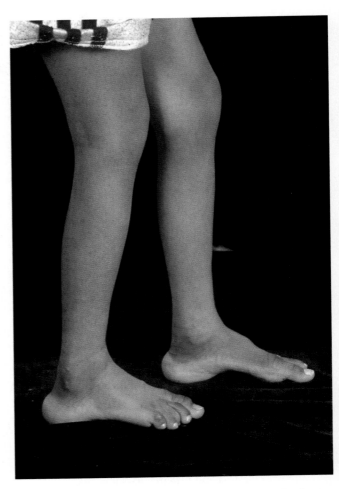

Fig. 32.2 Clinical photographs of a patient with bilateral calcaneo-cavus feet. Note that both medial and lateral longitudinal arches are raised off the ground. This patient had a positive "coin" sign

Treatment

Irrespective of the cause of the cavovarus foot, treatment demands that the flexibility of the forefoot and the hindfoot be assessed. It is most important that the primary site responsible for the deformity be identified. In most instances, the major problem resides in a rigid, plantar flexed fore-foot with the first and second metatarsals most affected. This effectively pronates the forefoot in relation to the hind-foot, and during standing the inflexible pronated forefoot forces the heel into varus as a result of the "tripod" effect (Fig. 32.1).

By careful physical examination, one can determine whether or not the hindfoot is flexible or rigid. This can be documented visually by placing the heel and fifth metatarsal on a raise or block of about 2–3 cm in width and allow-ing the remainder of the forefoot to fall into plantar flexion (Fig. 32.3). In a positive "block test," the heel goes into val-gus and hindfoot flexibility is present. Price and Price in 1997 [7] described another method of demonstrating hindfoot flex-ibility with the patient prone; this is a useful alternative to the block test. Alternatively, if the heel is held rigidly in varus or does not move into valgus when the block test is applied, both the forefoot and the hindfoot are rigid, a situation that requires a different therapeutic approach. In 2005, Aznaipairashvili et al. [8] described an imaging tech-nique which they called a Coleman block lateral radiographic view. This was used both to assess hindfoot flexibility and to determine the appropriate surgical treatment.

Non-Operative Treatment

Non-operative treatment such as shoes or orthotic devices can only support the cavovarus deformity, not correct it. In most patients, the deformity is progressive. If it becomes increasingly disabling despite conservative treatment, surgi-cal treatment is indicated.

Surgical Treatment

When the forefoot is rigidly plantar flexed and pronated and the hindfoot is flexible, the appropriate surgical procedure is a radical plantar release combined, if necessary, with proxi-mal first and sometimes second metatarsal osteotomy when there is fixed bony deformity at the first and second rays. It is important to remember that the growth plate of the first metatarsal is proximal and should not be damaged by the osteotomy. This should correct the forefoot and result in a plantigrade forefoot if the hindfoot is flexible. Serial changes of plaster may be necessary after the initial opera-tion to obtain the maximal effect. The plaster is retained for 6–8 weeks and then a decision can be made as to whether tendon transfers are necessary to prevent recurrence of the deformity. The degree of correction obtained can be assessed on the lateral weight-bearing radiograph by measuring the angle of Meary [9] (Fig. 32.4).

If both the hindfoot and the forefoot are inflexible, char-acterized by a negative block test, both components of the deformity must be treated. In young children, this may require a plantar release combined with a medial release. In older children in whom a medial release is not sufficient, the plantar release can be combined with a lateral wedge osteotomy [10], or simply a valgus displacement osteotomy of the calcaneus. In adolescents and adults, the forefoot cor-rection may require a wedge tarsectomy or even a full triple arthrodesis.

The place of tendon transfers is difficult to assess, par-ticularly if one is dealing with a progressive neurological condition such as HMSN. If there is significant forefoot inversion and overactivity of the tibialis posterior, transfer of this tendon to the dorsum has been advocated at the same time as the medial release. Full transfer of the tibialis ante-rior should be avoided, but a split transfer, or the procedure described by Fowler et al. [11] in which the tibialis anterior is transferred onto the dorsum of the base of the first metatarsal and combined with a wedge osteotomy of the base of the first cuneiform, may be undertaken.

Toe deformities are also a major problem. These patients, because of their disturbance of pain and temperature sen-sation, are liable to develop serious soft-tissue lesions, par-ticularly over the pressure areas on the toes. The typical Z deformity of the big toe can be treated by a classical Robert Jones tendon transfer, in which the extensor hallucis longus is transferred to the distal portion of the shaft of the first metatarsal and the interphalangeal joint of the big toe is either fused or tenodesed if the child still has significant growth left in the toe. Clawing of the lesser toes can cause serious problems with nail deformities and pressure sores. In the past, the so-called Girdlestone toe flexor to extensor transfer was recommended [12]. This transfer was described originally for victims of polio, but in the progressive forms of neurological disease the simple flexor tendon osteotomy described by Menelaus and Ross [13] is simpler and more effective.

Pes Calcaneocavus

This type of foot is characteristic of paralytic neurologi-cal conditions such as poliomyelitis, spinal muscular atro-phy, and the lower motor neurone type of spina bifida. Characteristically, both the medial and the lateral arches are raised, giving rise to a positive coin sign. The heel is in cal-caneus and the subtalar joint stiff, so that the block test is negative and is not applicable in this type of foot. A lateral radiograph shows the characteristic "pistol-grip" appearance of the calcaneus (Fig. 32.5).

Fig. 32.3 (**a**) Clinical photograph showing the block test assessing the right foot. The heel varus is corrected so this is a flexible cavovarus foot and the test is positive. (**b**) Line drawing of the block test showing the flexed pronated first and second rays, with the heel varus corrected

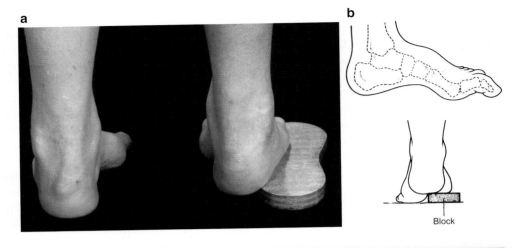

Fig. 32.4 (**a**) Lateral radiograph of the left, uncorrected cavovarus foot. (**b**) Lateral radiograph of the right foot after correction by radical plantar release. Meary's angle [9] between the long axis of the talus and the first metatarsal is substantially reduced

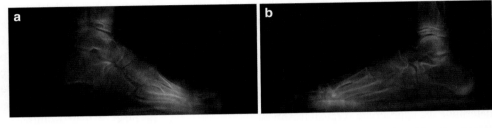

Fig. 32.5 (**a**) lateral radiograph of a calcaneocavus foot showing the so-called pistol-grip appearance of the calcaneus. (**b**) after calcaneal osteotomy

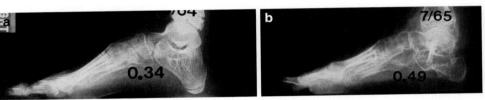

In younger children, a Steindler [14] soft-tissue release of the plantar fascia may be helpful. Once bony deformity becomes fixed, a Mitchell [15] posterior displacement osteotomy of the calcaneus combined with a plantar release can be used. For the rigid foot in adolescents or young adults, the Elmslie triple arthrodesis reported by Cholmeley [16] is effective. In this procedure, a posterior wedge is excised from the subtalar joint to correct the calcaneus of the heel, and subsequently a wedge tarsectomy is performed to bring the forefoot up on the corrected hindfoot. Attempts to restore power and "push-off" by the Robert Jones transfer, in which the dorsiflexors are transferred into the calf, have never been successful. Silver et al. [17] pointed out that the calf muscle is approximately six times stronger than the dorsiflexors of the foot as it has to lift the entire body weight and not just the foot. As a result, it is not surprising that transfers of the dorsiflexors into the calf are unlikely to reproduce good push-off. Westin et al. [18] described an unusual variant of this procedure. Instead of fixing the tendo-Achilles to the back of the tibia, the tendo-Achilles was transferred into the fibula.

This technique was used in a number of patients with calcaneus feet associated with spina bifida and appears to be useful in preventing progression of calcaneus and valgus in these patients.

References

1. Coleman SS, Chesnut WJ. A simple test for hindfoot flexibility in the cavovarus foot. Clin Orthop Rel Res 1977; 123: 60.
2. Price A, Maisel R, Drennan JC. Computer tomographic analysis of pes cavus. J Paedriatr Orthop 1993; 13: 646–653.
3. Deluca PA, Banta JB. Pes cavovarus as a late consequence of peroneus longus tendon laceration. J Paedriatr Orthop 1985; 5: 582–583.
4. Brewerton DA, Sandifer PH, Sweetnam DR. Idiopathic pes cavus, an investigation into its aetiology. Br Med J 1963; 2: 659.
5. Nagai MK, Chan G, Guile JT, et al. Prevalence of Charcot–Marie–Tooth disease in patients who have bilateral cavovarus feet. J Pediatr Orthop 2006; 26: 438–433.
6. Harding AE, Thomas PK. The clinical features of hereditary motor and sensory neuropathies types 1 and II. Brain 1980; 103: 259.

7. Price BD, Price CT. A simple demonstration of hindfoot flexibility in the cavovarus foot. J Paedriatr Orthop 1997; 17: 18–19.

8. Aznaipairashvili Z, Riddle EC, Savina M, et al. Correction of cavovarus foot deformity in Charcot–Marie–Tooth disease. J Pediatr Orthop 2005; 25: 360–365.

9. Meary R. On the measurement of the angle between the talus and the first metatarsal Symposium: Le Pied Creux Essentiel. Rev Chir Orthop 1967; 53: 389.

10. Dwyer FC. Osteotomy of the calcaneum for pes cavus. J Bone Joint Surg 1959; 41B: 80.

11. Fowler D, Brooks AL, Parrish TF. The cavovarus foot. J Bone Joint Surg 1959; 41A: 757.

12. Taylor RG. The treatment of claw toes by multiple transfers of flexor into extensor tendons. J Bone Joint Surg 1951; 35B: 539–542.

13. Menelaus MB, Ross ERS. Open flexor tenotomy for hammer toes and curly toes in children. J Bone Joint Surg 1984; 66B: 770.

14. Steindler A. Stripping of the os calcis. J Orthop Surg 1920; 2: 8.

15. Mitchell GP. Posterior displacement osteotomy of the calcaneus. J Bone Joint Surg 1977; 59B: 233.

16. Cholmeley JA. Elmslies' operation for the calcaneus foot. J Bone Joint Surg 1953; 35B: 46.

17. Silver RL, de la Garza J, Rang M. The myth of muscle balance. J Bone Joint Surg 1985; 67B: 432–437.

18. Westin GW, Dugeman RD, Gausewitz SH. The results of tenodesis of the tendo-Achilles to the fibula for paralytic pes calcaneus. J Bone Joint Surg 1988; 78A: 320–338.

Chapter 33

Congenital Vertical Talus (Congenital Convex Pes Valgus)

John A. Fixsen

This rare foot deformity has been given many different names depending on how various authors view the pathology and its clinical manifestations. The most commonly used names are congenital vertical talus or congenital convex pes valgus [1], but perhaps the most accurate term has been suggested by Tachdjian [2]—"teratologic dislocation of the talo-calcaneo-navicular joint." Irrespective of the term used, it is important to understand that this is a rigid foot deformity. Hamanishi [3], in a major review of 69 cases, suggested that, from the etiological point of view, these feet could be grouped according to an association with one of five disorders:

1. Neural defects/spinal anomalies.
2. Neuromuscular disorders.
3. Malformation syndromes.
4. Chromosomal aberrations.
5. Idiopathic.

Coleman [4] from a personal experience of 40 cases of congenital vertical talus reported that only two feet in one child were not associated with any other abnormality. It is most important, therefore, that the orthopaedic surgeon presented with a child with a congenital vertical talus examines the child thoroughly for any other problems and considers the treatment of the foot in relation to these other problems.

In infancy, the deformity superficially resembles a severe calcaneo-valgus or plano-valgus foot (Fig. 33.1). It is for this reason that the diagnosis is often delayed. The difference between the two, which is most important from a diagnostic and therapeutic point of view, is that the true congenital vertical talus is rigid and cannot be passively corrected. In older children, it must be distinguished from severe flat foot, paralytic flat foot, flat foot in cerebral palsy, and spuriously corrected or rocker-bottomed foot after treatment of club

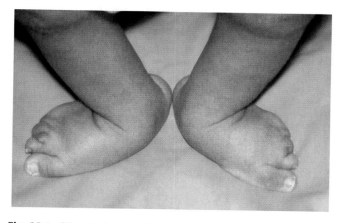

Fig. 33.1 Clinical photograph of an infant with bilateral congenital vertical talus. Note the valgus and eversion of the forefeet

foot [5]. A plantar flexion stress lateral radiograph (the Eyre-Brook view) shows that the relationships of the bones of the hindfoot do not change and that the navicular remains dorsally dislocated on the talar head [6]. It is important to remember that the navicular is the last bone to ossify in the foot, at the age of about 4 years. However, the position of the navicular can be determined in younger children by a line drawn through the longitudinal axis of the first metatarsal, which will run through the center of the navicular (Fig. 33.2).

The pathology of congenital vertical talus includes four basic abnormalities that involve the bones, joints, ligaments, and muscles of the foot. Although there is some variability in the degree of severity, certain abnormalities of anatomy are always present. These consist of the following:

- A complete, irreducible dorsal dislocation of the navicular on a vertically orientated talus.
- Abnormal displacement of the peroneus longus and posterior tibial tendons so that they function as dorsiflexors rather than plantar flexors.
- Subluxation of the talo-calcaneal joint.

J.A. Fixsen (✉)
Orthopaedic Department, Great Ormond Street Hospital for Sick Children, London, UK

M. Benson et al. (eds.), *Children's Orthopaedics and Fractures*,
DOI 10.1007/978-1-84882-611-3_33, © Springer-Verlag London Limited 2010

Fig. 33.2 Line drawing of the Eyre-Brook plantar flexion stress lateral radiograph of a normal and a congenital vertical talus foot. N=navicular, C=cuboid, CAL=calcaneus

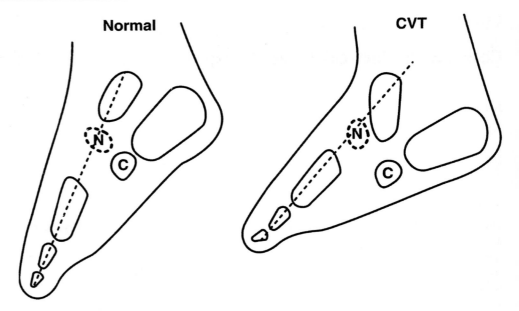

- Fixed equinus of the hindfoot as the result of a contracted heel cord and ankle capsule (Fig. 33.3); in some cases there is also a calcaneo-cuboid subluxation or dislocation [7].

Once the diagnosis has been established it is accepted that nonoperative treatment will not succeed. Manipulation of the foot into plantar flexion may stretch out the anterior structures, including the skin, but true restoration of the bony relationships rarely, if ever, occurs. Surgical correction is therefore necessary.

Over the years, many methods of surgical treatment have been proposed, but the basic principles remain the same, namely restoring the bones to their normal relationships and holding them there. Many different techniques have been described but the essential steps are as follows:

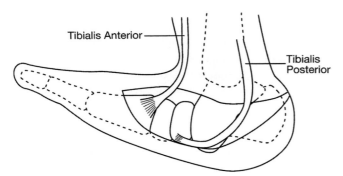

Fig. 33.3 Line drawing of the exposed medial side of a congenital vertical talus through a Cincinnati incision showing the dorsal dislocation of the navicular on the vertically orientated talus, the calcaneus in equinus, and the position of the tibialis anterior and posterior tendons

1. The talo-navicular dislocation must be reduced and stabilized.
2. The hindfoot equinus must be corrected and the normal talo-calcaneal relationships restored.
3. The forefoot, which is in calcaneus and frequently everted, must be reduced and stabilized on the corrected hindfoot.

These steps comprise, in essence, an open reduction of the three major deformities present in the foot.

In the past, two-stage reduction was commonly advocated [8]; the forefoot was reduced on the hindfoot at the first stage, and at the second stage the hindfoot was corrected. Stone and Lloyd-Roberts [8] also advised removing the navicular, to shorten the medial column of the foot. This procedure was also reported by Clark et al. [9]. More recently, the importance of a full release of the contracted peroneal tendons and reduction of the calcaneo-cuboid subluxation that lengthens the lateral column of the foot has made excision of the navicular and shortening of the medial column unnecessary. Finally, Stone and Lloyd-Roberts [8] advised transfer of the tibialis anterior to the neck of the talus to help in supporting the talus in its corrected position. The results of using this technique were reported in 1999 by Duncan and Fixsen [10] (Fig. 33.4). Although minimal access surgical release is also being advocated, coupled with regular stretching casts, the results of this approach have yet to be published and the recurrence rate is unknown.

Nowadays, the majority of surgeons prefer a single, one-stage complete reduction of the triple deformity without any tendon transfers [11]. It is probably best to perform this operation when the child is between the ages of 6 months and 2 years; many of these children have multiple other problems

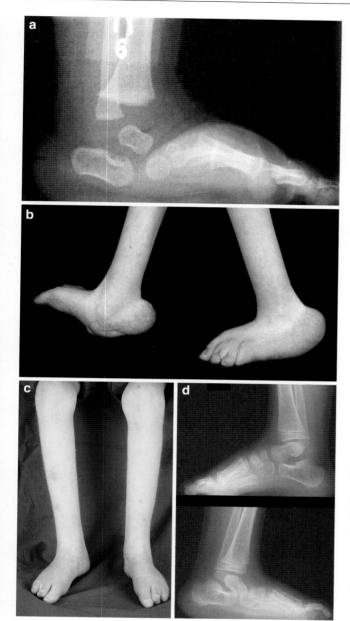

Fig. 33.4 (**a**) Preoperative clinical photograph of bilateral congenital vertical talus in a patient with arthrogryposis. (**b**) Clinical photograph 3 years postoperatively showing satisfactory correction of the deformity bilaterally

release is important to correct the heel equinus, and a lateral release to reduce the calcaneo-cuboid displacement and elongate the peroneal tendons. In order to allow satisfactory correction of the forefoot upon the hindfoot, the tibialis anterior and the dorsiflexors of the foot, which are always tight, require lengthening. In patients older than 3–4 years it may be difficult to stabilize the talus satisfactorily on the calcaneum, because of the deformation of the subtalar joint. In this situation, Coleman [4] advises a subtalar arthrodesis to secure the unstable talo-calcaneal joint.

Congenital vertical talus is a rare but fascinating condition. It is important to establish the diagnosis clearly and not confuse it with other conditions and milder forms of "rocker-bottom" feet. The majority of these children will have other major problems and it is very important that the treatment of the foot deformity is seen in relation to these and not in isolation. Inevitably, with such a rare condition, most reports are small and anecdotal. Dodge et al. in 1987 [12] published a useful long-term retrospective review of 36 feet followed up for an average of 14 years. A number of surgical techniques had been used but none produced significantly better results than others. They confirmed the high incidence of other problems in these children and found that the majority did well after surgery. Kodros and Dias in 1999 [11] reviewed 32 patients (42 feet) in whom a one-stage complete reduction was performed using the Cincinnati incision. They reported no wound complications and no incidence of avascular necrosis of the talus. The Cincinnati incision apparently provided excellent exposure for this complex procedure, but 10 feet had required further operations. Overall functional result in many of their patients was determined as much by the underlying condition from which they suffered as by the quality of the result of their foot operation.

References

1. Lamy L, Weissman L. Congenital convex pes valgus. J Bone Joint Surg 1939; 21: 79–91.
2. Tachdjian MO. Paediatric Orthopaedics. Congenital Convex Pes Valgus. Philadelphia: WB Saunders; 1983:2557–2576.
3. Hamanishi C. Congenital vertical talus. Classification with 69 cases and new measurement system. J Pediatr Orthop 1984; 4: 318.
4. Coleman SS. Complex Foot Deformities in Children. Philadelphia: Lea & Febiger; 1983.
5. Lloyd-Roberts GC, Spence AJ. Congenital vertical talus. J Bone Joint Surg 1958; 40B: 336.
6. Eyre-Brook L. Congenital vertical talus. J Bone Joint Surg 1967; 49B: 618–627.
7. Coleman SS, Stelling FH, Jarrett J. Pathomechanics and treatment of congenital vertical talus. Clin Orthop Rel Res 1970; 70: 62.
8. Stone KH, Lloyd-Roberts GC. Congenital vertical talus. A new operation. Proc Royal Soc Med 1963; 56: 12.
9. Clark MW, D'Ambrosia RD, Ferguson QB Jr. Congenital vertical talus. Treatment by open reduction and navicular excision. J Bone Joint Surg 1977; 59A: 816.

and it is reasonable to delay surgery until the child's development has been assessed and other problems are dealt with. The deformity, although unsightly, is unlikely to severely hinder the establishment of walking. Complete reduction of the deformity requires medial surgery to reduce the talo-navicular dislocation, which is normally stabilized with a K-wire passed along the first ray and fixing the navicular in its corrected position on the reduced talus. A posterior

10. Duncan RDD, Fixsen JA. Congenital convex pes valgus. J Bone Joint Surg 1999; 81B: 250–254.

11. Kodros SA, Dias LS. Single stage correction of congenital vertical talus. J Paedriatr Orthop 1999; 19: 42–48.

12. Dodge LD, Ashley RK, Gilbert RJ. Treatment of the congenital vertical talus; a retrospective view of 36 feet with long term follow up. Foot Ankle 1987; 7: 326.

Chapter 34

Congenital Disorders of the Cervical Spine

Robert N. Hensinger

Radiological interpretation of the infant's spine may be difficult and a clear understanding of its appearance at different ages is essential if deformity and malalignment are to be recognized. Normal development of the cervical spine is discussed in the section on cervical trauma.

In 1912, Klippel and Feil [1] published the first description of various congenital disorders of the cervical spine. The "Klippel–Feil syndrome" in its present usage refers to all patients with congenital fusion of the cervical vertebrae, whether it involves two segments, congenital block vertebrae, or the entire cervical spine. As radiographic techniques improved, it became apparent that certain anomalies of the occipito-cervical junction, atlanto-occipital fusion, basilar impression, and abnormalities of the odontoid should be considered separately from the original syndrome. Although they occur commonly in conjunction with fusion of the lower cervical vertebrae, their significance depends upon their influence on the atlanto-axial joint. Their prognostic and therapeutic implications are distinctly different and they occur with sufficient frequency to warrant individual analysis.

Basilar Impression

Basilar impression (or basilar invagination) is a deformity of the bones of the base of the skull at the margin of the foramen magnum, The floor of the skull appears to be indented by the upper cervical spine. The tip of the odontoid is more cephalad, sometimes protruding into the opening of the foramen magnum, and it may encroach upon the brain-stem. This increases the risk of neurological damage from injury, circulatory embarrassment, or impairment of cerebrospinal fluid flow. There are two types:

1. Primary basilar impression. A congenital abnormality often associated with other vertebral defects such as atlanto-occipital fusion, hypoplasia of the atlas, bifid posterior arch of the atlas, odontoid abnormalities, and the Klippel–Feil syndrome.
2. Secondary basilar impression. A developmental condition attributed to softening of the osseous structures at the base of the skull, with deformity developing later in life. This occurs in conditions such as osteomalacia, rickets, Paget's disease, osteogenesis imperfecta, renal osteodystrophy, rheumatoid arthritis, neurofibromatosis, and ankylosing spondylitis.

Clinical Features

Patients with basilar impression frequently have a deformity of the skull or neck; however, these physical findings are also often found in patients without such impression (Klippel–Feil syndrome, occipitalization) and are not considered pathognomonic.

Basilar impression is often associated with conditions such as the Arnold–Chiari malformation and syringomyelia, which may cloud the clinical picture. Symptoms are generally caused by crowding of the neural structures (particularly the medulla oblongata) at the level of the foramen magnum. The dominant complaints of symptomatic patients are weakness and paresthesia of the limbs. In contrast, those who are symptomatic with pure Arnold–Chiari malformation are more likely to have cerebellar and vestibular disturbances (unsteadiness of gait, dizziness, and nystagmus). In both conditions, there may be impingement of the lower cranial nerves as they emerge from the medulla oblongata. The trigeminal (V), glossopharangeal (IX), vagus (X), and hypoglossal (X1I) nerves may be affected. Headache and pain in the nape of the neck in the distribution of the greater occipital nerve is a common finding. Posterior encroachment may cause blockage of the aqueduct of Silvius and the presenting symptoms may be caused by increased intracranial pressure [2].

R.N. Hensinger (✉)
Department of Orthopaedic Surgery, University of Michigan, Ann Arbor, MI, USA

M. Benson et al. (eds.), *Children's Orthopaedics and Fractures*,
DOI 10.1007/978-1-84882-611-3_34, © Springer-Verlag London Limited 2010

There is an increased incidence of vertebral artery anomalies in basilar impression, atlanto-occipital fusion, and absence of the C1 facet. In addition, the vertebral arteries may be compressed as they pass through the crowded foramen magnum, causing symptoms suggestive of vertebral artery insufficiency, such as dizziness, seizures, mental deterioration, and syncope. These symptoms may occur alone or in combination with those of spinal cord compression. Erbengi and Oge [3] have noted that the preoperative evaluation of these patients needs special care as many have an unrecognized low vital capacity with chronic alveolar hypoventilation as a result of chronic slow progressive brainstem neurological injury. The gag and cough reflexes are often depressed.

Although this condition is congenital, many patients do not develop symptoms until the second or third decade. This may be due to a gradually increasing instability from ligamentous laxity. Patients with this malformation have been mistakenly diagnosed as having multiple sclerosis, posterior fossa tumors, amyotrophic lateral sclerosis or traumatic injury. It is therefore important to survey this area whenever such a diagnosis is considered and whenever this malformation is suspected.

Imaging Features

Basilar impression is difficult to assess radiographically and many measurement schemes have been proposed. The most commonly used are those described by Chamberlain [4], McGregor [5], and McRae [2]. McRae's line [2] defines the opening of the foramen magnum and is derived from his observation that "if the tip of the odontoid lies below the opening of the foramen magnum, the patient will probably be asymptomatic." It proves a helpful guide in the radiological assessment of patients with basilar impression (Fig. 34.1).

With the development of computed tomography (CT) reconstruction and, more recently, magnetic resonance imaging (MRI), it is now possible to view the relationship at the occipital-cervical junction in much greater detail [6, 7]. Clinically, the lateral reference lines [2, 5] are still important for screening. CT reconstruction and MRI are generally reserved for the patient whose routine examination or clinical findings suggest the presence of an occipito-cervical anomaly. Rouvreau et al. [8] found that occipital and atlas abnormalities were often associated with neurological risk. MRI with lateral flexion/extension views seems the best method of detecting spinal impingement on the spinal cord, especially in patients with odontoid dysplasia and basilar impression.

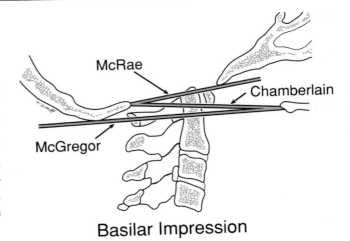

Basilar Impression

Fig. 34.1 Lateral craniometry. The drawing indicates the three lines used to determine basilar impressions. Chamberlain's line (1939) is drawn from the posterior lip of the foramen magnum (opisthion) to the dorsal margin of the hard palate. McGregor's line [5] is drawn from the upper surface of the posterior edge of the hard palate to the most caudal point of the occipital magnum. McGregor's line is the best method for screening, because the bony landmarks can be clearly defined at all ages on a routine lateral radiograph

Occipito-Cervical Fusion

Occipito-cervical fusion, which may be partial or complete, is a congenital union between the atlas and the base of the occiput. Synonyms include assimilation of the atlas, occipito-cervical synostosis, and occipitalization of the atlas. The condition ranges from total incorporation of the atlas into the occipital bone, to a bony or even fibrous band uniting one small area of the atlas to the occiput. Basilar impression is commonly associated with occipito-cervical synostosis. Other associated anomalies include the Klippel–Feil syndrome, occipital vertebrae, and condylar hypoplasia.

Clinical Features

Most patients have an appearance similar to the Klippel–Feil syndrome, with a short broad neck, low hairline, torticollis [6], high scapula, and restricted neck movements. Kyphosis and scoliosis are frequent. Other associated anomalies occasionally seen include dwarfism, funnel chest, pes cavus, syndactylies, jaw anomalies, cleft palate, congenital ear deformities, hypospadias, and genitourinary tract defects.

Neurological symptoms do not usually occur until middle life but they may present in childhood. They progress in a slow, unrelenting manner which may be initiated by trauma or an inflammatory process. Gholve et al. [6] recommend continued periodic clinical and radiographic evaluation because instability may occur with aging. McRae [2] suggested that the odontoid is the key to the development of a neurological lesion and that its position indicates the degree of actual or relative basilar impression. If the odontoid lies below the foramen magnum, the patient is usually asymptomatic. However, with decreased vertical height of the atlas, the odontoid may project well into the foramen magnum and produce brain-stem pressure. In children and adolescents with the Klippel–Feil syndrome, superior migration of the odontoid does not always correlate with symptoms. Those with four or more fused segments and, to a lesser degree, the female sex may have a higher risk of severe odontoid migration [9]. Fusion should be considered for those with instability and when signs of impingement on the spinal cord, nerve roots, or cranial nerves occur.

Anterior compression of the brain-stem from the posteriorly unstable odontoid is the most common problem. The neurological findings depend on the location and degree of pressure. Pyramidal tract symptoms and signs (spasticity, hyperreflexia, muscle weakness and wasting, and gait disturbances) are most common; cranial nerve involvement (diplopia, tinnitus, dysphagia, and auditory disturbances) is less common. Compression from the posterior lip of the foramen magnum or a constricting band of dura may disturb the posterior columns, resulting in loss of proprioception, vibration, and tactile discrimination. Nystagmus, a common occurrence, is probably due to posterior cerebellar compression. Vascular disturbances from vertebral artery involvement may occasionally result in syncope, seizure, vertigo, and unsteady gait among other signs and symptoms of brain-stem ischemia.

Imaging

Standard radiographs of this area can be difficult to interpret. CT reconstruction may be necessary to clarify the pathology. Most commonly, the anterior arch of the atlas is assimilated into the occiput, usually in association with a hypoplastic posterior arch. Congenital anomalies of the atlantal arch are usually incidental findings in asymptomatic patients. Congenital defects in the posterior arch are more common than those in the anterior arch [10]. There is varying loss of height of the atlas, allowing the odontoid to project upward into the foramen magnum and creating a primary basilar impression (Fig. 34.2). Gholve et al. [6] reviewed patients with occipitalization and identified four patterns of fusion:

- Zone 1—fused at the anterior arch
- Zone 2—fusion of the facets (lateral masses)
- Zone 3—fused at the posterior arch
- and a combination of these zones

There is a high association (up to 70%) with congenital fusion between C2 and C3, which can put added strain on the C1–C2 articulation (associated atlanto-axial instability has been reported to develop eventually in 50% of patients). CT reconstructions and MRI are important in establishing the diagnosis, assessing the zone of fusion, and measuring the encroachment [6].

Anomalies of the Ring of C1

In 1986, in the first large study, Dubousset [11] called attention to a previously barely recognized problem with the ring of C1, the hemi-atlas. The absence of one facet of C1 leads to a severe progressive torticollis in the young child. Initially, the deformity is flexible and can be passively corrected. As the child ages, the torticollis becomes more severe and eventually fixed. Radiographic diagnosis using tomograms or CT has helped to identify this deformity (Fig. 34.3), which may accompany the Klippel–Feil syndrome. Dubousset [11] found some of these children had associated anomalies of the vertebral vessels. He suggested arteriographic evaluation

Fig. 34.2 A 10-year-old male with the Klippel–Feil syndrome. The lateral CT scan (**a**) and MRI (**b**) of the cervical spine and base of the skull demonstrate a C2–C3 fusion and odontoid protrusion into the opening of the foramen magnum. Patients with this pattern of fusion are at great risk. With aging the odontoid may become hypermobile, and the space available for the spinal cord may be compromised

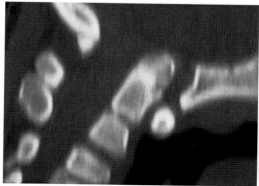
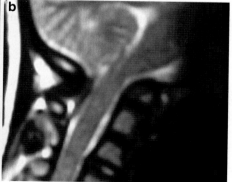

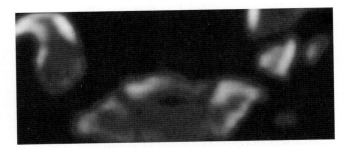

Fig. 34.3 Absent facet of C1: anteroposterior CT scan in a 5-year-old with a hemi-atlas that has led to a progressive torticollis. The deformity is initially flexible and passively correctible. Note that the left C1 facet is fused to the occiput

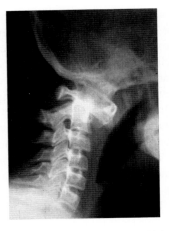

Fig. 34.4 The cervical spine of an 11-year-old with Down's syndrome and gross atlanto-axial instability. The gait was clumsy and physical examination revealed poor coordination of the extremities. There was no other evidence of motor or sensory impairment or of pathological reflexes. The patient has no symptoms referable to the cervical spine 2 years after surgical stabilization

before traction or surgical intervention, which could further compromise a precarious blood supply to the midbrain and spinal cord.

Laxity of the Transverse Atlantal Ligament

This is a diagnosis of exclusion suggested by the clinical occurrence of chronic atlanto-axial dislocation without a predisposing cause. There is no history of trauma, congenital anomaly, infection, or rheumatoid arthritis to account for the radiological finding. Most patients discovered (excluding those with Down's syndrome) have the typical symptoms of atlanto-axial instability and require surgical stabilization.

Laxity of the transverse atlantal ligament is common in patients with Down's syndrome, with a reported incidence of 15% [12] (Fig. 34.4). The lesion may be found in all age groups, without any age preponderance [12]. These patients rupture or attenuate the transverse atlantal ligament, with encroachment of the "safe zone of steel," but at least initially are protected from spinal cord compression by the "check-rein" of the alar ligaments. In other words, many have excessive motion, but relatively few are symptomatic. The majority are discovered only by radiological survey. If radiographs of the upper cervical spine indicate an atlantal-dens interval of more than 4.5 mm, instability is considered to be present. Usually, if symptoms are present, instability of greater than 7 mm or even 10 mm is found. Recent reports suggest an increased incidence of occiput-C1 instability also.

We still know very little about the natural history of atlanto-axial instability in Down's syndrome despite the radiographic examination of hundreds of children. Some studies have suggested that some children become looser with time; others that those with small degrees of instability can, on occasion, become stable [12]. Currently, routine radiographic examination for children with Down's syndrome is recommended only if they plan to compete in

athletics. Any Down's affected child with a musculoskeletal complaint such as subluxating patellae, dislocating hips, or a wide-based ataxic gait should be investigated. Similarly, if a child with Down's syndrome needs a general anesthetic, cervical spine stability should be evaluated because head and neck positioning during the procedure could lead to neurological injury. With our present knowledge, prophylactic stabilization does not appear to be indicated.

Those with a minor degree of hypermobility or instability should be followed regularly with flexion–extension radiographs. They should not engage in contact sports, somersaults, trampoline exercises, or other activities which encourage neck flexion and the potential risks should be discussed with the parents. Any child who has persisting neck symptoms caused by instability or a history of neurological problems should have surgical stabilization [12].

Odontoid Anomalies

The anomalies of the odontoid range from aplasia and hypoplasia to os odontoideum. A congenital or developmental etiology has always been assumed. Hypoplasia and os odontoideum can be acquired secondary to trauma or, rarely, infection [13]. This has led to the suggestion that some cases of os odontoideum or hypoplasia follow an unrecognized fracture of the base or damage to the epiphyseal plate of the odontoid in the first few years of life [13]. The insult could compromise the developing dens blood supply, resulting in partial failure, complete absorption, or an os odontoideum. Sankar et al. [14] support the concept that both trauma and congenital deficiency may be etiologically responsible. It is important to recognize that children who have syndromes which involve the cervical spine such as spondyloepiphyseal dysplasia or Down's syndrome, may develop os odontoideum without a history of previous trauma.

Clinical Features

Odontoid hypoplasia and os odontoideum present with similar clinical findings, caused by instability and displacement of the atlas on the axis. Patients usually present in young adult life and problems are rare in infancy [13], although we have seen cases in children under 3 years.

Congenital odontoid anomalies may be incidental findings in patients who have neck radiographs taken after trauma. This trauma may initiate the atlanto-axial instability or precipitate symptoms in an already compromised, previously asymptomatic joint. Patients may present with no symptoms (incidental diagnosis), local neck symptoms (neck pain, torticollis, and headache), transitory paresis after trauma, or myelopathy (cord compression). Neurological manifestations are recognized with increasing frequency. Although accurate statistics are not available, it is believed that more than 50% of patients either have or will develop neurological problems. These are varied: weakness and loss of balance are common complaints. Upper motor neurone signs, proprioceptive and sphincter disturbances are relatively common. Children with odontoid aplasia and an altered vertebral circulation may suffer a stroke [15].

Imaging

Odontoid aplasia is extremely rare. It is best seen in the open-mouth view. The diagnostic feature is the absence of the basilar portion of the odontoid, which normally dips down into and contributes to the body of the axis. The most common form of hypoplasia presents with a short, stubby peg of odontoid projecting just above the lateral facet articulations. Matsui et al. [16] found that the "round type," which appears to be a very flat C2, has more instability and a greater risk of severe myelopathy. This often causes a Brown-Sequard lesion suggesting a more lateral instability by comparison with the blunt stubby or "cone-shaped" os odontoideum. Watanabe et al. [17] developed an instability index to help evaluate children with an os odontoideum. They defined it as the percentage change in the space available for the cord from neck flexion to extension. Watanabe noted that children with a sagittal plane rotation angle of over 20° or an instability index of more than 40% are likely to have spinal cord signs.

However, the instability associated with os odontoideum is often multidirectional and lateral instability is more likely to cause a neurological problem [16].

Os odontoideum may be overlooked if tomograms or CT are not taken (Fig. 34.5). It appears as a radiolucent oval or round ossicle with a smooth, dense bone border. The size varies but it is usually located in the position of the normal odontoid tip or near the basioccipital bone where it may fuse with the clivus. The dens base is almost invariably hypoplastic.

It may be difficult to differentiate an os odontoideum from non-union after an odontoid fracture. With odontoid non-union, a narrow line separates the odontoid at its base. This may have either irregular or smooth edges of variable cortical thickness. The preservation of the normal shape and size of the dens on the anteroposterior view is an important distinguishing feature. Fagan et al. [18] observed that the C1 anterior arch was intimately related to the os odontoideum in a pattern they termed the "jigsaw sign". The surface interdigitation and narrowed cartilage space suggested a congenital rather than posttraumatic etiology. With os odontoideum, the gap between the os and the hypoplastic dens is wide and usually lies well above the level of the superior articular facets of the axis. The os generally does not preserve the normal shape or size of the odontoid, usually being half the size, rounded or oval, and having a smooth uniform cortex. If the os is in the area of the foramen magnum, there is little diagnostic problem.

The free ossicle of the os odontoideum usually appears fixed to the anterior arch of the atlas and moves with it in flexion and extension. The C1–C2 articulation is usually most unstable in flexion, less often so in extension, and only occasionally unstable in all directions [13]. In one series of patients, the average displacement of those undergoing surgical stabilization was 1.1 cm [13].

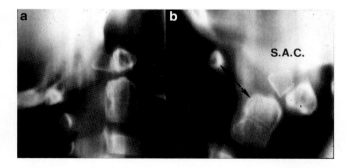

Fig. 34.5 Lateral flexion–extension radiograph of an os odontoideum: (**a**) extension; (**b**) flexion. The odontoid ossicle is fixed to the anterior ring of the atlas and moves with it in flexion and extension and lateral slide. The space available for the spinal cord (SAC) decreases with flexion and the ossicle moves into the spinal canal with extension. From Fielding et al. [13], used with permission

Treatment

Patients with congenital anomalies of the odontoid lead a precarious existence. A trivial insult superimposed on an already weakened and compromised structure may be catastrophic.

Patients with local symptoms or transient myelopathy may expect recovery, at least temporarily. Surgical stabilization is indicated for:

1. neurological involvement (even if transient);
2. instability of 10 mm or greater in flexion and extension;
3. progressive instability;
4. persistent neck complaints associated with instability.

Controversy exists as to the role of prophylactic stabilization in the asymptomatic patient with instability [13]. The possible complications of surgery must be weighed against the dangers of instability with secondary spinal cord pressure. In the paediatric age group, it may be difficult or impossible to curtail activity, even when instability is marked [13]. When fusion is undertaken, regardless of the indication, preoperative halo traction is often required to achieve reduction. This may need to be retained during surgery and postoperatively until converted to a suitable immobilization device [13].

Generally, a posterior approach is sufficient for atlanto-axial arthrodesis by the Gallie technique [19] (Fig. 34.6). When there are associated bony anomalies at the occipito-cervical junction, the fusion may need extension to the occiput. Koop et al. [20] have reported excellent results with stabilization, using a technique of flapping the occipital periosteum to the ring of C1, and external stabilization. Posterior fusion using wiring techniques and/or transarticular screw fixation may avoid the need for postoperative

halo immobilization. C1–2 transarticular screws are the first choice whenever possible [21] (Fig. 34.7). They demonstrate resistance to all three planes of movement. In adults, this construct has provided excellent outcomes and C1–2 transarticular screws have been successful in a large number of children and adolescents. However C1–2 transarticular screws cannot always be used. In 7–22% of patients, the variable location of the foramen transversarium and vulnerability of the vertebral artery make them unsafe [21–24]. The alternatives, which have been less well studied, are C1 lateral mass screws and C2 pars screws combined in a rod-cantilever construct, "the Harms construct" [21].

For irreducible deformity, anterior decompression in conjunction with posterior C1–C2 or occipito-cervical fusion, coupled with internal fixation, has given satisfactory results [25]. Patients with an os odontoideum without neurological deficit and no instability at C1–C2 can be managed without operative intervention. Nonetheless, in these patients, longitudinal clinical and radiographic surveillance is recommended [25].

Klippel–Feil Syndrome

Congenital cervical fusion is the result of failure of the normal segmentation of the cervical somites during the third to eighth weeks of life. With the exception of a few patients in whom this condition is inherited, the etiology is as yet undetermined. It is important to note that the effect of this embryological abnormality is not limited to the cervical spine. Patients with the Klippel–Feil syndrome, even those with minor cervical lesions, may have defects in the genitourinary, nervous, and cardiopulmonary systems, and even hearing impairment [26]. Many of these "hidden" abnormalities may be more detrimental to the patient's general well-being than the obvious deformity in the neck.

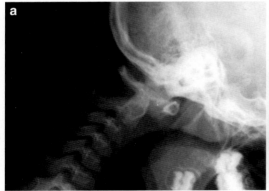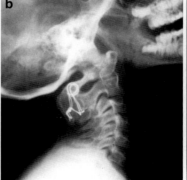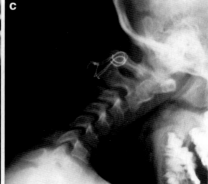

Fig. 34.6 This 7-year-old had a 1-year history of peculiar posturing and stiffness of the neck. (**a**) Flexion and (**b**) Extension and (**c**) flexion radiographs taken after posterior stabilization. Reduction must be accomplished before surgery, and if wire stabilization is selected, care must be taken to avoid further flexion of the neck during passage of the wire under C1

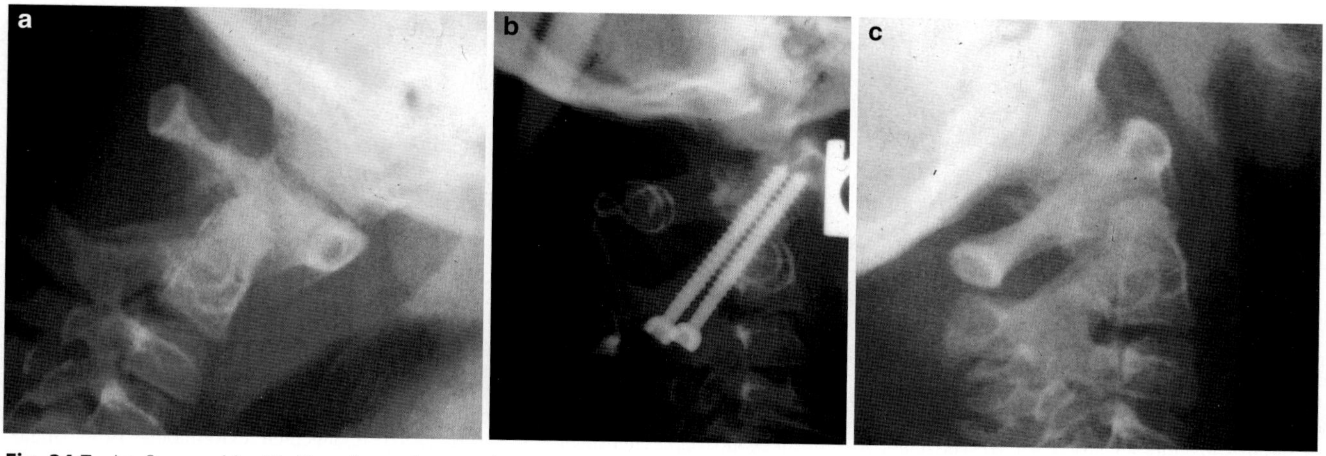

Fig. 34.7 An 8-year-old with Down's syndrome with C1–C2 instability secondary to os odontoideum. (**a**) Flexion view demonstrates instability with significant compromise in the space available for the spinal cord. (**c**) Extension view demonstrates that the C1 ring reduces satisfactorily with C2. (**b**) Postoperative view demonstrates transarticular screws and posterior wire fixation of C1–C2. The patient fused quickly, is asymptomatic, and fully active

In the review by Hensinger et al. [26], a high incidence of related congenital anomalies was reported, emphasizing that all patients with the Klippel–Feil syndrome should be thoroughly investigated.

Symptoms

With the exception of the anomalies that involve the atlantoaxial joint, there are no symptoms that can be directly attributed to the fused cervical vertebrae. All symptoms commonly associated with the Klippel–Feil syndrome originate at the open segments, where the remaining free articulations may show compensatory hypermobility. Symptoms may then arise from two sources:

1. Mechanical symptoms caused by irritation of the joints.
2. Neurological symptoms caused by root irritation or spinal cord compression.

The majority of patients who develop symptoms are in the second or third decade of life, suggesting that the instability is in part a function of time, with increasing ligament laxity.

Clinical Features

The classical clinical description of the syndrome is a triad of low posterior hairline, short neck, and limitation of neck motion (Figs. 34.8a, b), but fewer than 50% of the patients have all three signs. Clinically, the most consistent finding is limitation of neck movement. Shortening of the neck, unless extreme, is a subtle finding. Similarly, the low posterior hairline is not constant. Fewer than 20% of patients with the Klippel–Feil syndrome have obvious facial asymmetry, torticollis, or webbing of the neck.

Sprengel's deformity (Chapter 22) occurs in 17–33% of patients [27]. Other clinical features are occasionally found: ptosis of the eye, Duane's contracture (contracture of the lateral rectus muscle), lateral rectus palsy, facial nerve palsy, and a cleft or high arched palate. Abnormalities of the upper extremities include syndactyly, thumb hypoplasia, supernumerary digits, and hypoplasia of the upper extremity. Abnormalities of the lower extremities are infrequent [26].

Imaging Features

In the severely affected child, adequate radiographic evaluation can be difficult. Fixed bony deformities frequently prevent proper positioning, and overlapping shadows from the mandible, occiput, or foramen magnum may obscure the upper vertebrae. CT scanning coupled with flexion–extension radiographs of the cervical spine (Figs. 34.8c, d) can delineate more precisely the presence or absence of spinal cord compression. MRI is also useful. Apart from vertebral fusion, flattening and widening of the involved vertebral bodies and absent disc spaces are the most common findings (Figs. 34.9 and 34.10).

Narrowing of the spinal canal, if it occurs, usually manifests in adult life and is due to degenerative changes (osteoarthritic spurs) or hypermobility. Enlargement of the cervical canal is uncommon and, if found, may

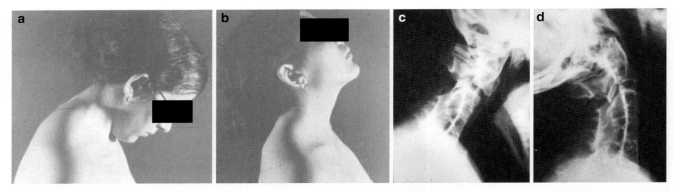

Fig. 34.8 An 18-year-old female with the Klippel–Feil syndrome demonstrating flexion–extension of the cervical spine, both clinically (**a** and **b**) and radiologically (**c** and **d**). The majority of the neck motion is occurring at the C3–C4 disc space. Clinically, the patient is able to maintain adequate range (90°) of flexion–extension. At the time of these examinations, she was asymptomatic, but with aging this hypermobile articulation may become unstable. This article was published in: Hensinger RN, MacEwen GD. Congenital abnormalities of the spine. In: Rothman RH, Simeone FA, eds. The Spine. Philadelphia: Elsevier; 1982:219. Copyright Elsevier; 1982

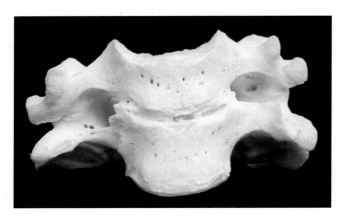

Fig. 34.9 Anterior view of a postmortem specimen of a congenital block vertebra of C3–C4. The specimen demonstrates complete fusion, but remnants of the cartilaginous vertebral endplates can still be seen

indicate the presence of conditions such as a syringomyelia, hydromyelia, or the Arnold–Chiari malformation.

All these defects may extend into the upper thoracic spine, particularly in the severely affected patient. A disturbance of the upper thoracic spine on a routine chest radiograph may be the first clue to an unrecognized cervical synostosis. When a high thoracic congenital scoliosis is being assessed, the radiographic evaluation should routinely include lateral flexion–extension views of the cervical spine. In a group of 33 patients with the Klippel–Feil syndrome, occipitalization occurred in nearly half and fusion in the C2–C3 segment was noted in 72% [7]. When these are combined, there is a great propensity for instability at the atlanto-axial joint. However, the authors found that minor degrees of hypermobility at the atlanto-axial junction were not necessarily associated with an increased risk of symptoms or neurological signs.

Associated Conditions

Scoliosis/Kyphosis

Scoliosis is the most frequent anomaly found in association with the syndrome [26], with 60% of patients having a significant curve.

Renal Abnormalities

In the Klippel–Feil syndrome, more than 33% of the children can be expected to have a significant urinary tract anomaly, which is often asymptomatic in the young.

Sprengel's Deformity

Sprengel's deformity occurs in 17–33% of Klippel–Feil patients. There is no specific correlation with fusion patterns, gender, the number of fused segments, or the degree of cervical scoliosis [27].

Cardiovascular Abnormalities

Up to 14% of patients have congenital heart disease.

Deafness

The otology literature has reported hearing impairment and deafness in more than 30% of patients with Klippel–Feil syndrome. Other defects include absence of the auditory canal

Fig. 34.10 (**a**) Radiographs of a 7-year-old demonstrating posterior fusion of the laminae and spinous process, but incomplete fusion of the vertebral bodies anteriorly. (**b**) Same patient at age 20 years, now demonstrating complete fusion of the vertebral bodies C1–C2 and C3–C7. In children, narrowing of the cervical disc spaces cannot always be appreciated, as ossification of vertebral bodies is not completed until adolescence. The unossified cartilage endplates can give a false impression of a normal disc space

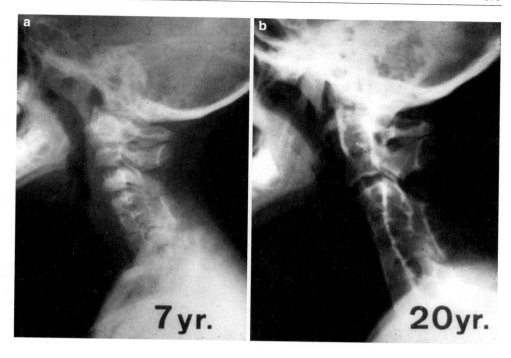

and microtia. There is no characteristic audiological anomaly and all types of hearing loss have been described.

Mirror Motions (Synkinesia)

Synkinesia consists of involuntary paired movements of the hands and, occasionally, the arms. It was first described by Bauman [28], who found it to be present in four of six patients with the Klippel–Feil syndrome. Approximately 20% demonstrate mirror motions clinically [26].

Treatment

The minimally affected patient with the Klippel–Feil syndrome can be expected to lead a normal active life, with no or only minor restrictions. Many severely affected patients will enjoy the same good prognosis if early and appropriate treatment is instituted when needed. This is particularly applicable in the area of associated Sprengel's deformity, scoliosis, and renal abnormalities. Prevention of further deformity or complications can be of great benefit to the patient. Those patients with major areas of cervical synostosis or high-risk patterns of cervical spine motion should be strongly advised to avoid activities that place stress on the cervical spine. Theiss et al. [29] found that 22% of the patients with the Klippel–Feil syndrome and congenital scoliosis developed cervical symptoms on long-term follow-up. Some fusion patterns put them at particular risk. There was a greater

likelihood of neck symptoms with fusion at the cervicothoracic junction and congenital cervical stenosis. Pizzutillo et al. [30] reported on long-term follow-up that individuals with Klippel–Feil syndrome who had hypermobility of the upper cervical segments were at risk of neurological sequelae. Those with alteration in motion in the lower cervical segment were more likely to develop degenerative disease. Sudden neurological compromise or death after minor trauma has been reported in the Klippel–Feil syndrome and is usually the result of disruption at the hypermobile articulation. The role of prophylactic surgical stabilization in the asymptomatic patient has not yet been defined.

Differential Diagnosis of Torticollis

Torticollis, or wry-neck, is a common childhood complaint. The etiology is diverse and identifying the cause can be difficult.

Congenital muscular torticollis is the most common cause in the infant and young child, but there are other problems that lead to this unusual posture. Head tilt and rotatory deformity of the head and neck (torticollis) usually indicate a problem at C1–C2, whereas head tilt alone indicates a more generalized problem in the cervical spine. If the posturing of the head and neck is noted at or shortly after birth, congenital anomalies of the cervical spine, particularly those that involve C1–C2, typically present as a rigid deformity, and the sternocleidomastoid muscle is not contracted or in spasm.

Approximately 20% of patients with the Klippel–Feil syndrome have associated torticollis [26, 31]. With asymmetric development of the occipital condyles or the facets of C1, the head tilt may result in a torticollis unless compensated for by a tilt of the lower cervical spine such as occurs in the milder forms [11].

Inflammatory conditions such as cervical lymphadenitis may cause a wry-neck tilt. A less frequent cause is a retropharyngeal abscess complicating posterior pharyngeal inflammation or tonsillitis. Children with polyarticular juvenile idiopathic arthritis often develop cervical joint involvement: torticollis and limited neck movement may be the only clinical signs. Spontaneous atlanto-axial rotatory subluxation may follow acute pharyngitis [31]. A rare inflammatory cause is acute calcification of a cervical disc, which can be seen on plain radiographs.

Trauma should always be considered and carefully excluded. If unrecognized it may have serious neurological consequences. In general, torticollis most commonly follows injury to the Cl–C2 articulation. Minor trauma can lead to spontaneous C1–C2 subluxation. Fracture or dislocation of the odontoid may not be apparent on the initial radiographs and, consequently, a high index of suspicion and careful follow-up are required.

Children with bone dysplasia, Morquio's syndrome, spondyloepiphyseal dysplasia, and Down's syndrome have a high incidence of Cl–C2 instability and should be evaluated routinely.

Intermittent torticollis can occur in the young child. A seizure-like disorder called benign paroxysmal torticollis of infancy is due to many neurological causes, including drug intoxication. Similarly, Sandifer's syndrome, involving gastro-esophageal reflux with sudden posturing of the trunk and torticollis, is being recognized more often, particularly in the neurologically handicapped child, for example, with cerebral palsy [32].

Neurological disorders, particularly space-occupying lesions of the central nervous system, such as tumors of the posterior fossa or spinal column, chordoma and syringomyelia, are often accompanied by torticollis. Generally, there will be additional neurological findings such as long-tract signs and weakness in the upper extremities. Uncommon neurological causes include dystonia musculorum deformans and problems of hearing and vision that can result in head tilt. Although uncommon, hysterical and psychogenic causes exist, but should be diagnosed only after other causes have been excluded.

Radiographs

All children with torticollis should be evaluated with radiographs to exclude a bony abnormality or fracture.

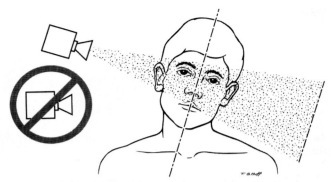

Ring of C1 stays with the Occiput

Fig. 34.11 Obtaining a satisfactory radiograph may be hampered by the patient's limited ability to cooperate, fixed bony deformity, and overlapping shadows from the mandible, occiput and foramen magnum. A helpful guide is that the atlas moves with the occiput, and if the X-ray beam is directed 90° to the lateral of the skull, a satisfactory view of the occipito-cervical junction usually results

Radiographic interpretation of congenital torticollis may be difficult because of the fixed abnormal head position and restricted motion. In those with a painful wry-neck, it may be impossible to position the child appropriately for a standard view of the occipito-cervical junction. A helpful guide is that the atlas moves with the occiput, so that if the X-ray beam is directed 90° to the lateral skull, a satisfactory view of the occipito-cervical junction is usually obtained (Fig. 34.11). Flexion–extension stress films, laminograms, or cineradiography may be necessary to confirm atlanto-axial instability.

Atlanto-Axial Rotary Displacement

The onset of the problem may be spontaneous, associated with trivial trauma, or may follow an upper respiratory tract infection. Typically, the child awakes with a "crick" in the neck and, with little or no treatment, this resolves within 1 week. Rarely, these deformities persist and the child presents with a resistant, unresolving torticollis, best described as atlanto-axial rotary fixation or fixed atlanto-axial displacement.

This problem can occur within the normal range of motion or with anterior shift of the atlas on the axis as a result of fractures of C1 and C2 or ligamentous deficiency, leading to atlanto-axial instability. Neurological deficits may rarely be associated with rotary displacements, particularly with anterior displacement.

The etiology of this type of displacement remains theoretical, because insufficient anatomical and postmortem evidence is available. The obstruction is probably capsular and synovial interposition, which produces pain in the

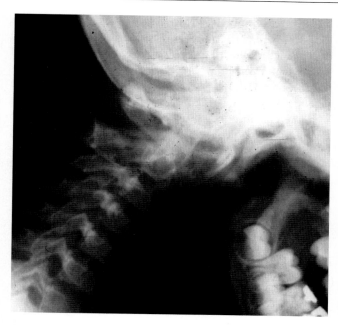

Fig. 34.12 Marked anterior displacement of C1 on C2 found in a patient with atlanto-axial rotatory fixation of 2 months' duration

initial stages, with resultant muscle spasm. The spasm holds the neck in flexion and may aggravate forward displacement of C1 on C2 (Fig. 34.12).

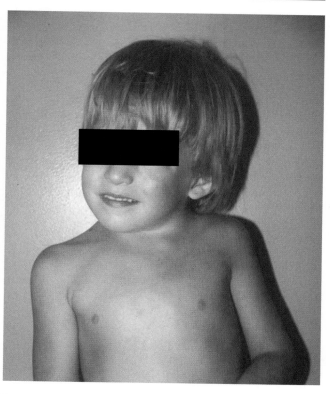

Fig. 34.13 Typical torticollis position of atlanto-axial rotatory displacement (cock robin), with the head rotated in one direction and tilted to the opposite side, with slight flexion

Clinical Features

The torticollis position is likened to a robin listening for a worm or the "cocked robin" position (Fig. 34.13). The head is tilted to one side and rotated to the opposite side, with slight flexion. When the condition is acute, the child resists attempts to move the head, complaining of marked pain with any passive attempts to do so. Associated muscle spasm, unlike muscular torticollis, is predominantly on the side of the "long" sternocleidomastoid, because this muscle is attempting to correct the deformity. If the deformity becomes fixed, the pain will subside but the torticollis will persist, associated with a diminished range of neck motion. In long-standing cases, particularly in younger children, facial asymmetry with flattening may develop.

Imaging Features

In the acute stages, the diagnosis depends primarily on history and clinical evidence, because plain radiographs are not diagnostic. In the open-mouth anteroposterior and lateral projections, the lateral mass of C1 that has rotated forward appears wider and closer to the midline (medial offset), whereas the opposite lateral mass is narrower and away from the midline (lateral offset). One of the facet joints may be obscured because of apparent overlapping.

On the lateral projection, the wedge-shaped lateral mass of the atlas lies anteriorly, where the oval arch of the atlas normally lies. The posterior arches of the atlas fail to superimpose because of head tilt. This may suggest assimilation of the atlas to the occiput because head tilt allows the skull to obscure C1. Flexion–extension stress films rule out the anterior displacement of atlas on axis that is occasionally seen with rotary displacement.

Type I rotary displacement is by far the most common form seen in children (Fig. 34.14). It is more benign and may be managed expectantly. The type II deformity is potentially more dangerous needs carefully management. Type III and IV deformities are rare, but neurological involvement or even instant death may follow and demand very careful treatment. CT has largely replaced cineradiology as the radiological technique of choice for this condition (Fig. 34.15). In children with suspected atlanto-axial rotary displacement, Been et al. [33] recommend CT scanning under general anesthesia. Patients improve if the examination is normal.

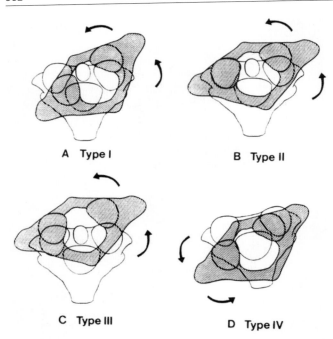

Fig. 34.14 Classification of rotatory displacement. From Fielding and Hawkins [31], used with permission

Treatment

Many cases of atlanto-axial rotary displacement prove transitory. The stiff neck and slightly twisted head resolve in a few days. If the complaints are mild and have been present for less than 1 week, we advise a simple soft collar and analgesics. If there is no spontaneous improvement or the symptoms persist, more aggressive treatment should be instituted. When simple measures fail, we suggest bed rest, halter traction, muscle relaxants, and analgesics. If the atlas is displaced anteriorly on the axis, gradual reduction should be obtained, followed by immobilization in the corrected position in a Minerva cast for 6 weeks to allow ligamentous healing. Careful follow-up is necessary because of the potential for continued atlanto-axial instability.

If the condition has been present for 1–3 months, halo traction is often necessary to achieve reduction. However, the C1–C2 articulation may not stabilize after immobilization and then needs surgical correction and fusion. If the condition has been present for over 3 months, the deformity typically is fixed. In those whose spinal canal is compromised by anterior C1 displacement, a further insult could be catastrophic. C1–C2 fusion is indicated to achieve stability and to maintain correction.

Congenital Muscular Torticollis (Congenital Wry-Neck)

Torticollis is common in the first 6–8 weeks of life. The deformity is caused by contracture of the sternocleidomastoid muscle, with the head tilted toward the involved side and the chin rotated toward the contralateral shoulder (Fig. 34.16). If the infant is examined within the first 4 weeks of life, a mass or "tumor" is usually palpable in the neck (Fig. 34.17). It is generally a non-tender, soft enlargement that is mobile beneath the skin and attached to or located within the body of the sternocleidomastoid. The mass attains maximum size within the first 1 month of life and then gradually regresses. If the child is examined after 4–6 months of age, the mass is usually absent, and contracture of the

Fig. 34.15 Dynamic CT scan of the upper cervical spine in atlanto-axial rotatory subluxation. (**a**) The head is rotated approximately 45° to one side, with the contralateral lateral mass of C1 moving forward on the facet of C2. (**b**) The head cannot be rotated past the midline, and the relationship of C1–C2 is unchanged. From Phillips WA, Hensinger RN. The management of rotatory atlanto-axial subluxation in children. J Bone Joint Surg 1989; 71A:665. Used with permission

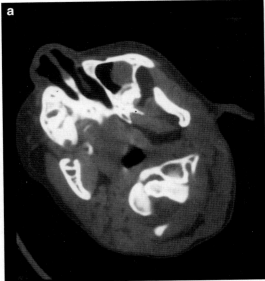
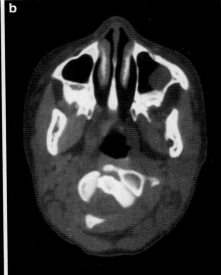

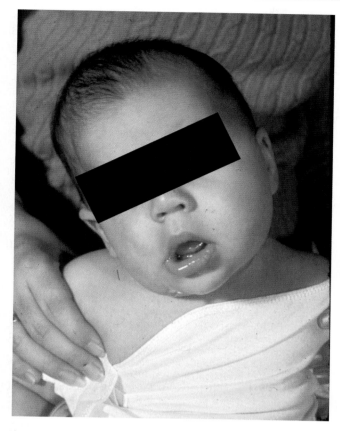

Fig. 34.16 A 6-month-old infant with right-sided congenital muscular torticollis. Note the rotation of the skull and asymmetry and flattening of the face on the side of the contracted sternocleidomastoid

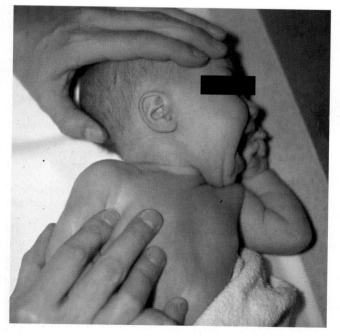

Fig. 34.17 Six-week-old infant with swelling in the region of the sternocleidomastoid muscle. The mass is usually soft, non-tender, and mobile beneath the skin, but is attached to the muscle

sternocleidomastoid muscle and the torticollis posture are the only clinical findings (Fig. 34.16).

If the condition is progressive, deformities of the face and skull can result, and they are usually apparent within the first year. Flattening of the face on the side of the contracted sternocleidomastoid muscle may be marked (Fig. 34.16). If the condition remains untreated during the growth years, the level of the eyes and ears becomes distorted and may result in considerable cosmetic deformity.

Etiology

Birth records of affected children demonstrate a preponderance of breech or difficult deliveries or primiparous births [34]. However, the deformity may occur with normal delivery and in infants born by Cesarean section [34]. In one study, half the patients had a difficult delivery, 7% were born by Cesarean section and 44% by uncomplicated vaginal delivery [35]. Difficult deliveries included breech presentation, vacuum extraction and forceps instrumentation. Microscopic examination of resected surgical specimens and experimental work suggest that the lesion is caused by occlusion of the venous outflow of the sternocleidomastoid muscle. This leads to edema, muscle fiber degeneration and eventually, fibrosis. The problem may be caused by uterine crowding or "packing" because in 75% of children in one study the lesion was right sided [34]. In addition, 20% of children with congenital muscular torticollis have congenital dysplasia of the hip, similarly associated with restricted infant movement in the tight maternal space. In a more recent publication, 6% of children with developmental dysplasia of the hip (DDH) were diagnosed subsequently with congenital muscular torticollis [35]. Infants less than 1 month at diagnosis were at greater risk (9%) and boys were at greater risk of having both conditions.

Imaging

It is probably unnecessary to take radiographs of all neonates with a typical sternomastoid tumor. Radiographs of the cervical spine should be taken to exclude bony anomaly if infants fail to respond to simple stretching or if the torticollis, is atypical. Tatli et al. [36] found cervical ultrasound to be helpful in the diagnosis of congenital torticollis, identifying a fusiform enlargement of the muscle. They identified two clinical groups, one with (85%) and one without (15%) the swelling. In considering a compartment syndrome, MRI was inconsistent, did not alter treatment, and is not therefore recommended in assessment [37].

Treatment

Conservative

Most respond to a range of motion exercises supervised by a physiotherapist and carried out by the family [34, 38]. Ninety-five percent of children treated at a mean age of 2.3 months resolved with early aggressive treatment [36]. If treatment begins before 6 weeks and the infant has no neck mass, the prognosis is excellent. If the neck mass persists for more than 6 weeks, persistent deformity may follow [36].

Additional treatment measures include positioning the crib and toys so that the neck will be stretched when the infant reaches and grasps. Using a "sleeping helmet" to reduce deformity and hasten face and skull remodeling [39] is rarely necessary.

Operation

If the condition persists beyond 1 year, non-operative measures rarely succeed [38]. Similarly, established facial asymmetry and movement limited by more than 10° usually preclude a good result and operation is needed to prevent further facial flattening and poor cosmesis [38]. However, a good (but not perfect) cosmetic result may be obtained as late as 12 years of age. Asymmetry of the skull and face will improve as long as adequate growth potential remains once the deforming pull of the sternocleidomastoid is removed.

The operation should completely section the distal insertion of the sternocleidomastoid muscle. It is important to release fascial bands. In the older child it may be necessary to divide the muscle proximally at its mastoid origin in addition. Recently, endoscopic release has been used to reduce scarring and the risk of injuring the spinal accessory nerve or greater auricular nerve [40]. The entire muscle should not be excised, because this may lead to reverse torticollis [34] or additional deformity. The postoperative regimen includes passive stretching exercises in the same manner as those performed preoperatively. The night use of halter traction at home may help. Bracing or cast correction may be necessary if the deformity is long-standing. The results of surgery are uniformly good with a low incidence of complications or recurrence [34, 38]. If the patient is young, the facial asymmetry can be expected to resolve completely [34].

References

1. Klippel M, Feil A. Un cas d'absence des vertebras cervicales avec cage thoracique. remontant jusqu'à la base du crane. Nouvelle Iconographie de la Salpetrière. 1912; 25:223–250.

2. McRae DL. The significance of abnormalities of the cervical spine. Am J Roentgenol 1960; 84:3–25.

3. Erbengi A, Oge HK. Congenital malformations of the cranioverte-bral junction: classification and surgical treatment. Acta Neurochir (Wien) 1994; 127:180–185.

4. Chamberlain WE. Basilar impression (platybasia): bizarre developmental anatomy of occipital bone and upper cervical spine with striking and misleading neurologic manifestation. Yale J Biol Med 1939; 11:487–496.

5. McGregor M. The significance of certain measurements of the skull in the diagnosis of basilar impression. Br J Radiol 1948; 21:171–181.

6. Gholve PA, Hosalkar HS, Ricchetti ET, et al. Occipitalization of the atlas in children. Morphologic classification, associations, and clinical relevance. J Bone Joint Surg Am 2007; 89:571–578.

7. Shen FH, Samartzis D, Herman J, et al. Radiographic assessment of segmental motion at the atlantoaxial junction in the Klippel-Feil patient. Spine 2006; 31:171–177.

8. Rouvreau P, Glorion, C, Langlais, J, et al. Assessment and neurologic involvement of patients with cervical spine congenital synostosis as in Klippel–Feil syndrome: study of 19 cases. J Pediatr Orthop 1998; 7B:179–185.

9. Samartzis D, Kalluri P, Herman J, et al. Superior odontoid migration in the Klippel-Feil patient. Eur Spine J 2007; 16:1489–1497.

10. Senoglu M, Safavi-Abbasi S, Theodore N, et al. The frequency and clinical significance of congenital defects of the posterior and anterior arch of the atlas. J Neurosurg Spine 2007; 7:399–402.

11. Dubousset J. Torticollis in children caused by congenital anomalies of the atlas. J Bone Joint Surg Am 1986; 68:178–188.

12. Burke SW, French HG, Roberts JM, et al. Chronic atlanto-axial instability in Down syndrome. J Bone Joint Surg Am 1985; 67:1356–1360.

13. Fielding JW, Hensinger RN, Hawkins RJ. Os odontoideum. J Bone Joint Surg Am 1980; 62:376–383.

14. Sankar WN, Wills BP, Dormans JP, et al. Os odontoideum revisited: the case for a multifactorial etiology. Spine 2006; 31:979–984.

15. Phillips PC, Lorentsen KJ, Shropshire LC, et al. Congenital odontoid aplasia and posterior circulation stroke in childhood. Ann Neurol 1988; 23:410–413.

16. Matsui H, Imada K, Tsuji H. Radiographic classification of Os odontoideum and its clinical significance. Spine 1997; 22:1706–1709.

17. Watanabe M, Toyama Y, Fujimura Y. Atlantoaxial instability in os odontoideum with myelopathy. Spine 1996; 21:1435–1439.

18. Fagan AB, Askin GN, Earwaker JW. The jigsaw sign. A reliable indicator of congenital aetiology in os odontoideum. Eur Spine J 2004; 13:295–300.

19. Stabler CL, Eismont FJ, Brown MD, et al. Failure of posterior cervical fusions using cadaveric bone graft in children. J Bone Joint Surg Am 1985; 67:371–375.

20. Koop SE, Winter RB, Lonstein JE. The surgical treatment of instability of the upper part of the cervical spine in children and adolescents. J Bone Joint Surg Am 1984; 66:403–411.

21. Anderson RC, Ragel BT, Mocco J, et al. Selection of a rigid internal fixation construct for stabilization at the craniovertebral junction in pediatric patients. J Neurosurg 2007; 107:36–42.

22. Brockmeyer DL, York JE, Apfelbaum RI. Anatomical suitability of C1–2 transarticular screw placement in pediatric patients. J Neurosurg 2000; 92:7–11.

23. Igarashi T, Kikuchi S, Sato K, et al. Anatomic study of the axis for surgical planning of transarticular screw fixation. Clin Orthop Rel Res 2003; 408:162–166.

24. Madawi AA, Casey AT, Solanki GA, et al. Radiological and anatomical evaluation of the atlantoaxial transarticular screw fixation technique. J Neurosurg 1997; 86:961–968.

25. Os odontoideum. Neurosurgery 2002; 50:S148–155.
26. Hensinger RN, Lang JE, MacEwen GD. Klippel–Feil syndrome; a constellation of associated anomalies. J Bone Joint Surg Am 1974; 56:1246–1253.
27. Samartzis D, Herman J, Lubicky JP, et al. Sprengel's deformity in Klippel–Feil syndrome. Spine 2007; 32:E512–516.
28. Bauman G. Absence of the cervical spine: Klippel–Feil syndrome. JAMA 1998; 98:129–132.
29. Theiss SM, Smith MD, Winter RB. The long-term follow-up of patients with Klippel–Feil syndrome and congenital scoliosis. Spine 1997; 22:1219–1222.
30. Pizzutillo PD, Woods M, Nicholson L, et al. Risk factors in Klippel–Feil syndrome. Spine 1994; 19:2110–2116.
31. Fielding JW, Hawkins RJ. Atlanto-axial rotatory fixation. (Fixed rotatory subluxation of the atlanto-axial joint). J Bone Joint Surg Am 1977; 59:37–44.
32. Sutcliff J. Torsion spasms and abnormal postures in children with hiatus hernia: Sandifer's syndrome. Prog Pediatr Radiol 1969; 2:190–197.
33. Been HD, Kerkhoffs GM, Maas M. Suspected atlantoaxial rotatory fixation-subluxation: the value of multidetector computed tomography scanning under general anesthesia. Spine 2007; 32:E163–167.
34. MacDonald D. Sternomastoid tumour and muscular torticollis. J Bone Joint Surg Br 1969; 51:432–443.
35. von Heideken J, Green DW, Burke SW, et al. The relationship between developmental dysplasia of the hip and congenital muscular torticollis. J Pediatr Orthop 2006; 26:805–808.
36. Tatli B, Aydinli N, Caliskan M, et al. Congenital muscular torticollis: evaluation and classification. Pediatr Neurol 2006; 34:41–44.
37. Parikh SN, Crawford AH, Choudhury S. Magnetic resonance imaging in the evaluation of infantile torticollis. Orthopedics 2004; 27:509–515.
38. Canale ST, Griffin DW, Hubbard CN. Congenital muscular torticollis. A long-term follow-up. J Bone Joint Surg Am 1982; 64:810–816.
39. Clarren SK, Smith DW, Hanson JW. Helmet treatment for plagiocephaly and congenital muscular torticollis. J Pediatr 1979; 94:43–46.
40. Swain B. Transaxillary endoscopic release of restricting bands in congenital muscular torticollis—a novel technique. J Plast Reconstr Aesthet Surg 2007; 60:95–98.

Chapter 35

Back Pain in Children

Robert A. Dickson

Introduction

Back pain in childhood, while uncommon, is often associated with serious underlying pathology. In one series of 210 cases [1], infection or neoplasia proved to be the underlying cause in more than 40% of patients younger than 12 years of age. After this age, there is a relative increase in non-specific causes of backache. Adolescent back pain is associated with decreased mobility of the lumbar spine and stiffness of the hip and knee joints [2]. Back pain in the adolescent age group is more common in girls and also exhibits a familial pattern [3]. During later adolescence, trauma, mechanical, and early degenerative disorders are more frequent causes of back pain, and serious pathology affects only a small proportion.

In young children, back pain tends to be vague and poorly localized. Consequently spinal or paraspinal pathology in the young may be easily missed or incorrectly diagnosed, with adverse effects upon subsequent treatment and outcome. Careful clinical evaluation, appropriate investigation, and a grasp of the likely causes for each age group minimize the likelihood of that unsatisfactory state of affairs.

Assessment of the Child

While older children and adolescents can often give a clear history of their back pain, localizing it well and describing neurological symptoms, this is not so in the infant or younger child who may just be irritable, with a stiff back and a reluctance to move or weight-bear. In this very young age group meaningful examination can be difficult, so it is best to assess the child on mother's lap in a warm quiet environment. It is often only possible to observe the presence or absence of movement of major muscle groups and, perhaps, muscle wasting since an irritable young child often prevents any further neurological examination. When assessed prone, muscle spasm, swelling, and abnormal alignment may be seen; it is very important to palpate for spinal tenderness (only present with infection or fresh injury). With infection, especially if associated with a psoas abscess, abdominal pain and tenderness are common and may mimic renal or retroperitoneal sepsis.

The older child and adolescent can be more meaningfully assessed and both kyphotic and scoliotic deformities are best visualized in the forward bending position. When a thoracic kyphosis is present, forward bending demonstrates either a smooth hyperkyphosis with postural, roundback deformity or an angular one in association with Scheuermann's disease or localized pathology.

Idiopathic scoliosis is not usually painful except for a fatigue-type discomfort over the rotational prominence. If pain is severe, particularly at night, or if there is an atypical curve pattern such as a progressive left thoracic curve in a male then underlying pathology (tumor or syrinx) must be excluded. In the case of lumbosacral pain (with or without a local step), spondylolysis, spondylolisthesis, or adolescent disc syndrome should be suspected, particularly if associated with significant lumbosacral stiffness, tight hamstrings, or neurological deficit. Ankylosing spondylitis is another, but unusual, cause of back stiffness. It is important to differentiate between spine and hip movement particularly during the composite, forward flexion of back movement.

A more adequate neurological assessment can be carried out in the older child and adolescent. Power in all muscle groups and sensation in all lower limb dermatomes should be examined along with all reflexes, including the abdominals which may be suppressed or asymmetrical in the presence of a syrinx.

R.A. Dickson (✉)
Academic Unit of Orthopaedic Surgery, Leeds General Infirmary, Leeds, UK

M. Benson et al. (eds.), *Children's Orthopaedics and Fractures*,
DOI 10.1007/978-1-84882-611-3_35, © Springer-Verlag London Limited 2010

Congenital Spinal Anomalies

Be wary of blaming troublesome back symptoms on a congenital malformation: it may be a coincidental finding. The various types of congenital scoliosis and kyphosis, even when associated with dysraphism, rarely cause pain unless they produce secondary mechanical effects. The child or adolescent with a painful scoliosis should be assumed, until proven otherwise, to have an underlying tumor (such as osteoid osteoma) or infection.

Spinal Trauma

In general, the paediatric spine is remarkably resistant to trauma because of its suppleness and spinal cord injuries are therefore rare. However, Kewalramani and Tori [4] found a much higher incidence of cord injury in children under 15 years of age, accounting for one-tenth of all spinal cord injuries. They also reported a preponderance of cervical injuries. In this age group about 50% suffer incomplete or complete paralysis.

Spinal cord injury without obvious radiographic abnormality (SCIWORA) is encountered frequently in the elderly, whose pre-existing degenerative neck disease and spurs of bone already indent the spinal cord and render it vulnerable to, for example, a whiplash flexion injury. It not uncommonly occurs also in children with pristine but hypermobile neck joints and is peculiar to the cervical spine. Consequently neck radiographs can be entirely normal, but physiological displacements, curvatures, and variations in ossification are the subtle features that point to the diagnosis [5].

Most children, particularly younger ones, sustain spinal trauma as a result of a road traffic accident, while older children are usually injured in a sporting mishap [4]. The upper cervical spine is greatly over-represented in children as the site of injury [6], the atlanto-axial level being notorious. A central cord pattern of spinal cord injury is usually produced. The problem is discussed in detail in Chapter 52.

In infancy back trauma raises the possibility of non-accidental injury. Cullen in 1975 demonstrated that vertebral collapse particularly in the thoraco-lumbar region can be part of the battered baby syndrome [7]. Therefore a lateral view of the thoraco-lumbar spine is recommended as part of the non-accidental injury radiograph series [8] (Fig. 35.1).

With thoraco-lumbar spinal injuries, after the initial acute pain subsides, the symptoms can persist or worsen if a traumatic kyphosis develops. There is usually some increase in kyphosis from compression of the cancellous bone of the affected vertebral body but significantly progressive kyphosis suggests a Salter type V injury to the growth plate. Eventually the pain does tend to settle but a considerable post-traumatic kyphosis may warrant surgical correction, as does severe Scheuermann's disease.

The growing spine can be traumatized iatrogenically by way of laminectomy, undertaken surgically to deal with spinal cord tumors or other problems (Fig. 35.2). The tension band function of the posterior column is lost, leading to progressive kyphosis. A combined approach from a neurosurgeon and an orthopaedic spinal surgeon, the latter instrumenting and fusing the spine after laminectomy, guards against subsequent deformity.

Spinal Infection

While spinal infection still represents a problem in the developing world, only 2–4% of infections in the developed world involve the spine [9]. Two-thirds are pyogenic and one-third

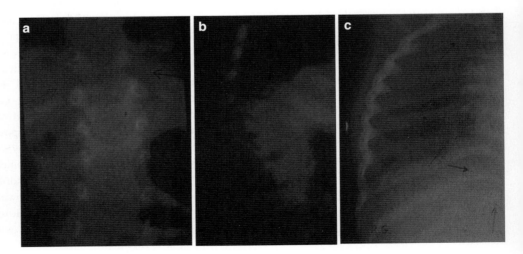

Fig. 35.1 The spine in child abuse. (**a**) Anteroposterior (AP) view showing soft tissue shadowing (*arrows*) at the T11/12 level. (**b**) Lateral radiograph showing a wedge compression fracture. (**c**) AP radiograph of right ribs showing multiple healing fractures (*arrows*)

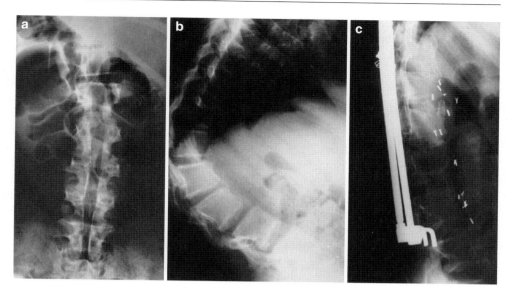

Fig. 35.2 Post-laminectomy kyphosis in a growing child. (**a**) AP view of the lumbar spine showing a decompressive laminectomy for spinal stenosis in a 15-year-old boy with achondroplasia. (**b**) Lateral radiograph of the lumbar spine 2 years later. With loss of the posterior tension band the spine has collapsed into 90° of kyphosis. (**c**) Lateral radiograph of the lumbar spine after anterior release and interbody grafting and posterior instrumentation

tuberculous, but the initial presentation is often very similar and in both there is commonly a delay or failure in making the correct diagnosis which leads to chronicity [10].

More than 50% of pyogenic infections are due to the *Staphylococcus aureus*, the remainder being caused by *Streptococci, Escherichia coli, Pseudomonas, Pneumococcus, Meningococcus, Salmonella, Brucella*, and fungi. With an increasing number of human immunodeficiency virus (HIV)-positive patients unusual organisms are being detected with more mixed growth patterns and increased antibiotic resistance. Previous antibiotic administration makes it difficult to isolate the offending organism. Tuberculosis is now universally caused by the human rather than the bovine bacillus.

The final common pathway for organisms tracking into the vertebra is by way of the rich vascular supply to the spine and, in particular, Batson's plexus of veins. This communicates freely with the valveless vertebral veins which spread from the occiput to the coccyx [11]. However, it is thought that the rich arterial route to the spine is probably the more important, organisms entering the vertebral bodies by the anterior and posterior nutrient foramina [12]. Here they flourish in the richly vascular metaphyseal region close to the end plate. This increased blood supply in the immature spine probably accounts for the greater prevalence of infection in the young. The relatively avascular nucleus may suffer infarction as a result of pressure from local pus or toxins and from vascular spasm. Disc resorption is particularly common in pyogenic infection as the discs are much more resistant to tuberculous infection.

As the infection gains momentum there is vertebral collapse on each side of the disc region with end plate perforation (Fig. 35.3). Abscess formation is much more obvious

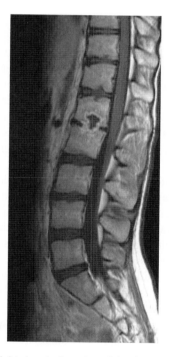

Fig. 35.3 T2-weighted sagittal section of the thoraco-lumbar spine of a teenager showing pyogenic osteomyelitis with disc space narrowing and end plate perforation

in tuberculous infection, and this can spread anteriorly in the lumbar region to the psoas muscle sheath and posteriorly into the epidural space. Compression of the spinal cord results not only from the abscess but also from locally sequestrated bone and disc fragments and an increasing kyphotic deformity. Cord compromise in tuberculosis is caused by spasm of the arterial supply, bacterial meningitis, or fibrotic constriction of the meninges.

Magnetic resonance imaging (MRI) is diagnostic in more than 95% of cases, but plain films are useful for assessing bone destruction and overall spine alignment [9].

Pyogenic Infection

Fever, back pain, and tenderness constitute the classical triad. Of these, back pain is the most common presenting feature. There can also be extreme stiffness and muscle spasm of the spine and sometimes radicular pain. The white blood cell count is seldom less in 10,000 per milliliter and the erythrocyte sedimentation rate (ESR) not usually less than 20 mm in the first hour (plasma viscosity 1.7). A raised ESR has been found to be the most reliable laboratory test [13]. It is important that diagnostic material be submitted for aerobic, anaerobic, tuberculous, and fungal examination as well as samples being sent for pathological examination in case the cultures prove negative. In the presence of significant pyrexia blood cultures may yield the organism, but needle biopsy of the spine under computed tomography (CT) guidance is becoming more widely used. Because 40% of patients in one series had received antibiotics before biopsy, an organism was only isolated in 40%, but the result of biopsy led to a change in management in more than a third of patients [14]. Molecular biological techniques are increasingly used to determine the precise organism.

The mainstay of treatment for pyogenic infections is antibiotic therapy according to the culture and sensitivity of the bacteriological examination. Inpatient intravenous antibiotic administration should be prescribed until the general condition of the patient and blood inflammatory markers improve to the point when antibiotics can be administered orally and the patient may be mobilized and discharged. Spinal infection can be very painful, and a thoraco-lumbar orthosis may have a potent analgesic effect.

Most pyogenic infections develop spontaneous interbody fusion and so late instability is uncommon. In addition the recurrence rate is less than 5%. Pyogenic infection is not usually accompanied by significant abscess formation but, if it is, and particularly with cord pressure signs, then anterior decompression is required. Laminectomy is of no value.

Tuberculous Infection

Just as the febrile infant with septicemia, pyogenic spinal infection and failure to thrive has become uncommon, so too has the old-fashioned Potts' tuberculous kyphosis in the young become rarer in the developed world. Notwithstanding this, tuberculous spinal infection remains common, particularly in those who are, or have come, from developing countries. In addition, vaccination for tuberculosis is only being taken up by a minority of families. Tuberculosis worldwide still causes more deaths than all other notifiable infectious diseases combined. Spinal disease accounts for almost 60% of all musculoskeletal tuberculosis, and the L1 vertebral body is the most commonly affected. The T10 vertebral body is the most common level for the development of paralysis [15].

Tuberculous spinal infection tends to have an insidious onset with more significant local deformity so that the gibbus in an untreated individual is diagnostic. Paralysis as a presenting feature is also much more common than with pyogenic infection. Inflammatory markers are generally only modestly raised. Biopsy is essential and, as with pyogenic infection, the diagnosis can be clinched either by bacteriological assessment or by examination of histological specimens which, in tuberculosis, demonstrate granulomata, giant cells, and caseation. It is particularly important from the bacteriological point of view to identify the organism and its sensitivities so that appropriate chemotherapy can be prescribed.

Tuberculous spinal infection is particularly rife in countries where acquired immunodeficiency syndrome (AIDS) is prevalent and lowers the resistance of the host to infection. Moreover, resistant mycobacteria are increasingly emerging, making the prescription of appropriate antibiotics more difficult. The drugs available for treatment of tuberculous spinal infection are listed in Table 35.1. Some centers use a combination of four drugs but many centers will use just two drugs for 9 months (Rifampicin and Isoniazid), others adding Streptomycin for the first 3 months [9].

Unfortunately drug treatment is often unsuccessful and patient/parent compliance may be a major problem. Significant abscess formation, cord compression, and increasing kyphosis are the indications for anterior decompression, debridement, and strut grafting (the Hong Kong procedure described by Hodgson and Stock in 1960) [16]. Over the past three decades or so it has become apparent that the presence of a metal implant in the tuberculous spine carries with it no morbidity and so it is now routine for internal fixation to be used when operating on the tuberculous spine.

Table 35.1 Anti-tuberculous drugs

Rifampicin 10–600 mg/kg/day
Isoniazid 5–300 mg/day
Ethambutol 25 mg/day for 2 months then reduce
Pyrazinamide 25 mg/kg/day (max. 2.5 g/day)
Streptomycin 0.75–1.0 g/day 60–90 days, then 1.0 g 2–3 times/week
(See also Chapter 11)

For whatever reason, and unlike many other causes of paralysis such as tumor, Potts' paraplegia is much more amenable to surgical intervention with a much greater potential for neurological recovery.

Juvenile Discitis

This is a very interesting condition which tends to affect young children after infancy. The lumbar spine is nearly always the site of disease and the child complains of severe low back pain with a rigid lumbar hyperlordosis, often laterally deviated into a mild scoliosis. No movement of the lumbar spine is possible. The child is miserable but not systemically unwell. There is usually no pyrexia, the white blood cell count is normal but the erythrocyte sedimentation rate/plasma viscosity (ESR/PV) may be modestly raised. The earliest plain film findings are slight narrowing of the disc space at the relevant level with some blurring

of the adjacent vertebral margins (Fig. 35.4). Technetium bone scanning is strongly positive in the region of the adjacent vertebral bodies. However, this does not appear to be an infectious condition and biopsies invariably fail to grow organisms.

The term "discitis" was first coined by Menelaus [17] to describe this disorder characterized by disc inflammation but no primary bone involvement. The Mayo Clinic group also recognized that this was a non-infective condition and thought it might be an autoimmune reaction [18].

With time, further disc space narrowing occurs, but this seldom goes on to spontaneous fusion. Symptomatic treatment consists of initial bed rest, followed by a thoracolumbar orthosis (in the ambulatory child). Stiffness and pain may take several months to settle, a frustrating period for child, parents, and doctor.

Arthritis

Early-onset ankylosing spondylitis is very uncommon. The disease appears to be pursuing a more benign course quite naturally. In the 1997 classification of the childhood arthritides, two types may affect the spine, enthesitis-related arthritis and psoriatic arthritis [19]. The childhood form of enthesitis-related arthritis is similar clinically to the adult form and is also strongly linked to the HLA B27 antigen (Fig. 35.5). Sacroiliitis is not diagnostic and only a small minority (15%) have spinal symptoms early on. The condition occurs more frequently in boys with a typical age of onset at about 11 years. It is not uncommon for the first symptom to be hindfoot pain and stiffness.

With psoriatic arthritis, the arthritis tends to appear before the psoriasis. Girls are affected more than boys with age of onset generally under 11 years.

Adolescent Disc Syndrome

This describes disc prolapse in the second decade. It is a similar process of disc degeneration to that which occurs in adults

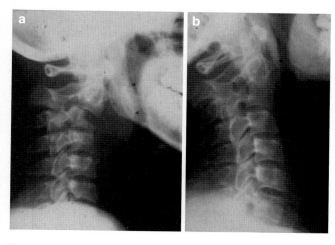

Fig. 35.4 Tuberculosis of the spine. (**a**) Lateral radiograph of the neck of a quadriparetic teenage girl immigrant showing destruction of the third cervical vertebra and a huge retrophalangeal abscess (*arrowheads*) causing spinal cord compression. (**b**) Lateral radiograph of the neck 2 years after anterior debridement, cord decompression, and strut grafting. There was complete resolution of the neurological signs and a solid fusion

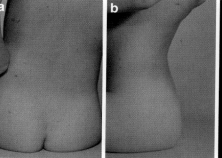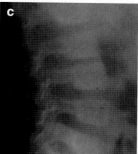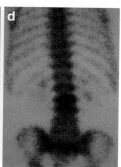

Fig. 35.5 Juvenile discitis. (**a**) Back and (**b**) side views of a 6-year-old boy with a typical rigid hyperlordosis and slight scoliosis produced by muscle spasm. (**c**) Lateral radiograph of the lumbar spine showing L2/3 disc space narrowing. (**d**) Isotope bone scan showing increased uptake in L2 and L3

with dehydration and increasing disc stiffness. There is seldom a discrete herniation, but rather bulging of the nucleus within a contained annulus [20].

In the mid-1990s Battié and his colleagues in Finland looked at the Finnish identical twin cohort, all of whose spines were MRI scanned. There was a remarkably similar distribution of degenerative disease in each of the twins' spines but very importantly, when they were divided into discordant groups as regards physical activity (heavy jobs or contact sports versus a sedentary lifestyle), there was no difference in the severity of degenerative disease between each set of twins [21].

There have been several case reports of children with degenerative disc disease, one involving a girl of 12 whose lumbar spine symptoms were so severe that they warranted an MRI scan which showed multi-level disc degeneration and herniation. Her identical twin sister volunteered for a MRI and it showed similar multi-level disc disease, demonstrating the genetic etiology of the condition [22]. The youngest child we have treated in Leeds was a boy of 4 years.

In the adolescent the predominant symptom is low back pain. Radicular pain and paraesthesia are seldom early symptoms. There is marked lumbar stiffness and very often a sciatic tilt (Fig. 35.6). Otherwise the back pain is mechanical, being worsened by activity and being eased by rest. Forward bending is markedly restricted and often produces a sciatic scoliosis; straight leg raising is also very limited but would appear to be due to hamstring tightness rather than a truly positive straight leg raise test. These clinical features can produce a most unusual gait and it is not at all uncommon for an adolescent to present with all the above features and yet deny severe pain or even have no pain at all. A prolapse in this age group does not produce marked neurological loss in the compromised nerve roots. Sphincter symptoms are very rare. Plain films are normal although spinal posture indicates spasm. The diagnosis is clinched by MRI which shows diffuse bulging of the disc rather than a focal hernia (Fig. 35.7).

Treatment is expectant but recovery is slow and may take 18 months to 2 years. Unless the case is unusually associated with significant neurological dysfunction operative treatment should be withheld. If nerve root decompression is required then the same sort of results can be expected as in the adult. A microsurgical approach should yield an excellent result in 90%.

Sometimes in the adolescent a very large disc prolapse can be seen to resorb as symptoms improve and finally settle.

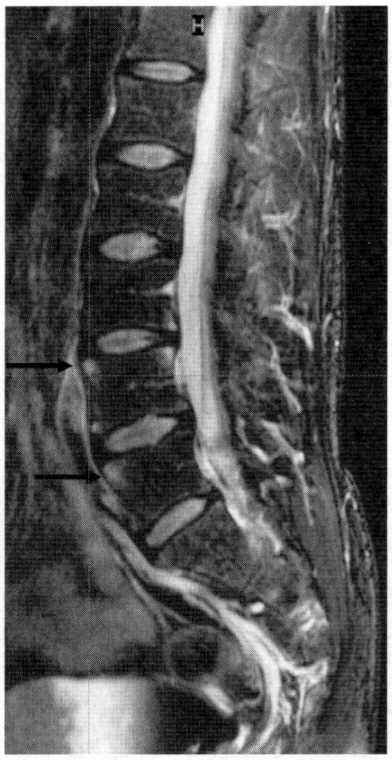

Spondylolisthesis

Spondylolysis and spondylolisthesis are by far the commonest causes of low back pain in childhood and adolescence [23].

Fig. 35.6 Ankylosing spondylitis. T2-weighted sagittal image of the lumbar spine of a teenage boy showing the oedematous Romanus lesions typical of early disease

Isthmic Spondylolisthesis

The incidence of spondylolysis (stress fracture in the pars interarticularis) has increased over the past decades as more sophisticated diagnostic radiographic techniques have been used for the child with low back pain. By far the majority of spondylolyses occur at L5 and consequently the slip occurs at the L5/S1 level. Plain films reveal spondylolyses in about 5% of children in the population (Fig. 35.8) with a slippage of about half that rate [24]. If CT scanning with an oblique gantry angle is utilized then the prevalence rate doubles (Fig. 35.9). The defect can also be seen on MRI (Fig. 35.10).

The pain is well localized to the low back, although it may radiate to the buttocks and thighs. Symptoms tend to be worsened by extension of the spine and activity, and reciprocally relieved by rest. There would appear to be a much higher incidence in gymnasts, athletes, ballet dancers, trampolinists, and other flexible athletes, reflecting increased repetitive cyclical movement of the low back during sporting activities [25]. The incidence rises to almost 50% in Eskimos which strongly suggests a genetic factor [26]. Recent research has demonstrated that when lyses occur

Fig. 35.7 Adolescent disc syndrome. (**a**) Back view of a teenage boy with a sciatic scoliosis. Note the erythema ab igne over the left lumbar region due to the application of a hot water bottle for pain relief. (**b**) Axial MRI image of his L5/S1 disc showing a large central disc hernia

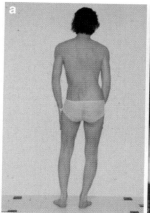

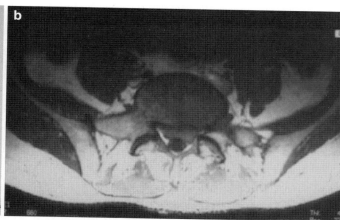

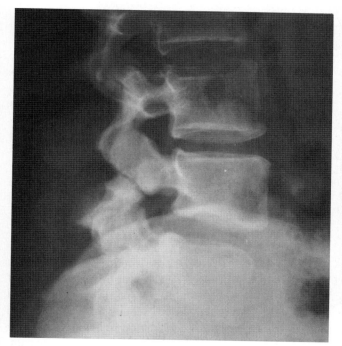

Fig. 35.8   Lateral radiograph of the lumbar spine showing bilateral L4 lyses with a slight L4/5 slip

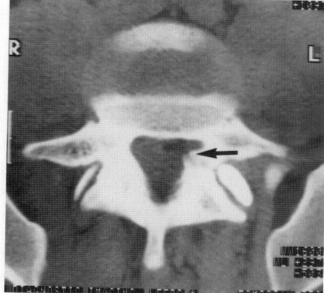

Fig. 35.9   Axial CT scan of L5 showing a lysis on the left side (*arrow*) and sclerosis of the pedicle on the right side, a common combination

either unilaterally or bilaterally the facet joint orientation is significantly more coronal, and this would therefore allow a pincer effect, particularly in spinal extension, thus leading to fatigue failure across the pars [27].

Treatment is expectant and symptoms usually settle with a period of rest from sporting activity or perhaps the intermittent use of a lumbosacral orthosis. Injections of the lytic region under radiographic control using a local anesthetic and a water soluble steroid can also be helpful in more recalcitrant cases. Slippage very seldom exceeds 20–30% and never becomes complete (the isthmic form of spondylolisthesis). Only in the most recalcitrant cases should spinal fusion be necessary.

Dysplastic Spondylolisthesis

This form of spondylolisthesis is more likely to slip progressively, although it is much less common than the isthmic form. The primary problem is hypoplasia or aplasia of the L5/S1 facet joints and so the deformity always occurs at the L5/S1 level. It is not so much a forward slippage but a forward rolling of the L5 vertebra on the top of the sacrum (Fig. 35.11). This can sometimes progress to complete spondyloptosis with L5 sitting on the front of the sacrum and it is in these very progressive slips that prophylactic fusion has a place. Despite the fact that there is no lysis of L5 to leave the back of the spine behind, neurological compromise is rare (see Chapter 37).

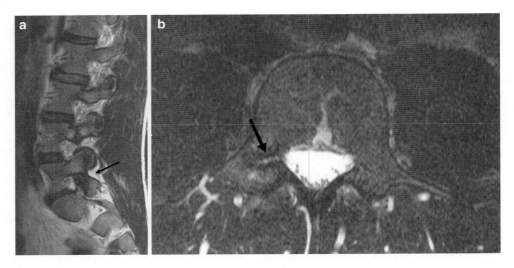

Fig. 35.10 Sagittal and axial MRI views through the fourth lumbar vertebra showing a unilateral lysis (*arrowed*)

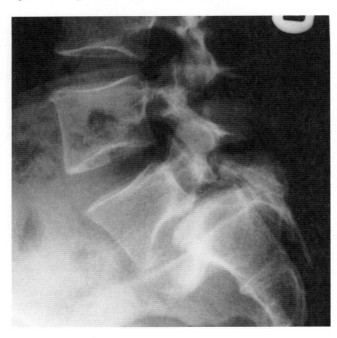

Fig. 35.11 Lateral radiograph of the lumbar spine showing a dysplastic spondylolisthesis with a lordotic-shaped L5 body, reciprocal rounding of the top of the sacrum, and secondary lyses in the back of L5

Tumors

Spinal neoplasms may be grouped into those that occur in bone, in neurological tissue, or in paravertebral tissues.

Intradural Tumors

When spinal cord dysfunction in the child occurs subacutely or chronically, it is most often due to tumor. Tachdjian

and Matson [28] have written the most informative article on the subject of intraspinal tumors in children which should be compulsory reading for all orthopaedic surgeons who treat children. They reported on 30 years of experience in Boston. In children the most common intradural neoplasms are gliomas, including astrocytomas and ependymomas. Neuroblastoma is the second commonest neoplasm but the commonest cause of spinal cord compression in the infant. Boys are affected twice as commonly as girls and 50% occur in the first 4 years of life. Slightly more lesions are benign than malignant.

Limp and leg weakness are the chief presenting features; back pain is present in one-third and torticollis in one-fifth. The most important physical findings in order of frequency are pathological reflexes, spastic paralysis, flaccid paralysis, a sensory level loss, a scoliosis in one-third, and muscle spasm. Tachdjian and Matson found an alarmingly high rate of wrong initial diagnosis, these tumors being commonly attributed to poliomyelitis, brachial plexus lesions, muscular dystrophy, and postural torticollis [28]. Fraser et al. [29] found sphincter disturbance in one-fifth. In children under the age of 6, 75% are malignant, falling to 30% over the age of 6.

Back pain tends not to be episodic but characteristically continuous and steadily worsening. Typically, inactivity increases the pain so that patients tend to pace the room at night. Tumors involving the cord tend to have upper motor neurone features and a progressive sensory disturbance, while cauda equina lesions have lower motor neurone features with painless leg wasting. Intramedullary lesions produce a characteristic, suspended disassociated sensory loss with reduction in pain and temperature but normal appreciation of touch; this physical sign is common also in syringomyelia. Vertebral column signs include reduced straight leg raising, decreased lumbar lordosis, and a scoliosis.

Syringomyelia has some similarities with intradural neoplasms and is a chronically progressive degeneration of the spinal cord and medulla, resulting in cavitation and gliosis within the substance of the cord. The condition was first described by Duchenne [30] and there are two pathological varieties: communicating and non-communicating. In the former there is communication between the cavity and the posterior fossa, while in the latter the fluid has another origin, usually from tumor or traumatic paraplegia. Typically, there is sensory dissociation with pain and temperature sensation involved but not touch at the level of the lesion, and weakness and wasting of the muscles of the involved segments. The commonest presenting symptom is pain in the head, neck, trunk, or limbs increased by straining. The cervical spine is the most commonly affected area.

With intradural tumors and syringes plain radiographs may show interpedicular widening and erosion of both neural arches and vertebral bodies locally (Fig. 35.12). Untreated cases can develop intrinsic muscle wasting and clawing of the hands as well as pes cavus. Treatment is by way of posterior fossa decompression (communicating) or cerebrospinal fluid shunting (non-communicating).

Laminectomy with tumor excision and additional radiotherapy for those which are malignant is the treatment of choice and microsurgical techniques are essential, often with a deep and wide laminectomy. It is important that this should be carried out by a neurosurgeon in combination with an orthopaedic spinal surgeon who can then stabilize the spine to prevent the inevitable progressive kyphosis (Fig. 35.2). The prognosis is not appreciably reduced by incomplete excision if radiation treatment is given post-operatively and the 5 year survival for malignant disease is better than 60%.

Tumors of Bone

The common bone-forming tumors in childhood and adolescence are the osteoid osteoma/osteoblastoma and the aneurysmal bone cyst.

Osteoid osteomas and osteoblastomas have the same histological appearance of vascularized osteoid tissue with a central nidus. Osteoid osteomas are cortical or subcortical, surrounded by an area of sclerotic bone, the nidus being about 1 cm in diameter. In contrast, osteoblastomas are medullary and the reactive zone is greater than 2 cm in diameter (Fig. 35.13). They tend to occur in the spine and flat bones. These lesions are painful because of the release of prostaglandins, so symptoms are relieved by prostaglandin inhibitors.

Plain films may appear normal with osteoid osteomas as they are cortical. Radiographs are always abnormal with

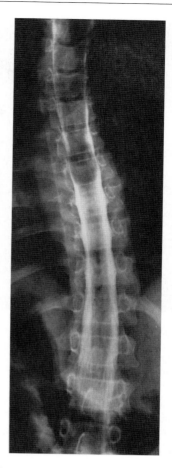

Fig. 35.12 Myelogram of a 12-year-old boy with a mild scoliosis and severe pain, particularly at night. There is marked pedicular widening in the upper thoracic spine going through to the neck and the syrinx extends down into the lumbar region. It proved to be secondary to a malignant glioma

osteoblastoma, particularly enlargement and expansion of the base of the adjacent transverse process. Both lesions are intensely positive on technetium bone scanning.

Delay in diagnosis is common and in one series averaged almost 18 months [31]. The natural history for these lesions is to settle spontaneously but persistence and severe pain merit treatment. Osteoid osteomas can be ablated under radiographic control but the larger osteoblastomas require complete surgical removal.

Aneurysmal bone cysts are of unknown pathogenesis but their large blood-filled spaces are separated by fibrous septa which contain both osteoblasts and osteoclasts. They were thought to be variants of giant cell tumors, but any spinal lesion that looks as though it might be a giant cell tumor is almost always an aneurysmal cyst.

Radiographically they have a "blow-out" appearance with soap-bubble trabeculation (Fig. 35.14), and while their growth may be so rapid as to imply malignancy, they are benign and recurrence is not common. One-fifth of

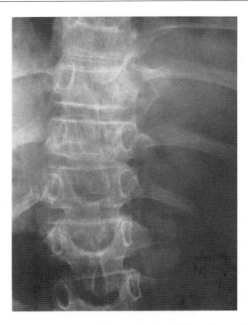

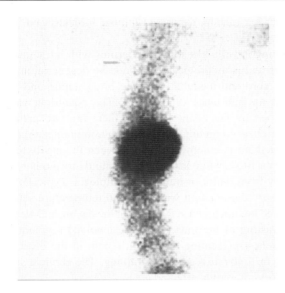

Fig. 35.14 Technetium bone scan showing intense uptake, characteristic of this lesion

Fig. 35.13 Osteoblastoma. Posteroanterior (PA) radiograph of the thoraco-lumbar region in a 14-year-old boy with a mild scoliosis and severe pain at night. The pedicle at T10 on the right side is missing and the lesion extends into the transverse process, the typical site for an osteoblastoma

all aneurysmal cysts are in the vertebral column, most commonly the lumbar region (Fig. 35.15). They tend to occur between the ages of 10 and 15 years [32]. The current

preferred treatment is complete excision of the lesion which may require total vertebrectomy and a strong anterior strut graft.

Eosinophilic granuloma of the spine produces back pain and muscle spasm, tenderness, local spinal rigidity, and often a mild kyphosis. The condition was described first by Calvé [33] in 1925 and in those days the important differential

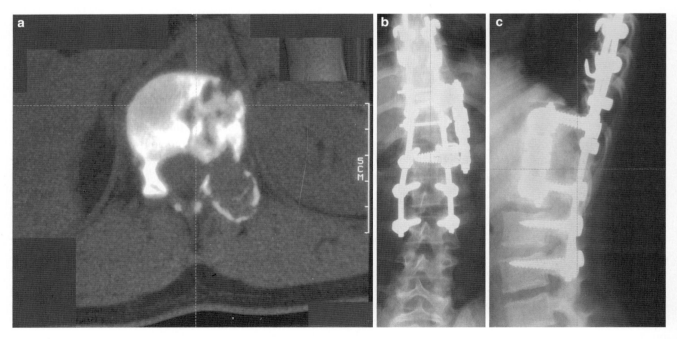

Fig. 35.15 Aneurysmal bone cyst. (**a**) CT scan of a 15 year old boy with severe constant back pain showing the typical blow-out appearance of an aneurysmal bone cyst. (**b**) AP and (**c**) lateral radiographs 2 years after combined anterior and posterior total vertebrectomy with a strut graft and anterior and posterior fixation. At this stage we removed the posterior metalwork; he resumed playing rugby and grew to a height of 6' 6"

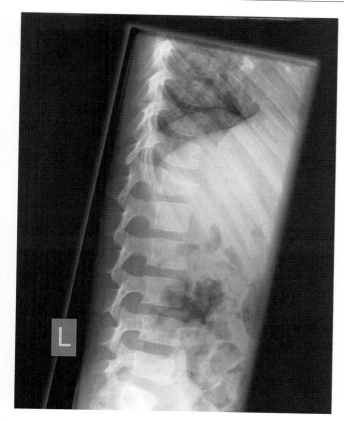

Fig. 35.16 Lateral radiograph showing an eosinophilic granuloma of T12 in the early stages of collapse

diagnosis was Pott's disease. It was not until 1953 that Lichtenstein [34] gave the lesion the name "Histiocytosis X" and integrated eosinophilic granuloma of bone with Letterer–Siwe disease and Hand–Schüller–Christian disease, similar lesions with a common histological pattern [34]. Lesions of the vertebral bodies go through stages of an initial lytic appearance followed by collapse (Fig. 35.16) and then increased sclerosis before recovery to normal height which may take 1–3 years. Radiographically there is a typical vertebra plana appearance of a silver dollar on its edge. Treatment is not indicated but biopsy may be required to distinguish it from osteomyelitis, Ewing's tumor, or malignancy.

References

1. Burgoyne W, Edgar M. The assessment of back pain in children. Curr Paediatr 1998; 8:173–179.
2. Fairbank JCT, Pynsent PB, Poortvleit JAY, Phillips H. Influence of anthropometric factors and joint laxity in the incidence of adolescent back pain. Spine 1984; 9:461–464.
3. Balagué F, Troussier B, Salminen JJ. Non-specific low back pain in children and adolescence: risk factors. Eur Spine J 1999; 8: 429–438.
4. Kewalramani LS, Tori JA. Spinal cord trauma in children; neurological patterns, radiologic features and pathomechanics of injury. Spine 1980; 8:11–18.
5. Bohlmann HH. Acute fractures and dislocations of the cervical spine; analysis of 300 hospitalised patients and review of the literature. J Bone Joint Surg 1979; 61A:1119–1142.
6. Henrys P, Lyne ED, Lifton C, Salciccioli G. Clinical review of cervical spine injuries in children. Clin Orthop 1977; 129:172–176.
7. Cullen JC. Spinal lesions in battered babies. J Bone Joint Surg 1975; 57B:364–366.
8. Dickson RA, Leatherman KD. Spinal injuries in child abuse; case report. J Trauma 1978; 18:811–812.
9. Wilson-Macdonald J. Management of spinal infection. Cur Orthop 2003; 16:462–470.
10. Wedge JH, Oryshak AF, Robertson DE, Kirkaldy-Willis WH. A typical manifestations of spinal infections. Clin Orthop 1977; 123:155–163.
11. Batson OV. The function of the vertebral veins and their role in the spread of metastases. Ann Surg 1940; 112:138–149.
12. Wiley AM, Truator J. The vascular anatomy of the spine and its relationship to pyogenic vertebral osteomyelitis. J Bone Joint Surg 1959; 41B:796–809.
13. Griffin PH, Hooper JC. Vertebral osteomyelitis. J Bone Joint Surg 1976; 58B:258.
14. Rankine JJ, Barron DA, Robinson P, et al. Therapeutic impact of percutaneous spinal biopsy in spinal infection. Postgrad Med J 2004; 80:607–609.
15. O'Brien JP. Kyphosis secondary to infectious disease. Clin Orthop 1977; 128:56–64.
16. Hodgson AR, Stock FE. Anterior spine fusion for the treatment of tuberculosis of the spine. J Bone Joint Surg 1960; 42A: 295–310.
17. Menelaus MB. Discitis—an inflammation affecting the intervertebral discs in children. J Bone Joint Surg 1965; 46B:16–23.
18. Boston HC, Bianco AG, Rhodes KH. Disc space infections in children. Orthop Clin North Am 1975; 6:953–964.
19. Edmonds SE. Juvenile arthritis. In Bulstrode C, Buckwalter J, Carr A, et al., eds. Oxford Textbook of Orthopaedics and Trauma. Oxford and New York: Oxford University Press; 2002:2427.
20. Taylor TK, Akeson WH. Intervertebral disc prolapse: a review of morphologic and biochemic knowledge concerning the nature of the prolapse. Clin Orthop 1971; 76:54–79.
21. Battié MC, Videman T, Gibbons LE, et al. 1995 Volvo award in clinical sciences. Determinants of lumbar disc degeneration. A study relating lifetime exposures and magnetic resonance imaging findings in identical twins. Spine 1995; 20(24): 2601–2612.
22. Obukhov SK, Hankenson L, Manka M, Mawk JR. Case report. Multilevel lumbar disc herniation in 12 year old twins. Childs Nerv Syst 1996; 12:169–171.
23. Dickson RA. Spondylolisthesis. Curr Orthop 1998; 12(4): 273–282.
24. Bailey W. Observations on the etiology and frequency of spondylolisthesis and its pre-cursors. Radiology 1947; 48:107–112.
25. Jackson DW, Wiltse LL, Cirincioner J. Spondylolysis in the female gymnast. Clin Orthop 1976; 117:68–73.
26. Stewart TD. The age incidence of neural arch defects in Alaskan natives, considered from the standpoint of etiology. J Bone Joint Surg 1953; 35A:937–950.
27. Rankine JJ, Dickson RA. An investigation of the facet joint anatomy in spondylolysis. Musculoskeletal Scientific Session 1. Proceedings of the UK Radiology Congress 2008. British Institute of Radiology.
28. Tachdjian MO, Matson DD. Orthopaedic aspects of interspinal tumors in infants and children. J Bone Joint Surg 1965; 47A: 223–248.

29. Fraser RD, Paterson DC, Simpson DA. Orthopaedic aspects of spinal tumors in children. J Bone Joint Surg 1977; 59B:143–151.

30. Duchenne GBA. De l'electrisation localisée, 3rd ed. Paris: JB Bailliere et Fils, Paris; 1872:493.

31. Marsh BW, Bonfiglio M, Brady LP, Enneking WF. Benign osteoblastoma: range of manifestations. J Bone Joint Surg 1975; 57A:1–9.

32. MacCarty CS, Dahlin DC, Doyle JB, et al. Aneurysmal bone cysts of the neural axis. J Neurosurg 1961; 18:671–677.

33. Calvé J. A localized infection of the spine suggesting osteochondritis of the vertebral body, with a clinical aspect of Pott's disease. J Bone Joint Surg 1925; 7A: 41–46.

34. Lichtenstein L. Histiocytosis X; integration of eosinophilic granuloma of bone, Letterer-Siwe disease, and Schüller-Christian disease as related manifestations of a single nosologic entity. AMA Arch Pathol 1953 56: 84–102.

Chapter 36

Spinal Deformities

Robert A. Dickson

Basic Principles

Definitions and Terminology

The spine is normally straight in the frontal (coronal) plane. If it is not, a lateral curvature or scoliosis is present. Scolioses are subdivided into structural and non-structural, according to whether the spine is additionally twisted [1]. Thus structural scoliosis is defined as a lateral curvature with rotation. The important attribute of a structural scoliosis is that it is intrinsic to the spine and may progress with growth to produce a serious deformity that may threaten health and quality of life. By contrast, non-structural curves are secondary to some other factors such as leg length inequality or muscle spasm from a painful focus (e.g., disc prolapse, infection, tumor). Significant progression is seen only occasionally in some curves associated with spinal cord tumor. Other non-structural curves tend to resolve when the underlying problem is dealt with.

In the sagittal plane, it is normal to have lordotic spinal curvatures (curves convex anteriorly) in the cervical and lumbar regions and an intervening kyphosis (a curve convex posteriorly) in the thoracic region. Only if these natural curves are exaggerated or reduced can they become pathological. For instance, the thoracic kyphosis is increased in Scheuermann's disease, otherwise known as idiopathic hyperkyphosis. The lumbar lordosis is characteristically increased in paralytic conditions such as muscular dystrophy or cerebral palsy.

Distinguishing between structural and non-structural scoliosis is not always easy on initial inspection. Most non-structural curves occur lower down in the spine, where the lateral profile is naturally lordotic. If a lateral curvature

develops here, for example, secondary to the pelvic tilt produced by leg length inequality, then the presence of a spinal curvature in two planes (lordosis plus lateral curvature) will impose a deformity in the third plane, with resultant spinal rotation (Fig. 36.1). It is for this reason that non-structural lumbar scolioses, secondary to a leg length inequality, are found in large numbers during school screening programs that focus upon minor alterations in spinal shape.

It is conventional to describe scolioses according to their site, direction, and the number of curves present. The site of a curve is determined by the position of its apical vertebra or vertebrae, and thus curves can be, for example, thoracic or lumbar. Curves with apices at T12 or L1 are called thoraco-lumbar and those at C7 or T1 are cervico-thoracic. The direction of curve convexity determines the side of the

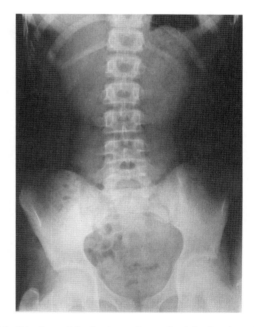

Fig. 36.1 PA view of the lumbar spine and pelvis showing a lumbar scoliosis due to pelvic obliquity secondary to a leg length inequality. There is mild rotation in the upper lumbar region

R.A. Dickson (✉)
Academic Unit of Orthopaedic Surgery, Leeds General Infirmary,
Leeds, UK

M. Benson et al. (eds.), *Children's Orthopaedics and Fractures*,
DOI 10.1007/978-1-84882-611-3_36, © Springer-Verlag London Limited 2010

curve: right thoracic and left lumbar curve patterns are common. Multiple curves are more common than single ones, with the combined right thoracic and left lumbar pattern the most common.

Structural and Non-Structural Scoliosis

When Adams in 1865 [2] described his "forward-bending test," he recognized that the rotational component of the three-dimensional deformity increased with spinal flexion (Fig. 36.2). This remains the favored position for examining patients in scoliosis clinics and in community screening programs. Because the deformity is less evident in the erect position, a mechanical event must take place when the spine flexes to enhance rotation. This provides an important clue to the nature of the underlying deformity of structural scoliosis.

When a postero-anterior (PA) radiograph of a structural scoliosis is examined the lateral curvature is obvious, but the vertebrae within the curve are also rotated, and this direction of rotation is constant: the posterior elements turn into the concavity and the vertebral bodies into the convexity, irrespective of the type or spinal level of the scoliosis. If the spinous processes and the centers of the vertebral

bodies are marked on a PA radiograph, it can be seen that the line joining the spinous processes is shorter than the line joining the vertebral bodies, and thus the back of the spine is shorter than the front (Fig. 36.3). If the back of the spine is shorter than the front in every case of structural scoliosis, then all these deformities are lordotic and there is no such deformity as kyphoscoliosis. This fundamental point was obvious to Adams in the mid-nineteenth century before radiographs were discovered, and his careful cadaver dissections demonstrated the essential lordosis beautifully. The overlong front of the spine readily buckles to the side on flexion, to produce a positive Adams' forward-bending test. It is the three-dimensional nature of this deformity, particularly with reference to the abnormal lateral profile, that holds the key to understanding the clinical features, behavior, and treatment of idiopathic scoliosis.

"Structural" scolioses resulting from solitary congenital hemivertebrae tend to exist in the coronal plane only and exhibit no rotational prominence on forward bending and no rotation on the PA radiograph: the sagittal profile is not affected. Similarly a true lordoscoliosis is produced by leg length inequality, by the combination of coronal and sagittal plane curvatures, but the sagittal profile is not abnormal and progressive buckling does not develop.

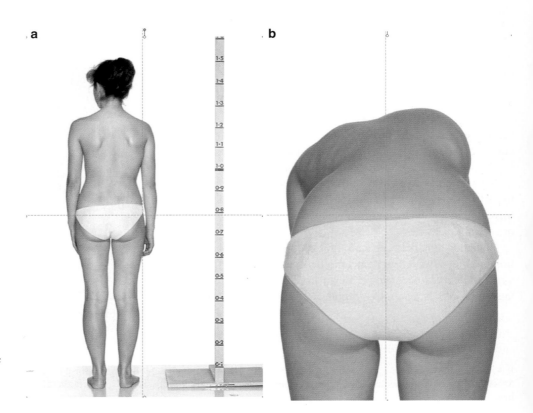

Fig. 36.2 (**a**) Erect and (**b**) forward-bending views of a teenage girl with a right thoracic idiopathic scoliosis. The rib hump is much bigger in the forward-bending position

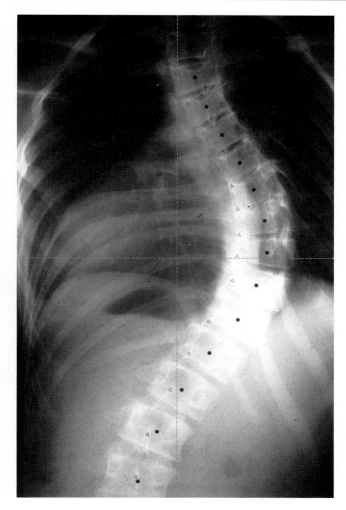

Fig. 36.3 PA radiograph of a right thoracic idiopathic scoliosis. The center of the vertebral bodies has been marked with *solid dots* while the tips of the spinous processes have been marked with *hollow triangles*. It can be seen that a *line* down the back of the spine would be shorter than a *line* down the front confirming the presence of a lordosis

The Size of the Deformity

Because the deformity exists in three dimensions each vertebra occupies a different position in space relative to its neighbors. *Planes are two-dimensional, and there is therefore no one plane that adequately describes the deformity.* By contrast, if the spine is straight in the coronal plane, a lateral radiograph can be used to measure the amount of cervical or lumbar lordosis and the amount of thoracic kyphosis. Angles are planar measurements and, as no one plane can assess structural scoliosis, the deformity cannot be described by an angular measurement [3]. Cobb [4] was aware of this, but in an effort to assess his patients and their response to treatment he devised the angle that bears his name. If a PA

radiograph of a structural scoliosis is examined and the vertebrae that are maximally tilted at the top and bottom of the deformity are selected, lines can be drawn along their upper and lower borders, respectively. These lines subtend an angle referred to as the Cobb angle, and it is a standard practice to measure the deformity of structural scoliosis in this way (Fig. 36.4).

If the deformity is only in two planes, e.g., a solitary hemivertebra, then this angle accurately reflects the shape of the spine. However, the more the spine has twisted the less satisfactory it becomes because the vertebrae within the structural scoliosis are rotated and the PA projection becomes an oblique view of the deformity, with each vertebra being portrayed in a different degree of obliquity (Fig. 36.5). Of course, the direction of rotation of the posterior elements indicates that the deformity is unquestionably lordotic, but it does not say by how much. Meanwhile, the lateral view is another oblique view of the same deformity, this time spuriously suggesting a kyphosis, which is really the scoliosis seen in another plane. In simple terms, therefore, altering the plane of projection changes our perception of a curve's magnitude and shape.

This can be simply verified by inspecting, say, a coat hanger (Fig. 36.6). If the long side (hypotenuse) is vertical, and the hook points due east or west, the angle subtended will be maximal (if we look in a north–south direction), whereas if the hook points north or south the appearance is that of a straight line—i.e., there is no deformity present. As the hook is moved from either due east or west round to north or south,

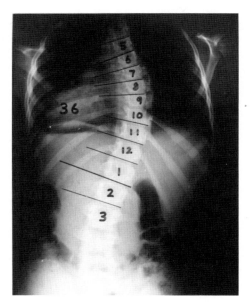

Fig. 36.4 Measuring the Cobb angle. PA radiograph of a right thoracic curve. It can be seen that the sixth thoracic vertebra and the first lumbar vertebra are maximally tilted. These are the end vertebrae. The *lines* along these vertebrae subtend the Cobb angle which in this case is 36°

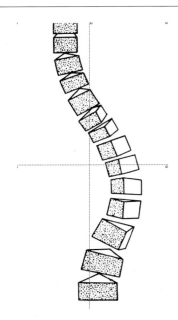

Fig. 36.5 A diagram to show that each vertebra within the structural curve is tilted and rotated and so there is no one plane that can register the entire deformity

the angle subtended steadily decreases. Stagnara was aware of this and devised a radiograph to be taken truly PA to the apical vertebra [5]. If, for example, the apical vertebra was rotated 30° from neutral about a vertical axis, then the radiograph beam was similarly rotated to ensure that this vertebra appeared truly PA. This *plan d'election* is the plane of projection illustrating the largest deformity. A 90° rotated film reveals the true curve apex lateral and unmasks the essential lordosis (Fig. 36.7). Using Stagnara's principle, it is possible only to obtain true PA and lateral projections of one vertebra at a time and excessive radiation would be needed to build up a three-dimensional radiographic picture of a growing child's deformity.

With these limitations, there is much to learn qualitatively if not quantitatively from the PA projection of the patient's spine. In the coronal plane, above and below the structural curve, there are compensatory curves that straighten the spine. These are convex the opposite way to the structural curve and are referred to as "compensatory scolioses." If we consider the direction of rotation of the primary structural scoliosis and its two compensatory curves, it will be seen that for a single curve—e.g., a right thoracic curve—the spinous

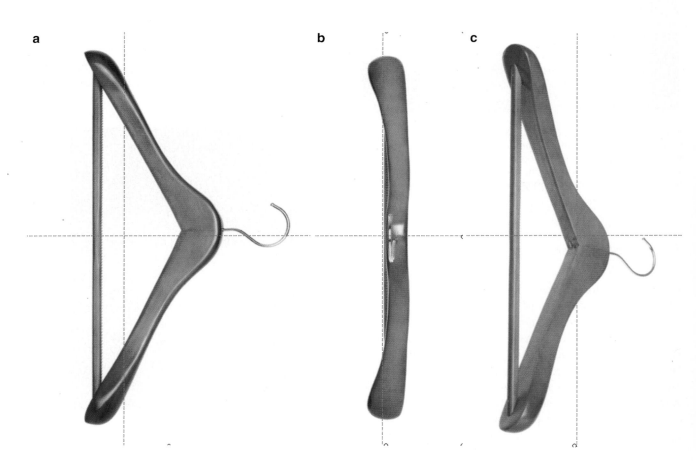

Fig. 36.6 Three views of a coat hanger showing how the angle varies according to the plane of projection

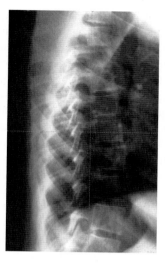

Fig. 36.7 True lateral radiograph of the apical vertebra of a thoracic scoliosis demonstrating the lordosis

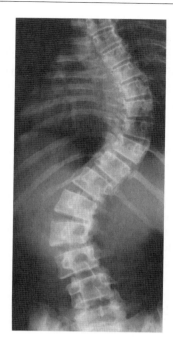

Fig. 36.8 PA radiograph of a right thoracic and left lumbar double-structural scoliosis. The neutral vertebra is T11 and above and below the direction of rotation indicates the presence of lordoses

processes are rotated toward the left in the region of the structural curve in addition to the first segment or two of the compensatory curves above and below (Fig. 36.4). Bearing in mind that posterior element rotation into the curve concavity implies lordosis, and the reverse kyphosis, the direction of rotation in the compensatory curves is now the opposite of the structural curve—i.e., the compensatory curves are convex left and the posterior elements are also rotated to the left. Thus these so-called compensatory scolioses are kyphoses. This is not surprising because the structural curve is a lordoscoliosis and ought to be balanced in three dimensions above and below by asymmetric kyphoses.

On the PA radiograph of a double-structural right thoracic and left lumbar curve there is no intervening kyphosis between the two structural curves (Fig. 36.8), but there are kyphoses above the upper and below the lower one. Triple- or multiple-curve patterns also exist, and the PA radiograph then shows that the entire spine from top to bottom is lordotic. Thus much about the three-dimensional shape of the spine in structural scoliosis can be inferred from a single PA spinal radiograph.

Classification of Spinal Deformities

The following is a brief classification based upon the recommendations of the Scoliosis Research Society [6]:

1. Idiopathic
2. Congenital
3. Neuromuscular
4. Neurofibromatosis
5. Mesenchymal disorders
6. Trauma
7. Infection
8. Tumors
9. Miscellaneous

Idiopathic spinal deformities are divided into two broad categories: scoliosis and kyphosis. Idiopathic scoliosis is further subdivided into two types according to the patient's age at disease onset—early onset (before the age of 5 years) and late onset (after the age of 5 years). The age distinction is important because it is only with early-onset deformities that health can be jeopardized [7]. Late-onset scoliosis gives cause for concern about appearance rather than health, although there may be social and psychological disadvantages.

Idiopathic kyphosis is Scheuermann's disease, and there are two types according to site. Type I is typically mid-lower thoracic hyperkyphosis, apical about T8–T9, whereas type II Scheuermann's disease is in the thoraco-lumbar or upper lumbar spine and is referred to as "apprentice's spine" as it can be associated with a more vigorous lifestyle.

Congenital spinal deformities are broadly divisible into two groups: bone and spinal cord deformities. Congenital bone deformities are produced by congenital bony anomalies—either failures of formation (hemivertebrae or wedged vertebrae) or failures of segmentation (congenital fusions or bars across disc spaces). When there is a hemivertebra on one side and a unilateral bar on the other, the prognosis is particularly bad because growth leads inexorably to severe progression.

Congenital spinal cord deformities include the spina bifida and myelodysplasia syndromes. The underlying anomaly is present before birth, but the prognosis for deformity depends heavily on the degree of paralysis. Congenital kyphosis in myelomeningocele is always associated with complete paralysis from the waist down, whereas the time of onset and ultimate severity of the more common paralytic-type lordoscoliosis with pelvic obliquity are proportional to the level and severity of paralysis.

These congenital spine deformities are often associated with spinal dysraphism (e.g., diastematomyelia, tethered filum, spino-cutaneous fistula), which may further jeopardize spinal cord function (see Chapter 17).

Neuromuscular spinal deformities include conditions such as cerebral palsy, poliomyelitis, Friedreich's ataxia, and the muscular dystrophies. The typical paralytic lordoscoliosis with pelvic obliquity occurs in proportion to the severity of the neurological problem.

Neurofibromatosis deformities are either scoliosis or kyphosis and can be of early onset and very progressive.

Mesenchymal disorders refer to those heritable disorders of connective tissue (e.g., brittle bone disease and Marfan's syndrome), mucopolysaccharidoses, skeletal dysplasias, and metabolic bone diseases in which spinal deformities occur.

Traumatic spinal deformities can be produced by trauma to the spine itself (fracture, fracture-dislocation, or secondary paralysis) or can result from extra-spinal trauma such as damage to the chest or abdominal wall from surgery, burns, or retroperitoneal fibrosis.

Infection, which may be pyogenic or tuberculous, typically produces kyphotic deformities.

Deformities associated with tumors may be caused by the tumor itself or by its treatment. Non-structural deformities are produced by associated muscle spasm, whereas idiopathic-type scolioses are produced by intradural tumors, probably by a neuropathological mechanism. The widespread laminectomy used to excise the neoplasm can produce progressive kyphosis in the growing spine.

A number of other conditions, such as congenital anomalies of the upper extremity, juvenile idiopathic arthritis, and congenital heart disease, are also associated with a higher prevalence of spinal deformities.

The Pathogenesis of Structural Spinal Deformities

As with all musculoskeletal deformities, structural scoliosis develops as a consequence of both biological and biomechanical factors [8]. Innumerable scoliosis screening programs have shown (as anatomists centuries ago described) that a degree or two of lateral spinal curvature can hardly be considered abnormal. Epidemiological surveys have demonstrated that 10% of normal teenagers have a scoliosis measuring 5° or more. Forty percent of these are due to leg length inequality, but that still leaves a substantial number (6% of all normal children) with a structural scoliosis somewhere in their spine. However, with increasing curve size the prevalence rate diminishes exponentially: 2% have curves of 10° or more and 0.5% a curve of 20° or more [9]. Clearly, something has to be added to "schooliosis" to make it scoliosis, and not surprisingly this problem exists in the sagittal plane. What is perhaps surprising is that the importance of the lateral profile has been largely ignored, despite the pioneering work of Adams [2] and Somerville [10].

More than 20 years ago in Leeds an epidemiological survey involving 16,000 schoolchildren commenced, paying particular attention to the lateral spinal profile. Every year during this 5-year longitudinal survey, measurements such as standing height and bone age were recorded and PA and lateral low-dose radiographs of the spine were taken. A number of children with straight spines at study outset developed idiopathic scoliosis. Analysis of their initial lateral profiles demonstrated that the lordotic sagittal plane abnormality preceded the lateral spinal curvature, so confirming its crucial etiological significance [11] (Fig. 36.9).

When a true lateral radiograph of the apex of an idiopathic thoracic scoliosis is compared with a lateral view of the apical region of a patient with type I Scheuermann's hyperkyphosis, the deformities in the sagittal plane would appear to be exactly the opposite of idiopathic scoliosis (Fig. 36.10): in Scheuermann's disease the anterior vertebral height is *reduced* in comparison with posterior height and Schmorl node formation is situated anteriorly in the growth plate. Idiopathic scoliosis and Scheuermann's disease have therefore considerable similarities: both develop in otherwise normal, healthy children with a similar community prevalence and familial trend [12].

The thoracic kyphosis varies during late childhood and adolescence: in the prepubertal phase it reduces appreciably, only to be regained a year or two before maturity. It is while the kyphosis is reducing in the prepubertal phase, when girls are at their peak adolescent growth, that they are most prone to develop idiopathic scoliosis. Boys, with their constant growth velocity at this age, are relatively protected. However, when their thoracic kyphosis increases just before maturity boys are at their peak adolescent growth period. This may explain why girls are more prone to scoliosis and boys to Scheuermann's disease. Clinically, idiopathic scoliosis presents during adolescence or even childhood while Scheuermann's disease presents a year or two before maturity.

Fig. 36.9 (**a**) PA radiograph of a mild idiopathic scoliosis which developed 2 years into a prospective epidemiological survey. (**b**) PA radiograph at the start of the study showing a straight spine. (**c**) Lateral radiograph at the start of the study showing the primary lordosis

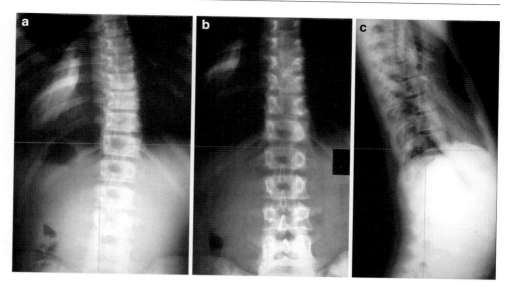

Fig. 36.10 (**a**) True lateral radiograph of the apex of an idiopathic thoracic curve showing vertebral bodies longer at the front than at the back. (**b**) Lateral tomogram of the apex of a Scheuermann's deformity showing reduced height at the front of the vertebrae

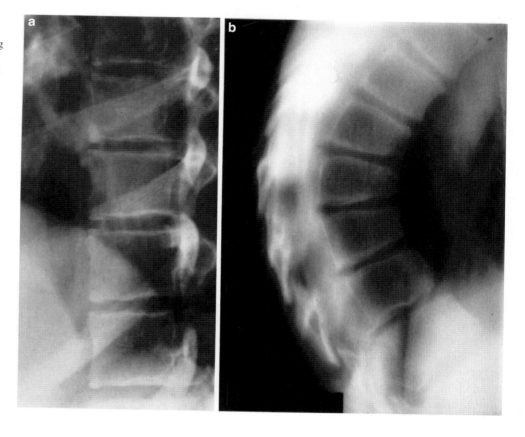

Interestingly, two-thirds of all patients with type I thoracic Scheuermann's disease also have coexistent idiopathic scoliosis, but several segments lower down in the compensatory lumbar hyperlordosis (Fig. 36.11). As the thoracic hyperkyphosis increases, so does the compensatory lumbar hyperlordosis, and the latter readily buckles to the side to produce the scoliosis. Two similar deformities in one adolescent, differing only by their sagittal plane direction, are most unlikely to have different etiologies. The deformities of idiopathic scoliosis and Scheuermann's disease represent the extreme ends of the spectrum of lateral profile, with so-called normal individuals somewhere between.

Fig. 36.11 (**a**) Lateral radiograph of the spine of a patient with thoracic Scheuermann's disease. (**b**) PA radiograph of the same patient showing an idiopathic lumbar scoliosis

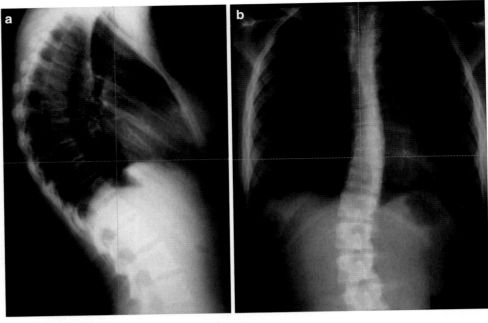

The orientation of the posterior facet joints in the transverse plane allows an axis of spinal column rotation in the sagittal profile of the spine to be constructed (Fig. 36.12). This axis runs behind the cervical and lumbar lordoses, but in front of the thoracic kyphosis. In the transverse plane, vertebral shape is interesting: the cervical and lumbar vertebrae are broad from side to side and short from front to back; the thoracic vertebrae are heart-shaped—much longer from front to back than from side to side and almost pointed anteriorly (Figs. 36.13 and 36.14). Thus the cross-sectional shape of the vertebral column can be considered as triangular or prismatic, with the apex of the prism posterior in the cervical and lumbar regions but anterior in the thoracic region. When a prismatic-shaped structure flexes toward an apex, it buckles much more readily than when it flexes toward a base.

The spine does not stop growing until the middle of the third decade when vertebral endplate growth cartilage can no longer be seen. Therefore, although the spine does not grow appreciably in vertical height after fusion of the long-bone epiphyses, any tendency toward spinal deformity can be accommodated by an alteration of vertebral shape. This accounts for spinal deformities progressing, albeit slowly, after apparent cessation of growth.

Meanwhile, the vulnerable cervical and lumbar lordoses, being in front of the axis of spinal column rotation, have inbuilt protection mechanisms to resist buckling. The bases of the prisms are anterior and the flexibility of the neck and low back allows them to become frankly kyphotic before the limit is reached. They are also protected by the pay-out of powerful paraspinal muscles although, when that fails as in paralytic disorders, a typical collapsing lordoscoliosis is rapidly produced. Finally, the cervical and lumbar lordoses

are top and bottom of the column and buckling tends to occur in the middle, which is precisely where idiopathic thoracic scoliosis and type I Scheuermann's disease occur.

Established engineering laws (Euler's laws) govern column buckling: in this respect, critical load, the modulus of elasticity of the column, the beam length, and the end conditions are all important. For example, both epidemiological and clinical studies have shown that a curve of, say, 40° is more likely to progress than a curve of 20°, all else being equal. This has nothing to do with biology but is purely biomechanical: the more a column has buckled the more likely it is to continue doing so. Similarly, the taller a column the more readily it will buckle, and it is interesting to note that children with idiopathic scoliosis are significantly taller than their straight-backed age- and sex-matched counterparts. There is also evidence that their spines are more slender [13].

The question of critical load is very important. In simple terms, if the spine has any inherent weakness it will buckle more readily, earlier, and more severely. This is recognized in the etiological classification. In conditions such as brittle bone disease or neurofibromatosis, bone is characteristically dystrophic and less strong. In brittle bone disease, bone fractures readily, whereas in Von Recklinghausen's disease bone characteristically grows dystrophically (vertebral scalloping, widened intervertebral foraminae, penciled ribs). The critical load to the spine is therefore increased at bone level and, not surprisingly, in both these disorders there is an earlier onset of spinal deformity and a greater potential for progression. The deformity produced is, however, the same as that occurring in idiopathic cases—i.e., either a lordoscoliosis or a kyphosis.

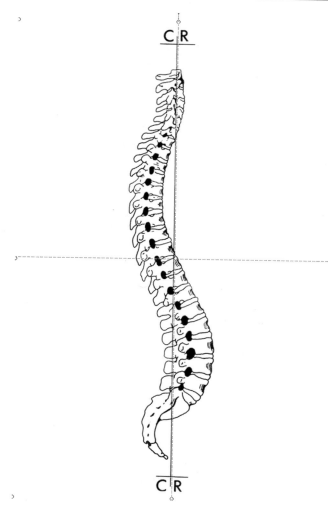

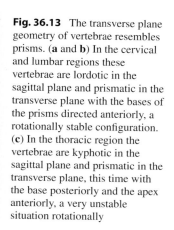

Fig. 36.12 The axis of spinal column rotation (CR) runs in front of the thoracic kyphosis and behind a lumbar lordosis

Euler's laws allow failure at the soft tissue level also: in Marfan's and Ehlers–Danlos syndromes, ligamentous laxity

promotes the development of severe spinal deformities of the idiopathic type. Failure may be at neuromuscular level, i.e., the spinal guy ropes become inadequate, and the weaker they are the more evident is the spinal deformity. In cerebral palsy, the incidence and extent of the paralytic spinal deformity increase with the severity of the neuromuscular deficit.

The spinal column therefore obeys the laws of elementary mechanics but biological factors account for the variability in clinical response [14].

Idiopathic Scoliosis

Idiopathic scoliosis can develop at any time during spinal growth. There are two phases when skeletal growth is particularly rapid—infancy and adolescence—while in the intervening juvenile period growth velocity is relatively constant. Idiopathic scoliosis is thus most prevalent during infancy and adolescence. James in 1954 [15] subdivided idiopathic scoliosis into infantile, juvenile, and adolescent types according to the time of onset but few of his patients belonged to the juvenile-onset group. Long-term follow-up studies of untreated idiopathic scoliosis show considerable disadvantage for those with large deformities not only because of cardiopulmonary morbidity and mortality [16] but also because of social and psychological deprivation [17]. Management of these patients became focused on the concept that curve size must not be allowed to progress excessively with growth: a Cobb angle threshold of 60° became the norm and surgical treatment imperative if this was exceeded.

While the data from these long-term follow-up studies were not flawed, the inferences drawn sometimes were: the size of the deformity attracted attention rather than the age of onset. For example, if one 16-year-old girl has a 50° and another a 100° deformity then, all things being equal, the

Fig. 36.13 The transverse plane geometry of vertebrae resembles prisms. (**a** and **b**) In the cervical and lumbar regions these vertebrae are lordotic in the sagittal plane and prismatic in the transverse plane with the bases of the prisms directed anteriorly, a rotationally stable configuration. (**c**) In the thoracic region the vertebrae are kyphotic in the sagittal plane and prismatic in the transverse plane, this time with the base posteriorly and the apex anteriorly, a very unstable situation rotationally

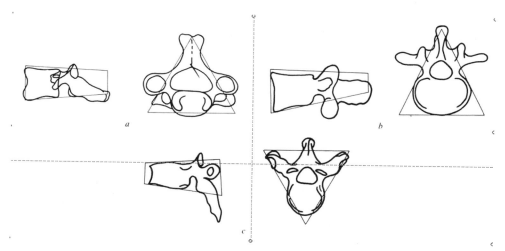

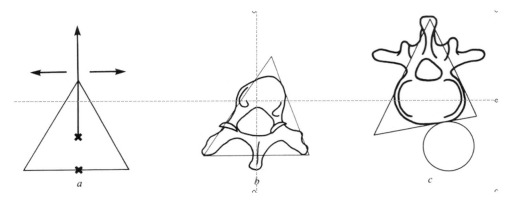

Fig. 36.14 (**a**) If a symmetrical prism was flexed toward its apex it could rotate to either direction. (**b**) The thoracic prisms are not however symmetrical, being constantly grooved on the left side by the pulsations of the descending thoracic aorta such that the apex of the prism is to the right of the median sagittal plane and therefore the prismatic column will tend to rotate to the right. (**c**) In the lumbar region the abdominal aorta is to the left of the median sagittal plane and thus rests against the left side of the base of the lumbar prism. This favors left-sided rotation of the lumbar spine

greater deformity probably started earlier: the age of onset is the crucial issue. The cardiopulmonary implications of scoliosis illustrate this well. At birth the lungs are not simply mini-versions of the adult: rather, they comprise a small number of alveoli which reduplicate until the adult number is achieved by the age of 5 years (Fig. 36.15). Should anything interfere with this process, permanent pulmonary damage can result, leading later to cardiopulmonary dysfunction. A significant thoracic scoliosis with its attendant chest asymmetry may be a critical damaging factor. Branthwaite in 1986 [7] showed that, if the onset of the deformity occurred after the age of 5 years, there was no significant cardiopulmonary compromise no matter how large the Cobb angle. By contrast, the younger the child with scoliosis the greater

is the susceptibility to subsequent heart and lung problems. Clinically, therefore, it is better to consider only two types of idiopathic scoliosis: early onset (before the age of 5 years) and late onset (after the age of 5 years) [1].

Late-Onset Idiopathic Scoliosis (After 5 Years of Age)

This is largely a question of deformity and appearance as there are few health consequences. It is not associated with an increased prevalence or severity of back pain, although when the scoliotic back does become painful, symptoms

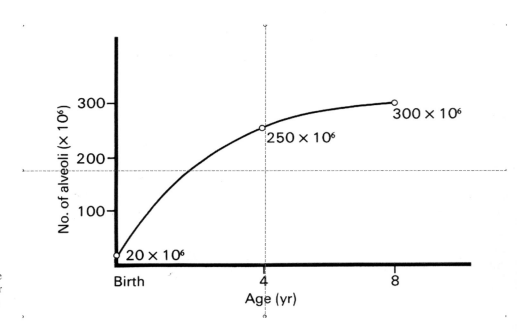

Fig. 36.15 Graph showing the reduplication of the alveolar tree from birth. Almost the full adult complement is reached by the age of 4 but it is the increased number in the first year or two of life that is crucial

are more recalcitrant than with a straight back. The condition, however, should not be regarded simply as cosmetic, as the deformity may have a major impact on the quality of life [17]. It is particularly distressing when an adolescent presents with a deformity so severe that, even with optimal treatment, a significant residual deformity remains for life. Although nowadays fewer such cases attend scoliosis clinics for the first time, curve size at presentation remains a concern and continues to fuel the debate about the value of routine school screening.

When screening was introduced curve size was the dominant consideration. Routine screening has been used for a variety of medical conditions, from which much has been learnt and guidelines and criteria laid down [18]. An important prerequisite is that the natural history of the condition should be adequately understood. Screening for scoliosis has major financial implications and it is pointless to identify thousands of minor cases if progression can neither be anticipated nor prevented. Recent years have shown a progressive loss of confidence in any form of conservative treatment, with many studies struggling to differentiate the effects of treatment from the natural history.

Some countries still insist upon regular routine school screening for scoliosis using some quick measure of rotational asymmetry of the torso on forward bending, such as the scoliometer, but there is a move away from compulsory screening until the natural history is better understood. However, early detection is clearly important, and national orthopaedic associations and scoliosis societies have a responsibility to increase awareness among both lay and medical colleagues of the need for early recognition and prompt referral [9].

An important by-product of school screening programs has been a better understanding of normality and abnormality, of incidence and prevalence rates, curve patterns, and familial trends [19]. Some evidence suggests that the condition is pursuing a more benign course, with lower prevalence and less likelihood to progress [11].

Clinical Features

Patients with late-onset idiopathic scoliosis present with truncal asymmetry and the rotational deformity is usually the most obvious: thoracic deformities present as a rib hump (Fig. 31.8) and thoraco-lumbar or lumbar deformities as a loin hump. Lower curves are associated also with waist asymmetry, an increased flank recession on the concave side, and a flattening of the waist on the convex side. As a result, the hip on the concave side appears unduly prominent and this can be as cosmetically obvious as a rib hump (Fig. 36.16).

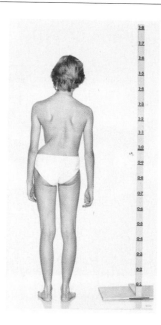

Fig. 36.16 Back view of a teenage girl with an idiopathic lumbar curve showing marked waist asymmetry

Most patients referred to scoliosis clinics are adolescent females. There is a fairly even sex ratio for very small curves detected by screening, but a steep rise in the female/male ratio with increasing curve magnitude. Patients and parents are frequently alarmed by a Cobb angle of 30–40°, and many feel a sense of guilt that they did not recognize the problem earlier. There are two principal reasons for this. First, adolescence is an emotional time and, whereas parents are used to seeing their infants and young children nearly naked, they seldom so see their adolescent children. Although adolescent girls rarely see their own backs, they notice the more prominently developing breast on the side opposite the curve convexity associated with a twisting torso. Second, curve size is more appreciable radiographically: the spinal column has to undergo a certain amount of buckling before this adversely affects the shape of the outer surface of the body. Although this may delay presentation, it has a surgical advantage. If the deformity does not significantly alter surface shape until the Cobb angle reaches 30°, the surgeon does not have to reduce the deformity to much less to make it cosmetically acceptable.

Pain is not a feature of idiopathic scoliosis, although some fatigue discomfort over the rotational prominence may occur. Any suspicion of more significant pain demands further investigation, particularly if there is any suggestion of night pain when neoplasm or a syrinx must be excluded (see Chapter 35). The use of magnetic resonance imaging (MRI) in progressive idiopathic deformities has shown a syrinx to be much more common than previously thought (Fig. 31.12). The usual curve patterns of single right thoracic, single left thoraco-lumbar or lumbar, or double right thoracic and left

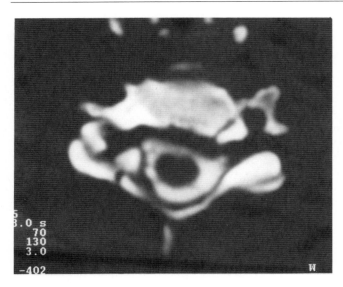

Fig. 36.17 Axial MRI scan through the cervical spine showing a large syrinx in the spinal cord

thoraco-lumbar/lumbar (Fig. 36.8) are those we generally see, and any unusual curve pattern, such as a progressive left thoracic curve in a teenager, should arouse suspicion of a possible underlying lesion. If there is any doubt about etiology an MRI must be performed. This is particularly important if surgery is considered because altering spinal shape in the presence of an intradural tumor or syrinx is a recipe for neurological disaster, with a very high rate of paraplegia.

In idiopathic scoliosis, the neurological examination should be normal. In congenital scoliosis there may be additional spinal dysraphism and the overlying skin in the midline may be the site of a dimple, sinus, nevus, hemangioma, or hairy patch. Furthermore, spinal dysraphism may cause a short so that wasted leg on one side so that a full neurological assessment is essential.

At the conclusion of the history and physical examination, it is useful to obtain a permanent record of surface shape (Fig. 36.18). The deformity buckles further on forward bending and patients should be assessed in flexion as well as upright.

Radiographic Assessment

Too many radiographs are taken of patients with idiopathic scoliosis. At presentation, the patient should have one full set of spinal films, including antero-posterior (AP) and lateral views of the spine from C1 to S1 inclusive. Their principal purpose is to exclude a congenital spine deformity or other relevant feature. As patients present with problems of surface shape, the only certain way of excluding a congenital scoliosis is radiographic. Patients with an intradural tumor or syrinx may appear to have an idiopathic deformity and only radiographs of the whole spine will reveal widening of the interpedicular distance or flattening of the internal pedicular surface. Syrinxes tend to be cervical, reinforcing the need to view the cervical spine. Although emphasis is placed upon isotope scanning for painful scoliosis to exclude

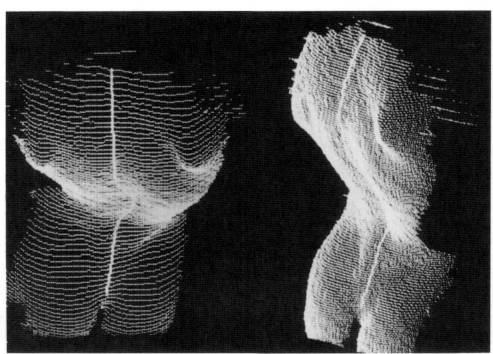

Fig. 36.18 Three-dimensional surface shape measurements recording torso asymmetry in a thoracic scoliosis

osteoid osteoma or benign osteoblastoma, these lesions are usually visible on plain radiographs as an expansion of bone, often with a central lucency, at the junction of pedicle and transverse process on the concave side of the curve apex. A PA view of the left hand and wrist should be obtained in the immature patient to assess bone age.

Measuring the deformity by radiography is controversial, although most scoliosis surgeons continue to use the Cobb angle [4] (Fig. 36.4). Perhaps the most useful single measure on an AP radiograph is the amount of apical rotation at the curve apex. This is a much more accurate index of the patient's chief problem (the rotational component of the deformity). Perdriolle in 1979 [20] introduced his technique using a transparent template over the apical vertebra, with particular reference to the pedicle on the concave side, which is sited more and more toward the concave side, with more and more apical rotation. The amount of rotation is read off in degrees from the template. This measurement of rotation can then be repeated with clinical progression or after surgical intervention. Any differences accurately reflect real change better than the Cobb angle [3]. Unless obscured by metalwork, the convex pedicle is still easily seen after a spinal fusion as it was before.

Radiograph dosage should be kept to a minimum and low-dose techniques are readily available. Good-quality normal-dose radiographs are required at presentation for diagnostic purposes but subsequent radiographs need only be of low dose. Wherever possible, measurement of surface shape should be used in place of radiographs (Fig. 36.18). Although sophisticated techniques are available, they still cannot offer a single overall figure for the patient's deformity.

Treatment

Late-onset idiopathic scoliosis is principally a question of deformity and appearance. What is acceptable depends much more upon the patient and family than the surgeon. Patients' perceptions change during adolescence and "acceptability" may also change with time. This means that, if the deformity were not to change in future, at that moment the patient and family would be happy with the situation. Wise counsel from the scoliosis surgeon is crucial to this decision. Although the surgeon cannot and should not state whether the patient's deformity is acceptable, the advice and information given is essential in helping the family reach a decision [21].

The only way in which spinal shape can be appreciably improved is by major spinal surgery, which may require both anterior and posterior stages. Despite improvements in anesthesia, high dependency care, spinal cord monitoring, and the routine "wake-up" test, there are still definite risks of damaging the spinal cord. Thus acceptability is a balance of risks and rewards; the rewards are a much-improved

spinal shape but the risks include catastrophic neurological deficit. "Acceptability" therefore varies very considerably from deformity to deformity and from family to family as the balance of risk and reward is interpreted differently. A 40° Cobb angle deformity may be so distressing for one patient and family that they would accept significant risks to have it improved, whereas a 70° deformity might be acceptable to another whose concern about one or two major operations and possible paralysis overrides any thought of cosmetic improvement. Although our knowledge of natural history is incomplete, it should be explained that bigger deformities tend to progress more than smaller ones, and more immature patients have a greater progression potential than those approaching maturity. As the spine does not stop growing until the middle of the third decade, it is unwise to consider that progression potential is exhausted when the bones of the hand and wrist reach maturity. Under the responsible guidance of the surgeon and with repeat consultations, often over many years, it is usually possible for the patient, family, and surgeon to reach the correct joint therapeutic decision.

Once acceptability has been decided upon, the management of late-onset idiopathic scoliosis is relatively straightforward. If the deformity is acceptable, then the objective is to preserve this acceptability through the remainder of growth by conservative management. If the deformity is unacceptable, the objective is to restore acceptability and maintain it through the rest of growth by operation.

Conservative Treatment

From the time of Hippocrates various orthotic devices have been worn in the belief that progression of an idiopathic scoliotic deformity could be slowed or prevented. The first popular orthosis was the Milwaukee brace, a cervico-thoraco-lumbar-sacral orthosis introduced by Blount [22] for the postoperative management of poliomyelitic curves. The Milwaukee brace was believed to work by three-point fixation—above, below, and over the apex of the deformity. There was a pelvic mold below, with vertical metal uprights going initially to a ring, which exerted upward pressure on the mandible in front and the occipital condyles behind. Problems with dentition and malocclusion led to the use of a simple cervical choker in later models. Slung between the uprights was a pad held just below the apex of the curve posteriorly to complete the three-point fixation. An important feature was that, for thoracic curves, the lumbar lordosis should be obliterated in the brace and consequently some "correction" could be seen when radiographs were taken without and then with the brace on.

However, the brace did not address the three-dimensional nature of the deformity. Nevertheless, it rapidly became the accepted method of treatment and, in its heyday, it would have been almost heretical to suggest a controlled trial of its efficacy. It was also empirical for the brace to be worn for 23 h a day, from diagnosis until after the vertebral ring apophyses had fused. As spinal growth continues, albeit very slowly, after limb growth, has ceased for a sustained effect to be achieved, the brace would have to be worn until the age of 25 years [23]! Furthermore, it was assumed that children wore their braces assiduously until Houghton et al. [24] showed, by using compliance meters, that they only wore them for a small fraction of the prescribed time: a major disappointment for brace protagonists!

Thresholds for treating idiopathic scoliosis evolved: those with a Cobb angle under 20° were observed; those with an angle 30–50° were braced; those with an angle of greater than 50–60° degrees were operated upon. That brace wearing did not modify natural history was not challenged until recently, when a retrospective study showed that no significant benefit was conferred on brace wearers [25]. The same "corrective effect" had been previously achieved with plaster casts, and flattening of the lumbar lordosis in the cast was considered a very important point. When the need for superstructure was challenged and the Boston underarm thoraco-lumbar-sacral orthosis was introduced, the point of flattening the lumbar lordosis to induce thoracic hyperextension was reinforced, as there was now only two-point fixation rather than the previous three-point fixation [26]. There is, however, no doubt that temporary "correction" by brace wearing can be achieved by flattening the lumbar lordosis.

Electro-stimulation of the convex paraspinal muscles was introduced in the 1970s in an attempt to treat idiopathic scoliosis conservatively. Rather like orthotic treatment, it principally addressed the coronal plane and, not surprisingly, no evidence proved its effectiveness.

A prospective randomized controlled trial was needed to determine whether bracing altered the natural history of late-onset idiopathic scoliosis. Unfortunately, a number of logistical reasons prevented this: bracing proponents would not stop bracing and those who had abandoned bracing would not resume it. Randomization was therefore impossible but centers in America and Europe made their cases available so that at least a prospective comparison could be made between bracing, electrical spinal stimulation, and untreated controls [27]. If a Cobb angle increase of 6° was considered a "failure," then failure occurred in 36% of those braced, 52% of the observed group, and 63% of those electrically stimulated. These differences were statistically significant.

However, in the subsequent paper from this study predicting curve progression [28] there was clear evidence that thoracic curves had a much worse prognosis than thoraco-lumbar or lumbar curves. In reviewing the original brace trial paper [27] we found that the more benign thoraco-lumbar curves were much more prevalent in the braced group (32%) but occurred in only 19% of those observed,

seriously undermining the trial's validity. A further in-depth review of bracing for idiopathic scoliosis was carried out [29] which revealed no significant benefit from bracing, questioning again whether the natural history of the deformity could be influenced non-operatively in any way. In simple terms if a thoracic hyperkyphosis needs extension (for which extension bracing is very effective), then a lordoscoliosis needs flexion which as we have seen makes the deformity buckle further (Fig. 36.2).

At present patients with acceptable curves are reviewed regularly; if their curves become unacceptable the only effective treatment is surgical. The majority of curves under 30° will either remain the same or improve somewhat; only about one-third progress to unacceptability. Clinical and epidemiological experience suggests that the proportion which proves unacceptable is smaller than 20 years ago and that the condition is becoming more benign. What is required is a careful contemporaneous longitudinal study of natural history to allow us to identify early the group of patients whose curve will progress; early operation could then be tailored. Similarly, the parents of a young child with a benign 20° curve could be reassured that there was little or no risk of progression. Despite much epidemiological work, we are still far from this ideal.

Surgical Treatment

For almost half a century after Hibbs introduced spinal fusion for scoliosis in 1911 [30] correction was achieved by using pre- and postoperative localizer or turn-buckle casts. In the early 1950s Harrington [31] developed the instrumentation that bears his name and operative management gained considerable momentum. Plaster treatment was not required before operation, although casts or braces were prescribed postoperatively for a period of about 6 months. It would be tempting to think that inserting metalwork would enhance correction. However, when Moe in 1958 [14] compared the results of Harrington instrumentation with localizer cast correction, he found no evidence in favor of the instrumentation. Perhaps this is not surprising, as both localizer casting and Harrington instrumentation seek to correct principally by distraction.

In favor of instrumentation, Moe found a much lower rate of pseudarthrosis and a reduction in the duration of cast treatment and bed rest. The pseudarthrosis rate was so high in the early development of spinal fusion surgery that the American Orthopaedic Association demanded an audit review [32], which confirmed the very high rates of pseudarthrosis and loss of correction in 425 cases. Proper selection of the fusion area, the addition of bone graft [4], and facet fusion [30] reduced the pseudarthrosis rate from just over 50% to a much more acceptable 7%.

The strategy of Harrington's instrumentation was to insert on the concave side of the curve a longitudinal distraction rod that was attached to the spine by hollow hooks. The upper hook was inserted under the facet and the lower hook under the lamina. The upper part of the rod was fashioned into a series of consecutive ratchets that would catch on the margin of the hole in the upper hook so that distraction effected a lengthening of the scoliosis (Fig. 36.19). At the same time,

Harrington insisted upon the insertion of a compression system on the convex side, whereby smaller hooks sliding on a threaded rod compressed above and below the curve apex, thus seeking to shorten the convex side while lengthening the concavity.

By alternate distraction and compression, the deformity was corrected and in addition made rigid, thus favoring fusion and reducing the pseudarthrosis rate. Because an

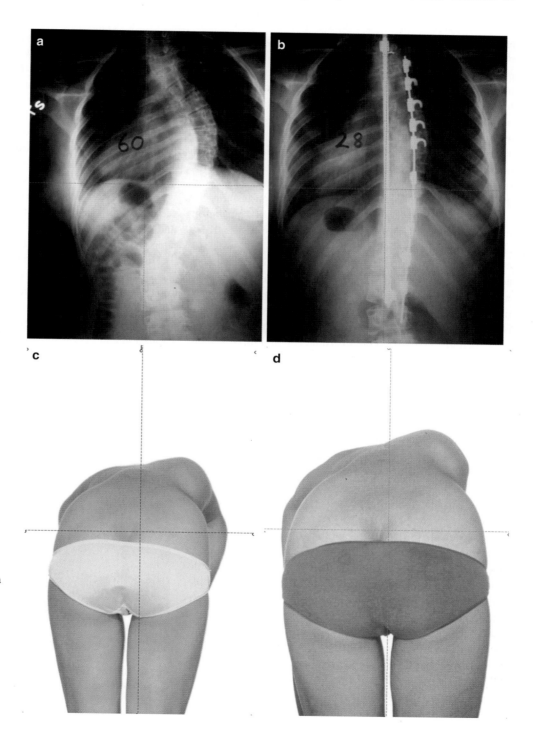

Fig. 36.19 Harrington instrumentation. (**a**) PA view of a thoracic curve measuring 60°. (**b**) Two years after Harrington instrumentation showing a solid fusion and a good correction in the frontal plane. (**c**) Forward-bending view before surgery. (**d**) Forward-bending view 2 years after surgery showing no correction at all in the transverse plane

important part of the deformity was rotational, it was necessary to insert the upper and lower distraction hooks into neutral, non-rotated vertebrae above and below the curve. If the hooks were inserted into the maximally tilted upper and lower end vertebrae then segments of the deformity would be omitted above and, more commonly, below the instrumentation: subsequent growth could lead to buckling beyond the limits of the fusion, so-called adding on. In young children, it was wise to instrument from parallel vertebra to parallel vertebra, thus encompassing not only the scoliosis itself but also the compensatory curves above and below. Combined with meticulous decortication out to the tips of the transverse processes, facet joint excision, and the application of copious autogenous iliac crest bone grafts to induce a massive fusion, this technique became the gold standard of operative scoliosis management, although many surgeons relegated the compression system to an optional extra.

Double curve patterns, e.g., right thoracic and left lumbar, or double thoracic major curves, were dealt with by extending the distraction rod from above the upper curve to below the lower curve, crossing the spine in dollar-sign fashion.

Based upon their considerable experience of Harrington instrumentation, the Minneapolis group devised the King classification of curve patterns to better define the lower end of the fusion, to maintain balance, and to mitigate against adding on [32]. This defines five curve patterns—types 1 and 2 double thoracic and lumbar curves; types 3 and 4 thoracic curves; type 5 double thoracic curve. If a vertical line is drawn upward from the center of the sacrum on an AP view then the lowest vertebra instrumented and fused should be that bisected by this line. They pointed out that the lowest vertebra which needed inclusion in the fusion was often below the lowest neutral vertebra.

However, this King classification is based upon the older Harrington instrumentation and the notion that the postoperative curve size cannot better that measured on preoperative lateral-bending films. Considerably greater correction can now be achieved with modern instrumentation. Furthermore neither the lateral profile nor rotation is taken into account and the classification applies only to adolescent idiopathic scoliosis.

Lenke et al. [33] devised another classification placing greater emphasis on the sagittal plane deformity. This classification has six curve types—(1) single thoracic, (2) double thoracic, (3) double major (thoracic and lumbar), (4) triple major, (5) and (6) thoraco-lumbar and lumbar. This primary classification is modified by the presence and severity of any lumbar curve (based upon the relationship of the lumbar spine to the central sacral line). An additional sagittal thoracic modifier depends upon the lateral profile (the Cobb angle measured on a lateral radiograph). This of course reflects the size of the scoliosis in another plane: the bigger this lateral angle, the bigger the Cobb angle in the frontal

plane. However, the Lenke classification is reproducible, appears reliable, and is in wide current use.

In 1982 Luque [34] in Mexico reintroduced the concept of supplementing rods with wires. This technique developed and was practiced extensively early in the twentieth century in Portugal. Sublaminar wires were added to a Harrington distraction rod before Luque realized that the longitudinal rods did not need to be hooked into the spine and developed his twin L-rod system wired at each level on both sides of the spine. His first cases were patients with early paralytic deformities (Fig. 36.20), but the system was subsequently used for idiopathic scoliosis. The addition of sublaminar wires meant that postoperative external support was unnecessary and introduced the concept of segmental correction.

Harrington's instrumentation was a key advance in spinal surgery but it principally addressed the lateral curvature of the spine. Although the patient complained of a rib hump, it was the lateral spinal curvature seen on the radiograph that attracted most attention to the exclusion of the deformity in the other two planes. There were two fundamental problems with this distraction and posterior fusion approach: first, it did not significantly improve the transverse plane deformity and second, in a deformity where the back of the spine is shorter than the front, posterior fusion does not seem logical.

However, as most patients were not far from maturity, they were not penalized by having the shorter side of their spines converted to solid bone, particularly as vertebral bodies are half their adult size at 2 years and virtually full size by 10 years. Most teenagers after Harrington instrumentation and fusion showed an improved Cobb angle, little

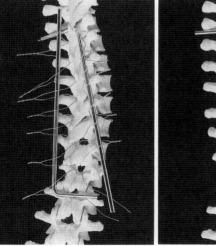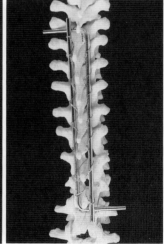

Fig. 36.20 The Luque twin L-rod system. (**a**) The rods are loosely attached with sublaminar wires at each level. The convex L-rod is then cantilevered down to correct the curve. (**b**) A straight spine after final wire tightening

change in their rotational prominence (Fig. 36.19), and little subsequent deterioration.

The situation was very different in the less mature patients: Harrington instrumentation provided only a temporary correction of the Cobb angle, and the posterior tethering fusion of the immature spine led to subsequent buckling with further growth [35]. Adding segmental sublaminar wires to a straight longitudinal rod may not be as advantageous as was initially believed: while providing more rigidity, the sideways pull of the wires behind the axis of spinal column rotation may make rotation worse even though the Cobb angle improves.

Throughout the last two decades further attempts have been made to understand and to rationalize the three-dimensional deformity of idiopathic scoliosis. It was appreciated that there were two essential prerequisites of a surgical procedure: to de-rotate the spine (rather than simply improve the Cobb angle) and to recreate the thoracic kyphosis (to minimize the likelihood of further buckling).

After much experimental work, Dubousset, Cotrel, et al. [36] introduced their intriguing concept of applying a scoliotic rod to the coronal plane of the patient and then turning it through 90° to recreate thoracic kyphosis, while at the same time de-rotating the spine. A second rod on the curve convexity, plus two transverse cross-link metal connections above and below, added considerable stability (Fig. 36.21). In the Cotrel–Dubousset system, the longitudinal rods have a rough outer surface and multiple hooks are used, rather than the simple upper and lower hook of the Harrington assembly. The upper and lower hooks are closed, so that the rod is fitted through a hole in the hook while the intermediate hooks are open, thus allowing easier communication between rod and hook. The multiple hooks allow compression and distraction at different points along the same longitudinal rod. The bulky system reduces the surface bone area available for fusion and is only used to secure the spine temporarily until the associated fusion consolidates. The rigidity of the fixation avoids the need for any postoperative spinal support.

A similar approach was developed in Leeds: if a simple longitudinal Harrington rod with a square-ended lower hook was bent into about 20° kyphosis, then concave sublaminar wires at each level would pull the spine backward, rather than simply sideways. This should permit spinal de-rotation as the thoracic kyphosis is recreated. A pilot study in 50 patients over a 2-year period tested this hypothesis. The initial correction of apical rotation was of the order of 50% and this was sustained at 2 years with no loss of correction [37]. Further experience in 200 cases confirms these excellent results.

It is important to note that the Harrington rod is not distracted after prebending and wire tightening. If the rod were distracted, the deformity would be under tension and the wires could not easily approximate the vertebrae to the rod. Furthermore, injudicious tension could be applied to the contents of the spinal canal. The technique therefore segmentally de-rotates and shortens the spine (Fig. 36.22).

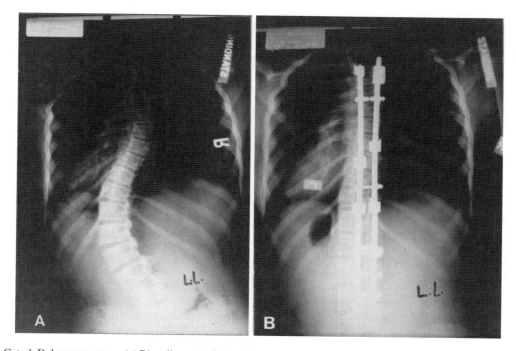

Fig. 36.21 The Cotrel–Dubousset system. (**a**) PA radiograph of a double-structural curve. (**b**) PA radiograph of Cotrel–Dubousset instrumentation

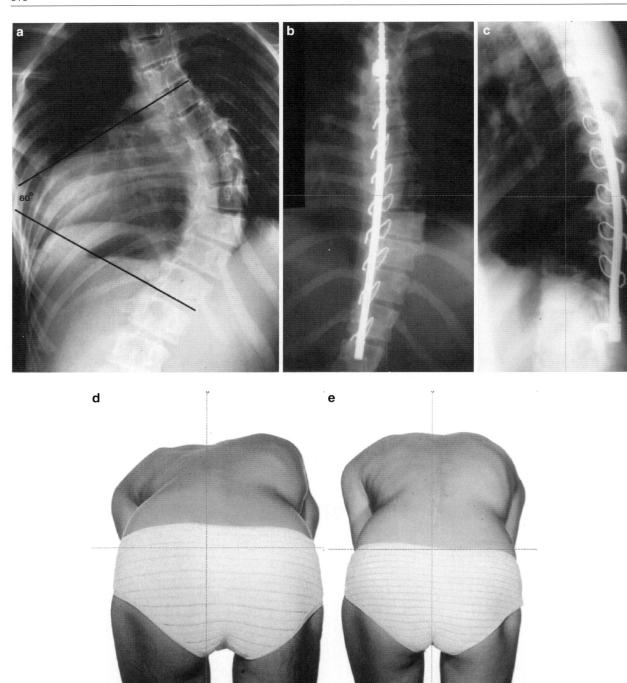

Fig. 36.22 (**a**) PA radiograph of a 60° right thoracic idiopathic scoliosis. (**b**) PA radiograph after the Leeds procedure showing a good correction particularly of rib asymmetry. (**c**) Lateral radiograph postoperatively showing that the sublaminar wires have pulled the concavity back to a kyphotic rod thereby de-rotating the spine. (**d**) Forward-bending view before surgery showing a sizeable rib hump. (**e**) Forward-bending view 2 years after surgery showing an excellent and sustained correction of the reason the patient presented in the first place

These original techniques have since been superseded by third-generation instrumentation systems such as the AO Universal spine system and the Moss-Miami spine system and with rods being connected to the spine using mainly transpedicular screws, usually in the lower half of the spine downward, but also sometimes involving the upper thoracic spine (Fig. 36.23).

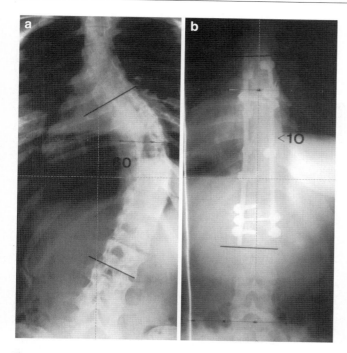

Fig. 36.23 Modern generation posterior instrumentation. (**a**) PA radiograph of a right thoracic curve measuring 60°. (**b**) Postoperative radiograph showing a virtually straight spine

Currently in the United States all idiopathic scolioses at any site and of any severity are dealt with by transpedicular fixation bilaterally from end vertebra to end vertebra. Correction of Cobb angle with these powerful systems is impressive and while some address segmental apical derotation, there is little emphasis on kyphosis restoration to protect the spine from subsequent buckling.

Not only can thoraco-lumbar and lumbar curves be corrected anteriorly but so can thoracic deformities through a thoracotomy, mini-thoracotomy, or indeed thoracoscopically. Anterior fusion is achieved by removing the intervertebral discs at each level to promote interbody fusion: it is important to remove the whole intervertebral disc right back to the posterior longitudinal ligament, not generally possible by mini-thoracotomy or thoracoscopic techniques.

If there is still a residual rib hump at the end of this procedure, it can be further improved by dividing the apical five or six ribs on the curve convexity, just beyond the transverse process. By tucking the lateral cut end under the medial, considerable further cosmetic improvement occurs; this can easily be performed extrapleurally, although a routine pleural drain for 24 h is a good safety measure.

For curves lower in the spine or for double-structural thoracic and thoraco-lumbar/lumbar curves, careful thought is required to decide whether surgery is necessary and which technique is best. Straight posterior metalwork in the lumbar spine may produce an ugly flat-back deformity with a tendency for patients to lean forward and develop considerable pain. Fusion down to the fifth lumbar vertebra leads to stress concentration on the L5–S1 motion segment and the likelihood of premature degenerative disease at this level. Lordotic contouring of longitudinal metalwork does avoid the flat-back deformity, but a long instrumentation and fusion are still required. Anterior instrumentation and fusion in the low back can avoid flat-back deformity and spare motion segments.

In 1969, Dwyer et al. [38] devised an anterior segmental instrumentation system of transverse vertebral body screws with hollow heads that could receive a braided cable down the curve convexity. When the intervertebral discs and endplates were excised, the convex screw heads could be approximated and then crimped over the cable, thus shortening the long antero-convex side of the deformity. As a result, considerable correction in all three planes was achieved. This system became popular for collapsing paralytic lordoscolioses, but it was not easily accepted for idiopathic thoraco-lumbar or lumbar curves, even though these were the deformities for which the apparatus was devised (Fig. 36.24).

More recently, Zielke's group in Germany markedly improved both the quality of the implants and the instruments used to insert them. His segmental instrumentation and fusion technique is currently favored for thoraco-lumbar or lumbar idiopathic curves [39]. The entire spine may be balanced by applying four apical Zielke screws, so facilitating short fusions. The system utilizes screw heads which are conjoined to a threaded rod; antero-convex shortening is achieved by nut chasing.

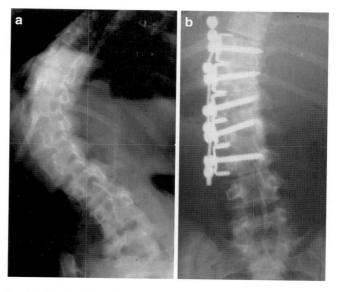

Fig. 36.24 (**a**) PA radiograph of a 90° idiopathic thoraco-lumbar curve. (**b**) PA radiograph showing an excellent correction after anterior Dwyer instrumentation

Fig. 36.25 (**a**) PA radiograph showing a right lower idiopathic thoracic scoliosis with spinal imbalance. (**b**) Postoperative PA radiograph showing an excellent correction of both the curve size and the spinal imbalance

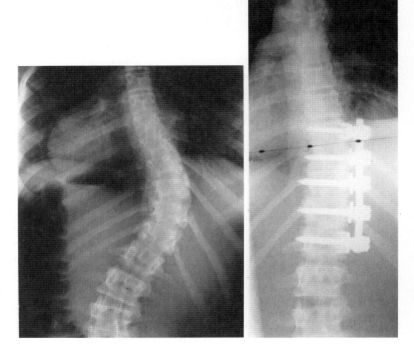

Modern universal spine systems which utilize both anterior and posterior surgical approaches allow excellent correction but are very expensive (Fig. 36.25).

For double thoracic and thoraco-lumbar/lumbar curves, different problems need different solutions. Often either the upper or lower deformity predominates, in which case it should be dealt with as if it were the sole deformity. If the two curves are of similar severity there is merit in dealing only with the lower curve anteriorly, as the upper curve usually improves reciprocally if there is appreciable growth remaining. When the patient is at or near maturity, anterior instrumentation of the lower curve alone may not effect adequate correction of the upper curve (although preoperative traction or side-bending films indicate flexibility). In the mature patient, therefore, it may be best practice to fuse the lower curve anteriorly and the upper curve posteriorly.

As with all other orthopaedic implant procedures prophylactic antibiotics should be used. The risk of neurological injury when correcting major spinal deformity makes it essential to monitor the spinal cord electrophysiologically during the operation, in addition to carrying out routinely a "wake-up test" immediately after tightening or tensioning the instrumentation.

Postoperatively, patients can be mobilized when their wounds are stable. They are usually discharged from hospital within 2 weeks, but it is wise to insist upon 1 month's convalescence at home. Children should be able to return to school 6 weeks after operation, but physical exercise and games should be avoided for 6 months. Swimming and noncontact are then allowed but full mechanical stability should not be assumed before 12 months.

The concept of curve flexibility/rigidity is crucial in scoliosis surgery. For flexible curves up to 60°, a single instrumented posterior fusion usually gives a satisfactory result. Once a curve exceeds 60°, flexibility reduces and, as correction becomes progressively less satisfactory, the risk of inducing tension neurological problems increases appreciably. Understanding the geometry of curve progression helps this fundamental point to be understood. As the primary lordosis buckles out of the sagittal plane, it is progressively more accommodated in the coronal plane, and thus both the lordosis and the true secondary scoliotic deformity increase. Each vertebra in the region of the curve apex becomes progressively more asymmetrically wedge-shaped in three dimensions. As this occurs, flexibility is lost and rigidity increases. True lateral radiographs of the apical vertebra in mild, moderate, and severe curves demonstrate this beautifully (Fig. 36.26). If these asymmetrically wedged vertebrae were to be removed and given to the surgeon as pieces of blocks to stack as a column, they would not readily stack in any position other than that from which they were removed. Curve rigidity really means "unstackability": the greater the deformity, the more deformed the constituent vertebrae.

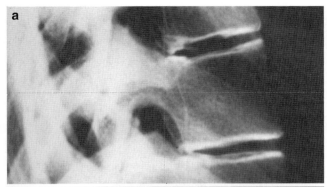
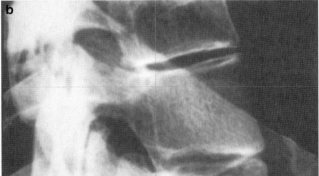
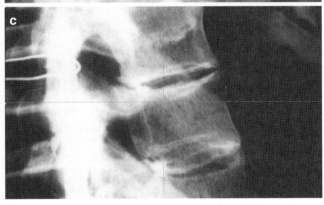

Fig. 36.26 True lateral radiographs of the apical vertebrae of idiopathic thoracic curves. (**a**) A mild curve. (**b**) A moderate curve. (**c**) A severe curve. With increasing curve magnitude the vertebrae are increasingly wedged in three dimensions so that the vertebral body endplates become less linear and more ellipsoid

This means that for curves over 60°, some additional maneuver is needed. For moderate 60–90° deformities, sufficient space for restacking can be achieved by performing multiple anterior discectomies over the apical five or six levels [40]. This allows the deformity to collapse into itself, so that not only is correction facilitated in the second stage but also the spine is not unduly lengthened in the process (Fig. 36.27). The second stage is the same posterior segmental instrumentation and fusion that would be performed as a one-stage procedure for a milder flexible curve. Such staged surgery is an important concept in scoliosis surgery and is key to achieving a safe and satisfactory correction.

There is a trend emerging of "two-in-one" surgery whereby both stages are performed under the same anesthetic. Proponents suggest that one long operation may have fewer complications than two shorter ones separated by a week or two. This may be so, but considerable deformity correction is often seen in the interval between operations, which may make the second posterior fusion safer. Spinal deformity surgery is very much a matter of risks and rewards, and while the rewards of a new and pleasing shape are considerable, risks should be kept to a minimum.

Early-Onset Idiopathic Scoliosis (Before 5 Years of Age)

Like progressive congenital scoliosis this can give rise to serious health problems such as cardiopulmonary compromise. Although the age divide for heart and lung troubles in later life is 5 years [7] the really worrying cases are the infantile idiopathic "malignant" progressive curves which, untreated, may exceed 100° in the first 2 years. The resulting disturbed alveolar reduplication can lead to severely hypoplastic lungs.

Clinical Features

Interestingly, when this condition was first reported from Holland by Harrenstein [41] the great majority of cases proved progressive, with only a minority resolving spontaneously. This state of affairs persisted for two or three decades. James [15] reported that only 4 of 33 cases resolved. The Oxford group reported that four times more progressed than resolved [42] but, for whatever reason, the proportions changed quite dramatically, and by the mid-1960s Lloyd-Roberts and Pilcher [43] reported 92 of 100 cases resolving. By 1968, only 5% progressed [44] and this remains the situation. In the 500 babies with early-onset idiopathic scoliosis we have treated in Yorkshire, we prescribe treatment in about 20%, in order to err on the safe side.

How is the deformity produced? One school of thought favors intrauterine and the other postnatal molding caused by the baby habitually lying in the oblique lateral decubitus position. There is more support for the latter theory as plagiocephaly develops only after birth. The "skew" baby with eccentric shape of head, thorax, and pelvis, together with unilateral bat ear, wryneck, and an adducted hip is linked to persistent sleeping on one side. There is also a greater incidence of mental retardation, congenital heart disease, inguinal hernia, breech delivery, low birth weight, older mothers, congenital hip dislocation, and familial predisposition [45].

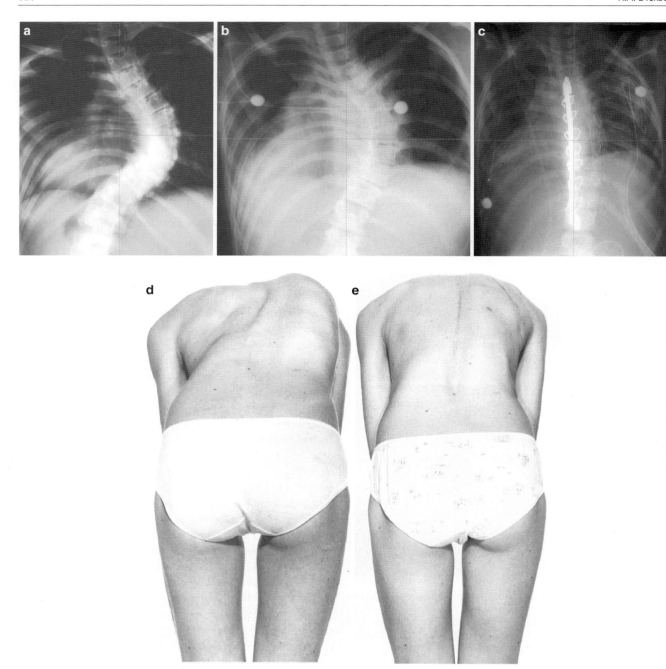

Fig. 36.27 Two-stage anterior and posterior corrections of a severe idiopathic thoracic curve. (**a**) PA radiograph showing a 90° right thoracic deformity. (**b**) PA radiograph in recovery just hours after anterior multiple discectomy. The deformity has lessened to a third of its original size simply by taking out five intervertebral discs and growth plates and allowing the leading edge to collapse. (**c**) PA radiograph a week later after posterior instrumentation showing an excellent correction of the deformity but more importantly an excellent correction of the chest wall asymmetry. (**d**) Forward-bending view before surgery showing a grotesque and rigid deformity. (**e**) Forward-bending view 6 months postoperatively showing a virtually complete correction in all planes

Males are affected more commonly than females, in a ration of 3:2, and thoracic curves are more common than thoraco-lumbar and double curve patterns. Most thoracic curves are to the left, and females with right-sided curves have a worse prognosis.

Mehta [46] described the rib vertebra angle difference (RVAD), recognizing it as a useful parameter in early-onset idiopathic scoliosis in helping to differentiate progressive from resolving scoliosis. On a PA radiograph of a thoracic curve the apical vertebra is located and its vertical axis drawn; lines are drawn along the necks of the associated ribs. The angles between these are the rib vertebra angles (RVAs), and when the smaller is subtracted from the larger the RVAD is calculated (Fig. 36.28). Mehta noted that when the RVAD exceeded 20° there was a significant risk of progression. The RVAD is probably a measure of the amount of rotation or torsion at the apex of the curve.

Some clinical factors are crucial in assessing these babies. A normal baby of 3.64 kg (8 lb), which reaches its milestones quickly, invariably has a mild deformity that will resolve. By contrast, a low birth weight, floppy, hypotonic baby which is slow to reach normal milestones has all the hallmarks of progression. Curve flexibility is important: this is best assessed by laying the baby gently over the examiner's knee, convex side downward, with the curve apex on the leg. If the shoulders and pelvis are allowed to sag, flexibility can be assessed. If the curve does not correct during this maneuver it is very likely to be progressive. These clinical and radiological evaluations ensure that no time is lost in managing the child with progressive deformity: curve deterioration can occur at an alarming rate.

Management

If the clinical and radiological evaluation suggests the likelihood of spontaneous resolution no treatment is required, but the child should be re-examined in 2–3 months. In the hypotonic, floppy, low birth weight baby treatment should start immediately, regardless of the radiological parameters. Borderline cases should also be dealt with as if they were progressive.

The only type of scoliosis that is really helped by non-operative treatment is early-onset idiopathic scoliosis, for which serial elongation–de-rotation–flexion (EDF) casting is very successful [47]. The casts are applied under a light general anesthetic on a traction table and take advantage of the young, malleable skeleton. By exerting pressure on the convex ribs in an effort to untwist the spine while the plaster sets, one can achieve correction. The casts usually last for a period of 3 months before replacement. Such casts are surprisingly well tolerated by babies and mothers (Fig. 36.29).

If curve resolution occurs quickly, casting can be discontinued and observation maintained; otherwise serial casting should be continued until the age of 4 years, when infantile growth velocity has abated. At the pubertal growth spurt, careful observation is again important. Long-term follow-up has shown the remarkable success of EDF casting [48].

If curve progression continues despite casting or the patient presents with major deformity, operative treatment is required. This can be a daunting prospect as the very young spine is more cartilaginous than bony. These are lordoscolioses just like late-onset idiopathic curves and anterior overgrowth is the main driving force; posterior fusion is contraindicated and some form of instrumented "subcutaneous" spinal procedure is necessary. Lifting the periosteum

Fig. 36.28 The rib vertebra angle distance. (**a**) PA radiograph of an infantile idiopathic curve of 18° Cobb angle and only 9° rib RVAD. This might suggest a resolving curve but observe that the lumbar compensatory curve is indeed structural and, in particular, the 12th rib on the right side droops more than the left (a negative RVAD). This indicates that this is a double-structural curve and these have much greater progression potential than single curves. (**b**) PA radiograph of the same child a year later. He was not treated, the RVAD is now 30°, and the Cobb angle 40°. The double-structural curve pattern is more clearly visible

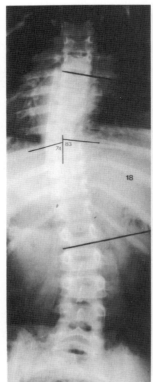
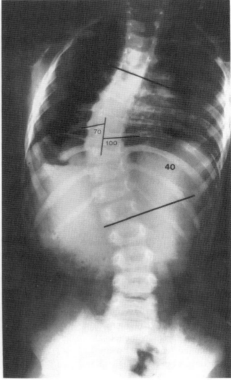

Fig. 36.29 (**a**) Applying an EDF cast for an infant with progressive infantile idiopathic scoliosis. An hour well spent. (**b**) PA radiograph of a boy of 4 years at presentation to the scoliosis clinic showing a thoracic deformity in excess of 100°. In the radiograph packet there was a film taken 2 years earlier showing a deformity of only 30°. Urgent referral and treatment is essential

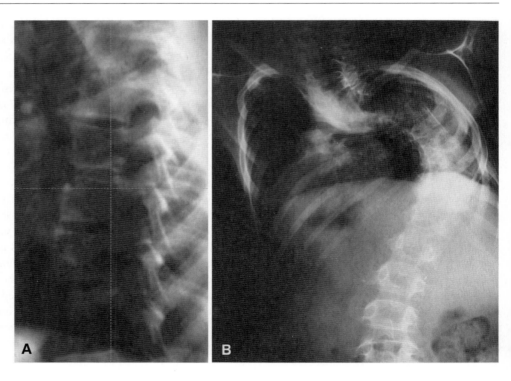

might produce osteogenesis and so, although the hooks at top and bottom will be subperiosteal, the intervening rod must be extraperiosteal [49]. It may be possible to manage the child throughout skeletal growth with posterior subcutaneous instrumentation, extending or replacing the rod as necessary. However, anterior growth ablation is often required by anterior discectomy and removal of the growth plates over the

middle one-third to two-fifths of the curve to control anterior overgrowth.

This gives rise to an anterior fusion over the operated segments but leaves several segments above and below the subcutaneous rod for growth throughout childhood (Fig. 36.30) until definitive posterior spinal fusion is necessary if it does not occur spontaneously.

Fig. 36.30 (**a**) PA radiograph of a severe infantile idiopathic progressive thoracic scoliosis in a boy aged 5 years, despite EDF casting. (**b**) PA radiograph 10 years after anterior growth ablation over the apical region and 10 posterior growing rod lengthenings/replacements. An excellent correction has been achieved. A posterior fusion has spontaneously developed

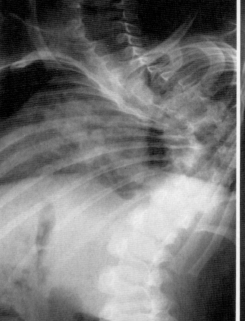
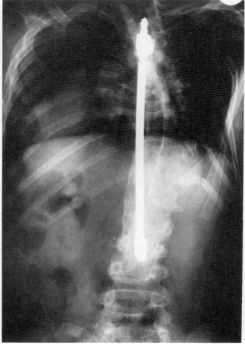

Newer generation metalwork systems have been developed in which one or two longitudinal rods are connected with a domino in the middle. By loosening the domino, distracting, and retightening, the construct can be lengthened with growth.

Roaf in 1963 [50] tried to control the growth of early-onset idiopathic curves by an antero-convex hemiepiphysiodesis. Unfortunately, while this worked for coronal plane deformities such as a solid hemivertebra, it did not work for the rotational lordoscoliosis of infantile idiopathic scoliosis [51]. Epiphysiodesis may alter growth but cannot counter the unfavorable buckling biomechanics of the underlying lordosis.

Recently there has been a resurgence of interest in restraining growth on the antero-convex side of the spine by stapling but no long-term results are available. Elevating the periosteum may not be as osteogenic as is generally believed, and the Luque segmental wire fixation system may be an option for posterior metalwork: as the back of the spine grows, the wires can migrate down the L-rods (the "Luque trolley") [1]. It also allows the correction to occur in kyphosis rather than lordosis (Fig. 36.31).

To avoid tackling the spine in severe deformity, the ribs have recently been the target of instrumentation with the vertical expandable prosthetic titanium rib procedure (VEPTR) [52] (Fig. 36.32). These need regular replacement surgically and long-term results are not yet available.

With EDF casting most scolioses either resolve or can be held relatively static until the adolescent growth spurt; management then is similar to late-onset idiopathic scoliosis. For those that resolve, it is the rotational component that may take several years to untwist, long after the spine appears straight on the AP radiograph.

Idiopathic Hyperkyphosis (Scheuermann's Disease)

Type I thoracic Scheuermann's disease is the opposite condition to idiopathic thoracic scoliosis (Figs. 36.10b and 36.33). It tends to occur in males and, although it has a community prevalence and familial trend similar to idiopathic

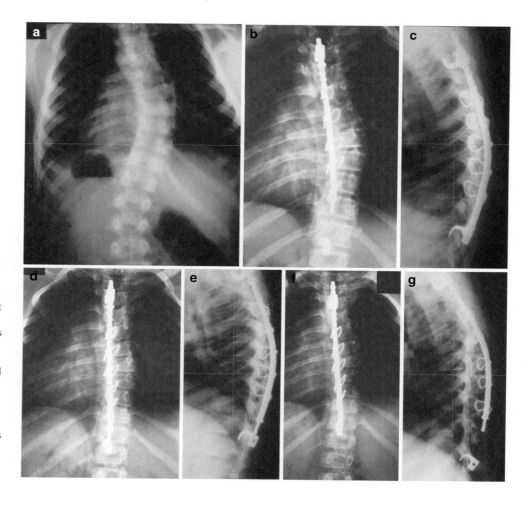

Fig. 36.31 Harrington–Luque trolley. (a) PA radiograph of a 5-year old whose curve could not be controlled by EDF casting. (b) PA and (c) lateral radiographs after recreation of the thoracic kyphosis using a Harrington rod and sublaminar wires. (d) PA and (e) lateral radiographs 3 years later showing that the lower end of the rod has almost grown out of the lower hook. (f) PA and (g) lateral radiographs taken 10 years later show that the spine has remained corrected and grown more than 2 inches

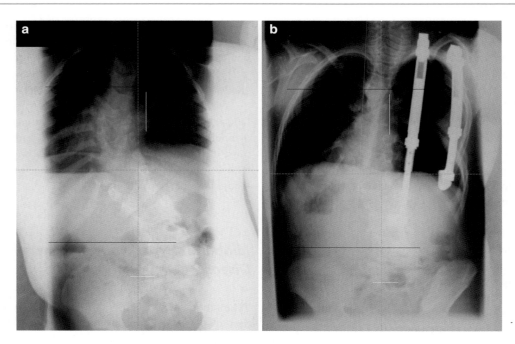

Fig. 36.32 (**a**) PA radiograph of a progressive early-onset case. (**b**) PA radiograph after insertion of the VEPTR apparatus to distract the ribs on the concave side

thoracic scoliosis, it has a later age of onset: most patients present about 2 years before skeletal maturity [12]. The condition is frequently painful, although the pain is usually fatigue discomfort over the lower part of the kyphosis, rather than significant night pain, is suggestive of a more

sinister lesion. Patients present with either increasing thoracic round back, pain, or both. Unlike the benign postural round back deformity, which is fully flexible on extension, type I Scheuermann's disease is characteristically rigid: on forward bending there is an angular apex to the kyphosis

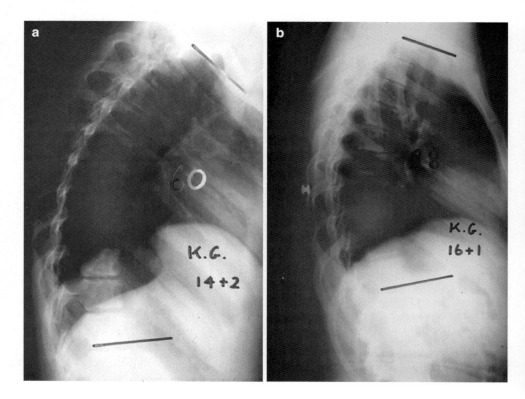

Fig. 36.33 (**a**) Lateral radiograph of a boy with a 60° thoracic Scheuermann's kyphosis. (**b**) After extension bracing 2 years later a normal kyphosis has been restored

rather than the smooth hyperkyphosis of the postural round back deformity. Pressure on this angular apex demonstrates its rigidity. Pectus carinatum or other deformity of the anterior chest wall is common and becomes more obvious with larger kyphoses. There is also characteristic and considerable hamstring tightness. Lower-limb neurological abnormalities are rare and occur only with very severe angular deformity when the spinal cord is tightly stretched. Two-thirds have a mild idiopathic scoliosis below the hyperkyphosis (Fig. 36.11).

Lateral radiographs of the spine show vertebral wedging with a reduced anterior versus posterior height. There is often evidence of anterior Schmorl node formation or endplate irregularity (Fig. 36.10b). The AP view may show a slight scoliosis with no rotation in the region of the kyphosis if the anterior growth plate is affected asymmetrically.

Unlike idiopathic thoracic scoliosis, thoracic Scheuermann's disease is treatable conservatively, provided the spine is not too kyphotic and that some spinal growth remains. Because the deformity exists in the sagittal plane and is rotationally stable, extension bracing or casting generally restores an acceptable sagittal profile within a year or so (Fig. 36.33). This should then be followed by extension exercises until spinal maturity is reached in the early to mid-twenties. Even if a patient is beyond general skeletal maturity worthwhile improvement may follow conservative management by extension.

For severe deformities correction can be achieved only by operation. Even with extensive surgery only a 40% correction is possible and not without risk to the patient. Although two-stage anterior multiple discectomy and interbody grafting followed by posterior segmental instrumentation is favored, it is possible to achieve a reasonable correction by posterior surgery alone. The pseudarthrosis rate, however, is much greater than in idiopathic scoliosis, because the posterior fusion is on the tension side of the kyphosis. In the balance between risks and rewards, the rewards are less obvious than in idiopathic thoracic scoliosis.

With the exceptional case of neurological dysfunction in the lower limbs, confirmed by imaging as due to the angular hyperkyphosis, the only satisfactory surgical solution is anterior dural decompression by apical vertebral body resection and anterior strut grafting.

Type II Scheuermann's disease, "apprentice's spine" (Fig. 36.34), nearly always presents as local thoraco-lumbar pain rather than deformity. However, sometimes patients present with mechanical low back pain because of the high prevalence of associated lower lumbar spondylolyses, which may be multiple. As the hypertrophic callus around these lyses can irritate local nerve roots, a careful history and neurological examination of the lower extremities are essential. The radiographs should also include oblique views of the lower lumbar spine to search for lyses. The pain of type II

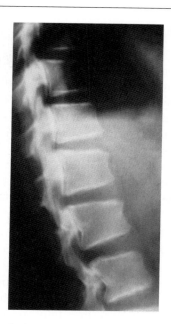

Fig. 36.34 Lateral thoraco-lumbar myelogram showing thoraco-lumbar type 2 Scheuermann's disease with significant vertebral body kyphotic wedging. There were intermittent neurological symptoms but no myelographic abnormality

Scheuermann's disease generally settles with conservative measures, which may include rest in a spinal support.

Congenital Deformities

Congenital deformities of the spine comprise two basic types—congenital bone deformities and congenital spinal cord deformities—although coexistence is common. Congenital spinal cord deformities are those of spina bifida and myelodysplasia (see Chapter 17), whereas congenital bony deformities are failures of vertebral formation or segmentation. Embryologically, mesenchyme migrates to surround the notochord; a breakdown of the medial surface of the somites leads to bony deformities. The segmental pattern of sclerotomal mesenchyme is staggered relative to the part of the somite left behind, so forming segmental muscle blocks. As a result the spinal nerves and muscles are segmental, whereas the vertebrae are intersegmental.

The re-segmentation theory was formulated to explain this complex, staggered arrangement, but this has been challenged by Verbout [53], who demonstrated clearly that all the elements of the future vertebral column develop in their definitive positions and that re-segmentation was neither required nor occurred. In any event, as early as the fourth week of intrauterine life, spinal structure and shape are developing and interference with this delicate process results in a variety of congenital spinal deformities.

Congenital Bony Deformities

Congenital bony deformities derive either from failures of formation or from failures of segmentation (Fig. 36.35); both probably relate to abnormalities of the intersegmental arteries leading to abnormal differential growth of mesenchymal cells at different sites in the developing spinal column—i.e., lateral, anterior, posterior, or at disc level. Lateral defects produce scoliosis, anterior defects kyphosis, and posterior defects lordosis, but defects commonly exist in at least two planes, producing a three-dimensional deformity.

Failures of Formation

Failures of formation are either wedge-shaped vertebrae or hemivertebrae. Furthermore, the hemivertebra can be segmented to varying degrees, from fully segmented (with disc spaces and growth plates both above and below) to nonsegmented (no disc space or growth plates above and below and the vertebra effectively fused to its adjacent neighbors). In simple terms, the more growth available, the more significant the potential deformity: the fully segmented hemivertebra is more likely to produce a progressive deformity than the non-segmented variety (Fig. 36.35). Nonetheless, even a fully segmented solitary hemivertebra generally has a benign prognosis. It tends to exist in the coronal plane and produces a lateral scoliosis with no significant rotation and generally requires observation only. However, in the lumbosacral region, a solitary hemivertebra with an oblique lumbosacral

takeoff can produce an ugly and progressive list of the trunk (Fig. 36.36). Of course, when double or multiple hemivertebrae occur on the same side, progressive and unacceptable deformities may develop.

In the sagittal plane, dorsal hemivertebrae produce progressive angular kyphoses. With growth, the hemivertebra can be squeezed out posteriorly into the front of the spinal canal and lead to impending paraplegia with hyperreflexia and clonus. Careful follow-up with neurological assessment is essential.

Failures of Segmentation

Failures of segmentation mean that one or more adjacent vertebrae fail to develop normal discs and growth plates. Complete failure of segmentation gives rise to a block vertebra—adjacent vertebrae with no disc space between. These are often found as routine radiological anomalies in otherwise healthy individuals. Partial failures of segmentation, with discs and growth plates on one side only of the spine (unilateral bars), progress more aggressively than their failure of formation counterparts. There are two reasons for this: first there is no growth on the other side, so that progression is the rule; second, unilateral bars in the coronal plane tend to involve the sagittal plane with a lordosis and thus superimpose a biomechanical buckling akin to idiopathic scoliosis. Indeed, such patients can present with a similar rotational prominence, and only the radiograph

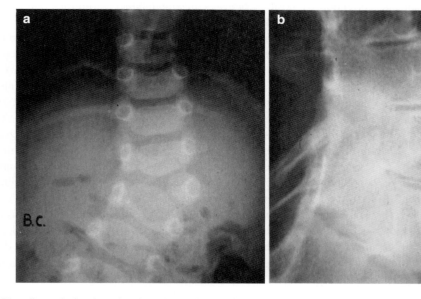

Fig. 36.35 (**a**) PA radiograph showing a hemivertebra (unilateral failure of formation). This is well segmented with growth plates above and below. A progressive deformity can develop. (**b**) PA radiograph showing a unilateral bar (unilateral failure of segmentation) extending over four vertebrae. There is no growth on the concave side and so a progressive deformity of significance will develop

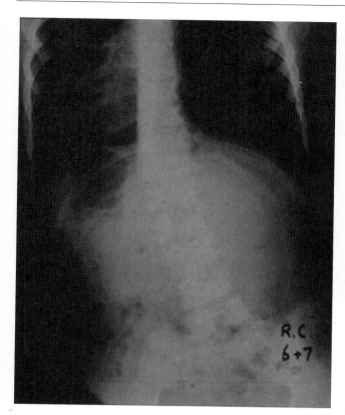

Fig. 36.36 PA radiograph of a lumbar spine showing a lumbosacral hemivertebra producing a marked torso list

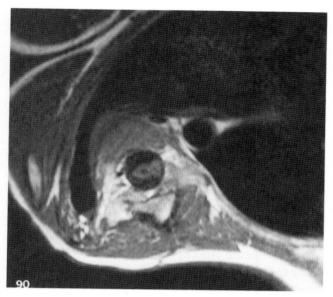

Fig. 36.37 Axial MRI slice showing two spinal cords split by a diastematomyelia

demonstrates the underlying congenital deformity. A particularly sinister combination is a unilateral bar on one side with a hemivertebra on the other: inexorable progression is the rule.

Failures of segmentation also occur in the sagittal plane: an anterior bar causes progressive kyphosis but, unlike a dorsal hemivertebra, which is squeezed into the spinal canal, neurological problems are rare. Patients present with progressive deformity, which tends to be less angular and less severe than that caused by a dorsal hemivertebra.

Treatment

If the child is referred to the orthopaedic surgeon by a paediatrician, systems other than the locomotor system have usually already been assessed. If, however, the orthopaedic surgeon is the first examiner, he must organize appropriate investigations, including abdominal ultrasound to assess the renal tract (there is a high incidence of congenital urological malformations in association with congenital spinal anomalies). In addition, the full length of the spine should be evaluated by radiograph, MRI, and/or computed tomography (CT) myelography because of the high incidence of

spinal dysraphism (Fig. 36.37). In spinal dysraphism, however, the spine column is never normal on plain films: there is widening of the interpedicular distance at the level of the diastematomyelia (midline bony or fibrous spur cleaving the spinal cord sagittally). A diastematomyelia or a low conus secondary to a tethered filum must be excluded before operation to avoid tension paralysis (a tight filum may need division or a diastematomyelia excision before tackling the spinal deformity).

As with idiopathic scoliosis, conservative treatment is of no value: treatment is surgical for both scoliosis and kyphosis. The general indications for operation are similar to those for idiopathic scoliosis. Significant deformities of early onset require treatment to mitigate against subsequent cardiopulmonary problems; later-onset deformities are more a question of appearance than of function. The anomaly associated with the most severe progression—the unilateral bar on one side with a failure of formation on the other—is sufficiently sinister to consider early prophylactic fusion. This is easier said than done; posterior fusion may make matters worse by tethering the back of the spine. Logic suggests a combined anterior and posterior fusion, but this is a formidable undertaking, particularly in the young cartilaginous spine and no published evidence testifies to its prophylactic benefit. Indeed, despite prophylactic anterior and posterior fusions, the deformity may progress inexorably, presumably as the result of plastic deformation of the fusion mass from biomechanical buckling. Furthermore, if anterior and posterior prophylactic fusions fail to halt progression, subsequent corrective surgery is made difficult or even impossible because of pleural adhesions from previous surgery.

Moreover, the natural history of congenital scoliosis is not always predictable and not all potentially serious growth asymmetries produce unacceptable deformities. When definite progression does occur operation should be advised to avoid irreversible chest problems. Otherwise it is sensible to review regularly as all anomalies do lead to unacceptable deformity [54].

When deformity is unacceptable the only safe way to alter spinal shape significantly is by two-stage wedge resection of the curve apex, so that correction is not accompanied by tension lengthening of the spinal cord. Roaf's concept of antero-convex hemiepiphysiodesis was sound biologically but is only reliable for the solitary hemivertebra, which seldom progresses to unacceptability [50]. It is ineffective for failures of segmentation as the underlying lordotic deformity has driven further deformity before the biological effect of epiphysiodesis can occur with growth [51]. Leatherman and Dickson [55] concluded that it is better to wait for the deformity to declare itself and to carry out a two-stage closing wedge resection once serious progression has taken place. Removing the apical keystone vertebra (Fig. 36.38) with prophylactic anterior fusion of the levels above and below is a much more certain way of controlling asymmetric spinal growth at a young age than prophylactic fusion. Isolated removal of a hemivertebra is usually only indicated for a lumbosacral hemivertebra causing progressive imbalance and trunk list. At other sites, prophylactic posterior fusion at an earlier stage may be preferable to hemivertebra excision to reduce the risk of cord dysfunction.

Congenital kyphosis needs surgical treatment if any abnormal neurological signs develop in the lower limbs.

Operation entails anterior dural decompression by excision of the dorsal hemivertebra, interbody strut grafting, and posterior instrumental support.

Congenital Spinal Cord Deformities

This refers to the spina bifida syndromes (see Chapter 17). More significant myelodysplasia is linked with more severe spinal deformity: patients with total neurological loss in the lower extremities are most likely to develop the most severe deformities. The majority of these are long C-shaped paralytic lordoscolioses with pelvic obliquity (Fig. 36.39).

Progressive trunk imbalance imperils walking and sitting, and undue pressure on the lower buttock may produce recurrent pressure sores with serious even life-threatening effects. These are difficult deformities to manage: the extensive anterior and posterior surgery necessary has a high complication rate and the risk/benefit equation needs careful evaluation.

For those with sufficient lower-limb function to walk, spinal surgery is contraindicated because a rigid lumbar spine can send them off their feet and make them permanent wheelchair users. Some patients who are wheelchair sitters with no lower-limb function can be managed by the provision of a total contact "Derby" seat in their wheelchair. However, for the patient with a progressive trunk list compelled to use upper limbs for support in the wheelchair, surgical correction and fusion are indicated.

The objective is to provide a square pelvis with a balanced spine above. This requires anterior and posterior instrumentation and fusion down to the sacrum. Anterior segmental instrumentation is favored for the first stage and posterior

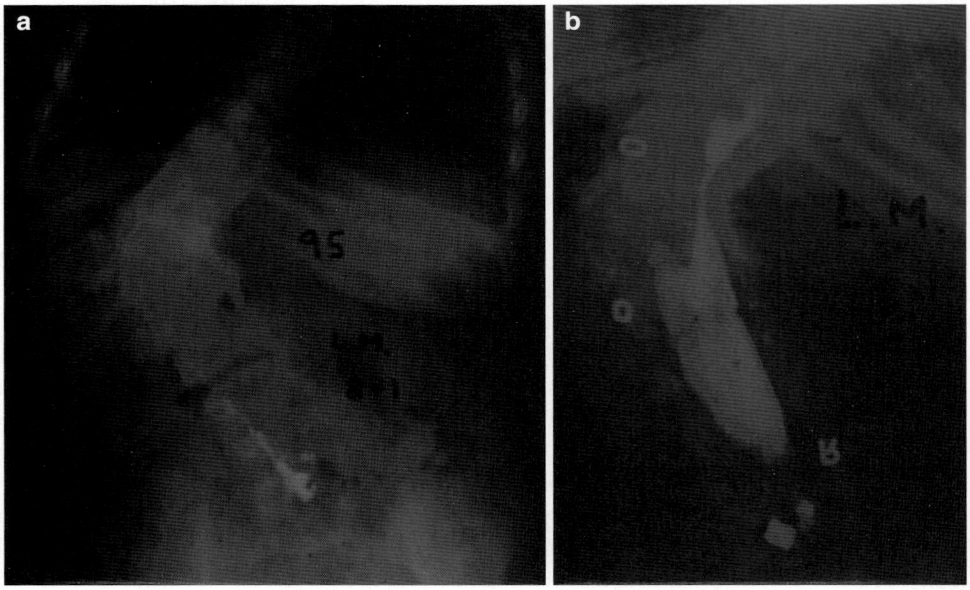

Fig. 36.38 Wedge resection for a severe congenital spinal deformity. (**a**) PA radiograph of an 8-year-old girl with a 95° rigid thoraco-lumbar scoliosis. (**b**) Preoperative myelogram demonstrating a split spinal cord due to a diastematomyelia. (**c**) PA radiograph after two-stage wedge resection showing an excellent correction. During the second posterior stage the diastematomyelia was removed

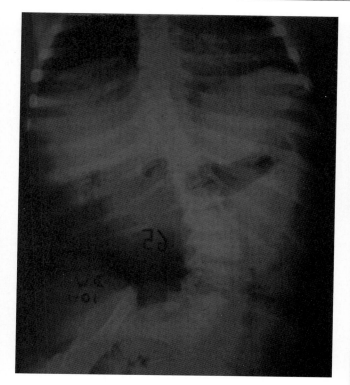

Fig. 36.39 PA radiograph of a spina bifida patient showing the typical C-shaped thoraco-lumbar deformity with severe pelvic obliquity

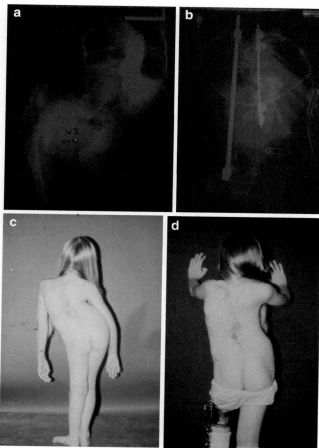

Fig. 36.40 (**a**) PA radiograph of a spina bifida patient with a congenital bony failure of segmentation in the thoracic spine above posterior element deficiency in the lumbar spine and a significantly tilted pelvis. The pelvic tilt is caused principally by the upper congenital bony deformity decompensating the spine. There was also a shortened, weakened, and attenuated left lower extremity. (**b**) After two-stage wedge resection of the upper congenital bony anomaly and then posterior instrumentation extending down to the pelvis, an excellent correction has been achieved. Note the old Harrington instrumentation as most scoliosis clinics have not seen a spina bifida patient for two or three decades. (**c**) Posterior view of this patient who was "going off her feet." (**d**) Postoperative view of this patient. Surgery put her back into balance although she required a knee brace and foot raise for the left lower extremity

instrumentation for the second. This must vary in accordance with the local anatomy. Areas with wide posterior element deficiency can be managed by transpedicular instrumentation but the spine above can be dealt with by hooks or segmental wires.

Careful preoperative assessment is important as up to 40% of patients with paralytic lordoscolioses also have a significant congenital bony anomaly (e.g., a hemivertebra or bar) in the thoraco-lumbar region above the spina bifida that can produce torso imbalance (Fig. 36.40).

Some severely affected children also have a congenital deficiency of the anterior spinal column in the lumbar region and develop progressive lumbar kyphoses. They are eventually drawn so far forward that the anterior chest wall rests on the anterior thighs (Fig. 36.41). All the anterior structures, even the anterior abdominal wall, contract secondarily and may need to be surgically released if the deformity is to be effectively straightened.

Congenital Spinal Deformity Syndromes

Congenital spinal deformities are encountered in a number of generalized conditions such as Goldenhar's syndrome (hemifacial dysplasia), Treacher-Collins syndrome (mandibulo-facial dysostosis), Crouzon's syndrome (craniofacial dysostosis), Apert's syndrome (craniofacial dysostosis plus syndactyly), and Larsen's syndrome (multiple congenital dislocations with a characteristic facies). Progressive deformities are not uncommon in these children but other major clinical considerations may take precedence over the spinal deformity.

Klippel–Feil syndrome incorporates congenital bony anomalies in the cervico-thoracic region with a short neck, low hairline, and restricted cervical movement (Fig. 36.42; see Chapter 34). Progressive deformity, associated wryneck, facial asymmetry, and Sprengel's shoulder (see Chapter 22)

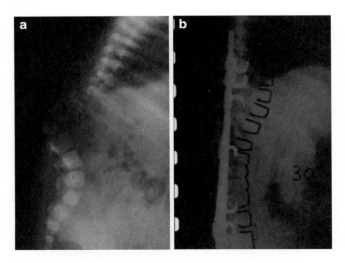

Fig. 36.41 The congenital kyphosis of myelomeningocele. (**a**) Preoperative lateral radiograph. (**b**) Lateral radiograph 5 years after radical anterior soft tissue release and discectomy followed by posterior instrumentation; sitting stability has been restored

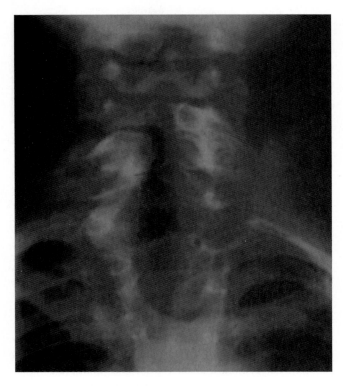

Fig. 36.42 PA radiograph of the cervico-thoracic region showing the typical multiple congenital abnormalities of Klippel–Feil syndrome

can produce a very unfavorable appearance, but corrective surgery in the cervico-thoracic region is difficult, dangerous, and not recommended. Congenital intervertebral fusions reduce the number of motion segments and the resulting

instability particularly in the upper cervical spine may lead to neurological problems. Limited simple fusion then has an important role.

In the lumbosacral spine the bony skeleton may completely or partially fail to form resulting in lumbosacral agenesis. With complete lumbar absence, the appearance is that of a "sitting Buddha"; however, more often, the lesions are partial. Many patients have significant urogenital or alimentary tract problems, which override the spine in priority, but for those with spino-pelvic instability, fusion may be necessary.

Other Spinal Deformities

Neuromuscular Deformities

The true neuromuscular diseases of childhood are those which affect the spinal cord, peripheral nerves, neuromuscular junctions, and muscles [56]. They include spinal muscular atrophy, the peripheral neuropathies, Friedreich's ataxia, arthrogryposis, and the muscular dystrophies. It is convenient also to include in this section cerebral palsy and poliomyelitis.

The common denominator is the spinal column buckling associated with inadequate neuromuscular control. Not surprisingly, the most severe neuromuscular problems usually cause the most severe progressive spinal deformities. Thus, in cerebral palsy those at the milder end of the spectrum, with minimal brain dysfunction, may develop no spinal deformity, whereas those with total body involvement almost invariably develop a significant scoliosis. In general two types of scoliosis are encountered:

1. An idiopathic-type deformity above a square and stable pelvis.
2. A collapsing C-shaped lordoscoliosis associated with the more severe forms of paralysis.

The idiopathic-type curves above a stable pelvis tend to appear in less-affected individuals, whereas the collapsing paralytic curves are more prevalent in those more severely affected.

Management of the spinal deformity must not be considered in isolation: it is essential to assess the whole patient. Nevertheless broad therapeutic generalizations can be made accepting that they may sometimes need radical changes.

Patients with a mild neuromuscular problem and idiopathic-type curves above a stable pelvis can be treated like those with idiopathic scoliosis. Patients with collapsing paralytic deformities with pelvic obliquity must to be assessed with regard to function rather than shape. If the patient is a walker, surgical treatment is contraindicated because interference with a mobile lumbar lordosis can stop walking and render the patient wheelchair-bound. However, as many deformities prove progressive and walking ability is lost, surgery if necessary can then be undertaken. When, to achieve wheelchair stability, the patient needs upper limbs for support the arms cannot be used for other purposes and corrective spinal surgery is functionally very helpful.

Many collapsing paralytic scolioses remain remarkably flexible despite their size in the sitting position. Most can therefore be dealt with by posterior instrumentation. Although two-rod systems using transpedicular metalwork have become popular, sublaminar wiring to L-rods is still an acceptable option (Fig. 36.43).

Cerebral Palsy

Considerable judgment is required to assess whether a patient with a seemingly treatable deformity has the overall ability to complete safely and successfully a difficult and lengthy treatment program. Even in specialized centers complications are the rule rather than the exception. Although lost function is the prime indicator for operation, only a minority of patients demonstrate improved function. Probably, only those who are losing sitting stability should be treated surgically [57] (Fig. 36.44).

Poliomyelitis

After the convalescent phase, when recovery can still occur, the residual deformities can be widespread and may include scoliosis and pelvic obliquity. Understanding the causes

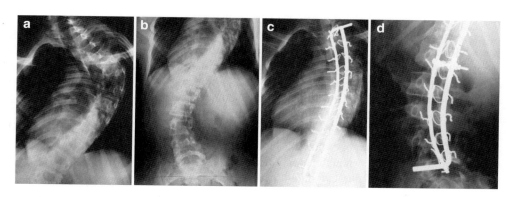

Fig. 36.43 (**a** and **b**) Preoperative supine radiographs of a wheelchair-bound teenager with Friedreich's ataxia. He was losing sitting stability. (**c** and **d**) Postoperative PA radiographs following Luque sublaminar wiring

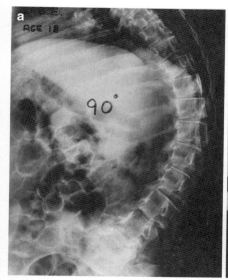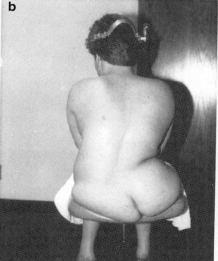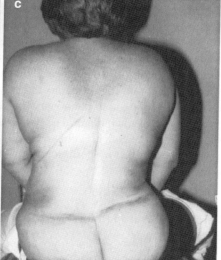

Fig. 36.44 (**a**) PA radiograph of a severe scoliosis with pelvic obliquity in an 18-year-old boy with cerebral palsy. He was bed-bound and in no pain. There was no indication for treatment. (**b**) Preoperative back view of a young teenage girl with a scoliosis and severe pelvic obliquity threatening sitting stability. (**c**) Back view 5 years after anterior and posterior instrumentation and fusion. Sitting stability has been restored

of pelvic obliquity is important in assessing spinal deformity. There are three types: infrapelvic, suprapelvic, and transpelvic. Lower-limb length inequality or contracture cause *infrapelvic* obliquity; loss of trunk balance due to scoliosis causes *suprapelvic* obliquity and unequal contracture of the ilio-psoas muscles (which alone span the pelvis) causes *transpelvic* obliquity. Suprapelvic obliquity is much underrated: it is fruitless trying to prevent progressive hip subluxation by hip surgery in the presence of suprapelvic obliquity rather than by correcting and stabilizing the scoliosis. This reduces the pelvic obliquity and improves femoral head cover. As with other non-spastic neuromuscular disorders, the scoliosis of poliomyelitis is usually flexible and can be treated by powerful posterior segmental instrumentation and fusion.

Spinal Muscular Atrophy

This was previously subdivided into the early-onset Werdnig–Hoffmann and later-onset Kugelberg-Welander varieties but is better regarded as a continuum with severe, intermediate, and mild subgroups [58]. The severe infantile onset group dies within 2 years and orthopaedic treatment addresses only the intermediate and mild groups. This is an anterior horn cell problem and electromyography and muscle biopsy are required to differentiate it from the Becker or limb girdle dystrophies (see Chapter 16).

Although walking may be possible for many years, patients who live long enough become confined to a wheelchair. Again, spinal surgery should not be undertaken too early as it can impair walking ability. Many patients develop contractures of the lower limbs and around the hips, compounding the scoliosis and pelvic obliquity. If surgery is considered for the collapsing spine of a sitting patient, chest function may be the limiting factor: some degree of postoperative atelectasis or chest infection occurs in most patients and several days of endotracheal intubation or even preoperative tracheotomy are often necessary. Although the heart is not involved, reduced pulmonary function contraindicates operating via the diaphragm. The prime candidate for scoliosis surgery is the patient with a relatively flexible deformity that can be handled by posterior segmental instrumentation only [59].

Peripheral Neuropathies, Friedreich's Ataxia, and Arthrogryposis

Orthopaedic surgeons often encounter and first diagnose these patients. Pes cavus and a high-stepping gait typify the hereditary sensorimotor neuropathies, and a broad-based ataxic gait suggests Friedreich's ataxia. Cardiomyopathy is associated with Friedreich's ataxia and some forms of hypertrophic polyneuritis are also linked with heart problems [56]. Anterior spinal surgery should be avoided and it is important that affected children should undergo careful paediatric scrutiny before considering posterior segmental instrumentation and fusion (Fig. 36.43). The more rigid curves that sometimes occur in some forms of arthrogryposis require two-stage anterior and posterior instrumentation.

The Muscular Dystrophies

Patients with the milder Becker, limb girdle, and facioscapulo-humeral varieties of muscular dystrophy tolerate scoliosis operations well, but those with Duchenne dystrophy or congenital myopathies, although they may benefit the most, are at much greater risk (see Chapter 16). Anterior surgery is contraindicated because of the associated cardiomyopathy. One-stage posterior segmental instrumentation and fusion should be undertaken when these unfortunate patients lose walking ability because the inevitable progressive spinal deformation can be successfully prevented while they are in their best physical condition. Surgery is hazardous because of the cardiomyopathy and the tendency to excessive bleeding. Surgeons performing this type of surgery have to accept a mortality rate as high as 10% [60].

Deformities Associated with Von Recklinghausen's Disease

Neurofibromatosis (type NF-1) involves many tissues of the body—cutaneous, subcutaneous, nervous, skeletal, vascular, and lymphatic. Although an autosomal dominant, more than 50% of cases are new mutations. Any two of the following features are considered diagnostic:

- a positive family history
- a positive nodule biopsy
- six café au lait spots
- the presence of multiple nodules

As with many inherited conditions it is not so much the condition that matters as its individual severity of expression. Scoliosis is the most common skeletal manifestation, developing in almost 50% of patients. Its prevalence, progression potential, and the age of the child at onset are proportional to the degree of dystrophic bone change (Fig. 36.45) [61]. Thus attenuated "penciled" ribs, enlarged intervertebral foraminae, and vertebral scalloping are associated with early-onset curves with significant potential for progression. Moreover,

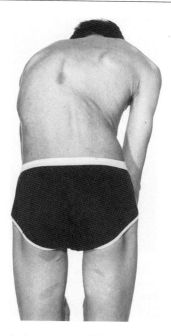

Fig. 36.45 The typical appearance of a boy with Von Recklinghausen's disease. There are multiple café au lait skin patches and a short sharp angular thoraco-lumbar curve with rotation

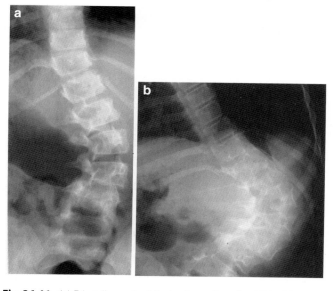

Fig. 36.46 (**a**) PA radiograph of the lumbar spine of a child with a typical dystrophic Von Recklinghausen curve. Unfortunately no treatment was offered. (**b**) PA radiograph 2 years later. Do not delay with Von Recklinghausen dystrophic curves

such curves are typically short, sharp, and angular with a lot of apical rotation. By contrast, less dystrophic bone change makes scoliosis less prevalent, and, if it occurs, less severe: the curves resemble straightforward idiopathic scoliosis.

Reports of patients with Von Recklinghausen's scoliosis frequently and erroneously call the deformity kyphoscoliosis. While these short, sharp, angular dystrophic curves can *look* kyphotic, with a posterior chest wall prominence on the convex side, the apical vertebral bodies are found immediately under the convex ribs: the front of the spine points backward or, in more simple terms, the lordosis has buckled all the way round, so that it now effectively points posteriorly (Fig. 36.45).

As with idiopathic and congenital scoliosis, the earlier the onset and the greater the progression potential, the more difficult it is to obtain a lasting correction. The Von Recklinghausen's curve is notorious, as bone graft is often rapidly resorbed rather than consolidated. A golden rule is that the dystrophic curve always requires anterior and posterior fusions with excision of the anterior growth plates. If the curve is acceptable, then early anterior and posterior fusions are required. If the deformity is unacceptable, less severe curves can be dealt with by anterior multiple discectomies, followed by posterior instrumentation and fusion. The most severe curves require wedge resection.

At the milder end of the spectrum, these deformities can be managed like their idiopathic counterparts, but if the patient is young and features suggest dystrophic change, an anterior stage should be performed.

Pure kyphoses, akin to early-onset severe angular Scheuermann's kyphosis, are much less common than scolioses but can produce progressive lower-limb paralysis. They should be treated by anterior decompression and strut grafting.

Cervical spine deformities are not uncommon in Von Recklinghausen's disease and can be extremely complex, with an area of lordoscoliosis at one level and angular kyphosis at another. Again, anterior and posterior fusions are necessary, although access can be difficult.

Heritable Disorders of Connective Tissue, Mucopolysaccharidoses, and Skeletal Dysplasias

About 70% of patients with osteogenesis imperfecta (see Chapter 7) develop a scoliosis (Fig. 36.47) [62]. Even in those who do not the spine is abnormal with changes similar to juvenile osteoporosis (multiple compression fractures and biconcave vertebrae). Patients with spinal deformity are nearly always those with severe disease. Like Von Recklinghausen's disease, the more dystrophic the bone the earlier the onset and the more progressive the spinal deformity. Because of the problems of bone quality and strength in relationship to instrumentation it has been said that progressive curves require stabilization or nothing. To spread the load segmental instrumentation is preferred. Adding

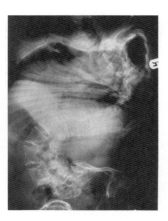

Fig. 36.47 PA radiograph of the spine in severe osteogenesis imperfecta. The main deformity is a huge right thoracic curve

methyl methacrylate cement to hook sites merely moves the weakness problem to another interface. The improved bone density following bisphosphonate treatment may make spinal surgery less hazardous.

Marfan's syndrome, homocystinuria, congenital contractural arachnodactyly, Ehlers–Danlos syndrome, and their various formes frustes, are all associated with a greater prevalence rate of the idiopathic type of scoliosis as the spinal column is disadvantaged at the soft tissue level by these inherited disorders of ligamentous laxity [63]. The resulting deformities should be dealt with like their idiopathic counterparts. The patient with Marfan's syndrome may have significant heart valve and aortic disease, but this seldom presents a problem in adolescent scoliosis surgery. With homocystinuria, however, vascular damage may lead to thrombosis and it is important to avoid unnecessary surgery in these patients. Similarly, it is important to differentiate the various types of Ehlers–Danlos syndrome, in order to avoid surgery in those with vascular fragility, in whom excessive bleeding is a serious problem.

Of the mucopolysaccharidoses, MPS4 (Morquio's syndrome) is the most important to the spinal surgeon because of its two common and major spinal problems—thoraco-lumbar kyphosis and atlanto-axial instability. The thoraco-lumbar kyphosis is associated with platyspondyly and the apical anteriorly beaked vertebra may gradually produce cord compression (Fig. 36.48). There is some evidence that an extension trunk brace can be helpful but once neurological signs develop anterior decompression becomes necessary.

Atlanto-axial instability results from a deficient odontoid and this is a significant source of mortality and neurological morbidity [64]. It is common also in the spondyloepiphyseal dysplasias. Untreated, most patients develop myelopathy. Thus C1–C2 fusion is generally recommended prophylactically in all cases by the age of 10 years. This can be performed posteriorly, with a supportive halo-vest.

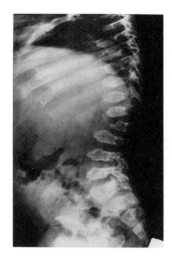

Fig. 36.48 Lateral radiograph of the thoraco-lumbar spine in a patient with Morquio's syndrome showing the typical platyspondyly and apical bullet-shaped vertebra

Achondroplasia

There are two important spinal problems that occur in these patients: thoraco-lumbar kyphosis and spinal stenosis [65]. Spinal stenosis, which tends to be more marked lower down the spine, is a problem of late adolescence and early adulthood and presents with claudication in the leg, weakness related to exercise, and gradually increasing neurological abnormalities in the legs. MRI confirms the diagnosis and decompressive laminectomy is required to prevent progressive paralysis and aid recovery. If this is performed on the immature spine, it is important to add a concomitant fusion to prevent progressive kyphosis (see Fig. 35.2).

Thoraco-lumbar kyphosis is a constant feature of achondroplasia, with a bullet-shaped apical vertebra. Seventy-five percent of these kyphoses resolve with growth, and treatment is only indicated if there are signs of impending paralysis. Occasionally there can be occipitalization of C1 with stenosis of the foramen magnum and secondary atlanto-axial instability: posterior C1–C2 fusion is then indicated.

Other Dysplasias

Spondyloepiphyseal dysplasia can also be associated with a thoraco-lumbar bullet-shaped vertebra, but posterior vertebral humping differentiates this from Morquio's syndrome. Kyphosis akin to Scheuermann's disease can also occur and is amenable to extension bracing, but if the bullet-shaped vertebra produces impending paralysis anterior cord decompression and grafting are required.

Scoliosis is not uncommon in diastrophic dysplasia and, again, the dystrophic bone favors buckling and anterior and posterior fusions are necessary. A particularly nasty deformity in this condition is cervical kyphosis. These patients require careful neurological monitoring and any tendency toward progressive kyphosis should be treated by anterior and posterior fusions.

Traumatic Spine Deformities

Trauma is a potent cause of deformity in the immature spine. It may be vertebral or extravertebral, accidental, non-accidental, or iatrogenic [1] (see Fig. 35.1) (see Chapters 52 and 53). The trauma of thoracoplasty or thoracotomy may cause spinal deformity, although it is nearly always very mild. Burns to the trunk, retroperitoneal fibrosis, or theco-peritoneal shunt syndrome can also cause deformity, the last usually a rather rigid hyperlordosis. It is, however, vertebral trauma that is most commonly associated with progressive deformity.

Deformities Caused by Infection

Infection in the immature spine is a potent cause of progressive kyphosis, with tuberculosis being much more serious than pyogenic infection (see Chapter 11). Most pyogenic infections produce a spontaneous interbody fusion with little in the way of spinal asymmetry but tuberculosis is quite different: there is much more disc and endplate destruction so that anterior spinal growth can be seriously impaired (Fig. 36.49). Thus, in the immature spine, progressive kyphosis is common, and, although anterior decompression and fusion may be required for the established disease or its neurological complications, anterior fusion itself produces further kyphosis.

Much has been learnt from the considerable experience of the tuberculous spine in Hong Kong [66]. The recommended treatment for tuberculous kyphosis is anterior discectomy above and below the kyphotic area with anterior strut and interbody grafting followed by second-stage segmental posterior stabilization.

Deformities Caused by Tumors

There are a number of ways in which tumors produce spinal deformities and in this respect intradural tumors, syringomyelia, extradural tumors, and the paravertebral tumors in childhood, plus the effect of their treatment, are all important considerations.

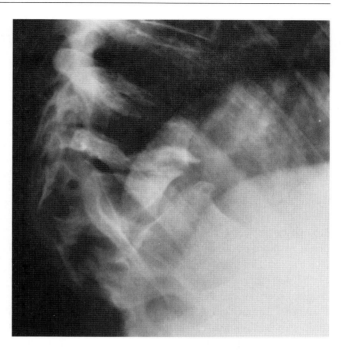

Fig. 36.49 Lateral radiograph showing long-standing tuberculous kyphosis since childhood. The owner is a distinguished orthopaedic surgeon!

Gliomas are the most common intradural neoplasm in children, followed by neuroblastomas and developmental hamartomas. Over half are benign and the cervical and thoracic spines are the sites of predilection. Back pain, limp, and leg weakness are common presenting symptoms and pathological reflexes, paralysis, and muscle spasm are common physical signs. Scoliosis is the presenting feature in 33% of cases. It is this combination of pain and scoliosis that should draw attention to the possibility of an underlying neoplasm (see Chapter 35).

Syringomyelia—pathological cavitation of the spinal cord—also commonly presents with a painful scoliosis, but headache is the most important associated symptom (see Fig. 35.12).

The spinal deformity which develops in association with intradural neoplasms and syringomyelia is of the idiopathic lordoscoliosis type and may be indistinguishable from true idiopathic scoliosis, although curve size and rotation are usually less obvious. Muscle spasm can make these deformities more rigid than would be expected. No particular side is favored and suspicion should be aroused by, for example, a progressive left thoracic deformity in a boy. With the more regular use of preoperative MRI scanning more and more syrinxes and cysts are being demonstrated although the pathological significance of some very small cysts is unknown. The message here is important: any painful or suspicious spinal deformity must be assessed by adequate imaging of the spinal canal contents (see Fig. 35.12).

Both syrinxes and intradural neoplasms require a posterior surgical approach by laminectomy which can produce a traumatic progressive kyphosis, particularly in the immature. Otherwise, decompression of the syrinx or excision of the tumor is generally accompanied by resolution of the idiopathic-type lordoscoliosis.

Extradural tumors such as aneurysmal bone cysts, giant-cell tumors, and eosinophilic granulomas tend not to produce a spinal deformity, or only a very mild kyphosis. However, osteoblastoma or its smaller equivalent, the osteoid osteoma, is generally associated with a mild idiopathic-type lordoscoliosis, with the lesion sitting at the junction of the pedicle and transverse process on the concave side of the curve apex. Isotope bone scan typically show a "hot spot." Tomography or CT scanning defines the lesion precisely (see Chapter 5) (see Fig. 35.13). Excision nearly always produces resolution of the deformity, although the posterior tethering effect of surgical scarring can sometimes induce further progression.

Wilms' tumor and neuroblastoma are the paravertebral tumors of childhood. Although they are paravertebral, radiation therapy can induce vertebral changes, particularly in the form of platyspondyly and a thoraco-lumbar kyphosis with a bullet-shaped vertebra. A true structural lordoscoliosis is, however, uncommon. Should progressive kyphosis require surgical treatment, previous spinal irradiation can increase the risk of pseudarthrosis after autogenous iliac crest grafting.

References

1. Leatherman KD, Dickson RA. Management of Spinal Deformities. Bristol: John Wright; 1988.
2. Adams W. Lectures on the Pathology and Treatment of Lateral and Other Forms of Curvature of the Spine. London: Churchill; 1865.
3. Dickson RA. Scoliosis: how big are you? Orthopaedics 1987; 10:881–887.
4. Cobb JR. Outline for the study of scoliosis. Am Acad Orthop Surg Instr Course Lect 1948; 5:261.
5. du Peloux J, Fauchet R, Faucon B, Stagnara P. Le plan d'election pour l'examen radiologique des cyphoscolioses. Rev Chirurg Orthop 1965; 51:517–524.
6. Goldstein LA, Waugh TR. Classification and terminology of scoliosis. Clin Orthop 1973; 93:10–22.
7. Branthwaite MA. Cardiorespiratory consequences of unfused idiopathic scoliosis. Br J Dis Chest 1986; 80:360–369.
8. Deacon P, Archer IA, Dickson RA. The anatomy of spinal deformity: a biomechanical analysis. Orthopaedics 1987; 10:897–903.
9. Dickson RA. Screening for scoliosis. Br Med J 1984; 289: 269–270.
10. Somerville EW. Rotational lordosis: the development of the single curve. J Bone Joint Surg 1952; 34B:421–427.
11. Stirling J, Howel D, Millner PA, et al. Late-onset idiopathic scoliosis in children six to fourteen years old. J Bone Joint Surg 1996; 78A:1330–1336.
12. Sorenson KH. Scheuermann's juvenile kyphosis. Copenhagen: Munksgaard; 1964.
13. Archer IA, Dickson RA. Stature and idiopathic scoliosis. A prospective study. J Bone Joint Surg 1985; 67B:185–188.
14. Moe JH. A critical analysis of methods of fusion for scoliosis. J Bone Joint Surg 1958; 40A:529–554.
15. James JIP. Idiopathic scoliosis: the prognosis, diagnosis, and operative indications related to curve patterns and the age at onset. J Bone Joint Surg 1954; 36B:36–49.
16. Nachemson AL. A long term follow up study of non-treated scoliosis. Acta Orthop Scand 1968; 39:466–476.
17. Bengtsson G, Fallstrom K, Jansson B, Nachemson A. A psychological and psychiatric investigation of the adjustment of female scoliosis patients. Acta Psychiatrica Scand 1974; 50:50–59.
18. Whitby LG. Screening for disease. Definitions and criteria. Lancet 1974; ii:819–821.
19. Mardia KV, Walder AN, Berry E, et al. Assessing spinal shape. J Bone Joint Surg 1999; 61B:36–42.
20. Perdriolle R. La scoliose—son etude tridimensionnelle. Paris: Maloine; 1979.
21. Dickson RA. Spinal deformity—adolescent idiopathic scoliosis: nonoperative treatment. Spine 1999; 24:2601–2606.
22. Blount WP, Moe JH. The Milwaukee Brace. Baltimore: Williams & Wilkins; 1973.
23. Howell FR, Mahood J, Dickson RA. Growth beyond skeletal maturity. Spine 1992; 17:437–440.
24. Houghton GR, McInerney A, Tew A. Brace compliance in adolescent idiopathic scoliosis. J Bone Joint Surg 1987; 69B:852.
25. Miller JA, Nachemson AL, Schultz AB. Effectiveness of braces in mild idiopathic scoliosis. Spine J 1984; 5:362–373.
26. Watts HG, Hall JE, Stanish W. The Boston brace system for the treatment of low thoracic and lumbar scoliosis by the use of a girdle without superstructure. Clin Orthop 1977; 126:87–92.
27. Nachemson AL, Peterson L-E. Effectiveness of treatment with a brace in girls who have adolescent idiopathic scoliosis. J Bone Joint Surg 1995; 77A:815–822.
28. Peters L-E, Nachemson AL. Prediction of progression of the curve in girls who have adolescent idiopathic scoliosis of moderate severity. J Bone Joint Surg 1995; 77A:823–827.
29. Dickson RA, Weinstein SL. Bracing (and screening)—yes or no? Review Article. J Bone Joint Surg 1999; 81B:193–198.
30. Hibbs RA. An operation for progressive spinal deformities. NY Med J 1911; 93:1013–1016.
31. Harrington PR. Surgical instrumentation for management of scoliosis. J Bone Joint Surg 1960; 42A:1448.
32. American Orthopaedic Association Research Committee. End result study of the treatment of idiopathic scoliosis. J Bone Joint Surg 1941; 23:963–977.
33. Lenke LG, Betz RR, Harms J, et al. Adolescent idiopathic scoliosis: a new classification to determine extent of spinal arthrodesis. J Bone Joint Surg Am 2001; 83-A(8):1169–81.
34. Luque ER. The anatomic basis and development of segmental spinal instrumentation. Spine 1982; 7:256–259.
35. McMaster MJ, Macnicol MF. The management of progressive infantile idiopathic scoliosis. J Bone Joint Surg 1979; 61B:36–42.
36. Dubousset J, Graft H, Miladi L, Cotrel Y. Spinal and thoracic derotation with CD instrumentation. Orthop Trans 1986; 10:36.
37. Archer IA, Deacon P, Dickson RA. Idiopathic scoliosis in Leeds—a management philosophy. J Bone Joint Surg 1986; 68B:670.
38. Dwyer AF, Newton NC, Sherwood AA. An anterior approach to scoliosis: a preliminary report. Clin Orthop 1969; 62:192–202.
39. Griss P, Harms J, Zielke K. Ventral derotation spondylodesis (VDS). In: Dickson RA, Bradford DS, eds. Management of Spinal Deformities. London: Butterworths International Medical Reviews; 1984:193–236.
40. Dickson RA, Archer IA. Surgical treatment of late-onset idiopathic thoracic scoliosis. The Leeds procedure. J Bone Joint Surg 1987; 69B:709–714.

41. Harrenstein RJ. Die Skoliose bei Saueglingen und ihre Behandlung. Z Orthop Chir 1930; 52:1–40.

42. Scott JC, Morgan TH. The natural history and prognosis of infantile idiopathic scoliosis. J Bone Joint Surg 1955; 37B: 400–413.

43. Lloyd-Roberts GC, Pilcher MF. Structural idiopathic scoliosis in infancy. J Bone Joint Surg 1965; 47B:520–523.

44. Mau H. Does infantile scoliosis require treatment? J Bone Joint Surg 1968; 50B:881.

45. Wynne-Davies R. Infantile idiopathic scoliosis. J Bone Joint Surg [B] 1975; 57:138–141.

46. Mehta MH. The rib vertebra angle in the early diagnosis between resolving and progressive infantile scoliosis. J Bone Joint Surg 1972; 54B:230–243.

47. Mehta MH, Morel G. The non-operative treatment of infantile idiopathic scoliosis. In: Zorab PA, Siegler D, eds. Scoliosis. London: Proceedings of the Sixth Symposium Academic; 1979: 71–84.

48. Mehta MH. Growth as a corrective force in the early treatment of progressive infantile scoliosis. J Bone Joint Surg 2005; 87B: 1237–1247.

49. Moe JH. A critical analysis of methods of fusion for scoliosis. J Bone Joint surg 1958; 40A:529–554.

50. Roaf R. The treatment of progressive scoliosis by unilateral growth arrest. J Bone Joint Surg 1963; 45B:637–651.

51. Andrew TA, Piggott H. Growth arrest for progressive scoliosis. J Bone Joint Surg 1996; 67B:193–197.

52. Thompson GH, Akbarnia BA, Campbell RM Jr. Growing rod techniques in early-onset scoliosis. J Pediatr Orthop 2007; 27(3): 354–361.

53. Verbout AJ. The Development of the Vertebral Column. Berlin: Springer; 1985.

54. McMaster MJ, Ohtsuka K. The natural history of congenital scoliosis. A study of 251 patients. J Bone Joint Surg 1982; 64A:1128–1147.

55. Leatherman KD, Dickson RA. Two-stage corrective surgery for congenital deformities of the spine. J Bone Joint Surg 1979; 61B:324–328.

56. Shapiro F, Bresnan MJ. Orthopaedic management of childhood neuromuscular disease. Part II: Peripheral neuropathies, Friedreich's ataxia, and arthrogryposis multiplex congenital. J Bone Joint Surg 1982; 64A:949–953.

57. Lonstein JE, Akbarnia BA. Operative treatment of spinal deformities in patients with cerebral palsy or mental retardation. J Bone Joint Surg 1983; 63A:43–55.

58. Shapiro F, Bresnan MJ. Orthopaedic management of childhood neuromuscular disease. Part I: Spinal muscular atrophy. J Bone Joint Surg 1982; 64A:785–789.

59. Aprin H, Bowen JR, MacEwen GD, Hall JE. Spine fusion in patients with spinal muscular atrophy. J Bone Joint Surg 1982; 64A:1179–1187.

60. Weimann RL, Gibson DA, Moseley CF, Jones DC. Surgical stabilization of the spine in Duchenne muscular dystrophy. Spine 1983; 8:776–780.

61. Winter RB, Moe JH, Bradford DS, et al. Spine deformity in neurofibromatosis. A review of 102 patients. J Bone Joint Surg 1979; 61A:677–694.

62. Benson DR, Donaldson DH, Millar EA. The spine in osteogenesis imperfecta. J Bone Joint Surg 1978; 60A:925–929.

63. Robins PR, Moe JH, Winter RB. Scoliosis in Marfan's syndrome, its characteristics and results of treatment in 35 patients. J Bone Joint Surg 1975 57A:358–368.

64. Kopits SE, Perovic MN, McKusick V, Robinson RA. Congenital atlanto-axial dislocations in various forms of dwarfism. J Bone Joint Surg 1972; 54A:1349–1350.

65. Nelson MA. Orthopaedic aspects of the chondrodystrophies. The dwarf and his orthopaedic problems. Ann Royal Coll Surg England 1970; 47:185–210.

66. Hodgson AR. Correction of kyphotic spinal deformities. J Bone Joint Surg 1973; 55B:211–212.

Chapter 37

Spondylolisthesis

Robert A. Dickson

Introduction

Spondylolisthesis is the slipping forward of one vertebra and the spine above it upon the vertebra immediately below. When the condition first received orthopaedic attention in the latter half of the twentieth century, it was believed to be of congenital origin, but now it is recognized that several varieties exist, most being acquired.

The International Society for Study of the Lumbar Spine proposed a classification that is now generally accepted [1]. Five types are recognized :

- dysplastic
- isthmic
- degenerative
- traumatic
- pathological

Degenerative spondylolisthesis affects the over 50-year-old age group and is attributable to instability of arthritic posterior facet joints. It is much more common in women, particularly at the L4–L5 level, and because the back of the spine is not left behind, it can lead to spinal stenosis.

Traumatic spondylolisthesis refers to forward subluxation of one vertebra upon another as the result of a fracture in a region other than the pars interarticularis, such as the pedicle. Taillard questioned whether this should be called spondylolisthesis, rather than simple traumatic vertebral subluxation [2].

Pathological spondylolisthesis may complicate a number of underlying conditions such as tuberculosis, giant cell tumor, Paget's disease, rheumatoid disease, Albers-Schönberg disease, arthrogryposis, syphilis, and metastases.

In childhood and adolescence only the dysplastic and isthmic varieties are encountered. Both forms are strongly familial, with almost one-third of first-degree relations having the same lesion [3].

Isthmic Spondylolisthesis

The isthmus or pars interarticularis is the posterolateral bony element between the upper and the lower articular processes. There are three subtypes of isthmic spondylolisthesis classified as

- lytic
- attenuation of the pars
- acute pars fracture

However, there is little convincing evidence that acute fractures of the pars ever occur, and attenuation and elongation of the pars is seen only with dysplastic spondylolisthesis [4]. Therefore, for practical purposes, "isthmic spondylolisthesis" and "lytic spondylolisthesis" are interchangeable terms.

The defect in the pars interarticularis is referred to as a spondylolysis and slippage in lytic spondylolisthesis is the consequence of this defect (Fig. 37.1; see also Figs. 34.8, 34.9, and 34.10). The development of this defect was originally believed to be congenital, but lyses have been shown to be fatigue or stress fractures in what has been shown biomechanically to be the weakest part of the neural arch [5]. Although lyses have been noted in children younger than 2 years, these lesions do not generally develop until after the age of 5 years, with an increasing prevalence rate from 1 to 2% at this young end of the age spectrum to a constant 6–7% in the adult population, except in Eskimos who have a prevalence rate in excess of 50% [6]. Slippage (spondylolisthesis) probably only occurs in 10–20% of lyses. These fatigue fractures are much more common in those who pursue a particularly active life. Among gymnasts lyses occur in

R.A. Dickson (✉)
Academic Unit of Orthopaedic Surgery, Leeds General Infirmary, Leeds, UK

M. Benson et al. (eds.), *Children's Orthopaedics and Fractures*,
DOI 10.1007/978-1-84882-611-3_37, © Springer-Verlag London Limited 2010

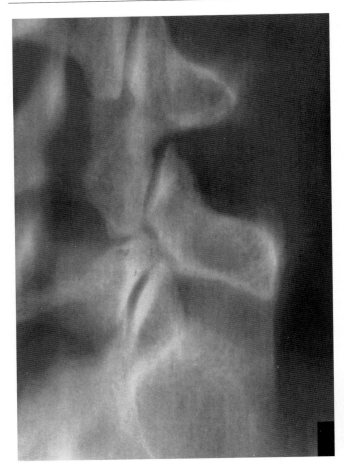

Fig. 37.1 Oblique lumbar tomogram showing a lysis in the pars interarticularis. The Scotty dog of LaChapelle has a collar

over 10% and spondylolisthesis in 6% [7]. Of course, these prevalence rates are derived from anteroposterior (AP) and lateral plain films of the spine and, if oblique tomograms or computed tomography (CT) were carried out, these rates would probably at least double. In contrast, the condition does not occur in those who, because of physical handicap, have never walked.

During childhood, the lytic region is filled with cartilage in which there are zones of endochondral ossification. Thus there is considerable potential for healing. Despite this, there is an increasing prevalence rate throughout growth. Once adulthood is reached, the nature of the spondylolysis changes toward that of a fracture non-union with hypertrophic callus (see Fig. 35.9), with little or no spontaneous healing potential. This explains the constant prevalence rate at maturity. In the adult, the appearance of the lytic defect should not therefore be misinterpreted as a gap, but rather as a mass lesion that may irritate the local nerve root. Radicular symptoms from lyses are not uncommon in the adult but are rare in the immature.

In the lumbar spine, forces are concentrated at the pars, particularly at the L5–S1 level, which is by far the most common site for spondylolisthesis [5].

Recently it has been shown that in the presence of a lysis the posterior facet joints are significantly more coronally orientated, thus producing a pincer-type effect, increasing forces across the pars [8] (Fig. 37.2).

Individuals with type II Scheuermann's disease (thoraco-lumbar kyphosis or apprentice's spine) have a much greater incidence of lower lumbar lyses, and these may be multiple.

When slippage occurs, the vertebral body in front of the lyses moves forward and leaves the back of the spinal arch behind. The spinal canal is therefore locally more capacious, quite unlike degenerative spondylolisthesis, and the step that is visible or palpable is at the junction of the slipped vertebra with the one above. Because the canal is large and the lyses cartilaginous, neurological symptoms and signs are very unusual.

As lytic spondylolisthesis is an acquired condition, both L5 and S1 are reasonably well formed and the slippage tends to be forward in the sagittal plane, without much in the way of local angular kyphosis (Fig. 37.3).

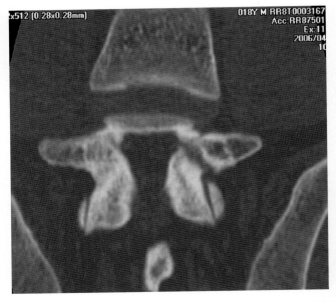

Fig. 37.2 Axial CT scan through the facet joints. On the side of the lysis the facet joint is more coronally orientated creating a pincer effect on movement

Dysplastic Spondylolisthesis

Originally termed "congenital," dysplastic spondylolisthesis is caused by hypoplasia or aplasia of the L5–S1 facet joints. The back of the spine is not left behind, so that the AP canal diameter is proportionately reduced. Interestingly, however,

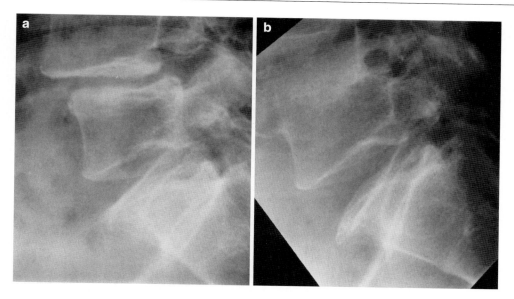

Fig. 37.3 (**a**) Lateral radiograph showing an L4/L5 lytic spondylolisthesis of long standing. These do not slip further after the attainment of maturity when they stabilize and produce no symptoms. (**b**) Over the course of the next year this man developed a septicemia and back pain. His L4/L5 discitis went on to spontaneous interbody fusion

only a modest degree of slippage occurs (usually not more than 25% of the sagittal width of the top of the sacrum) before a secondary spondylolysis develops in the pars of L5 which, although allowing further slippage to take place, does not further jeopardize the size of the spinal canal. Therefore, as with lytic spondylolisthesis, neurological symptoms and signs are unusual. It is only when secondary spondylolysis complicates dysplastic spondylolisthesis that attenuation of the pars can be seen before a frank spondylolysis develops [4] (Fig. 37.4).

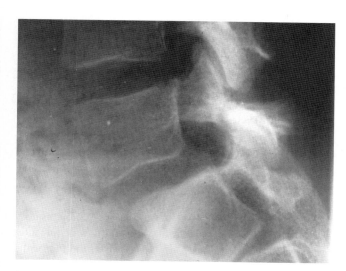

Fig. 37.4 Lateral radiograph of the lower lumbar spine with an L5/S1 dysplastic spondylolisthesis (note the lordotic-shaped L5 and the reciprocal rounding of the upper border of the sacrum anteriorly). The pars on each side have stretched and a secondary lysis has developed

Because the condition is congenital and develops at an earlier age than lytic spondylolisthesis, the body of L5 and the upper sacrum may be considerably deformed. The L5 vertebra becomes increasingly wedge shaped and the upper sacrum rounds off. Furthermore, in dysplastic spondylolisthesis there is always a spina bifida occulta of L5 or S1 and the sacrum appears more open than normal. It is these radiographic features on both AP and lateral projections that clearly differentiate the dysplastic from the lytic variety (Fig. 37.5). Because the L5 and S1 vertebrae are reciprocally misshapen, the slippage in dysplastic spondylolisthesis is very much more a progressive kyphosis than a simple slip forward in the sagittal plane.

Measurement

It has become the accepted standard to measure the degree of spondylolisthesis on a standing lateral radiograph [9]. Although a variety of measurements have been described, two are of particular value:

1. The extent of anterior displacement or slip.
2. The angle of sagittal rotation, also known as the sagittal roll, slip angle, or lumbo-sacral kyphosis (Fig. 37.6).

The extent of anterior displacement is the distance between the posterior cortex of L5 and the posterior cortex of S1, expressed as a percentage of the anteroposterior diameter of S1.

Fig. 37.5 AP radiograph of the lumbo-sacral junction in a severe dysplastic spondylolisthesis. Note the upside down appearance of Napoleon's hat as the sacrum overlaps L5. Observe the obligatory spina bifida occulta

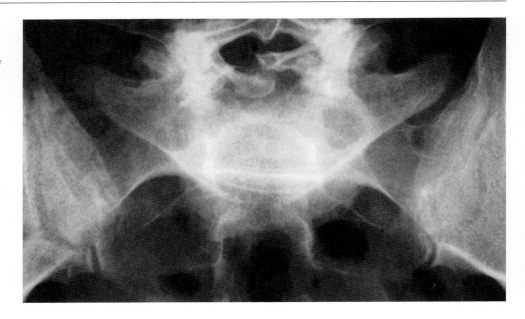

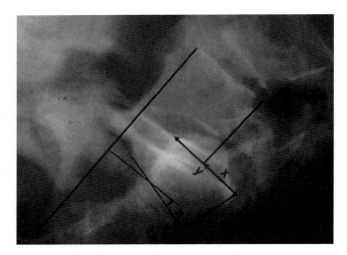

Fig. 37.6 Radiological measurement of spondylolisthesis. (i) Anterior displacement—the degree of slip forward of L5 is expressed as a percentage, $x/y \times 100$. (ii) Sacral inclination—angle a (the tilt of the sacrum from the vertical). (iii) Sagittal rotation—angle b (the angle subtended by L5 and S1 in the sagittal plane)

A more important clinical correlation is the angle of sagittal rotation, which is the relationship between L5 and S1 as subtended by lines drawn parallel to the anterior cortex of L5 and the posterior cortex of S1. The important clinical deformity in spondylolisthesis is lumbo-sacral kyphosis. The angle of sagittal rotation more accurately defines the clinical problem as a very considerable lytic spondylolisthesis with, say, a 75% slip purely in the sagittal plane may produce no clinical deformity whatever.

Clinical Features

Patients present with pain, deformity, neurological symptoms, hamstring tightness, and gait abnormality. The low back pain is mechanical, being worse during activity and hyperextension and relieved by rest. The pain is often referred to the buttock and thigh, but rarely with radicular distribution into the leg. Hamstring spasm or contracture is commonly associated with the more severe degrees of spondylolisthesis, particularly of the dysplastic variety, in which progressive lumbo-sacral kyphosis leads to relative flexion of the hip and knee; in severe degrees of slippage, there is frank hamstring contracture over and above any spasm induced by local discomfort. As the lumbo-sacral kyphosis progresses and the hips and knees take up a Z-deformity, posture becomes increasingly more distressing. Occasionally, with spondyloptosis, the L5 body finishes anterior to the first sacral segment, allowing the upper posterior corner of S1 to indent the canal, producing symptoms of spinal claudication and leg fatigue (Fig. 37.7). Otherwise, the only other neurological symptom encountered is occasional radicular pain in the same nerve root as the slipping vertebra (i.e., L5 for an L5–S1 slip and L4 for an L4–L5 slip).

Above the lumbo-sacral kyphosis, a compensatory thoraco-lumbar hyperlordosis may develop, with an anterior skin crease at umbilical level. Thus from the top of the spine down to the feet a gradually increasing Z-deformity can occur. Neurological examination is usually normal, but attention should be directed to the relevant nerve root. During adolescence, these children may suffer a spondylolisthetic

Fig. 37.7 (**a**) Lateral radiograph of the lumbo-sacral region showing a spondyloptosis with L5 lying in front of S1. (**b**) Sagittal MRI slice showing that, as usual, despite the severe deformity the spinal canal is capacious because secondary lyses have left the back of the spine behind. (**c**) Side view of this girl showing no significant deformity. (**d**) Front view showing the abdominal skin crease because severe dysplastic spondylolisthesis is effectively a kyphosis. (**e**) Forward bending view revealing the obvious kyphosis. She was in no pain and had normal function

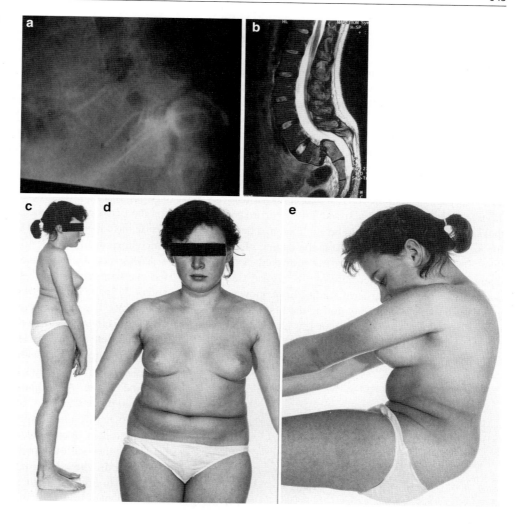

"crisis" [4], with profound muscle spasm such that patients can be deformed in the frontal plane in addition to their lateral profile. Lesions at the L4–L5 level tend to have a worse prognosis than those at the L5–S1 level, in terms of both irritability and progression.

Treatment

As with most orthopaedic conditions, there is a considerable divergence of opinion as to how patients should be treated. Recent years have seen an exponential increase in the use of operative surgery, particularly in the nature of attempted reduction with transpedicular instrumentation in addition to biological fusion. In many countries, such techniques are currently accepted as standard, but there is no convincing evidence that patients fare better.

There is a place for both conservative and operative management. For the immature patient with a spondylolysis and considerable potential for healing, an expectant policy should

be pursued. The child presenting with mechanical low back pain whose plain radiographs indicate no obvious abnormality and in whom there is no suspicion of any underlying bone destructive lesion (e.g., absence of night pain) should have oblique films taken of the lumbar spine. If necessary, CT scanning with the gantry angle appropriate for the pars (see Fig. 35.9) rather than the intervertebral disc is useful for demonstrating spondylolyses. Spondylolyses with active cartilaginous endochondral ossification zones can be detected with isotope bone scanning.

Many patients with mechanical low back pain do not have a satisfactory diagnosis even after exhaustive investigation, and it is important to bear in mind the possibility of a spondylolysis. As patients approach maturity, they are also vulnerable to intervertebral disc derangements and the two frequently coexist. Therefore in the older adolescent it is important to take a careful history, with particular reference to nerve root compression. Exuberant tissue around the spondylolysis may compress the local nerve root (L5 for the L5–S1 level) (see Fig. 35.9), the same root that will be affected by an L4–L5 disc prolapse. It is therefore quite wrong to rush in to surgical treatment at the level of the spondylolisthesis without careful imaging of the adjacent motion segments.

As the majority of spondylolyses heal, or at least become asymptomatic with the passage of time, the condition should be treated symptomatically. Many patients are sporting individuals and a period of rest which, if unsuccessful, can be followed by injecting the lysis with painkiller and anti-inflammatory drugs can often be successful. For particularly recalcitrant cases the lyses can be fused with screws or compression hooks (Fig. 37.8). Wiltse has a very considerable experience of spondylolysis and spondylolisthesis and advises that treatment of a spondylolysis or a spondylolisthesis of less than 25% should be confined to a period of rest for the acute exacerbation [10]. If the degree of slip is less than 50%, sporting activities are not restricted. A concern to many is the risk of further slippage if surgical treatment is not carried out, but long-term studies have shown that progressive slippage occurs only during the first few years [10]. If the degree of slippage is 30% or less at presentation, then further slipping is unusual.

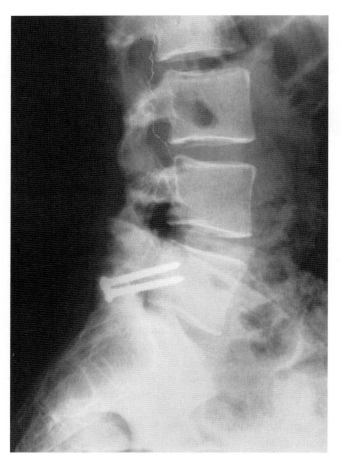

Fig. 37.8 Lateral radiograph of the lumbar spine showing a Buck's fusion for bilateral lyses

If a child has a slip of more than 50% or intractable local symptoms, spinal fusion is indicated (Fig. 37.9). Wiltse and Jackson advise bilateral intertransverse fusion in situ without instrumentation and have reported excellent results in 90% of cases [10]. Bilateral intertransverse fusion is preferred to either anterior or posterior fusion, for both biomechanical and clinical reasons [11]. The fusion rate is greater and further slippage after surgery is unusual. For those with neurological symptoms, nerve root decompression and removal of the loose, "rattle" fragment can be performed, but Wiltse and Jackson state that these symptoms always resolve with a solid fusion [10]. Interbody fusion should be reserved for the occasional patient in whom bilateral intertransverse fusion has failed; although usually performed anteriorly, this procedure can also be performed posteriorly [12].

Wiltse and Jackson also demonstrated clearly that lumbar and hamstring muscle spasm resolves with solid fusion, and body shape improves without the need for reduction [10] (Fig. 37.9). The more severe the slip, and the more severe the clinical disability, the more tempting is the desire to correct the condition surgically. However, with lytic spondylolisthesis the deformity is seldom significant, and what muscle spasm exists in the erector spinae or hamstrings settles with a sound fusion. As lumbo-sacral kyphosis is more important than percentage slip, reduction is particularly attractive in significant dysplastic spondylolisthesis. In 1932, Capener first attempted open reduction of a spondylolisthesis [13], and since then various open and closed techniques have been advanced. In 1969, Harrington used his scoliosis instrumentation in an effort to reduce spondylolisthesis and designed and implanted transpedicular screws attached to his rods in an unsuccessful attempt to correct the position of the displaced vertebrae [14]. Segmental wiring techniques became popular and were followed by staged anterior and posterior multiple procedures, some of which corrected the slippage at the expense of the L5 nerve root [15].

It would seem logical to try closed reduction first and, if that fails and reduction is still considered important, to proceed to operative reduction. The Scaglietti closed cast system can be very effective, although it is time-consuming for the patient [16]. A localizer cast similar to that used for scoliosis is applied under traction on a Risser–Cotrel table, with the spine extended at the lumbo-sacral region as much as can be tolerated. The addition of a spica round one thigh maintains the spine–pelvis relationship. Lateral radiographs taken before and after casting demonstrate whether a reduction is being achieved. Further casts are applied over the ensuing weeks until no further correction is obtained. Bilateral intertransverse fusion is then performed in the cast, which is retained until the fusion consolidates.

Should this technique be unsuccessful, operative reduction can be achieved, but it is necessary to visualize clearly

Fig. 37.9 (**a**) Lateral radiograph of the lumbo-sacral region showing a dysplastic spondylolisthesis on the point of going in front of the sacrum. (**b**) Side view of this 15-year-old boy. He had severe pain and spasm with no back movements at all. This is called the adolescent crisis.
(**c**) PA radiograph of the lumbar spine showing a scoliosis secondary to muscle spasm. (**d**) Lateral radiograph taken a year after Scaglietti cast treatment showing a good correction and a sound posterior fusion.
(**e**) PA radiograph 1 year after surgery. All pain and spasm had been completely relieved. Note the sound ala-transverse fusion. There is no need for metalwork

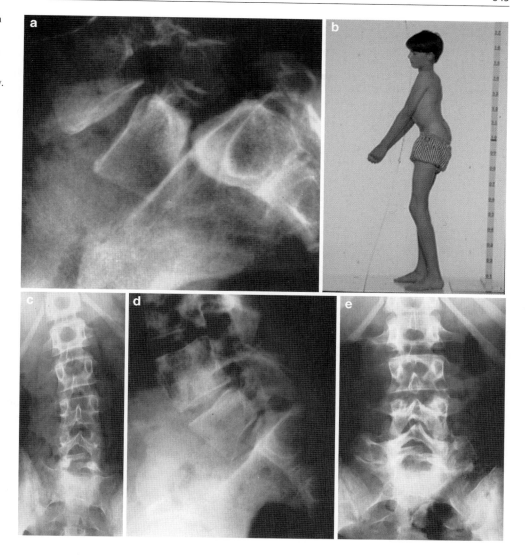

the L5 nerve roots during the procedure. In fact, the instability produced locally by thorough visualization of the L5 roots from cauda equina to foramen allows a degree of reduction to occur spontaneously on the operating table.

The end point of surgical treatment for spondylolisthesis has to be a sound spinal fusion, and the addition of rigid internal fixation may enhance the fusion rate. While there are distinct advantages in rigidly fixing the spine internally, from the point of view of earlier mobility without a cumbersome cast, it has to be asked whether, if a Wiltse-type fusion in situ without metalwork allows successful fusion in over 90%, can the addition of metalwork be regarded as either justified or advantageous?

References

1. Wiltse LL, Newman PH, Macnab I. Classification of spondylolysis and spondylolisthesis. Clin Orthop Rel Res 1976; 117:23–29.
2. Taillard WF. Etiology of spondylolisthesis. Clin Orthop Rel Res 1978; 117:30–39.
3. Wynne-Davies R, Scott JHS. Inheritance and spondylolisthesis. A radiographic family survey. J Bone Joint Surg 1979; 61B:301–305.
4. Scott JHS. Spondylolisthesis. In: Dickson RA, ed. Spinal Surgery: Science and Practice. London: Butterworths; 1990:353–367.
5. Shah JS, Hampson WGJ, Jayson MIV. The distribution of surface strain in the cadaveric lumbar spine. J Bone Joint Surg 1978; 60B:246–251.
6. Stewart TD. The age incidence of neural arch defects in Alaskan natives, considered from the standpoint of etiology. J Bone Joint Surg 1953; 35A:937–950.
7. Jackson DW, Wiltse LL, Cirincione RJ. Spondylolysis in the female gymnast. Clin Orthop 1976; 117:68–73.
8. Rankine JJ, Dickson RA. An investigation of the facet joint anatomy in spondylolysis. Musculoskeletal Scientific Session 1.

Proceedings of the UK Radiology Congress 2008. British Institute of Radiology.

9. Wiltse LL , Winter RB. Terminology and measurement of spondylolisthesis. J Bone Joint Surg 1983; 65A:768–772.

10. Wiltse LL, Jackson DW. Treatment of spondylolisthesis and spondylolysis in children. Clin Orthop Rel Res 1976; 117:92–100.

11. Lee CK, Langrana NA. Lumbosacral spinal fusion. A biomechanical study. Spine 1984; 9:574–581.

12. Cloward RB. Lesions of the intervertebral disks and their treatment by interbody fusion methods. Clin Orthop Rel Res 1963; 27:51–77.

13. Capener N. Spondylolisthesis. B J Surg 1932; 19:374–386.

14. Harrington PR, Tullos. Spondylolisthesis in children. Observations and surgical treatment. Clin Orthop Rel Res HS 1971; 79:75–84.

15. Bradford DS. Treatment of severe spondylolisthesis. A combined approach for reduction and stabilisation. Spine 1979; 4:423–429.

16. Scaglietti O, Frontino C, Bartolozzi P. Technique of anatomical reduction of lumbar spondylolisthesis and its surgical stabilisation. Clin Orthop Rel Res 1976; 117:164–175.

Part V
Fractures

Chapter 38

Principles of Fracture Care

Malcolm F. Macnicol and Alastair W. Murray

Introduction

In childhood, bone has certain characteristics that are qualitatively different from those of the adult. First, the modulus of elasticity is relatively high and the thick periosteal sleeve adds further resistance to complete fracturing. Hence buckle (torus) and greenstick fractures are relatively common, although they may be more extensive than plain radiographs suggest. Second, it should be appreciated that bone tends to give way before ligament in the prepubertal child: apophyses and other bony points of soft tissue attachment avulse before the tendon ruptures or the ligament tears.

The etiology of paediatric fractures is discussed by Landin (see Chapter 39) and Ibrahim and Abdul-Hamid (see Chapter 12); to some extent, it is culturally determined. The incidence of skeletal injury varies geographically and between urban and rural communities while increased social deprivation is associated with a greater likelihood of skeletal injury in childhood. In temperate countries, seasonal variations and alteration in the hours of daylight also affect fracture patterns. Epidemiological studies are important, as they identify trends and hazards and have led to significant improvements in child safety such as the mandatory use of child car seats in many countries and safer surfaces in play parks. In the first year of life, the frequency of fracturing is equivalent in the two sexes, but boys are twice as likely to fracture during late childhood and adolescence, just as they are more than twice as likely to die from severe injury. Pathological changes in the skeleton may predispose to fracture and are dealt with later in this chapter.

The psychological impact of trauma in childhood should also be considered. Anxiety and depression following accidents is well recognized in children of all ages and often not considered by clinicians [1]. Minimizing the stress of the hospital experience and having access to counseling for children and adults can be helpful.

Characteristics of Fractures

The sites of bony injury in the child differ from those in the adult, the most important difference relating to the fact that the bones of a child are actively growing. A paediatric fracture possesses greater potential to unite quickly and to remodel deformity. Whereas approximately one in six fractures are initially angulated more than 20° after reduction and splintage, 5 years after the injury this figure reduces to approximately 1 in 40. This capacity to realign depends principally upon the reorientation of the epiphysis and growth plate as the bone elongates.

In addition to the trophic changes in physeal growth (Fig. 38.1), which accounts for the majority of the correction, differential periosteal activity produces remodeling of the shaft, but does not supplement the growth realignment [2].

Successful remodeling of the malalignment is more likely

- in the younger child;
- the nearer the fracture is to the epiphyseal plate;
- if the deformity is angulated in the plane of the adjacent joint movement.

The history of growth and correction of malalignment is of interest. The monographs of Poland [3], Konig [4], Aitken [5], and Blount [6] recorded the pathophysiology of epiphyseal injury and the subsequent physeal response. The speed of correction is exponential rather than linear and appears to be the result of redistribution of loading through the growth plate. Little correction occurs if the primary angulation is

M.F. Macnicol (✉)
University of Edinburgh, Edinburgh, UK; Royal Hospital for Sick Children, Edinburgh, UK; Edinburgh and Murrayfield Hospital, Edinburgh, UK; Royal Infirmary, Edinburgh, UK

M. Benson et al. (eds.), *Children's Orthopaedics and Fractures*,
DOI 10.1007/978-1-84882-611-3_38, © Springer-Verlag London Limited 2010

Fig. 38.1 The growth plate gradually realigns the epiphysis if anatomical reduction is not achieved. This process will not correct the deformity fully if the angulation is excessive

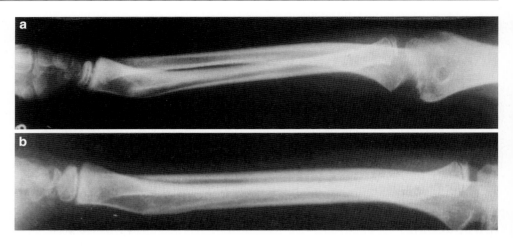

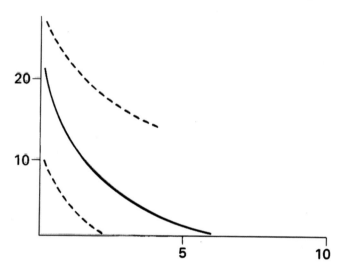

Fig. 38.2 Growth plate correction of malalignment is maximal in the first year, proceeding at a rate of approximately 1° per month (*y*-axis labeled "degrees of malalignment" and *x*-axis labeled "years")

Management

Management of the injured child must begin with the examining physician ensuring that life-threatening pathology has been successfully treated or excluded. The next priority is to prevent further damage to the soft tissues of the injured limb. Most importantly, this requires a prompt evaluation of the neurovascular integrity distal to the injury and early, effective action to alleviate ischemia or neuropathy. Urgent reduction of gross fracture displacement will usually restore an adequate blood supply if acute ischemia is encountered. If general anesthesia is likely to be delayed then it is quite appropriate to carry out a provisional reduction and splintage of a child's limb under sedation in the emergency department. The same applies when the degree of fracture displacement is leading to severe tenting of the soft tissues and blanching of the overlying skin. Undue delay in alleviating the pressure on the soft tissues will lead to soft tissue necrosis and possible skin breakdown at the fracture site. This is as true in children as it is in adults.

Early, adequate, and appropriate analgesia must be provided as this will lessen both the child's and the parent's distress and anxiety and make assessment easier. Intravenous opiate is often required for long bone fractures and early advice from colleagues expert in providing analgesia to children can be very useful. It should not be forgotten, however, that most fractures can be rendered significantly less painful by application of sufficient splintage at an early stage. Children with an unsupported fracture should not be made to wait for long periods for radiographs.

Open fractures in children require the same initial management as those encountered in the adult. Superficial lavage in the emergency department with removal of obvious, accessible contaminants is indicated. This should be followed

less than 5°; in contrast, malalignment of more than 20° will usually not correct completely (Fig. 38.2). The correction is about 1 degree per month but the precise method of this trophic change is unknown. Pauwels [7] considered that increased pressure on the growth plate results in a stimulus to growth. This may explain the correction of genu varum in the toddler and the eventual lessening of valgus after a proximal tibial metaphyseal fracture. However, it is also known that longitudinal tension across the plate will decrease its growth rate, and Crilly [8] suggested that the periosteal sleeve may control axial growth by reining in the physis. Whatever the mechanism, the epiphysis tends to realign until it lies at 90° to the axial forces passing up the limb and this phenomenon is referred to as the Hueter–Volkmann principle.

by application of a sterile dressing which should then be left undisturbed until definitive treatment in the operating theater. The temptation to re-examine the wound prior to theater should be resisted as this increases the risk of infection and the distress of the child. The child's immunization status should be clarified and appropriate tetanus prophylaxis ensured. Administration of a broad spectrum, intravenous antibiotic should be carried out prior to leaving the emergency department. There is evidence that a delay of greater than 6 hours to definitive treatment of open fractures in children can be tolerated [9] but each case should be judged on its merits and rapid access to theater may be indicated in situations of severe soft tissue compromise. Adequate operative stabilization of significant open fractures should be the aim and can be achieved with internal or external fixation. Intramedullary stabilization of open diaphyseal fractures with titanium elastic nails appears to be safe and may have some advantages over external fixation [10]. The modified Gustilo classification (Table 38.1) [11] is often used to classify open fractures in children and has the benefit of facilitating a common understanding of the severity of a particular injury. It should be noted, however, that the Gustilo classification was developed from studying predominantly diaphyseal fractures in adults and, although commonly used, its prognostic value may not apply to children's fractures.

Compartment syndrome can develop in children and communication difficulties may lead to a delay in the diagnosis. Clinicians must be attentive for the cardinal symptom of increasing pain despite adequate immobilization and usual analgesia. Pain on passive stretching of involved muscles is a relatively early sign but development of altered sensation or circulation indicates that hypoxic damage to the compartment has been ongoing for some time [12]. Compartment pressure monitoring should be considered in children with high-risk fractures and impaired consciousness. Interpretation of the results is, however, hindered by the limited knowledge of normal values for children [13].

Effective management of musculoskeletal injury in children must also include early identification of conditions beyond local expertise or facilities. Early communication with a specialist center used to dealing with childhood injuries is recommended if any uncertainty exists.

Although paediatric fractures unite rapidly and are rarely associated with major complications, several management problems may be encountered. The young child, in particular, may be fretful and difficult to examine fully. Worried parents and a crying child pose problems for even the most experienced clinician.

Many fractures are difficult to see and therefore imaging must be of good quality. In addition to standard anteroposterior (AP) and lateral radiographs of the injured site, oblique views may be useful in cases of uncertainty. Reference to atlases of normal variants and the use of more advanced imaging has largely replaced the requirement for comparison radiographs of the opposite limb but this may still occasionally have a place. Computed tomography (CT) scans can provide highly detailed views of ossified tissue and are particularly useful in managing periarticular and complex physeal injuries. Magnetic resonance imaging (MRI) can aid in the diagnosis of osteochondral and soft tissue injury but is hampered by the frequent need to sedate or anesthetize the younger child.

Once a fracture has been identified, its site, degree of displacement, and the age of the patient determine whether reduction and possibly fixation are required. No firm prescription can be given in terms of acceptable angulation or malposition for defined age groups. However, as a general rule, mid-diaphyseal angulation of more than 10° is unacceptable, particularly in the older child. Rotational malalignment should be corrected fully but the overgrowth that follows long bone fracture may make a modest overlap at the fracture site desirable in some situations.

The three "R's" of management are

1. realign the fracture
2. respect the soft tissues
3. remember the patient

These apply to children as much as to adults, although the alignment of long bone fractures can be slightly less precise and still allow good function ultimately.

Disruptions of the growth plate (physis) account for 15–20% of all paediatric fractures. This proportion is an underestimate because metaphyseal cracks may propagate

Table 38.1 Classification of open fractures [11]

Grade	Definition
1	Open fracture with a clean wound of less than 1 cm
2	Open fracture with a wound of greater than 1 cm but minimal soft tissue damage
3a	High-energy injury or heavily contaminated wound but with sufficient tissue to achieve soft tissue cover
3b	High-energy injury with periosteal stripping and bone exposure with insufficient soft tissue cover
3c	Any open fracture with limb threatening vascular injury

into the growth plate but be missed on the radiograph. Growth plate injury is very common in the phalanges or the distal radius, so that approximately 70% of all these fractures occur in the upper limb. The distal tibia accounts for just under 10% of the total and the distal femur 1–2%.

A fracture through the growth plate occurs at the zone of hypertrophy: shear produces varying degrees of displacement at the weakest site in the physis where the matrix is minimal and the cells largest [14]. The resistance to shearing or angulation is enhanced by the surrounding tissues, principally the periosteum and the musculoligamentous cuff. Of greater importance is the intrinsic structure of the growth plate including the mammillary (small, cone-shaped) projections that interdigitate with the metaphysis and the overlapping edge (lappet) of the peripheral physis which fits like a cap upon the ossified metaphysis. Surrounding the physis is the groove of Ranvier, which consists of undifferentiated cells capable of increasing the circumference of the growth plate and of anchoring the plate to the perichondrial sheath. A further fibrous band, the perichondrial ring of Lacroix, attaches to the groove of Ranvier [15] and acts as a protective sleeve; this weakens as the skeleton matures. The combination of the Salter–Harris classification and the identification of mechanisms of injury, such as the Lauge-Hansen [16] classification for ankle fractures, allows greater appreciation of the three-dimensional displacement and the best technique for closed reduction [17].

Reduction of paediatric fractures can make use of the more abundant periosteum of childhood which is often intact on the compression side of a long bone fracture. Simple angulation can be corrected with three-point bending with over-correction prevented by the intact periosteum. Translated or off-ended fractures must initially have the deformity exaggerated to relax the intact periosteum on the compression (concave) side of the bone. This will allow careful apposition of the fracture ends before the residual angulation is corrected with bending. Maintenance of the intact periosteum allows effective three-point molding to be applied to support the reduction. This is one of the factors, in combination with the remodeling potential and speed of healing in children, which reduces the need for internal fixation in many paediatric fractures. Management of fractures in a cast should not, however, be considered a simple option. Due vigilance must be given to the technique of cast application to ensure ridges and pressure points are avoided. Care must also be taken to avoid unnecessary restriction of movement of adjacent joints such as the elbow or metacarpal joints by a badly applied forearm cast. Following cast application, the limb should be elevated and observed for signs of evolving neurovascular compromise due to swelling within the cast. Worsening pain, swelling, or pallor of the digits despite elevation mandates splitting of the cast and bandages down to skin without

delay. Loss of fracture reduction should be a secondary concern to preservation of soft tissue and neurovascular integrity. Patients discharged with a recently applied cast should be provided with verbal and written advice regarding the signs of evolving soft tissue problems. The same degree of caution is required after application of a "backslab" splint as these can be just as restrictive as a complete cast.

Potentially unstable fractures treated in a cast require radiographic surveillance until time and radiological appearance reassure that no redisplacement will occur. Weight bearing should be encouraged as soon as possible after lower limb fracture since there is no evidence that this increases the likelihood of displacement or angulation. Complex regional pain syndrome (algodystrophy) and psychological difficulties occasionally complicate limb fractures in children and satisfactory function is by no means assured where there has been extensive soft tissue injury and vascular impairment.

Overgrowth after a long bone fracture is a well-known problem, particularly in the lower limb. Reynolds [18] considered that this was due to increased vascularity at the time of healing and that the compensatory mechanism thereafter was minimal. The stimulus occurs principally in the first 18 months after trauma, although a further 25% of overgrowth may occur in the subsequent 18 months. Shapiro [19] found that there was a continual, slight overgrowth until maturity, or certainly for the first 4 years after the fracture. There is no clear influence from the dominant limb, and anatomical reduction with internal fixation does not appear to increase the overgrowth. Boys appear to produce a greater degree of overgrowth than girls, although this is an inconstant feature. It is best to allow a 1 cm overlap at the time of femoral fracture splintage or traction in children under 10 years of age in order to accommodate overgrowth of around 1–2 cm. A certain amount of overgrowth will also occur in the ipsilateral uninjured bone of the leg, whether tibia or femur.

Throughout the convalescent period, the parents and child should be kept fully informed of any developments, particularly the concern that further manipulation or even internal fixation may be required. Epiphyseal plate injuries should be reviewed carefully for subsequent growth arrest, which may be either temporary or permanent. The Salter–Harris [20] type V, or sometimes type II, fracture may appear innocent initially, but the effects of growth arrest become increasingly obvious with time.

The problem of growth arrest is dealt with in Chapter 41. Displaced type III and IV fractures should be treated with open reduction and internal fixation, as late as 5 or 7 days after the fracture if necessary. Transepiphyseal fixation with smooth wires is safe and it is advisable to excise the periosteum in order to prevent peripheral bridging. When growth

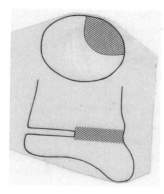

Fig. 38.3 Radiographic projections of a growth tether (osseous bar) will tend to exaggerate the size of the bridge. CT affords a more accurate portrayal of the tether

arrest occurs from a bridging bar of bone, the periphery is involved in 60% of cases (type I), whereas the central (type II) tether occurs in approximately 20% of cases. A combination of patterns (type III) occur in a further 20%.

Surgical procedures to excise the bar must be carried out with precision after preliminary imaging with CT or MRI. At least 50% of the growth plate should be normal, although radiographic projections of the area may exaggerate the bulk of the bar (Fig. 38.3). If the surgery is to be effective, it should be carried out with at least 2 years of potential growth available. Langenskiold and Osterman [21] pointed out that bone shortening maybe treated by a

lengthening procedure or contralateral epiphysiodesis and that angular deformity can be realigned by osteotomy or frame distraction. However, these procedures do not prevent deformation of the joint, which always follows partial closure of the growth plate if the malalignment is allowed to progress (Fig. 38.4a, b).

Baeza Giner and Oliete Sanz [22] studied the use of interposition materials after the excision of an osseous bar. They considered that fat was far more effective than the silastic sheet promoted by Bright [23] and also stated that methylmethacrylate cement [24] caused growth disturbance in its own right.

Indications for Internal Fixation

While the place for internal fixation of fractures in adults is well understood, the indications in children's fractures are more contentious. The existence of multiple variables in childhood fractures such as the age of the child, remodeling potential, and involvement of growth plates has contributed to a lack of large, well-controlled trials. There are, however, broad principles which can guide the decision to treat a fracture surgically.

Three fundamental criteria should be considered:

- the condition of the child
- the age of the child
- the nature of the fracture

Fig. 38.4 (**a**) Distal fibula physeal arrest has significantly affected ankle alignment. (**b**) Disproportionate growth of the forearm bones after physeal injury (7/11/90) may be checked by distal radial epiphysiodesis (22/5/91) but a later ulnar lengthening is the only means of improving the radio-ulnar relationship

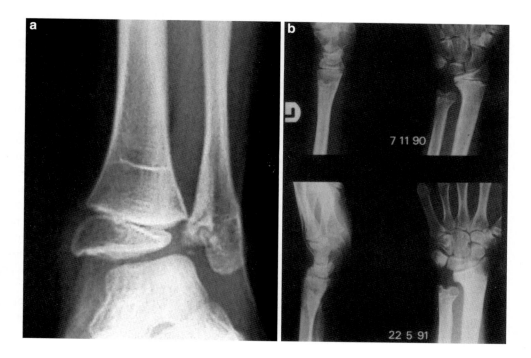

Condition of the Child

The clinical condition influences the decision about internal fixation, either because the injuries pose problems in effective nursing and rehabilitation (e.g., in polytrauma) [25] or severe head injury with behavioral disturbance or because a pre-existing disorder makes conservative management difficult. Some children with skeletal dysplasias, including osteogenesis imperfecta and fibrous dysplasia, cerebral palsy with gross muscle spasm, and mental impairment, are better managed if the fracture is securely fixed at the outset. Pathological fractures of any sort should be considered for operative treatment: This subject is dealt with later in the chapter. Occasionally, social circumstances or concerns about compliance with conservative methods may determine, in part, whether surgical treatment is appropriate.

Age of the Child

Internal fixation is indicated more often in the adolescent, particularly if growth plates are closing when fracture management becomes more akin to the adult situation. In practice, this means that girls older than 12 years and boys older than 14 years may be considered as adults, particularly when dealing with difficult long bone fractures.

Nature of the Fracture

The clinical characteristics of a fracture are determined by

- its site in the bone
- its behavior

Before discussion of the specific anatomical sites at which fixation is often advisable, factors affecting fracture behavior should be considered. Oblique, comminuted, or pathological fractures are usually unstable, and their control may only be achieved with internal fixation. If there is additional bone loss or type III compounding, external fixation with or without subsequent conversion to internal fixation may be required. A fracture may be irreducible by closed means necessitating open reduction which may lower the surgeon's threshold for proceeding to internal fixation. Fracture reduction may be impeded by

- buttonholing through muscle or fascia (lower femoral shaft, proximal humeral shaft, and supracondylar humerus)

- periosteal entrapment (proximal or distal tibia)
- joint incarceration (medial humeral condyle, talus)

Nerve entrapment in the fracture site should also be suspected, particularly in the upper limb at the mid-humeral level, around the elbow, and in the mid-forearm where nerve trunks in relatively anchored sites are close to bare areas of bone between muscle attachments [26]. Muscle contraction may displace fractures producing an unacceptable gap (olecranon and other avulsion injuries) or malalignment (single or double forearm fractures, subtrochanteric femoral fractures).

Primary or delayed internal fixation should therefore be considered for the following reasons, where suitable local expertise allows

- impractical or failed manipulative reduction
- redisplacement of the fracture
- multiple injuries, particularly ipsilateral femoral and tibial fractures (the floating knee)
- significant arterial, neurological, or soft tissue damage where a stable limb facilitates repair
- rare instances of delayed union such as the lateral condyle of the humerus
- displaced intra-articular fractures such as the Tillaux or "triplane" fractures of the distal tibia

Internal Fixation

A wide variety of options exists for the internal fixation of children's fractures. The most common method remains the use of smooth wires. These have the advantages of minimal soft tissue violation and the ability to cross the physis with no noticeable damage. Disadvantages include migration, damage to neurovascular structures, and occasionally infection if used percutaneously. They also have limited stability and require skilful placement to avoid complications and achieve maximal benefit.

Cannulated screw fixation can be very effective for intra-articular fractures such as lateral condylar fractures of the humerus. Plate osteosynthesis remains an option for some long bone fractures. Removal of plates carries a recognized risk of complications as dissection of scarred tissue can lead to neurovascular damage and refracture following plate removal. Some choose to leave plates in situ for these reasons but the susceptibility to subsequent fracture at the ends of the plate should be considered.

Elastic nailing of diaphyseal fractures has become increasingly common. For children aged 6–13 years they are the treatment of choice for many types of femoral diaphyseal fractures. They have the advantages of minimally invasive insertion and relatively easy extraction, but their success relies upon good surgical technique and the experience of the user (see Chapters 48 and 49). They may not be appropriate in highly unstable diaphyseal fractures with a likelihood of shortening. This is particularly the case in the treatment of lower limb fracture in older, heavier children (>40 kg). Rigid intramedullary nailing of femoral shaft fractures carries the risk of causing avascular necrosis of the femoral head in skeletally immature children. In adolescents very near skeletal maturity use of a rigid nail with a lateral trochanteric entry point appears to be safe [27].

The use if internal fixation for specific fractures is considered in more detail in later chapters.

Pathological Fractures

Pathological fractures in childhood may occur at any site in the long bones, vertebrae, or pelvis, although they are extremely rare in flat bones. Relatively minor injuries produce the fracture. Characteristically there is no history of convincing trauma, or the incident may be relatively trivial. The child complains of pain, which is usually persistent and sufficient to limit walking if the lower limb is involved. Although the periosteal tube usually prevents significant displacement, the effects of the fracture cannot be ignored.

Internal fixation (see above) will be indicated in specific cases, particularly femoral or tibial fractures. Surgical treatment of fractures associated with conditions of generalized osteopenia such as osteogenesis imperfecta has the advantage of avoiding prolonged immobilization and hence minimizes further loss of bone density from disuse.

Skeletal alterations leading to pathological fracture may be considered as follows:

- generalized
- localized to one limb
- localized to the lesion

The skeletal changes will be either congenital or acquired. The biochemical and biomechanical changes vary, affecting both the composition and the architecture of the bone.

Generalized Conditions

Generalized conditions may be present at birth. Osteogenesis imperfecta [28] is an autosomal recessive disease that may result in multiple fractures at birth and a significantly shortened life span. Birth fractures will be described in Chapter 42 and may be caused by other congenital conditions such as hypophosphatasia and the Silverman syndrome. The child with arthrogryposis who has stiff joints (see Chapter 20) may also present with a long bone fracture (Fig. 38.5). Proximal femoral pseudarthrosis associated with congenital short femur and pseudarthrosis of the femur may prove confusing.

In later childhood, pathological fractures occur in association with congenital insensitivity to pain (Fig. 38.6), and in osteogenesis imperfecta (Figs. 38.7 and 38.8), whether inherited as autosomal recessive or dominant. Certain of the other skeletal dysplasias such as polyostotic fibrous dysplasia, pycnodysostosis, and osteopetrosis (Fig. 38.9) predispose to pathological or stress fractures, as does osteoporosis of adolescence or the rare juvenile form (Fig. 38.10a, b). The metabolic bone disease associated with end-stage renal or

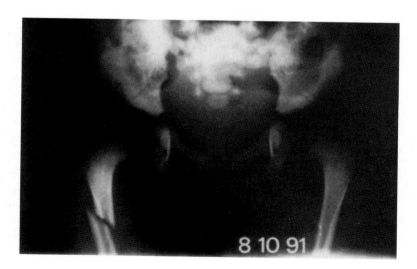

Fig. 38.5 Oblique fracture of the right femoral shaft after the difficult delivery of an arthrogrypotic child

Fig. 38.6 Radiographs of a swollen but painless elbow in a child who was found to be suffering from congenital insensitivity to pain

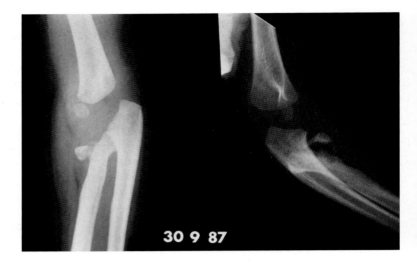

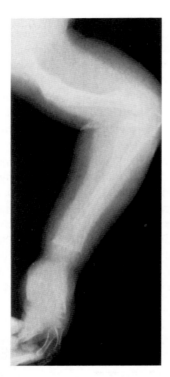

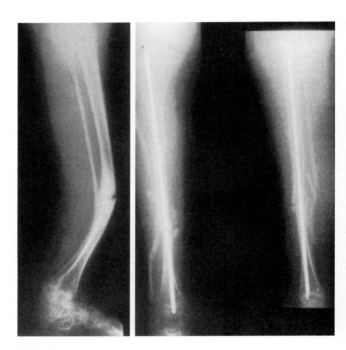

Fig. 38.8 Tibial fracture in osteogenesis imperfecta before and after intramedullary rodding

Fig. 38.7 Upper limb deformity after multiple fracture in osteogenesis imperfecta

hepatic failure is also associated with an increased incidence of fracture, particularly in the convalescent phase after organ transplantation, when steroid therapy and immunosuppression are required. Unusual metabolic conditions such as Bartter's syndrome [29] may be encountered (Fig. 38.11).

Acquired diseases that affect the entire skeleton include leukemias, renal osteodystrophy, hyperparathyroidism, pituitary dysfunction, and infiltrative disorders such as Langerhans' cell histiocytosis. Malnutrition leads to rickets, scurvy, and the wasting diseases (kwashiorkor and marasmus), with concomitant weakening of the skeleton and a predisposition to fracture. These children with their acquired systemic disease are unwell, and the diagnosis must be established if the underlying condition is to be treated effectively. Multiple fractures should also arouse suspicion that the injuries are non-accidental (Chapter 42).

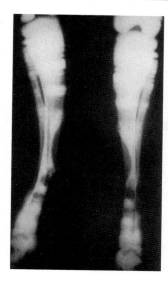

Fig. 38.9 Pathological tibial fractures in a child with osteopetrosis

Single-Limb Involvement

Fractures localized to one limb may be secondary to congenital conditions affecting one or more bones of the limb, such as fibrous dysplasia or Ollier's disease. More commonly, the pathological fracture occurs when disuse osteoporosis results from congenital or acquired conditions. Immobilization or paralytic conditions cause significant bone loss, and rehabilitation must always be graduated and carefully supervised. Myelodysplasia, poliomyelitis, severe cerebral palsy, and arthrogryposis are associated with an increased incidence of fractures, as are chronic osteomyelitis, tuberculosis, septic arthritis, juvenile idiopathic arthritis, post-irradiation osteoporosis, and chemotherapy.

Fractures occur in up to 30% of children with spina bifida [30] and may involve the diaphysis, metaphysis, or growth plate [31]. The diagnosis is often delayed, as the child may not feel pain. Local warmth, erythema, swelling, and progressive deformity should alert the surgeon to the likelihood of pathological fracture. It is easy to confuse the finding with infection. The radiographic appearances may be quite alarming and mimic chronic osteomyelitis [32] or tumor. Congenital insensitivity to pain [33] and post-traumatic neurological loss may also lead to repeated fractures of the weight-bearing bones and to osteolysis. However, blood tests are usually normal and the temptation to take a biopsy of the lesion should be resisted.

The healing of these fractures may be delayed [34], but orthotic support and graduated weight bearing will usually ensure a satisfactory outcome. However, recurrent stress may promote further pathological fracture and a hypertrophic callus response may lead to thickening and deformity around the knee and ankle together with altered growth

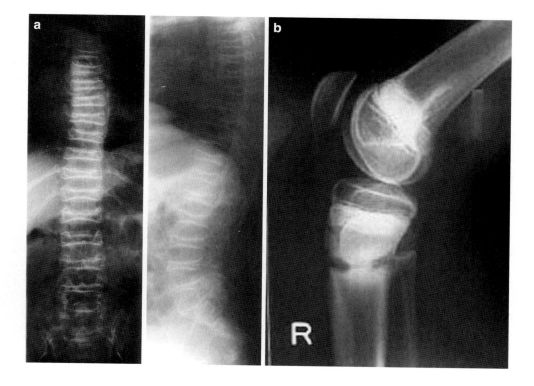

Fig. 38.10 (a) Compression fractures of the vertebrae in idiopathic osteoporosis. (b) Stress fracture of the proximal tibia in a child with idiopathic osteoporosis. Note the sclerotic metaphyseal bands secondary to bisphosphonate treatment

Fig. 38.11 Stabilization of a
stress fracture of the tibia in
Bartter's syndrome

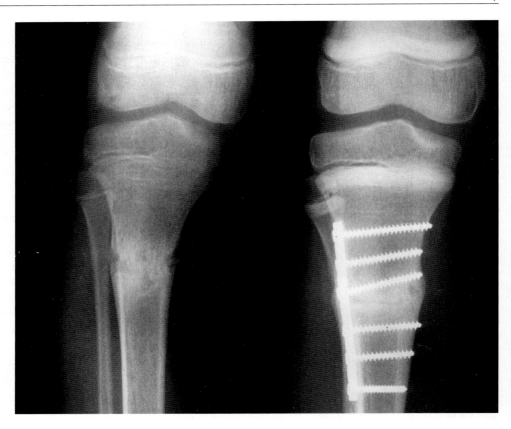

(see Chapter 41). Epiphysiolysis typically produces an initial widening of the growth plate before major slipping occurs. If stress is minimal, the displacement will not progress and the type I epiphyseal fracture [20] will heal slowly.

Monostotic Lesions

Benign cystic conditions of bone are the most common cause of single pathological fracture, which occurs most often in the upper humerus (Fig. 38.12). Although the fracture itself may cause the underlying lesion to heal, needle decompression and injection with steroid or the insertion of bone marrow or cancellous bone graft (Fig. 38.13) may be required before the condition resolves. Splintage may be sufficient in some patients, but a unicameral bone cyst or fibrous dysplasia involving the proximal femur should be fixed in order to prevent varus deformity.

Benign and malignant neoplasms (see Chapter 14) and infection (see Chapter 10) may cause pathological fracture if cortical destruction exceeds 50% of normal bone strength. A metastatic deposit from nephroblastoma or neuroblastoma (Figs. 38.14 and 38.15) should be included in any

differential diagnosis. Fractures may also occur where the bone has been weakened by the insertion or removal of a screw, pin, or plate, or if blood supply has been impaired by previous trauma, with resultant scarring of the soft tissues.

The typical radiographic appearances include a transverse fracture with little comminution and a relatively indistinct

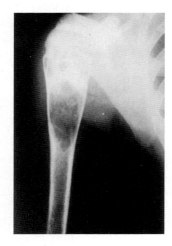

Fig. 38.12 Unicameral cyst of the proximal humerus

Fig. 38.13 A minor pathological fracture through a proximal phalangeal cyst (*left*) was treated by neighbor strapping to the adjacent digit. The cyst healed subsequently (*right*)

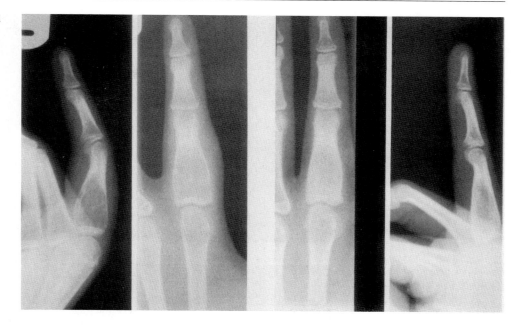

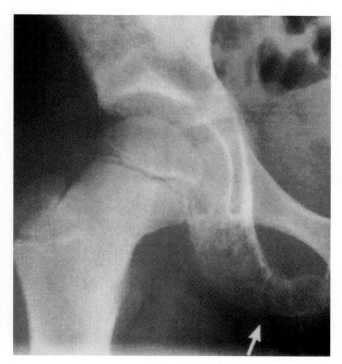

Fig. 38.14 Neuroblastoma metastasized to the inferior pubic ramus

femoral condyles, also produce a form of pathological fracture when the ischemic trabeculae are revascularized during the healing process. Finally, congenital pseudarthrosis may sometimes mimic the localized form of pathological fracture, particularly in the absence of cutaneous neurofibromatosis.

Stress Fractures

Stress fractures, while not in themselves "pathological," may also be confusing if a history of repetitive, relatively minor trauma is not sought. In the adolescent, stress fracture of the femoral neck (Fig. 38.16) may occur transversely across the inferior or superior aspects of the neck [35]. The inferior, compression fracture is less likely to displace, but varus deformity resulting from delayed union and persisting symptoms are indications to fix the lesions internally. Stress fractures of the tibia (Fig. 38.17), fibula [36], patella, ulna, and metatarsal have also been described. Chronic epiphyseal and apophyseal changes can be seen in adolescent athletes (Fig. 38.18). Spondylolysis secondary to pathological changes in the pars inter-articularis and spondylolisthesis are discussed in Chapter 37, and chronic stress lesions of the neck, humerus, and ulna are also recognized as rare pathological conditions in childhood.

The tibia usually develops a linear shadow in the proximal metaphysis, and the posteromedial or posterolateral border eventually shows a resorptive fracture line. The midshaft may also thicken anteriorly, similar to the shin splint fracture in the adult. As the fracture line is difficult to see by conventional radiography in the early stages, isotope bone scanning, CT, or MRI are helpful.

fracture line. Displacement is usually minimal and significant soft tissue wounding is rare. The fracture is usually missed because radiographs are not obtained, although it may be difficult to discern at certain sites, particularly in the spine and ribs. Perthes' disease (see Chapter 27) and other examples of osteonecrosis, such as osteochondritis of the

Fig. 38.15 CT scan of the pelvic lesion seen in Fig. 38.14

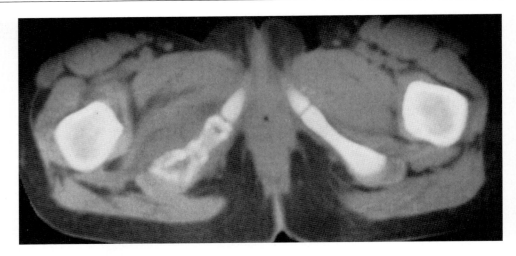

Fig. 38.16 Inferior stress fracture of the right femoral neck

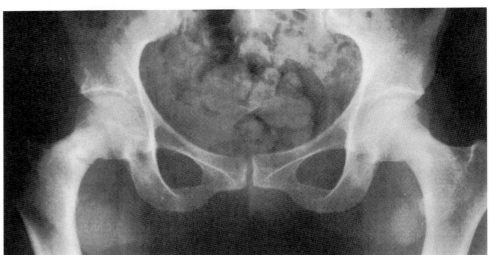

Fig. 38.17 Stress fracture of the proximal tibia in an athletic boy

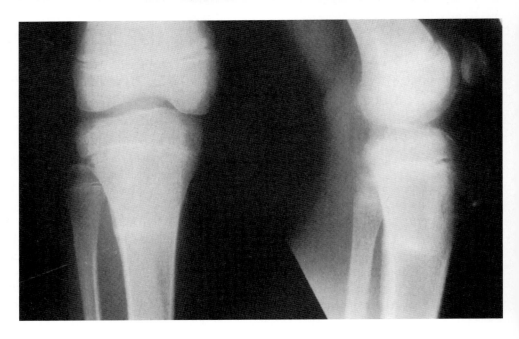

Fig. 38.18 Widened physes and tibial apophyseal fragmentation seen in the knee of a female gymnast

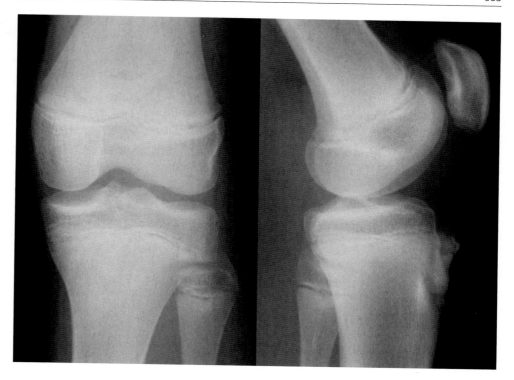

References

1. Jonovska S, Franciskovic T, Kvesic A, et al. Self-esteem in children and adolescents differently treated for locomotor trauma. Coll Anthropol 2007; 31(2): 463–9.

2. Friberg S. Remodeling after distal forearm fractures in children: correction of residual angulation in fractures of the radius. Acta Orthop Scand 1979; 50: 731–9.

3. Poland J. Traumatic separation of the epiphysis. London: Smith Elder; 1898.

4. Konig F. Die spateren Schicksale deform-geheiter Knochenbruche, besonders bei Kindern. Arch Klin Chirurg 1908; 85:187–211.

5. Aitken AP. The end results of the fractured distal radial epiphysis. J Bone Joint Surg 1935:17:302–8.

6. Blount WP. Fracture care in children. Baltimore: Williams & Wilkins; 1954.

7. Pauwels F. Eine Klinische Beobachtung als Beispiel und Beweis fuer funktionelle anpassung des Knochens durch Laengenwachstum. Zeitschrift Orthop 1975; 113:1–5.

8. Crilly RG. Longitudinal overgrowth of chicken radius. J Anat 1972; 112:11–8.

9. Skaggs DL, Friend L, Alman B, et al. The effect of surgical delay on acute infection following 554 open fractures in children. J Bone Joint Surg Am 2005; 87(1):8–12.

10. Ramseier LE, Bhaskar AR, Cole WG, Howard AW. Treatment of open femur fractures in children: comparison between external fixator and intramedullary nailing. J Pediatr Orthop 2007; 27(7):748–50.

11. Gustilo RB, Mendoza RM, William DN. Problems in the management of type III (severe) open fractures: a new classification. J Trauma 1984; 24:742–6.

12. Bae DS, Kadivala RK, Waters PM. Acute compartment syndrome in children: contemporary diagnosis, treatment, and outcome. J Pediatr Orthop 2001; 21(5):680–8.

13. Staudt JM, Smeulders MJC, Van der Horst CM. Normal compartment pressures of the lower leg in children. J Bone Joint Surg Br 2008; 90(2):215–9.

14. Haas SL. Retardation of bone growth by a wire loop. J Bone Joint Surg 1945; 27:25–36.

15. Rang MC. The growth plate and its disorders. Edinburgh: Churchill Livingston; 1969.

16. Lauge-Hansen N. Fractures of the ankle II. Arch Surg 1950; 60:957–985.

17. Dias LS, Giergerich CR. Fractures of the distal tibial epiphysis in adolescence. J Bone Joint Surg 1983; 65-A:438–44.

18. Reynolds DA. Growth changes in long-bones: a study of 126 children. J Bone Joint Surg 1981; 63-B:83–8.

19. Shapiro F. Fractures of the femoral shaft in children: the overgrowth phenomenon. Acta Orthop Scand 1981; 52:649–55.

20. Salter RB, Harris RW. Injuries involving the epiphyseal plate. J Bone Joint Surg 1963; 45-A:587–622.

21. Langenskiold A, Osterman K. Surgical elimination of post-traumatic partial fusion of the growth plate. In: Houghton GR, Thompson GH, eds. Problematic Musculoskeletal Injuries in Children. London: Butterworth; 1983: 14–31.

22. Baeza Giner V, Oliete Sanz V. Profilaxis de los puentes osseous del cartilago de crecimiento. Estudio experimental. Rev Orthop Traumatol 1980; 24: 305–20.

23. Bright RW. Operative correction of partial epiphyseal closure by osseous-bridge resection and silicone rubber implant. J Bone Joint Surg 1974; 56-A:655–64.

24. Mallet J. Les epiphysiodeses patielles traumatique de l'extremite inferieure du tibia chez l'enfant. Rev Chirurg Orthop 1975; 61: 5–16.

25. Loder R. Polytauma in children. Orth Trauma 1987; 1:48–54.

26. Macnicol MF. Roentgenographic evidence of median nerve entrapment in a greenstick fracture. J Bone Joint Surg 1978; 60-A: 998–1000.

27. Kanellopoulos AD, Yiannakopoulos CK, Soucacos PN. Closed, locked intramedullary nailing of pediatric femoral shaft fractures through the tip of the greater trochanter. J Trauma 2006; 60(1):217–22.

28. Sillence DO, Senn A, Danks DM. Genetic heterogeneity in osteogenesis imperfecta. J Med Genetics 1979; 16:101–16.

29. Gill JR. Batter's syndrome. In: Gonick HC, Buckalen VM, eds. Renal Tubular Disorders: Pathophysiology, Diagnosis and Management. New York: Marcel Dekker; 1985.

30. Menelaus MB. The Orthopaedic Management of Spina Bifida Cystica, 2nd ed. Edinburgh: E&S Livingston; 1971:63–65.

31. Parsch K. Origin and treatment of fractures in spina bifida. Eur J Pediatr Surg 1991; 1:298–306.

32. Townsend PF. Cowell HR, Steg NL. Lower extremity fractures simulating infection in myelomeningocele. Clin Orthop Rel Res 1979; 144:256–9.

33. Kuo R, Macnicol MF. Congenital insensitivity to pain: orthopaedic implications. J Pediatr Orthop B 1996; 5:292–5.

34. Wenger DR. Jeffcoat BT, Herring JA. The guarded prognosis of physeal injuries in paraplegic children. J Bone Joint Surg 1980; 62-A:241–6.

35. Devas MB. Stress fractures in children. J Bone Joint Surg 1963; 45-B: 528–41.

36. Griffiths AL. Fatigue fracture of the fibula in childhood. Arch Dis Child 1952; 27:552–7.

Chapter 39

Fracture Epidemiology

Lennart A. Landin

The purpose of fracture epidemiology, as of epidemiology in general, is to identify and describe the etiology of disease in a population, with the ultimate goal of finding methods of prevention. The planning of medical services is also facilitated and made more accurate from epidemiological data. By tradition and out of necessity, the interest of orthopaedic surgeons has focused on diagnosis and therapy but it is also our duty to participate in preventive programs to reduce accidents and to recognize any new hazards that may affect the children in our society. Therefore it is important to have some knowledge of what, why, when, and how the fractures occur in children.

In surveys of paediatric trauma, fractures are found to contribute 10–25% of all injuries in childhood and adolescence [1, 2]. In a series of 23,915 patients seen at four major hospitals for injury-related symptoms in the United States, 17.8% had fractures; thus close to one fifth of children who present to hospitals with injuries have a fracture [3].

Definitions

Incidence is the number of new cases occurring in a defined population during a certain time interval. Thus, the age-specific annual incidence is the risk for an individual or a group of individuals of a certain age of catching a disease or incurring an accident during 1 year.

Prevalence is the total number of persons with a disease or a condition at a certain time in a defined population.

Frequency or *rate* is the percentage of a specific disease or fracture in relation to the total number of cases in a series.

The incidence is dependent upon the accuracy of the sampling procedure and a knowledge of the size of the population at risk; minor fractures can escape diagnosis, and severe fractures might be referred to other centers and thus not be recorded. These sources of error should be estimated and non-residents in the population excluded in order to arrive at as precise an incidence as possible. The ultimate goal is to produce reliable data, allowing comparison with other populations, and to detect secular changes. The term incidence is unfortunately often confused with frequency but they are two different entities.

Incidence

The risk of sustaining a fracture, or the incidence, is closely related to age [4]. The incidence of childhood fractures has been calculated in studies from Malmö, Sweden [5, 6], covering 8682 fractures between 1950 and 1979, and 1673 fractures between 1993 and 1994. The risk of fracture increased in children of both sexes up to the age of 11–12 years and then decreased in girls but further increased in boys until the age of 13–14 years (Fig. 39.1). Boys are more commonly represented in all age groups, accounting for 62% of all fractures. From the incidence figures in the Malmö studies, it can be calculated that the cumulative risk of having at least one fracture from birth to the age of 16 years is 42% for boys and 26% for girls, which means that nearly every second boy and every fourth girl will sustain a fracture during the period from birth to the age of 16 years.

The overall annual incidence of fractures was 193 per 10,000, which means that approximately 2% of the children in the population sustain a fracture each year. In a recent study during the year 2000 from Edinburgh, Scotland, the annual incidence of fractures in children was 20 per 1000 and 61% of these fractures occurred in boys [7]. Thus, the incidence and sex distribution are almost identical in these two studies from western Europe.

L.A. Landin (✉)
Department of Orthopaedics, Malmö University Hospital, Malmö, Sweden

M. Benson et al. (eds.), *Children's Orthopaedics and Fractures*,
DOI 10.1007/978-1-84882-611-3_39, © Springer-Verlag London Limited 2010

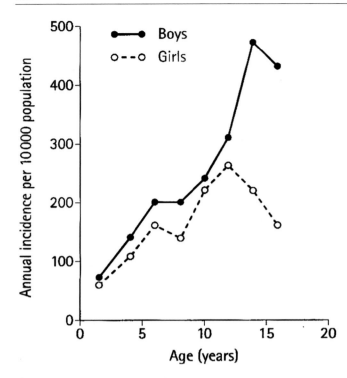

Fig. 39.1 Age- and sex-specific incidence of fractures among children in Malmö, Sweden. (From [5], with permission)

Table 39.1 The frequency of various fracture types

Type	Malmö 1996 (%)	Edinburgh 2000 (%)
Distal forearm	22.7	32.9
Hand (phalanges)	18.9	15.3
Carpus or metacarpal (scaphoid excluded)	8.3	7.6
Clavicle	8.1	7.3
Ankle	5.5	3.5
Tibial shaft	5.0	2.5
Tarsus or metatarsal (talus, os calcis excluded)	4.5	0.3
Foot (phalanges)	3.4	3.0
Forearm shaft	3.4	5.4
Supracondylar region of the humerus	3.3	7.4
Proximal end of the humerus	2.2	1.8
Femoral shaft	1.6	0.7
Vertebrae	1.2	0.35

Frequency

The unique mechanical properties of the growing skeleton, characterized by increased mineralization with age, the function of the periosteum, the presence of the growth plate, physical activity, and psychomotor development, make the fracture pattern in children different from that seen in adults or in the elderly, in whom the loss of bone mass causes the typical patterns of fragility fractures.

In addition, the frequency of the different fracture types, and the incidence of fractures, will be influenced by factors such as age, cultural and environmental factors, and the climate.

The frequencies of the different fracture types in a series of fractures in an urban population in Malmö, Sweden, are shown in Table 39.1 and compared to the Edinburgh data. The most common skeletal injury in children is the fracture of the distal end of the forearm, which contributes to 25% of all fractures, followed by fractures of the hand phalanges and of the carpal and metacarpal regions. Overall, the hand is the most common location of skeletal injury, although many fractures are minor avulsions of little consequence. During the last decade there seems to be an increased incidence and frequency of wrist fractures, accounting for 33% of all fractures in the Edinburgh study. Paediatric fracture patterns are similar in different parts of the world with some exceptions.

In developing countries, road traffic accidents are a much more common cause of fractures as are falls from heights. In a study from Nigeria (1999–2003), femoral shaft fractures accounted for 34%, supracondylar fractures of the humerus 17%, and distal radial factures only 15%. Access to medical services influences the sampling procedure of the data and many minor fractures are likely to be undetected [8].

When the different fracture types are related to age, some patterns can be discerned (Fig. 39.2). The *late peak pattern* is mostly sport and equipment related. The *bimodal pattern* includes an early increase in incidence as a result of low-energy trauma, followed by a late incidence peak, attributable to high- or moderate-energy trauma and again from sport or road accidents. The *decreasing pattern* is typical of skull fractures only. The *rising pattern* is closely related to sports, skateboarding, cycling, and similar activities, which increase with age, particularly in boys. Finally, the *early peak* of the supracondylar fracture of the humerus, mostly caused by falling from a height, and the *irregular pattern* of the tibial shaft are unique for those particular fractures.

Etiology

Environmental Factors

In the Edinburgh study, falls from below bed height accounted for 37%, falls from above bed height 17%, sports-related trauma 12%, and road traffic accidents 6% of all fractures.

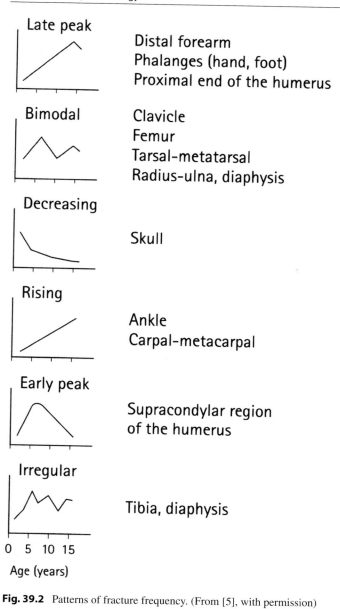

Late peak
Distal forearm
Phalanges (hand, foot)
Proximal end of the humerus

Bimodal
Clavicle
Femur
Tarsal-metatarsal
Radius-ulna, diaphysis

Decreasing
Skull

Rising
Ankle
Carpal-metacarpal

Early peak
Supracondylar region
of the humerus

Irregular
Tibia, diaphysis

0 5 10 15
Age (years)

Fig. 39.2 Patterns of fracture frequency. (From [5], with permission)

New Trends

For several decades, trampolines have been popular as part of playground equipment. In Europe, the recreational use of trampolines has increased during the last 15 years, with an associated increase in the number of children presenting with injuries caused by trampoline use. In a study from Dublin [9], these injuries accounted for 1.5% of the total attendances to the emergency department. Of these, 20% required admission to hospital. Trampolines carry a significant risk of severe orthopaedic injury, the worst being head and spine injuries. In the Irish study, 35% of the patients were on a trampoline with at least one other person. Clear guidelines have been

issued for the safe use of trampolines (Fig. 39.3): only one

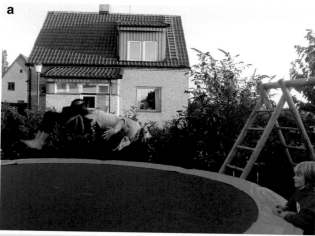

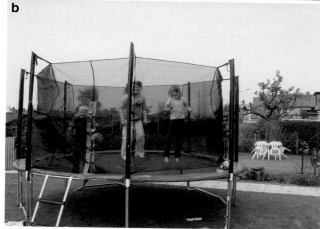

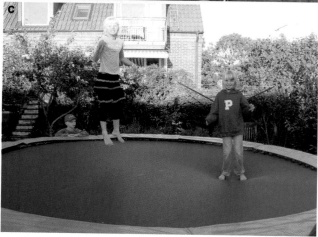

Fig. 39.3 (a) Trampoline carry a significant risk of spine and head injuries. (b) Trampoline should be fitted with a protective net to prevent falling to the ground and trapping between the trampoline and its frame. (c) The smallest child should not be on the trampoline at the same time as the older and heavier ones

person should be on the trampoline at a time and if a number of children are using the trampoline simultaneously, the youngest child is most likely to get hurt. Also, trampolines should be fitted with a peripheral protective net to avoid falls to the ground or trapping between the springs and the frame.

Distal radial fractures have recently been named "the young goalkeeper's fracture." Boyd et al. found that the risk of sustaining a distal radial fracture while goalkeeping was related to the size of the ball [10]. Significantly more injuries were sustained when an adult-sized ball was used instead of a junior ball. One recommendation is also that the goalkeeper should not be younger or smaller than the players in the opposing team.

Other new gadgets are kick boards, motorized scooters, heelies, or street gliders. In a study of injuries caused by using heelies or street gliders, 20% of the injuries happened while using the gliders for the first time and 36% of the injuries occurred while learning how to use them [11]. A similar risk attends the use of skateboards. Most of these injuries are upper extremity fractures and it seems sensible to use wrist protection although the beneficial effects are not scientifically proven.

Endogenous Factors

There has been much debate about whether the etiology of accidents among children reflects not only environmental hazards but also personality traits and social factors. In some investigations, injured children have been found to be impulsive, overactive, impatient, and energetic [12, 13], whereas other studies have shown no personality differences between accident-prone children and control group. It is realistic to accept that "all children are accident-prone sometimes" [14].

Recently, attention deficit hyperactivity disorder (ADHD) has been assessed as a contributing factor to fractures in children. The condition is characterized by permanent and continuous attention deficit with inappropriate hyperactivity or impulsivity, impacting upon all aspects of social life. The conclusions to be drawn from investigations into ADHD and trauma in children are inconsistent, Lam [15] confirming an association while Ford et al. [16] did not.

Children aged 3–6 years and 13–14 years who have sustained one fracture have an increased risk of an additional fracture compared with the overall incidence [5]. Boys are more likely than girls to be "fracture repeaters," which supports the theory that psychological factors are influential.

Children with an evidently fragile skeleton as a result of osteogenesis imperfecta, neurological disorders (such as cerebral palsy, epilepsy, and myelomeningocele), juvenile idiopathic arthritis, and renal osteodystrophy sustain fractures more often than expected, but the scarcity of these conditions makes their contribution to the total number of fractures small. This is in contrast to fractures in the elderly, among whom the majority of patients are osteoporotic or present with associated conditions such as metabolic bone disease, neurological disorders with impaired balance, or rheumatoid arthritis.

In recent decades, the issue of low bone density in children has caused much concern. Landin and Nilsson [17] found that bone mineral content was reduced in 8% of those children who sustained fractures from low-energy trauma, whereas there was no difference in children who sustained their fractures from moderate- or high-energy trauma. In a recent review, Bianchi et al. [18] found an association between reduced bone density and fractures in children. However, there is no distinct pattern of fragility fractures in children as in adults although the quality of the skeleton or the degree of mineralization probably is of importance.

Secular Trends

From 1950 to 1979, the incidence of fractures in children in Malmö, Sweden, almost doubled. The increase was due to a greater number of fractures caused by minor trauma, such as sports-related accidents, whereas high-energy trauma, such as road traffic accidents, decreased over the period. The recorded increase over the years was not explained by improved medical care and access, as the rate of minor avulsions compared with diaphyseal fractures remained constant over the years [5]. A fracture incidence similar to that in Malmö for 1975–1979 was found in children from Nottingham in 1981 [4].

To investigate any further changes in the epidemiology of children's fractures in Malmö, a study covering the years 1993–1994 was performed [6]. The data collection procedure and the organization of the medical facilities were the same as for the study in 1950–1979, allowing an analysis over half a century of paediatric fracture epidemiology in an urban population of western Europe. An overall reduction of 9% in the incidence since 1979 was recorded (Fig. 39.4). It could not be attributed to any single type of skeletal injury or group of fractures. Since the late 1970s, participation in organized sports has increased, whereas unsupervised play has decreased [19]. By 1992, not many more than 50% of 15-year-old Swedish youths engaged in jogging or a corresponding physical effort at least once a week. Although these observations do not constitute direct proof, they can be regarded as circumstantial evidence of the effects of a more sedentary life style upon the risk of fracture. Another explanation could be the effects of safety programs and an increasing awareness of safety among the public in

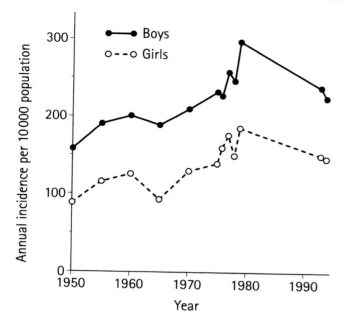

Fig. 39.4 Changes in the incidence of fractures in boys and girls in Malmö, Sweden, from 1950 to 1979 and in the early 1990s

western Europe, exemplified by the use of protective equipment in sports and safety belts in the back seats of cars. The latter, together with the extensive use of specially designed children's seats in cars, have resulted in a threefold reduction in the number of children killed in traffic accidents annually, comparing the periods 1975–1979 and 1993–1994 [20]. However, after 1994 there has been no further reduction; the incidence of lethal traffic accidents in Sweden for individuals 0–17 years in 2007 was per 100,000 annually.

The Future

The incidence of fractures in children seems to mirror the affluence of our society, with sport activities increasing the risk of injury, against a background lifestyle that is more protective and sedentary, governed by video games and computers.

The future will certainly bring new toys, sports, and equipments with associated risks of injuries. Although physical activity is necessary and beneficial for the normal development of the growing child, it is the duty of the paediatric orthopaedic community to act as a whistle blower and initiate preventive measures if fractures and other injuries amass from new devices.

References

1. Sibert JR, Maddocks GB, Brown BM. Childhood accidents—an endemic of epidemic proportions. Arch Dis Child 1981; 56: 225–234.
2. Nathorst Westfelt JAR. Environmental factors in childhood accidents. A prospective study in Göteborg, Sweden. Acta Paediatr Scand Suppl 1982; 53:291.
3. Wilkins KE. The incidence of fractures in children. In: Rockwood CA, Wilkins KE, Beaty JH, eds. Fractures in Children. Philadelphia: Lippincott-Raven; 1996:3–17.
4. Worlock P, Stower M. Fracture patterns in Nottingham children. J Pediatr Orthop 1986; 6:656–660.
5. Landin LA. Fracture patterns in children. Analysis of 8682 fractures with special reference to incidence, etiology and secular changes in a Swedish urban population 1950–1979. Acta Orthop Scand Suppl 1983; 202:1–109.
6. Tiderius CJ, Landin LA, Düppe H. Decreasing incidence in fractures in children. An epidemiological analysis of 1673 fractures in Malmö, Sweden 1993–1994. Acta Orthop Scand 1999; 70: 622–626.
7. Rennie L, Court-Brown CM, Mok JYQ, Beattie TF. The epidemiology of fractures in children. Int J Care Injured 2007; 38:913–922.
8. Nwadinigwe CU, Ihezie CO, Iyidiobi EC. Fractures in children. Niger J Med 2006; Jan-Mar; 15(1):81–84.
9. McDermott C, Quinlan JF, Kelly IP. Trampoline injuries in children. J Bone Joint Surg Br 2006; Jun; 88(6):796–798.
10. Boyd KT, Brownson P, Hunder JB. Distal radial fractures in young goalkeepers: a case for an appropriately sized soccer ball. Br J Sports Med 2001; Dec; 35(6):409–411.
11. Vioreanu M, Sheehan E, Glynn A, et al. Heelys and street gliders injuries: a new type of pediatric injury. Pediatrics 2007; 119(6):e1294–e1298.
12. Mechem Fuller E. Injury prone children. Am J Orthopsychiatr 1948; 18:708–723.
13. Bijur PE, Stewart-Brown S, Bather N. Child behaviour and accidental injury in 11 966 preschool children. Am J Dis Child 1986; 140:487–492.
14. Gustafsson LH. Childhood accidents. Three epidemiological studies on the etiology. Scand J Soc Med 1977; 5–13.
15. Lam LT. Attention deficit disorder and hospitalization due to injury among older adolescents in New South Wales, Australia. J Atten Disord 2002; 6(2):77–82.
16. Ford JD, Racusin R, Daviss WB, et al. Trauma exposure among children with oppositional defiant disorder and attention deficit-hyperactivity disorder. J Consult Clin Psychol 1999; 67(5): 786–789.
17. Landin LA, Nilsson BE. Bone mineral content in children with fractures. Clin Orthop Rel Res 1983; 178:292–296.
18. Bianchi ML. Osteoporosis in children and adolescents. Bone 2007; (41):486–495.
19. Engström LM. Sweden. In: De Knop, P, Engström LM, Skirstad B, Weiss MR, eds. Worldwide Trends in Youth Sport. Champaign IL: Human Kinetics; 1996:231–243.
20. Swedish National Road Administration. Annual Statistics. Borlänge, Sweden: Vägverket Trafikantavdelningen; 1998.

Chapter 40

Polytrauma in Children

Peter P. Schmittenbecher and Cathrin S. Parsch

Introduction

Trauma is still the most common cause of mortality in children, even in countries with the most advanced medical services. Severe head injury carries a high morbidity and mortality, whether isolated or in association with other trauma. However, a fatal outcome is usually the consequence of combinations of injuries. We define "real" polytrauma as two or more system injuries, involved at the same time endangering life as a result of one single or a combination of several injuries. Multiple trauma is always more than the sum of the single injuries; it should be considered as a systemic disease. Orthopaedic injuries account for a high proportion of the damage incurred by the polytraumatized child but are rarely life-threatening in their own right [1].

Scoring Systems

Numerous methods have been developed to classify trauma in adults as well as in children. Anatomical scores, physiological scores, and combined classifications have been promoted. Some authors have concluded that trauma scores especially conceived for use in children fail to show any superiority compared to general trauma scores [2]. Scores seem to be more helpful in the retrospective evaluation of treatment, allowing comparison on a comprehensible basis. They have no crucial influence upon the initial management of patients, although early classification and potential triage on the base of a validated score is still a matter for debate.

The most widely used and accepted scoring systems for children are the modified injury severity score (MISS) and the paediatric trauma score (PTS) [3]. The MISS captures five anatomical body areas with five severity rates (minor to critical), including the Glasgow Coma Scale (GCS) as part of neurological examination (Table 40.1). The score is the sum of the squares of the three most severely injured body areas. More than 25 points indicates an increased risk of permanent disability, and more than 40 points predicts a lethal outcome [4].

The PTS includes six anatomical or physiological components and assigns these severity grades: −1 (major injury), +1 (minor injury), or +2 (minimal or no injury) (Table 40.2). With more than eight points, no deaths have occurred, with less than zero points the mortality rate was 100%. A linear relationship exists between the PTS and the MISS, but the former can be obtained more easily either at the scene of the accident or in the emergency room and is therefore of use for triage purposes [5].

Epidemiology

It is difficult to obtain reliable data on the incidence of polytrauma in childhood because definitions are vague and the data refer to restricted urban or rural areas. Prospective and obligatory nationwide paediatric trauma registries unfortunately do not exist.

Data from the United States show that 15,000 children (14 years or younger) die each year from accidental injuries, 19 million need some form of medical care, and 100,000 are permanently crippled [6]. The bimodal age distribution has one peak in the first year of life and another during adolescence. The incidence increases with the child's interaction in the outside world (traffic and other accidents) as life moves from the home to out of doors.

In Central Europe, children represent 10–20% of all polytrauma victims. The incidence is estimated to be 360 per 100,000 children. The mortality rate is about 12%. In the German trauma registry, including 17,000 polytrauma cases with an ISS of >16, approximately 6.1% ($n = 1,032$) are children or adolescents under 17 years of age. Every year

P.P. Schmittenbecher (✉)
Department of Pediatric Surgery, Municipal Hospital, Karlsruhe, Germany

M. Benson et al. (eds.), *Children's Orthopaedics and Fractures*,
DOI 10.1007/978-1-84882-611-3_40, © Springer-Verlag London Limited 2010

Table 40.1 Modified injury severity score (MISS) [4, 5]

Body area	1 Minor	2 Moderate	3 Severe	4 Life-threatening	5 Critical
Neural	GCS 13–14 Abrasion Contusion	GCS 9–12 Undisplaced facial #	GCS 9–12 Loss of eye Optic nerve avulsion	GCS 5–8 Bone/soft tissue injury with minor destruction	GCS <5 Injuries with airway obstruction
Face and neck	Vitreous or conjunctival hemorrhage Fractured teeth	Laceration of eye Retinal detachment	Displaced facial # Blow-out #		
Chest	Muscle ache Chest wall stiffness	Simple rib # Sternal #	Multiple rib # Hemo-/pneumothorax Diaphragmatic rupture Pulmonary contusion	Open chest wounds Pneumomediastinum Myocardial contusion	Tracheal, aortic, myocardial laceration Hemomediastinum
Abdomen	Muscle ache Seat belt abrasion	Major abdominal wall contusion	Organ contusion Retroperitoneal hematoma Extraperitoneal bladder rupture Thoracic or lumbar spine #	Organ laceration Intraparietal bladder rupture Spine # with paraplegia	Rupture or severe laceration of organs or vessels
Limbs, pelvic girdle	Minor sprains Simple #	Non-displaced # long bones or pelvis	Displaced long bone # Multiple hand/foot # Displaced pelvic # Major nerve/vessel laceration	Multiple closed long bone # Amputations	Multiple open long bone #

= *fracture*

Table 40. 2 Paediatric Trauma Score (PTS) [5, 6]

	+ 2	+ 1	−1
Size	>20 kg	10–20 kg	<10 kg
Airway	Normal	Maintainable	Unmaintainable
CNS	Normal	Obtunded	Comatose
Systolic blood pressure	>90 mmHg	90–50 mmHg	<50 mmHg
Open wounds	None	Minor	Major, penetrating
Skeletal	None	Closed #	Open or multiple #

33,000 patients suffer from an injury with an injury severity score (ISS) greater than 16; about 2,000 of them are children or adolescents. Males account for 66%, and the incidence mounts with age [7, 8].

Every polytraumatized child should be taken as a warning to reduce accident risks at home, to lobby for the prevention of road traffic accident injuries (e.g., including the use of bicycle helmets), and to ensure that the care of the critically injured child is a clinical priority.

Injuries

Child abuse is the most important cause of polytrauma in the first year of life. In younger children (1–4 years old) falls from a height at home or in the playground are the principal concern. With increasing age road traffic is the main danger. Motor vehicle collisions with pedestrians and bicyclists are common, yet children are also affected as car passengers if safe seating is not provided or its use enforced.

Principal Patterns of Injuries

Younger children suffer different injury patterns compared to adults. Head injuries and lower limb trauma are more common than thoracic, abdominal, and pelvic injuries (Fig. 40.1). The upper extremity is less often affected. Facial injuries may implicate the cervical spine. First rib and multiple rib fractures are markers for severe trauma and should promote a further search for undetected injuries. Thoracic or lumbar spine trauma suggests additional abdominal injuries. A displaced pelvic fracture warns of other trauma, especially to the abdominal and pelvic cavities.

Falls from a height result in head injuries and a variety of fractures. A typical pattern in a child pedestrian hit by a car comprises head trauma, femoral shaft fracture, and lung contusion. In car passengers 3- or 4-point restraint systems (but not the pelvic restraint belt alone) prevent the characteristic lap-belt injuries: flexion-distraction trauma to the lumbar vertebral column (Chance fracture), disruption of small bowel, and post-traumatic pancreatitis.

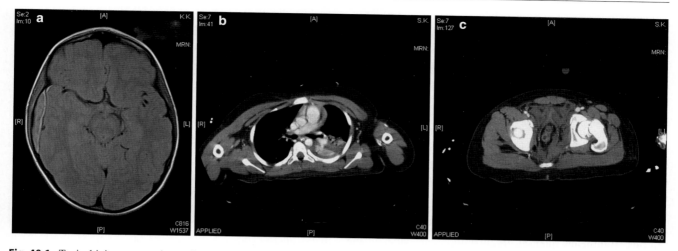

Fig. 40.1 Typical injury pattern in a polytraumatized child with (**a**) an epidural hematoma, (**b**) thoracic (pulmonary) contusion, and (**c**) femoral neck fracture

Generally complications occur in a third of cases, mainly pneumonia and other infections. Mortality is highest with head, thoracic, and abdominal injuries, and the child with an injured cervical spine is at particular risk. Although head and abdominal injuries are often more severe than in adults thoracic trauma carries less hazard than in the adult [9].

Specific Physiological and Anatomical Characteristics

Children differ in many physiological and anatomical aspects from adults. The body proportions are quite different, depending on and changing with age. The head occupies a much larger percentage of the body surface and mass compared to adults. The inability of young children to communicate poses an unique challenge in the setting of multisystem trauma.

Airway and Cervical Spine

Recognition and management of airway obstruction and protection of the cervical spine are paramount. The larynx is in a more superior and anterior position, the tongue is larger. The cartilages and soft tissues are softer and more easily compressed. Combined with overall smaller airways especially in the subglottic region, these factors can easily lead to airway obstruction in the setting of an altered conscious state due to head/facial/neck trauma, hypoxia, and hypoperfusion. Post-traumatic mucosal swelling or foreign body obstruction needs additional attention.

A child's neck is short and supports the large head. Due to the flexible spinal column and soft attachments, spinal cord damage and neurological impairment are not necessarily associated with radiological abnormalities. Physiological C2/C3 pseudo-subluxation has to be differentiated radiologically from traumatic spinal injuries.

Breathing

Hypoventilation is the most common cause of cardiac arrest in children. Compared to adults, the chest wall is more compliant and compressible and the overlying skin and muscles are thin and provide little protection. The elasticity of the cartilaginous ribs allows efficient transmission of a traumatic impact onto the intrathoracic organs. Therefore lung contusions, hemothorax, or diaphragmatic rupture with catastrophic ventilatory and hemodynamic consequences can occur without the rib fractures or clinically obvious external signs of chest trauma. The short, fat neck makes assessment of neck veins and the position of the trachea difficult.

Circulation

Circulatory failure in the setting of multitrauma is mostly due to hypovolemia and blood loss. Other causes are obstruction of venous return (tension pneumothorax and pericardial tamponade) or sympathetic failure (spinal cord injury). In young children in particular the total blood volume is smaller, the stroke volume is fixed, and therefore cardiac output is determined by the heart rate. Tachycardia is usually present but may also be due to pain and anxiety. The age-dependent range for vital signs has to be taken into consideration. Knowledge about age-specific values is important (the normal heart rate for a preschooler is 100–130 beats/min), relative bradycardia for age is a sign of impending cardiac arrest. Other signs of hypoperfusion are decreased central capillary refill, weak pulse pressure, and a decreased level of consciousness due to cerebral hypoperfusion. Blood loss is compensated satisfactorily in the early stages of hemorrhage by vasoconstriction, but decompensation may occur rapidly (talk and die). A decrease in blood pressure is a late sign and resuscitation aims at its prevention.

Abdominal organs are more likely to be injured, as ribs and muscles provide much less protection. Similar to chest injuries, significant internal organ trauma can occur in the absence of obvious external signs. The thoracic spine is seldom affected but lumbar spine (Chance) fractures may occur as part of the lap-belt injury. Chance fractures are usually associated with intra-abdominal injuries. The elasticity of the pelvis prevents severe, unstable disruptions of the ring with severe bleeding.

Disability

The main differences when assessing neurological function relates to preverbal age group. The Paediatric Glasgow Coma Scale has incorporated age-related modifications. Small and seriously ill or injured children are prone to hypoglycemia, which may contribute to the altered conscious state. Sympathetic and adrenal mechanisms as well as relative insulin resistance may cause hyperglycemia, which has been shown to contribute to worse outcomes in the setting of severe head injury.

Exposure/Endocrine

The higher ratio of surface area to volume makes the child vulnerable to hypothermia. Thermal energy loss can occur very quickly and complicate the management of any critically ill or injured paediatric patient.

Furthermore, polytrauma is a systemic disease with a systemic response. Children respond differently to metabolic and physiological stress than adults. The systemic response is reinforced by hypotension, hypovolemia, hypothermia, hypoxemia, pain, and tissue damage and includes a neuroendocrine response (catecholamines, adrenocorticotropic hormones, endorphins, and other local mediators), endotheliopathy, compromised hemostasis, and further dysfunction of temperature regulation. This may be followed by the

release of more mediators, which in turn induce multiple organ failure. But immunological competence and reactive synthesis of cytokines is limited in children. This is the explanation for the low number of systemic inflammatory response syndromes (SIRS) and multiple organ failures (MOF) [8, 10, 11].

Fracture Patterns

Fracture patterns of the limbs in children change with age. In polytrauma minor and incomplete fractures such as greenstick fractures are less frequent because of the higher traumatic energy, but open fractures are more common than usual. The complexity of the soft tissue damage is not a predictor of fracture severity as it is in adults.

Initial Assessment and Management

A structured approach to the seriously injured child enables the timely recognition and management of life-threatening injuries [11–13]. The initial assessment includes

- Primary survey (commences pre-hospital)
- Resuscitation (commences pre-hospital)
- Adjuncts to primary survey (in-hospital)
- Secondary survey
- Emergency treatment and ongoing monitoring
- Definitive care

First Aid, Transport, and Hospital Facilities

The importance of treatment in the pre-hospital phase is well documented since most deaths occur shortly after trauma. As in adults, the most common causes of immediate death are hypoxia, massive hemorrhage, and overwhelming central nervous system (CNS) injury. Scene time should be as short as possible, but during these critical initial minutes, a systematical *primary survey* is vital in identifying life-threatening injuries. The first priority in pre-hospital care is the provision of adequate oxygenation. Multiple attempts at gaining intravenous access should be avoided. Alternative routes such as intraosseous access if available in the pre-hospital environment can be time and life saving.

It is debated whether one should "stay and play" (substitution of volume and intubation) or "load and go" (scoop and run). The decision is influenced by the individual situation.

The child should be managed according to the internationally established principles such as those taught by PALS (Pediatric Advanced Life Support) or APLS (Advanced Pediatric Life Support) courses [11, 13]. Polytraumatized children need a sophisticated and integrated trauma management system specifically focused upon the child. Rapid transport to a dedicated paediatric trauma facility as soon as safely possible is recommended. This means that paediatric intensive care unit (PICU) facilities are required and that experienced paediatric, orthopaedic, and general surgeons are available to assist the emergency team. Paediatric trauma centers have lowered the mortality and morbidity rates, although high costs and geographical restrictions have limited the number of such centers [1, 14, 15]. If this is not possible, then temporary stabilization in a smaller hospital and secondary transfer to a trauma center may be necessary. Communication from the scene or en route enables the receiving facility to mobilize an adequate trauma team, theater, equipment, and blood products as required.

A—Airway

Signs and symptoms of a life-threatening airway or chest injury may be subtle initially, but children can deteriorate rapidly. Supplemental oxygen of around 12 l/min should be supplied. The pharynx is cleared and the neck stabilized in-line with a collar, sandbags, or a tape in neutral position.

Indications for endotracheal intubation are

- inability of the child to protect its airway to prevent aspiration
- inability to ventilate the child with a self-inflating bag-mask system
- altered conscious state or cerebral irritability to protect the airway and prevent further cervical spine injury
- need for controlled ventilation in the context of severe head injury
- ventilatory failure due to severe chest wall and lung injury, e.g., flail chest with paradoxical breathing, pain, exhaustion, and hypoxemia

If intubation is indicated, proper preparation is mandatory. Pre-oxygenation with 100% oxygen, airway opening and clearance (jaw thrust, gentle suction, and airway adjuncts such as an oropharyngeal airway if necessary), as well as preparation of the age/size appropriate instruments and pre-calculated drugs (rapid sequence induction). Manual in-line stabilization of the cervical spine still provides protection from excessive neck movement.

B—Breathing

After airway maintenance and patency has been secured, acutely life-threatening chest injuries need to be identified and addressed. Asymmetrical chest movement may be difficult to identify in children, as they have small tidal volumes. Signs of increased work of breathing such as accessory muscle use, chest wall retractions, and increasing respiratory rate have to be taken very seriously.

Unilaterally decreased/absent breath sounds, hyperresonant percussion, and tracheal deviation to the opposite side indicate an expanding and tensioning pneumothorax, which has to be decompressed immediately via needle thoracocentesis followed by a large caliber intercostal drain. When aeromedical transfer is undertaken, a Heimlich valve instead of an underwater seal drain is required if tube thoracostomy has been performed.

Unilaterally decreased breath sounds with dull percussion in the context of acute ventilatory and respiratory failure are indicative of a massive hemothorax. The treatment consists of intercostal drainage and fluid resuscitation (including blood transfusion). Thoracotomy may be required.

Flail chest causes paradoxical breathing and is usually accompanied by severe underlying lung contusions. Ventilatory support is generally required.

Pericardial tamponade is rare in blunt trauma. Beck's triad of muffled heart sounds, distended neck veins, and poor perfusion may be difficult to detect in a noisy environment and in the presence of hypovolemia. Immediate pericardiocentesis is followed by emergency thoracotomy. An open pneumothorax (sucking chest wound) is fortunately not a common occurrence. Emergency treatment consists of a bandage taped on three sides followed by a chest drain.

C—Circulation and Hemorrhage Control

Circulatory efficiency depends on the integrity of the "3 Ps"[16]:

- pump (myocardium):
  - Threat: hypoxia and ischemia from hypovolemia

- pipes (integrity of the vascular system)
  - Threat: disruption, organ hypoperfusion due to vasoconstriction

- prime (circulating volume)
  - Threat: hypovolemia due to blood loss or obstruction of venous return (tension pneumothorax and pericardial tamponade)

Indicators of poor perfusion are tachypnea, tachycardia, prolonged capillary refill time, pallor, anxiety, and restlessness. Hypotension occurs late and the child may be obtunded from a combination of intracranial injury as well as cerebral hypoperfusion.

Severe external blood loss is managed by direct manual pressure. Traction splints can also assist in hemorrhage control. Tourniquets should be restricted to exceptional circumstances such as traumatic amputations and are a last resort. Occult blood loss may occur into the thoracic and abdominal cavities, along fractured bones, and into the retroperitoneal space.

Recognizing hemorrhagic shock is essential to ensure good outcomes. Children have an amazing physiological reserve and demonstrate few obvious signs of hypovolemia even when severe volume depletion has occurred. Tachycardia is usually the earliest noticeable response. As mentioned before, knowledge of normal vital signs appropriate for the age of the child is important.

Venous access has to be established before the circulation deteriorates. The insertion of two large bore cannulae is recommended. However, gaining peripheral intravenous access in a child can be difficult, particularly in the presence of shock. After 90 s or 3 failed attempts intraosseous access in a non-fractured extremity should be established. The anterior tibial marrow can usually be cannulated quickly and complications during short-term use are rare. Crystalloids are appropriate for volume substitution (20 ml/kg body weight). If perfusion remains poor after this initial fluid bolus, another bolus of 20 ml/kg is given. If there is still no improvement, O negative blood or group-specific blood, if available (10 ml/kg), must be transfused immediately. Ongoing and repeated assessment of the indicators of adequate perfusion is critical and surgical consultation should be sought early. Although fluid administration should be judicious in the head-injured child, cerebral hypoperfusion due to hypovolemia must be avoided. Once circulatory stability has been achieved, weight-based calculation of maintenance fluids, which should contain glucose, can be ensured whilst monitoring ongoing losses. If the child is moved with an intraosseous needle in place, the flow has to be stopped temporarily before the needle is checked again by aspiration. An unnoticed displacement of the needle tip may cause a compartment syndrome and more importantly prevent further fluid resuscitation, at least temporarily.

D—Disability

CNS injury is the leading cause of death and a presenting GCS of 8 carries a high mortality. However, a rapid assessment of neurological function is performed at the end of the primary survey, because hypoxia, hypoventilation, and hypotension need to be proactively treated to prevent secondary brain damage. Evaluation can include a GCS with age-related modifications, a very quick "AVPU" score (Alert, response to Voice, response to Pain, Unconscious) and a pupillary assessment. A more detailed neurology examination comprises part of the secondary survey.

E—Exposure

Exposure to ambient temperatures and wet weather often render trauma victims hypothermic in the pre-hospital phase.

The patients should be undressed for a full examination and wet garments should be removed immediately as they add to thermal losses. The treating team however has to be aware of the potential heat loss and embarrassment of the child. Warming blankets and devices and (particularly in small children) a heat lamp may be used. If the trauma team receives timely warning about an emergency admission the overall resuscitation room temperature can be raised to prevent further heat loss from the child. Hypothermia, acidosis, and coagulopathy due to hypovolemia comprise the so-called lethal triad [10].

Management of the Multi-injured Child

Adjuncts to the Primary Survey

Full cardiorespiratory monitoring should be established as soon as possible. Radiographic evaluation of the cervical spine, chest, and pelvis is an integral part of the initial assessment of seriously injured children. The interpretation of cervical spine views can be challenging. Depending upon the mechanism of trauma and clinical findings further imaging such as computed tomography (CT) scans may be required. If available a rapid total body projection for the severely injured and unstable child is recommended (Fig. 40.2) [17]. Focused abdominal sonography in trauma (FAST) is gaining more acceptance as a bedside assessment tool in paediatric trauma victims as well. It is mainly useful in the unstable trauma patient where it can reveal free abdominal fluid or pericardial tamponade. In small children ultrasound scans can even identify intracranial injuries.

Bedside glucose (DEFG = Don't Ever Forget Glucose), hemoglobin, and venous blood gas analysis as well as cross/match testing should be obtained as soon as possible.

Aerophagia and manual bag-mask ventilation can cause significant gastric distention. This impedes lung expansion,

Fig. 40.2 Polytrauma CT scan of a pedestrian after collision with a motorcycle. (**a**) An inconspicuous CT, (**b**) pulmonary contusion, (**c**) splenic rupture, (**d**) pelvic fracture, (**e**) open ankle fracture, and (**f**) subcapital humerus fracture

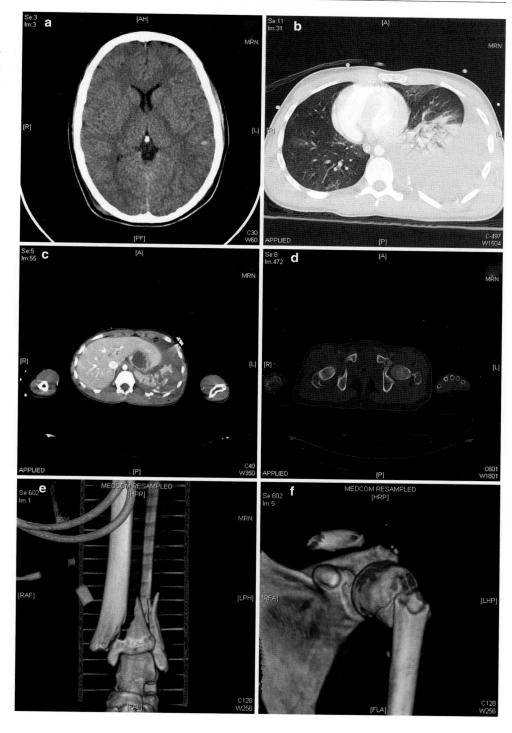

decreases the functional residual capacity, and increases the aspiration risk. Decompression with a nasogastric (in the absence of facial or head trauma) or orogastric catheter can facilitate ventilation. After pelvic fractures and/or urethral injuries have been excluded, a bladder catheter can be inserted. This assists in monitoring the adequacy of fluid resuscitative measures.

Secondary Survey

The secondary survey is a detailed evaluation from head to toe and does not begin until the primary survey is completed and resuscitative measures have been established. If at any stage during the secondary survey there is clinical deterioration, it is important to reassess ABCDE. Neurological deterioration may have led to airway compromise or a simple pneumothorax may have become a tension pneumothorax; these conditions have to be addressed immediately.

It is very important to document all findings as each system is in a state of flux. Most trauma centers have templates that aid in the assessment and documentation of the examination findings.

The secondary survey of paediatric emergency medicine resource [16] includes SAMPLE history

S Signs and symptoms
A Allergies
M Medications and if immunizations are up to date
P Last medical conditions
L Last meal
E Events before the injuries occurred.

Physical Examination

Head including orifices: Loose teeth and oral bleeding pose an inhalational hazard and can cause airway compromise. As yet unrecognized lacerations, facial injuries including epistaxis and surgical emphysema or ocular damage are important findings. Signs and symptoms of basilar skull fractures, such as hemotympanum, Battle sign, or cerebrospinal fluid otorrhea/rhinorrhea may be detected. Gentle palpation of the head and cranial vault may reveal a boggy scalp hematoma or an underlying skull fracture.

Neck and cervical spine: Without compromising cervical immobilization gentle examination of the neck is important. Midline tenderness and step-offs may indicate underlying bony injury. Increasing swelling, stridor, and surgical emphysema suggest injury to the upper gastrointestinal tract.

Chest: Frequent re-examination of the thorax has to be undertaken so that early signs of deterioration and ventilatory compromise can be detected and reversed. Palpation of the entire bony chest wall as well as looking and listening for symmetry of chest expansion and air entry are mandatory. It has to be remembered that children may sustain major intrathoracic injury with minimal external signs due to the elasticity of the chest wall.

Abdomen: Ecchymosis of the abdominal wall and signs of peritoneal irritation suggest intra-abdominal injuries [18]. About 25% of children with multisystem trauma have a significant abdominal injury. The mortality following blunt abdominal trauma is related to the level of organ involvement: it is less than 20% in isolated solid organ injury and rises to 20% with hollow organ damage. If major vessels are involved, the mortality rises to 50%. External signs may be subtle, and evidence of intra-abdominal blood loss may be masked by the significant ability of children to compensate. Repeated examination (preferably by the same experienced

person) and careful review of ventilatory effort must be ensured.

Pelvis: External palpation will establish tenderness and instability. Perineal bruising or wounds and urethral bleeding are important indicators of major pelvic trauma.

Limbs: The limbs should be examined for deformity, bleeding, and neurovascular dysfunction. Fractured limbs should be temporarily splinted. Frequent re-examination with particular attention to the neurovascular status and skin appearance is important. A high index of suspicion for impending compartment syndrome should mean that this limb-threatening condition is identified early. The effects of extensive soft tissue contusion or lacerations should not be underestimated (Fig. 40.3).

Log roll/examination of the back: Rolling the patient en bloc with the help of several members of the team prevents dangerous movements of the spine. The examiner should look for bruising and open wounds and palpate the spine for abnormal steps, crepitation, and surgical emphysema. In the severely injured child, particularly with lower abdominal/back or pelvic injuries, a rectal examination may be necessary to assess the sphincter tone and the integrity of the rectal wall.

Neurologic examination: During the secondary survey a detailed neurological examination includes motor and sensory examination and reflexes as well as examination of the cranial nerves, orientation, and conscious state. Lumbosacral plexus and sciatic, femoral, or obturator nerve damage may coexist in cases of suspected pelvic fractures.

Adjuncts to the Secondary Survey

The urgency and order of investigations depend on the findings of the primary and secondary surveys. Basic blood tests, plain radiology, and FAST scans can usually be performed whilst resuscitation is being undertaken. Diagnostic peritoneal lavage has been largely abandoned. If emergency surgery is required, some imaging may need to be deferred. Transporting an unstable child out of the resuscitation room into the CT scanner is fraught with danger. This has to be weighed against the need for a definitive diagnosis and anatomical knowledge of injuries present. A team approach involving the surgeon, emergency physician, intensivist, and anesthetist helps to categorize risks and priorities.

Monitoring, Re-evaluation and Analgesia

The severely injured child has to be frequently re-assessed and continuously monitored. Urine output as an indicator of adequate perfusion should be measured by the hourly urine

Fig. 40.3 (**a**) Soft tissue
contusion produced by collision
with a bus with (**b**) a secondary
soft tissue defect

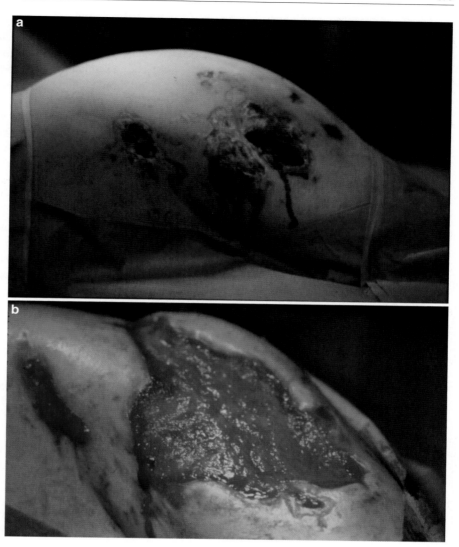

output (provided it is safe to insert a bladder catheter) and
1 ml/kg/h of urine is desirable. Even minor deterioration in
vital signs such as relative tachycardia or increase in respiratory rate is significant, as they precede decompensation
if not addressed early. Pain relief plays an important part
in the management of trauma [19]. Sufficient analgesia and
sedation are very important to the child under physical and
psychological duress. Intravenous doses of opiates (such as
morphine 0.05–0.1 mg/kg using a closely monitored pain
protocol) offer effective analgesia without over-sedation and
respiratory depression.

Radionuclide scans are useful to identify fractures of different age in cases of non-accidental injury but do not play
a role in the emergency setting in a severely injured child.
Magnetic resonance (MR) scanning has yet to find a place in
the initial evaluation but is of value in later assessment.

Definitive Care

Effective treatment recognizes the control of "threat to
life" factors first, followed by the "limitation of disability." So-called damage-control surgery [10] comprises four
steps:

1. Control of any significant hemorrhage by compression,
   ligation, or packs; thorough removal of any contamination; closure of débrided, open wounds; and limb
   immobilization. These interventions should be completed
   within 3 h. If emergency operations are necessary, mortality increases in proportion to the time needed for this
   surgical intervention.

2. Stabilization of the patient in the PICU, including rewarming, correction of coagulopathy, reversal of acidosis, and the monitoring of abdominal and pelvic organ function.
3. Primary phase of definitive surgery within 72 h (for the pelvis, spine, femur, and severe soft tissue injuries)
4. Secondary and tertiary phases of surgery some 10 days after the trauma.

Principles of Treatment

Head Injury

Head injuries are the most common cause of death or long-term disability in children after polytrauma. The severity of head injury correlates with mortality and residual deficits in those who survive, although children often make remarkable recoveries from apparently severe cerebral damage.

A 30° elevation of the head or of the bed, fluid restriction, and slight hyperventilation are the cornerstones of head injury management. Hydration of the patient for volume deficiency or shock has to be achieved carefully in severe brain injury as mentioned previously, yet uncorrected hypovolemia and hypoxemia may also induce secondary brain damage. Diffuse brain edema complicates 30% of cases and if clinical and/or CT signs of head injury or severe edema develop in the unconscious patient intraparenchymatous or intraventricular cerebral pressure monitoring is essential to exclude or confirm significant pressure elevation. The monitoring, fluid management, and ventilation procedures of the severely head-injured child are beyond the scope of this chapter but represent a vital prevention of further brain injury. Early extensive bitemporal craniotomy may be helpful in individual cases if uncontrollable, high cerebral pressure persists. An additional MRI investigation is ensured later to detect brainstem or long-tract injuries if the clinical course is worse than anticipated from the initial CT appearances.

Approximately 10% of children develop post-traumatic seizures after head injuries and prophylactic medication will then be required [20].

The orthopaedic surgeon may be peripheral to many of these therapeutic interventions but still offers an important service in the judicious fixation of fractures, thus minimizing pain and its secondary effects upon intracranial pressure [21].

Spinal Cord Injuries

In multiple trauma a spinal cord injury should be presumed until ruled out. Statistically, 2% of patients have spinal injuries with some element of spinal shock. Cervical spinal cord trauma may occur in typical whiplash injuries and thoracolumbar trauma in lap-belt injuries. A careful examination pays attention to the vertebral column, the surrounding muscle groups, the prevertebral cervical soft tissue, and the peripheral neuromuscular and autonomic function, thus differentiating complete from incomplete lesions. If spinal shock is diagnosed the use of steroids seems to be effective in improving neurologic recovery. Chapter 52 deals with these details. In up to 66% of patients with spinal trauma SCIWORA lesions (spinal cord injury without obvious radiological abnormality) are found with stretching or distraction of the spinal cord in conjunction with the increased elasticity, hypermobility, ligamentous laxity, and immature vascular supply of the spine seen especially in the younger child. Clinical symptoms can develop after a 4-day delay, MR scanning offering an accurate means of assessing the extent of the trauma [1].

Thoracic Injury

The incidence of thoracic injuries is high in polytrauma. Mortality rises to 39% if thoracic trauma is combined with brain and abdominal injury. Although head injury is the main contributor to mortality, morbidity in survivors is influenced by cerebral hypoxia caused by pulmonary deficit.

A first rib fracture or multiple rib fractures are poor prognostic signs because they are indicative of severe trauma. But even without rib fractures, significant intrathoracic injuries may be present. Direct airway injury is rare but is lethal in up to one third of cases. Aortic or diaphragmatic rupture occurs in high-velocity injuries and may be diagnosed from the chest radiograph or the CT scan (Fig. 40.4).

Pulmonary contusion is the most common form of thoracic trauma in paediatric polytrauma and tends to be underestimated on the chest radiograph. If suspected, CT imaging is important because the clinical course of this condition typically deteriorates after a delay, interim extubation and spontaneous breathing worsening matters (Fig. 40.5) [22].

The lung and the kidney are the most significant target organs of secondary damage. Endothelial injury, impaired vascular response, pulmonary vasoconstriction, capillary leak, and interstitial edema are common. In the lung the result is an increase in alveolar capillary permeability, surfactant inactivation, and increased dead space ventilation secondary to intrapulmonary shunts. Respiratory support comprises a limited use of oxygen to prevent toxicity and an adequate positive airway pressure to reduce ventilation/perfusion imbalance.

Fig. 40.4 (**a**) Diaphragmatic rupture with (**b**) peripheral fracture of pelvis

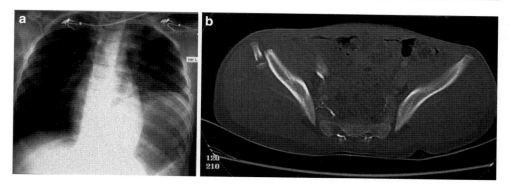

Fig. 40.5 (**a**) Radiograph of the lung with pulmonary contusion compared with (**b**) the CT scan

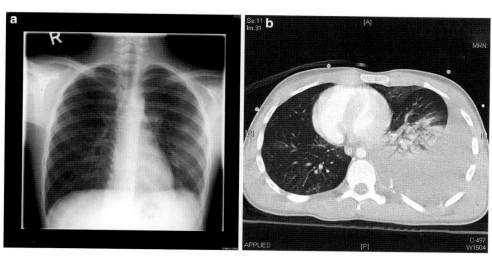

Abdominal Injury

Abdominal injuries occur in one third of polytrauma cases. Trunk ecchymosis is a sign of serious visceral injury, kidney, spleen, and liver being the most often affected. Ultrasound and CT diagnose and classify the injuries accurately. Today most parenchymatous injuries are treated conservatively, but 15% of traumatized kidneys need exploration and reconstruction for renal pelvis laceration or nephrectomy for central disruption [23]. Spleen and liver trauma are stabilized by dealing with the hemorrhage using volume substitution and catecholamine infusions, provided that the blood pressure is stabilized with no more than 40 ml blood transfusion per kilogram body weight per 24 h. With this approach laparotomy is rarely required and the number of splenectomized children is significantly reduced. Even the exploration of an injured liver is seldom indicated, being confined to severe central lacerations or retrohepatic caval tears which make packing essential. The serum transaminase values are a reliable monitor of progress such that abdominal lavage is rarely indicated [24].

Pancreas and gastrointestinal tract are hardly ever involved. Pancreatic contusions are treated like acute pan-

creatitis. Organ ruptures and lesions of the pancreatic duct are rarely mentioned in case reports. Post-traumatic pseudo-cysts often resolve spontaneously but large, single cysts may need percutaneous or endoscopic drainage. An enlarging or ruptured cyst, pain, or infection may make an internal surgical drainage via cysto-jejunostomy necessary [25]. Gastrointestinal injuries are found in less than 5% of cases. An obstructing duodenal hematoma is vented by a gastric tube. Perforation of small bowel or colon presents with the signs of peritonitis, and a pneumo-peritoneum is seen on an abdominal radiograph. Bowel rupture should be sutured or resected, followed by anastomosis or enterostomy. This injury is often found in lap-belt injuries and is sometimes identified late since most other parenchymatous organ injuries are now managed without surgery [26].

Orthopaedic Injuries

Skeletal injuries occur in approximately three quarters of polytraumatized children. An emergency intervention is unnecessary except for certain open fractures, vascular damage or a compartment syndrome, and an unstable pelvic or spine fracture. All other cases can be temporarily stabilized, with later elective and definitive management, preferably within 72 h as this improves recovery and rehabilitation [27]. If possible primary definitive fracture care should be achieved at the time of intervention.

The pulmonary benefits of fracture stabilization are not as certain as they are in adults, but longer immobilization undoubtedly increases general complications and an abdominal examination is difficult if a spica cast has been applied. Preliminary fixation with an external fixator during emergency room resuscitation represents a valuable advance in specific cases.

Initially a neurovascular examination is necessary to exclude the necessity of any urgent intervention. In the unconscious child, Doppler studies and possibly compartmental monitoring are appropriate. If vascular repair is necessary, fracture stabilization is essential concurrently or beforehand. In open fractures sterile dressings are applied and tetanus prophylaxis given if the status is unknown.

Femur Fractures

In closed shaft fractures elastic stable intramedullary nailing (ESIN) and external fixator (EF) are the preferred techniques (Figs. 40.6 and 40.7). Both methods are adequate and effective if the surgeon is familiar with the systems. If there is sufficient contact between the main fragments a biomechanically correct insertion of intramedullary elastic nails guarantees correct axis of the limb with enough stability for movement and intensive care and with rapid callus formation. Formation of callus is abundant, particularly in those with head injury. If fractures of the lower limb are at risk of shortening because of a long spiral fracture or a butterfly fragment, end caps can be screwed over the nail ends in the cortical bone and enhance axial stability [28]. When there is bone loss and likely shortening, or a juxta-articular fracture, external monolateral or ring fixators are indicated. In most instances these do not require to be changed before bone union, although occasionally a fixator may be changed to internal fixation later during the recovery period.

Epiphyseal/Metaphyseal Fractures

Metaphyseal fractures are not a major problem but may occasionally merit fixation to aid in nursing care. Epiphyseal fractures are seldom seen with polytrauma. Humeral condylar or ankle fractures are the most common and can be treated with K-wires or screws. In cases of severe, periarticular injury minimal osteosynthesis can be combined with a transarticular, external fixator. Late physeal arrest may

be seen following polytrauma and the details of management are presented in the next chapter.

Open Fractures

Open fractures in children differ from adults' fractures because the degree of soft tissue damage does not predict the complexity of the fracture. Compound fractures can be treated even after a delay of 6–8 h, following the standard principles of copious normal saline irrigation and debridement. Intramedullary fixation with ESIN is effective in first- or second-degree open fractures, reserving external fixation for grade three open fractures, especially degloving injuries of the foot and ankle. Antibiotics are given for 2–3 days or longer depending upon the clinical situation. Wounds are drained and left open if necessary, and in extensive soft tissue loss a temporary coverage is beneficial. Intraoperative cultures correlate poorly with ultimate wound infection and are optional. Soft tissue viability improves with time and facilitates the decision for or against local or free muscle flaps. If an amputation is inevitable, every effort should be made to preserve length and physeal function.

Pelvic Fractures

In pelvic fractures the greater plasticity of bones and the flexibility and elasticity of the sacro-iliac joints and symphysis pubis explain why so much more force is required to produce a fracture than in the adult. These fractures are an indicator of very high-energy injuries (see Chapter 46) and warn about the presence of associated injuries. Retro- and intraperitoneal bleeding from the cancellous bone and disrupted vessels or urogenital trauma are indicated by the presence of a hematoma beneath the inguinal ligament or within the scrotum or by a palpable rectal bony prominence or hematoma. Since pelvic fractures are often stable, they can be managed non-operatively and allow early function. Surgical stabilization is required in horizontal or vertical, unstable pelvic disruption, for rotatory instability or for large, displaced fragments (Fig. 40.8). External fixation reduces bleeding, facilitates transport, and can often be used as the definitive management. Acetabular fractures with displaced fragments and loss of hip joint stability need surgical intervention. Only half of pelvic fractures seen on CT were identified on plain films.

In 9–24% of pelvic fractures genitourinary injury occurs, especially in anterior pubic disruptions. Males are more often affected and urethral disruption is found in the majority of cases (Fig. 40.9). It should be remembered that there is a much bigger symphyseal distance in small children

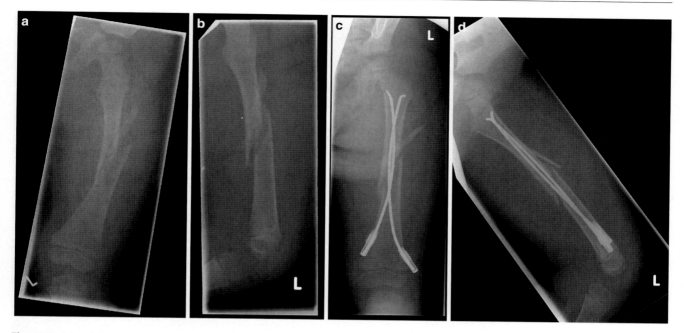

Fig. 40.6 (**a**) and (**b**) Femoral shaft fracture with (**c**) and (**d**) intramedullary nailing using stabilizing end caps

Fig. 40.7 (**a**) Femoral shaft fracture with (**b**) external fixator in place

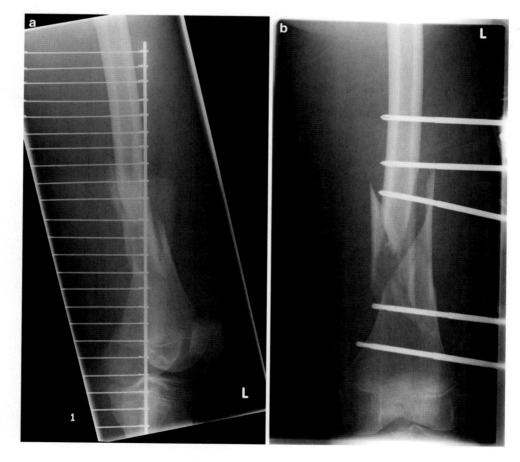

Fig. 40.8 Example of (**a**) and
(**b**) unstable pelvic and femoral
neck fracture (**c**) and (**d**) after
stabilisation with external fixator
and femoral neck and sacro-iliac
screw fixation

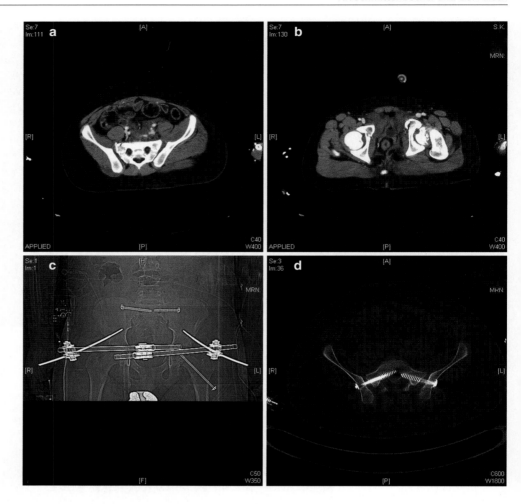

Fig. 40.9 Stabilization of a
pelvic fracture with external
fixator and reconstruction of
urethral disruption

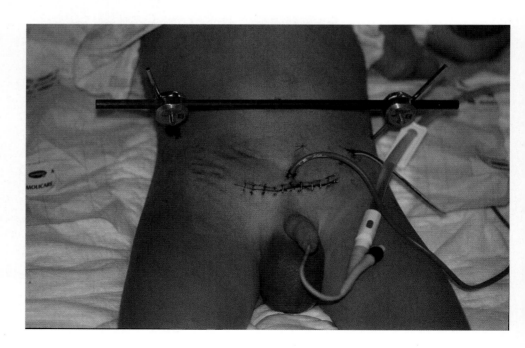

(10–12 mm) compared with adolescents (6 mm) or adults (2–4 mm) [29]. Late diagnosis is common if initial symptoms are not obvious. Care should be taken when inserting a bladder catheter.

Fractures of the Spine

As previously mentioned, the spine is more mobile than in adults and this allows force to be dissipated over a greater number of segments. Hence CT or MR scans show bony contusion and edema over a number of vertebral bodies. Only 1% of paediatric fractures occur in the spine and compression fractures of the thoracic and lumbar segments are more often seen than distraction injuries. Limited spinal fusion is the treatment of choice for the unstable lesion [30].

It is well known that a significant number of skeletal injuries are not identified during the first examination. Therefore repeated and thorough clinical examination is necessary 2–3 days later, augmented by coned radiographs to detect additional skeletal injuries.

A special indication for stabilization is the development of post-traumatic convulsions. Early limb spasticity following severe head injury also makes long bone fracture fixation advisable. In polytrauma, unconventional or atypical surgical interventions may help in the child's recovery, so the surgeon needs to be adaptable.

Psychological Problems

Polytrauma inflicts significant stress upon the child and his family. Emotional shock is followed by denial or depression before recovery takes place. During the first post-traumatic phase psychiatric manifestations may develop and persist throughout a potentially long convalescence.

Outcome, Rehabilitation, and Long-Term Course

The prognosis depends upon the extent of the brain injury [31]. The majority of deaths take place during the first hour and a second peak is found after 48 h. Of those who are not dead on arrival, the mortality rate is approximately 17%.

Long-term disability is seen in 19–28% of all children involved in polytrauma, declining to 12% during the next decade. Nearly half of the relevant functional impairment is the result of brain injury. Five years after the trauma, the signs of focal neurological loss are apparent in one third

of the patients. Neuropsychological and psychosocial problems persist for 6 months in 24% of cases while 42% of brain-injured children following polytrauma exhibit cognitive impairment. The musculoskeletal injuries account for one third of the cases with long-term disability [32–34].

Institutions caring for polytraumatized children need a protocol on how to manage the withdrawal of care for those unfortunate children who cannot be salvaged. Ethical principles must play a part in that very personal and painful decision. The complex problem of organ donation and the dignity of dying require an informed and professional approach.

References

1. Kay RM, Skaggs DL. Pediatric polytrauma management. J Pediatr Orthop 2006; 26:268–277.
2. Ott R, Kramer R, Martus P, et al. Prognostic value of trauma scores in pediatric patients with multiple injuries. J Trauma 2000; 49:729–736.
3. Yian EH, Gullahorn LJ, Loder RT. Scoring of pediatric orthopaedic polytrauma: correlations of different injury scoring systems and prognosis for hospital course. J Pediatr Orthop 2000; 20:203–209.
4. Mayer T, Matlak ME, Johnson DG, et al. The modified injury severity scale in pediatric multiple trauma patients. J Pediatr Surg 1980; 15:719–726.
5. Wilber JH, Thompson GH. The multiply injured child. In: Green NE, Swiontkowski MF, eds. Skeletal Trauma in Children, 3rd ed. Philadelphia: Saunders; 2003.
6. Tepas JJ, Ramenofsky ML, Mollitt DL. The pediatric trauma score as a predictor of injury severity: an objective assessment. J Trauma 1988; 28:425–429.
7. Meier R, Krettek C, Grimme K, et al. The multiply injured child. Clin Orthop Relat Res 2005; 432:127–131.
8. Navascues del Rio JA, Ruiz RMR, Martin JS, et al. First Spanish trauma registry: analysis of 1500 cases. Eur J Pediatr Surg 2000; 10:310–318.
9. Husain B, Kuehne C, Waydhas C, et al. Incidence and prognosis of organ failure in severely injured children and adult patients. Eur J Trauma 2006; 32:548–554.
10. Wetzel RC, Burns RC. Multiple trauma in children: critical care overview. Crit Care Med 2002; 30:468–477.
11. Mackway Jones K, ed. Advanced Pediatric Life Support (APLS), 4th ed. Carlton, Victoria: BMJ Books, Blackwell Publishing Asia; 2005.
12. American College of Surgeons, Committee on Trauma. Advanced Trauma Life Support (ATLS), 7th ed. Chicago: American College of Surgeons; 2002.
13. National Association of Emergency Medical Technicians (U.S.), Pre-Hospital Trauma Life Support Committee; American College of Surgeons Committee on Trauma. PHTLS Prehospital Trauma Life Support, 6th ed. St. Louis MO: Elsevier; 2006.
14. Biaret D, Bingham R, Richmond S, et al. European resuscitation council guidelines for resuscitation, section 6. Pediatric life support. Resuscitation 2005; 67S1:S97–S133.
15. Hall JR, Reyes HM, Meller JF, et al. The outcome for children with blunt trauma is best at a pediatric trauma center. J Pediatr Surg 1996; 31:72–76.
16. American College of Emergency Physicians. The Pediatric Emergency Medicine Resource, revised 4th ed. 2007.
17. Kloppel R, Brock D, Kosling S, et al. Spiral computerized tomography diagnosis of abdominal seat belt injuries in children. Akt Radiol 1997; 7:19–22.

18. Lutz N, Nance ML, Kallan MJ, et al. Incidence and clinical significance of abdominal wall bruising in restrained children involved in motor vehicle crashes. J Pediatr Surg 2004; 39:972–975.

19. O'Donnell J, Ferguson LP, Beattie TF. Use of analgesia in a pediatric accident and emergency department following limb trauma. Eur J Emerg Med 2002; 9:5–8.

20 Morris KP, Forsyth RJ, Parslow RC, et al. UK pediatric traumatic brain injury study group, pediatric intensive care society study-group. Intracranial pressure complicating severe traumatic brain injury in children: monitoring and management. Intensive Care Med 2006; 32:1606–1612.

21. Loder RT, Gullahorn LJ, Yian EH, et al. Factors predictive of immobilization complications in pediatric polytrauma. J Orthop Trauma 2001; 15:338–341.

22. Balci AE, Kazez A, Erern S, et al. Blunt thoracic trauma in children: review of 137 cases. Eur J Cardiothorac Surg 2004; 26:387–392.

23. Delarue A, Merrot T, Fahkro A, et al. Major renal injuries in children: the real incidence of kidney loss. J Pediatr Surg 2002; 37:1446–1450.

24. Stylianos S. Compliance with evidence-based guidelines in children with isolated spleen or liver injury: a prospective study. J Pediatr Surg 2002; 37:453–456.

25. Jobst MA, Canty TG, Lynch FP. Management of pancreatic injury in pediatric blunt abdominal trauma. J Pediatr Surg 1999; 34:818–824.

26. Nance ML, Keller MS, Stafford PW. Predicting hollow visceral injury in the pediatric blunt trauma patient with solid visceral injury. J Pediatr Surg 2000; 35:1300–1303.

27. Magin MN, Erli HJ, Mehlhase K, et al. Multiple trauma in children: pattern of injury—treatment strategy—outcome. Eur J Pediatr Surg 1999; 9:316–324.

28. Dietz H-G, Schmittenbecher P, Slongo T, et al. AO Manual of fracture management. Elastic stable intramedullary nailing (ESIN) in children. Stuttgart: Thieme; 2005.

29. Vitale MG, Kessler MW, Choe JC, et al. Pelvic fractures in children—an exploration of practice and patient outcome. J Pediatr Orthop 2005; 25:581–587.

30. Hasler C, Jeanneret C. Wirbelsäulenverletzungen im Wachstumsalter. Orthopaede 2002; 31:65–73.

31. Rupprecht H, Mechlin A, Ditterich D, et al. Prognostic risk factors in children and adolescents with craniocerebral injuries with multiple trauma. Kongressbd Dtsch Ges Chir 2002; 119: 683–688.

32. Nau T, Ohmann S, Ernst E, et al. Psychopathologic deficits after polytrauma in childhood and adolescence. Wien Med Wochenschr 2003; 153:526–529.

33. Schalamon J, von Bismarck S, Schober PH, et al. Multiple trauma in pediatric patients. Pediatr Surg Int 2003; 19:417–423.

34. van der Sluis CK, Kingma J, Eisma WH, et al. Pediatric polytrauma: short-term and long-term outcomes. J Trauma 1997; 43:501–506.

Chapter 41

Management of Growth Plate Injuries

Franck Accadbled and Bruce K. Foster

Introduction

Treatment of acute growth plate injuries is determined by a prognostic evaluation of the radiographs. The Salter and Harris classification [1] is the most widely used and has been modified by Ogden [2] and more recently by Peterson [3]. The present Ogden classification includes nine major types with subclassifications. For practical purposes the intra-articular fracture line and the degree of initial chondroepiphyseal displacement determine management, as originally proposed by Poland in 1898 [4].

Once there is established growth plate injury, the treatment available is interpositional physiolysis after the method of Langenskiöld [5] with either fat, methyl methacrylate [6], or silastic [7]. Historically, established growth plate deformity with angulation and shortening of the bone has been treated by repeated corrective osteotomy, although transphyseal lengthening [8, 9] and callus distraction [10] can also be considered.

Embryology and Development

Mesenchyme condensations occur in the sixth week of intrauterine life. By the seventh week the condensations become cartilaginous and form anlages that resemble the bones that they will become. The matrix of the cartilage anlage begins to undergo calcification centrally. The periosteal bony cover also starts to be laid down through the process of intramembranous ossification [11].

During the ninth week, vessels invade the newly calcified matrix and begin to remodel the center of the cartilage anlage into bone. The process continues by forming two cartilage plates, one at each end of the bone [11]. The cartilage plates are called the growth plates (physes) and here the process of endochondral ossification responsible for longitudinal bone growth from 9 to 10 weeks' gestational age through to skeletal maturity takes place. The cartilaginous epiphysis at each end of the forming bone also undergoes calcification at a time specific for each bone. It ranges from near birth (e.g., head of the humerus and the proximal tibial epiphysis) to 10–11 years for the lateral epicondyle of the humerus [12].

Endochondral ossification is the process by which bone forms via a cartilaginous intermediary. The growth plate can be divided into at least three zones. The reserve zone is situated on the epiphyseal side of the plate and contains small, spherical cells randomly distributed throughout the zone. It is thought that these cells represent the stem cells which give rise to the chondrocytes in the proliferative zone. In their adjacent proliferative zone, chondrocytes undergo mitosis and are organized into elongated stacks of cells running parallel to the axis of bone growth [13]. Cells in the proliferative zone mature and eventually increase their volume many times in the hypertrophic region. The differentiation and maturation of the chondrocytes together with the associated changes within the matrix surrounding the cells is geared toward producing a microenvironment which encourages mineralization. This culminates in mineralization of the longitudinal septum around the terminal hypertrophic chondrocytes. The mineralized cartilage is then remodeled into true bone in the metaphysis (Fig. 41.1). Much of the process is controlled by growth factors, hormones, and binding proteins, which have the potential to activate or inactivate the growth factors.

Growth hormone has a global effect on physeal function throughout the body, but many growth factors act locally. Of particular interest are parathyroid hormone and parathyroid hormone-related protein (PTHrP) as they can inhibit the maturation of chondrocytes. It is postulated that physeal chondrocytes regulate the local production of PTHrP by secreting a protein (Indian Hedgehog). Indian Hedgehog protein stimulates the chondrocyte to produce PTHrP, which slows the maturation of proliferative chondrocytes to their hypertrophic form [14, 15].

F. Accadbled (✉)
Service de Chirurgie Orthopédique, Hôpital des Enfants, Toulouse, France

M. Benson et al. (eds.), *Children's Orthopaedics and Fractures*,
DOI 10.1007/978-1-84882-611-3_41, © Springer-Verlag London Limited 2010

Fig. 41.1 A diagrammatic view of the physis and similar histological view. Fractures occur at the weakest level between the hypertrophic and mineralization zones

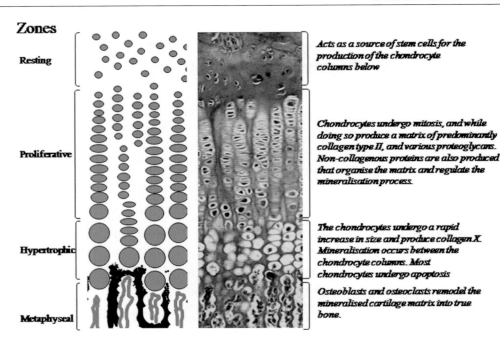

Zones

Resting — *Acts as a source of stem cells for the production of the chondrocyte columns below*

Proliferative — *Chondrocytes undergo mitosis, and while doing so produce a matrix of predominantly collagen type II, and various proteoglycans. Non-collagenous proteins are also produced that organise the matrix and regulate the mineralisation process.*

Hypertrophic — *The chondrocytes undergo a rapid increase in size and produce collagen X. Mineralisation occurs between the chondrocyte columns. Most chondrocytes undergo apoptosis*

Metaphyseal — *Osteoblasts and osteoclasts remodel the mineralised cartilage matrix into true bone.*

Blood Supply

Each growth plate is supplied by the epiphyseal artery from the epiphyseal side and by the main nutrient artery from the metaphyseal side [16].

The epiphyseal artery enters near the capsular insertion point, branches and feeds the numerous capillaries that terminate at the resting side of the physis [17]. While the epiphyseal artery is critical for physeal survival, the metaphyseal vessels are only required for physeal function. Ischemia resulting from damage or destruction of the epiphyseal vessels causes necrosis of the portion of the physis affected [18]. Depending upon the proportion involved, physeal growth can be abolished or differentially slowed leading to angular deformity.

The main nutrient artery enters the diaphysis and branches in the metaphysis to form many small capillaries whose terminal branches invade the matrix between the hypertrophic cells. Interruption to the metaphyseal supply results in a growth plate that can still synthesize cartilage, although mineralization of the cartilage is delayed until the vascular supply has recovered. Upon revascularization the physeal function often returns to normal [18].

Hence, minimizing epiphyseal vasculature injury is important during closed or open fracture reduction and during Langenskiöld procedures. As few pins and screws as possible should be inserted in the epiphysis.

Clinical Condition

Etiology

The junction between hypertrophic and mineralizing cartilage near the metaphysis is biomechanically the weakest point of an adolescent long bone and is therefore the most vulnerable to shearing injury [19]. However, uniform separation does not necessarily occur at that level as the fracture can propagate through different levels of the growth plate. At particular sites, such as the proximal femur, periosteal thinning toward the end of skeletal growth may also predispose to pathological fracture, allowing the upper femoral epiphysis to displace [20]. Hormonal imbalance, irradiation and, in the rat, experimental lathyrism are also contributory factors.

The propagation of the fracture line can occur at different sites through the growth plate, upon which the following classification proposed by Salter and Harris is based [1, 21] (Fig. 41.2).

Type I

There is complete separation of the epiphysis from the metaphysis without any osseous fracture. The growing cells of the physis remain with the epiphysis.

Fig. 41.2 Salter and Harris classification of a physeal fracture. Included here is the important type VI peripheral physeal lesion described by Rang (Reproduced from Rang [21])

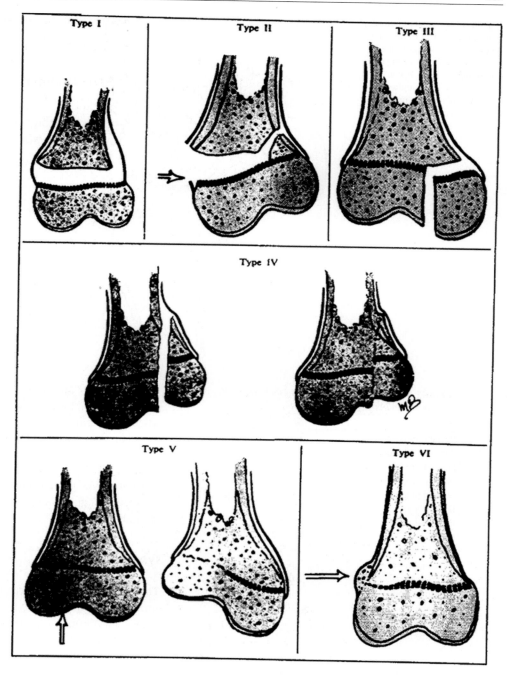

This type of injury occurs in early childhood when the physis is thick. It is also seen in pathological conditions with physeal separation, for example, scurvy, rickets, osteomyelitis, and endocrine imbalance [22]. Wide displacement is uncommon because the periosteal attachment remains intact. Reduction is not difficult, and the prognosis concerning future growth is excellent unless the epiphysis is intra-articular [23], when the blood supply may be damaged and lead to premature closure of the physis (Fig. 41.3).

Type II

The line of separation extends a variable distance along the physis and out through a triangle of metaphyseal bone (the Thurston-Holland sign radiographically). It is the most common type of fracture occurring in 73% of cases [24] (Table 41.1), usually in children over the age of 10 years. The periosteum is torn on the side opposite to the angulation but is intact on the concave side.

Fig. 41.3 Blood supply to the epiphysis. (**a**) The intra-articular epiphysis and physis of the proximal femur are prone to a vascular injury. (**b**) Epiphysis covered only by articular cartilage such as the proximal tibia is less prone to a vascular injury

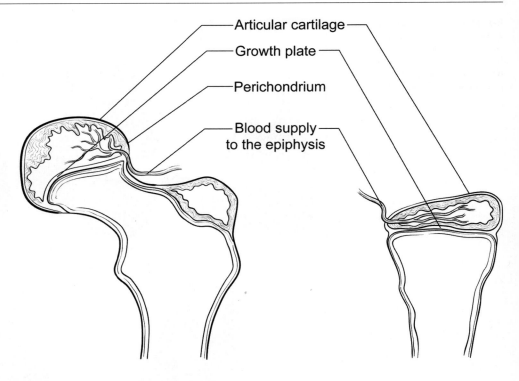

Articular cartilage

Growth plate

Perichondrium

Blood supply to the epiphysis

Table 41.1 Relative frequency of physeal injuries in each location [24]

Physis	No. of injuries (%)
Distal radius	100 (28.3)
Phalanges (fingers)	91 (25.8)
Distal tibia	33 (9.4)
Phalanges (toes)	25 (7.1)
Distal humerus	24 (6.8)
Distal ulna	16 (4.5)
Proximal radius	16 (4.5)
Metacarpals	15 (4.2)
Distal fibula	12 (3.4)
Proximal humerus	7 (2.0)
Metatarsals	5 (1.4)
Proximal tibia	4 (1.1)
Lateral clavicle	3 (0.9)
Proximal ulna	1 (0.3)
Distal femur	1 (0.3)
Total	353 (100.0)

The growing cartilage cells of the physis remain with the epiphysis. The prognosis concerning growth is excellent, provided the circulation to the epiphysis remains intact, which is usually the case.

Type III

The fracture, which is intra-articular, extends from the joint surface to the level of the hypertrophic cells of the physis, and then along the growth plate to its periphery.

The injury is uncommon, but when it occurs it is usually at the upper or lower tibial physis and is caused by intra-articular shearing forces.

Accurate reduction is essential to prevent osseous bar formation across the physis, and to restore a smooth joint surface.

As with type I and II injuries, provided the blood supply to the separated epiphysis is intact, the prognosis is good after accurate reduction.

Type IV

The fracture, which is intra-articular, extends from the joint surface through the epiphysis across the full thickness of the physis and through a portion of the metaphysis, producing complete discontinuity of epiphysis, physis, and metaphysis.

Perfect reduction of a type IV physeal injury is essential if growth and a smooth joint surface are to be restored.

Unless the fracture is undisplaced, open reduction is usually necessary. The physis must be accurately realigned to prevent bony union across the plate with resultant local premature cessation of growth. These fractures occur commonly at the lateral condyle of the humerus, the distal femoral physis, and the distal tibia (Fig. 41.6).

Type V

This relatively rare injury results from a severe crushing force applied through the epiphysis to one area of the physis. It occurs in joints that normally move in one plane only, such as the ankle or knee. At the ankle a severe abduction or adduction force may be applied to the foot, which normally only flexes or extends. The physis is crushed but displacement is unusual, so that the initial radiograph gives little indication of a fracture. The injury may be dismissed as a sprain but where there is localized physeal tenderness, compression of the physis should be suspected. It is postulated but unproven that the risk of premature cessation of growth may be reduced by protection from weight-bearing for 3 weeks.

Rang added the peripheral Ranvier zone injury [21]. This so-called type VI lesion is most commonly associated with a shearing or abrading open injury to the limb such as from a lawn mower or bicycle spoke (Fig. 41.2).

Pathology

Although growth arrest is most common following direct physeal trauma there are many other causes of premature arrest. Idiopathic or pathological avascular necrosis may predispose to growth arrest. For example, patients with Perthes' disease have a 17% incidence [25]. Avascular necrosis secondary to septic arthritis or traumatic hemarthrosis may predispose to growth arrest, as may frostbite, severe burns, irradiation, osteomyelitis, and cannulation injury [26]. The pathology of the growth plate lesion has been defined by experimental work [27]. Bone bridges span the physis with effects similar to the Phemister technique [28] for inducing growth arrest. Fibrous metaplasia may cause the specialized hyaline physeal cartilage to become non-functional fibrocartilage, particularly after avascular necrosis, and this makes treatment of the lesion by interposition methods more difficult.

Incidence

Traumatic and infective physeal injuries do not have a genetic basis. However, Rubin [29] classified the bone dysplasias based upon a dynamic appreciation of their specific structure and function, and observed that heredity did influence both growth and alignment in these conditions.

In reviewing our own experience, the incidence of physeal fractures has been estimated at 17.9% of all fractures that occur in children. They are more common in older children with a peak incidence at 11–12 years of age. Salter-Harris type I displacements made up 8.5% of injuries, type II fractures 73%, type III fractures 6.5%, type IV fractures 12%, and type VI fractures less than 1%. Complication rates are dependent upon the type of fracture, the actual physis involved, and the age of the patient. With accurate open

reduction the complication rate for premature union is in the order of 1–2% [24]. Salter-Harris type IV, V, and VI fractures are much more likely to cause bone bridge formation than types I–III. The distal femur and the proximal tibia account for only 3% of physeal fractures but are responsible for the majority of bone bridges [30]. Rohmiller et al. reported a premature physeal closure rate (PPC) of 39.6% in Salter-Harris II fractures of the distal tibial physis, if there had been insufficient reduction [31]. The site and mechanism of injury therefore can be as important as the degree of severity of the causative violence (Table 41.2).

Table 41.2 The incidence of physeal injuries among 353 children according to the Salter-Harris classification (reproduced from Mizuta et al. [24])

Physis	Salter-Harris type (Figures in parentheses are open fractures)					
	I	II	III	IV	V	Total
Distal radius	7	90 (1)	1	2	0	100
Phalanges (fingers)	7 (1)	74 (2)	8 (1)	2	0	91
Distal tibia	2 (1)	12	8	11	0	33
Phalanges (toes)	1	21 (2)	2	1	0	35
Distal humerus	0	0	0	24	0	24
Distal ulna	2 (1)	12	2	0	0	16
Proximal radius	3	13	0	0	0	16
Metacarpals	0	14	0	1	0	15
Distal fibula	4 (1)	8	0	0	0	12
Proximal humerus	2	5	0	0	0	7
Metatarsals	0	2	2	1	0	5
Proximal tibia	1	2	0	0	1	4
Lateral clavicle	0	1	0	0	0	1
Proximal ulna	0	1	0	0	0	1
Distal femur	0	1	0	0	0	1
Total	30 (4)	257 (5)	23 (1)	42	1	353
Incidence (%)	8.5	73.0	6.5	12	< 1	100

Diagnosis and Differential Diagnosis

Plain anteroposterior and lateral radiographs are the basic investigation in acute growth plate injuries. For complex fractures such as the triplane fracture of the distal tibia, computed tomography (CT) and magnetic resonance imaging (MRI) will give a clearer picture of the fracture pattern. In the patient where there is doubt about the appearance of epiphyseal centers, radiographs of the contralateral side are helpful. For the type V crushing injury there is currently no reliable method of evaluation, although MRI scans may give the earliest indication of growth plate dysfunction [32–35].

Established growth plate injury may be demonstrated by fine-cut CT, which shows the extent of the growth plate arrest. MRI also defines bony bridges but the cortical signal

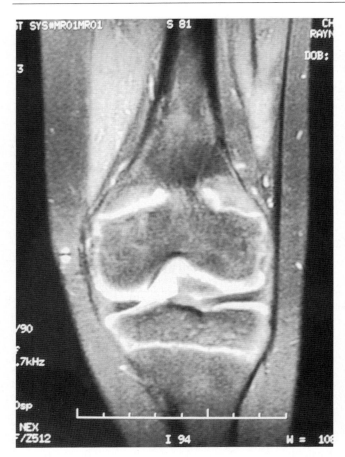

Fig. 41.4 Magnetic resonance image demonstrating central cancellous bone bridging of the distal femoral physis 2 years post injury (Courtesy of Professor Sales de Gauzy)

is similar to that of the cartilage signal and may be confusing (Fig. 41.4). It increases the sensitivity but for bone detail we still prefer CT examination.

The role of isotope bone scanning in determining the extent of growth plate injury is poorly defined. Initial experience suggested that it may be useful to use the bone scan apex view of the distal femur described by Howman Giles et al. [36]. In clinical practice today, however, isotope scanning is probably most helpful in establishing the diagnosis when a fracture is in doubt.

Treatment

Effect of Patient's Age

All patients with the same diagnosis have the same clinical management except for those at the end of their longitudinal growth. If longitudinal growth is almost complete, the need to rescue the physis is diminished. A clinical management flow diagram is presented in Fig. 41.5.

Time of Presentation

Early Presentation

The earlier guidelines of the Salter classification are appropriate. Closed reduction is recommended for all type I and II growth plate fractures. Closed reduction is indicated if the angular displacement is greater than 20° or if there is greater than 20% of epiphyseal displacement. If the child is less than 7 years of age, greater angulations and displacements may safely be accepted. As a working rule, if the limb looks deformed then reduction may be indicated. Follow-up at 1–2 weeks with radiographs is essential to confirm maintenance of reduction. Upper limb splintage is maintained for 4–6 weeks in an above-elbow cast and lower limb splintage for 6–8 weeks in an above-knee cast. Traditionally, weight-bearing is avoided for 2 weeks in the lower limbs.

Should closed reduction fail, judicious open reduction may be indicated. There are certain sites where remodeling is so great that open reduction is rarely indicated. The proximal humeral type II fracture, for example, rarely needs reduction unless there is skin tenting and soft tissue interposition.

Type III and IV injuries usually require open reduction, particularly if the intra-articular displacement is greater than 2 mm. CT, with or without three-dimensional reconstruction, may help to evaluate the displacement. During open reduction, particular care must be taken to prevent damage to the epiphyseal blood supply. Arthroscopically assisted reduction and minimal internal fixation therefore represent an interesting alternative [37]. Minimal internal fixation is best undertaken for 2–3 weeks using Kirschner wires that may or may not traverse the growth plate, or small compression screws placed transversely in the epiphyseal or metaphyseal fragments. Particular care should be taken to avoid damage to the zone of Ranvier. Obliquely placed wires or screws that cross the physis may induce bone bridge formation. Threaded pins or screws that traverse the physis will lead to bone bridge formation [30]. If there is a large metaphyseal fragment, 3.5 mm diameter screw fixation may be all that is required for the metaphyseal fragment. In the distal femur or the distal tibia particularly, intra-epiphyseal screws may provide the most rigid fixation. This is more clearly indicated toward skeletal maturity when avoiding plaster immobilization in addition to internal fixation diminishes joint stiffness (Fig. 41.6).

For comminuted type II, III, IV, and type VI physeal injuries, irrigation and debridement of grossly crushed physeal cartilage and interposition of fat at the time of open reduction and fixation may diminish the risk of bone bridging. The dissection should be restricted in order to reduce potential further damage that may in turn lead to instability

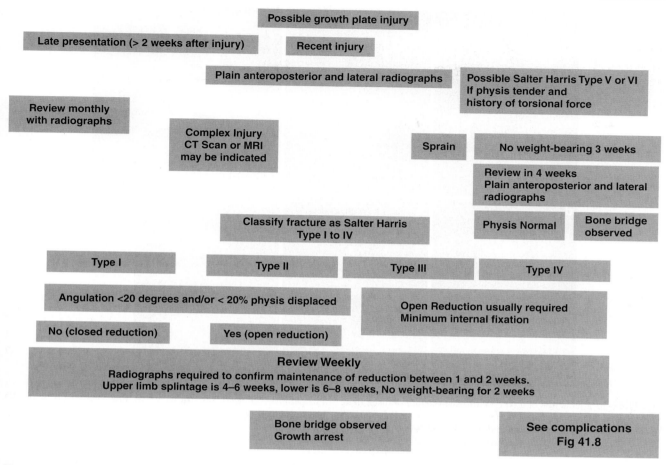

Fig. 41.5 The flow diagram covers the basics of the clinical management of physeal fractures

and deformity. In our experience, early surgical intervention is advisable. Later surgical procedures like osteotomies may need to be repeated until maturity (Fig. 41.7).[38].

Intermediate Presentation

The displaced growth plate fracture seen 2 weeks after injury always poses a management dilemma. Late closed manipulation may further injure the growth plate and it may be prudent to defer treatment and perform a realignment osteotomy later. However, if an open procedure is undertaken, a circumferential metaphyseal-periosteal release may allow gentle repositioning of the grossly displaced epiphysis.

Late Presentation

This is considered under "Salvage Procedures" below.

Complications

Early removal of Kirschner wires after open reduction and internal fixation should prevent pin track infection. For example, following lateral condylar elbow fractures the wires are removed after 2–3 weeks. Biodegradable implants made of synthetic polymers may obviate the need to remove implants but still prove problematical because of local inflammation or their mechanical characteristics. Nevertheless, biodegradable wires have been proved useful in animals and humans [39–46].

With fractures of the distal femoral and proximal tibial physes the risk of associated vascular injury needs to be emphasized. Similarly, compression of the median nerve may occur with markedly displaced distal radial injuries. The site of the growth plate injury is important prognostically. The distal femoral physis, for instance, is most at risk of bone bridge formation and significant premature arrest.

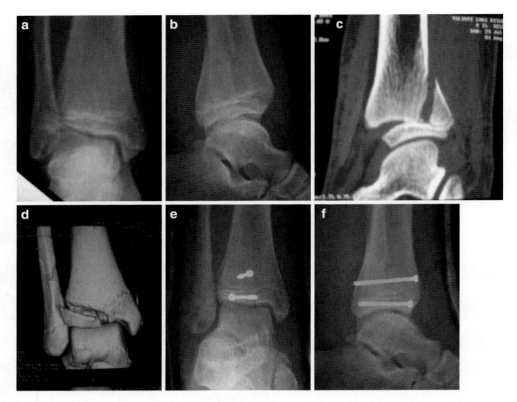

Fig. 41.6 Open reduction of a type IV triplane fracture of distal tibia. Preoperative planning assisted by CT evaluation. Interfragment screw fixation provides intra-epiphyseal and metaphyseal stable fixation. (**a**) Preoperative AP radiograph. (**b**) Preoperative lateral radiograph. (**c**) Preoperative CT scan, sagittal view. (**d**) Preoperative CT scan, 3D reconstruction. (**e**) Postoperative AP radiograph. (**f**) Postoperative lateral radiograph

Salvage Procedures

Once it has been established that bone growth is compromised, techniques used to correct the problem depend upon the physis involved and the age of the patient. Peterson has reviewed the treatment in detail [3, 30, 47]. A clinical flow diagram of the complications is presented in Fig. 41.8.

Possible treatment regimens are described below.

Conservative

If the physeal arrest has occurred near the end of skeletal growth, or in a physis whose contribution to the total length of the limb is minor, the need to excise the bone bridge is small. Limb-length discrepancy of upper limbs is very well tolerated and up to 2.5 cm is acceptable in the lower limbs [30].

Orthoses

Small disparities in lower limb length may be corrected with orthotic support.

Epiphysiodesis (Injured Physis)

Angular deformity in a limb that is almost at the end of skeletal growth may be reduced by destruction of the undamaged portion of the injured physis. This can be performed by placing a staple or screw across the physis. If the limb is already angulated, a corrective wedge osteotomy should be performed (see below).

Epiphysiodesis (Contralateral Physis)

Limb-length discrepancy can be reduced by premature closure of the corresponding physis on the adjacent leg. While this can be achieved by the placement of staples that span the physis on both the lateral and the medial side [48], percutaneous drill epiphysiodesis is now the favored procedure in our center. Screw fixation techniques are sometimes advocated.

Physiolysis

When the bone bridge is likely to lead to unacceptable deformity, the bone bridge itself can be surgically removed.

Fig. 41.7 (**a**) An illustrative case of a 6-year-old boy with a Gustillo compound grade 3 comminuted fracture of the right tibia and fibula sustained in a motor vehicle accident. The wound extended to the medial aspect of the ankle joint which was open. The growth plate of the distal medial tibia was abraded to the bone for 1 cm (*distal arrow*) as in a type VI Rang and Kessel physeal injury. (**b**) Initially the wound was debrided and the fracture stabilized with an external fixator. An acute Langenskiöld procedure was performed for the distal tibial growth plate injury. This included debridement of the exposed peripheral physis with a dental burr and fat interposition. Additionally a rectus abdominal free flap was carried out to cover the skeletal lesion, with splint thickness skin graft to the exposed muscles. The ruptured tibialis anterior tendon was repaired. (**c**) and (**d**) At 3 years 6 months after injury, radiograph confirmed ongoing physeal growth. (**e**) At 4 years and 6 months, CT showed peripheral growth plate repair. At final follow-up 5.5 years later there was no angular deformity of the leg. The distal tibial growth plate was open and the affected limb was 1.5 cm longer than the normal side [38]

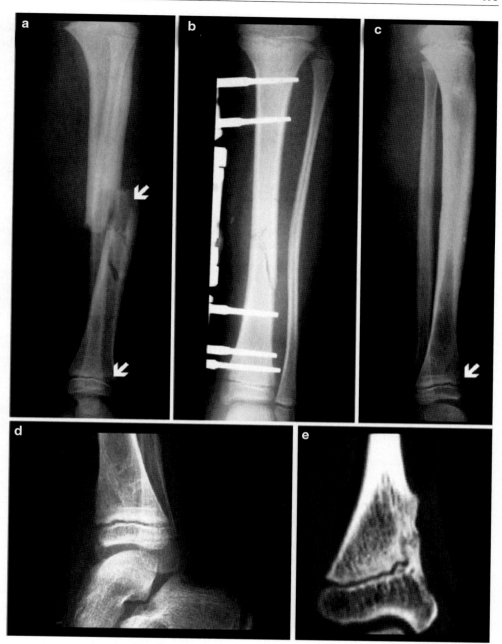

Angular deformity and shortening as a consequence of bone bridge formation can be substantially reduced by timely surgical intervention [24].

The management of growth arrest involves the assessment of angular deformity as well as the extent of the bone bridge. Langenskiöld recommends that, if angulation is greater than 25° at the time of the interpositional physiolysis, a concomitant osteotomy to correct the axis should be undertaken [49]. Interpositional physiolysis may be undertaken within 12 months of normal growth plate closure with an anticipation of correction of length and angulation.

In experimental peripheral growth arrest studies a bridge lesion of up to 17.2% of total physeal area can be treated successfully [50] (Table 41.3). With central lesions as much as 50% of the physeal area may be resected and still allow continued longitudinal growth [6, 49]. Growth arrest is reversed by creating a physiological non-union at the site of the tether so that the remaining physis continues to elongate. This is satisfactory if the critical area of physeal resection is not exceeded and the bone bridge does not reform.

Evaluation of the growth plate lesion is an essential part of the preoperative planning and is best undertaken by CT scans, and more recently by MRI. Physeal mapping using

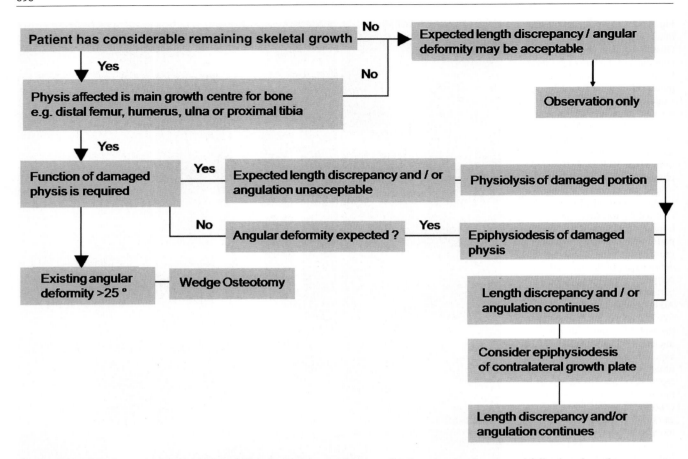

Fig. 41.8 The flow diagram covers the basics of clinical management of the complications that may be expected following physeal trauma

Table 41.3 Reversal by fat interposition in peripheral growth arrest (ovine model) [50]

Reversal groups	Entered	Completed	Sacrifice		Initial	Reversal success (%)
			CT % area of defect			
			3 Months	6 Months		
1 cm²	20	14	7	7	17.2 ± 2.2	85.7
2 cm²	15	11	7	4	28.4 ± 6.0	54.5
3 cm²	10	8	5	3	33.7 ± 7.2	50.0
			Not significant		P < 0.0001	

MRI has been demonstrated to be accurate and to offer excellent correlation with intraoperative findings [51–53].

Techniques of Surgery

For a peripheral lesion a longitudinal exposure is made at the anatomical site and, using image intensification, the lesion is identified from the metaphyseal side. After a subperiosteal dissection is made at that point the normal physis and Ranvier zone are identified (Fig. 41.9) using magnification and a dental burr. Damage to the normal growth plate is reduced by irrigation and the bone bridge is then resected completely. Usually fat can be taken from the wound edge to provide the interpositional material. To prevent migration, the fat is sutured to the epiphysis or the perichondrial ring [54]. Bone wax is placed on the bleeding metaphyseal and epiphyseal bone surfaces to reduce the hematoma. Klassen and Peterson [6] have recommended that methyl methacrylate be used as the interpositional material, and Bright [7] has recommended silastic anchored with Kirschner wires. The interpositional material should be anchored to the epiphysis to prevent recurrence [55].

The periosteum is excised at the level of the peripheral lesion to prevent peripheral bone bridge reformation. It is important to place a titanium wire or ball in the epiphysis and metaphysis for subsequent measurement of reconstitution of growth.

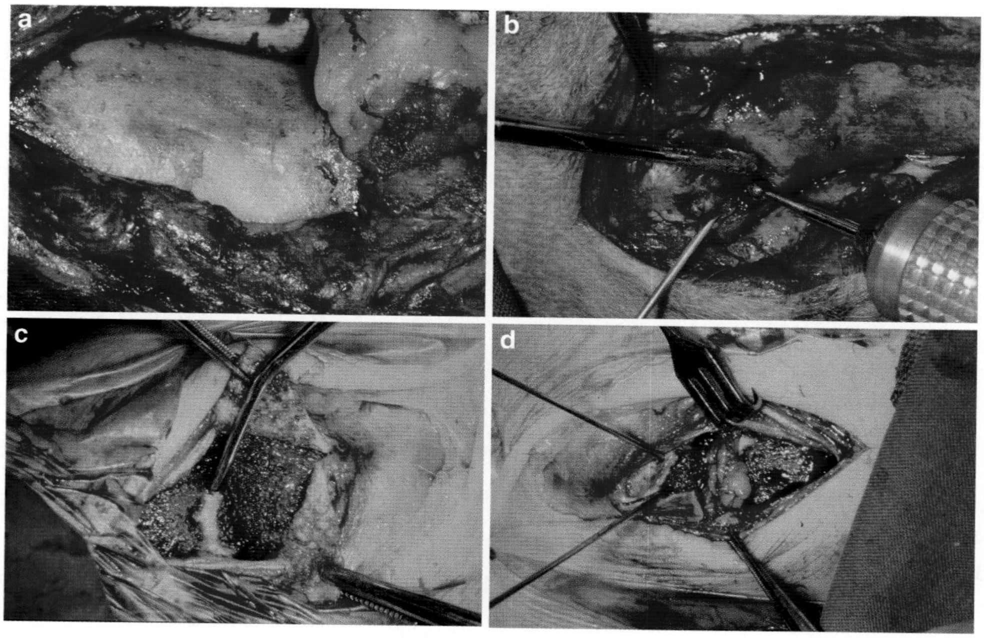

Fig. 41.9 Interpositional physeal surgery. Method of resection of physeal bar. (**a**) Identification of lesion. (**b**) Dental burr and irrigation resection. (**c**) Clear peripheral physeal line. (**d**) Fat transfer and suture to epiphysis

For central lesions the procedure is identical. A larger metaphyseal window is required and visualization of the central lesion is assisted greatly if a powerful light source is used. An arthroscopic cable will sometimes provide a good light source in the small cavity, combined with a dental mirror. Marsh et al. reported on the efficacy of alternating visualization with an arthroscope and burring under fluoroscopy[56].

The bone bridge, whether central or peripheral, may be of ivory cortical or of soft cancellous bone. An additional area that may be difficult to resect is a fibrocartilaginous, nonfunctional growth plate such as occurs after infection. The principal difficulty is to identify the normal ring of growth plate. Resection of the defect should be such that normal growth plate is left circumferentially. Immobilization in a plaster is unnecessary but weight-bearing should be reduced initially in order to prevent impaction fracture into the bone defect.

Limb Lengthening

The procedure of leg lengthening is tedious. It is reserved for the cases in which simple measures have failed. Its role is to regain limb function that is otherwise compromised due to length discrepancy and angular deformity. The procedure, which often takes months to complete, is prone to complications and is outlined in Chapter 24.

Conclusions and Future Developments

Physeal injury is common and usually easily diagnosed and treated. Failure to diagnose or to instigate the treatment can lead to significant clinical sequelae. The ability to predict which growth plate injury will lead to premature growth arrest and hence require more aggressive treatment remains a problem. The undiagnosed type V injury may present as a minor injury but may produce extensive arrest, such as a distal radial fracture with subsequent Madelung deformity.

Future developments will also depend upon biological interpositional materials, either physeal cell cultures or the transplantation of physeal cartilage into arrest locations.

Much research has been devoted to finding better ways to repair physeal injury. Most aim to replace the damaged portion with a new tissue.

This has been approached by physeal and chondrocyte transplantation [57–60]. Chondrocyte transplantation has also uncovered a need for better carrier substrates. Three-dimensional biocompatible matrices that enable chondrocyte embedding are slowly being established [61]. Although chondrocyte transplantation has had some success clinically, it still cannot replace large physeal defects. Some of the problems may arise from the inherent polarity of the physis. A physis that is rotated in its vascular bed will continue to produce "metaphyseal bone" on the epiphyseal side [62]. It is hard to envisage how a suspension of cells will determine its own polarity.

Lee et al. demonstrated the feasibility of muscle-based gene therapy and tissue engineering using direct adenovirus-mediated gene transfer to influence reconstruction in injured growth plates [63]. The release of IGF-1 protein after the direct transfer of the IGF-1 gene into the autologous muscle scaffold showed a supportive effect on the restoration of the injured growth plate. The application of mesenchymal stem cells (MSC) also demonstrated some promising results [64, 65].

Further research at the basic level is required. We believe that specific proteins such as growth factors may become key therapeutic tools in the treatment of physeal injuries. Proteins may be able to promote chondrocyte proliferation and migration into defectives zones. Other proteins may be able to inhibit bone bridge formation. However, although some growth factors such as the bone morphogenic proteins (BMPs) are being advocated in the treatment of non-union bone defects, none has yet been shown to aid healing of physeal defects.

References

1. Salter RB, Harris WR. Injuries involving the epiphyseal plate. J Bone Joint Surg [Am] 1963; 45-A: 587–622

2. Ogden JA. Skeletal growth mechanism injury patterns. J Pediatr Orthop.1982; 2:371–377.

3. Peterson H. Physeal injuries and growth arrest. In: Beaty JH, Kasser JR, eds. Rockwood and Wilkins' Fractures in Children. Philadelphia: Lippincott Williams & Wilkins; 2001:91–138.

4. Poland J. Separation of the epiphysis. London: Smith Elder; 1898.

5. Langenskiöld A. An operation for partial closure of an epiphysial plate in children, and its experimental basis. J Bone Joint Surg [Br] 1975; 57-B: 325–330.

6. Klassen RA, Peterson HA. Excision of physeal bars: The Mayo Clinic experience 1968–1978. Orthop Trans 1982; 6:65–75.

7. Bright RW. Operative correction of partial epiphyseal plate closure by osseous-bridge resection and silicone-rubber implant. An experimental study in dogs. J Bone Joint Surg [Am] 1974; 56-A: 655–664.

8. Monticelli G, Spinelli R. Distraction epiphysiolysis as a method of limb lengthening. III. Clinical applications. Clin Orthop Rel Res1981; 154:274–285.

9. De Bastiani G, Aldegheri R, Renzi Brivio L, et al. Chondrodiatasis-controlled symmetrical distraction of the epiphyseal plate. Limb lengthening in children. J Bone Joint Surg [Br] 1986; 68-B: 550–556.

10. Ilizarov GA, Soybelman LM. Some clinical and experimental data concerning bloodless lengthening of the lower extremities. Eksperimental'naya Khirurgiya i Anesteziologiya1969; 14:27–32.

11. Brighton CT. Longitudinal bone growth: the growth plate and its dysfunctions. Instruct Course Lect 1987; 36:3–25.

12. Kaufmann H. Appearance of secondary ossification centers. In: Lentner C, ed. Geigy Scientific Tables, Physical Chemistry, Composition of Blood, Hematology, Somatometric Data. Basle: Ciba-Geigy; 1984:316–318.

13. Johnstone EW, Leane PB, Kolesik P, et al. Spatial arrangement of physeal cartilage chondrocytes and the structure of the primary. J Ortho Sci 2000; 5:302–306.

14. Vortkamp A, Lee K, Lanske, B et al. Regulation of rate of cartilage differentiation by Indian hedgehog and PTH-related protein [see comments]. Science 1996; 273:613–622.

15. Kronenberg HM, Lanske B, Kovacs CS, et al. Functional analysis of the PTH/PTHrP network of ligands and receptors. Recent Prog Horm Res 1998; 53:283–301; discussion 301–303.

16. Harris W. Epiphysial injuries. AAOS Instruct Course Lect1958; 32B: 5.

17. Trueta J, Morgan JD. The vascular contribution to osteogenesis. I. Studies by the injection method. J Bone Joint Surg [Br] 1960; 42:97–109.

18. Trueta O, Amato VP. The vascular contribution to osteogenesis. III. Changes in the growth cartilage caused by experimentally induced ischaemia. J Bone Joint Surg [Br] 1960; 42:571–87.

19. Bright RW, Burstein AH, Elmore SM. Epiphyseal-plate cartilage. A biomechanical and histological analysis of failure modes. J Bone Joint Surg [Am] 1974; 56-A: 688–703.

20. Chung SM. The arterial supply of the developing proximal end of the human femur. J Bone Joint Surg [Am] 1976; 58-A: 961–970.

21. Rang M. The growth plate and its disorders. Edinburgh: Churchill Livingstone; 1969.

22. Salter RB. Textbook of Disorders and Injuries of the Musculoskeletal System. Baltimore: Williams and Wilkins; 1970.

23. Dale GG, Harris WR. Prognosis of epiphyseal separation. An experimental study. J Bone and Joint Surg [Br] 1958; 40:116–122.

24. Mizuta T, Benson W, Foster B, et al. Statistical analysis of the incidence of physeal injuries. J Pediatr Orthop 1987; 7:518–523.

25. Bowen JR, Schreiber FC, Foster BK, et al. Premature femoral neck physeal closure in Perthes' disease. Clin Orthop Rel Res1982; 171:24–29.

26. Macnicol MF, Anagnostopoulos J. Arrest of the growth plate after arterial cannulation in infancy [Br] 2000; 82-B: 172–175.

27. Johnson JTH, Southwick WO. Growth following transepiphyseal bone grafts. An experimental study to explain continued growth following certain fusion operations. J Bone Joint Surg [Am] 1960; 42-A: 1381–1395.

28. Phemister DB. Operative arrestment of longitudinal growth of bones in the treatment of deformities. J Bone Joint Surg [Am] 1933; 15:1–15.

29. Rubin P. Dynamic classification of bone dysplasias. Chicago: Year Book Medical Publishers; 1964.

30. Peterson HA. Partial growth plate arrest and its treatment. J Pediatr Orthop1984; 4:246–258.

31. Rohmiller MT, Gaynor TP, Pawelek J, et al. Salter-Harris I and II fractures of the distal tibia: does mechanism of injury relate to premature physeal closure? J Pediatr Orthop 2006; 26:322–328.

32. Smith BG, Rand F, Jaramillo D, et al. Early MR imaging of lower-extremity physeal fracture-separations: a preliminary report. J Pediatr Orthop 1994; 14:526–533.

33. White PG, Mah JY, Friedman L. Magnetic resonance imaging in acute physeal injuries. Skeletal Radio1994; 23:627–631.

34. Carey J, Spence L, Blickman H, et al. MRI of pediatric growth plate injury: correlation with plain film radiographs and clinical outcome. Skeletal Radiol 1998; 27:250–255.

35. Kamegaya M, Shinohara Y, Kurokawa M, et al. Assessment of stability in children's minimally displaced lateral humeral condyle fracture by magnetic resonance imaging. J Pediatr Orthop 1999; 19:570–572.

36. Howman Giles R, Trochei M, Yeates K, et al. Partial growth plate closure: apex view on bone scan. J Pediatr Orthop 1985; 5: 109–111.

37. Laffosse JM, Cariven P, Accadbled F, et al. Osteosynthesis of a triplane fracture under arthroscopic control in a bilateral case. Foot Ankle Surg 2007; 13:83–90.

38. Foster BK, John B, Hasler C. Free fat interpositional graft in acute physeal injuries. The anticipatory Langenskiöld procedure. J Pediat Orthop 2000; 20:282–285.

39. Bostman O, Vainionpaa S, Hirvensalo E, et al. Biodegradable internal fixation for malleolar fractures. A prospective randomised trial. J Bone Joint Surg Br 1987; 69:615–619.

40. Bostman O, Makela EA, Tormala P, et al. Transphyseal fracture fixation using biodegradable pins. J Bone Joint Surg Br 1989; 71:706–707.

41. Bostman O, Hirvensalo E, Partio E, et al. [Resorbable rods and screws of polyglycolide in stabilizing malleolar fractures. A clinical study of 600 patients]. Unfallchirurg 1992; 95:109–112.

42. Bostman O, Paivarinta U, Partio E, et al. Degradation and tissue replacement of an absorbable polyglycolide screw in the fixation of rabbit femoral osteotomies. J Bone Joint Surg Am 1992; 74: 1021–1031.

43. Makela EA, Bostman O, Kekomaki M, et al. Biodegradable fixation of distal humeral physeal fractures. Clin Orthop Relat Res 1992; 283:237–243.

44. Partio EK, Hirvensalo E, Bostman O, et al. [Absorbable rods and screws: a new method of fixation for fractures of the olecranon]. Int Orthop 1992; 16:250–254.

45. Partio EK, Hirvensalo E, Partio E, et al. Talocrural arthrodesis with absorbable screws, 12 cases followed for 1 year. Acta Orthop Scand 1992; 63:170–172.

46. Hara Y, Tagawa M, Ejima H, et al. Application of oriented poly-L-lactide screws for experimental Salter-Harris type 4 fracture in distal femoral condyle of the dog. J Vet Med Sci 1994; 56:817–822.

47. Peterson H. Treatment of physeal bony bridges by means of bridge resection and interposition of cranioplasty. In: Pablos J, ed. Surgery of the Growth Plate. Madrid: S.A Ediciones Ergon; 1998:299–307.

48. Zuege RC, Kempken TG, Blount WP. Epiphyseal stapling for angular deformity at the knee. J Bone Joint Surg Am 1979; 61:320–329.

49. Langenskiöld A. Surgical treatment of partial closure of the growth plate. J Pediatr Orthop 1981; 1:3–11.

50. Foster B. Epiphyseal plate repair using fat interposition to reverse physeal deformity. An Experimental study. MD, Paediatrics. Adelaide: The University of Adelaide; 1989.

51. Borsa JJ, Peterson HA, Ehman RL. MR imaging of physeal bars. Radiology 1996; 199:683–687.

52. Ecklund K, Jaramillo D. Patterns of premature physeal arrest: MR imaging of 111 children. AJR Am J Roentgenol 2002; 178: 967–972.

53. Sailhan F, Chotel F, Guibal AL, et al. Three-dimensional MR imaging in the assessment of physeal growth arrest. Eur Radiol 2004; 14:1600–1608.

54. Hasler CC, Foster BK. Secondary tethers after physeal bar resection: a common source of failure? Clin Orthop Relat Res 2002; 405:242–249.

55. Jouve JL, Guillaume JM, Frayssinet P, et al. Growth plate behavior after desepiphysiodesis: experimental study in rabbits. J Pediatr Orthop 2003; 23:774–779.

56. Marsh JS, Polzhofer GK. Arthroscopically assisted central physeal bar resection. J Pediatr Orthop 2006; 26:255–259.

57. Foster BK, Hansen AL, Gibson GJ, et al. Reimplantation of growth plate chondrocytes into growth plate defects in sheep. J Orthop Res 1990; 8:555–564.

58. Hansen AL, Foster BK, Gibson GJ, et al. Growth-plate chondrocyte cultures for reimplantation into growth-plate defects in sheep. Characterization of cultures. Clin Orthop Relat Res 1990; 256:286–298.

59. Boyer MI, Danska JS, Nolan L, et al. Microvascular transplantation of physeal allografts. J Bone Joint Surg Br 1995; 77:806–814.

60. Lee EH, Chen F, Chan J, et al. Treatment of growth arrest by transfer of cultured chondrocytes into physeal defects. J Pediatr Orthop 1998; 18:155–160.

61. Sims CD, Butler PE, Casanova R, et al. Injectable cartilage using polyethylene oxide polymer substrates. Plast Reconstr Surg 1996; 98:843–850.

62. Abad V, Uyeda JA, Temple HT, et al. Determinants of spatial polarity in the growth plate. Endocrinology 1999; 140:958–962.

63. Lee CW, Martinek V, Usas A, et al. Muscle-based gene therapy and tissue engineering for treatment of growth plate injuries. J Pediatr Orthop 2002; 22:565–572.

64. Mc Carthy R. Stem cell repair of physeal cartilage. PhD Thesis. Adelaide: The University of Adelaide; 2007.

65. Xian CJ, Foster BK. Repair of injured articular and growth plate cartilage using mesenchymal stem cells and chondrogenic gene therapy. Curr Stem Cell Res Ther 2006; 1:213–229.

Chapter 42

Birth and Non-accidental Injuries

Peter J. Witherow†, Michael K.D. Benson, and Jacqueline Y.Q. Mok

Part I: Birth Injuries

Peter J. Witherow and Michael K.D. Benson

General Considerations

Introduction

The fracture patterns in early infancy differ from those in later childhood and adult life [1]. A knowledge of the infant's bony anatomy helps in understanding how, where, and why fractures occur, particularly in the low-velocity, low-energy skeletal injuries seen in birth trauma and child abuse.

Anatomy

The physis or growth plate tends to be weakest in the hypertrophic and calcifying zones three and four except in infancy: the plane of greatest weakness is then through the ossifying calcified cartilage columns in the metaphysis rather than the deeper layers of the physis. *Fracture separations, therefore, tend to take off a thin shell of juxta-physeal bone.* Peripherally there is a small indentation around the resting and proliferating parts of the growth plate, the groove of Ranvier [2], which contains a zone of increased cellularity. This is associated with bone deposition at the interface between the perichondrium and the physis, producing a thin cuff of bone described by Lacroix as the perichondrial "bone bark" which extends a few millimeters beyond the physis–metaphysis junction, reinforcing it. There is then the zone of bone resorption to establish proper metaphyseal tubulation before laminar bone is deposited at the metaphyseal–diaphyseal junction.

This zone of resorption is associated with a honeycomb-like surface which, particularly in the young infant, represents a point of weakness [3].

The shafts of the neonate's long bones are composed largely of woven bone as Haversian systems are relatively under-developed at birth.

The child's periosteum is thick. It is continuous and densely adherent with the perichondrium of the chondroepiphysis. In the fenestrated area of metaphyseal remodeling, the periosteum is also quite adherent to the fibro-vascular tissue of the inter-trabecular marrow spaces. This stabilizes those metaphyseal fractures which follow the plane of weakness adjacent to the diaphyseal side of the physis so that they tend to heal with minimal subperiosteal new bone. Once this periosteal–bone bond at the metaphysis is broken, however, the loosely applied diaphyseal periosteum can be widely stripped and extensive subperiosteal new bone forms (Fig. 42.1).

Biomechanics

The bone of the neonate and infant is more flexible than that of the older child or adult, although it is not as strong. The load–deformation curve has a long plastic deformation region prior to failure, a characteristic that slows the rate of crack propagation [4]. In the metaphysis and also in the diaphysis of young children, there is relatively little dense lamellar bone and the surface of the propagating crack tends to be irregular rather than relatively smooth. Greater energy is required to drive the fracture line and this restricts its extent.

P.J. Witherow (✉)
Bristol Royal Hospital for Sick Children, Bristol, UK

† It is sad to record the death of Peter J. Witherow, an outstanding children's doctor.

M. Benson et al. (eds.), *Children's Orthopaedics and Fractures*,
DOI 10.1007/978-1-84882-611-3_42, © Springer-Verlag London Limited 2010

Fig. 42.1 Extensive periosteal reaction following reduction and pin fixation of distal femoral epiphysiolysis in a newborn. This is the post-operative radiograph of the little girl's injury shown in Fig. 42.6

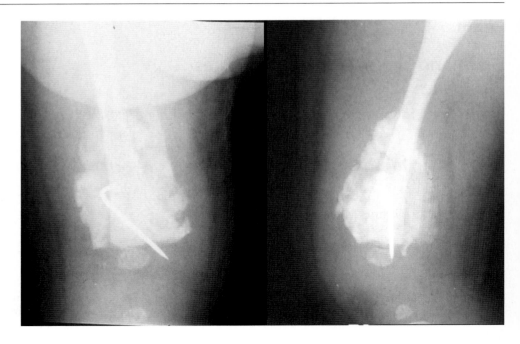

Fracture patterns

Transverse and spiral fractures of the shafts of the long bones occur as in adults and the majority are complete fractures. Incomplete spiral fractures can occur in toddlers, particularly in the tibia, but also sometimes in the femur.

Physeal fracture patterns change as chondroepiphyses mature (only the distal femur regularly has an ossific nucleus at the time of birth): Salter–Harris type I injuries are common in infants; types II, III, and IV become more likely as secondary ossification centers develop and plate undulations enlarge. After the neonatal period, a peripheral fragment which is backed up by the perichondral bone ring of Lacroix frequently remains, with the epiphysis forming the chip or bucket handle appearance seen on radiographs.

Greenstick fractures occur with low-velocity, low-energy injuries when there is failure in tension on one side with plastic deformation or buckling on the other. The woven bone of the young child can also fail largely in compression, which gives rise to metaphyseal torus or buckle fractures usually occurring at the junction between metaphysis and diaphysis, where the transition between the flexible fenestrated and the stiffer cortical bone produces stress concentration.

Healing

The rate of growth of long bones in the first year of life, although decaying, will not be approached again until puberty. Compared with the adult the young child's bones are more vascular and more porous with increased endosteal and periosteal osteogenic potential.

In the neonate, diaphyseal fractures are frequently sticky at a week and stable at three: a toddler may take twice as long to reach the same end points. Remodeling occurs by a combination of periosteal appositional growth and resorptive remodeling together with differential epiphyseal growth.

The potential for remodeling is greatest in the child's first year. Malalignment in the plane of the adjacent joint tends to be best corrected and rotational malalignment worst.

The metaphysis is well vascularized: it is a region of intense bone deposition and remodeling activity and fractures usually heal rapidly.

Birth Injuries

Introduction

Advances in obstetric practice, particularly the more widespread use of Caesarean section to deliver babies presenting by the breech and the better assessment of fetal maturity, have led to a decrease in both the number and the severity of birth injuries. Bruising and lacerations are associated with difficult delivery and episiotomy. Cephalhematoma is common after non-instrumental, vacuum, and forceps deliveries. Brachial plexus palsies may or may not be associated with clavicular fracture. Facial palsy, almost always transient, can follow forceps delivery. Some injuries may be serious and pose difficult problems of diagnosis and treatment.

Incidence

The combined incidence of fractures and brachial plexus injuries has fallen steadily in developed countries: 20 per thousand in the 1930s [5], 7 per thousand in the 1950s [6], and a current level of approximately 2–3 per thousand [7]. The clavicle is most commonly injured followed by the brachial plexus, the humerus, and the femur.

Cervical cord injuries are often present in fatal cases [8], but unidentified fractures of the cervical spine associated with more limited cord or root damage occur more frequently than is appreciated.

The risk of birth injury is increased if manipulation is needed at delivery, if the baby's weight is over 4.5 kg [7], and following breech delivery. Prolonged labor, dystocia, and prematurity are additional risk factors. Finally fractures are more likely in inflexible children such as those with arthrogryposis (Fig. 42.2).

Etiology

In vertex presentations cervical cord injuries can occur during instrumental rotation of the head from occipito-posterior to anterior in the mid-cavity. They can also result if strong head traction is used to deliver arrested shoulders or, in breech presentations, if heavy traction is used to deliver the after-coming head.

Forceful groin traction during delivery of the extended breech can result in femoral shaft fractures. Humeral fractures may be caused in breech babies when bringing down the arms by hooking a finger into the axilla, particularly when there is shoulder dystocia or the arms are in the nuchal position. Fractures can occur even during Caesarean section delivery [9].

It must be borne in mind that fractures or dislocations may develop in utero. The dislocated hip present at birth may have developed in the later stages of pregnancy, particularly if there were uterine abnormalities, more than one fetus,

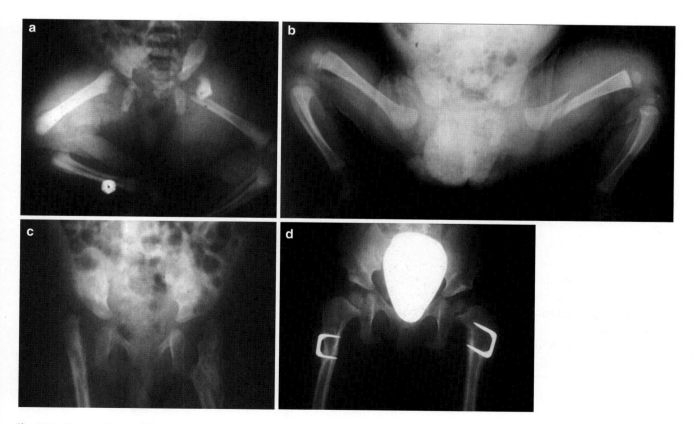

Fig. 42.2 Proximal femoral fracture in a neonate delivered by breech; the child has arthrogryposis and bilateral hip dislocation in addition. (**a**) Initial image. (**b**) In Pavlik harness. (**c**) Fracture union at 5 weeks. (**d**) Following bilateral open hip reduction and femoral shortening at 12 months

or deficient liquor. The dislocated knee similarly reflects a cramped intra-uterine breech position with the knees hyperextended. Fractures may occur antenatally, particularly with severe osteogenesis imperfecta, and are readily diagnosed with routine antenatal ultrasound scans.

Specific Injuries

Clavicle

Clavicular fractures account for 40–50% of all birth injuries. The fracture usually occurs in the mid-third of the bone and is commonly greenstick, although it may be complete and either transverse or oblique. Both shoulder dystocia and large birth weight are risk factors [10]. Most clavicle fractures follow vertex deliveries. Complete fractures of the clavicle are recognized by pseudoparalysis of the ipsilateral arm and pain on handling, but greenstick fractures may not become apparent until 2–3 weeks from the time of delivery when the fracture callus mass becomes obvious.

It is important to exclude an associated brachial plexus palsy because 5% of clavicular fractures are associated with plexus damage [10] and 13% of infants with brachial plexus palsy have a fractured clavicle [11]. It may be difficult to rule out neural injury in the first few days after birth as pain may produce pseudoparalysis or an asymmetrical Moro reflex. The diagnosis normally becomes clear by the end of the first week as the clavicular fracture firms up. Other conditions to be considered in the differential diagnosis of pain around the shoulder are upper humeral osteomyelitis and separation of the proximal humeral epiphysis. Both of these can be differentiated by careful clinical examination.

Congenital pseudarthrosis of the clavicle, although rare, should not be forgotten [12] (see Chapter 22). The abnormality may be noted shortly after birth or, more significantly, after discharge home when questions of undiagnosed birth trauma and of possible child abuse may be raised. The pseudarthrosis, unless very rarely bilateral, is on the opposite side to the heart, the bone ends are smooth on radiographs without callus formation, and there is no local tenderness.

Most fractured clavicles need no treatment apart from careful handling. If the fracture is displaced and the baby is in pain, a simple sling made from a crêpe bandage is all that is required.

Shoulder and Proximal Humerus

In the neonate and young infant the junction between the metaphysis and the physis is relatively weak and susceptible to rotational injury. The joint capsule and ligaments fail very infrequently so that dislocations are rare. Most apparent dislocations of the shoulder are therefore fracture separations between the cartilaginous head of the humerus and the metaphysis. This injury produces pain with pseudoparalysis, local swelling, and tenderness around the shoulder. Crepitus is often palpable [13].

The radiographic appearances mimic dislocation because the chondroepiphysis usually lacks an ossific center in the neonate. If there is any uncertainty, ultrasonography (Fig. 42.3) or arthrography can help to confirm that the humeral head is located in the glenoid [14].

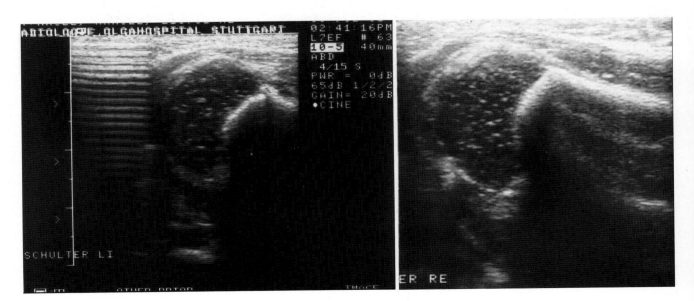

Fig. 42.3 US of proximal humeri in a newborn. Note the left-humeral epiphysiolysis

Treatment is by immobilizing the arm in internal rotation with a sling and swathe. Periosteal new bone appears between the sixth and tenth days and immobilization should be continued for 2–3 weeks.

Distal Humerus and Elbow

Again, dislocation is extremely uncommon, although medial dislocation of the radial head due presumably to forced pronation has been reported [15]. The apparent posterior dislocation is therefore a fracture separation of the distal chondroepiphysis [16, 17] (Fig. 42.4).

Local swelling, tenderness, and possibly crepitus are evident despite the normal relationship between the epicondyles and the tip of the olecranon. The radiologic appearances suggest a posteromedial dislocation but the proximal ends of the radius and ulna lie too close to the lower end of the humerus as the spacer effect of the chondroepiphysis is missing. Ultrasound or arthrography will confirm the diagnosis.

Treatment should be by re-alignment with splintage of the elbow in a sling and swathe or a posterior slab for 2–3 weeks. Recovery is usually very satisfactory.

Humeral and Femoral Shaft Fractures

Most fractures are mid-third, transverse, and complete (Fig. 42.5). For the humerus, immobilization with the forearm across the chest is needed for 2–3 weeks. For the femur, properly applied and supervised Bryant's traction can be used until the fracture is reasonably firm at about 1 week, followed by a further week or two in a plaster spica. Treatment is simple and satisfactory also in a Pavlik harness. If the fracture occurs in a baby who was in the extended breech position in utero, the proximal fragment tends to flex strongly and marked angular malunion will follow if this is not appreciated. Although angular malunions of up to 40° will normally correct quite rapidly with growth, this problem can be avoided by immobilizing the baby in the squat position in a spica cast after 5–7 days of traction.

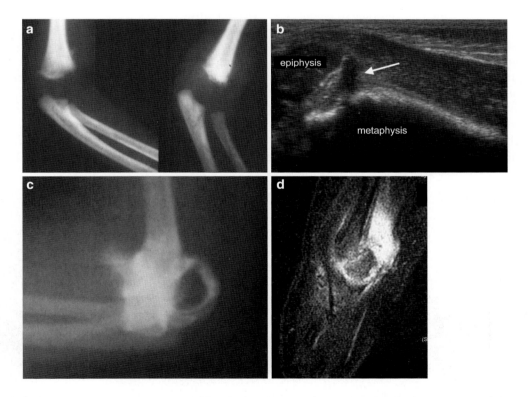

Fig. 42.4 Fracture-separation of distal humeral epiphysis at birth. (**a**) Plain radiograph at 6 days. Early subperiosteal ossification is developing. The alignment is wrong but the lack of epiphyseal ossification makes understanding difficult. (**b**) Ultrasound confirms the displaced epiphysis. (**c**) Lateral view of arthrogram: epiphyseal displacement is even clearer. MRI confirms displacement and demonstrates huge hematoma

Fig. 42.5 Short oblique humeral fracture seen shortly after birth. (**a**) The initial appearance. (**b**) Healing at 3 weeks

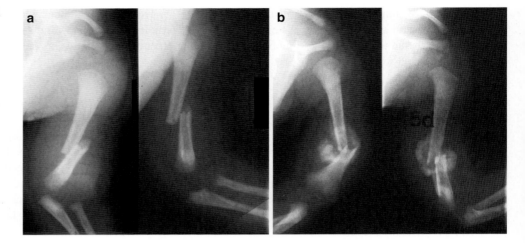

Overlap and angulatory malunion normally correct quite quickly and full functional recovery is the rule. However, rotational malalignment should be corrected whenever possible to prevent long-term abnormality [18].

Proximal Femur

Fracture separation of the upper femoral epiphysis is uncommon but can be confused with developmental dysplasia. The leg lies flexed, abducted, and externally rotated at the hip. There is local swelling and pain on gentle examination. The radiographic appearances suggest congenital dislocation or proximal femoral dysplasia. However, the acetabular appearance is normal (acetabular angle below 30°). The metaphysis tends to buttonhole anteriorly and laterally through the torn periosteum, leaving an intact posterior hinge [19]. Ultrasound will confirm that the femoral head is in the acetabulum and an arthrogram can be carried out if doubt

persists. The displacement can usually be reduced by putting the leg in abduction, internal rotation, and slight flexion. Immobilization in a spica in this position or treatment with overhead traction in abduction minimize the risk of late femoral neck retro-version and coxa vara.

Distal Femur

Separation of the distal chondroepiphysis can occur, particularly after breech delivery (Fig. 42.6). This is usually incomplete and produces a picture similar to that seen in child abuse with varying degrees of periosteal stripping. Assessment of the degree of displacement is easier at the knee than it is at the elbow because the epiphyseal ossific centre is present in most term infants [20]. Differentiation from congenital dislocation (see Chapter 29) is usually straightforward (Fig. 42.7).

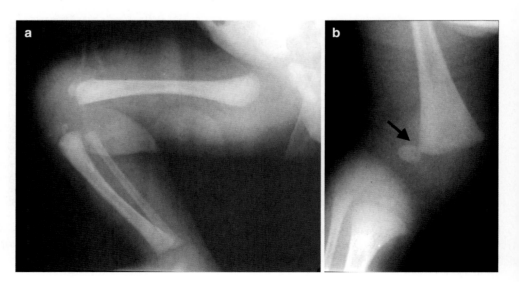

Fig. 42.6 Fracture separation of distal femoral epiphysis. Ossification makes it easier to appreciate the displacement. (**a**) Lateral and (**b**) AP knee radiographs demonstrate the shear injury

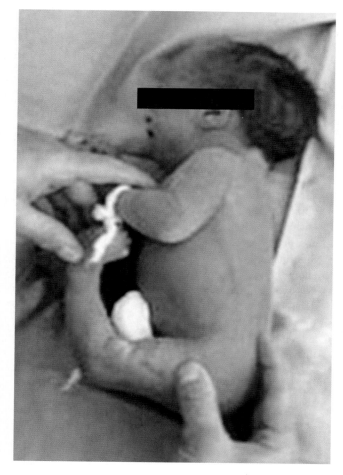

Fig. 42.7 Infant with knee dislocation related to intrauterine position and not to a birth injury

Distal Tibia

Posterior epiphyseal displacement occasionally occurs with hyperflexion of the foot. The deformity is apparent and is associated with swelling and tenderness. It should not be confused with simple equinus deformity. Plain radiographs demonstrate malalignment but the injury is better demonstrated by ultrasound which is also useful to monitor reduction. Healing is accompanied by extensive periosteal new bone. The prognosis is excellent.

Cervical Spine

Cervical cord and cervical vertebral injuries are most likely to occur during breech delivery when there is difficulty with the after-coming head or in vertex deliveries when there is a shoulder dystocia (see Chapter 52).

The historical experiments of Duncan [21] demonstrated that the cervical spine tends to fail when sustained loads of the order of 100 lb (45 kg) are applied. In traction the meninges and the cord usually fail before the vertebrae [22]. Cervical cord injury has been implicated in up to 10% of infant deaths which occur at the time of delivery. Cervical spine injuries are normally associated with marked dystocia and sometimes the obstetrician feels a snap or "give" during traction to deliver the after-coming head in breech deliveries or the shoulder in vertex presentations.

Vertebral injuries do occur [23] and may be associated with respiratory distress or brachial plexus palsy. The mode of vertebral failure is usually a fracture-separation between the body and the physis of the vertebral end plate. Because the facet joints are relatively horizontal in infancy, cervical fractures are both unstable and easily reduced in extension.

The normal failure mode is through the upper vertebral end plate with forward displacement of the more cephalad vertebra at this level. Rarely, the displacement may be posterior with a vertical separation at the body-arch synchondroses.

Because of the relative prominence of the occiput in the infant, babies with cervical spine injuries should be nursed supine on a sponge support with a hollow for the back of the head. If they are nursed on a flat surface, the cervical spine is brought into flexion and displacement at the fracture site increased (see Chapter 52).

Differential Diagnosis of Neonatal Injury

The neonate tends to lie in the fetal flexed posture and, when awake, normal limb mobility is evident. Abnormal immobility of arm or leg is due either to true weakness from brachial plexus or spinal cord injury or to pseudoparalysis which occurs when the limb is painful. In the first few days of life the diagnosis is between plexus injury and clavicular fracture or epiphyseal fracture separation, bearing in mind that both conditions can co-exist. After the first few days, osteomyelitis or septic arthritis must also be considered. Infantile osteomyelitis has a propensity to cause physeal damage with partial growth arrest so that prompt treatment is essential (see Chapter 10). Complete cervical spinal cord damage produces tetraplegia and the diagnosis is obvious. Incomplete cord damage may be mistaken for spinal muscular atrophy, myotonia congenita, or hypoxic—ischemic brain damage; it should be appreciated that radiographs are usually normal. Clearly limb weakness may also be caused by cerebral palsy.

Acknowledgment It is a pleasure to record my thanks to Klaus Parsch and David Wilson for some of the images and to Paul Cooper, exemplary photographer, at the Nuffield Orthopaedic Centre NHS Trust.

Part II: Non-Accidental Injuries

Jacqueline Y.Q. Mok

Introduction

Child abuse involves acts of commission or omission which directly or indirectly result in harm to the child and affect its normal development into healthy adulthood. The prevalence is difficult to measure as events tend to be unreported by children and some professionals are reluctant to recognize the nature of the injury. Neglect remains the commonest form of abuse. The phrase "non-accidental injury" (NAI) is used to describe physical abuse in children. Physical abuse includes hitting, shaking, throwing, poisoning, burning or scalding, drowning, and suffocating. It may also result from fabricating or inducing illness in the child.

Most children who have been physically abused present with cutaneous injuries and fractures. If non-accidental injury is not recognized, there is the risk of further injury with significant morbidity and mortality. The risk of subsequent injury may be as high as 20% and of death 5% [24]. Safeguarding children from harm and promoting their well-being is the responsibility of all doctors, whether or not they work directly with children. Therefore all doctors should be familiar with national and local child protection policies and procedures and act on them if there is any suspicion of abuse [25, 26]. Most errors are caused either by not sharing information or by not revising an assessment when new information becomes available.

Doctors working in Accident and Emergency (A & E) departments who see children with fractures regularly miss indicators of abuse. Taitz et al. [27] analyzed the medical records of all children below the age of 3 years who were treated for a long bone fracture in a tertiary children's hospital. The mean age of 100 children who presented with 103 fractures was 21.6 months, with 14 patients younger than 12 months. Thirty-one children were considered to have indicators suspicious of abuse, but only one child was referred to child protection services for further evaluation.

Diagnosis

Recognition

The history of the injury may be inappropriate and may change if the initial explanation is rejected or more injuries come to light. Factors that should alert the clinician to suspect non-accidental injury are the following:

- History which is vague, inconsistent, and discrepant with clinical findings or the child's developmental stage.
- History which is unexplained; the event happened in the absence of witnesses, or a sibling is blamed for the injury.
- Significant delay between injury and seeking medical attention, without credible explanation.
- Evasive or aggressive responses from the parent when details of injury are sought.
- Presence of other injuries.
- Evidence of frank neglect—e.g., non-organic failure to thrive, lack of hygiene.
- Previous concerns regarding child or sibling(s)—e.g., lack of care, unusual injuries, repeated attendances at A&E.

Risk Factors

Child abuse and neglect usually result from interplay between several risk and protective factors. The risk factors identified [28] are shown in Table 42.1. The risk of recurrence following an index incident is high. Hindley et al. [29] reviewed the evidence base for predicting those children at highest risk of recurrent maltreatment. Rates of recurrence were difficult to calculate due to differing follow-up times but ranged from 3.5 to 22.2% at 6 months. The time of greatest risk was the first month after an index episode. Important predictors of recurrence were the number of previous episodes of maltreatment, neglect, parental conflict, and parental mental health problems.

Cutaneous Injuries

Bruises

The commonest non-accidental injury to soft tissues is bruising. Any part of the body is vulnerable. Accidental bruises are related to increased mobility. A systematic review [30] reported accidental bruises in fewer than 1% of babies who were not independently mobile, 17% of infants who were just mobile, 53% of walkers, and the majority of school-aged

Table 42.1 Risk Factors for Child Abuse

Parental background	Socio-economic environment	Family environment	Child characteristics
Young parents	Poverty	High parity	Unintended pregnancy
Low educational attainment	Mother unemployed	Single mother	Low birth weight
Past psychiatric history	Poor social networks	Reported domestic violence	Few positive attributes reported
History of abuse in childhood		Re-ordered family	

Adapted from Sidebotham and Heron [5]

children. Abusive bruises tended to be found away from bony prominences were large, multiple, and occurred in clusters. Commonly affected sites were the head and neck, buttocks, trunk, and arms. Sometimes, a bruise may carry an imprint of the implement used. However, it is not possible to age a bruise accurately, from a description of its color alone, either in vivo or from a photograph [31, 32].

Bites

The characteristic bite mark consists of oval or circular marks which may form two opposing arcs. Teeth marks and ecchymoses may or may not be present. Bites are currently the only abusive injury where the perpetrator may be identified by using DNA technology and dental characteristics. It is therefore essential that clinicians recognize a human bite mark so that referral can be made to a forensic dentist. If there is a delay in obtaining a forensic dental opinion, the bite should be swabbed for saliva and DNA. Photographs should be taken, incorporating a right-angled ruler positioned parallel to the injury. Serial photographs taken at 12–24 h intervals are recommended to assess evolving bite marks [33]. The clinical characteristics which define abusive bites have not been defined [34].

Skeletal Injuries

Studies of the epidemiology of childhood fractures provide useful information on which to base a diagnosis of non-accidental injuries. In a retrospective analysis of 2,198 fractures presenting to one paediatric center in the year 2000, the commonest accidental fractures were found to involve the

distal radius and the ulna. [35] The overall mean age of children presenting with fractures was 9.7 years; the incidence increased with age (Table 42.2). Only 27 children (1.2%) sustained more than one fracture. Multiple and unusual fractures should alert the orthopaedic surgeon to the possibility of non-accidental injury.

Non-accidental fractures indicate a serious assault on a child. The prevalence of non-accidental fractures is between 11 and 55% of physically abused children, depending on the age of the population studied. In a comparative study of fracture patterns in accidental and non-accidental injuries, 80% of children with abusive fractures were found to be young (less than 18 months old), whereas 85% of accidental fractures occur in children more than 5 years old. The authors concluded that one in eight children under the age of 18 months who sustains a fracture may be a victim of abuse [36].

In a retrospective analysis of 467 children presenting or referred with a suspicion of non-accidental fractures, 91% were less than 2 years old. [37] The presenting features were often subtle, with medical non-traumatic features (drowsiness, decreased consciousness levels, breathing difficulties, apnea, seizures, vomiting, failure to thrive) and bruises being most common. Eleven children (8%) were brought in dead, mainly from non-accidental head injuries. A total of 1,689 non-accidental fractures were found in 408 children, affecting the long bones (36%), ribs (26%), metaphysis (23%), and skull (15%). About two-thirds of the children had multiple fractures. Isolated long bone fractures involved the femur (25, with 2 metaphyseal fractures), tibia (14, with 5 metaphyseal fractures), humerus (27, with 1 metaphyseal fracture), forearm (9), clavicle (2), and rib (11). Less common fractures involved the scapula, digits, spine, pelvis, and mandible. [37]

Table 42.2 The basic epidemiology of fractures in children by age group

Age group (years)	Prevalence (%)	Incidence/1000/year	Commonest fractures
0–1	2.1	3.6	Clavicle (22.2%) Distal humerus (22.2%)
2–4	11.6	12.9	Distal humerus (22.0%) Distal radius (21.3%)
5–11	51.3	23.2	Distal radius (40.3%) Finger phalanges (14.4%)
12–16	33.8	26.6	Distal radius (28%) Finger phalanges (20.3%)

Adapted from Rennie et al. [12]

Fig. 42.8 Transverse fracture in the midshaft of radius in a 6-week-old infant admitted with periorbital bruising

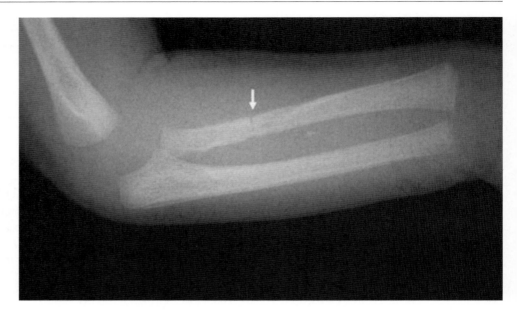

Diaphyseal (Long Bone) Fractures

These are the most common inflicted fractures. Typically there is a single rather than multiple fractures and the fracture is diaphyseal rather than metaphyseal [36]. Figs. 42.8, 42.9, and 42.10 show examples of inflicted fractures in infants.

Subperiosteal New Bone Formation (SNBF)

Periosteal elevation with subperiosteal new bone formation may be seen in child abuse [38] as part of the healing process following a fracture or as a non-specific finding in metabolic and infectious conditions. It may be difficult to differentiate from the "physiologic" periosteal reaction in infants. The "physiological" reaction is usually bilateral, often less than 2 mm in thickness and occurs around the femur. If in doubt, follow-up radiographs help to demonstrate significant changes in traumatic SNBF.

The Classic Metaphyseal Lesion (CML)

Also known as a "bucket handle," "chip," or "corner" fracture, this was regarded as pathognomonic for NAI. It is thought to be produced by shearing, such as when an infant is shaken with the limbs flailing and unsupported [39]. The injuries have been reported to occur accidentally at birth or during physiotherapy to neonates. The CML may be asymptomatic and recent fractures are difficult to visualize

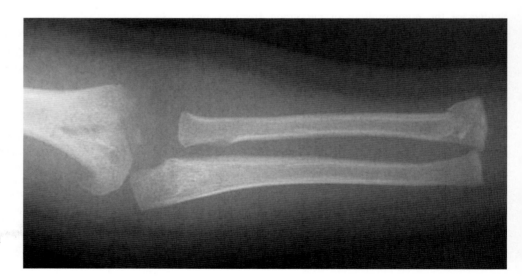

Fig. 42.9 Fractures in right arm—distal radius and ulna, distal humerus—in 20-month-old who presented with facial bruising

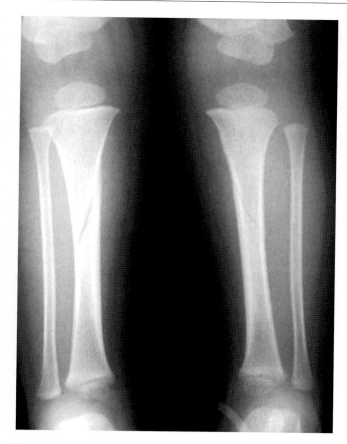

Fig. 42.10 Same infant as in Fig. 42.9, bilateral spiral fractures of tibia found on skeletal survey

radiologically. Appearances depend on the angle at which the radiograph was taken, as well as the stage of healing. Fig. 42.11 illustrates a distal femoral CML in a 6-week-old infant.

Rib Fractures

A systematic review [40] of fractures in child abuse has shown that rib fractures which are found in children without explicit explanation have the highest specificity of abuse. The fractures commonly occur posteriorly at the head–neck junction of the ribs. The detection of occult rib fractures is improved by asking for oblique rib views in the skeletal survey and by another set of views 10–14 days later. Cardio-pulmonary resuscitation (CPR) has often been used in defense argument to explain rib fractures in the young child found collapsed. Maguire and colleagues [41] reviewed 427 studies to establish the evidence base for this opinion. Only six studies met their strict methodological criteria and included 923 children who had had CPR performed by both medical and non-medical personnel. Rib fractures were found to be rare (<2%) after CPR. When they did occur, they were often multiple and found to be anterior.

Skull Fractures

Between 5 and 10% of children who have been abused have skull fractures, which tend to be complex (depressed,

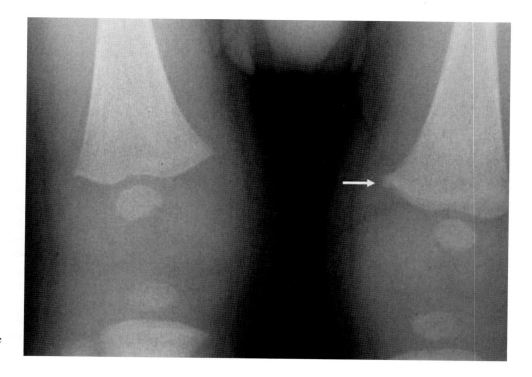

Fig. 42.11 Metaphyseal fracture at the distal end of the femur

compound, or comminuted) and involve more than a single cranial bone. Diastasis of fracture margins is sometimes seen ("growing" fracture), usually in association with an underlying dural injury [42]. Skull fractures are the result of a direct blow or part of shaking which ends with impact. Further neuroimaging [computed tomography (CT) or magnetic resonance imaging (MRI) brain scan] should always be considered in young infants who present with skull fractures.

Assessment

A fracture, like any other injury, should never be interpreted in isolation. It must always be assessed in the context of the medical and social history, developmental stage, and any explanation given. Child abuse should be suspected under the following circumstances:

- Child less than 18 months old.
- Fracture inconsistent with child's developmental stage.
- Multiple fractures of different ages in the absence of an adequate explanation.
- Rib fractures in children with normal bones and no history of major trauma.
- Fractured femur in a pre-mobile child.

The investigation and management of a possibly harmed child must be in the same systematic and rigorous manner as would be appropriate for the investigation and management of any other potentially fatal disease [43]. The doctor must be aware of the referral pathways to senior colleagues with the specialist skills necessary to help assess whether the child has been abused. However, it is not necessary to make a firm diagnosis of child abuse before referral to the statutory agencies (social services or police).

Record keeping is vital and must be contemporaneous, comprehensive, and legible. Negative as well as positive findings must be recorded. Any statements from the child or the parent must be written down verbatim. Body charts are helpful for documenting injuries. Photographs are useful.

Inter-Agency Cooperation

The mechanisms for investigating potential child abuse vary considerably around the world. A structured and validated approach is essential both to protect the child and to avoid inappropriate censure of the parents. When non-accidental injury is suspected, it is necessary to consider both the injuries themselves and co-existing forms of abuse. In the United Kingdom, the Child Protection Register should be checked by telephoning social services. Local as well as

national procedures and guidelines must be followed to ensure the child's safety [25, 26].

A multi-agency child protection enquiry should be commenced by contacting the social services department who should in turn discuss the case with the police. Referrals should be followed up in writing within 24 h. Social services have a statutory responsibility to make enquiries when concerns are expressed about a child, while police have a duty to investigate. In the United Kingdom, a multi-agency meeting (child protection conference), attended by the parents and all concerned, is the forum where professionals decide, based on the available information, whether the child has suffered harm. If so, the child is placed on the Child Protection Register and a Child Protection Plan agreed with the parents to ensure the safety and well-being of their child. Risks to other children living in the same household must also be considered during the case conference.

Differential Diagnosis

It is important to exclude other causes which might have contributed to the injury. An underlying medical condition might be responsible for fractures, such as the following:

- Normal variant/physiological finding, e.g., subperiosteal new bone formation.
- Accidental injury.
- Birth injury in a young infant. Most fractures sustained at birth heal within a few weeks. Obstetric and neonatal records should be checked.
- Bone disease, e.g., osteogenesis imperfecta, osteopenia of prematurity, rickets, copper deficiency, osteomyelitis, scurvy, and metastatic lesions.

However, it is important to remember that abuse may coexist with an underlying medical problem.

Investigations

High-quality radiographs and interpretation by a skilled paediatric radiologist will increase fracture detection rate. The British Society of Paediatric Radiology has established standards for skeletal imaging in cases of suspected non-accidental injury [44]. In children under 2 years of age where physical abuse is suspected, skeletal surveys should be mandatory. Predictive factors which might guide clinical practice include the age of the child (younger than 12 months) and the type of presenting injury (overt fracture or head injury) [45]. However, no single radiological investigation (skeletal survey or bone scan) has been found to identify all fractures. Bone scans will identify acute fractures not seen easily on skeletal surveys but may miss skull fractures. Diagnostic accuracy is increased if all skeletal surveys include oblique views of the ribs, with follow-up films to evaluate suspicious findings [46]. Criminal investigators often rely on the radiological dating of injuries to exclude or identify perpetrators. Didactic statements are often forthcoming on the date of a bone injury: the primary evidence for these statements is lacking. Although a recent fracture can be distinguished from an old one, the dating of the age of a fracture based on its pattern of healing is imprecise [47].

The two most common causes of bone fragility in infancy are osteopenia of prematurity and osteogenesis imperfecta. In pre-term infants, fractures associated with osteopenia tend to occur in the first two years of life. Risk factors which predispose to fractures are cholestatic jaundice, intravenous nutrition for more than 3 weeks, chronic lung disease, diuretic treatment for longer than 2 weeks, and physiotherapy [48]. The controversial entity of "temporary brittle bone disease" has been dismissed by the European Society of Paediatric Radiology as a possible explanation for fractures in children [49].

Apart from careful history taking and examination, blood must be taken to evaluate biochemical markers of bone disease (calcium, phosphate, alkaline phosphatase, copper, magnesium, fasting 25-hydroxyvitamin D, and parathyroid hormone levels). It is helpful to discuss with an experienced paediatric radiologist the need for further radiological investigations, e.g., special views and MRI scans. Where a non-accidental fracture is suspected in a child under 2 years of age, a full skeletal survey must be performed to exclude occult fractures. Repeat radiographs of doubtful areas should be obtained 1–2 weeks later to identify callus (which helps with approximate dating of injury) and to demonstrate previously occult injuries. While a laboratory diagnosis of osteogenesis imperfecta can be made from a skin biopsy (biochemical analysis of collagen species and mutation analysis of RNA) or from a blood sample (mutation analysis of DNA), both take a long time and are not readily available: adequate samples of skin in infants are technically difficult to obtain and the investigations are available only in specialist centers. No clear guidelines are available regarding the utility of these investigations in suspected non-accidental injury. Furthermore, the positive predictive value of these tests has not been defined.

Conclusion

Awareness that abuse may underlie injury is essential. Although more common in the financially deprived, it occurs throughout society and in communities world over. Nearly 50% occur in infants under 1 year. Toddlers, children, and adolescents are equally affected and in the last group neurological or psychiatric problems are common [50]. In the United States, child maltreatment is estimated to occur in 15–42 cases per 1,000 children and over one million children each year are the substantiated victims [51]. In the United Kingdom, a national study of young people estimated that 1 in 4 children experienced one or more forms of physical violence during childhood. Of this 25% of children, the majority had experienced some degree of physical abuse by parents or carers [52]. Although the history and findings may be suggestive of abuse, no fracture pattern is pathognomonic.

References

1. Xian CJ, Foster BK. The biologic aspects of children's fractures. In: Rockwood CA, Wilkins KE, Beaty JH, Kasser JR, eds. Rockwood and Wilkins' Fractures in Children, 6th ed. Philadelphia: Lippincott, Williams and Wilkins; 2006:21–50.
2. Shapiro F, Holtrop ME, Glimcher MJ. Organisation and cellular biology of the perichondrial ossification groove of Ranvier. A morphological study in rabbits. J Bone Joint Surg 1977; 59A: 703–23.
3. Marks SC Jr. The structure and developmental contexts of skeletal injury. In: Kleinman PK, ed. Diagnostic Imaging of Child Abuse, 2nd ed. St. Louis: Mosby; 1988:2–7.
4. Curry JD, Butler G. The mechanical properties of bone tissue in children. J Bone Joint Surg 1975; 57A: 810–14.
5. Thorndike A, Pierce FR. Fractures in the newborn. A plea for adequate treatment. New England J Med 1936; 215:1013–18.
6. Rubin A. Birth injuries: incidence, mechanisms and end results. Obstet Gynecol 1964; 23:218–21.
7. Wickstrom I, Axelsson D, Bergstrom R, Meirik O. Traumatic injury in large-for-dates infants. Acta Obstet Gynecol Scand 1988; 67:259–64.
8. Gresham EL. Birth Trauma. Ped Clin North Am 1977; 22:317–28.
9. Nadas S, Gudinchet F, Capasso P, Reinberg O. Predisposing factors in obstetric fractures. Skeletal Radiol 1993; 22:195–8.
10. Oppenheim WL, Davis A, Growden WA, et al. Clavicle fracture in the newborn. Clin Orthop 1990; 250:176–80.
11. Greenwald AG, Schute PC, Shively JL. Brachial plexus palsy. A 10 year report on the incidence and prognosis. J Ped Orthop 1984; 4:689–92.
12. Owen R. Congenital pseudarthrosis of the clavicle. J Bone Joint Surg 1970; 52B: 644–52.
13. Lemperg R, Liliequist B. Dislocation of the proximal epiphysis of the humerus in newborns: report of two cases and discussion of diagnostic criteria. Acta Ped Scand 1970; 59:373–80.
14. Broker FH, Burbach T. Ultrasonic diagnosis of separation of the proximal humeral epiphysis in the newborn. J Bone Joint Surg 1990; 72A: 187–91.
15. Bayne O, Rang M. Medial dislocation of the radial head following breech delivery: a case report and review of the literature. J Ped Orthop 1984; 4:485–7.
16. Downs DM, Wirth CR. Fracture of the distal humeral chondroepiphysis in the neonate. Clin Orthop 1982; 169:155–58.
17. Barrett WP, Almquist EA, Staheli LT. Fracture separation of the distal humeral epiphysis in the newborn. J Ped Orthop 1984; 4:617–19.

18. Hagglund G, Hansson LI, Wiberg G. Correction of deformity after femoral birth fracture. 16 year follow-up. Acta Orthop Scand 1988; 59:333–35.

19. Ogden JA, Lee KE, Rudicel SA, Pelker RR. Proximal femoral epiphysis in the neonate. J Ped Orthop 1984; 4:282–92.

20. Hensinger RN. Standards in Pediatric Orthopaedics. New York: Raven Press; 1986:284.

21. Byers RK. Spinal-cord injuries during birth. Dev Med Child Neurol 1975; 17:103–10.

22. Lanska MJ, Roessman U, Wiznitzer M. Magnetic resonance imaging in cervical cord birth injury. Pediatrics 1990; 85:760–5.

23. Stanley P, Duncan AW, Isaacson J, Isaacson JS. Radiology of fracture-dislocation of the cervical spine during delivery. Am J Radiol 1985; 145:621–5.

24. Morse CW, Sahler OJZ, Friedman SB. A three-year follow up study of abused and neglected children. Am J Dis Child 1970; 120:439–46.

25. Department of Health. Working together to safeguard children. London: The Stationery Office, 2006. At: http://www.everychild matters.gov.uk/_files/AE53C8F9D7AEB1B23E403514A6C1B17D. pdf. Accessed 15 October 2008.

26. Protecting Children and Young People. Framework for Standards. The Scottish Executive, Edinburgh 2004. At: http://www.scotland. gov.uk/Resource/Doc/1181/0008818.pdf. Accessed 15 October 2008.

27. Taitz J, Moran K, O'Meara M. Long bone fractures in children under 3 years of age: Is abuse being missed in Emergency Department presentations? J Pediatr Child Health 2004; 40:170–4.

28. Sidebotham P, Heron J. Child maltreatment in the "children of the nineties": A cohort study of risk factors. Child Abuse Negl 2006; 30:497–522.

29. Hindley N, Ramchandani PG, Jones DPH. Risk factors for recurrence of maltreatment: a systematic review. Arch Dis Child 2006; 91:744–52.

30. Maguire S, Mann MK, Sibert J, Kemp A. Are there patterns of bruising in childhood which are diagnostic or suggestive of abuse? A systematic review. Arch Dis Child 2005; 90:182–6.

31. Maguire S, Mann MK, Sibert J, Kemp A. Can you age bruises accurately in children? A systematic review. Arch Dis Child 2005; 90:187–9.

32. Munang LA, Leonard PA, Mok J. Lack of agreement on colour description between clinicians examining childhood bruising. J Clin Foren Med 2002; 9:171–4.

33. British Association of Forensic Odontology. Guidelines Bitemark Methodology. 2001. At: http://www.forensicdentistryonline. org/forensic_pages_1/bitemarkguide.htm. Accessed 15 October 2008.

34. Kemp A, Maguire SA, Sibert J, et al. Can we identify abusive bites in children? Arch Dis Child 2006; 91:951.

35. Rennie L, Court-Brown CM, Mok JYQ, Beattie TF. The epidemiology of fractures in children. Injury 2007; 38:913–22.

36. Worlock P, Stower M, Barbor P. Patterns of fractures in accidental and non-accidental injury in children: a comparative study. Br Med J 1986; 293:100–2.

37. Carty H, Pierce A. Non-accidental injury: a retrospective analysis of a large cohort. Europ Radiol 2002; 12:2919–25.

38. Kleinman PK. Skeletal trauma: general considerations. In: Kleinman PK, ed. Diagnostic Imaging of Child Abuse, 2nd edition. St. Louis: Mosby; 1998:8–25.

39. Kleinman PK, Marks SC, Blackbourne B. The metaphyseal lesion in abused infants: a radiologic–histologic study. Am J Roentgenol 1986; 146:895–905.

40. Kemp AM, Dunstan F, Harrison S, et al. Patterns of skeletal fractures in child abuse: systemic review. BMJ 2008; 337:a1518.

41. Maguire S, Mann M, John N, et al. Does cardiopulmonary resuscitation cause rib fractures in children? A systematic review. Child Abuse Negl 2006; 30:739–51.

42. Hobbs CJ. Skull fracture and the diagnosis of abuse. Arch Dis Child 1984; 59:246–52.

43. Report of an Inquiry into the death of Victoria Climbie. Lord Laming. London: The Stationery Office; 2003.

44. British Society of Paediatric Radiology. NAI standard for skeletal surveys. At: http://www.bspr.org.uk/nai.htm. Accessed 10 November 2008.

45. Day F, Clegg S, McPhillips M, Mok J. A retrospective case series of skeletal surveys in children with suspected non-accidental injury. J Clin For Med 2006; 13:55–9.

46. Kemp AM, Butler A, Morris S, et al. Which radiological investigations should be performed to identify fractures in suspected child abuse? Clin Radiol 2006; 61:723–36.

47. Prosser I, Maguire S, Harrison S, et al. How old is this fracture? Radiological dating of fractures in children: a systematic review. Am J Roentgenol 2005; 184:1282–6.

48. Bishop N, Sprigg A, Dalton A. Unexplained fractures in infancy: looking for fragile bones. Arch Dis Child 2007; 92:251–6.

49. Mendelson KL. Critical review of "temporary brittle bone disease." Pediatr Radiol 2005; 35:1036–40.

50. Loder RT, Feinberg JR. Orthopedic injuries in children with nonaccidental trauma. J Pediatr Orthop 2007; 27:421–6

51. Kocher MS, Kasser JR. Orthopaedic aspects of child abuse. J Am Acad Orthop Surg. 2000; 8:10–20.

52. Cawson P, Wattam C, Brooker S, Kelly G. Child maltreatment in the United Kingdom: a study of the prevalence of child abuse and neglect, 2000. London: NSPCC. ISBN: 1842280066.

Section 2
Fractures of the Shoulder, Upper Limb, and Hand

Chapter 43

Fractures Around the Shoulder and the Humerus

J. B. Hunter

Clavicle Fractures

Etiology

Fractures of the clavicle are seen extremely commonly in the children's fracture clinic. The vast majority are of the diaphysis and are caused by a fall on the outstretched hand. These low-energy fractures occur in children who have an excellent potential for remodeling. After 7–10 days a mass forms over the affected clavicle: this represents a healing fracture callus and disappears within another 2–3 weeks when the fracture has stabilized.

Treatment

Conservative management with a sling or a figure-of-eight bandage is the traditional treatment. The figure-of-eight bandage has some theoretical advantages in that it braces the shoulders back and preserves clavicular length. In practice the bandage and even the commercial varieties loosen easily and children find them rather uncomfortable. There is no evidence that the figure-of-eight bandage offers any superior analgesia and therefore our practice has been to use a simple sling worn underneath the clothes [1]. The sling or figure-of-eight bandage needs to be worn for 10–20 days depending on the age of the child and the configuration of the fracture. No further radiographs are required and we do not routinely follow these patients up. We allow them to remove their own sling or figure-of-eight bandage and return to normal activities 3 weeks after injury (Fig. 43.1).

Very occasionally diaphyseal fractures of the clavicle require internal fixation because of patient factors such as polytrauma, floating shoulder, or neurovascular injury. In these situations stabilization is advantageous, and may be done either by plating or more commonly with elastic stable intramedullary nailing [2].

Obstetrical Clavicle Fracture

In obstetric and neonatal practice fractures of the clavicle are associated with shoulder dystocia and brachial plexus palsy. The fracture itself rarely requires any active intervention but the child requires follow-up in order to establish that any tendency to underuse in the arm is related to the fracture rather than any underlying palsy [3].

Fracture Dislocations of the Medial and Lateral Ends of the Clavicle

Fractures and dislocations of the medial and distal ends of the clavicle are unusual. There are physes at each end of the clavicle. Increased mobility after trauma that appears to be caused by a dislocation is in fact a growth plate injury in which the metaphysis can rupture out of the periosteal sleeve. These need to be recognized because, although the fractures will heal protected by a figure-of-eight splint, there will be massive sub-periosteal new bone formation, which may or may not fully remodel. At the distal end of the clavicle the periosteal sleeve remains attached both to the capsule of the acromioclavicular joint and the coraco-clavicular ligament. In adolescents stabilization may be achieved by careful periosteal repair. K-wire fixation is never advised to avoid possible migration [4]. At the medial end of the clavicle reduction, periosteal suture is necessary if a fracture has displaced posteriorly and compressed underlying structures causing stridor and/or dysphagia [5].

J.B. Hunter (✉)
Departments of Trauma and Orthopaedics, Nottingham University Hospital, Nottingham, UK

M. Benson et al. (eds.), *Children's Orthopaedics and Fractures*,
DOI 10.1007/978-1-84882-611-3_43, © Springer-Verlag London Limited 2010

Fig. 43.1 Clavicle healing and remodeling. Courtesy of K. Parsch

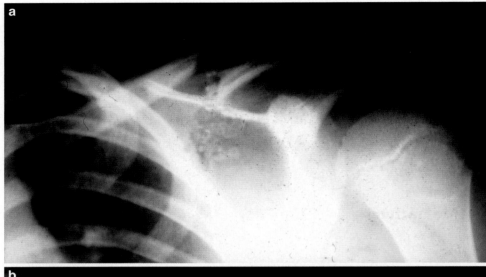

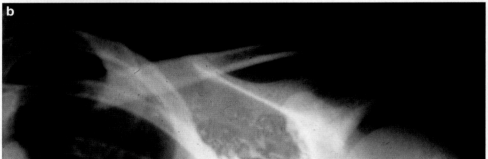

Fractures of the Scapula

Fractures of the scapula are unusual in paediatric practice and body fractures are virtually only seen in the multi-injured. There are multiple secondary ossification centers in the scapula, which can be mistaken for fractures, but are also potential sites of weakness, particularly in teenagers. Fractures at the junction of the body of the scapula and the coracoid process do occur and are frequently missed. Similarly, the apophyses around the acromion are occasionally diagnosed as fractures in cases of bruised shoulder.

Fractures of the Proximal Humerus

Fractures of the proximal humerus are fairly uncommon with an incidence of 1–2 per 1000 (about 5% of paediatric fractures) [6].

Classification

Fractures of the proximal humerus are best classified using the AO paediatric fracture classification [7], all classifiable within the sections 11 E. or 11 M. The different fracture types

are shown in Fig. 43.2. The epiphyseal fracture types follow the Salter–Harris classification (e.g., 11 E/2) but also have a category for flake fractures (11 E/8). For metaphyseal fractures only type 11 M/2 (torus, buckle, or greenstick fractures) and type 11 M/3 (complete fractures) are seen (Fig. 43.2).

Birth Fractures of the Proximal Humerus

Physeal fractures of the proximal humerus occur in obstetric practice and, because the ossification center of the humeral head has not appeared, tend to be misdiagnosed as congenital dislocations of the humerus. The diagnosis can be established either by arthrogram or more conveniently by ultrasound, which does not require an anesthetic [8]. Once it is established that the head is in the socket no treatment is required beyond a body bandage for analgesia (see Chapter 42).

Proximal Humerus Fracture of the Older Child

In older children direct or indirect trauma may cause the fracture. Because of the thick periosteum and the proximity to the physis there is an enormous potential for healing.

11-E Proximal epiphyseal fractures

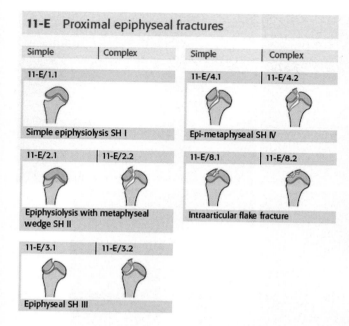

Simple	Complex	Simple	Complex
11-E/1.1		**11-E/4.1**	**11-E/4.2**
Simple epiphysiolysis SH I		Epi-metaphyseal SH IV	
11-E/2.1	**11-E/2.2**	**11-E/8.1**	**11-E/8.2**
Epiphysiolysis with metaphyseal wedge SH II		Intraarticular flake fracture	
11-E/3.1	**11-E/3.2**		
Epiphyseal SH III			

11-M Proximal metaphyseal fractures

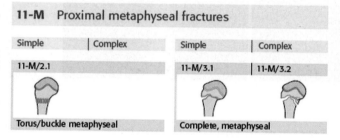

Simple	Complex	Simple	Complex
11-M/2.1		**11-M/3.1**	**11-M/3.2**
Torus/buckle metaphyseal		Complete, metaphyseal	

Fig. 43.2 Classification of proximal humeral fractures. From: Slongo T, Audigé L, AO Classification Group. AO Pediatric Comprehensive Classification of Long Bone Fractures (PCCF) Brochure. Davos, Switzerland: AO Publishing; 2007

Remodeling of the proximal humerus occurs more readily than in any other bone. Fractures of the proximal humerus have been described as the most overtreated fracture in the body: Mercer Rang stated that bayonet apposition of the fracture fragments could be accepted at all times, provided 2 years of growth remained [9].

In older children physeal fractures are most commonly Salter–Harris 1 or 2 fractures; intra-articular growth plate injuries are extremely rare. These latter need to be accurately reduced and fixed to allow early mobilization, but the more common extra-articular injuries rarely require operative treatment; there is some evidence that, far from improving the results, operation is associated with an increased rate of complications in the management of these fractures [10]. Although interposition of the biceps tendon has been described in children's fractures, this is rare [11]. More commonly the fracture heals and remodels perfectly, despite significant displacement. Displaced metaphyseal fractures of

the proximal humerus remodel as well as physeal fractures and a conservative approach is appropriate.

If fracture fixation is required because of associated injuries, then elastic nailing is much more elegant than percutaneous K-wire fixation, which risks migration and prevents early mobilization. However, just because this is an elegant technique does not mean that it should be used frequently. If elastic nailing is the chosen management, then technique preferred is retrograde. The starting point is on the lateral supracondylar ridge where two separate holes are made for the nails. The first nail is inserted in a C-shape, the second nail in an S-shape to allow the nail points to diverge in the humeral head. Reduction by the nails is controlled on the image intensifier. Pendulum movements are allowed immediately, with full active mobilization at 7–10 days [12, 13] (Fig. 43.3).

Fractures of the Humerus Shaft

Classification

Plastic deformation and greenstick fractures of the humeral shaft are rare. The main codes for these fractures are therefore 12 D/4 (transverse fractures) and 12 D/5 (oblique or spiral fractures). Fractures of the humeral shaft are rare in children but more common in adolescents with higher energy injuries.

In children the most important aspect of humeral shaft fractures to recognize is the non-accidental injury. A humeral shaft fracture in a child younger than 2 years has been identified as the fracture that is likely to be inflicted, particularly if the fracture pattern is spiral. This information came from a large study of children's fractures in Nottingham, and has been challenged since, but certainly a fracture of the humerus shaft in a non-walking child is highly abnormal and worthy of investigation [14–16].

Treatment

These fractures can generally be managed non-operatively as both healing and remodeling are excellent in children. Initial management should be with a collar and cuff or a hanging cast to allow the weight of the elbow to straighten the humerus. This can be augmented by a sugar tong splint or a coaptation splint. If the physes are open, remodeling is excellent and non-union unlikely. Conservative management of the humeral shaft requires immobilization and splintage for 3–6 weeks depending on the age of the child. Physiotherapy

Fig. 43.3 (**a** and **b**) Fully displaced fracture of the proximal humerus in a 14-year-old girl nearing skeletal maturity. (**c**) and (**d**) Similar fracture in another teenaged girl, stabilized by ESIN. Courtesy of K. Parsch

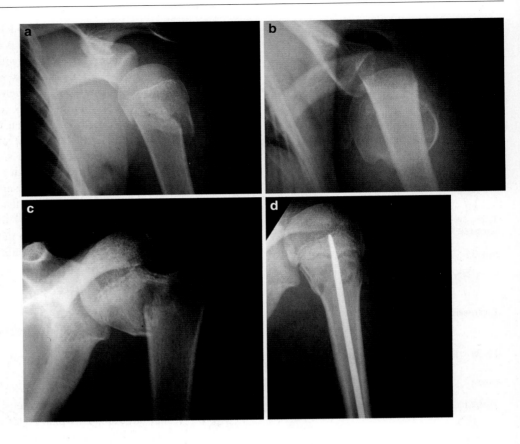

is rarely required, as stiffness of either shoulder or elbow is uncommon.

Injury to the radial nerve in conjunction with the humeral shaft fracture is less common in children than in adults; the norm is for spontaneous resolution and surgical exploration is generally not indicated. Exceptions might be fracture patterns highly suggestive of a laceration to the radial nerve and the onset of a nerve lesion following manipulation or closed surgery.

Indications for surgical stabilization of the humeral shaft are only relative: neurovascular injury, open fractures, and multiple injuries. Pathological fractures secondary to simple bone cysts are well treated by elastic nailing as it allows an earlier return to activities and promotes cyst healing. Fractures of the lower diaphysis or the junction of the shaft and metaphysis are also a relative indication of surgical treatment as residual angulation at this level can lead to functional problems. The most common surgical treatment is by elastic nailing. If the fracture is of the midshaft then elastic nailing should be done from the distal end of the humerus using the technique described above. If the fracture is off the distal third of the humerus, then the nailing should be antegrade from a start point in the region of the deltoid tuberosity [12, 13] (Figs. 43.4 and 43.5).

Fractures of the Distal Humerus

Supracondylar Fractures

The peak ages when supracondylar fractures occur is between 5–7 years. Traditionally, boys have a higher incidence for this fracture than girls, outnumbering girls by about 3:2 [17]. Almost all supracondylar fractures are caused by accidental trauma. A fall from a height such as a bed or furniture in small children or monkey bars or swings in kindergarten and school-age children is a common cause for the injury.

Classification

In the first instance supracondylar fractures should be classified as either extension or flexion types, depending on the angulation or displacement of the distal fragment. Only 5% of displaced supracondylar fractures are of the flexion type; they are difficult to manage and will be considered separately.

The supracondylar fracture is a metaphyseal fracture and the primary code in the AO classification is 13 M/3 (complete

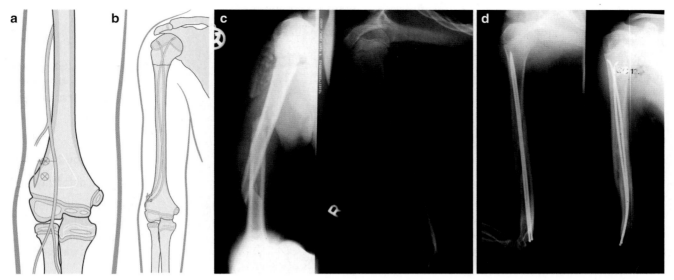

Fig. 43.4 (**a**) Start points for elastic nailing of the humeral shaft or neck. (**b**) Configuration of elastic nails in humeral nailing. From: Dietz H-G, Schmittenbecher P, Slongo T. AO Manual of Fracture Management: Elastic Stable Intramedullary nailing (ESIN) in Children. Davos, Switzerland: AO Publishing; 2006. (**c**) Spiral fracture of the humerus in a 12-year-old boy. Courtesy of K.Parsch. (**d**) Same fracture stabilized by ESIN and healing

Fig. 43.5 Pathological fracture through a simple bone cyst leading to cyst healing at 18 months

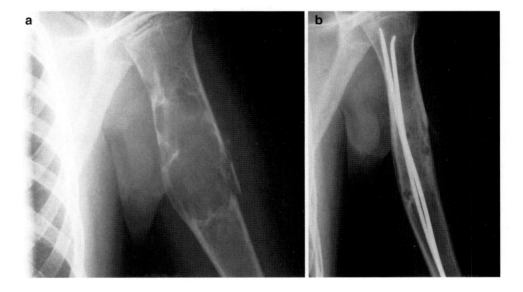

metaphyseal fracture of the distal humerus). The standard English language classification of extension supracondylar fractures is that of Gartland [18], most simply described in three types:

  I. Undisplaced fractures.
 II. Fractures that are angulated/displaced into extension with an intact posterior cortex.
III. Displaced fractures (Fig. 43.6)

This classification has been validated and shown to perform reasonably well in terms of inter- and intra-observer error. Over time, various authors have added to this classification. Mubarak and Davids described a variant of the undisplaced fracture with comminution or collapse of the medial column [19]. This fracture is certainly unstable with the potential to collapse into varus but is nearly always angulated at initial presentation and therefore not truly undisplaced.

Wilkins described two types of the displaced fracture, the postero-medial and postero-lateral, noting that the latter was much more likely to cause injury to the brachial artery and median nerve [20]. The distinction is more useful if the displacement is incomplete rather than complete, when the distal fragment is fully mobile in all directions.

Fig. 43.6 AO and Gartland classification methods for supracondylar fractures. From: Slongo T, Audigé L, AO Classification Group. AO Pediatric Comprehensive Classification of Long Bone Fractures (PCCF) Brochure. Davos, Switzerland: AO Publishing; 2007

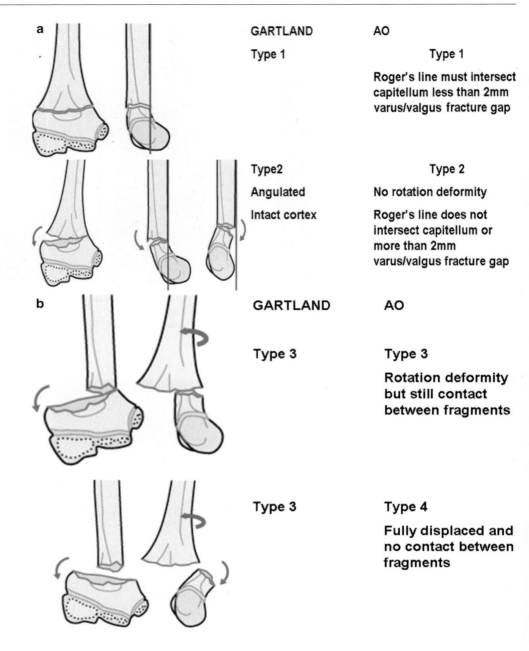

In Central Europe, von Laer introduced the concept of rotational failure [21]. In his classification, type 1 was undisplaced, type 2 angulated but with no rotation of the distal fragment, type 3 displaced by rotation of the distal fragment but still in contact between the main fragments, and type 4 fully displaced with no contact between the fragments. Initial attempts to validate this by the AO classification group showed poor reliability, interestingly because of the lack of definition of *undisplaced* [7]. Each modification, therefore, may make Gartland's classification less reproducible.

Treatment

The purpose of classification is mainly to guide treatment which allows Gartland's original classification to remain very useful.

Type I undisplaced supracondylar fractures can be treated in a sling or collar and cuff and need only 3 weeks treatment.

Type II fractures with posterior angulation (apex anterior) should be manipulated under general anesthesia and placed in full flexion. If the reduction is successful the fracture should be stabilized by crossed K-wires. Once stabilized, the position of full flexion can be avoided. Full flexion supposedly predisposes to elevated compartment pressures in the forearm [22], although compartment pressure studies performed by Clavert et al. suggest this may not be the case [23].

Type III fully displaced fractures should not be treated by manipulation and immobilization alone as the success rate is only just over 60%. Chinese authors have described treating the displaced fracture in an extension plaster, taking care to correct varus and valgus, but ignoring any posterior displacement [24]. Traction is still used successfully in some British hospitals [25, 26]. This is time-consuming, but avoids some of the complications associated with percutaneous pinning.

Reduction of the displaced supracondylar fracture is achieved by traction and disimpaction followed by the correction of any medial or lateral displacement. The distal fragment is "thumbed" into place as the elbow is flexed.

One of the controversies in managing these fractures is the configuration of the wires that should be used. Higher rates of ulnar nerve injury have been reported using the typical crossed wire configuration [27]. Multiple wires inserted from the lateral side avoid this complication but are less stable [28]. Excellent results have been reported using two or three lateral wires and obeying these rules [29] (Figs. 43.7 and 43.8):

(1) The wires should be at least 2 mm in diameter.
(2) The wires should diverge to engage both medial and lateral columns.
(3) The medial wire should engage all four cortices at the olecranon fossa.
(4) The construct should be tested for stability in rotation on the table [30].

Many surgeons continue to use crossed wires for stability [31]. Recently, ascending and descending wires inserted from a lateral approach have been shown to provide excellent stability [32]. Ulnar nerve injury can be avoided by inserting the medial wire with the elbow extended as recommended by Rang, and by examining the contralateral elbow for subluxation of the ulnar nerve in flexion and extension.

Alternative methods to stabilize supracondylar fractures include down-going elastic nailing and external fixation. Anterograde elastic nailing was described in Nancy [13]. It has the advantage that the implant is entirely internal and does not cross the joint. This minimizes the need for external protection and allows early mobilization [33]. The disadvantages are that the technique is technically demanding and almost impossible to achieve without two image intensifiers at 90° to each other. In very few units is this standard treatment but it is useful for fractures that are slightly more proximal at the diaphyseal/metaphyseal border. External fixation is a well-described method of stabilizing osteotomies

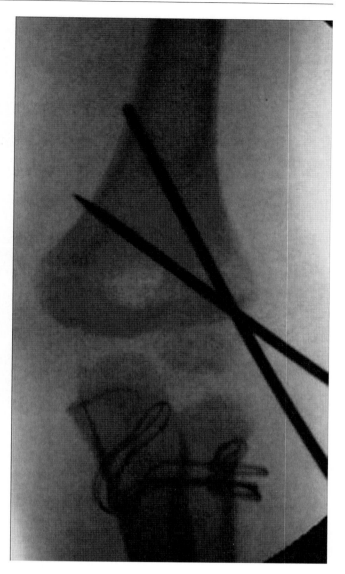

Fig. 43.7 Supracondylar fracture pinned with lateral wires. Courtesy Richard Reynolds

of the distal humerus and may be useful for very unstable or open fractures [34].

Neurovascular Injury

Supracondylar humeral fractures in children generate anxiety and excitement, particularly among trainees and adult surgeons who are exposed to the fracture infrequently. The feared complications are vascular and neural injury. Injury to the brachial artery can be direct laceration, interruption through kinking, vascular spasm, or intimal tear. The consequence of any of these injuries is a compartment syndrome of the flexor compartment of the forearm, which, if untreated,

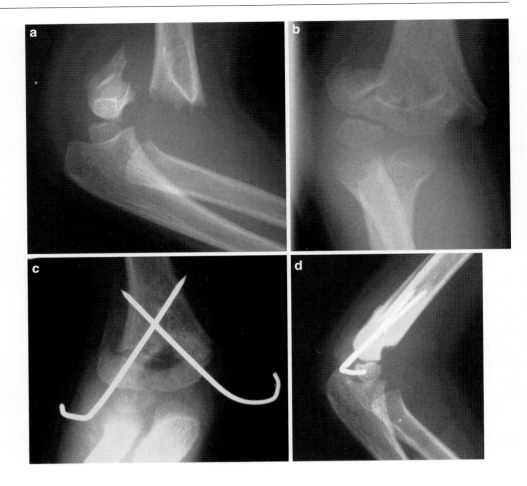

Fig. 43.8 Typical AO type 4 (Gartland 3) displaced supracondylar fracture, reduced and stabilized with crossed K-wires

leads to ischemic contracture and severe loss of function in the wrist and hand. Re-establishing the flow in the brachial artery is not the most important aspect of treatment as there is an excellent collateral circulation and symptoms of claudication of the forearm muscles are extremely rare in follow-up studies. The important thing is to monitor, diagnose, and if necessary treat the incipient compartment syndrome by fasciotomy [35].

Management of the Vascular Injury

Assessing vascular status following supracondylar fracture requires examination of three things: the pulse, the capillary return, and the amount of pain from and activity in the forearm muscles. The pulse and the capillary return give information on the state of circulation to the extremity.

If the hand is *white and pulseless* then circulation must be restored [36]. This situation arises most frequently either when the fracture is severely displaced prior to manipulation, or immediately after a reduction maneuver, indicating that the artery has been trapped in or close to the fracture

site. In the first circumstance the action should be gentle provisional reduction, straightening the arm without attempting to definitively reduce the fracture. This should be done in the emergency department under appropriate analgesia. In the second situation, the immediate action should be to re-displace the fracture to see if circulation is restored. Exploration of the artery is likely to be required to prevent it from being entrapped in the fracture when it is reduced for a second time. The white, pulseless hand is, however, fortunately quite rare.

The *pink pulseless* hand is, by contrast, much more common: in our series of supracondylar fractures treated on traction, the pink pulseless hand occurred in more than 10% of cases [37]. If the hand is pink with satisfactory capillary return then the circulation to the extremity is adequate. The necessity is then to prevent a compartment syndrome and ischemic contracture. The normal values of forearm compartment pressure in the young child are not well established. Therefore, the compartment syndrome can only be diagnosed clinically, waking the child up and assessing movements and stretch pain. The vast majority of patients (100% in our series) with a pink pulseless hand recover completely, without exploration of the artery [36]. Protocols that demand exploration of the artery are over-invasive [38]. Exploration is, however, warranted in some situations:

(1) There is a block to accurate reduction.
(2) There is a loss of pulse, accompanied by a nerve injury, particularly of the median or anterior interosseous nerves.
(3) There is severe, disproportionate pain with an accurately reduced and stabilized fracture.

Exploration of the artery may yield a variety of findings. In the most extreme situation, the artery is divided or lacerated, and there is severe local bleeding, which is a potent cause of the compartment syndrome. In this situation, the artery should be repaired using a vein graft [39]. This should be accompanied by forearm fasciotomies. An intimal tear may cause re-occlusion of the artery and the recommendation is that a vein patch be applied.

The more common situation is that the artery is found intact, but collapsed. The collapse may be secondary to vascular spasm caused by direct pressure or to an intimal tear. If the artery is collapsed over an extensive segment the child's blood pressure may not be sufficient to reinflate it. Direct re-inflation is recommended, using a syringe of saline [40].

Flexion Supracondylar Fractures

In this much rarer fracture type, the distal fragment is displaced anteriorly. Generally, the fracture is much more unstable, and conservative methods are difficult to pursue essentially because the elbow must be held fully straight to keep the fracture reduced. This makes closed reduction and pinning extremely difficult and open reduction is often necessary. A recent study suggests that these fractures occur in older children, that open reduction is three times more common, and that ulnar nerve injury is six times more common [41].

Complete Physeal Displacement

This variant of the supracondylar fracture occurs exclusively in children under the age of 2 years. Because the capitellar epiphysis is the first to appear at the age of 12 months these fractures can be difficult to diagnose, masquerading either as elbow dislocations or lateral condyle fractures. The fractures are high-energy injuries and child abuse must always be considered as a possible cause. Another recognized cause is birth trauma, and the injury may be misdiagnosed as an obstetric brachial plexus palsy [42].

The key to diagnosis is an index of suspicion. The best investigations to confirm the diagnosis are ultrasound and arthrography. Of these, ultrasound is superior because it can be used in the conscious infant. Arthrography is a useful adjunct to the operative procedure. Because the displacement is at the level of the physis, rather than in the thin metaphysis, where the conventional supracondylar fracture occurs, the fracture may be much more stable after closed reduction. Some authors therefore recommend closed reduction with traction and a cast, while others feel that this fracture should be pinned to prevent later deformity. Just as in the supracondylar fracture, deformity in the plane of the elbow joint remodels well, whereas valgus and varus do not.

Lateral Condyle Fractures

These fractures are the second most common children's elbow fracture to need operative treatment. The fracture is unusual for a child's fracture in that:
(1) The fracture heals slowly.
(2) Late deformity can occur.
(3) Non-union is a recognized complication.

The fracture crosses both the joint line and the physis. It should therefore be regarded as a Salter–Harris IV fracture, whether or not the fracture line transects the bony epiphysis. If the fracture line extends beyond the bony epiphysis of the capitellum toward the middle of the joint, then displacement is likely to be much more extensive and the injury is a fracture dislocation.

The diagnosis is made on plain X-rays. Pitfalls are that the films may be of poor quality and out of plane; the metaphyseal fragment can be very small; and displacement rather subtle. Ultrasound can be a useful aid to diagnosis, and several authors have described arthrography to confirm the diagnosis and decide whether operative stabilization is required [43, 44].

Treatment

Essentially *undisplaced lateral condyle fractures* are likely to have intact articular cartilage medially and therefore will not displace any further. These can be treated by immobilization in a sling with or without a split long arm cast. X-rays during and at the end of treatment should be taken to ensure that there is neither delayed displacement nor non-union.

Displaced fractures are likely to displace further due to the pull of the common extensors of the forearm, and therefore should be stabilized. There is general agreement that these fractures should be stabilized and there are two common techniques.

The first of these is open reduction through a lateral approach (Kocher) and stabilization with two divergent

Fig. 43.9 K-wire fixation of a displaced lateral condyle fracture

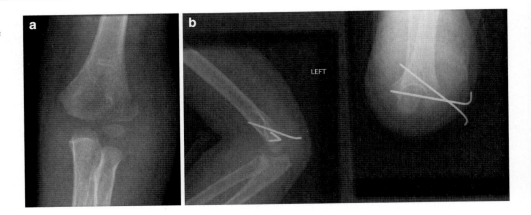

Fig. 43.10 Posterior screw fixation of displaced lateral condyle fracture

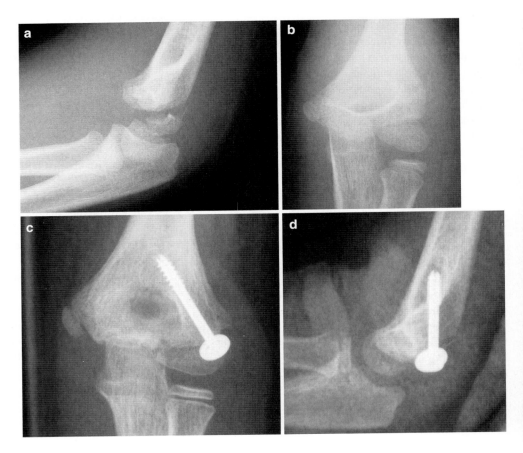

K-wires. Reduction of the joint is observed through an anterior arthrotomy, and no posterior dissection is undertaken in order to protect the blood supply to the fragment. The K-wires are buried under the skin and a long arm cast or a sugar tong splint is applied for immobilization. Healing is generally achieved in 5 weeks. The buried K-wires are removed under general anesthesia in a day clinic; if the wires are not buried they can be removed in the clinic (Fig. 43.9).

Some deformity of the lateral supracondylar ridge has been noted in follow-up studies of these cases [45].The alternative involves screw fixation of the fracture through the metaphyseal fragment [46] (Fig. 43.10). Provided the

common extensor origin is left attached to the fragment it will remain fully vascularized, and the screw can be inserted through the metaphyseal fragment, which is frequently quite large but not well seen from a lateral approach. The advantages of screw fixation are that mobilization can be begun quite early and deformity of the supracondylar ridge is less often seen [47]. The disadvantages are that the screw cannot be used in small children and that the implant removal is a more formal operation.

There is a group of fractures that present rather late. Controversy exists as to at when one should abandon attempts at anatomical reduction. Recent publications

Fig. 43.11 CT of incarcerated medial epicondyle after elbow dislocation and reduction

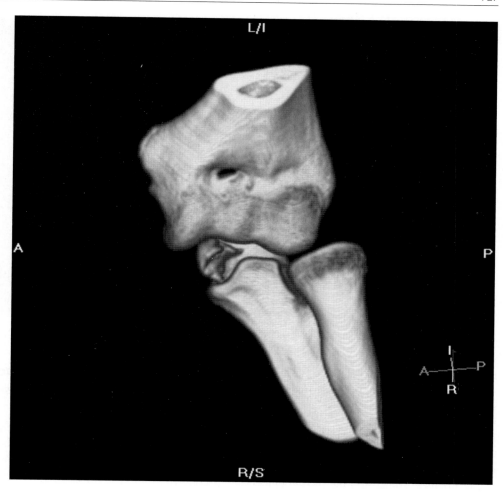

suggest that the window for treatment closes at 6–8 weeks. This seems unnecessarily conservative for a group of fractures that by definition are displaced and slow to heal. Even at 12 weeks the fracture line can be identified in delayed and mal-union and, provided the main soft tissue attachment of the common extensor is left attached, then repositioning is reasonable [48].

Treatment of Late Cases

Conservative treatment of a displaced lateral condyle fracture is usually not successful and leads to non-union. Late diagnosed cases of lateral condyle non-unions are characterized by surprisingly good function in terms of elbow movements. Children present with valgus deformity of the distal humerus and/or with tardy ulnar palsy. Union is achieved by open reduction, autologous bone grafting, pinning by several K-wires, or screw fixation, if the physis is about to terminate growth. Nerve compression often needs ulnar nerve transfer rather than simple decompression.

In very late cases, the objective should be to obtain union of the fracture and prevent further deformity, rather than attempt anatomical reduction which may cause the fragment to lose its blood supply. Having achieved union of the fragment, more proximal osteotomies may be required to achieve the correct alignment of the arm. The variety of different osteotomies described suggests that none is superior and corrective procedures may be accompanied by more residual deformity than operator or parents expect [49, 50].

Fractures of the Medial Epicondyle

Fractures of the medial epicondyle are exclusively associated with dislocations of the elbow joint. Few other injuries produce sufficient force to avulse the epicondyle. Fifty percent of these injuries have a dislocated elbow at the time of presentation. Most of the remainder will have suffered a transient dislocation or subluxation (Fig. 43.11).

The treatment of avulsion fracture of the medial epicondyle is controversial. Undisplaced fractures may be

Fig. 43.12 T-fracture of distal humerus fixed percutaneously

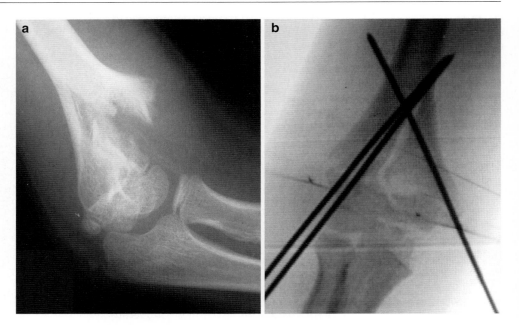

treated non-operatively, but there is little agreement as to what constitutes an undisplaced fracture. The most invasive will only accept 2 mm displacement. About 5–10 mm is commonly accepted, while a long-term follow-up study has suggested that the functional outcome is satisfactory even with 15 mm displacement. Poor results happen: the epicondyle may become stuck down to the medial aspect of the trochlea; sometimes the medial epicondyle becomes entrapped within the joint. This does require intervention, and although closed maneuvers to remove the epicondyle are described, open reduction and fixation are probably superior.

If operation is required, an approach sufficiently large to visualize the ulnar nerve is advisable. In young children two K-wires will be more appropriate to fix a displaced fragment. A long arm cast must be used for 3–5 weeks. If the patient is old enough the medial epicondyle is fixed with a screw as mobilization can then start as soon as the soft tissues have settled down. Mercer Rang recommended fixing these fractures with the patient prone and the affected arm behind the back as this makes reduction easier.

It is important to remember that medial epicondyle avulsions always occur in association with traumatic elbow dislocation and have a relatively high risk of impaired elbow function irrespective of whether they are treated conservatively or operatively. Elbow stiffness should be considered more as a sequel of the ruptured capsule than of the avulsed epicondyle. Parents should be warned about this.

Complete Articular Fractures of the Distal Humerus—T-Fractures

These unusual fractures require reconstitution of the articular surface and suitable re-attachment to the shaft. The treatment chosen depends on the patient's age and the fracture complexity. They usually occur in adolescents who are close to the end of growth, and the fracture patterns resemble those of adults. They should be treated like an adult fracture with precise open reduction and plate fixation. Slightly premature elbow closure will not cause any deformity or length discrepancy. Fractures that occur in the younger age group may have intact articular cartilage with the T being a metaphyseal split only. In that situation treatment should be as for supracondylar fractures although a medial wire is advisable. Preoperative CT scan or arthrography may aid the diagnosis [42]. In those rare cases when a younger child is injured, it may be possible to reduce and hold the fracture with percutaneous wires, thereby avoiding an extensive surgical approach [51] (Fig. 43.12).

References

1. Andersen K, Jensen PO, Lauritzen J. Treatment of clavicular fractures. Figure-of-eight bandage versus a simple sling. Acta Orthop Scand 1987; 58:71–74.
2. Kubiak R, Slongo T. Operative treatment of clavicle fractures in children: a review of 21 years. J Pediatr Orthop 2002; 22:736–739.

3. Al-Qattan MM, Clarke HM, Curtis CG. The prognostic value of concurrent clavicular fractures in newborns with obstetric brachial plexus palsy. J Hand Surg [Br] 1994; 19:729–730.

4. Ogden JA. Distal clavicular physeal injury. Clin Orthop Relat Res 1984; 188:68–73.

5. Waters PM, Bae DS, Kadiyala RK. Short-term outcomes after surgical treatment of traumatic posterior sternoclavicular fracture-dislocations in children and adolescents. J Pediatr Orthop 2003; 23:464–469.

6. Landin LA. Fracture patterns in children. Analysis of 8682 fractures with special reference to incidence, etiology and secular changes in a Swedish urban population, 1950–1979. Acta Orthop Scand Suppl 1983; 3:54

7. Slongo T, Audige L, Clavert JM, Lutz N, Frick S, Hunter J. The AO comprehensive classification of pediatric long-bone fractures: a web-based multicenter agreement study. J Pediatr Orthop 2007; 27:171–180.

8. Broker F, Burbach T. Ultrasonic diagnosis of separation of the proximal humeral epiphysis in the newborn. J Bone Joint Surg (Am) 1990; 72:187–191.

9. Rang M. Children's fractures. 2nd ed. Philadelphia: Lippincott; Philadelphia, Toront; 1983.

10. Chee Y, Agorastides I, Garg N, et al. Treatment of severely displaced proximal humeral fractures in children with elastic stable intramedullary nailing. J Pediatr Orthop B 2006; 15: 45–50.

11. Lucas JC, Mehlman CT, Laor T. The location of the biceps tendon in completely displaced proximal humerus fractures in children: a report of four cases with magnetic resonance imaging and cadaveric correlation. J Pediatr Orthop 2004; 24: 249–253.

12. Dietz H-G, Schmittenbecher PP, Slongo T, Wilkins K. AO Manual of Fracture Management—Elastic Stable Intramedullary Nailing (ESIN) in Children. Stuttgart. New York: Thieme; 2006.

13. Lascombe P. L'embrochage centromédullaire élastique stable Elsevier-Masson 2006; 107–123

14. Worlock P, Stower M, Barbor P. Patterns of fractures in accidental and non-accidental injury in children: a comparative study. Br Med J (Clin Res Ed) 1986; 293(6539):100–102.

15. Shaw BA, Murphy KM, Shaw A, Oppenheim WL, Myracle MR. Humerus shaft fractures in young children: accident or abuse? J Pediatr Orthop 1997; 17:293–297.

16. Loder RT, Feinberg JR. Orthopaedic injuries in children with non-accidental trauma: demographics and incidence from the 2000 kids' inpatient database. J Pediatr Orthop 2007; 27:421–426.

17. Kasser JR, Beaty JH. Supracondylar fractures of the humerus. In: Beaty JH and Kasser JR eds., Rockwood and Wilkins' Fractures in Children. 5th ed. Lippincott: Williams & Wilkins Philadelphia; 2002

18. Gartland JJ. Management of supracondylar fractures of the humerus in children. Surg Gyn Obstet 1959; 109:145–154.

19. Mubarak SJ, Davids J. Closed reduction and percutaneous pinning of the supracondylar fracture in the child. In: Morrey BF, ed. Master Techniques in Orthopaedic Surgery. The Elbow. New York: Raven Press; 1994: 37.

20. Wilkins KE. Supracondylar fractures: what's new? J Pediatr Orthop B 1997; 6:110–116.

21. von Laer L, Gunter SM, Knopf S, Weinberg AM. Supracondylar humerus fracture in childhood—an efficacy study. Results of a multicenter study by the Pediatric Traumatology Section of the German Society of Trauma Surgery—II: Costs and effectiveness of the treatment. Unfallchirurg 2002; 105:217–223

22. Skaggs DL, Sankar WN, Albrektson J, Vaishnav S, Choi PD, Kay RM. How safe is the operative treatment of Gartland type 2 supracondylar humerus fractures in children? J Pediatr Orthop 2008; 28:139–141.

23. Clavert JM, Lecerf C, Mathieu JC, Buck P. Retention in flexion of supracondylar fracture of the humerus in children. Comments apropos of the treatment of 120 displaced fractures. Rev Chir Orthop Reparatrice Appar Mot 1984; 70:109–116

24. Chen RS, Liu CB, Lin XS, Feng XM, Zhu JM, Ye FQ. Supracondylar extension fracture of the humerus in children. Manipulative reduction, immobilisation and fixation using a U-shaped plaster slab with the elbow in full extension. J Bone Joint Surg Br 2001; 83:883–887.

25. Gadgil A, Hayhurst C, Maffulli N, Dwyer JS. Elevated, straight-arm traction for supracondylar fractures of the humerus in children. J Bone Joint Surg Br 2005; 87:82–87.

26. Badhe NP, Howard PW. Olecranon screw traction for displaced supracondylar fractures of the humerus in children. Injury 1998; 29:457–460.

27. Skaggs DL, Hale JM, Bassett J, Kaminsky C, Kay RM, Tolo VT. Operative treatment of supracondylar fractures of the humerus in children. The consequences of pin placement. J Bone Joint Surg Am 2001; 83:735–740.

28. Skaggs DL, Cluck MW, Mostofi A, Flynn JM, Kay RM. Lateral-entry pin fixation in the management of supracondylar fractures in children. J Bone Joint Surg Am 2004; 86:702–707.

29. Reynolds RA, Jackson H. Concept of treatment in supracondylar humeral fractures. Injury 2005; 36(Suppl 1):A51–56.

30. Zenios M, Ramachandran M, Milne B, Little D, Smith N. Intraoperative stability testing of lateral-entry pin fixation of pediatric supracondylar humeral fractures. J Pediatr Orthop 2007; 27:695–702.

31. Zionts LE, McKellop HA, Hathaway R. Torsional strength of pin configurations used to fix supracondylar fractures of the humerus in children. J Bone Joint Surg Am 1994; 76:253–256.

32. Eberhardt O, Fernandez F, Ilchmann T, Parsch K. Cross pinning of supracondylar fractures from a lateral approach. Stabilization achieved with safety. J Child Orthop 2007; 1:127–133

33. Prevot J, Lascombes P, Metaizeau JP, Blanquart D. Supracondylar fractures of the humerus in children: treatment by downward nailing. Rev Chir Orthop Reparatrice Appar Mot 1990; 76:191–197.

34. Slongo T, Jakob RP. The small AO external fixator in paediatric orthopaedics and trauma. Injury 1994; 25(Suppl 4):S-D77–84.

35. Mubarak SJ, Carroll NC. Volkmann's contracture in children: aetiology and prevention. J Bone Joint Surg Br 1979; 61: 285–293.

36. Garbuz DS, Leitch K, Wright JG. The treatment of supracondylar fractures in children with an absent radial pulse. J Pediatr Orthop 1996; 16:594–596.

37. Lewis J, Monk J, Chandratreya A, Hunter J. Changing the management from olecranon screw traction to percutaneous wiring for displaced supracondylar fractures of the humerus in children. A justified decision? Eur J Trauma Emerg Surg 2007; 33: 256–261.

38. Luria S, Sucar A, Eylon S, et al. Vascular complications of supracondylar humeral fractures in children. J Pediatr Orthop B 2007; 16:133–143.

39. Lewis HG, Morrison CM, Kennedy PT, Herbert KJ. Arterial reconstruction using the basilic vein from the zone of injury in pediatric supracondylar humeral fractures: a clinical and radiological series. Plast Reconstr Surg 2003; 111:1159–1163; discussion 1164–1156.

40. Holden C. The pathology and prevention of Volkmann's ischaemic contracture. J Bone Joint Surg Br 1979; 61:296—300.

41. Mahan ST, May CD, Kocher MS. Operative management of displaced flexion supracondylar humerus fractures in children. J Pediatr Orthop 2007; 27:551–556.

42. Blane CE, Kling TF, Jr., Andrews JC, DiPietro MA, Hensinger RN. Arthrography in the posttraumatic elbow in children Am J Roentgenol 1984; 143:17–21.

43. Marzo JM, d'Amato C, Strong M, Gillespie R. Usefulness and accuracy of arthrography in management of lateral humeral condyle fractures in children. J Pediatr Orthop 1990; 10:317–321.

44. Mintzer CM, Waters PM, Brown DJ, Kasser JR. Percutaneous pinning in the treatment of displaced lateral condyle fractures. J Pediatr Orthop 1994; 14:462–465.

45. Thomas DP, Howard AW, Cole WG, Hedden DM. Three weeks of Kirschner wire fixation for displaced lateral condylar fractures of the humerus in children. J Pediatr Orthop 2001; 21:565–569.

46. Mohan N, Hunter JB, Colton CL. The posterolateral approach to the distal humerus for open reduction and internal fixation of fractures of the lateral condyle in children. J Bone Joint Surg Br 2000; 82:643–645.

47. Hasler CC, von Laer L. Prevention of growth disturbances after fractures of the lateral humeral condyle in children. J Pediatr Orthop B 2001; 10:123–130.

48. Wattenbarger JM, Gerardi J, Johnston CE. Late open reduction internal fixation of lateral condyle fractures. J Pediatr Orthop 2002; 22:394–398.

49. Tien YC, Chen JC, Fu YC, Chih TT, Hunag PJ, Wang GJ. Supracondylar dome osteotomy for cubitus valgus deformity associated with a lateral condylar nonunion in children. J Bone Joint Surg Amul 2005; 87:1456–1463.

50. Kim HS, Jahng JS, Han DY, Park HW, Kang HJ, Chun CH. Modified step-cut osteotomy of the humerus. J Pediatr Orthop B 1998; 7:162–166.

51. Ruiz AL, Kealey WD, Cowie HG. Percutaneous pin fixation of intercondylar fractures in young children. J Pediatr Orthop B 2001; 10:211–213.

Chapter 44

Fractures of the Elbow and Forearm

James B. Hunter and Klaus Parsch

Radial Neck

The radial head develops a secondary ossification center, the second to appear at the elbow during childhood, by the age of 3 years or slightly afterward. The radial head is therefore largely made of cartilage and intraarticular fractures are rare. In comparison, the radial neck is commonly fractured, either as a metaphyseal fracture, or as a growth plate injury (Salter Harris I or II). The typical mechanism of injury is a fall on the extended arm with the forces resolving to produce elbow extension and valgus. Radial neck fractures also occur in combination with elbow dislocation. It is vital to diagnose these since the reduction maneuver may otherwise result in full displacement of a previously undisplaced fracture.

The classification of radial neck fractures is somewhat unsatisfactory. Judet's classification has been most widely used but has proved unreliable [1]. Classifications have either concentrated upon the degree of angulation of the fracture, or on the amount of displacement. The key anatomical feature that determines functional outcome is the relationship between the radial head and the annular ligament. This is much more affected by displacement than by angulation, such that quite marked angulation can be accepted, while almost any displacement will need correction. The AO classification distinguishes between metaphyseal and growth plate injuries and uses a simple three-group system for severity (Fig. 44.1):

I. fracture with no angulation and no displacement
II. fracture with angulation and displacement, up to 50% of the bone diameter
III. fracture displaced more than 50% of the bone diameter

Treatment

Many angulated radial neck fractures require no treatment other than early mobilization. All authors would accept 30° of angulation, and some have suggested that more (up to 50°) can be treated conservatively provided there is no displacement [2].

Displaced fractures need to be reduced but closed reduction can be difficult, because of the problems of reducing the distal fragment to the proximal fragment. Manipulation involves the application a valgus force to the elbow and pressure over the radial head to reduce it. This maneuver needs to be accompanied by rotation of the forearm, but is frequently unsuccessful. Semi-closed methods, using a large diameter percutaneous K-wire, are frequently used. We prefer to use the flat end of a 3 mm wire to push against the radial head directly, rather than using the sharp end in the fracture gap, which can endanger the posterior interosseous nerve or the blood supply [3]. This method is frequently used in conjunction with the technique of Metaizeau in which an intramedullary elastic nail or K-wire is used both to reduce the fracture and to stabilize it, allowing early mobilization [4]. This is now the most popular method throughout Europe (Fig. 44.2).

The key steps are shown in Fig. 44.3:

1. Partially reduce using manipulation or K-wire.
2. Visualize maximum displacement under the image intensifier.
3. Direct bent nail into the head, disimpacting the fracture.
4. Rotate the nail to reduce the fracture.

Open reduction is only rarely required if the combination of the above techniques has failed. Generally, this only occurs if the radial head is fully displaced and lying parallel to the shaft. In some circumstances, the radial head may be flipped over, such that the articular surface is facing the fracture site. This occurs most frequently when radial neck fracture is associated with elbow dislocation, the

J.B. Hunter (✉)
Departments of Trauma and Orthopaedics, Nottingham University Hospital, Nottingham, UK

M. Benson et al. (eds.), *Children's Orthopaedics and Fractures*,
DOI 10.1007/978-1-84882-611-3_44, © Springer-Verlag London Limited 2010

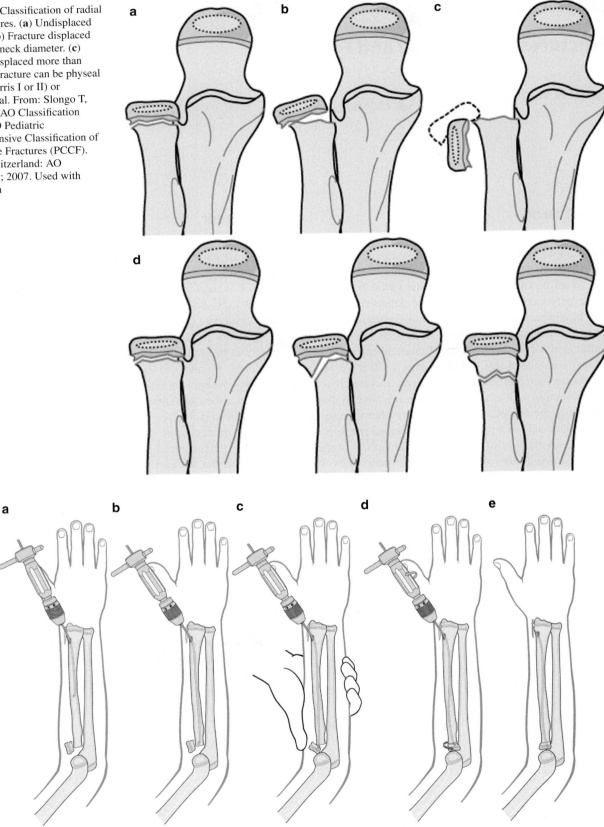

Fig. 44.1 Classification of radial neck fractures. (**a**) Undisplaced fracture. (**b**) Fracture displaced up to 50% neck diameter. (**c**) Fracture displaced more than 50%. (**d**) Fracture can be physeal (Salter–Harris I or II) or metaphyseal. From: Slongo T, Audigé L, AO Classification Group. AO Pediatric Comprehensive Classification of Long Bone Fractures (PCCF). Davos, Switzerland: AO Publishing; 2007. Used with permission

Fig. 44.2 Metaizeau technique for reduction and stabilization of radial neck fractures. From: Dietz H-G, Schmittenbecher P, Slongo T. AO Manual of Fracture Management: Elastic Stable Intramedullary nailing (ESIN) in Children. Davos, Switzerland: AO Publishing; 2006. Used with permission

Fig. 44.3 Radiographs of radial neck fracture treated by Metaizeau technique

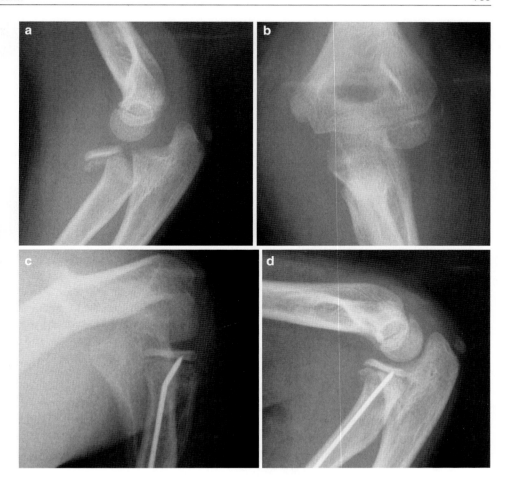

inversion occurring during attempted reduction. The surgical approach is determined by the position of the radial head, and sometimes an anterior approach (Henry) is appropriate. A sigmoid, transverse incision is much more cosmetic than a longitudinal incision crossing the elbow. If a lateral approach is used, then great care must be taken to preserve the periosteal sleeve that is attached to the radial head. This contains the blood supply so that an over-invasive open reduction is associated with avascular necrosis of the radial head and non-union of the fracture. Intramedullary stabilization is still preferable, even after open reduction, to allow forearm rotation during healing.

Olecranon Fractures

True olecranon fractures are relatively rare in children, especially when one considers how often they graze their elbows. This is because the olecranon is largely composed of cartilage during childhood. The proximal apophysis appears at around the age of 9 years, and fuses to the ulnar shaft at the end of the growth spurt after becoming bipartite and

enlarging. At this stage, it is somewhat vulnerable both to fracture and misdiagnosis. Olecranon fractures can be sleeve fractures in which a large portion of articular cartilage is contained within a fragment that appears to be extra-articular. Displaced olecranon fractures should be explored, reduced, and stabilized accurately. Tension band wiring, as used in adult practice, is the technique of choice; wires of appropriate diameter for the size of the child should be used, and the elbow mobilized early (Fig. 44.4).

More complex fractures of the proximal ulna are frequently associated with Monteggia injuries and are considered below.

Fractures of the Radial and Ulnar Shafts

These are the most common diaphyseal injuries of childhood. Generally, the mechanism is a simple fall, frequently from a modest height, such as a gate or playground equipment. All types of childhood diaphyseal injury are seen, often in combination. Thus a complete fracture of the radius may be seen with plastic deformity of the ulna, and the

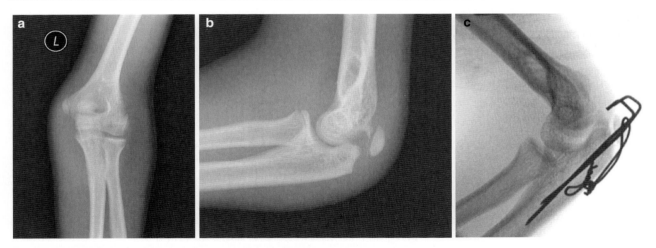

Fig. 44.4 Olecranon fracture treated by tension band wiring, although apparently extra-articular a large sleeve of articular cartilage was attached to the fragment

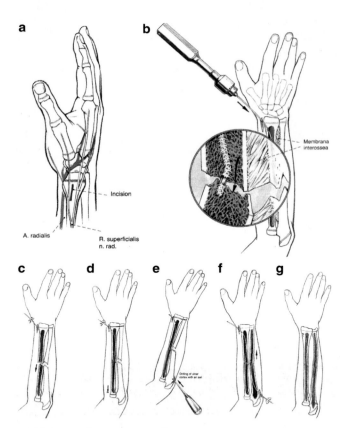

Fig. 44.5 Intramedullary elastic pinning with blunt K-wire From Parsch K. Morote pinning Orthopaedic Traumatologic operations 1992 Copyright © Urban and Vogel. Reproduced with permission **a)** Entry point for radial elastic wire. **b)** blunt prebent K-wire passes the fracture by rotating back and forth reducing the fracture. **c)** Radial wire is moving past the fracture. **d)** Radial wire has reached the radial neck, aligning the radial fracture. **e)** An awl opens the medullary canal of the proximal ulna distal to the olecranon. **f)** The ulnar wire is pushed past the ulna fracture by rotatory movements. **g)** The wire ends are cut 10 mm distal the entry point and bent 150 degrees and impacted into the periostium. The skin is closed

different behavior of these fracture types may affect management. The vast majority of these fractures are incomplete and undisplaced, although angulated sufficiently to require active management. The relationship between the radius and ulna must be accurately maintained to preserve forearm rotation. In adult practice, anatomical reduction is required for pronation and supination; in children this is not the case, because the periosteal sleeve and the interosseous membrane are generally intact, and because some remodeling will take place, albeit less than in the metaphyses.

Conservative Treatment

Angulation is the main cause of lost forearm rotation. Every 10° of angulation in the midshaft will lead to a loss of 20° of total forearm rotation (180°) [5, 6]. If forearm rotation is blocked, then remodeling will not occur satisfactorily. Therefore, 10° of angulation developing during follow-up is acceptable, but more is not. If angulation does develop, then it should be corrected, either by re-manipulation or by wedging of the cast, which can be achieved in the clinic under appropriate analgesia.

Displacement of forearm shaft fractures is important, because of the effect it has upon angulation. In younger children (8 years and under), bayonet apposition of the radius and the shaft is acceptable provided both bones have displaced in the same direction and the interosseous distance is maintained. In this situation, healing occurs quickly and rotation can resume before any permanent stiffness develops. If one fracture is reduced and the other displaced, the situation is unstable and likely to tip into angulation. If managed conservatively, the cast must be carefully molded into an oval shape to spread the interosseous membrane (as it must for all radial and ulnar fractures), and careful, weekly follow-up instituted as angulation may occur quite late.

Rotation at the fracture site is classically judged using the method of Evans, assessing the appearance of the bicipital tuberosity and comparing it with the appearance of the distal radius [7]. Use of this method has led to the recommendation that 30° of rotational mismatch can be accepted in the management of forearm shaft fractures [8]. From first principles this seems unlikely, particularly as Evans's method can be very difficult to use in the young child. Reductions in which there is obvious rotational mismatch of the diameter of the radius and ulna are unlikely to be correct, and re-reduction is recommended [6].

The main debate in the treatment of these fractures in children concerns how much angulation can be accepted in the expectation of remodeling, and how much morbidity actually results from residual angulation. Papers from the last decades of the 20th century suggested that there was little loss of movement as a result of conservative management of these fractures [6, 8]. A more critical analysis from Central Europe found a relatively high rate of malunion, and loss of motion associated with it [9]. Typical results were a re-reduction rate of 10%, visible residual deformity at follow-up in more than 10%, and a greater than 20° loss of forearm rotation in 7%. Some papers found loss of rotation to be greatest when the fractures were at the same level, while others found loss of function to be worst with proximal radial fractures [10]. Therefore, when treated conservatively forearm fractures require a relatively long period of immobilization and very careful follow-up.

Surgical Treatment

The combination of a moderately high risk of less than perfect results, the need for multiple visits, and the availability of a less invasive method of osteosynthesis (elastic stable intramedullary nailing, or ESIN) has led to more of these fractures being treated operatively in the last 25 years. Good results have been reported using both formal elastic nails and K-wires inserted by the same technique (Fig. 44.6) [11–14]. Our policy is to use elastic nails primarily for all fully displaced (off-ended) diaphyseal fractures of the radius and ulna, except for children under 6 years of age. The reason for this seemingly aggressive policy is that closed nailing is much more likely if the nails are used at the first operation rather than at any later procedure. The learning curve for nailing is such that in the third year of practice, 85% of these cases can be dealt with by closed nailing [14]. The infection rate is minimal and the main complication seems to be a slight increase in the incidence of compartment syndrome [15]. This probably results because any open reduction is normally done through a minimal approach in the line of the Thompson incision, insufficient to decompress the volar forearm compartments; secondly, elastic nails prevent loss of reduction by shortening which would normally lead to a reduction in compartment pressure.

The technique for intramedullary nailing of the radius and ulna is relatively simple [3, 13, 14] (Fig. 44.7). The conventional entry points in the distal radial metaphysis are either at the base of the radial styloid or Lister's tubercle. If the

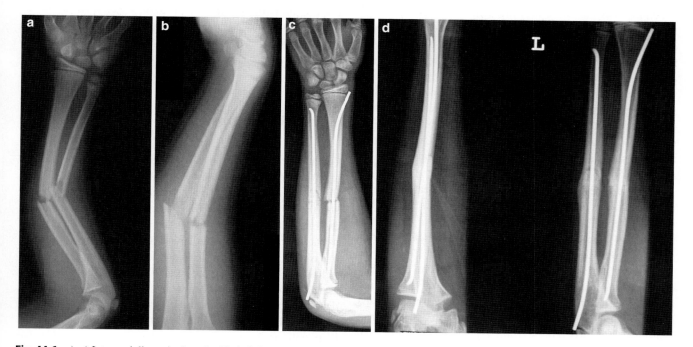

Fig. 44.6 a)–c) Intramedullary pinning of mid-shaft forearm fracture. **d)** follow-up at 3 months before pin removal

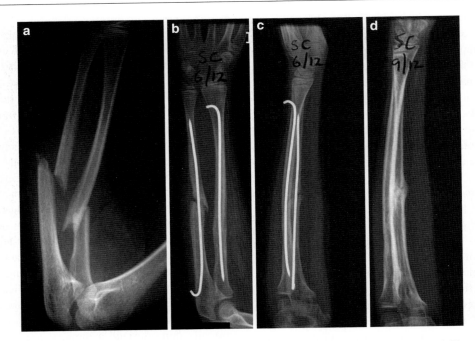

Fig. 44.7 **a**) dislocated mid-shaft forearm fracture in a 10-year-old boy. **b**) after 2 months low healing tendancy. **c**) Five months after fracture solid healing. **d**)The stainless steel wires have been removed

former is chosen, care must be taken to avoid the superficial branches of the radial nerve. If the latter is chosen it is the extensor tendons that are at risk. Damage to these can be avoided by an adequate incision to visualize the insertion point and by leaving the nail long so that the cut end is not in the same plane as the tendons but in the subcutaneous fat. If Kirschner wires are used they are bent over to form a "pig's tail" thus avoiding irritation to the soft tissues. The ulna is conventionally pinned from the lateral side of the proximal metaphysis, which is easily and safely accessible. This can be a little awkward with positioning and image intensification, so a start point in the distal metaphysis has been described [3]. The radial nail should be contoured to recreate the bow of the radius thus stretching the interosseous membrane. The ulnar nail is generally straight, or gently contoured to keep the ulna straight, preventing it from collapsing toward the radius.

The aftercare of fractures that have been treated by elastic nailing is to mobilize them early. No cast is required. A bandage and a broad arm sling for a few days are all that is required. Elbow, forearm, and wrist movements should be commenced as soon as symptoms permit.

Forearm shaft fractures are relatively slow to heal when compared to other paediatric fractures. Generally, 6 weeks in a cast is required for fractures that have been manipulated. Elastic nailing of these fractures is associated with slower healing, particularly if open reduction has been required [16]. Another factor implicated in slow healing may be the use of

nails that are too stiff, either because they are too broad or made of steel. Nail or K-wire diameters should be between 1.6 and 1.8 mm if they are made of stainless steel and 1.5 or 2 mm if they are made of titanium, depending upon age (Fig. 44.8).

The Nancy group recommend that the nails be left in situ for 6 months before retrieval [13, 17]. Retrieval is recommended in all cases. If secondary fractures occur with nails still in place these can either be bent straight and immobilized in a cast or, more usually, be replaced by new nails.

Galeazzi Fractures

Galeazzi fractures of the radius with dislocation of the distal radio-ulnar joint are less common than isolated fractures of the radius in children. They generally occur in adolescence shortly before maturity. This is because the ligaments and capsule of the joint are extremely strong. The principle of management is accurate reduction of the radius to allow healing of the joint capsule. The method of stabilization of the radius will depend upon the level of the fracture: diaphysis—elastic nail; junction of metaphysis and diaphysis—plate; distal radius—K-wires. Immobilization in pronation is recommended, but this should not be too prolonged as ligaments and capsule require movement for effective healing.

Fig. 44.8 Mid-shaft fracture in 9-year old boy treated with intramedullary Morote wires

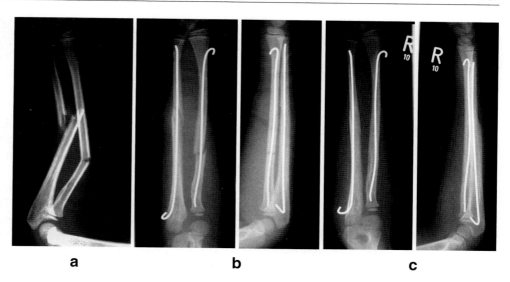

a   b   c

Monteggia Fracture Dislocation

In the early 19th century Giovanni Battista Monteggia, Professor of Surgery in Milan, described the clinical picture of a fracture of the proximal ulna in a young girl which, after healing, was followed by a hard and ugly prominence on the anterior surface of the elbow identified as a "jumping radius." [18].

The classification is detailed in Fig. 44.9. Bado from Montevideo defined the Monteggia lesion as an association of a radial head dislocation or fracture with a fracture of the middle or proximal ulna and described four types: [19]

- Type I: anterior dislocation of the radial head in combination with an anteriorly angulated, mid-shaft ulnar fracture. About 70% of Monteggia injuries belong to this group.
- Type II: posterior dislocation of the radial head in combination with a very proximal metaphyseal fracture of the ulna, angulated posteriorly. Bado type II lesions are rare and are more common in adults than in children, where they have a frequency of only 3% [20].
- Type III: the radial head is dislocated antero-laterally in association with a fracture of the ulnar metaphysis. This type accounts for 23% of these fractures in children [20].

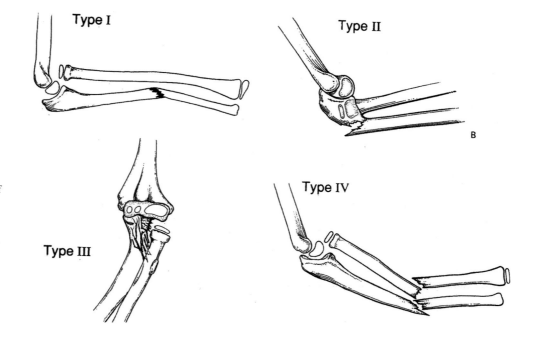

Fig. 44.9 Bado classification of Monteggia lesions. Reproduced with permission from Stanley EA, de la Garza JF. Monteggia fracture dislocations in children. Part III. In Rockwood And Wilkins' Fractures in children. 5th edition. Editors: JH Beaty and JR Kasser Philadelphia PA, Lippicott Williams & Wilkins 2001

- Type IV: an anterior dislocation of the radial head in combination with a fracture of both radius and ulna at the same level. This combination is rare, only 1% of the total [21, 22].

Monteggia Equivalent (Variant) Injuries

In addition to the classic Monteggia lesion, Bado classified certain injuries as Monteggia equivalents:

Type I equivalent (variant) is an isolated anterior dislocation of the radial head with a minimal plastic deformation of the ulna which might not be visible radiographically. The pulled elbow with radial head subluxation under the annular ligament is also classified as a Monteggia equivalent. Another type I equivalent is the combination of a fracture of the ulnar diaphysis with fracture of the radial neck.

Type II equivalent is an epiphyseal fracture of the radial head or radial neck.

Type III and type IV Monteggia equivalents are extremely rare.

Letts et al. [23] based their classification of Monteggia fractures upon both the direction of radial head displacement and the type of ulnar fracture. Bado type I lesions were subdivided into three groups:

Letts type A is a bowing fracture of the ulna with anterior dislocation of the radial head. Type B shows a greenstick fracture of the ulna, while type C has a complete ulnar fracture. Letts type D corresponds to Bado type II, while type E corresponds to Bado type III.

Mechanism of Injury

Three different mechanisms have been considered to cause Monteggia type I lesion:

- *The direct blow theory* is attributable to Monteggia himself in his description of the girl who was the index case [18]. A direct blow to the forearm can cause a transverse fracture of the ulna and anterior dislocation of the radial head.
- *The hyperpronation theory* has been favored by Bado [19]. The child falls on the pronated forearm in extension, fracturing the ulna and dislocating the radial head during further pronation in extension.
- *The hyperextension theory* described by Tompkins recognized the forward momentum caused by a fall on the outstretched hand, forcing the elbow into extension. Sudden biceps contraction forcibly dislocates the radial head. The forward momentum then fractures the ulna because the radius is no longer the weight transmitting

bone of the forearm. This theory combines dynamic and static forces [24].

Anatomy

The *annular ligament* provides stability for the radial head and its position within the radial notch of the ulna. In children the radial head pulls out of the intact annular ligament, while in adults the injury tears the ligament. This is one of the main reasons that the Monteggia lesion is more benign in children than in adults [25]. The *quadrate ligament* connecting the radial neck to the proximal ulna adds stability. Distal to the insertion of the biceps tendon the oblique ligament and the interosseous membrane tighten during supination of the radius.

The biceps muscle inserting into the radial tuberosity plays an important role in the pathomechanics of the Monteggia lesion. The posterior interosseous nerve also has a close anatomical relationship to the proximal radius such that acute anterior or lateral dislocation of the radius may cause paresis of this nerve. Recovery of function is usually complete in a few weeks.

Clinical Findings

Considerable swelling around the elbow and severe pain characterize the injury. The child cannot move the elbow in either flexion and extension or pronation and supination. As the swelling subsides a bump may be palpated in the cubital fossa, caused by the radial head.

Radiographic Findings

As in any forearm and elbow injury anteroposterior (AP) and lateral radiographs must always include the neighboring joints. Besides the ulnar fracture or bowing, the relationship of the radial head to the capitellum must be checked. On the AP view the radial head may look normally positioned but on the lateral view a line drawn through the center of the radial head and neck ceases to extend directly through the center of the capitellum [26]. It must be stressed that in suspected Monteggia lesion the radiocapitellar relationship must be very carefully assessed [27].

Treatment of Type I Lesions

Almost all acute type I Monteggia fractures can be treated conservatively; however, many benefit from operative ulnar stabilization. Conservative treatment entails three steps: reduction of the ulna, reduction of the radial head, and immobilization in a well-molded long arm cast.

Reduction of the ulna is achieved by longitudinal traction and manual pressure over the apex of the angular deformity. With greenstick fractures and plastic deformation of the ulna, reduction is equally necessary in order to gain length, allow for reduction of the radial head, and prevent loss of reduction. When the radius is intact it can be difficult to over reduce the plastically deformed ulna past its yield point, so the ulna may need to be osteotomized percutaneously by a drill and chisel technique.

Reduction of the radial head is possible only after restoration of the length and proper alignment of the ulna. The radial head can be located by a simple elbow flexion maneuver.

A well-molded long arm plaster or splint is needed in flexion of 110° in order to reduce the dislocating force of the biceps muscle. Repeated radiographic reviews are necessary to ensure that ulnar alignment and reduction of the radial head is preserved [28]. This approach works well with greenstick fractures but can be a problem in primarily unstable ulna fractures which may later develop malalignment of the ulnar fracture followed by redislocation or subluxation of the radial head.

In the past, unstable ulnar fractures have been fixed by plates [29–31], but intramedullary devices have a major advantage as pins or wires can be introduced with minimal invasiveness. There is a considerable advantage in stabilizing the fracture of the ulna with an intramedullary device under the same anesthetic [14]. The insertion of a K- wire or flexible nail is similar to the treatment of forearm shaft fractures (Fig. 44.10).

In Monteggia equivalent lesions, combining an ulnar fracture with a displaced fracture of the radial neck, the ulna fracture must be reduced and percutaneously pinned. The radial neck and head is then reduced according to the Metaizeau technique (Fig. 44.11).

Treatment of Type II Lesions

This fracture is more common in adults than in children, especially in those with osteoporosis after long-term therapy with corticosteroids [32]. Closed reduction of the ulnar fracture is usually possible by applying longitudinal traction with the elbow held at 60° of flexion. The radial head will reduce spontaneously or by applying local pressure against the posterior aspect of the elbow. If the fracture of the ulna is stable, immobilization in a long arm cast either in full extension or 80° of flexion is ensured for 4–6 weeks until the fracture has healed. In case of instability of the proximal ulna and the risk of repeated posterior dislocation, retrograde pinning is advised, or plate fixation, as in the adult.

Treatment of Type III Lesions

After the correct diagnosis is established, nonoperative treatment is advised and is effective in most cases. A valgus stress corrects the varus deformity of the metaphyseal fracture of the ulna. The radial head will slip back into its correct position during the same maneuver. Reduction of the fracture and of the radial head is monitored radiographically. When the ulna is stable after reduction and the radial head is well aligned, immobilization for 4 weeks in a long arm cast is necessary. If conservative treatment has failed, open reduction and internal fixation are necessary, possibly with repair of the annular ligament. The reduced ulna is either plated or secured by K-wires. A molded long arm cast with the elbow flexed is applied until union. Radiographs must confirm the reduced position of the radial head throughout the healing period.

Treatment of Type IV Lesions

Intramedullary stabilization with blunt K-wires or thin titanium nails is the treatment of choice [12, 14, 17]. After alignment of both ulna and radius the radial head will usually stay reduced. If the child is seen without delay closed reduction and percutaneous pinning are possible.

In delayed cases and larger adolescents open reduction may be necessary. The radius is internally fixed, the radiocapitellar relationship restored, and the ulna plated.

Differential Diagnosis—Congenital Dislocation of the Radial Head

If the radiocapitellar relationship is abnormal, congenital dislocation, with or without radio-ulnar synostosis, should be considered. Posterior radial head displacement can be confused with a Bado type II lesion. Congenital dislocations are often diagnosed quite late, when the child has developed restriction of forearm rotation. The extension deficit may be overlooked for years. True congenital dislocations are usually bilateral and seen in various syndromes like Larsen's or Ehlers–Danlos. Surgery to reduce the congenital dislocation of radial head is not advised; it is unlikely to produce a better range of motion because the radio-ulnar joint is incongruous.

Delayed Diagnosis of Monteggia Lesions

Monteggia lesions, especially the type I, may occur with only ulnar bowing or a greenstick fracture in the midshaft. If careful radiographic examination is omitted persistent dislocation

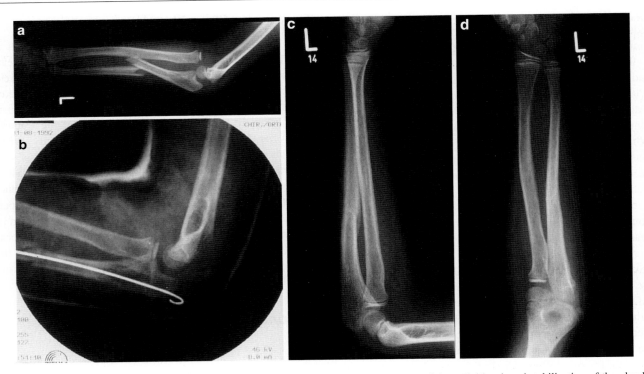

Fig. 44.10 **a**) Type I Monteggia fracture. **b**) Closed reduction of the ulna, closed reduction of the radial head, and stabilization of the ulna by intramedullary K-wire. **c**) and **d**) outcome 6 months after fracture dislocation

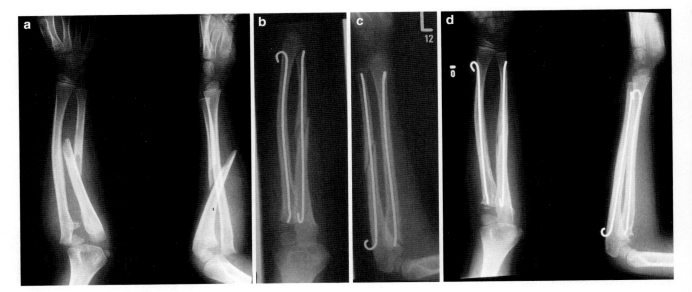

Fig. 44.11 Monteggia variant with displaced fracture of radial neck rather than dislocation. Closed reduction of the ulna and stabilization by intramedullary K-wire, closed reduction and stabilization of dislocated radial neck in the Metaizeau technique (see Fig. 44.3)

may be diagnosed at a later stage, manifest with a fullness in the lateral cubital fossa [33].

If the initial radiographic examinations do not include the elbow joint, most importantly a true lateral view, the dislocation of the radial head will be missed. Children presenting with persistent dislocation of the radial head usually present with insufficient previous radiographs.

Initially, an untreated Monteggia lesion with established radial head displacement is painless and movements are little restricted. In long-standing cases there is restricted motion, both pronation and supination and flexion (caused by impingement of the dislocated radial head). Pain, instability, degenerative joint disease, and late neuropathy may follow [25]. It is unclear how long after injury it is appropriate to attempt correction. Surgical reduction as late as 6 years after the injury has been reported [34].

Treatment of Persistent Dislocation of The Radial Head

Reduction of the Radial Head with Annular Ligament Reconstruction

Conservative methods have no chance of providing a stable radio-humeral joint. Although the annular ligament is not torn during the initial lesion, secondary atrophy occurs with time. Annular ligament reconstructions include reefing [25] or use of a strip of biceps tendon, triceps brachii tendon, or the lacertus fibrosus [35]. We have for many years used a strip taken from fascia lata. To support annular ligament reconstructions a transcapitellar K-wire has been recommended during the initial phase, thus keeping the radial head in the reduced position [33, 34]. Wire breakage and difficulty in implant retrieval are definite risks so a temporary, stabilizing oblique K-wire is safer, augmenting the use of a well-molded, long arm cast.

Osteotomy of The Ulna

An ulnar osteotomy is indicated if there is residual ulnar angulation on the lateral radiograph since radial head reduction will otherwise fail. Corrective osteotomy of the ulna, with or without lengthening, is then secured with a plate [36–39]. Combining this with open reduction and reconstruction of the annular ligament ensures more stability but bears a risk of loss of some pronation (Fig. 44.12). Closed or open reduction by gradual lengthening and angulation using an external fixator has also been suggested for the missed, chronic anterior dislocation of the radial head [40, 41].

Reconstructive surgery is fraught with complications, hence the debate about how late it can be undertaken. Residual radiocapitellar dislocation or subluxation, ulnar nerve palsy, heterotopic ossification, and fibrous synostosis with loss of pronation and supination may complicate the procedure [20, 42].

Summary

Paediatric Monteggia fracture-dislocations and Monteggia variants will do well after conservative treatment by closed reduction if recognized acutely. Fixation of the ulna reduces the risk of secondary malunion and redislocation of the radial head if there is concern about the durability of reduction. Late diagnosis is all too common, partly because the injury may be considered relatively trivial at presentation, but also because diagnostically important radiographs are not requested. The surgical treatment of a long-standing dislocation of the radial head is technically difficult. Angular and lengthening osteotomy of the ulna, with or without reconstruction of the annular ligament, leads to satisfactory results in most cases.

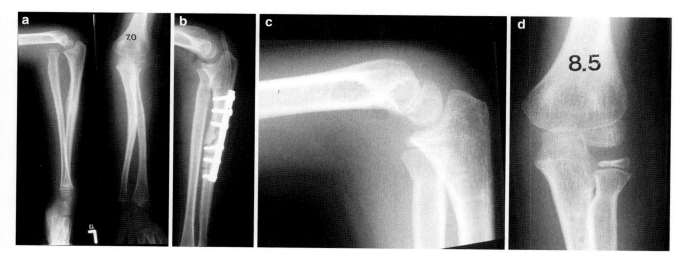

Fig. 44.12 Neglected Monteggia fracture treated by ulnar lengthening and flexion osteotomy, relocation of radial head, and reconstruction of the annular ligament using a fascia lata strip

References

1. Slongo T, Audige L, Clavert JM, Lutz N, Frick S, Hunter J. The AO comprehensive classification of pediatric long-bone fractures: a web-based multicenter agreement study. J Pediatr Orthop 2007; 27(2):171–180.

2. Vocke-Hell AK, von Laer L. Displaced fractures of the radial neck in children: long term results and prognosis with conservative treatment. J Pediatr Orthop Br 1997; 7(3):217–222.

3. Dietz H-G, Schmittenbecher PP, Slongo T, Wilkins K. AO Manual of Fracture Management—Elastic Stable Intramedullary Nailing (ESIN) in Children. Stuttgart, New York: Thieme; 2006.

4. Metaizeau JP, Lascombes P, Lemelle JL, et al. Reduction and fixation of displaced radial neck fractures by closed intramedullary pinning. J Pediatr Orthop 1993; 13(3):355–360.

5. Roberts JA. Angulation of the radius in children's fractures. J Bone Joint Surg Br 1986; 68(5):751–754.

6. Fuller DJ, McCullough CJ. Malunited fractures of the forearm in children. J Bone Joint Surg Br 1982; 64(3):364–367.

7. Evans EM. Fractures of the radius and ulna. J Bone Joint Surg Br 1951; 33:548–561.

8. Price CT, Scott DS, Kurzner ME, Flynn JC. Malunited forearm fractures in children. J Pediatr Orthop 1990; 10(6): 705–712.

9. Schmittenbecher PP, Dietz HG, Uhl S. [Late results of forearm fractures in childhood]. Unfallchirurg 1991; 94(4):186–190.

10. Holdsworth BJ, Sloan JP. Proximal forearm fractures in children: residual disability. Injury 1982; 14(2):174–179.

11. Perez-Sicilia J, Morote Jurado J, Corbacho Girones J. Osteosyntesis percutánea en fracturas diafisarias de antebrazo en ninos y adolescentes. Rev Esp Cir Ost 1977; 12:321–334.

12. Verstreken L, Delronge G, Lamoureux J. Shaft forearm fractures in children: intramedullary nailing with immediate motion: a preliminary report. J Pediatr Orthop 1988; 8(4):450–453.

13. Lascombes P, Prevot J, Ligier JN, et al. Elastic stable intramedullary nailing in forearm shaft fractures in children: 85 cases. J Pediatr Orthop 1990; 10(2):167–171.

14. Parsch K. Morote pinning for displaced midshaft forearm fractures in children. Orthop Traumatol 1992; 1:149–158.

15. Yuan PS, Pring ME, Gaynor TP, et al. Compartment syndrome following intramedullary fixation of pediatric forearm fractures. J Pediatr Orthop 2004; 24(4):370–375.

16. Schmittenbecher PP, Fitze G, Godeke J, et al. Delayed healing of forearm shaft fractures in children after intramedullary nailing. J Pediatr Orthop 2008; 28(3):303–306.

17. Lascombes P, Haumont T, Journeau P. [Centromedullary nailing for fracture of both forearm bones in children and adolescents]. Rev Chir Orthop Reparatrice Appar Mot 2006; 92(6):615–622.

18. Rang M. The story of orthopaedics. Philadelphia: WB Saunders; 2000:407–408.

19. Bado JL. The Monteggia lesion. Clin Orthop Relat Res 1967; 50:71–86.

20. Stanley E, de la Garzia J. Monteggia fracture dislocation in children. In: Beaty JH, Kasser JR, eds. Rockwood & Wilkins: Fractures in Children, 5th ed. Philadelphia: Lippincott Williams & Wilkins; 2002:529–562.

21. Wiley JJ, Galey JP. Monteggia injuries in children. J Bone Joint Surg Br 1985; 67(5):728–731.

22. Olney BW, Menelaus MB. Monteggia and equivalent lesions in childhood. J Pediatr Orthop 1989; 9(2):219–223.

23. Letts M, Locht R, Wiens J. Monteggia fracture dislocations in children. J Bone Joint Surg Br 1985; 67 :724–727.

24. Tompkins DG. The anterior Monteggia fracture: observations on etiology and treatment. J Bone Joint Surg Am 1971; 53(6):1109–1114.

25. Kalamchi A. Monteggia fracture-dislocation in children. Late treatment in two cases. J Bone Joint Surg 1986; 68(4):615–619.

26. Storen G. Traumatic dislocation of radial head as an isolated lesion in children. Acta Orthop Scand 1959; 116:144–147.

27. Miles KA, Finlay DB. Disruption of the radiocapitellar line in the normal elbow. Injury 1989; 20(6):365–367.

28. Dormans JP, Rang M. The problem of Monteggia fracture-dislocations in children. Orthop Clin of North Am 1990; 21(2):251–256.

29. Fowles JV, Sliman N, Kassab MT. The Monteggia lesion in children. Fracture of the ulna and dislocation of the radial head. J Bone Joint Surg 1983; 65(9):1276–1282.

30. Ring D, Waters PM. Operative fixation of Monteggia fractures in children. J Bone Joint Surg Br 1996; 78(5):734–739.

31. Ring D, Jupiter JB, Waters PM. Monteggia fractures in children and adults. J Am Acad Orthop Surg 1998; 6(4):215–224.

32. Haddad FS, Manktelow AR, Sarkar JS. The posterior Monteggia: a pathological lesion? Injury 1996; 27(2):101–102.

33. Lloyd-Roberts G, Bucknill T. Anterior dislocation of the radial head in children: aetiology, natural history and management. J Bone Joint Surg Br 1977; 59(4):402–407.

34. Best TN. Management of old unreduced Monteggia fracture dislocations of the elbow in children. J Pediatr Orthop 1994; 14(2):193–199.

35. Bell Tawse AJ. The treatment of malunited anterior Monteggia fractures in children. J Bone Joint Surg Br 1965; 47(4):718–723.

36. Bouyala JM, Chrestian P, Ramaherison P. [High osteotomy of the ulna in the treatment of residual anterior dislocation following Monteggia fracture (author's trans)]. Chir Pediatr 1978; 19(3):201–203.

37. Stoll TM, Willis RB, Paterson DC. Treatment of the missed Monteggia fracture in the child. J Bone Joint Surg Br 1992; 74(3):436–440.

38. Inoue G, Shionoya K. Corrective ulnar osteotomy for malunited anterior Monteggia lesions in children. 12 patients followed for 1–12 years. Acta Orthop Scand 1998; 69(1):73–76.

39. Lädermann A, Ceroni D, Lefèvre Y, et al. Surgical treatment of missed Monteggia lesions in children. J Child Orthop 2007; 1:237–242.

40. Exner GU. Missed chronic anterior Monteggia lesion. Closed reduction by gradual lengthening and angulation of the ulna. J Bone Joint Surg Br 2001; 83(4):547–550.

41. Hasler CC, von Laer L, Hell AK. Open reduction, ulnar osteotomy and external fixation for chronic anterior dislocation of the head of the radius. J. Bone Joint Surg Br 2005; 87:88–94.

42. Rodgers WB, Waters PM, Hall JE. Chronic Monteggia lesions in children. Complications and results of reconstruction. J Bone Joint Surg 1996; 78(9):1322–1329.

Chapter 45

Wrist and Hand Fractures

Malcolm F. Macnicol and Klaus Parsch

Children sustain fractures of the wrist and hand because they are vulnerable parts of the body during everyday activity, particularly in the older child. Distal forearm fractures account for 40% while phalangeal fractures account for 20% of all paediatric fractures [1]. Twenty-five percent of phalangeal fractures are physeal [2], second only to the distal forearm and wrist. Emergency staff will therefore find themselves dealing with these fractures on a regular basis, ideally with both efficient and knowledgeable help from orthopaedic and plastic surgical colleagues.

Distal Radial Fractures

These fractures dominate paediatric skeletal injury and may be associated with more proximal upper limb fractures, such as the supracondylar humeral [3], or with a scaphoid fracture. The distal ulna often fractures concomitantly, whether at the distal metaphysis, growth plate, or ulnar styloid. It is likely that many of the more minor distal fractures are passed off as a sprain and the child is never referred to hospital.

The different distal radial fractures are as follows:

The buckle or torus fracture resulting from axial compression through the dorsal cortex of the radius. By definition, these are little displaced and stable so treatment is symptomatic with a short arm cast or volar splint for 2–3 weeks.

A greenstick fracture describes a dorsal tilt (volar angulation) of the distal radial fragment, the dorsal cortex bending but remaining intact. In children under 10 years of age angulation of up to 30° can be accepted [4], as this will remodel substantially. However, this decision should be fully explained to the parents and may be unacceptable if the wrist looks obviously deformed.

No more than 10° of angulation is acceptable in a girl of 12–13 years or a boy of 14 years. If reduction is undertaken, under anesthesia, a long arm cast is applied with the elbow flexed to 90°. Careful, three-point molding of the cast in minimal palmar flexion and ulnar abduction should be ensured at the wrist and the plaster retained for 3 weeks. This is followed with a short arm cast for 2 weeks [5]. In a randomized study a comparison of short and long arm plaster casts showed equal effectiveness [6]. Radiographic monitoring of the fracture position is ensured for the first and second weeks.

Rupturing of the intact dorsal cortex and periosteum is unnecessary provided padding is minimized and the cast well molded. Forearm pronation is indicated if the fracture presents with volar angulation before reduction, supination for the dorsally angulated fracture.

The complete or "off-ended" fracture is difficult to reduce and 20% displace or angulate in the cast. Reduction relies on increasing the deformity (usually volar angulation) with the distal radius tilted 90° dorsally to allow the proximal and distal fragments to hinge at the fracture site dorsally. A so-called Bier's block (regional intravenous scandicain with tourniquet applied), regional, or general anesthesia is essential for adequate relaxation. Once the cortices are in precise contact the distal fragment is reduced by palmar flexing it, correcting any radial deviation by ulnar tilting.

If contact between the two fragments is anatomical and the reduction feels stable, a molded cast in palmar flexion and ulnar tilt is applied for 4 weeks in younger children, and for 6 weeks in adolescents. Well-molded sugar tong splints are an alternative [7]. The reduction is reviewed radiographically in routine fashion. If there is any doubt about stability following reduction, particularly in the older patient, or if any of the factors detailed below are relevant, retrograde K-wire fixation percutaneously through the radial styloid will secure reduction [5].

Indications for K-wire fixation are as follows:

- bilateral fractures or multilevel upper limb fractures
- open fractures, possibly complicated by neurovascular deficit

M.F. Macnicol (✉)
University of Edinburgh, Edinburgh, UK; Royal Hospital for Sick Children, Edinburgh, UK; Edinburgh and Murrayfield Hospital, Edinburgh, UK; Royal Infirmary, Edinburgh, UK

M. Benson et al. (eds.), *Children's Orthopaedics and Fractures*,
DOI 10.1007/978-1-84882-611-3_45, © Springer-Verlag London Limited 2010

- compartment syndrome where a cast will interfere with review
- soft tissue obstruction and unstable reduction
- redisplacement after closed reduction (Fig. 45.1)

Distal Radial Epiphyseal Fractures

The most common is the Salter-Harris type 2, peaking at 12 years of age. The distal ulna is often fractured too. As with metaphyseal fractures, a "dinner fork deformity" is produced, similar to the *Colles fracture* in the adult; less commonly the tilt is volar, akin to the *Smith's fracture*. Small fracture lines may propagate into the metaphysis from the growth plate but are of no significance.

Reduction is usually stable if undertaken early and therefore internal fixation is unnecessary. A well-molded cast in mild palmar flexion is used for 4 weeks. Remodeling is rapid and effective, so residual angulation of 10° is of no concern unless the patient is a year or two from skeletal maturation. As with all wrist fractures the alignment of the radius must be monitored radiographically (Fig. 45.2). Late manipulation of recurrent angulation and displacement is seldom effective after 10–14 days and may be injurious. Salter-Harris types 3 and 4 physeal fractures are rare and may require K-wire fixation after reduction.

Neurovascular complications, largely median nerve compression and compartment syndrome, require acute and effective management. Early recognition and decompression are the responsibilities of the orthopaedic staff. Anatomical reduction and fixation of the fragments are important in preventing this complication.

Premature growth plate closure is unusual, 7–10% according to Lee et al. [8], and possibly iatrogenic if manipulation is forced or delayed. Excision of a bone tether (see Chapter 41), distal ulnar epiphysiodesis, or ulnar shortening

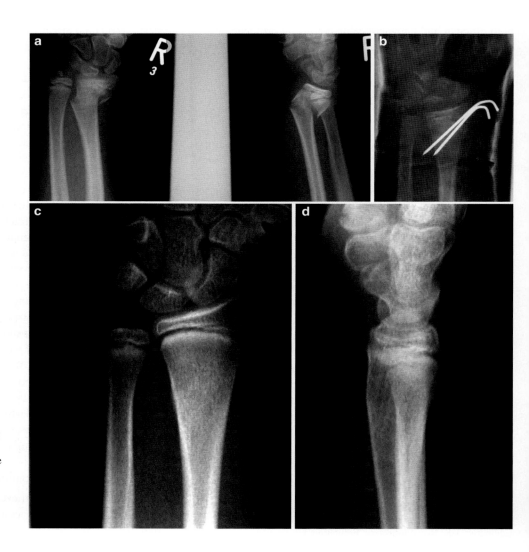

Fig. 45.1 Nine-year-old girl. (**a**) AP and lateral view of distal radial (off-ended) metaphyseal fracture. (**b**) AP view of fracture after closed reduction and stabilization with two K-wires. (**c**) AP and (**d**) lateral views at follow-up after 1 year with normal function of wrist

Fig. 45.2 Thirteen-year-old boy.
(**a**) AP radiograph of distal
Salter-Harris type 2 fracture of
radius and fracture of distal shaft
of the ulna. (**b**) Lateral view
shows extension fracture
dislocation. (**c**) AP radiograph
after reduction in cast. (**d**) Lateral
view of reduced physeal fracture
in a long arm cast, molded with
three-point pressure and some
palmar flexion. (**e**) AP view of
the distal forearm 1 year after the
fracture and lateral view of the
distal forearm at follow-up

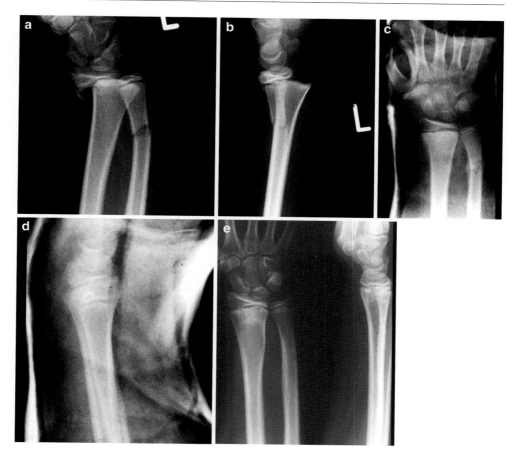

with plate fixation should aim to normalize distal radio-ulnar relationships, function, and range of movement. For late deformity radial osteotomy and possibly radial lengthening may improve function although symptomatic and cosmetic improvement is not assured. Carpoulnar impingement and triangular fibrocartilage tears can be defined by magnetic resonance (MR) scanning. Repair or debridement of the fibrocartilaginous disc may benefit long-term function.

Radial physeal stress fractures (see Fig. 38.18) may develop in gymnasts or from other repetitive upper limb activity. The affected wrist aches and is diffusely tender after exertion, later becoming swollen. Radiographs reveal physeal widening and reactive bone formation. In extreme cases growth arrest occurs.

Distal Ulnar Physeal Fractures

These can occur in isolation but more commonly accompany a distal radial fracture [9]. The displacement is rarely significant [10] and only requires reduction in the older child. Premature growth arrest produces ulnar deviation of the wrist which should be corrected by ulnar lengthening if severe.

Distal Radio-ulnar Subluxation

Forced supination or pronation of the wrist may cause capsular and ligamentous rupture, leading to palmar or dorsal dislocation of the distal ulna, respectively [11]. Reduction is achieved by pronation for the palmar displacement and supination for the dorsal dislocation, maintaining this position of reduction for 4 weeks in a long arm cast with the elbow in 90° of flexion.

Carpal Bone Fractures

The great majority involve the scaphoid (87%), the other carpal bones being injured by crushing or severe disruptions of the wrist [12]. Hyperdorsiflexion may very rarely fracture the capitate. Hamate and hook of hamate fractures may present in athletic adolescents who play a great deal of golf or racquet sports. Lunate fracture-dislocation and lunatomalacia have been reported very rarely in childhood.

Provided the carpal bones are normally aligned on antero-posterior (AP), lateral, and oblique views of the wrist, a short arm cast for 3–4 weeks is sufficient treatment if there is no gapping at the fracture. The wrist should be splinted in slight dorsiflexion and the thumb partially incorporated in the cast, leaving its interphalangeal joint to flex and extend.

Scaphoid Fractures

These are rarely sustained by the younger child but may coexist with a distal radial fracture [13]. Clinical features include the usual history of a fall on the outstretched hand, wrist pain worsened by gripping, and acute tenderness over the anatomical "snuff box." Four-view radiographs of the wrist should be obtained and, even if they appear normal, a precautionary plaster cast is indicated, as for a wrist sprain.

In case of suspicion radiographs should be repeated 10–14 days later if the initial radiological examination did not detect the fracture; occasionally, comparative views of the opposite wrist are justifiable. Failure to splint the undisplaced scaphoid fracture may lead to non-union. However, non-union is more common when the scaphoid fragments are separated and therefore most likely to be recognized on the initial films.

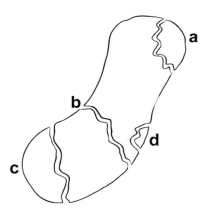

Fig. 45.3 The sites of scaphoid fracture. (**a**) Distal pole, (**b**) waist (*middle third*), (**c**) proximal pole, and (**d**) avulsion

Proximal pole fractures are rare, the majority (75%) involving the distal pole (Fig. 45.3), whether extra-articular or the larger intra-articular fragment, and 25% the waist or middle third of the scaphoid [14]. The incidence rises with age, being negligible under the age of 12 but progressively more common during adolescence. Scaphoid cast support for 4 weeks in the child and 6 weeks in the adolescent almost invariably results in healing (Fig. 45.4). Non-union characterizes late or inadequate splintage in most cases and merits screw fixation via a proximal approach. Additional cancellous bone grafting is essential for the established non-union with separation at the fracture site [15].

Proximal pole avascular necrosis is very rare in childhood [16] and usually progresses to localized osteoarthritis. Regional pain syndrome may complicate the recovery period.

Metacarpal Fractures

Diaphyseal

These are increasingly common as the child matures, usually involving the first, second, and fifth metacarpals. In the shaft the fracture line is transverse, oblique, or spiral and some degree of dorsal angulation and rotation occurs. Angulation of up to 30° is only acceptable at the fifth metacarpal as it is more mobile than the radial metacarpals. Remodeling will eventually correct knuckle recession and prominence of the metacarpal head in the palm.

Mid-shaft angulation of 15–20° leaves functional and cosmetic impairment in the adolescent, unlike the neck fracture, so reduction and transverse K-wire fixation are appropriate.

Reduction is achieved by flexing the metacarpophalangeal (MCP) joint to 90°, then pressing the digit dorsally with counterpressure at the fracture line using regional or general anesthesia. Rotational deformity is unacceptable and must be carefully avoided by reviewing the alignment of the fingers when flexed into the palm. In a few instances open reduction and K-wire or screw fixation are advisable.

Fig. 45.4 Eleven-year-old-boy. (**a**) Scaphoid waist fracture, (**b**) after 4 weeks in a long arm cast with scaphoid immobilization, and (**c**) after 7 weeks the fracture of the scaphoid has united

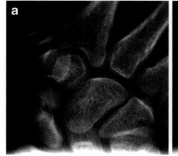
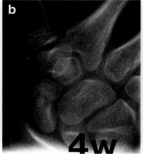
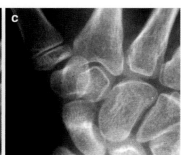

Distal Physeal

These fractures produce dorsal and lateral deviations, usually of the fourth and fifth metacarpals. The type 2 Salter-Harris fracture is the most common; types 3 and 4 carry a poorer prognosis. If the metacarpal head splits, K-wire fixation is advisable.

Reduction is achieved by flexing the MCP joint to 90° and then applying volar pressure to the metacarpal head. This is only applicable to angulations of more than 70° at the fifth or more than 40° at the second and third since remodeling is usually excellent [17, 18]. Avascular necrosis has been reported to result from the intracapsular tamponade [19].

Basal Fractures

These high-energy injuries are accompanied by soft tissue disruption so neurovascular deficit and compartment syndrome should be suspected. If the fracture is extra-articular and involves the thumb, reduction is rarely required. Intra-articular fractures, particularly the Salter-Harris type 3 of the first metacarpal, merit careful reduction and fixation to preserve pain-free motion of the affected joint [20, 21]. The type 2 physeal fracture and minimally displaced fractures involving the other metacarpals can be managed with a 3-week period of volar plaster slab splintage.

Proximal (and Middle) Phalangeal Fractures

These occur when an axial and rotational stress is applied, generally fracturing the proximal phalanges of the index and little fingers. In addition to proximal physeal (types 2, 3, and 4) fractures, the proximal metaphysis, shaft, neck, and distal condyles can be injured (Fig. 45.5). Angulation of the type 2 basal physeal fracture commonly affects the little finger, the so-called extra-octave fracture (coined by the late Mercer Rang, Toronto). Reduction is achieved by a corrective, angulatory force against a fulcrum, such as a pencil in the relevant web space. Although the fracture is relatively stable post-reduction, a volar splint or plaster slab should be applied for 2 weeks, with the MPJ flexed to 70–90° and the interphalangeal joints extended. A further fortnight of buddy taping to the neighboring digit is of value to control malrotation and to initiate movement.

In the adolescent age group avulsion of the ulnar collateral ligament can occur as a skiing injury. Anatomic reduction and fixation by K-wires or a miniscrew are indicated (Fig. 45.6).

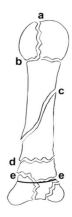

Fig. 45.5 The sites of phalangeal fracture. (**a**) Condylar or head splitting, (**b**) transverse neck, (**c**) spiral, oblique, or transverse shaft, (**d**) proximal shaft, and (**e**) basal condylar or avulsion with growth plate involvement

Shaft fractures are transverse, oblique, or spiral. Any resultant angulation tends to be volar due to the musculotendinous forces. Soft tissue interposition and rotational deformity should be suspected in the more displaced fracture. Reduction should be anatomical followed by the same splintage as detailed above.

Neck fractures are more common than intra-articular condylar fractures. The distal fragment may angulate significantly dorsally [22] so a true lateral radiographic view is essential. K-wire fixation rather than external splintage is appropriate as the post-reduction position is highly unstable and malunion is common [23].

Condylar fractures may involve one or both condyles. Displacement proximally and rotation necessitate accurate reduction of the condyle, often by surgical exposure and internal fixation (Fig. 45.7). Comminution of the fracture poses problems in reduction. Residual malunion leaves angulatory deformity and stiffness of the affected joint.

Distal Phalangeal Fractures

These may be transverse, longitudinal splitting or comminuted tuft fractures, generally produced by a crushing injury and therefore often open. Forced flexion produces mallet finger variants: Salter-Harris types 1, 2, 3, and 4 basal physeal fractures [24] with very occasional extensor tendon avulsion in the adolescent. Forced hyperextension (the "jersey fracture") causes the flexor digitorum profundus tendon to avulse a bone fragment from the volar aspect of the distal phalangeal shaft. Forced hyperflexion may cause a physeal fracture of the distal phalanx, a mallet finger (Fig. 45.8).

A major injury should be suspected when a mallet-type 1 or 2 physeal fracture coexists with a compounding wound. Most commonly encountered in children under the age of 12, a laceration of the nail bed means that the germinal matrix (ungual lamina) is incarcerated at the fracture site. A careful

Fig. 45.6 Twelve-year-old girl.
(**a**) Ulnar collateral ligament
avulsion from the base of the
proximal phalanx of the thumb.
(**b**) The fragment was openly
reduced and fixed by two 0.8-mm
K-wires

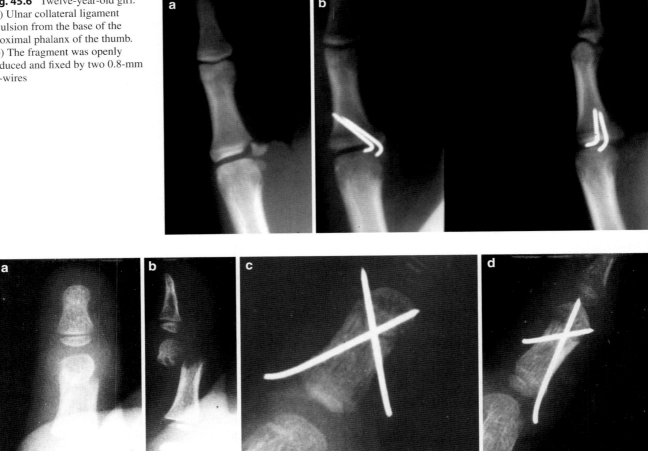

Fig. 45.7 Three-year-old boy. (**a**) AP view of displaced, open phalangeal shaft fracture, (**b**) lateral view confirming complete displacement, (**c**) AP view after reduction and crossed K-wire fixation, and (**d**) lateral view after reduction and crossed K-wire fixation

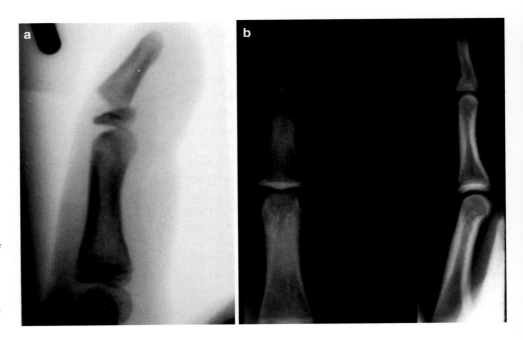

Fig. 45.8 Twelve-year-old-boy.
(**a**) Lateral view of mallet-type
physeal fracture of the base of the
proximal phalanx of the middle
finger. (**b**) The radiographic
appearance of the injury after
reduction, temporary K-wire
fixation, and union of the fracture

a

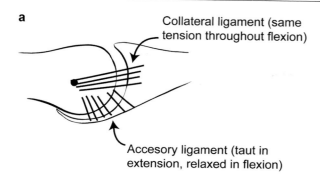

Collateral ligament (same
tension throughout flexion)

Accesory ligament (taut in
extension, relaxed in flexion)

b

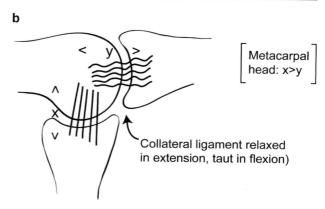

[Metacarpal
head: x>y]

Collateral ligament relaxed
in extension, taut in flexion)

Fig. 45.9 (**a**) At the interphalangeal joint the collateral ligament maintains the same tension throughout the flexion arc, but the accessory ligament is taut in extension and relaxed in flexion as the volar plate infolds slightly into the joint. Edema will lead to contracture of the accessory ligament if the injured joint is splinted in flexion. (**b**) At the MCP joint the collateral ligament is taut in flexion owing to the cam shape of the metacarpal head ($x>y$), which is also broader in its volar dimension. As there is no accessory collateral structure of concern, the collateral ligament is taut in flexion but not in extension and therefore may shorten pathologically if the injured joint or hand is splinted or bandaged with the joint extended

extrication and repair of this important soft tissue structure is vital [15]. Equally, a subungual hematoma spreading under more than 50% of the nail suggests the presence of a distal phalangeal fracture, possibly complicated.

Volar splintage is effective for most of these fractures once normal anatomical relationships have been assured. The nail should be preserved as a splint and post-reduction radiographs scrutinized. For the unstable reduction or when a Salter-Harris type 3 or 4 fragment remains out of position, K-wire fixation is merited. Contamination of the compound fracture leads to a risk of infection so internal fixation should be used sparingly. When soft tissue loss is of concern a variety of soft tissue reconstructions have been described but are beyond the scope of this chapter.

Interphalangeal Joint Dislocations

These are rare in childhood and usually occur at the proximal interphalangeal joint, the middle phalanx dislocating dorsally. Closed reduction may be achieved by flexion of the joint under regional or general anesthesia, thumbing the middle phalanx back over the condyles of the proximal phalanx. Traction is ineffectual.

Volar plate interposition may require open reduction. This structure spans the joint from the basal epiphysis distally to the volar metaphysis proximally. Damage to the associated accessory collateral ligaments or post-traumatic edema may lead to flexion contracture, so the interphalangeal joints should be splinted in slight rather than major flexion after injury (Fig. 45.9a). In contrast, the injured MCP joint (Fig. 45.9b) should be held in 60–90° of flexion after fracture or significant soft tissue disruption.

Conclusion

Fractures of the hand and wrist are highly visible and disturbing injuries for the child and family. Although many fractures are relatively trivial, experience is needed in deciding when to reduce angulatory and rotational deformities. Internal fixation should be used sparingly and can be avoided if reduction is timely, accurate, and effectively controlled by carefully applied splints and plasters.

References

1. Landin LA. Epidemiology of children's fractures. J Pediatr Orthop B 1997; 68: 79–83.
2. Mizuta T, Benson WM, Foster BK, et al. Statistical analysis of the incidence of physeal fractures. J Pediatr Orthop 1987; 7:518–23.
3. Biyani A, Gupta SR, Sharma JC. Ipsilateral supracondylar fracture of humerus and forearm bones in children. Injury 1989; 20:203–7.
4. Kasser JR. Forearm fractures. In: MacEwen GD, et al., eds. A Practical Approach to Assessment and Treatment. Baltimore: William and Wilkins; 1993:165–90.
5. McLaughlan GJ, Cowan B, Annan IH, Robb JE. Management of completely displaced metaphyseal fractures of the distal radius in children. A prospective, randomised controlled trial. J Bone Joint Surg [Br] 2002; 84:413–7.
6. Webb GR, Galpin RD, Armstrong DG. Comparison of short and long arm plaster casts for displaced fractures in the distal third of the forearm in children. J Bone Joint Surg [Am] 2006 ; 88:9–17.
7. Denes AE Jr, Goding R, Tamborlane J, et al. Maintenance of reduction of pediatric distal radius fractures with a sugar-tong splint. Am J Orthop. 2007; 36:68–70.
8. Lee BS, Esterhai JL, Das M. Fracture of the distal radial epiphysis. Clin Orthop Relat Res 1984; 185:90–6.
9. Bley L, Seitz WH Jr. Injuries of the distal ulna in children. Hand Clin 1998; 14:231–7.
10. Golz RJ, Grogan DP, Greene TL. Distal ulnar physeal injury. J Pediatr Orthop 1991; 11:318–26.

11. Mansat M, Mansat C, Martinez C. L'articulation radio-cubitale inferieur. Pathologie traumatique. In: Razemon JP, Fisk GR, eds. Le poignet. Paris: Expansion Scientifique Francaise; 1983:187–95.

12. Nafie SA. Fractures of the carpal bones in children. Injury 1987; 18:117–9.

13. Greene WB, Anderson WJ. Simultaneous fracture of the scaphoid and radius in children. J Pediatr Orthop 1982; 2:191–4.

14. Vahvanen V, Westerlund M. Fractures of the carpal scaphoid in children. A clinical and roentgenological study of 108 cases. Acta Orthop Scand 1980; 51:909–13.

15. Greene MH, Hadied AM, Lamont RL. Scaphoid fractures in children. J Hand Surg (Am) 1984; 9:536–41.

16. Larson B, Light TR, Ogden JA. Fracture and ischemic necrosis of the immature scaphoid. J Hand Surg (Am) 1987; 12:122–7.

17. Ford DJ, Ali MS, Steel WM. Fractures of the fifth metacarpal neck: is reduction or immobilisation necessary? Hand Clin 1989; 14:165–7.

18. Sanders RA, Frederick HA. Metacarpal and phalangeal osteotomy with miniplate fixation. Orthop Rev 1991; 20:449–56.

19. Prosser AJ, Irvine GB. Epiphyseal fracture of the metacarpal head. Injury 1988; 19:34–47.

20. Kjaer-Peteresen K, Junk AC, Petersen LK. Intra-articular fractures at the base of the first metacarpal. J Hand Surg (Br) 1992; 17: 144–7.

21. Dartee DA, Brink PR, Von-Houte HP. Iselin's operative technique for thumb proximal metacarpal fractures. Injury 1992; 23:370–2.

22. Dixon GL, Moon NF. Rotational supracondylar fractures of the proximal phalanx in children. Clin Orthop Relat Res 1972; 83:151–6.

23. Vandenberk P, De Smet L, Fabry G. Finger fractures in children treated with absorbable pins. J Pediatr Orthop [part B] 1996; 5: 27–30.

24. Seymour N. Juxtaepiphyseal fractures of the terminal phalanx of the finger. J Bone Joint Surg [Br] 1966; 48:347–9.

Section 3
Fractures of the Pelvis, Femoral Neck, Lower Limb, and Foot

Chapter 46

Fractures of the Pelvis

Peter W. Engelhardt

Frequency and Mechanism of Injury

Pelvic fractures are uncommon in children [1]. They account for only 1–2% of fractures seen by paediatric orthopaedic surgeons [2]. Their rarity is due to the greater volume of cartilage which provides a buffer for energy absorption. Case reports of pelvic fractures in early childhood are infrequent. Usually fractures of the pelvis are seen in polytraumatized children who have been struck by a motor vehicle. High-energy trauma is often life-threatening because of associated soft-tissue injuries and massive hemorrhage. These take priority over the fracture.

Uncomplicated fractures include all kinds of avulsions of the apophyses of the pelvis. These avulsions occur in children and adolescents playing soccer or football and result from sudden contraction of the muscle which inserts into the apophysis. Fractures of the acetabulum are even more rare and account for 5% of the pelvic fractures in children [3].

Classification

The classification of Torode and Zieg [4] is simple and follows a logical progression of injury status from mild to severe (Fig. 46.1). For practical purposes, fractures of the acetabulum need special attention due to potential injury of the growth cartilage, leading to incongruency of the hip and subsequent subluxation [5].

Type I

Avulsion of parts of the anterior iliac apophysis, the ischial tuberosity (Fig. 46.2) or the anterior inferior iliac spine (Fig. 46.3) represents a chondro-osseous injury, especially in the adolescent athlete.

Type II

Iliac wing fractures occur as a result of direct force against the pelvis.

Type III

Simple pelvic ring fracture, usually involving the pubic rami or disruption of the pubic symphysis.

Type IV

Instability of the pelvis is the result of a fracture or joint disruption creating abnormal motion when stressed or loaded. Included here are bilateral pubic rami fractures, fractures involving either the right or the left pubic ramus or the symphysis, and additional fracture-dislocation of the posterior elements of the pelvis (Fig. 46.4).

Assessment

Fractures of the pelvis need a multidisciplinary approach. Additional injuries of the genitourinary system, the abdomen, and the central nervous system must be ruled out

P.W. Engelhardt (✉)
Department of Orthopedic Surgery, Hirslanden Clinic Aarau, Aarau, Switzerland

M. Benson et al. (eds.), *Children's Orthopaedics and Fractures*,
DOI 10.1007/978-1-84882-611-3_46, © Springer-Verlag London Limited 2010

Fig. 46.1 Torode and Zieg's classification of pelvic fractures in children. See text for details

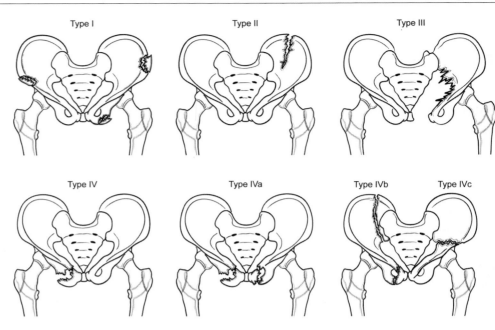

and properly treated. A computed tomography (CT) scan is indicated when there is suspicion of posterior element disruption particularly around the sacro-iliac joint (Type IV). Possible hemorrhage merits consultation with a vascular surgeon.

Treatment

It is generally accepted that children have greater potential for healing and remodeling skeletal injuries. Conservative treatment of fractures of the pelvis is the rule with protected weight bearing and a gradual return to activity [1–4]. External fixation is necessary for pelvic ring displacement of more than 2 cm [2] (Fig. 46.5).

Avulsion Fractures of the Ischial Tuberosity (Type I)

Sudden tension in the hamstrings during a fall, for example, in skiing accidents, can cause avulsion of the ischial tuberosity (Fig. 46.2). Initial bed rest is followed by crutch-supported walking. Abundant callus formation can form a pseudotumor, causing diagnostic concerns. Excessive callus formation can be painful and may require excision. Widely dislocated avulsions of the ischial tuberosity should be fixed by a lag screw [6].

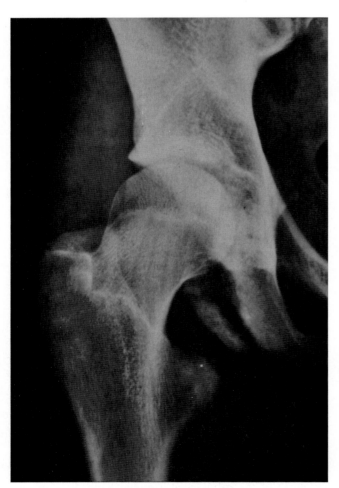

Fig. 46.2 Avulsion of the ischial tuberosity in a 16-year-old skier

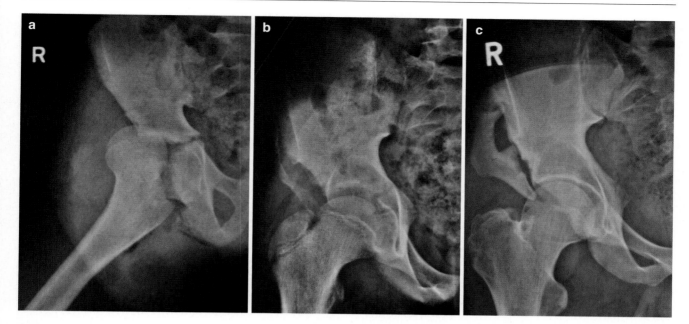

Fig. 46.3 (**a**) Anterior hip dislocation in a 12-year-old boy. The avulsed anterior inferior iliac spine is not visible on the plain film taken immediately after the injury because it is still cartilaginous. (**b**) Ossification of the displaced anterior component of the pelvis after 3 months. (**c**) After cessation of growth a large, ossified fragment persists in the groin, causing symptoms

Avulsion Fractures of the Anterior Superior and Anterior Inferior Iliac Spines (Type I)

Typically, these are sports injuries, for example, when playing soccer or hurdling. The fragment is larger than estimated on the radiograph because of the additional chondal component (Fig. 46.3). In cases with minimal displacement, bed rest with the hip flexed is sufficient. Near the end of growth a severely displaced apophysis may be openly reduced and fixed with strong sutures or with a lag screw.

Marginal Fractures of The Pelvic Ring (Type II)

The strength and rigidity of the pelvis is not affected. Cracks in the iliac wing heal without sequelae. Bed rest until the pain subsides is sufficient.

Anterior and Posterior Fractures of the Pelvic Ring, Malgaigne Fractures (Type III/IV)

Rotational and vertical instability should be analyzed by radiograph or under image intensification. Anterior disruption of the ring heals conservatively. Additional posterior lesions need to be carefully checked by CT scan.

Occasionally, open reduction and the application of an anterior external fixation frame are indicated (Fig. 46.5a). Intraabdominal trauma or bladder and urethral disruption (Fig. 46.4b) should always be considered and one must beware of misinterpreting a widened symphysis or sacro-iliac joint since the thicker growth cartilage layer makes the interval proportionally wider than in adults. Disruption through the sacro-iliac joint (Fig. 46.5b) can result in severe growth disturbance of the whole pelvis [7, 8].

Fractures of the Acetabulum

These fractures are best seen on CT scans. The potential hazard of premature closure of the triradiate cartilage (Fig. 46.6) must be kept in mind, but may not be prevented by open reduction. Often there is a delay in recognizing compression of the growth cartilage. In Salter-Harris Type V lesions, premature fusion may occur with progressive subluxation of the hip. Thickening of the medial acetabular wall is also observed (Fig. 46.6b). It is doubtful if the adult approach to fractures of the acetabulum should be applied to children. Secondary reconstructive procedures, such as a shelf operation or Chiari and intertrochanteric osteotomies, may be necessary to contain the femoral head [9]. In a survey of 34 patients, 16 were treated surgically because of incongruence or instability [3]. A common cause of acetabular fracture was dislocation of the femoral head, predominantly in a

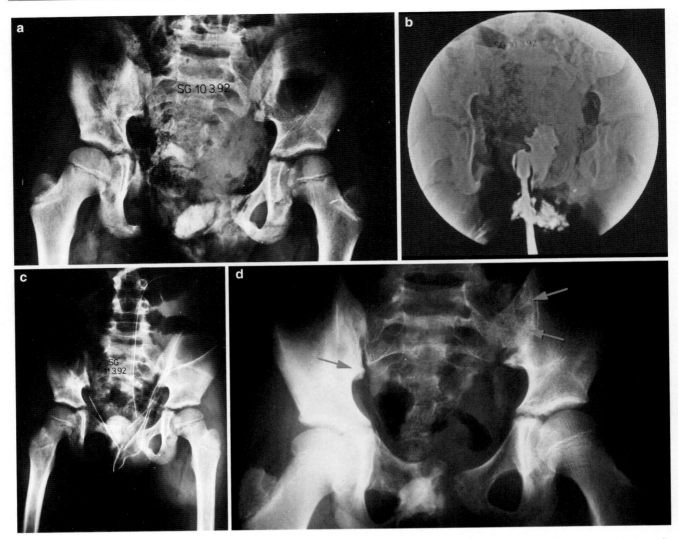

Fig. 46.4 (**a**) A 9-year-old boy was run over by a car causing severe fracture-dislocation of the pelvis with additional intra-abdominal trauma. (**b**) A urethrogram reveals a ruptured urethra. (**c**) Fixation of the pelvic fragments was achieved with heavy-duty sutures via a transabdominal approach. (**d**) Outcome 3 years post-injury. Fusion of the left sacro-iliac joint has not led to problems as yet

posterior direction. The indications for operative treatment were unstable posterior or central fracture dislocations and the presence of intra-articular fragments. Depending upon the fracture type and associated injuries, an anterior or a posterior approach was used.

Outcome

Outcome studies focus mainly on mortality rates with an average of 7.2% due to associated polytrauma. Type I, II, and III fractures usually heal without long-term disability. Initially they need close observation in the presence of additional genitourinary and other soft tissue injury. Disruption of the symphysis pubis heals even in the presence of diastasis because the lesion does not interfere with the growth potential of the cartilage.

Depending on the severity of the skeletal lesion, particularly if combined with vertical instability, permanent disability may result. Injury of the growth cartilage may lead to deformity of the pelvis, with leg length discrepancy and pelvic obliquity as well as fusion of the sacro-iliac joint [9]. In the case of triradiate cartilage damage, a shallow acetabulum can be expected, with the need for secondary reconstructive procedures [5]. Excellent results correlate with the eventual congruence of the reduction. Post-traumatic acetabular dysplasia differs from the morphology of developmental dysplasia of the hip as central acetabular wall thickening is more marked and the acetabulum is retroverted rather than anteverted [5].

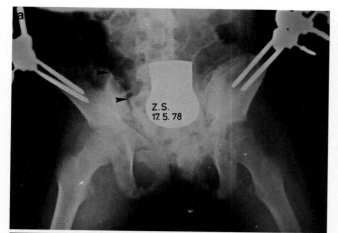

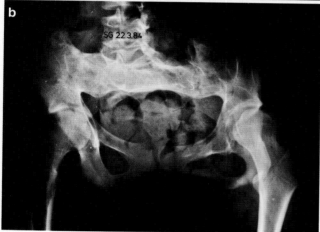

Fig. 46.5 (a) External fixator to close the "open book" injury of the pelvis in an 8-year-old child. (b) At the age of 15 years, major deformity of the pelvis had developed due to multiple growth plate arrest (including both sacro-iliac joints)

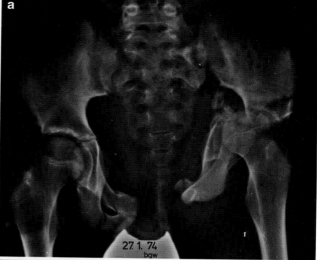

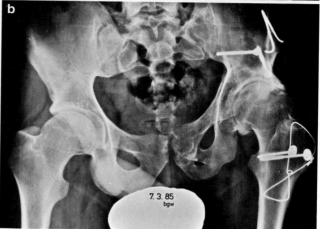

Fig. 46.6 (a) High-velocity trauma due to a motorcycle accident in a 15-year-old patient. Major disruption of the left hemipelvis with gross displacement of the fractured acetabulum. Open reduction was undertaken. (b) At the age of 27 years, leg length discrepancy and extrusion of the femoral head developed due to injury to the triradiate cartilage. Metal implants have been partially removed

References

1. Widman RF. Fractures of the pelvis. In: Beaty JH, Kasser JR, eds. Rockwood and Wilkins: Fractures in Children, 6th ed. Philadelphia, PA: Lippincott Williams Wilkins; 2006:850–860.
2. Holden CP, Holman J, Herman MJ. Pediatric pelvic fractures. J Am Acad Orthop Surg 2007; 15:172–177.
3. Heeg M, de Ridder V, Tornetta P, et al. Acetabular fractures in children and adolescents. Clin Orthop Rel Res 2000; 376:80–86.
4. Torode I, Zieg D. Pelvic fractures in children. J Pediatr Orthop 1985; 5:76–84.
5. Trousdale RT, Ganz R. Post-traumatic acetabular dysplasia. Clin Orthop Rel Res 1994; 305:124–132.
6. Stiletto RJ, Baacke M, Gotzen L. Comminuted pelvic ring disruption in toddlers: Management of a rare injury. J Trauma 2000; 48:161–166 .
7. Garvin K, McCarthy R, Barnes C, et al. Pediatric pelvic ring fractures. J Pediatr Orthop 1990; 10:577–582.
8. Engelhardt P. Die Malgaigne-Beckenringverletzung im Kindesalter. Orthopaede 1992; 21:422–426.
9. Schwarz N, Posch E, Mayer J, et al. Long term results of unstable pelvic ring fractures in children. Injury 1998; 29:421–433.

Chapter 47

Femoral Neck Fractures

Peter W. Engelhardt

Frequency and Mechanism of Injury

Fractures around the hip joint result from violent force such as high-energy trauma or less frequently in association with pathological conditions [1]. Femoral neck fracture as an atypical presentation of child abuse has also been presented recently [2]. The overall incidence of femoral neck fractures in children is less than 1% [3]. They occur in children of all ages, but the highest incidence is in 11- and 12-year-olds, with 60–75% occurring in boys, about the same age as slipped upper femoral epiphysis (SUFE) has its peak incidence. It is mandatory to identify additional injuries in the polytraumatized child (Fig. 47.1). Age-related differences in the mechanical property of bone account for the greater frequency of hip fractures among adults than among children, the ratio of adult to childhood fracture frequency being 130:1 [4].

A fracture of the femoral neck may be caused by a force applied to the greater trochanter, producing valgus angulation, or from axial loading directed along the shaft of the femur, causing varus deformity. A fracture caused by relatively minor trauma may be indicative of pathological conditions such as a cyst, disuse osteopenia, or neurological disorders. Large series of femoral neck fractures in children have been published [4–6]. Improvements in management and fixation techniques have significantly reduced complication rates over time.

A stress fracture of the femoral neck in a patient with an open physis is rare, so investigations should rule out any underlying disease. The youngest case is reported in a child of 10 years [7].

Classification

Hip fractures in children are classified according to their location and morphology. The AO Classification Supervisory Committee (CSC) coordinated by AO Clinical Investigation and Documentation (AOCID) has set a new standard for the classification of paediatric fractures [8] including proximal epiphyseal fractures (31-E) and the proximal metaphyseal femoral neck fracture (31-M).

The morphology of the fracture (Fig. 47.2) is classified according to the AO method which closely resembles the older system of Colonna and Delbet [9] (Table 47.1).

Assessment

The child is fearful of any passive limb motion and unable to move actively. The diagnosis is confirmed by radiographs, preferably in two planes if this is not too painful. Sonography is useful in doubtful conditions of hip pain in the child. A fracture line or intracapsular hematoma can be detected by ultrasound. With an undisplaced fracture of the femoral neck, the radiograph may not be diagnostic initially. Computed tomography (CT) can be used to assess the degree of displacement and any intracapsular hematoma (Fig. 47.3). A bone scan at 3 months post-injury is also helpful in detecting femoral head necrosis, the most common complication. Magnetic resonance imaging (MRI) detects avascularity earlier (see complications).

Treatment

The principles of management include

- Minimizing potential complications of avascular necrosis (AVN)
- Avoiding injury to the physeal plate

P.W. Engelhardt (✉)
Department of Orthopedic Surgery, Hirslanden Clinic Aarau, Aarau, Switzerland

M. Benson et al. (eds.), *Children's Orthopaedics and Fractures*,
DOI 10.1007/978-1-84882-611-3_47, © Springer-Verlag London Limited 2010

Fig. 47.1 (**a**) A 1-year-old
polytraumatized boy run over by
a tractor. Type I fracture of the
femoral neck (epiphysiolysis).
Closed reduction was followed by
premature closure of the growth
plate with subsequent coxa vara.
(**b**) Coxa vara as a result of the
fracture (epiphysiolysis)

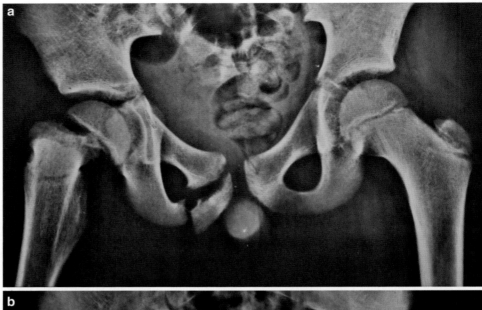

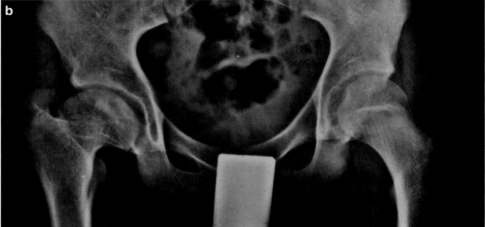

Fig. 47.2 Classification of
proximal femoral fractures in the
child, according to Colonna and
Delbet [9]

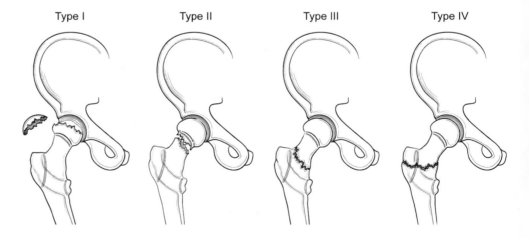

Type I   Type II   Type III   Type IV

- Anatomical reduction of the fragments
- Stabilization with pins or screws allowing early protected
  weight bearing.

Decompression of the hemarthrosis and stable internal fixation are essential aspects of treatment for all fractures
with displacement [3, 5, 7, 8]. Undisplaced fractures may

Table 47.1 Classification of Proximal Femoral Fractures

Classification	Location	AO classification	AVN risk	Urgency of treatment	Treatment undisplaced	Treatment displaced	Fixation
Type I	Epiphysiolysis	31-E/1.1–7.1	Very high	Emergency	Eventually conservative	Operative	K-wires, cannulated screws
Type II	Mid-cervical	31-M/2.1	High	Emergency	Eventually conservative	Operative	K-wires, cannulated screws
Type III	Basocervical	31-M/2.1–3.1	High	Emergency	Eventually conservative	Operative	K-wires under 3 years or cannulated screws
Type IV	Transtrochanteric	31-M/2.1–3.2	Low	Delay possible	Conservative	Operative	K-wires or blade plate

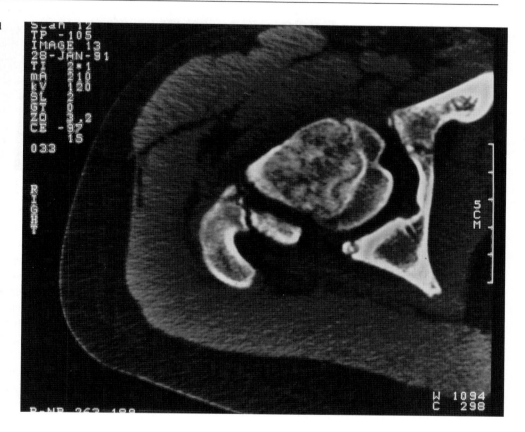

Fig. 47.3 CT Scan for improved analysis of the fracture morphology. Swelling and intracapsular hemarthrosis are mild. Planning of implant size and position is facilitated but a scan is not mandatory

be treated conservatively with cast immobilization using a hip spica. Some authors consider that decompression of the intracapsular hematoma reduces the incidence of AVN [10], particularly the frequency of AVN in displaced fractures [11].

Minimally invasive surgery has a place in undisplaced fractures. Under image intensifier control cannulated screws are inserted over a guide wire in order to maintain reduction. In all other cases the fracture site is exposed using the Watson–Jones' anterolateral approach. An anterior capsulotomy exposes the fragments and their orientation. A K-wire is inserted laterally below the greater trochanter and advanced to the fracture site using an image intensifier in two planes. After carefully checking the accuracy of reduction

the K-wire is driven across the fracture. In type 31-E (epiphyseal) fractures K-wires are inserted into the capital epiphysis and left there while the fracture unites.

In 31-M (metaphyseal) fracture two lag screws are inserted parallel to the K-wire, securing firm and compressive fixation of the fragments without crossing the growth plate (Fig. 47.4a, b). Cannulated screws of appropriate size may also be inserted directly over the guide wires. Shortly before skeletal growth ceases (from the age of 15 onwards) the thread of the screw may be inserted into the capital epiphysis without the risk of major leg length discrepancy from premature growth arrest [12]. The use of several small diameter pins may be sufficient in many cases [6, 13] but can lead

Fig. 47.4 (a) Ten-year-old boy with type III (basocervical) fracture of the femoral neck. (b) At follow-up 1 year after screw fixation solid union of the femoral neck is proven. The epiphyseal plate was not crossed by the thread of the screws

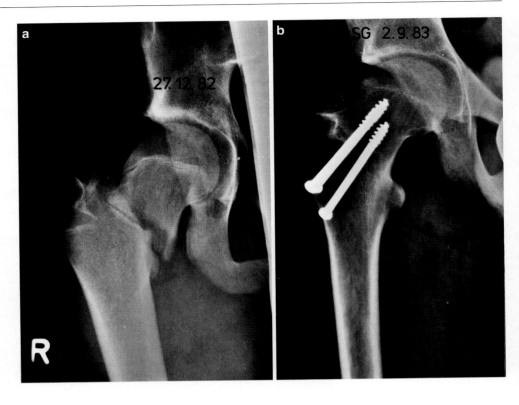

to distraction of the fragments. The large Smith-Petersen nail is no longer recommended for hip fractures in children. It may fail to penetrate the hard bone of the proximal fragment, causing wide separation or comminution at the fracture site. Closure of the joint capsule is not necessary. Immediate post-operative partial weight bearing is possible in the older child. The younger child is kept in bed for 2 weeks and a single hip spica cast can be used to control rotation if there is any concern about stable fixation. Full weight bearing should not be attempted before 8 weeks postoperatively.

Complications

The following complications may arise and determine the late outcome:

- AVN
- Growth arrest
- Coxa vara
- Nonunion
- Osteoarthritis
- Other untoward sequelae.

Avascular Necrosis

AVN, first described in 1927 [14], is the most feared complication because it leads to a very unfavorable result (Fig. 47.5). AVN was seen in as many as 9 of 19 fractures (47%) before the present treatment regimen was established [15]. It is presumed to result from rupture or tamponade of one or both circumflex arteries.

The amount of initial displacement is an important prognostic factor when considering its effect upon the vascular supply of the femoral head and neck but it does not explain AVN after fissure (undisplaced) fracture of the femoral neck. Several authors have suggested that femoral head ischemia results from the hip joint tamponade, which in turn prevents venous drainage [16, 17].

The necrosis can affect the epiphysis alone, the whole proximal fragment, or only the portion of the neck of the femur between the fracture and the growth plate [4]. Epiphyseal ischemia resembles that seen in Perthes' disease [18] and its treatment therefore follows principles that are established for this disease. However, healing and remodeling after post-traumatic AVN in children is usually prolonged and never complete (Fig. 47.5c, d). Decompression and stable internal fixation are the cornerstones of prevention of AVN [19].

Fig. 47.5 (**a**) Transcervical femoral neck fracture with only minimal displacement in an 8-year-old boy. Long-term follow-up after conservative treatment. (**b**) Lateral view of the femoral neck demonstrates the fracture morphology better. (**c**) Thirty months later AVN is clearly evident with collapse of the femoral head which gives a Legg-Calvé-Perthes-like appearance. (**d**) Thirty years after the initial fracture secondary osteoarthritis grade 2 is evident. (Adapted from the archives of the Balgrist Orthopedic University Hospital at Zürich, Switzerland. Used with permission)

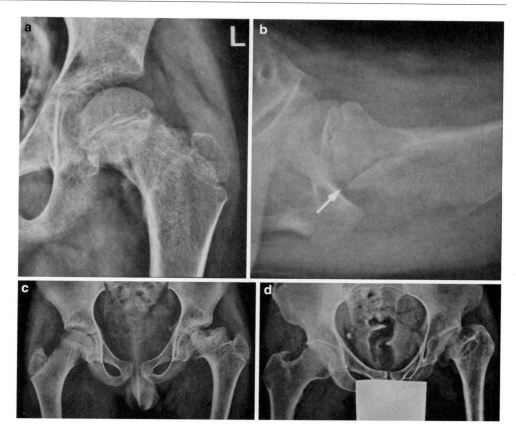

Growth Arrest/Coxa Vara

Coxa vara is caused by premature physeal fusion or by inadequate reduction (Fig. 47.1b). It occurs in about 15% of cases [7].

Nonunion

Delayed healing and nonunion are rarely encountered now that open reduction and stable, compressive internal fixation are recommended.

Osteoarthritis

Secondary osteoarthritis of the hip joint develops as a result of incongruity. Complications in early childhood are usually better compensated for by remodeling than those shortly before skeletal maturity. Deterioration of the hip joint in the

form of degenerative joint disease and impaired function may occur insidiously over a period of many years (Fig. 47.5d).

Other Complications

Subtrochanteric fractures at the level of screw insertion are a potential complication if the femoral cortex has been weakened by drilling or after screw removal. Poorly positioned implants may compromise function either as a result of proximal penetration or from prominence of the distal end of the fixation device.

Traumatic Dislocation of the Hip

Traumatic hip dislocation is a rare injury, accounting for 2–5% of all dislocations [20]. Usually, severe violence is required, but sometimes minor trauma can be the cause of dislocation of the immature hip joint up to the age of 10 years [20, 21]. Posterior dislocation is the most common,

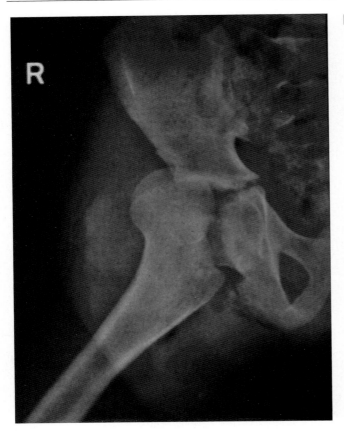

Fig. 47.6 Anterior hip dislocation in a 12-year-old boy (bicycle accident) with avulsion of the chondral physis of the anterior inferior iliac spine (see also Fig. 46.3)

whereas anterior dislocation is rare (Fig. 47.6) [22]. Habitual hip dislocation is reported as a cause of the rare snapping hip syndrome [23] and may occur in Down's syndrome [24, 25].

The leg is held in internal rotation, adduction, and flexion in cases of posterior dislocation. Radiographs should include the whole femur in order to rule out an associated fracture of the ipsilateral femoral shaft.

The dislocation is usually reducible by closed methods. Interposition of small fragments or button-holing of the head through the capsule may necessitate open reduction. Intra-articular fragments are best detected by CT scanning. Post-reduction treatment includes skin traction or even a spica cast if there is concern about stability [20]. The best prognosis results from an immediate closed reduction in the absence of bony or soft tissue interposition. AVN is more likely after violent injury and is less frequent in younger children if the dislocation occurs after minor trauma. Late-diagnosed cases are still encountered in some parts of the world.

References

1. Krieg A, Speth B, Won H, et al. Conservative management of bilateral femoral neck fractures in a child with autosomal dominant osteopetrosis (ADO). Arch Orthop Trauma Surg 2007; 127: 967–970.
2. Gholve P, Arkader A, Gaugler R, et al. Femoral neck Fracture as an atypical presentation of child abuse. Orthopedics 2008; 31: 271–273.
3. Canale ST. Fractures of the hip in children and adolescents. Orthop Clin North Am 1990; 21: 341–352.
4. Ratliff AH. Fractures of the neck of the femur in children. J Bone Joint Surg Br 1962; 44: 528–542.
5. Boitzy A. La fracture du col du femur chez l'enfant et l'adolescent. Paris: Masson; 1971.
6. Canale ST. Fracture of the neck and intertrochanteric region of the femur in children. J Bone Joint Surg Am 1977; 59: 431–433.
7. Ratliff AH. Complications after fractures of the femoral neck in children and their treatment. J Bone Joint Surg Br 1970; 52: 175–181.
8. Slongo T, Audigé L, AO Pediatric Classification Group. AO Pediatric Comprehensive Classification of Long-Bone Fractures (PCCF). Brochure AO Education, Switzerland: AO Publishing; 2007.
9. Colonna PC. Fracture of the neck of the femur in children. Am J Surg 1929; 6: 793–797.
10. Song KS, Kim YS, Sohn SW, Ogden JA. Arthrotomy and open reduction of he displaced fracture of the femoral neck in children. J Pediatr Orthop part B 2001; 10: 205–210.
11. Ng GP, Cole WG. Effect of early hip decompression on the frequency of avascular necrosis in children with fractures of the neck of the femur. Injury 1996; 27: 419–421.
12. Engelhardt P. Epiphyseolysis capitis femoris und die "gesunde" Gegenseite. Z Orthop 1990; 128: 262–265.
13. Miller WE. Fractures of the hip in children from birth to adolescence. Clin Orthop Rel Res 1973; 92: 155–188.
14. Johansson S. Über Epiphysennekrose bei geheilten Collumfrakturen. Zentralblatt Chir 1927; 54: 2214–2222.
15. Davison BL, Weinstein SL. Hip fractures in children: a long term follow-up study. J Pediatr Orthop 1992; 12: 355–358.
16. Kay SP, Hall JE. Fracture of the femoral neck in children and its complications. Clin Orthop Rel Res 1971; 80: 53–71.
17. Soto-Hall R, Johnson LH, Johnson RA. Variations of the intraarticular pressure oft he hip joint in injury and disease. J Bone Joint Surg Am 1964; 46: 509–512.
18. Ogden JA. Skeletal injury in the child, 3rd ed. Berlin: Springer; 2000.
19. Cheng JC, Tangh N. Decompression and stable internal fixation of femoral neck fractures in children can affect the outcome. J Pediatr Orthop 1999; 19: 338–343.
20. Rieger H, Pennig D, Klein W, et al. Traumatic dislocation of the hip in young children. Arch Orthop Trauma Surg 1991; 110: 114–117.
21. Pearson DE, Mann RJ. Traumatic hip dislocation in children. Clin Orthop Rel Res 1973; 92: 189–194.
22. Macnicol MF. The Scottish incidence of traumatic dislocation of the hip in childhood. J Pediatr Orthop [B] 2000; 9: 212–216.
23. Stuart PR, Epstein HP. Habitual hip dislocation. J Pediatr Orthop 1991; 11: 541–542.
24. Aprin H, Zink WP, Hall JE. Management of dislocation of the hip in Down's syndrome. J Pediatr Orthop 1985; 5: 428–431.
25. Greene WB. Closed treatment of hip dislocation in Down's syndrome. J Pediatr Orthop 1998; 18: 643–647.

Chapter 48

Femoral Shaft Fractures

Klaus Parsch

Incidence and Mechanism of Injury

Fractures of the shaft of the femur including the sub-trochanteric and the supracondylar regions account for 1.6% of all fractures in children. The boy-to-girl ratio is 2.3:1, a ratio which may change in the future as girls participate in contact sports like soccer. The incidence seems to have a bimodal distribution with one peak in young children and another in young teenagers [1–3]. The annual rate of femoral shaft fractures has been calculated as 19 per 100,000 children [4].

The etiology of femoral fractures is age-dependent. In the infant, the femoral bone is relatively weak and may break under the load condition of normal tumbles. At kindergarten and school age, about half of femoral shaft fractures are caused by low-velocity accidents like falls from a height, from a bicycle, tree, ladder, or after stumbling and falling on the same level with or without a collision. Due to the rising strength of femoral bone, with maturation in later childhood and adolescence, high-velocity trauma is needed to fracture the femur. Motor vehicle–pedestrian accidents were responsible for these fractures in children from 6 to 9 years and motor vehicle accidents in teenagers. Firearm injuries accounted for 15% of femoral fractures in African-American teenagers in Baltimore. Adverse socioeconomic conditions were significantly associated with higher rates of fracture [5].

Fractures of the femoral shaft from *birth trauma* are rare, with the exception of those encountered in *arthrogryposis multiplex congenita*, myelomeningocele, and osteogenesis imperfecta. Rigid contractures of hips and knees in arthrogrypotic children may cause a femoral shaft fracture during delivery or during later handling (see Chapter 20). The other risk groups are newborns with neuromuscular disease such as myelomeningocele, osteopenia, and *osteogenesis imperfecta* causing multiple fractures (see Chapters 7 and 8).

Femoral shaft fractures during the first 12 months of life are rare. As many as 30–50% may be *non-accidental* from child abuse [6]. It is easy to underestimate this cause and initial assessment by a designated doctor in child protection is important [7]. This risk drops considerably after walking age, with only 2.6% in the pre-school age group [8] (see Chapter 42).

Classification

Paediatric femoral shaft fractures are spiral, oblique, or transverse; they can be comminuted or non-comminuted, closed or open. An AO paediatric comprehensive classification of long bone fractures has been developed. The diagnosis includes the distinction between epiphyseal (E), metaphyseal (M), or diaphyseal (D) fractures as well as the identification of child-specific features. The new paediatric comprehensive classification allows exact documentation and comparison of methods of treatment in clinical practice as well as prospective clinical studies (Fig. 48.1). A complete midshaft fracture of the femur has the following codes: 33-D/3.1 bone 3 (femur), segment 3 (midshaft), type D (diaphysis), child code 3 (complete), severity code 1 (simple) [9].

Clinical Findings

The common signs of femoral shaft fracture are pain, shortening, angulation, swelling, and crepitus. A child with a fresh femoral fracture is unable to stand or walk. The whole child must be examined including the lower leg and pelvic ring and the abdomen so as not to overlook tibial, pelvic, abdominal, or kidney trauma.

K. Parsch (✉)
Orthopaedic Department, Pediatric Centre Olgahospital, Stuttgart, Germany

M. Benson et al. (eds.), *Children's Orthopaedics and Fractures*,
DOI 10.1007/978-1-84882-611-3_48, © Springer-Verlag London Limited 2010

Fig. 48.1 AO comprehensive classification of paediatric long bone fractures [9]: bone 3 (femur), segment 3 (midshaft), type D (diaphysis), child code 3 (complete), severity code 1 (simple). A complete midshaft fracture of the femur has the code: 33-D/3.1

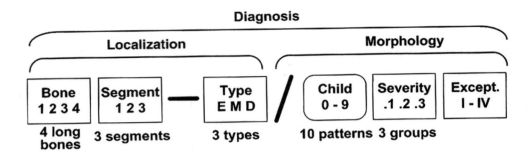

Radiographic Findings

The radiographic examination should include the whole length of the femur in two planes and the adjacent pelvic ring as well as the knee joint. If there is any doubt, the lower leg should be included in the examination. Computed tomography (CT) or magnetic resonance imaging (MRI) scans are not normally needed. The indication for an MRI would be a suspected occult or stress fracture, or a ligament injury of the knee.

Treatment

Femoral shaft fractures are treated according to the child's age and size, concomitant injuries such as head injury or polytrauma, or the presence of open lesions with vessel and nerve injury. Compliance with treatment and socioeconomic factors should be considered.

Femoral Shaft Fracture During the First Year of Life

In the postnatal period a simple cotton bandage or a harness used for dysplastic hips can be applied for a period of 2 weeks.

Bilateral overhead traction has been the treatment of choice for many years. The child has to be in hospital for about 10–14 days. The average transverse fracture heals with a shortening of several millimeters. In a case of suspected non-accidental injury, hospitalization offers the opportunity to investigate the social situation of the child.

Our Preferred Treatment

A *spica cast* after closed reduction of the femoral fracture is the treatment of choice for most paediatric orthopaedic surgeons. The position of the fractured leg is controlled by 90°

of hip and knee flexion [4]. The author prefers a well-padded spica cast with 60° hip and 60° knee flexion. In order to avoid secondary varus deformity, the fractured leg is kept in neutral abduction, while the contralateral side can be in abduction to allow nappy changes to take place. Routine radiographs in two planes after application of the cast are advised. If the mother or the family is well informed about the care of a baby in a spica cast, the child does not need to stay in hospital. During a visit to the clinic after 1 week, routine radiographs will detect angular deviation. Wedging of the cast may be necessary. Due to rapid callus formation consolidation occurs within 2–3 weeks (Fig. 48.2). After removal of the cast restoration of function is rapid.

The *Pavlik harness* used for a period of 3–5 weeks is an alternative treatment for the very small baby. The application does not need general anesthesia and hospitalization time can be minimized. Compliance problems seem to be rare [10].

Vertical traction for femoral fractures in this age group is popular in many places. However, it is less convenient for the child and the family and adds to the cost of hospitalization [11].

Femoral Shaft Fracture from 1 to 4 Years

Traction is still widely used for femoral shaft fractures in pre-school and early for school age children. Hospital stays of 4–6 weeks are usually necessary. Overhead skin traction has the risk of adverse effects on limb circulation [12]. Proximal tibial skeletal traction avoids too much shortening. Pins must be placed horizontally to avoid differences of the intercondylar angle [13, 14]. Traction can be started in the hospital and continued at home but compliance problems and economic considerations are important [15].

Elastic intramedullary nails or intramedullary Kirschner wires are occasionally used for femoral fractures in the pre-school age group. The main indication is failed conventional treatment in a spica cast [16]. Two millimeter-diameter titanium nails are introduced from the medial and lateral metaphysis of the distal femur in order to achieve an intramedullary stabilization of the fracture. The main advantage of this treatment is the opportunity of early mobilization

Fig. 48.2 (**a**) A 6month-old girl with left mid-shaft transverse fracture. (**b**) Child in a 60/60° spica cast with cyclist pants on non-fractured side. (**c**) fractured left femur in the cast. (**d**) Left femur at age 7 months with good callus formation (**e**) Standing X-ray at 18 months. There is minor varus and equal leg-length

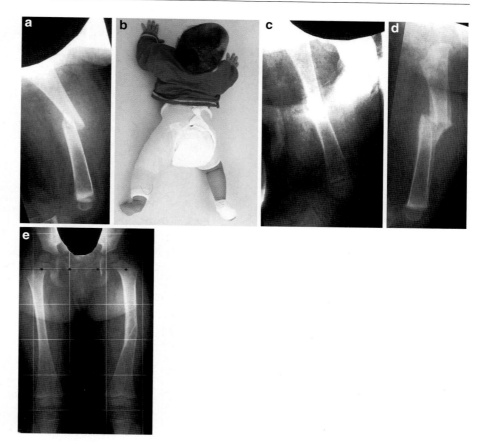

and weight bearing. The consolidation time is short, ranging from 2 to 5 weeks depending on the age of the patient. The implants are removed 3–6 months after introduction. As a sequel to anatomical reduction following the use of intramedullary nails, overgrowth of the involved side of 6–12 mm is common in transverse and oblique fractures.

External fixators are the treatment of choice for open fractures in poly-traumatized patients or for segmental fractures, also in this age group [17]. There is a risk of re-fracture after early removal of the fixator with a lack of callus formation. As in all other fixator use, pin tract infections are common and are treated by local skin care and antibiotics. We do not advise treatment by external fixation for isolated and closed femoral shaft fractures in pre-school children.

Our Preferred Treatment

Spica casts as an immediate treatment have gained wide support as the most efficient and well tolerated in any type of femoral shaft fractures in pre-school children [18, 19]. The cast must be carefully applied. Reduction of a transverse or an oblique fracture should be undertaken under general anesthesia, while spiral fractures can sometimes be reduced only with the help of an analgesic. Care is taken to achieve good alignment axially and to avoid malrotation. This is controlled by anteroposterior (AP) and lateral radiographs after cast application. Gortex or cotton linings can be used to avoid problems from urine or feces. Shortening of up to 15 mm can be accepted [4]. Generally the cast is worn for 4–6 weeks depending on the type of fracture and the age of the patient. Overgrowth after consolidation will compensate for most or all of the initial shortening (Fig. 48.3).

Femoral Shaft Fractures from 5 to 15 Years

Traction is still widely used mainly in places where there is no economic problem with prolonged hospitalization. Skeletal traction through a distal femoral pin on the fractured side is a low-risk treatment. Traction for 6–8 weeks exclusively and traction for 3–4 weeks followed by a period of 2–3 weeks in a spica cast are the alternatives [4, 20]. Traction with pins through both distal femurs and the child lying on a frame has been popular in Europe during the second part of the last century. Treatment on the *Weber frame* allowed optimal control of rotation, but meant an average period of 4 weeks in the hospital followed by another 2 weeks in a spica before mobilization was started [21].

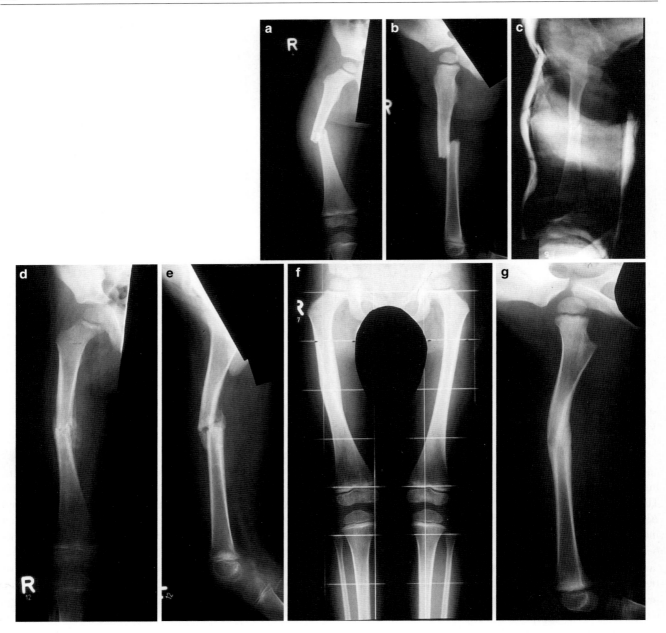

Fig. 48.3 (**a**) and (**b**) Right midshaft transverse fracture of a three-year-old boy. (**c**) AP view of fracture after closed reduction immobilized in a spica cast. (**d**) and (**e**) AP and lateral view of the fracture, slight varus and antecurvatum. sufficient callus formation. (**f**) Standing X-ray of both femora showing residual varus. (**g**) Side view of left femur with good alignment after remodelling of antccurvatum

Immediate spica cast application is a low-risk treatment used in some centers, at least in the age group up to 7 years [22] or up to 10 years [23]. Application of a well-fitting and well-functioning spica cast in a school child is not an easy task. A spica table must be available. Malposition in varus and/or external malrotation must be avoided. Flexion of 45° at the hip and knee joint is sufficient for the older child. The contralateral side needs abduction for toilet care, while the fractured side is positioned in neutral or only minor abduction. Post-reduction the fracture must be radiographed

in two planes. In case of malposition, wedging of the cast may be necessary. Transverse and oblique fractures may develop some shortening [24]. The cast is removed after 6–8 weeks. Most children do not require physical therapy after the removal of the cast and can return to normal activities after 3–4 weeks [25]. There may be compliance problems for some children and parents, especially if they hear about the alternatives of early mobilization with other protocols.

An alternative to cast treatment has been the use of a *cast brace* [26] and a *three-point fixation walking spica* [27]. Both

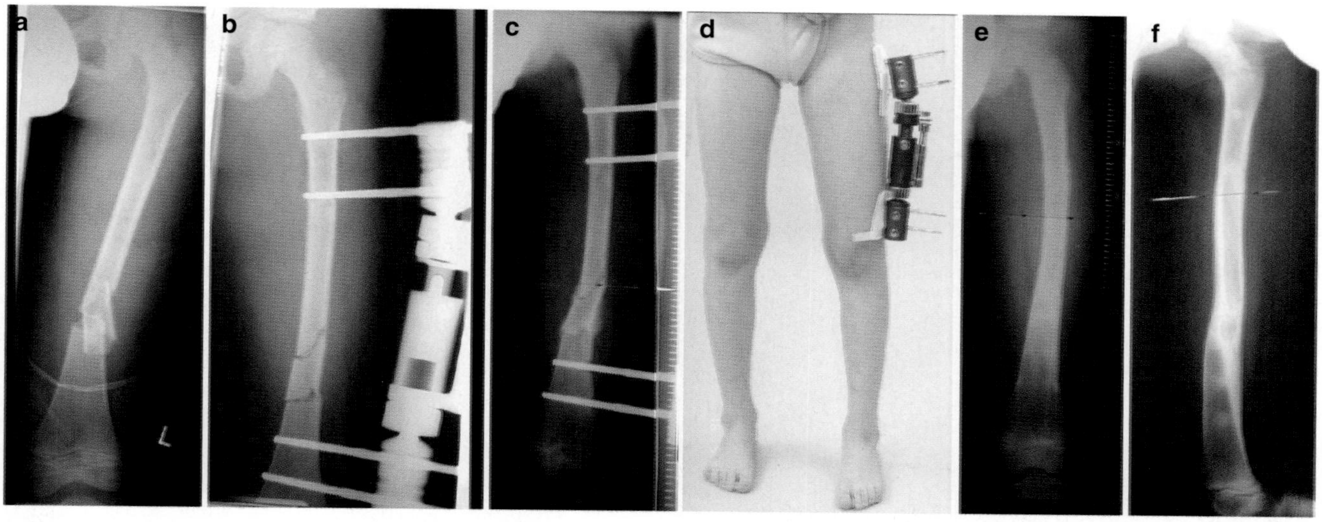

Fig. 48.4 (**a**) Eight-year-old boy with comminuted fracture of left femur and large third fragment. (**b**) After closed reduction of the fracture and fixation with external fixator. (**c**) Left femur after 4 weeks in the fixator. Some callus formation. (**d**) the patient 4 weeks later standing with his Orthofix external fixator. Eight months after trauma and 4 months after the removal of external fixator. (**e**) and (**f**) AP and lateral view of the left femur 8 months after injury. Minimal varus and overgrowth of 7 mm

methods avoid prolonged hospitalization and allow treatment at home.

External fixators of different design (AO, Orthofix, and others) have become popular around the world during the past 15 years (Fig. 48.4). Stable fixation of the fracture allows early weight bearing and return to school [28, 29].

There can be compliance problems in connection with screws and pins. Pin tract infections are less common than when using external fixators for leg lengthening. In transverse fractures the fixator must remain in place for 3 months, while spiral fractures are stable after 2 months or less. Re-fracture after fixator removal may occur in up to 10% of cases causing a second period of morbidity [30–32]. With the advantages seen in the use of intramedullary titanium nails for femoral shaft fractures in children, external fixators have lost ground during the past 10 years, at least for "simple" closed fractures [33].

External fixation still has a place in the extremely rare Gustilo 2 and 3 open fractures of the femur in children, for example, after gun shot or explosion injuries, while Gustilo 1 injuries are better treated with intramedullary nails. [34].

Plate fixation with dynamic compression has been used for many years, especially for polytrauma patients but also in simple closed fractures [17, 35, 36]. With the introduction of intramedullary elastic nails and external fixators, plate fixation of shaft fractures has become less popular and indicated only if other devices are not available.

Submuscular bridge plating as a minimally invasive method has been introduced for complex paediatric shaft fractures but mainly in adolescents [37, 38].

Our Preferred Method

In some centers *elastic intramedullary titanium or stainless steel nails* have become the treatment of choice for standard femoral shaft fractures in school children. The French paediatric orthopaedic schools of Nancy and Metz introduced the so-called elastic stable nails to stabilize femoral shaft fractures, also called "Nancy nails" or ESIN (elastic stable intramedullary nailing) [39–41]. The system spread to Europe [41–45] and North America and is now the treatment of choice around the world [46, 47].

When using elastic nails the child should be placed on a traction table with boots that can be adjusted to the size of the patient's foot. For closed manipulation an image intensifier is necessary. The fracture is reduced by gentle traction and manipulation. In a retrograde manner the two nails are pushed up the medullary canal, the medial nail into the femoral neck, and the lateral nail into the greater trochanter (Fig. 48.5). The retrograde method is satisfactory for all midshaft and proximal shaft fractures, while antegrade insertion is best for distal fractures. The intramedullary system offers axial and rotatory stability [40, 41].

Early mobilization after ESIN fixation of the femoral shaft fracture is possible. After correct implantation of titanium nails assisted walking can start immediately. Full weight bearing is encouraged as soon as the child is able to do so. This varies from 2 to 3 weeks and up to 10 weeks in other centers [48].

Distal femoral shaft fractures are best treated by antegrade titanium elastic stable nails [41]. After reduction of the fracture on the orthopaedic table, two nails are passed distally

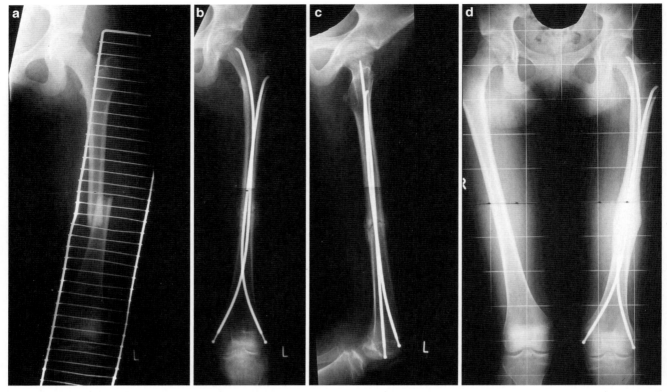

Fig. 48.5 (**a**) Thirteen-year-old girl with left midshaft transverse fracture with shortening. (**b**) Two months after intramedullary titanium pinning. Callus formation on AP view. (**c**) Two months after intramedullary titanium pinning. Callus formation on lateral view. (**d**) Scanogram of the femora at 14 years of age. Full stability from callus before pin removal. The left femur had been shorter before the accident. It is 1 cm short after fracture healing

Fig. 48.6 (**a**) Nine-year-old boy with distal transverse fracture. (**b**) After anterograde pinning with two 3.5 mm titanium nails. AP and lateral views. (**c**) Six months later complete union of the distal femoral fracture, before pin removal

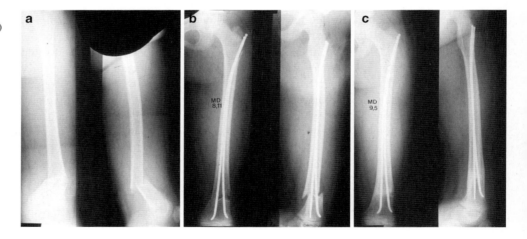

from a subtrochanteric entry point aligning the distal fracture. The distal end of the nails should spread out medially and laterally in order to secure stability inside the marrow space (Fig. 48.6).

Comminuted fractures benefit from additional immobilization in a spica cast, at least in the early phase until some callus has formed. In comminuted fractures, we advise delayed weight bearing in order to avoid secondary malposition and further intervention.

Consolidation is amazingly fast as fracture callus is stimulated by the elastic stability of the nails. The nails are removed after 4–6 months depending on the age of the child. Overgrowth of the fractured femur is common and averages 0.6 cm. The highest rate of overgrowth is seen in midshaft transverse fractures in the younger age group around 7 years. The lowest is encountered in long spiral fractures.

Complications in ESIN treated children are associated with the learning curve of the surgeon [47].

Skin and subcutaneous irritations around the knee, even nail erosions, have been encountered. Problems around the knee account for about half of the complications in titanium elastic nail (TEN) treatment of femoral shaft fractures [49–51]. Skin irritation at the insertion area above the knee can be lessened and even avoided by using a second-generation Nancy nail with olive-like rounded ends (Depuy Orthopedics, Inc.) which will not poke into the subcutaneous tissue, like the cut-off ends of other nails. Olive-ended titanium nails must be inserted with premeasured length [44]. A large assortment of different diameters and lengths must therefore be available. The rounded end is helpful to obtain a hold at the time of removal to obtain a hold on the nail.

Mismatched diameters of the nail, especially the insertion of nails with too thin a diameter, can be the cause of postoperative loss of alignment. The two nails should fill two-thirds of the diameter of the medullary canal. Mismatched diameters may cause secondary malposition and the need for further intervention [50].

Obese children have a higher rate of complications no matter what fixation is used [52]. In a study of 234 femur fractures, children weighing less than 49 kg had a significantly better outcome than those who were overweight [51]. The largest possible nail diameter should be chosen in obese patients [49]. Mobilization, but delayed weight bearing, must be considered in very heavy children.

The use of TENs is widely accepted and has replaced external fixation or plates in most centers. In a prospective randomized study, fractures fixed by flexible nails had a better outcome compared to those treated by external fixation [33]. The complication rate associated with nailing compares favorably with that following traction and application of a spica cast [53].

Flexible steel nails (Ender nails) introduced from below the greater trochanter into the distal metaphysis or by a retrograde approach, from the distal medial and lateral metaphysis into the femoral neck and greater trochanter, have their proponents [54–56].

Intramedullary stable nails with or without an interlocking mechanism have been introduced in the treatment of femoral shaft fractures in adolescents. They can be compared to the Küntscher nails used in the 1950 s and the 1960 s. In addition they offer an antirotatory locking mechanism with screws set in the trochanter and the distal femur [57–60]. Interlocking nails allow early weight bearing. Nail removal is undertaken on an average of 14 months post-injury. A risk of partial or segmental avascular necrosis (AVN) of the femoral head of approximately 10% has been reported. This is caused by injury to the posterior superior ascending branch of the

medial circumflex artery [61, 62]. We are in agreement with those who advise that rigid intramedullary rodding should be reserved for skeletally mature patients [63]. They can be used for the very heavy adolescent, where elastic nails may be too weak.

References

1. Landin LA. Fracture patterns in children. Analysis of 8682 fractures with special reference to incidence, etiology and secular changes in Swedish urban population 1950–1979. Acta Orthop Scand Suppl 1983; 202: 1–109.
2. Hedlund R, Lindgren U. The incidence of femoral shaft fractures in children and adolescents. J Pediatr Orthop 1986; 6: 47–50.
3. Cooper C, Dennison EM, Leufkens HG, et al. Epidemiology of childhood fractures in Britain: a study using the general practice research database. Bone Mineral Res 2004; 19: 1976–1981.
4. Kasser JR, Beaty JH. Femoral shaft fractures. In: Beaty JH, Kasser JR, eds. Rockwood and Wilkins' Fractures in Children, 5th ed. Philadelphia: Lippincott-Williams & Wilkins; 2001: 941–980.
5. Hinton RY, Lincoln A, Crockett MM, et al. Fractures of the femoral shaft in children. Incidence, mechanisms, and sociodemographic risk factors. J Bone Joint Surg 1999; 81: 500–509.
6. Taitz J, Moran K, O'Meara M. Long bone fractures in children under 3 years of age: is abuse being missed in Emergency Department presentations? J Paediatr Child Health 2004; 40: 170–174.
7. Banaszkiewicz PA, Scotland TR, Myerscough EJ. Fractures in children younger than age 1 year: importance of collaboration with child protection services. J Pediatr Orthop 2002; 22: 740–744.
8. Schwendt RM, Werth C, Johnson A. Femur shaft fractures in toddlers and young children: rarely from child abuse. J Pediatr Orthop 2000; 20: 475–481.
9. Slongo T, Audigé L, Clavert JM, et al. The AO comprehensive classification of pediatric long-bone fractures: a web-based multicenter agreement study. J Pediatr Orthop 2007; 27: 171–180.
10. Stannard JP, Christensen KP, Wilkins KE. Femur fractures in infants: a new therapeutic approach. J Pediatr Orthop 1995; 15: 461–466.
11. Nork SE, Hoffinger SA. Skeletal traction versus external fixation for pediatric femoral shaft fractures: a comparison of hospital costs and charges. J Orthop Trauma 1998; 12: 563–568.
12. Nicholson JT, Foster RM, Heath RD. Bryant's traction. A provocative cause of circulatory complications. J Am Med Ass 1955; 157: 415–418.
13. Aronson DD, Singer RM, Higgins RF. Skeletal traction for fracture of the femoral shaft in children. J Bone Joint Surg 1987; 69A: 1435–1439.
14. Dwyer AJ, Mam MK, John B, et al. Femoral shaft fractures in children—a comparison of treatment. Int Orthop 2003; 27: 141–144.
15. Newton PO, Mubarak SJ. Financial aspects of femoral shaft fracture treatment in children and adolescents. J Paediatr Orthop 1994; 14(4): 508–512.
16. Simanovsky N, Porat S, Simanovsky N, et al. Close reduction and intramedullary flexible titanium nails fixation of femoral shaft fractures in children under 5 years of age. J Pediatr Orthop Part B 2006; 15: 293–295.
17. Tolo VT. Orthopaedic treatment of fractures of the long bones and pelvis in children who have multiple injuries. J Bone Joint Surg 2000; 82A: 272–280.

18. Czertak DJ, Hennrikus WL. The treatment of pediatric femur fractures with early 90–90 spica casting. J Pediatr Orthop 1999; 19: 229–232.

19. Infante AF, Albert MC, Jennings WB, et al. Immediate hip spica casting for femur fractures in pediatric patients. A review of 175 patients. Clin Orthop Relat Res 2000; 376: 106–112.

20. Sullivan JA, Gregory P, Hemdon WA, et al. Management of femoral shaft fractures in children ages 5 to 13 by traction and spica cast. Orthopedics 1994; 2: 567–571.

21. Weber BG. Fractures of the femoral shaft in childhood. Injury 1969; 1: 65–68.

22. Berne D, Mary P, Damsin JP. Femoral shaft fracture in children: treatment with early spica cast. Rev Chir Orthop Repar Appar Mot 2003; 89: 599–604.

23. Ferguson J, Nicol RO. Early spica treatment of pediatric femoral shaft fractures. J Pediatr Orthop 2000; 20: 189–192.

24. Thompson JD, Buehler KC, Sponseller PD, et al. Shortening in femoral shaft fractures in children treated with spica cast. Clin Orthop Rel Res 1997; 338: 74–78.

25. Hughes BF, Sponseller PD, Thompson JD. Pediatric femur fractures: effects of spica cast treatment on family and community. J Pediatr Orthop 1995; 15: 457–460.

26. Gross RH, Davidson R, Sullivan JA, et al. Cast brace management of the femoral shaft fracture in children and young adults. J Pediatr Orthop 1983; 3: 572–582.

27. Guttmann GG, Simon R. Three-point walking spica cast: an alternative to early or immediate casting of femoral shaft fractures in children. J Pediatr Orthop 1988; 8: 699–703.

28. Aronson J, Tursky EA. External fixation of femur fractures in children. J Pediatr Orthop 1992; 12: 157–163.

29. Davis TJ, Topping RE, Blanco JS. External fixation of pediatric femoral fractures. Clin Orthop Relat Res 1995; 318: 191–198.

30. Hull JB, Bell MJ. Modern trends for external fixation of fractures in children: a critical review. J Pediatr Orthop B 1997; 6: 103–109.

31. Weinberg AM, Hasler CC, Leitner A, et al. External fixation of pediatric femoral shaft fractures. Europ J Trauma 2000; 1: 25–32.

32. Hedin H, Hjorth K, Rehberg L. External fixation of displaced femoral shaft fractures in children: a consecutive study of 98 fractures. J Orthop Trauma 2003; 17: 250–256.

33. Bar-On E, Sagiv S, Porat S. External fixation or flexible intramedullary nailing for femoral shaft fractures ion children. J Bone Joint Surg 1997; 79 B: 975–978.

34 Ramseier LE, Bhaskar AR, Cole WG, et al. Treatment of open femur fracture in children: comparison between external fixator and intramedullary nailing. J Pediatr Orthop 2007; 27: 748–750.

35. Ward WT, Levy J, Kaye A. Compression plating for child and adolescent femur fractures. J Pediatr Orthop 1992; 12: 626–632.

36. Kregor PJ, Song KM, Routt MLC, et al. Plate fixation of femoral shaft fractures in multiply injured children. J Bone Joint Surg 1993; 75 A: 1774–1780.

37. Kanlic EM, Anglen JO, Smith DG, et al. Advantages of submuscular bridge plating for complex pediatric femur fractures. Clin Orthop Relat Res 2004; 426: 244–251.

38. Sink EL, Hedequist D, Morgan SJ, et al. Results and technique of unstable pediatric femoral fractures treated with submuscular bridge plating. J Pediatr Orthop 2006; 26: 177–181.

39. Ligier JN, Metaizeau JP, Prévot J, Lascombe P. Elastic stable intramedullary nailing of femoral shaft fractures in children. J Bone Joint Surg 1988; 70B: 74–77

40. Metaizeau JP. L'ostéosynthèse chez l'enfant. Embrochage centromédullaire élastique stable. Sauramps, Montpellier 1988: 77–84.

41. Lascombe P, Métaizeau JD. Fracture du femur. In: Lascombe P, ed. Embrochage centromédullaire élastique stable. Issy-les-Moulineaux: Elsevier Masson SAS; 2006: 207–240.

42. Dietz HG, Schmittenbecher PP, Illing P. Intramedulläre Osteosynthese am Oberschenkel. In: Intramedulläre Osteosynthese im Wachstumsalter. München: Urban & Schwarzenberg; 1997: 135–168.

43. Mazda K, Khairouni A, Pennecot GF, et al. Closed flexible intramedullary nailing of the femoral shaft fractures in children. J Pediatr Orthop B 1997; 6: 198–202.

44. Parsch K. Modern trends in internal fixation of femoral shaft fractures in children. A critical review. J Pediatr Orthop Part B 1997; 6: 117–125.

45. Till H, Huettl B, Knorr P, et al. Elastic stable intramedullary nailing (ESIN) provides good long-term results in pediatric long bone fractures. Eur J Pediatr Surg 2000; 10: 319–322.

46. Carey TP, Galpin RD. Flexible intramedullary nail fixation of pediatric femoral fractures. Clin Orthop Relat Res 1996; 332: 110–118.

47. Flynn JM, Hresko T, Reynolds RA, et al. Titanium elastic nails for pediatric femur fractures: a multicenter study of early results with analysis of complications. J Pediatr Orthop 2001; 21: 4–8.

48. Ho CA, Skaggs DL, Tang CW, et al. Use of flexible intramedullary nails in pediatric femur fractures. J Pediatr Orthop 2006; 26: 497–504.

49. Luhmann SJ, Schootman M, Schoenecker, et al. Complications of titanium elastic nails for pediatric femoral shaft fractures. J Pediatr Orthop 2003; 23: 443–447

50. Narayanan UG, Hyman JE, Wainwright AM. Complications of elastic stable intramedullary nail fixation of pediatric femoral fractures, and how to avoid them. J Pediatr Orthop 2004; 24: 363–369.

51. Moroz LA, Launay F, Kocher MS, et al. Titanium elastic nailing of fractures of the femur in children. Predictors of complications and poor outcome. J Bone Joint Surg 2006; 88 B: 1361–1365.

52. Leet AI, Pichard CP, Ain MC. Surgical treatment of femoral fractures in obese children: does excessive body weight increase the rate of complications? J Bone Joint Surg 2005; 87A: 2609–2613.

53. Flynn JM, Luedke LM, Ganley TJ, et al. Comparison of titanium elastic nails with traction and a spica cast to treat femoral fractures in children. J Bone Joint Surg 2004; 86A: 770–777.

54. Heinrich SD, Drvaric DM, Darr K, et al. The operative stabilization of pediatric diaphyseal femur fractures with flexible intramedullary nails: a prospective analysis. J Pediatr Orthop 1994; 14: 501–507.

55. Linhart WE, Roposch A. Elastic stable intramedullary nailing for unstable femoral fractures in children: preliminary results of a new method. J Trauma 1999; 47: 372–378.

56. Rathjen KE, Riccio AI, de la Garza D. Stainless steel flexible intramedullary fixation of unstable femoral shaft fractures in children. J Pediatr Orthop 2007; 27: 432–441

57. Beaty JH, Austin SM, Warner WC, et al. Interlocking intramedullary nailing of femoral shaft fractures in adolescents: preliminary results and complications. J Pediatr Orthop 1994; 14: 178–183.

58. Canale ST, Tolo VT. Fractures of the femur in children. J Bone Joint Surg 1995; 77A: 294–315.

59. Gordon JE, Khanna N, Luhmann SJ, et al. Intramedullary nailing of femoral fractures in children through the lateral aspect of the greater trochanter using a modified rigid humeral intramedullary nail: results of a new technique in 15 children. J Orthop Trauma 2004; 18: 416–422.

60. Kanellopoulos AD, Yiannakopoulos CK, Soucacos PN. Closed locked intramedullary nailing of pediatric femoral shaft fractures through the tip of the greater trochanter. J Trauma 2006;60 217–222.

61. Mileski RA, Garvin KL, Crosby LA. Avascular necrosis of the femoral head in an adolescent following intramedullary nailing of the femur. J Bone Joint Surg 1994; 76A; 1706–1708.

62. O'Malley DE, Mazur JM, Cummings RJ. Femoral head necrosis associated with intramedullary nailing in an adolescent. J Pediatr Orthop 1995; 15: 21–23.

63. Letts M, Jarvis J, Lawton L, et al. Complications of rigid intramedullary rodding of femoral shaft fractures in children. J Trauma 2002; 52: 504–516.

Chapter 49

Fractures of the Knee and Tibia

Carol-C. Hasler

Extra-Articular Fractures of the Distal Femur

Incidence and Mechanism of Injury

Distal femoral extra-articular physeal fractures account for 1% of all fractures in children and 5% of physeal injuries. In *hyperextension injuries* the epiphysis is displaced anteriorly while the metaphysis is displaced into the popliteal fossa. The more frequent *varus–valgus fractures* result from abduction or adduction force in the coronal plane. Only a few are Salter–Harris I lesions (Fig. 49.1); the vast majority are Salter–Harris II fractures [1]. In children 2–11 years old these fractures are inevitably caused by severe trauma. In the adolescent, Salter–Harris I and II lesions are caused by less extensive trauma, usually sports injuries [2].

Treatment

In hyperextension injuries the epiphysis is displaced anteriorly; the popliteal surface of the metaphysis is separated only by a thin layer of fat from the popliteal artery. Posterior displacement of the metaphysis carries a greater risk of neurovascular injury. Any severe displacement in the coronal or sagittal plane should be reduced if possible as an emergency bearing in mind the risk of neurovascular injury from the metaphysis in the popliteal fossa [1].

In Salter–Harris type I or II valgus or varus lesions, closed reduction can be attempted by longitudinal traction along the axis of the deformity. Without stable fixation secondary displacement can occur and be the cause of secondary growth disturbance [3]. If there is no substantial metaphyseal fragment, smooth crossed K-wires are used for fixation [4]. If the metaphyseal (Thurston-Holland) fragment is large, one or two cannulated screws with a washer are inserted transversely to fix the fragment anatomically [5]. If periosteal infolding blocks reduction, open release should be performed followed by screw fixation. The limb should then be immobilized for 6 weeks in a split long leg cast or a splint. The vascular status must be carefully checked both before and after reduction (Fig. 49.2).

Prognosis

If the neurovascular supply is uninjured and compartment syndrome does not develop, the prognosis of distal Salter–Harris I and II fractures is usually good. There is however a high incidence of physeal growth disturbance after distal femoral epiphyseal fractures which may lead to asymmetry of length, angulation, or both (Fig. 49.3). The distal femoral physis has a complex contour which can cause shearing of the fracture line across the physis even in "benign" fractures. If the fracture is sustained toward the end of growth, the risk of post-traumatic angulation or shortening will not be significant. However, if it happens in a younger child the risks of malalignment and shortening are greater. Growth arrest of part or all distal femoral growth plate has been reported in up to 50% of injuries [6–10].

To detect post-traumatic deformity children must be followed closely until maturity [1, 11]. Femoral lengthening with correction of the angular deformity is necessary for children whose deformity becomes unacceptable.

Intra-articular Fractures of the Distal Femur

Fracture Types

Salter–Harris type III, IV and transitional fractures of the distal femur are rare. Salter–Harris type III fractures show a vertical fracture line extending from the physis into the

C.-C. Hasler (✉)
Department of Orthopaedics, University Children's Hospital Basel, Basel, Switzerland

M. Benson et al. (eds.), *Children's Orthopaedics and Fractures*,
DOI 10.1007/978-1-84882-611-3_49, © Springer-Verlag London Limited 2010

Fig. 49.1 (**a**) Salter–Harris type
I fracture of the distal femoral
epiphysis of an 11-year-old boy, a
pedestrian hit by a motorcycle.
The extension fracture was
reduced as an emergency. No
neurovascular compromise.
(**b**) Follow-up at age 13 years.
Two years after injury there is
premature growth arrest of the
right distal femur with $1\frac{1}{2}$ cm
shortening. Epiphysiodesis of the
opposite distal femur equalized
leg length discrepancy. Courtesy
of Dr. Klaus Parsch, Stuttgart

Fig. 49.2 (**a**) Salter–Harris type
II lesion of an 8-year-old girl who
had fallen from a tree. (**b**) Lateral
view shows posterior
displacement of the distal
metaphysis. The fracture was
reduced as an emergency and
fixed with two transverse screws.
(**c**) Standing femoral films with
the screws still in place.
(**d**) Radiological follow-up 4
years later: no sequelae. Courtesy
of Dr. Klaus Parsch, Stuttgart

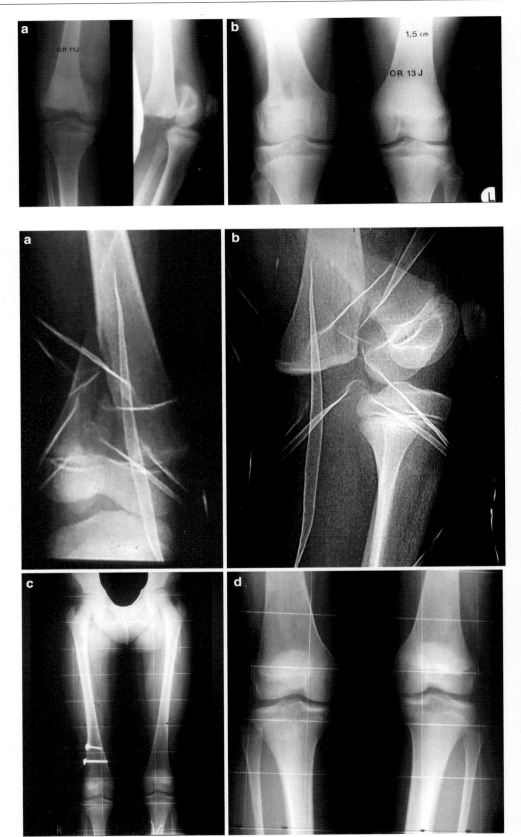

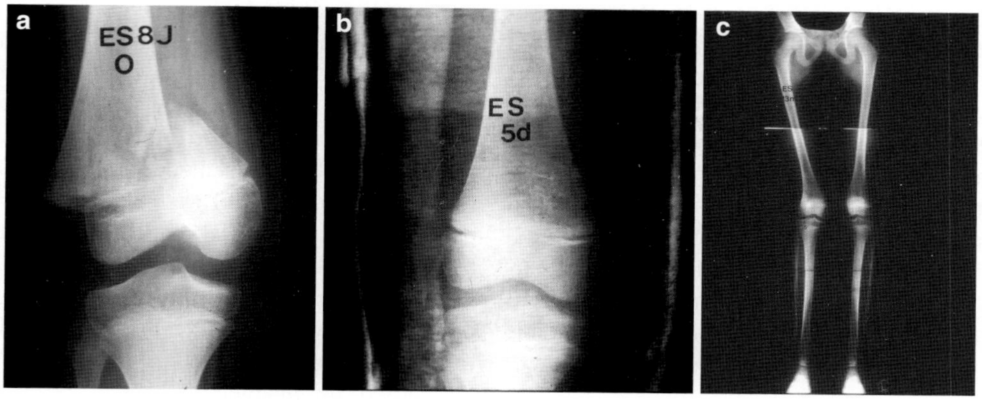

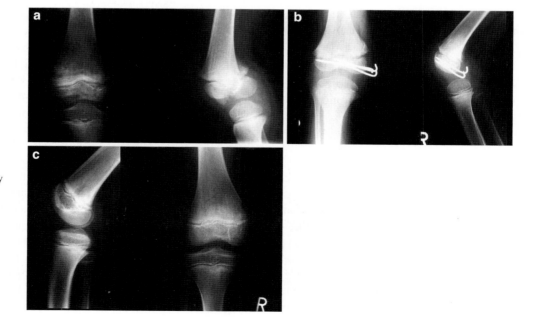

Fig. 49.3 (**a**) Salter–Harris type II fracture of distal femur of an 8-year-old girl run over by a car. (**b**) Following closed reduction in a long leg cast after 5 days. (**c**) Standing radiograph shows shortening and valgus deformity 13 months later. This was treated later by supracondylar varus osteotomy with lengthening. Courtesy of Dr. Klaus Parsch, Stuttgart

joint usually through the intercondylar notch. Type IV fractures run from the metaphyseal cortex, cross the physis, and extend into the joint. As the fracture can reduce spontaneously, it may be overlooked or mistaken for a ligamentous injury. The combination with a physeal injury of the proximal tibia (floating knee) is rare in children. Transitional fractures occur during adolescence when the physis has already partially closed. The asymmetrical closure may allow the non-fused part of the epiphysis to break off with a sagittal epiphyseal and a horizontal physeal fracture line (two-plane fracture) or an additional frontal metaphyseal plane (three-plane fracture). Careful inspection of the lateral radiograph helps to differentiate a transitional fracture from a Salter–Harris type I epiphysiolysis. Correct imaging by radiographs

in two planes and additional oblique planes is mandatory. If available, computed tomography (CT) scans add significantly to understanding the intra- and extra-articular parts of the fracture.

Treatment

Intra-articular displacement is always associated with considerable hemarthrosis and requires anatomical reduction and stable internal fixation with K-wires or screws. Emergency surgical intervention with anatomic reduction may give a satisfactory result (Fig. 49.4), but delayed

Fig. 49.4 (**a**) Four-year-old boy who had fallen 7 m. Displaced Salter–Harris type IV fracture. (**b**) Open reduction and K-wire fixation of the three fragments. Articular cartilage gap closed anatomically. (**c**) Follow-up 2 years later: full range of motion and intact growth plate. Courtesy of Dr. Klaus Parsch, Stuttgart

treatment has a reduced chance of anatomical reconstruction. Although the risk of an inhibiting growth disturbance is significantly diminished by an anatomical "waterproof" osteosynthesis, partial growth arrest and persistent intra-articular damage may cause secondary incongruence followed by a variable joint stiffness.

The transitional fractures of adolescents should be treated by open reduction and internal fixation. Post-traumatic stiffness caused by incongruence depends on the amount of cartilage damaged by trauma. As these fractures occur toward the end of growth post-traumatic shortening or angulation is less likely [1].

Acute Traumatic Dislocation of the Patella

Epidemiology and Mechanism of Injury

One in 1000 children has a first acute dislocation of the patella per year [12]. It is caused by an indirect external rotation and valgus stress on the flexed knee with the foot fixed on the ground and occurs predominantly during adolescence with a peak at the age of 15 years. Vigorous sports activities, muscular imbalance, relative weakness, and shortening of the thigh muscles as well as proprioceptive deficits during the growth spurt may be responsible. The patient's history allows differentiation of permanent, habitual, or recurrent instability as well as chronic patellofemoral instability from a first episode of true dislocation. In children, patellar dislocation is the commonest cause of acute traumatic hemarthrosis; it accounts for almost half and is also the most likely source of osteo-chondral fragments in the knee joint. Although medial and superior dislocations are described, lateral displacement is by far the most common. Treatment comprises

- immediate reduction of the patella
- recognition and repair of osteo-chondral lesions
- prevention of recurrent dislocation

Clinical Findings

Patients show painful fixed knee flexion and a laterally fully displaced, externally rotated patella. Usually it is easily reducible without anesthesia by gradual passive extension of the knee with the hip flexed to relax the quadriceps muscle. However, most patients present with a spontaneously relocated patella and are unaware of what happened. Some are convinced of medial displacement since the patella-free

medial femoral condyle looks prominent. Anterior cruciate ligament (ACL) rupture with subsequent pivoting may give the same impression and needs to be ruled out. Even when the knee cap has spontaneously relocated and the history of trauma is unclear, a thorough clinical examination should reveal the correct diagnosis. Since the medial patellofemoral ligament (MPFL) is invariably damaged by lateral patellar dislocation, local tenderness between the adductor tubercle and the superomedial patella is almost pathognomonic. In addition cartilaginous contusion or fracture at the lateral trochlear border and avulsion fractures at the medial patellar facet may be symptomatic. The hemarthrosis caused by ligamentous and/or osteochondral lesions may be slight or major and develop immediately or slowly over hours.

Radiological Findings

Imaging should include anteroposterior (AP) and lateral radiographs and an axial view (skyline view) of the patella in 30–45° knee flexion if pain allows. Assessment of the patello-femoral spatial relationship is not reliable as long as post-traumatic effusion elevates and lateralizes the patella and delayed imaging is more reliable. Osteochondral lesions may be found at the medial border of the patella as an extra-articular avulsion of the medial rim of the patella (avulsion of the medial patello-femoral ligament), intra-articular at the lateral femoral condyle, and as loose bodies anywhere in the joint. The size of this osteochondral fragment is usually underestimated since only the small osseous part is visible radiologically. The magnetic resonance imaging (MRI) findings are similar to adults and reflect the ligamentous injuries caused by the lateral dislocation and the trochlear damage suffered by the relocating patella: injuries of the medial patellar restraints are found in 81%, simple bone bruises and cartilaginous injuries at the infero-medial patella and at the lateral femoral condyle in 81% and 38%, respectively, and osteochondral fragments of various sizes in 42% [13].

Associated Injuries

The osteochondral lesions are half intra- and half extra-articular. In a prospective study intra-articular fragments were only found after spontaneous relocation when the medial patellar facet hits the lateral femoral condyle on the way back to the sulcus [12] (Fig. 49.5). Arthroscopy is indicated if there are signs of loose *intra*-articular fragments. Some of them are big enough to need open or arthroscopy-controlled fixation. Rarely a large soft tissue gap

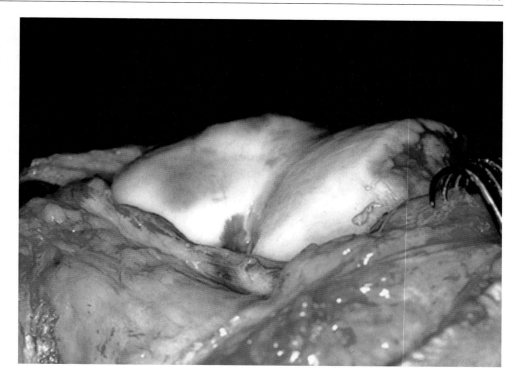

Fig. 49.5 Osteochondral shear fracture of lateral trochlear border after recurrent dislocations of the left patella. Finding at open trochleo-plasty for dysplasia

proximo-medial to the patella indicates avulsion of the vastus medialis muscle warranting open fixation.

MRI, a prerequisite for patients with a first episode of acute dislocation if recurrent dislocation is to be avoided by realignment (See Chapter 29).

Predisposing Factors

In most children under 10 years who present after a first patellar dislocation, an underlying abnormality of their static and dynamic soft tissue constraints is found (MPFL, ligamentum patella, patella alta, and dysplasia of the oblique vastus medialis muscle). Bony, ligament, and muscular anatomical factors may predispose to recurrence: Nearly all patients show some radiological signs of patello-femoral dysplasia such as a shallow cartilaginous sulcus, a positive crossing sign on the lateral radiograph or pathologic shape and distribution of the articular cartilage on MRI with consequent false tracking in early flexion [14, 15]. In patients with general ligamentous laxity contralateral patellar hypermobility is typical. It may be associated with hereditary conditions (Down syndrome, Ehlers-Danlos syndrome, osteogenesis imperfecta, Rubinstein–Taybi syndrome, and nail-patella syndrome), poor psychomotor abilities, and contractures of the lateral or central structures of the extensor mechanism. Genu valgum, genu recurvatum, increased femoral anteversion, or increased external torsion of the tibia may also contribute to patellofemoral instability. In most patients there is a unique combination of these factors. Their precise clinical assessment is best evaluated by CT or

Treatment

Aspiration quickly relieves the pain of a minor effusion. The fat drop sign in the aspirated fluid as an indicator of an associated osteochondral lesion should not be overestimated. It may also be caused by contusion of Hoffa's fat pad. For the first-time dislocation primary arthroscopy is indicated only if there is radiological or clinical evidence of an osteochondral fragment. After 7–10 days when pain, swelling, and effusion have subsided, a careful examination of the knee joint should be performed to rule out associated injuries of the cruciate ligaments, menisci, and the collateral ligaments.

Immobilization in a cylinder cast or a patella-stabilizing brace for 4 weeks with full weight-bearing will allow healing of the torn medial patellar retinaculum. Early functional rehabilitation with physiotherapy should include range of motion and strengthening exercises, proprioceptive training, and sports-specific exercises for active athletes supplemented by an individual home program. Return to stressful activities including contact sports is allowed when full range of motion and satisfactory quadriceps/vastus medialis (greater than 80% of contralateral side) strength is regained, if there is no longer a knee effusion and no sign of instability.

Operation should be considered for those with osteochondral fractures or persistent laterally subluxated patellae in spite of appropriate rehabilitation [16].

Prognosis

Primary surgical repair or autologous reconstruction of the torn MPFL, medial reefing of retinacular structures, and transposition of the patellar ligament or the oblique vastus medialis muscle do no better than conservative treatment in preventing recurrent dislocation or chronic patello-femoral instability. In a randomized controlled treatment trial in both the conservative and the early surgical realignment groups the rate of recurrent instability was reported to be 46% at 2-year follow-up. By the seventh year, there was a 22% risk of recurrent dislocation and instability episodes were reported as 40 and 45%, respectively [17]. Regression analysis defined the following risk factors for recurrence: young age, female gender, bilaterality, and osteochondral lesions. Recurrent dislocations are therefore most common in immature girls. Half of the re-dislocations occur within 2 years of the first injury [18]. Patients and parents need to be informed accordingly. Chronic post-traumatic anterior knee pain seems to be related to the degree of patello-femoral chondromalacia and warrants further assessment by MRI.

Osteochondral Fractures of the Knee

Mechanism of Injury

Shearing forces on the cartilage may cause osteochondritis dissecans or, if major and acute, a chondral or osteochondral fracture. In acute dislocations of the patella osteochondral fragments may be displaced as the patella strikes the lateral femoral condyle in relocation. Accordingly the lesions are found at the lateral trochlea or at the medial margin of the patella. The latter should be differentiated from an avulsion fracture of the medial patellar retinaculum which is extra-articular. Rarely, a direct fall on the knee or a flexion-rotation injury with major shearing forces involves the weight-bearing surface of the medial or lateral femoral condyle.

Clinical and Radiological Findings

Symptoms may be minimal and a high index of suspicion is required to prevent delayed diagnosis [19]. Clinical findings depend on the severity of the trauma, the size and origin of the fragment, and concomitant menisco-ligamentous injuries. A large osteochondral fragment leads to a significant hemarthrosis, swelling, and pain. If standard AP and skyline radiographs are not conclusive, a tunnel view better depicts the intercondylar area. Radiographs are searched for lesions at the condylar and patellar margins and for free fragments. Small pieces and those with little subchondral bone attached may go unrecognized. The differential diagnosis includes acute osteochondral fractures, impression fractures, chondral flaps, and separations as well as osteochondritis dissecans [20].

Late Presentation

The initial clinical and radiological examination may not reveal a fragment, the fragment is overlooked, or patients present much later. A history of intermittent pain on weight-bearing, mainly during sports, swelling, and transitory locking of the knee should raise suspicion of a meniscal problem or a loose body after an osteochondral fracture, the latter being more frequent during growth. Large, floating fragments are often palpable at different sites, even by the patient, and are visible on radiograph. If the diagnosis is not clear and the radiograph negative, MRI with intra-articular contrast medium (Gadolinium) helps to define the size, depth, origin, and stability of any fragment.

Treatment

Arthroscopic examination and clinical assessment of ligament stability under anesthesia give precise information about the size and origin of the fragment as well as additional injuries. Undisplaced lesions will heal with conservative treatment or, in very active young people, with temporary immobilization. In the fresh injury, fixation should be considered for vital fragments over 1 cm which consist of enough bone and arise from a weight-bearing area. Stable fixation with the implant buried beneath the cartilage can be performed with a Herbert screw, an AO mini-fragment screw, or biodegradable pins or screws inserted either arthroscopically or through a lateral or medial mini-arthrotomy [21]. Smaller fragments (under 1 cm) are removed. After several weeks or months osteochondral fragments lose their original size and shape which renders fixation difficult. Of course removal of the fragment prevents further locking and effusion of the knee. However, if there is a large crater in a weight-bearing area, a procedure to reconstruct the cartilaginous surface should be considered (e.g., osteochondral grafts and microfracturing). The value of those procedures during growth is unclear at the moment and it should be remembered that even large defects may undergo chondral regeneration with satisfactory results in children and adolescents [19].

Fractures of the Patella

Mechanism of Injury

The high proportion of shock-absorbing cartilage explains why fractures of the patella are rare in children. They either occur from a direct blow, mostly a fall on the bent knee, or a forceful contraction of the quadriceps muscle (avulsion fractures and sleeve fractures) followed by pain, swelling, and the inability to straight leg raise.

Fracture Types

The most frequent type is an osteochondral avulsion fracture of the medial border after a patella dislocation. Longitudinal fractures are usually undisplaced and in most cases only visible on an axial view. Transverse fractures and sleeve fractures (sleeve of articular cartilage, periosteum, and various amounts of bone pulled off) at the inferior or rarely at the superior pole show varying amounts of displacement due to the tension of the extensor muscles (Fig. 49.6). They correspond to a patellar tendon disruption in adults.

Sleeve fractures account for half (excluding patella dislocations) of all patella fractures and are therefore the most common during growth. This almost adolescence-specific event should be regarded as an avulsion injury and needs to be discriminated from a Sinding-Larsen–Johansson lesion. Indirect signs such as hemarthrosis, local tenderness, a palpable gap, and an unusually proximal position of the patella

(patella alta) define the injury. Radiographs may look normal if there is only a periosteal degloving without bony involvement. Ultrasound is a quick and safe way to assess periosteal and cartilaginous avulsions. If left untreated the displaced periosteum will continue to form bone and lead to apparent elongation or even duplication of the patella [22]. Avulsion may also occur from the superior and medial margins [23]. Comminuted fractures are rare. They follow a direct fall on the flexed knee and are therefore often open fractures. Transverse stress fractures occur exceptionally either in cerebral palsy and spina bifida patients or in athletes [24]. Anterior knee pain in cerebral palsy patients may also be due to chronic inferior pole fractures with subsequent irritating osseous spurs in the proximal part of the patella tendon [25]. A bipartite patella with an accessory ossicle in the superolateral quadrant should not be confused with a fracture: it is differentiated by its typical localization, its rounded margins, and its usual bilaterality.

Treatment

The pain of significant hemarthrosis is relieved by aspiration. For undisplaced fractures, 4–5 weeks in a cylinder cast with weight-bearing as tolerated is recommended. For displaced fractures the articular surface and the extensor tendon should be reconstructed and fixed by tension-band wiring to prevent osteoarthrosis; functional aftercare is helped by early passive motion [26]. In avulsion fractures the treatment depends on the severity of fragment separation and the amount of bone attached to the avulsed periosteum and cartilage. The surgeon chooses between osteochondral sutures, tension-band wiring, and more rigid types of fixation of larger bone fragments. Pole resection should be avoided [27].

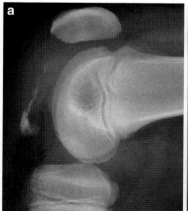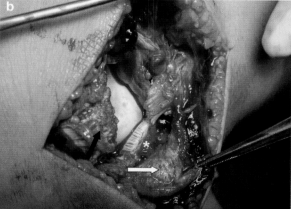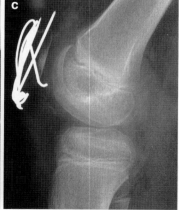

Fig. 49.6 Eleven-year-old boy who jumped from a 2-m wall and sustained a distal patellar sleeve fracture. (**a**) Lateral radiograph: high-lying patella (patella alta)—inferior pole fragments. (**b**) Open reduction: periosteal sleeve (*white arrow*) and inferior pole cartilage (asterisk) opposite cancellous bone of the main patella (*black arrow*). (**c**) Internal fixation with K-wires, tension-band wiring, and osteochondral sutures

Fractures of the Tibial Spine

Mechanism of Injury

The ACL inserts into the medial spine of the proximal tibia. No structure attaches to the lateral spine. Fractures of this tibial eminence are the most common childhood intra-articular fractures of the proximal tibia. Biomechanically they correspond to the ruptured ACL in adults. In children the tibial spine is less resistant to tensile stress than the ACL. However, prior to avulsion of the tibial spine, the ACL stretches due to sequential failure of ligament fibers [28]. A fall from a bicycle with a direct blow on the distal femur with the knee flexed is the most frequently cited cause of injury, followed by hyperextension/rotation trauma sustained during athletic activities (e.g., football or alpine skiing).

Clinical and Radiological Findings

Patients usually present with a painful hemarthrosis and inability to bear weight. Clinically they show a pathological Lachman and anterior drawer test. According to Meyers and McKeevers [29] fractures of the intercondylar eminence can be classified radiologically on a standard lateral view as type I (undisplaced), II (partially displaced, anterior gap but preserved posterior hinge), or III (fully displaced). Zaricznyj [30] suggested an additional type IV for comminuted fractures. Their relative frequency is about 12% (type I), 44% (type II), and 44% (type III) [31–33]. When the physis is still wide open, the whole eminence is avulsed; when it is partially closed, only one of the tubercles may be avulsed. The fragment is usually a single piece with varying amounts of subchondral bone attached, but it may be purely cartilaginous or comminuted. As the fracture often runs through the subchondral plate, the fragment size is easily underestimated on radiograph or even invisible if cartilaginous. Associated injuries to the medial collateral ligament and the menisci (lateral more often than medial) occur mainly with type III fractures but are rare [34]. Arthroscopy may reveal associated injuries, but there seems to be some potential for spontaneous healing as it is rare for non-arthroscoped patients to need secondary operation [35].

Treatment

A painful hemarthrosis is aspirated under sterile conditions. Type I lesions should be immobilized in a cylinder cast for 4 weeks. For type II fractures, closed reduction should be attempted by extending the knee and applying a cylinder cast. Anatomy studies have shown that ACL tension in extension does not prevent fracture reduction [36]. For the failed type II and III lesions, arthroscopic or open reduction is recommended. An interposed meniscal anterior horn and the transverse meniscal ligament are the commonest blocks to reduction and are more likely if the fragment is large. The displaced fragment may be fixed with a trans-epiphyseal suture, wire, wire suture, or crossed retrograde trans-physeal wire according to the surgeon's preference (Fig. 49.7) [31, 37]. The fragment should be anatomically reduced or even countersunk to compensate for the plastic ACL elongation.

Prognosis

A trans-epiphyseal screw may cause a partial growth arrest of the proximal tibial physis [38]. Despite consolidation of the fracture in an anatomical position, chronic anterior instability and loss of full extension are the most frequently reported long-term problems. In 38–70% of patients with a type II or III injury, there was objective evidence (Lachman test, KT 1000 arthrometer) of anterior cruciate laxity. However, only few have subjective complaints if the secondary restraints remain intact [32, 33, 39–41]. It is possible that post-traumatic overgrowth of the tibial spine helps to prevent instability. Obviously the ACL remains elongated with further growth and anatomical reduction does not necessarily prevent ACL laxity. Accordingly, the results of open and closed treatment are similar, provided the fragment consolidates anatomically. Knee laxity does not lead to functional impairment if there is no gross pivot shift. It remains to be seen how functional status and secondary meniscal and osteochondral pathology develop in the long term in post-traumatic lax knees. For the late-presenting patient with a non-united tibial spine associated with pain, giving way, or locking, fixation may still prove successful [42]. Lost extension caused by malunion warrants anatomic fixation if conservative treatment has failed.

Ruptures of the Anterior Cruciate Ligament

Ruptures of the ACL in skeletally immature patients are rare but have become more frequently recognized and reported. The mechanisms of injury are identical to those seen in adults. The site of failure is most commonly at the tibial insertion. Skeletally immature patients with ACL injuries have a narrower intercondylar notch than those with avulsion fractures of the tibial spine [43]. Most patients are male and keen sportsmen involved in contact sport. Thus, they are usually reluctant to consider long periods

Fig. 49.7 Thirteen-year-old boy with a type III avulsion fracture of the ACL. (**a**) Lateral radiograph not conclusive in differentiating between incomplete (type II) and complete (type III) avulsion. (**b**) CT reveals full displacement. (**c** and **d**) Anatomic reduction and wire fixation [28]. Courtesy of Dr. Klaus Parsch, Stuttgart

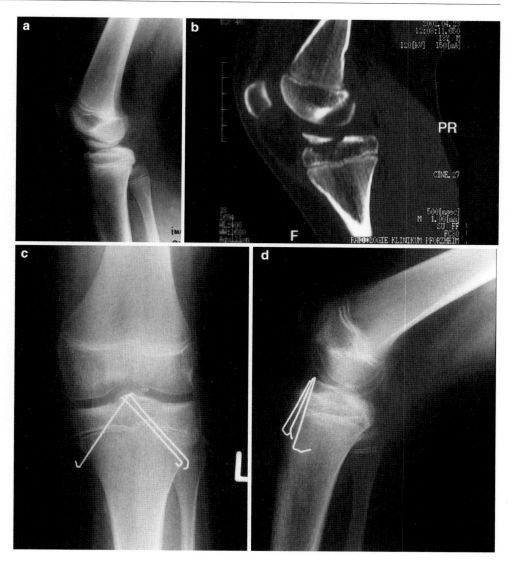

of conservative treatments with physiotherapy, rehabilitation, bracing, and activity modification; they worry about the unpredictable outcome. In addition ACL ruptures during growth are not benign: the natural history is of giving way, pain, and swelling; furthermore, persistent instability may cause meniscal or osteochondral damage.

Treatment

Children generally are highly active and are significantly impaired by ACL rupture. Conservative treatment, direct repair, and extra-articular reconstruction have poor outcomes. Intra-articular reconstruction should be considered when instability prevents participation in sport, conservative treatment has not helped, or if there are associated meniscal or osteochondral injuries [44]. The likelihood of associated meniscal injuries makes primary operative treatment an early

option for many [45, 46]. The gold standard technique of ACL reconstruction in adults, the central one-third bone-patellar-bone graft, may be used in adolescents with only little growth left [47, 48]. Intra-articular reconstruction with a low risk of a growth disturbance is possible if the physis is not damaged [49] or if reconstruction utilizes a soft tissue graft only (e.g., semitendinosus, gracilis, or quadriceps tendon) and is performed through a small diameter tibial drill hole combined with an over-the-top position of the femoral graft. Holes should be drilled perpendicular to the femoral physis or with a physeal-sparing technique (Fig. 49.8) [45].

Prognosis

In patients with an open physis, harvesting of the graft as well as the drill holes may injure the tibial and/or femoral physis with subsequent risk of growth disturbances [50].

Fig. 49.8 Fifteen-year-old soccer player 1 year after arthroscopically assisted replacement of the ACL by a quadriceps tendon graft. The graft fills a trans-epiphyseal tibial drill hole and a physeal-sparing distal femoral canal

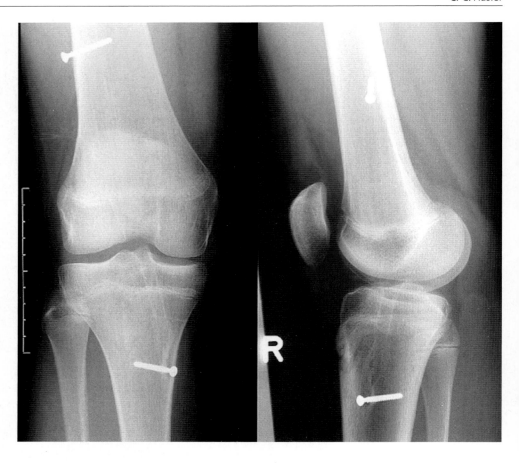

The close anatomic relation of the posterior distal femoral physis and the perichondral ring to the ACL origin has to be considered [51]. Regular review until the end of growth is necessary to detect any axial deviation or leg length discrepancies. Objective and subjective knee stability and re-rupture rates after ACL reconstruction are poorer in children than in adults. This may be attributable to ligamentous laxity during growth and more vigorous sports activities. However, long-term results of knee stability, meniscal degeneration, osteochondral problems, and development of osteoarthritis have so far not been reported.

Intra-articular Physeal Fractures of the Proximal Tibia

Salter–Harris type III, IV and transitional fractures are even rarer than those at the distal femur and, when they do occur, do so in late adolescence. Fracture patterns and treatment are basically the same as for distal intra-articular femoral fractures. Special attention should be paid to associated ligamentous injuries to prevent later instability, osteochondral injuries, as well as meniscal entrapment in the fracture

Fig. 49.9 Fifteen-year-old boy: 20° lack of extension and knee effusion after valgus right knee injury in a fall from a bicycle. (**a**) AP view: possible tibial plateau fracture. (**b**) Repeat radiograph in internal rotation: clear fracture gap. Knee arthroscopy showed meniscus trapped in the gap

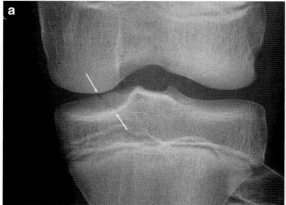
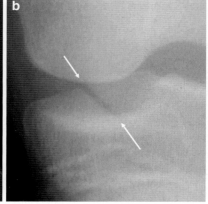

(Fig. 49.9). Arthroscopy helps to assess and fix these fractures.

Avulsion of the Tibial Tuberosity

Mechanism of Injury

This fracture—bony avulsion of the patellar ligament (or tendon), insertion—occurs mainly in adolescent athletes, after either acute forceful contraction of the quadriceps muscle or with acute knee flexion against the contracted quadriceps (e.g., landing after a jump). An association with pre-existing Osgood–Schlatter disease is possible [52]. Bilateral occurrence is reported [53]. Growth disturbances are rare, but in younger patients a genu recurvatum may develop after premature growth arrest [54].

Clinical and Radiological Findings

Patients present with marked pain and a local hematoma over the tuberosity. They are often unable to straight leg raise, to stand, or walk. A high-riding patella is seen with severe displacement and a joint effusion with intra-articular fractures. Severe pain over the anterior lower leg may indicate a compartment syndrome in displaced intra-articular fractures. A lateral radiograph confirms the suspected diagnosis and demonstrates any intra-articular involvement, the size, and displacement of the fragment (which is often much larger than the film suggests). The avulsion fractures of the tibial tuberosity are either extra- or intra-articular (Salter–Harris type III) (Fig. 49.10). The former are regarded as displaced if the tuberosity is elevated more than 5 mm; the latter, as with all intra-articular fractures, if there is a dehiscence or step-off of more than 2 mm. Sleeve avulsion fractures of the patella are well recognized; a similar morphology has been described for the proximal tibia [55]: It is important to be aware of the injury as the patella tendon disrupts with its apophyseal attachment and a sleeve of periosteum. Both may be free of bone and therefore overlooked on the radiograph. The combination of a high-riding patella and local swelling and pain is suspicious. Ultrasound or MRI is the diagnostic investigation of choice. There may be associated injuries like patellar and quadriceps avulsions, meniscal tears, tibial plateau rim fractures, and ligamentous injuries.

Treatment

Undisplaced fracture receives conservative treatment in a cylinder cast for 5–6 weeks. Displaced fractures are treated by open reduction and internal fixation with lag screws performed through a midline vertical incision lateral or medial to the tuberosity (Fig. 49.10). Sometimes an interposed periosteal flap is found under the avulsed fragment. Once this is pulled out, anatomical reduction and fixation of the fragment is easy when the knee is extended. At the end the torn periosteum is sutured over the fracture site. For the isolated bony lesion aftercare is cast free with partial weight-bearing for 6 weeks. If the lesion is an avulsion of the soft tissues (periosteum, patellar ligament) a cylinder cast for 6 weeks provides healing. Consolidation at 6 weeks is confirmed by radiograph. Patients should be followed-up until skeletal maturity.

Epiphysiolysis at the Proximal Tibia

Mechanism of Injury

Separation of the proximal tibial epiphysis (Salter–Harris type I and II fractures) is extremely rare. The tibial tuberosity is part of the proximal tibial epiphysis and will therefore dislocate. The mechanism of injury is an indirect valgus force. Forceful hyperextension with severe anterior displacement of the epiphysis puts the popliteal vessels at risk.

Clinical and Radiological Findings

Signs of circulatory or neurological impairment (peroneal nerve) should be looked for carefully. Undisplaced fractures, mainly simple Salter–Harris type I, may be overlooked if indirect clinical and radiological signs are not considered: pain and swelling over the proximal tibia, an associated fracture of the proximal fibula, and callus formation at the proximal tibia after 4–6 weeks. On the initial radiograph, the angle between the epiphysis and the diaphysis of the tibia should be measured to avoid missing any frontal plane angulation as remodeling is poor.

Treatment

Undisplaced fractures are treated in a long leg plaster cast. Displaced fractures are reduced under anesthesia. The primary goal is to correct any malrotation and angulation in the frontal plane. Only rarely is open reduction necessary and then mainly when soft tissue such as the pes anserinus or periosteum is interposed [56]. Closed or open reduction is stabilized by percutaneous crossed Kirschner-wire pinning and immobilization in a long leg cast for 4–5 weeks.

Radiological follow-up after 8–10 days is recommended; any secondary displacement of up to 20° may be corrected

Fig. 49.10 Fourteen-year-old
boy: displaced avulsion fracture
of tibial tuberosity with extension
into the joint. Anatomic open
reduction and internal fixation
with two cancellous lag screws.
AP (a) and lateral (b) radiographs
prior to fixation and after
fixations (c) and (d)

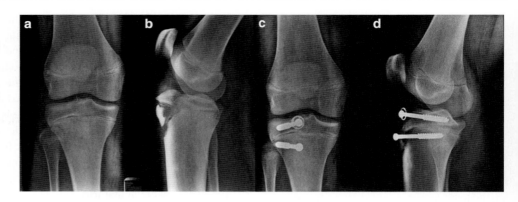

by simple cast wedging. Clinical and radiological review to
assess alignment and length should continue 6 monthly for 2
years.

Growth Disturbances

Transient stimulation of the proximal tibial physis with consecutive slight overgrowth of the tibia is the rule but of minor
clinical significance. Total or partial growth arrest is rare but
may follow even simple Salter–Harris type I or II fractures
[57]. It is related to the primary injury and is not preventable:
the risk should be discussed with the family before treatment.

Torus Fractures

The compression fractures show no displacement or angulation. They can be treated by immobilization in a long
leg plaster for 4–5 weeks. As they are stable, secondary
angulation is not a risk. After cast removal consolidation is
confirmed clinically by absence of local tenderness. Serial
review is unnecessary since growth disturbances do not occur
[58].

Bending Fractures of the Proximal Tibia

Mechanism of Injury and Complications

Forces acting upon the lateral aspect of the proximal tibia
may either result in a complete metaphyseal fracture of the
tibia and fibula or in a partial fracture of the medial cortex of
the proximal tibia with or without fibula fracture (greenstick
fracture).

The inherent risk of a progressive valgus deformity was
first described by Cozen in 1953 [59]. There are two theories
to explain post-traumatic valgus deformity:

- Mechanical reasons: entrapment of soft tissues in the
  fracture gap (periosteum, medial collateral ligament, and
  the pes anserinus) and loss of medial tethering by avulsion of pes anserinus in combination with ongoing lateral
  tethering of the intact fibula.
- Asymmetric growth: lack of compression on the fractured
  medial cortex independent of any interposition leads to
  a delayed union, a well-known phenomenon in greenstick fractures. The associated and persistent increased
  local blood supply stimulates the adjacent proximal tibial growth asymmetrically as demonstrated by bone scans
  [60].

Treatment

Parents must be warned that asymmetric growth may follow
this fracture.

Two important and easy steps may prevent the post-
traumatic valgus deformity:

1. Recognize even minor valgus deformity on the initial
   radiograph.
2. Compress the fracture gap at the medial cortex: Under
   general anesthesia an above-knee cast is applied with the
   knee in extension and stressed into varus. Patients should
   be warned further that the cast may slip with the knee
   extended; after 8 days the cast is wedged. The lateral half
   of the cast is cut transversely at the level of the fracture
   and opened with a cast spreader; a spacer is placed into the
   gap and the cast is completed. This wedging compresses
   the medially fractured cortex. If the fracture gap can be
   fully closed valgus deformity can be avoided, while the

tibia will be 5–10 mm longer. Only 4 weeks in plaster is needed. The child should be reviewed for 2 years to detect possible valgus deformity.

If these rules of treatment are not followed significant valgus deformity commonly develops within 1 year of injury (Fig. 49.11) [61]. In children below 5–6 years at injury, the tibia remodels to an S-shaped "serpentine" tibia (proximal tibia in valgus—distal tibia in varus—knee and ankle joint lines parallel) and over the years may grow almost straight [62, 63]. As an alternative to early osteotomy with its inherent risk of deformity recurrence or "wait and see" nihilism in expectation of spontaneous remodeling, hemiepiphysiodesis of the proximal tibia deferred for at least a year after trauma effectively and safely leads to correction within 1 year [64]. Mild rebound valgus deformity after removal occurs in 25% but responds well to re-stapling. The unpredictable further growth and remodeling make it important to review the fracture until skeletal maturity as angular deformity

and tibial overgrowth of up to 10 mm are common (See Chapter 29).

Stress Fractures of the Tibia

Pain with weight-bearing (but little night pain) in the absence of trauma, an insidious onset, local tenderness at the proximal tibia in a 10–15-year-old child should make the surgeon suspect a stress fracture. The symptoms may be bilateral. Radiographs may initially be normal, but periosteal reaction and cortical radiolucency at the fracture are visible 2–3 weeks later. A technetium bone scan or an MRI allows early diagnosis. The patient is usually a young athlete, typically a long-distance runner, or has recently changed activity patterns. In girls, one should be alert to the triad of disordered eating, amenorrhea, and osteoporosis. Questions should focus on eating and training habits as well as concomitant symptoms like fatigue, loss of concentration, and cold intolerance.

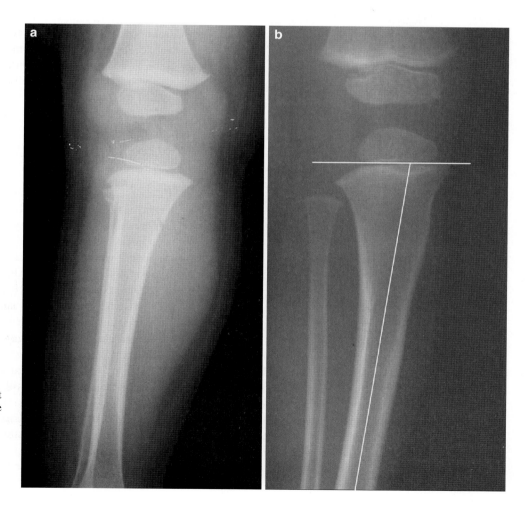

Fig. 49.11 Eighteen-month-old girl with bending fracture of right proximal tibia. (**a**) Bending of the lateral cortex, complete fracture of the medial cortex but no obvious valgus deformity at injury. (**b**) One year later, 12° valgus deformity has developed slowly

Treatment of a stress fracture consists of activity modification, or, if difficult to achieve, a long leg plaster for 3–4 weeks. Preventing recurrence should involve examining the psychosocial environment; liaising with trainers, parents, and teachers; and trying to address all underlying issues such as training hours and intensity, equipment usage, and the pressures placed on the young athlete. When osteoporosis occurs, a team approach with endocrinologist, psychologist, etc., is essential (See Chapter 8).

Diaphyseal Fractures of the Lower Leg

The treatment and prognosis of diaphyseal fractures of the lower leg depend on the bones involved. One should distinguish between tibial fractures with and without an intact fibula: the ratio is about 2:1. Isolated fractures of the fibula are rare and usually due to direct trauma.

Clinical and Radiological Findings

Mild to severe pain and swelling at the fracture site lead to a straightforward clinical diagnosis. With obvious severe deformity which clearly needs reduction, a single radiograph is sufficient to avoid unnecessary positioning in the radiology department. Although disruption of the posterior tibial artery is rare in children with closed fractures, both dorsalis pedis and posterior tibial pulses should be checked clinically and, if absent, by Doppler examination. Unusual severe pain may be the first sign of a compartment syndrome particularly after direct, high-impact, and rollover trauma in adolescents.

Isolated Tibial Fractures

Mechanism of Injury, Fracture Pattern, and Remodeling Capacity

Isolated tibial fractures are the commonest lower limb fracture. They follow indirect rotational forces. They are usually long oblique or spiral fractures at the junction between the middle and the distal thirds, starting anteromedially distally and spiraling up to the proximal postero-lateral cortex. They are seen most often in children below 10 years. Incomplete torus or greenstick fractures account for only about 10% of all tibial fractures. As they are stable they can always be treated conservatively by simple plastering with subsequent wedging to correct minor angular deformities.

In the isolated complete tibial fracture the intact fibula prevents significant shortening, but leads to lateral splinting: While initial tibial angulation rarely exceeds 10°, the more medially directed forces of the posterior flexor muscles cause progressive varus deformity of the tibia in 50%. This usually occurs within 2–3 weeks of injury [65]. Subsequent remodeling is age-dependent: Below 10 years, varus deformities of 10–15° reliably correct themselves. In older children the remodeling capacity is smaller and less predictable. The sagittal plane is the main plane of motion of the adjacent joints. Spontaneous remodeling of up to 20° of recurvatum can be expected in patients younger than 8 years. Procurvatum of the tibia is rare. Rotational deformities (usually external rotation) will persist [66]. They are cosmetically disturbing and, as they are not fully compensated at the knee and ankle, may cause functional impairment if they exceed 10°.

The more pronounced the deformity at consolidation, the longer the remodeling process, and prolonged stimulation of the tibial physis leads to tibial overgrowth of 0.5–1 cm in children under 10 years. In older patients the physis may close prematurely and even result in slight shortening. In summary most initial deformities in the sagittal and frontal plane remodel with time. Nevertheless, one should not accept them if post-traumatic leg length differences are to be avoided [67]. Furthermore, deformities of the tibia are easily visible and cosmetically disturbing due to the lack of medial musculature.

Treatment

Casting is the mainstay of treatment for isolated diaphyseal tibial fractures in children. Even if closed reduction under anesthesia is necessary, the long leg cast can usually be applied as an outpatient. The bimalleolar axis should be compared with the uninjured leg to ensure correct axis and rotation regardless of age. Alignment of the fracture should be monitored 1 week later. If the cast needs to be wedged to correct angulation, this is best performed 8–10 days after injury when the patient is pain free, swelling has subsided, and there is already some fibrous callus (Fig. 49.12). Technically an *open* wedging technique (as described above) is easier, avoids pinching the skin, and carries less risk of increasing compartment pressure:

- Undisplaced or slightly displaced fractures: initially split long leg cast, completed after 4 days and changed 2 weeks after trauma.
- Displaced fractures: closed reduction and posterior long leg split cast which is closed after 4 days. Wedge if greater than 10° deformity at radiological follow-up after 1 week.

Fig. 49.12 Isolated diaphyseal tibial fracture; secondary varus deformity corrected by simple wedging 10 days later

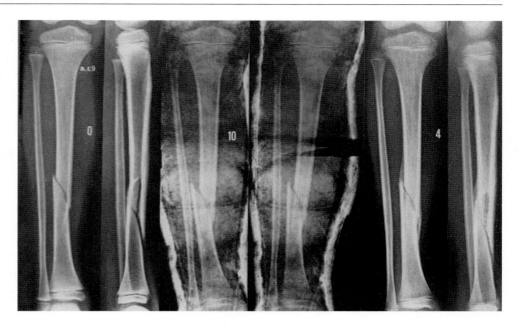

In older children or adolescents with undisplaced fractures a patellar tendon-bearing cast (Sarmiento cast) may be an alternative to allow immediate full weight-bearing [68]. The plaster is removed after 4–5 weeks but re-applied for a further 2–3 weeks if the fracture site is still tender.

- Completely displaced and therefore unstable transverse fractures of the tibia as well as open fractures, patients at risk for a compartment syndrome or poly-traumatized children should be stabilized by intramedullary elastic stable nails [69] or external fixation [70]. Both minimally invasive methods offer short operation times, minimal blood loss, aesthetic scars, preservation of a biologic environment around the fracture site, early mobilization, a low complication rate, and easy metal ware removal. External fixation should be reserved for highly comminuted and/or high-degree open fractures.

Diaphyseal Fractures of Tibia and Fibula

Mechanism of Injury—Remodeling Capacity

These are usually the result of direct trauma to the lower leg (e.g., pedestrian versus car). In contrast to isolated tibial fractures, the muscles of the anterior compartment act as lateral flexors leading to valgus deformity. Spontaneous remodeling should *not* be expected for valgus deformities which should be prevented by proper monitoring during treatment.

Treatment

Basically, stable fractures should be treated conservatively by cast and additional wedging whereas unstable fractures should be stabilized by elastic intramedullary nails or, if these are not available, by external fixation:

- Stable fractures (greenstick fractures, transverse fractures with angulation): after closed reduction split long leg cast which is closed after 4 days. Wedging or new long leg cast if angular deformity at radiological follow-up after 10 days. Non-weight-bearing for 4 weeks followed by a walking cast for another 2 weeks until radiographic consolidation.
- Unstable fractures (fully displaced fractures, oblique fractures with shortening) and polytrauma (Fig. 49.13): stabilization with antegrade descending elastic intramedullary nails or an anteromedial monolateral external fixator [69, 70]. In highly comminuted fractures in adolescents with open growth plates, ring fixation may be a better choice than monolateral fixation which has a significant rate of lost reduction, leading to malunion if not re-manipulated [70].

Prognosis

After open fractures union is usually delayed in younger patients. Patients over 14 years, following both open and closed fractures, show a substantially delayed healing after elastic stable intramedullary nailing (ESIN) [71].

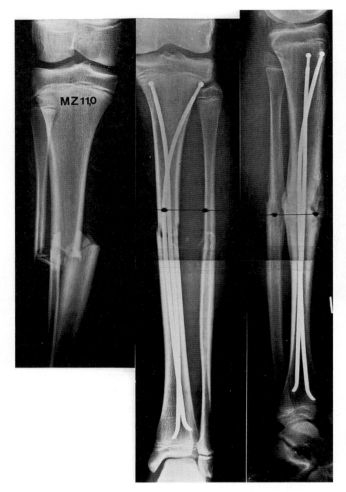

Fig. 49.13 Eleven-year-old boy: unstable diaphyseal fracture of his right tibia and fibula stabilized by antegrade intramedullary flexible nailing. Courtesy of Dr. Klaus Parsch, Stuttgart

Severe direct impacts, butterfly fragments, age-related borderline indications for ESIN (upper limit at closure of the physis), or technical errors may underlie delayed consolidation or malalignment. The technical principles which need to be considered include adequate nail diameter (usually 2.5–3.5 mm), identical nail diameters, and symmetric prebending of the nails with the maximal curve at the fracture site. Since the tibia is triangular in shape, anatomical stabilization may make it necessary to rotate the nails, sometimes both into valgus if the fibula is intact or vice versa in complete lower leg fractures to counteract the deforming varus forces (isolated tibial facture) or valgus forces (fracture of both tibia and fibula) [72]. Pseudarthrosis after pediatric shaft fractures of the tibia is extremely rare and seen only after high-energy open trauma with or without subsequent osteomyelitis or open reduction followed by unstable fixation [73].

Metaphyseal Fractures of the Distal Tibia

As in the proximal tibia, a variety of injury patterns affect the distal metaphysis. Most fractures are incomplete, leaving at least one cortex intact or both impacted.

Torus and Greenstick Fractures

Simple torus fractures (Fig. 49.14) show some recurvatum but no angulation in the frontal plane. True greenstick fractures with impaction of the anterior border and complete fracture of the posterior cortex result in a slight recurvatum. The latter may increase if the deformity is not controlled by applying a below-knee plaster in ankle *plantar flexion* to compress the posterior fracture site. Recurvatum may be combined with valgus deformity and procurvatum with varus [74]. Four weeks in plaster is usually sufficient and bone healing is usually uneventful.

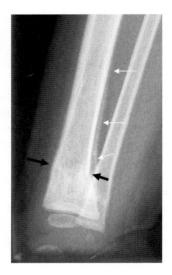

Fig. 49.14 Three-year-old girl with torus fracture (*black arrows*) of her left distal tibia presenting with a history of limping over 4 weeks. Radiographs revealed an old fracture with periosteal reaction along the posterior border of the tibia (*white arrows*). No further action was required

Bending Fractures

Distal bending fractures pose the same problems as those at the proximal tibia, although the subtalar joint may compensate for some mild deformities in the frontal plane. In patients older than 10 years, every malangulation in the frontal plane should be corrected; if not, asymmetric growth stimulation leads to progressive and persistent deformity. In younger patients, spontaneous correction of up to 20° valgus, varus, and recurvatum may be expected. Procurvatum is rare. A below-knee plaster is applied for 4 weeks.

Toddlers' Fractures

These fractures occur in children under 2 years by external rotation of the foot. This causes minimally displaced, short spiral or oblique fractures without fibular involvement. These "toddler fractures" may not be recognized on the initial radiograph but will be discovered at follow-up. It is important that they be considered in the differential diagnosis of limping in otherwise healthy toddlers. Immobilization in a long leg cast for 2–3 weeks sometimes followed by a below-knee cast for 2 weeks is sufficient.

References

1. Sponseller PD, Stanitski CL. Fractures and dislocations about the knee. In: Beaty JH, Kasser JR, eds. Rockwood & Wilkins' Fractures in Children, 5th ed. Philadelphia: Lippincott-Williams & Wilkins; 2001:981–1076.
2. Riseborough EJ, Barrett IR, Shapiro F. Growth disturbances following distal femoral physeal fracture-separations. J Bone Joint Surg Am 1983; 65:885–893.
3. Edmunds I, Nade S. Injuries of the distal femoral growth plate and epiphysis: should open reduction be performed? Aus NZ J Surg 1993; 63:195–199.
4. Lombardo SJ, Harvey JP. Fractures of the distal femoral epiphyses. J Bone Joint Surg Am 1977; 59:742–751.
5. Beaty JH, Kumar A. Fractures about the knee in children. Current concept review. J Bone Joint Surg Am 1994; 76:1870–1880.
6. Czitrom AA, Salter RB, Willis RB. Fractures involving the distal epiphyseal plate of the femur. Int Orthop 1981; 4:269–277.
7. Beck A, Kinzl L, Rüter A, Strecker W. Fractures involving the distal femoral epiphysis. Long-term outcome after completion of growth in primary surgical management. Unfallchirurg 2001; 104:611–616.
8. Eid AM, Hafez MA. Traumatic injuries of the distal femoral physis. Retrospective study on 151 cases. Injury 2002; 33:251–255.
9. Ilharreborde B, Raquillet C, Morel E, et al. Long-term prognosis of Salter-Harris type 2 injuries of the distal femoral physis. J Pediatr Orthop B 2006; 15:433–438.
10. Arkader A, Warner WC Jr, Horn BD, et al. Predicting the outcome of physeal fractures of the distal femur. J Pediatr Orthop 2007; 27:703–708.
11. Stephens DC, Louis E, Louis DS. Traumatic separation of the distal femoral epiphyseal cartilage plate. J Bone Joint Surg Am 1974; 56:1383–1390.
12. Nietos N, Nietosvaara Y, Aalto K, Kallio PE. Acute patellar dislocation in children: Incidence and associated osteochondral fractures. J Pediatr Orthop 1994; 14:513–515.
13. Zaidi A, Babyn P, Astori I, et al. MRI of traumatic patellar dislocation in children. Pediatr Radiol 2006; 36:1163–1170.
14. Nietosvaara Y. The femoral sulcus in children. An ultrasonographic study. J Bone Joint Surg Br 1994; 76:807–809.
15. Yamada Y, Toritsuka Y, Yoshikawa H, et al. Morphological analysis of the femoral trochlea in patients with recurrent dislocation of the patella using three-dimensional computer models. J Bone Joint Surg Br 2007; 89:746–751.
16. Stefancin JJ, Parker RD. First-time traumatic patellar dislocation. Clin Orthop Rel Res 2007; 455:93–101.
17. Nikku R, Nietosvaara Y, Aalto K, Kallio PE. Operative treatment of primary patellar dislocation does not improve medium-term outcome: A 7-year follow-up report and risk analysis of 127 randomized patients. Acta Orthop 2005; 76:699–704.
18. Palmu S, Kallio P, Donell ST, et al. Acute patellar dislocation in children and adolescents: a randomized clinical trial. J Bone Joint Surg Am 2008; 90:463–470.
19. Schillians N, Baltzer AWA, Liebau CH, et al. Osteochondrale Abscherfrakturen bei Kindern. Zentralbl Chir 2001; 126:233–236.
20. Bradley J, Dandy DJ. Osteochondritis dissecans and other lesions of the femoral condyles. J Bone Joint Surg Br 1989; 71:518–522.
21. Dines JS, Fealy S, Potter HG, et al. Outcomes of osteochondral lesions of the knee repaired with a bioabsorbable device. Arthroscopy 2008; 24:62–68.
22. Hunt DM, Somashekar N. A review of sleeve fractures of the patella in children. Knee 2005; 12:3–7.
23. Grogan DP, Carey TP, Leffers D, et al. Avulsion fractures of the patella. J Pediatr Orthop 1990; 10:721–730.
24. Brunner R, Doederlein L. Pathological fractures in patients with cerebral palsy. J Pediatr Orthop 1996; 5:232–238.
25. Senaran H, Holden C, Dabney KW, et al. Anterior knee pain in children with cerebral palsy. J Pediatr Orthop 2007; 27:12–16.
26. Maguire JK, Canale ST. Fractures of the patella in children and adolescents. J Pediatr Orthop 1993; 13:567–571.
27. Kastelec M, Veselko M. Inferior patellar pole avulsion fractures: osteosynthesis compared with pole resection. J Bone Joint Surg Am 2004; 86:696–701.
28. Noyes FR, Delucas JL, Torvik PJ. Biomechanics of anterior cruciate ligament failure: an analysis of strain-rate sensitivity and mechanisms of failure in primates. J Bone Joint Surg 1974; 56-A:236–253.
29. Meyers MH, McKeever FM. Fracture of the intercondylar eminence of the tibia. J Bone Joint Surg 1959; 41-A:209–220.
30. Zaricznyj B. Avulsion fracture of the tibial eminence: treatment by open reduction and pinning. J Bone Joint Surg Am 1977; 59:1111–1114.
31. Grönkvist H, Hirsch G, Johansson L. Fracture of the anterior tibial spine in children. J Pediatr Orthop 1984; 4:465–468.
32. Janarv PM, Westblad P, Johansson C, et al. Long-Term Follow-up of anterior tibial spine fractures in children. J Pediatr Orthop 1995; 15:63–68.
33. Willis RB, Blokker C, Stoll TM, et al. Long-term follow-up of anterior tibial eminence fractures. J Pediatr Orthop 1993; 13:361–364.
34. Ishibashi Y, Tsuda E, Sasaki T, et al. Magnetic resonance imaging aids in detecting concomitant injuries in patients with tibial spine fractures. Clin Orthop Rel Res 2005; 434:207–212.
35. Molander ML, Wallin G, Wikstad I. Fracture of the intercondylar eminence of the tibia. J Bone Joint Surg Br 1981; 63:89–91.
36. Hallam PJB, Fazal MA, Ashwood N, et al. An alternative to fixation of displaced fractures of the anterior intercondylar eminence in children. J Bone Joint Surg 2002; 84-B:579–582.
37. Mauch F, Parsch K. Internal fixation of intercondylar eminence avulsion in children. Operat Orthop Traumatol 2004; 16:418–432.
38. Mylle J, Reynders P, Broos P. Transepiphyseal fixation of anterior cruciate avulsion in a child. Report of a complication and review of the literature. Arch Orthop Trauma Surg 1993; 112:101–103.

39. Baxter MP, Wiley JJ. Fractures of the tibial spine in children. An evaluation of knee stability. J Bone Joint Surg 1988; 70-B:228–230.

40. Kocher MS, Foreman ES, Micheli LJ. Laxity and functional outcome after arthroscopic reduction and internal fixation of displaced tibial spine fracture in children. Arthroscopy 2003; 19:1085–1090.

41. Smith JB. Knee instability after fractures of the intercondylar eminence of the tibia. J Pediatric Orthop 1984; 4:462–464.

42. Kawate K, Fujisawa Y, Yajima H, et al. Seventeen-year follow-up of a reattachment of a nonunited anterior tibial spine avulsion fracture. Arthroscopy 2005; 21:760.

43. Kocher MS, Mandiga R, Klingele K, et al. Anterior cruciate ligament injury versus tibial spine fracture in the skeletally immature knee: a comparison of skeletal maturation and notch width index. J Pediatr Orthop 2004; 24:185–188.

44. Janarv PM, Nyström A, Werner S, Hirsch G. Anterior cruciate ligament injuries in skeletally immature patients. J Pediatr Orthop 1996; 16:673–677.

45. Aichroth PM, Patel DV, Zorilla P. The natural history and treatment of rupture of the anterior cruciate ligament in children and adolescents. J Bone Joint Surg Br 2002; 84:38–41.

46. Arbes St, Resinger C, Vécsei V, et al. The functional outcome of total tears of the anterior cruciate ligament (ACL) in the skeletally immature patient. Int Orthop 2007; 31:471–475.

47. Kannus P, Järvinen M. Knee ligament injuries in adolescents. J Bone Joint Surg Br 1988; 70:772–776.

48. McCarroll JR, Shelbourne KD, Porter DA, et al. Patellar tendon graft reconstruction for midsubstance anterior cruciate ligament rupture in junior high school athletes. Am J Sports Med 1994; 22:478–484.

49. Nakhostine M, Bollen SR, Cross MJ. Reconstruction of midsubstance anterior cruciate rupture in adolescents with open physis. J Pediatr Orthop 1995; 15:286–287.

50. Kocher MS, Saxon HS, Hovis WD, et al. Management and complications of anterior cruciate ligament injuries in skeletally immature patients: a survey of the Herodicus Society and The ACL Study group. J Pediatr Orthop 2002; 22:452–457.

51. Kocher MS, Hovis WD, Curtin MJ, et al. Anterior cruciate ligament reconstruction in skeletally immature knees: an anatomical study. Am J Orthop 2005; 34:285–290.

52. Ogden JA, Tross RB, Murphy MJ. Fractures of the tibial tuberosity in adolescents. J Bone Joint Surg Am 1980; 62:205–215.

53. Neugebauer A, Muensterer OJ, Buehligen U, Till H. Bilateral avulsion fractures of the tibial tuberosity: a double case for open reduction and fixation. Eur J Trauma Emerg Surg 2008; 34:83–87.

54. Christie MJ, Dvonch VM. Tibial tuberosity avulsion fracture in adolescents. J Pediatr Orthop 1981; 1:391–394.

55. Davidson D, Letts M. Partial sleeve fractures of the tibia in children: an unusual fracture pattern. J Pediatr Orthop 2002; 22:36–40.

56. Harries TJ, Lichtmann DM, Lonon WD. Irreducible Salter Harris II fracture of the proximal tibia. J Pediatr Orthop 1983; 3:92–95.

57. Burkhart SS, Peterson HA. Fractures of the proximal tibial epiphysis. J Bone Joint Surg Am 1979; 61:996–1002.

58. Von Laer L, Jani L, Cuny T, et al. The proximal fracture of the lower leg in adolescence. Cause and prophylaxis of the posttraumatic genu valgum. Unfallheilkunde 1982; 85:215–225.

59. Cozen L. Fracture of proximal portion of tibia in children followed by valgus deformity. Surg Gyn Obstet 1953; 97:183–188.

60. Zionts LE, Harcke HAT, Brooks KM, et al. Post-traumatic tibia valga: a case demonstrating asymmetric activity at the proximal growth plate on technetium bone scan. J Pediatr Orthop 1977; 7:458–462.

61. Parsch K, Manner G, Dippe K. Genu valgum nach proximaler Tibiafraktur beim Kind. Arch Orthop Unfall-Chir 1977; 90:289–297.

62. Brammar TJ, Rooker GD. Remodeling of valgus deformity secondary to proximal metaphyseal fracture of the tibia. Injury 1998; 29:558–560.

63. Tuten R, Keeler KA, Gabos PG, et al. Posttraumatic tibia valga in children. A long-term follow-up note. J Bone Joint Surg Am 1999; 81:799–810.

64. Stevens PM, Pease F. Hemiepiphysiodesis for posttraumatic tibial valgus. J Pediatr Orthop 2006; 26:385–392.

65. Teitz CC, Carter DR, Frankel VH. Problems associated with tibial fractures with intact fibulae. J Bone Joint Surg Am 1980; 62:770–776.

66. Shannak AO. Tibial fractures in children: a follow-up study. J Pediatr Orthop 1988; 8:306–310.

67. Von Laer L, Kaelin L, Girard T. Late results following shaft fractures of the lower extremities in the growth period. Z Unfallchir Versicherungsmed Berufskr 1989; 82:209–215.

68. Austin RT. The Sarmiento tibial plaster: a prospective study of 145 fractures. Injury 1981; 13:10–22.

69. Ligier JN, Metaizeau JP, Prevot J, et al. Elastic stable intramedullary nailing of femoral shaft fractures in children. J Bone Joint Surg Br 1988; 70:74–77.

70. Gordon JE, Schoenecker PL, Oda JE, et al. A comparison of monolateral and circular external fixation of unstable diaphyseal tibial fractures in children. J Pediatr Orthop B 2003; 12: 338–345.

71. Gordon JE, Gregush RV, Schoenecker PL, et al. Complications after titanium elastic nailing of pediatric tibial fractures. J Pediatr Orthop 2007; 27:442–446.

72. Lascombes P, Haumont T, Journeau P. Use and abuse of flexible intramedullary nailing in children and adolescents. J Pediatr Orthop 2006; 26(6):827–834.

73. Lewallen RP, Peterson HA. Nonunion of long bone fractures in children: a review of 30 cases. J Pediatr Orthop 1985; 5: 135–142.

74. Domzalski ME, Lipton GE, Lee D, et al. Fractures of the distal tibial metaphysis in children. Patterns of injury and results of treatment. J Pediatr Orthop 2006; 26:171–176.

Chapter 50

Ankle Fractures

Klaus Parsch and Francisco Fernandez Fernandez

Incidence and Mechanism of Injury

Injuries of the ankle joint are common. According to Peterson [1] physeal injuries of the distal tibia and fibula account for 25% of all physeal fractures. About 60% of physeal ankle fractures occur during sports activities and are more common in males than in females [2]. In his monograph Poland [3] pointed out that children's ligaments are stronger than physeal cartilage. Where adults would sustain ligamentous injuries the same forces will cause fractures of the physis in children.

Classification

After Poland [3] and Aitken [4], Salter and Harris coined a classification for physeal injuries in the ankle joint (Fig. 50.1) [5].

The classification of physeal injuries in the distal tibia and fibula of Dias and Tachdjian follows the injury mechanism shown in Fig. 50.2 [6].

Treatment

General Aspects

Non-displaced fractures can be simply immobilized in a cast. Displaced fractures can be treated by closed reduction and cast immobilization. If closed reduction cannot be *maintained* internal fixation is necessary. If closed reduction is

not possible, open reduction and internal fixation are indicated. The anatomic type of the fracture defined by the Salter and Harris (SH) classification, the mechanism of injury following Dias and Tachdjian, and the amount of displacement, especially the intraarticular lesion, must be considered. The status of the skin and the neurovascular function/integrity may require emergency treatment in some cases.

Salter and Harris Type I

These are rare injuries. The majority will have some metaphyseal fragments discovered classifying them SH type II. True displaced SH type I lesions should be reduced as an emergency for protection of the soft tissues and the skin. Complete reduction may be possible by closed means; if not open reduction and crossed K-wire fixation are indicated. Immobilization for 4 weeks in a non-weight bearing above-knee cast is followed by a weight bearing one for another 3 weeks [7].

Salter and Harris Type II

SH type II fractures can be undisplaced or displaced. The majority result from a pronation-eversion mechanism, but some have the supination-inversion mechanism [6]. SH type II fractures are the most common injuries [2].

Treatment

We treat *non-displaced fractures* with a below-knee cast for 3 weeks, followed by a short walking cast for another 3 weeks. Some prefer to use a long above-knee cast initially [2].

Displaced SH type II fractures should be reduced. We recommend a closed reduction under general anesthesia. If that is successful an above-knee cast should be applied.

K. Parsch (✉)
Orthopaedic Department, Pediatric Olgahospital, Stuttgart, Germany

M. Benson et al. (eds.), *Children's Orthopaedics and Fractures,*
DOI 10.1007/978-1-84882-611-3_50, © Springer-Verlag London Limited 2010

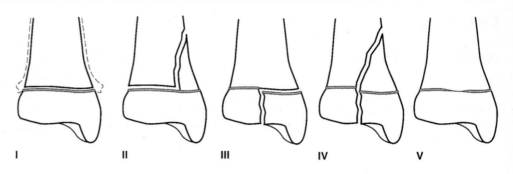

Fig. 50.1 Classification of Salter and Harris. I: Separation of the distal tibial metaphysis from the epiphysis; II: Separation of the distal tibia with metaphyseal fragment; III: Intraepiphyseal fracture of the distal tibia; IV: Fracture separation of distal tibial meta- and epiphysis; V: Crush injury of the distal tibial physis. From Cummings [7]. Used with permission

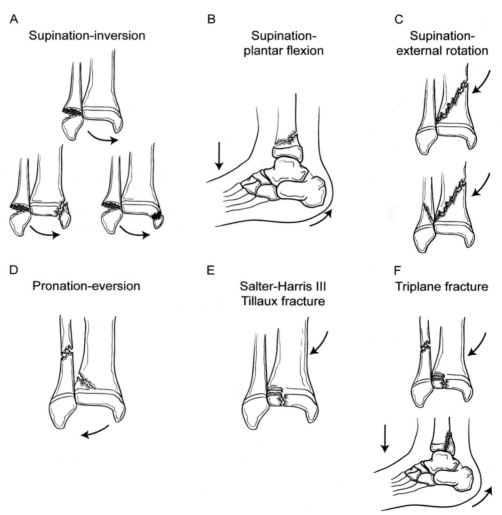

Fig. 50.2 Classification of Dias and Tachdjian. (**A**) *Supination-inversion:* Grade 1 adduction force causes avulsion of the distal fibular epiphysis, while grade 2 with further inversion produces additional Salter–Harris IV or III injury of the distal medial tibia. (**B**) *Supination-plantar flexion:* The plantarflexion forces displace the tibial epiphysis directly posteriorly producing a Salter–Harris I or II lesion. (**C**) *Supination-external rotation:* In grade I the external rotation forces result in a Salter–Harris II fracture. The distal fragment is displaced posteriorly. In grade II with more external rotation a spiral fracture of the distal tibia is produced. (**D**) *Pronation-eversion external rotation* forces cause a distal fibular fracture and a distal tibial fragment displaced later-

ally and possibly a lateral or posterolateral Thurston Holland fragment. (**E**) *Juvenile Tillaux fracture:* Salter–Harris III fracture involving the anterolateral part of the distal tibia. (**F**) *Triplane fracture* is produced by a combination of external rotation and plantar flexion forces. The fracture consists of three major fragments: the anterolateral quadrant of the distal tibial epiphysis, the medial and posterior portions of the epiphysis, and the tibial metaphysis. Triplane fractures can have two parts, three, or even four parts. Triplane fractures have the appearance of a Salter–Harris type III on the AP radiograph and of a Salter–Harris type II fracture on the lateral view. From Dias and Tachdjian [6]. Used with permission

Fig. 50.3 Fifteen-year-old boy after trampoline accident with pronation external rotation injury. (**a**) AP view of Salter–Harris II injury and distal fracture of fibula. (**b**) AP view after unsuccessful attempt at closed reduction. (**c**) AP view after open reduction, infolding of periosteal entrapment. (**d**) AP view after 4 months. Anatomic healing of tibia

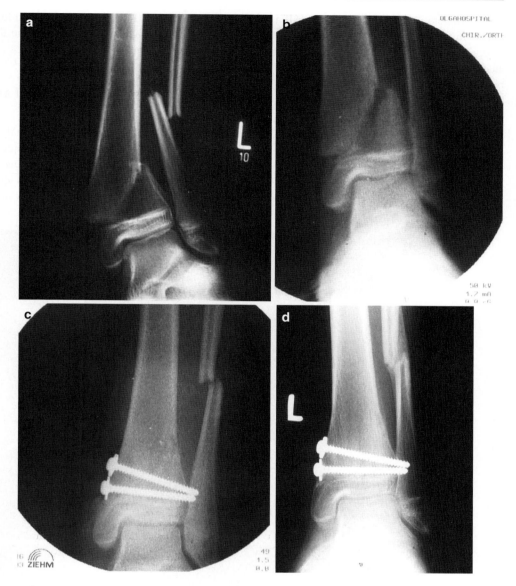

There is controversy as to how much residual displacement should acceptable after closed reduction. If the fracture gap is more than 2 mm, periosteum may be trapped and one should proceed to open reduction followed by internal fixation (Fig. 50.3).

Premature Physeal Closure

Wirth et al. [8] showed in their experimental studies on sheep that implantation of periosteum resulted in inhibition of longitudinal growth and the formation of bony bridges. Ablation of physeal cartilage combined with periosteal insertion results in dramatic injury that cannot be corrected [9]. Barmada et al. [10] noted the importance of entrapped periosteum causing a gap. If a residual gap is not closed the incidence of premature physeal closure (PPC) is increased to 60%, while the incidence decreased to 17% in those where no gap was present. Anatomic reduction must be achieved at all costs to decrease the risk of PPC [11].

Our Preferred Method

In SH type II fractures with displacement we recommend closed reduction under general anesthesia. The patient must be fully relaxed to allow the reduction manoeuvre, which will be noticed by a palpable click which can also be heard. Complete reduction should be confirmed on the image intensifier. Radiographic documentation is advised in two planes. The patient is immobilized in an above-knee long leg cast for 3 weeks followed by a short walking cast for another 3 weeks.

If complete reduction is not achieved, as revealed on the image intensifier, during the same anesthesia we proceed to open reduction. As soon as the entrapped periosteum is anatomical reduction is easy most of the time. The metaphyseal fragment is fixed by one or two screws inserted horizontally to provide a stable retention of the fragments (Fig. 50.3). As an alternative crossed K-wires can be used (Fig. 50.4). Postoperative immobilization is achieved by a below-knee cast for 3 weeks, followed by a below-knee walking cast for another 3 weeks.

If the rules concerning non-acceptance of incomplete reduction caused by periosteal entrapment are followed, SH type II fractures are a benign lesion and the outcome will be satisfactory. If a gap of more than 2 mm persists, there is a high risk of PCC [10].

Salter–Harris Types III and IV

Types III and IV distal tibial epiphyseal fracture are very demanding. The most frequent one is after supination-inversion injury. As described by Dias and Tachdjian [6] lesser supination force will cause a distal fibular epiphyseal avulsion, while stronger deforming forces will cause an

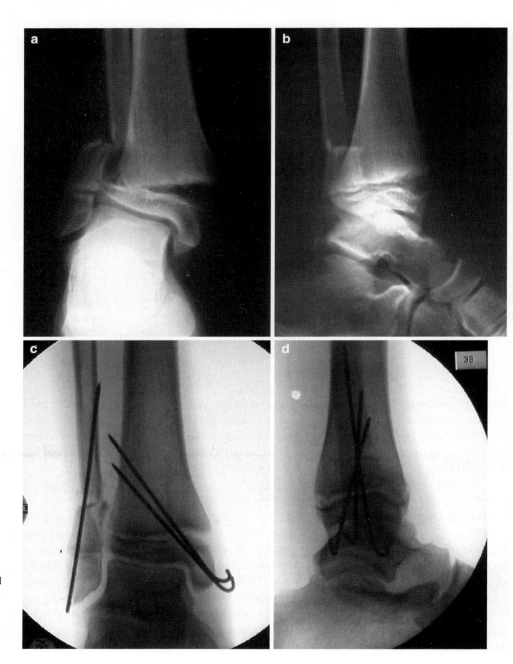

Fig. 50.4 Fifteen-year-old female athlete after pronation-eversion trauma playing soccer. (**a**) AP view of Salter–Harris II lesion and distal fibular fracture. (**b**) Lateral view of Salter–Harris II fracture with gapping. (**c**) AP view after closed reduction which was not stable. Crossed Kirschner wires provide stable fixation. (**d**) Lateral view after percutaneous pinning of Salter–Harris II fracture

avulsion of the medial malleolus, rarely type III (intraepiphyseal), more frequently type IV including a metaphyseal fragment.

Treatment

Anatomic reduction is necessary in to avoid, if possible, premature physeal closure. Even with a near perfect reduction small fragments from local crush injury can cause partial growth arrest. The age of the child is important: the young child will have a higher risk than the more mature patient shortly before the physes close. All type III and IV injuries must be followed for at least 2 years after injury in order to recognize any physeal damage followed by growth arrest in the young patients until maturity.

Undisplaced type III and IV lesions can be treated conservatively. This treatment is indicated only if the gap is 1 mm or less. Some prefer a computed tomography (CT) scan before initiating conservative treatment and also for control in the cast [7]. One must be sure that a close follow-up is guaranteed with review at 2, 4, and 6 weeks after injury. Secondary displacement can occur inside a cast as soon as posttraumatic swelling of the ankle has subsided. Immobilization time is 4 weeks in an above-knee cast followed by 3 weeks in a below-knee walking cast. Clinical and possibly radiological controls are obligatory for at least 2 years after the trauma, so that PCC is not overlooked (Fig. 50.5).

Displaced type III and type IV injuries must be correctly diagnosed by radiographs in two planes; oblique radiographs may be helpful to obtain a correct diagnosis. If available CT scan or magnetic resonance imaging (MRI) can contribute to an exact diagnosis similar to imaging in triplane fractures [12].

Surgical treatment is indicated in all displaced type III and IV lesions with more than 1 mm gap. Big epi-metaphyseal fragments have to be reduced anatomically. After provisional coaption with one or two K-wires the fragments are fixed by two transverse screws. The diameter of the intraepiphyseal screw must be according to the size of the epiphysis and should not interfere with the growth plate, while the metaphyseal screw can be larger (Fig. 50.6).

In younger children with small fragments several K-wires can be used in an attempt to fix the pieces of bone and cartilage in their anatomic position. If the fibular physis is displaced a longitudinal K-wire will help retain that part of the problem. The young children with a severe crush of the medial malleolus plus adjacent metaphysis carries a high risk of PPC, even if seemingly anatomical reduction is achieved. Follow-up reviews are mandatory until maturity, in order to recognize and treat the dreaded medial growth arrest causing deformity (Fig. 50.7). If medial growth arrest causes varus deformity, supramalleolar corrective osteotomy is indicated (Fig. 50.8).

Transitional Fractures

An asymmetric pattern of closure of the distal tibial physis during the last 18 months produces a special fracture pattern not seen in younger patients, where the physes are still wide open. This group of fractures has been labeled transitional fractures because they occur during the transition from

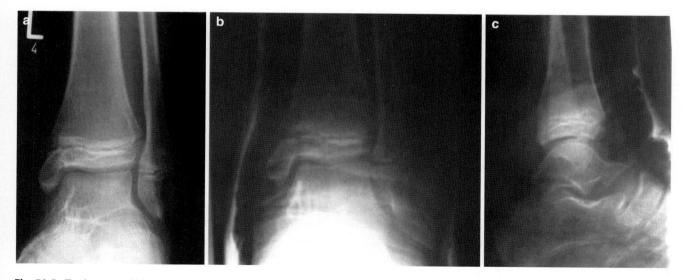

Fig. 50.5 Twelve-year-old boy after supination inversion injury playing football. (a) AP radiograph of non-displaced Salter–Harris III fracture. (b) AP view, after conservative treatment and immobilization in a below-knee cast. (c) Lateral view of undisplaced fracture in the cast

Fig. 50.6 Eleven-year-old girl had fallen from a horse with supination-inversion trauma. (**a**) Displaced Salter–Harris IV fracture seen on an oblique view of the ankle joint. Impaction trauma on the medial dome of talus. (**b**) AP and lateral view after open reduction, fixation with two transverse screws. (**c**) AP radiograph at age 15, 4 years post–trauma, showing anotomical (**d**) Lateral view at age 15, 4 years posttrauma

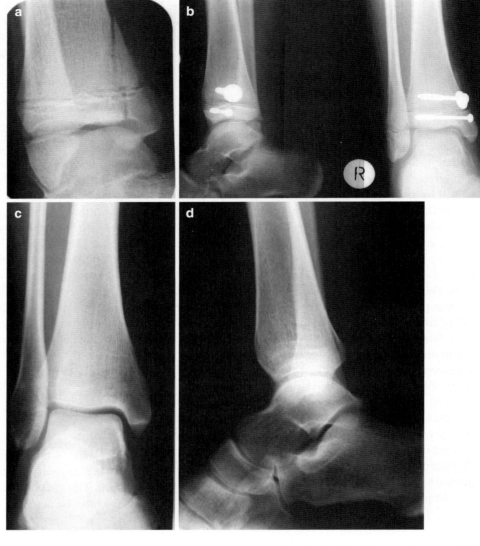

Fig. 50.7 Fifteen-year-old female athlete with severe supination inversion injury. (**a**) AP view of Salter–Harris IV fracture dislocation. Complete displacement of medial malleolus. (**b**) AP view after tension-band osteosynthesis of the medial malleolus and fibula. (**c**) Ankle joint in two planes 16 months later

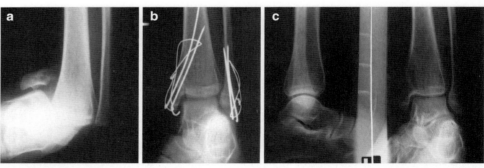

a skeletally immature to a skeletally mature ankle. There is the SH type III *Tillaux fracture* and a variety of triplane fractures. While the Tillaux fracture type was described for adults in the late nineteenth century [13] the triplane fractures were identified as a separate entity in the late twentieth century by Marmor [14] and Lynn [15]. They seem to be caused by external rotation, with stage I causing Tillaux fractures and further external rotation triplane fractures, while grade II will cause additional fracture of the distal fibula [16].

Fig. 50.8 Nine-year-old girl who had fallen off a ladder. (**a**) AP view of Salter–Harris IV with medial crush zone. (**b**) AP view after open reduction and K-wire fixation. (**c**) AP view 6 years later with medial growth arrest and varus deformity. (**d**) AP view at $16\frac{1}{2}$ years, 1 year after supramalleolar corrective osteotomy using a medial bone graft

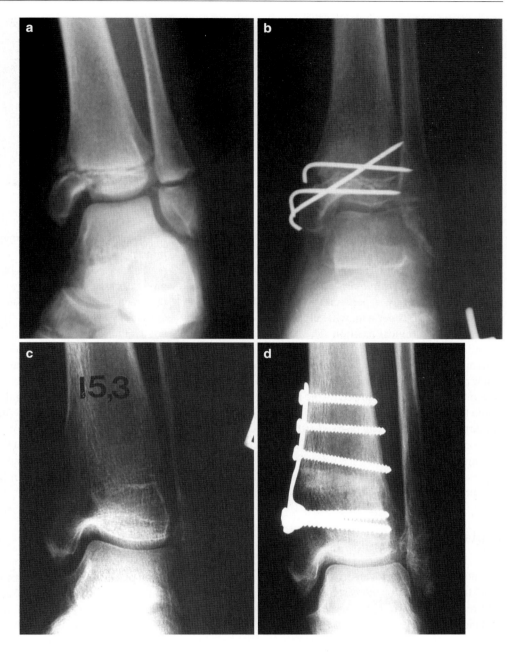

Tillaux Fracture

This SH type III fracture occurs with external rotation of the foot. The anteroinferior tibiofibular ligament through its attachment avulses an anterolateral fragment of the tibial physis. The position of the fibula prevents major displacement of the Tillaux fragment. Clinically local tenderness and swelling is present at the anterolateral aspect of the joint. In uncertain cases, when anteroposterior (AP) radiograph is not clear, an oblique view of the ankle joint will be helpful. If available, CT scan or MRI will show the fracture line clearly [12].

Treatment

For Tillaux fractures which are undisplaced or have a gap of less than 2 mm, we immobilize the patient in a below-knee cast with the ankle joint in neutral dorsiflexion. Secondary

Fig. 50.9 Fifteen-year-old girl after external rotation trauma during track event. (**a**) AP radiograph of displaced Tillaux fracture. (**b**) CT scan reveals a two-part distal tibial fracture fracture with two fragments. (**c**) AP radiograph after open reduction and insertion of cannulated screw

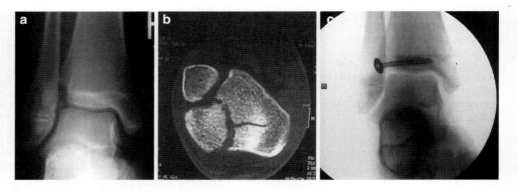

displacement is possible, CT controls after a few days are indicated, as on plain film control a change might not be noted. So CT scans are indicated after a few days as any displacement may not be seen radiographically.

Displacement of over 2 mm should be reduced and fixed. This can be done by a percutaneous cannulated screw. A percutaneous Kirschner wire will help to manipulate the fracture into its anatomical position. The screw has its diameter according to the size of the physis and should be inserted horizontally, parallel to the growth plate. If closed reduction is not possible, open reduction is performed through a small anterolateral incision, followed by the insertion of a lag screw inside the physis, parallel to the growth plate (Fig. 50.9). The intraarticular fragment can be fixed arthroscopically [17, 18].

Prognosis of reduced and fixed Tillaux fractures is good as long as the articular surface has been restored. Premature physeal closure is not a problem, because this fracture occurs only in patients who are about to close their physis.

Triplane Fracture

Marmor [14] described an irreducible ankle fracture in a child that at operation consisted of three fragments. Lynn [15] reported on two additional cases and coined the name triplane fracture.

Triplane fracture may consist of two parts, a large posterolateral epiphyseal fragment with its posterior metaphyseal fragment attached to it.

It may consist of three parts with a large epiphyseal fragment and its metaphyseal component. In addition there is a smaller anterolateral epiphyseal fragment.

In the four-part lateral triplane fracture there is an anterior split of the epiphyseal fragment into two, while the posterior fragment is the larger one with its metaphyseal component attached to it.

Intramalleolar triplane fracture as described by von Laer [19] is a rare extraarticular variant [20, 21] of the standard intraarticular triplane fracture.

Triplane fractures occur most frequently in adolescents, the main cause being sports injuries. Swelling and pain are

more on the lateral aspect of the ankle joint and because of the fixed fibula there is no major visible deformity in these injuries.

Radiography in the AP plane does show the intraepiphyseal fracture line, while the metaphyseal segment of the fracture is better seen on the lateral plane radiograph. Oblique views are helpful, if other imaging methods are not available. While most acute distal tibial fractures can be well diagnosed by plain radiographs, the complex status of intraarticular damage is better diagnosed with the help of a CT scan or MRI [22].

CT scans are recommended in suspected triplane fracture, in order to identify the intraepiphyseal and intraarticular situation [19, 23]. MRI is an ideal tool to identify epi- and metaphyseal injury as well as the damage to the soft tissues [12]. MRI can visualize entrapped periosteum from the metaphyseal fragment, which can be a major obstacle to closed reduction.

Treatment

Undisplaced triplane fractures with a gap smaller than 2 mm and extraarticular type D fractures can be treated with a below-knee cast in neutral position. Immobilization is 3 weeks in a long leg cast without weight bearing followed by another 3 weeks in a weight bearing below-knee cast.

Any intraarticular displacement of more than 2 mm needs surgical reduction. Preoperative CT scans provide a clear picture and shows whether one is treating a two- three- or four-segmented triplane tibial epiphyseolysis (TPE) [24]. The three-segmented type is well described by the "Mercedes star" [25].

Surgical reduction in two-segment TPE is done by an anteromedial incision. The fracture site is irrigated to remove debris. Most often entrapped periosteum has to be removed in order to be able to reduce the metaphyseal segment which will allow easier reduction of the intraepiphyseal lesion. A second anterolateral incision is sometimes needed for removal of the interposed periosteum. The reduced fracture is stabilised by provisional K-wires. Satisfactory reduction

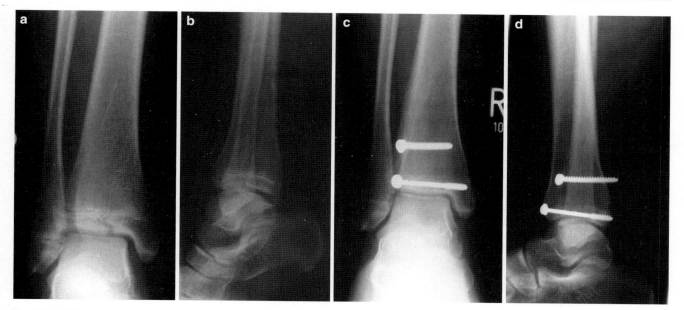

Fig. 50.10 Thirteen-year-old girl after fall from her bicycle with eversion trauma. (**a**) AP radiograph of two-part triplane fracture with 4 mm intraarticular gap. (**b**) Lateral view of the fracture shows displacement within the joint. (**c**) AP view after open reduction, removal of periosteum entrapment, and fixation with an epiphyseal and metaphyseal screws. (**d**) Lateral view with complete closure of the intraarticular fracture gap inside the joint

must be controlled on the image intensifier in both planes. Two cancellous screws are inserted horizontally from medial to lateral, or from anterior to posterior depending on the fracture pattern (Fig. 50.10).

Arthroscopy-assisted reduction and percutaneous fixation are described for triplane fractures (Fig. 50.11), at least taking care of the intraarticular part of that injury. The published data are small series or single case reports [17, 18, 26, 27].

Immobilization after surgical reduction, open or arthroscopically assisted, is needed for a 6-week period in a below-knee cast, the first 3 weeks without and the second 3 weeks with weight bearing.

The outcome after surgical treatment of triplane fractures is satisfactory as long as anatomical reduction of the intraepiphyseal and intraarticular lesion has been complete (Fig. 50.12). If steps of more than 2 mm are left behind osteoarthrosis will develop later.

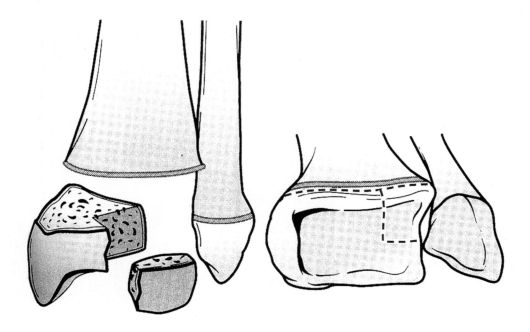

Fig. 50.11 Three-part triplane fracture. From Cummings [7]. Used with permission

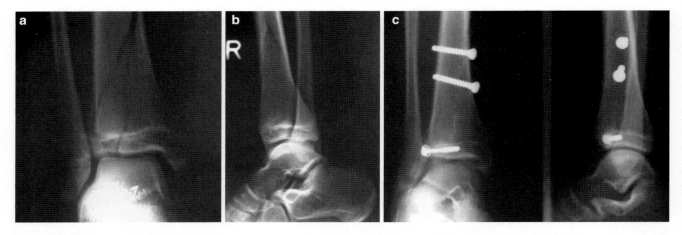

Fig. 50.12 Thirteen-year-old girl who fell during volleyball game. (**a**) AP view of triplane fracture (three fragments). (**b**) Lateral view of triplane fracture. (**c**) AP and lateral view 4 months after open reduction and fixation with one epiphyseal screw and two metaphyseal screws

Lateral Ankle Sprain

Sprained ankles are common lesions. After a phase of surgical treatment of ligamentous injuries of the ankle in the past it became obvious that conservative treatment achieved the same good results. It is widely accepted today that purely ligamentous injuries are treated with in 3 weeks a below-knee walking cast. Sprained ankles with an avulsed fragment of the distal fibula are a separate entity and need active treatment [28].

Avulsion Fractures of the Distal Fibula

Avulsion fractures of the distal fibula rarely occur in young children, but may be seen occasionally in adolescents, where ankle sprains are more common. Radiographic identification is not always obvious and sometimes needs a close-up view and a special technique [29].

Treatment

Radiologically visible fragments are avulsions from the distal fibula. The avulsed fragments are fixed with two Kirschner wires in younger patients (Fig. 50.13), and with a

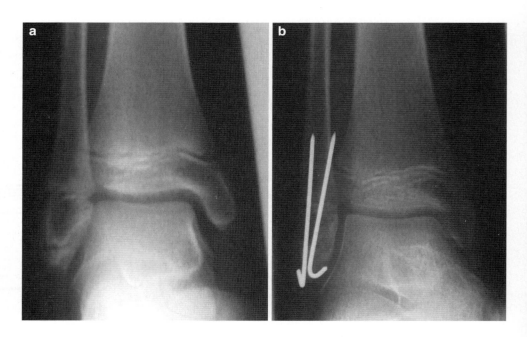

Fig. 50.13 Twelve-year-old female volleyball player injured during game. (**a**) Distal fibular fracture, not yet displaced. (**b**) AP view after fixation with two K-wires buried under the skin

screw in the almost mature adolescents. If these fragments are not recognized they may cause chronic pain, less frequently instability. In a small series of adolescent athletes, removal of a bony fragment gave relief from pain. The symptoms seemed to have come more from the bony fragment than from the ligamentous injury [30, 31].

References

1. Peterson HA, Madhog R, Benson JT, et al. Physeal fractures: Part 1. Epidemiology in Olmsted County Minnesota. J Pediatr Orthop 1994; 14: 423–430.
2. Spiegel PG, Cooperman DR, Laros GS. Epiphyseal fractures of the distal ends of the tibia and fibula. J Bone Joint Surg Am 1978; 60: 1046–1050.
3. Poland J. Traumatic separation of the epiphysis. Smith, Elder and Co, 1898 (Portions reprinted). Clin Orthop Relat Res 1965; 41: 7–18.
4. Aitken AP. The end result of the fractured distal tibial epiphysis. J Bone Joint Surg 1936; 18: 685–691.
5. Salter RB, Harris WB. Injuries involving the epiphyseal plate. J Bone Joint Surg Am 1963; 45: 587–622
6. Dias LS, Tachdjian MO Physeal injuries of the ankle in children. Clin Orthop Relat Res 1978; 136: 230–233.
7. Cummings RJ. Distal tibial and fibular fractures. In: Beaty JH, Kasser JH, eds. Rockwood and Wilkins' Fractures in Children 6th ed. Philadelphia: Lippincott Williams and Wilkins; 2001: 1077–1128.
8. Wirth T, Byers S, Byard RW, et al. The implantation of cartilaginous and periostal tissue into growth plate defects. Intern Orthop (SICOT) 1994; 18: 220–228.
9. Gruber HE, Phieffer LS, Wattenbarger JW. Physeal fractures, Part II: Fate of interposed periostium in a physeal fracture. J Pediatr Orthop 2002; 22: 710–716.
10. Barmada A, Gyanor TP, Mubarak SJ. Premature physeal closure following distal tibia physeal fractures. A new radiographic predictor. J Pediatr Orthop 2003; 23: 733–739.
11. Rohmiller MT, Gaynor TP, Pawalek J, et al. Salter-Harris I and II fractures of the distal tibia: Does mechanism of injury relate to premature physeal closure? J Pediatr Orthop 2006; 26: 322–328.
12. Seifert J, Matthes G, Hinz P, et al. Role of magnetic resonance imaging in the diagnosis of distal tibia fractures in adolescents. J Pediatr Orthop 2003; 23: 727–732.
13. Tillaux PJ. Traite d'anatomie topographique avec applications à la chirurgie, 2nd ed. Paris: Asselin and Houzeau; 1878.
14. Marmor L. An unusual fracture of the tibial epiphysis. Clin Orthop Relat Res 1970; 73: 132–135.
15. Lynn MD. The triplane distal tibial epiphyseal fracture. Clin Orthop Relat Res 1972; 86: 187–190.
16. Dias LS, Giegerich CR. Fractures of the distal tibial epiphysis in adolescents. J Bone Joint Surg Am 1983; 65: 439–433.
17. Whipple TL, Martin DR, McIntyre LF, et al. Arthroscopic treatment of triplane fractures of the ankle. Arthroscopy 1993; 9: 456–463.
18. Jennings MM, Lagaay P, Schuberth JM. Arthroscopic assisted fixation of juvenile intra-articular epiphyseal ankle fractures. Foot Ankle Surg 2007; 46: 376–386.
19. Von Laer L. Classification, diagnosis, and treatment of transitional fractures of the distal part of the tibia. J Bone Joint Surg Am 1985; 67: 687–698.
20. Feldman DS, Otsuka NY, Hedden DM. Extra-articular triplane fractures of the distal tibial epiphysis. J Pediatr Orthop 1995; 15: 479–481.
21. Shin AY, Moran ME, Wenger DR. Intramalleolar triplane fractures of the distal tibial epiphysis. J Pediatr Orthop 1997; 17: 352–355.
22. Petit P, Panuel M, Faure F. Acute fracture of the distal tibial physis: role of gradient-echo MR imaging versus plain film examination. Am J Roentgenol 1996; 166: 1203–1206.
23. Kärrholm J, Hansson LI, Laurin S. Computer tomography of intraarticular supination-eversion fractures of the ankle in adolescents. J Pediatr Orthop 1981; 1: 181–187.
24. Cooperman DR, Spiegel PG, Laros GS. Tibial fractures involving the ankle in children. J Bone Joint Surg Am 1978; 60: 1040–1046.
25. Rapariz JM, Ocete G, Gonzalez-Herranz P, et al. Distal tibial triplane fractures: long term follow-up. J Pediatr Orthop 1996; 16: 113–118.
26. Imeda S, Takao M, Nishi H. Arthroscopically-assisted reduction and percutaneous fixation for triplane fracture of the distal tibia. Arthroscopy 2004; 20: e123–128.
27. McGillion S, Jackson M, Lahoti O. Arthroscopically assisted percutaneous fixation of triplane fractures of the distal tibia. J Pediatr Orthop Part B 2007; 16: 313–316.
28. Vahvanen V, Westerlund M, Nikku R. Lateral ligament injury of the ankle in children. Follow-up results of primary surgical treatment. Acta Orthop Scand 1984; 55: 21–25.
29. Haraguchi N, Kato F, Hayashi H. New radiographic projections for avulsion fractures of the lateral malleolus. J Bone Joint Surg Br 1998; 80: 684–688.
30. Danielsson LG. Avulsion fracture of the lateral malleolus in children. Injury 1989; 12: 165–167.
31. Busconi BD, Pappas AM. Chronic, painful ankle instability in skeletally immature athletes. Ununited osteochondral fractures of the distal fibula. Am J Sports Med 1996; 24: 647–651.

Chapter 51

Fractures and Dislocations of the Foot

Francisco Fernandez Fernandez

Introduction

Ninety percent of all fractures of the foot occur in the metatarsals and phalanges. Fractures of the tarsal bones are rare and have an incidence of about 4%.

The child's foot has a different growth pattern to other parts of the body. Fifty percent of the total growth in length is present by 1 year in girls and 18 months in boys. Ninety-six percent of the total growth is present by 12 years in girls and 88% in boys [1]. This pattern of growth must be considered when treating injuries of the foot in children [2, 3].

Talus

Epidemiology

The reported incidence of talar fractures is 0.08% of all fractures in children [4]. However, with increasing numbers of children participating in high velocity sports the incidence of fractures of the talus is increasing.

Mechanism of Injury

Axial trauma is the most common mechanism of fracture of the talus. It can also be the result of a direct crushing injury [5].

Blood Circulation

A major problem in talar fractures is the nature of the blood supply of the tarsal bone. Three-fifths of the talar surface is covered with cartilage and the main blood supply is through the non-cartilage covered talar neck. There is a centripetal blood supply via the sinus and tarsal canal [5]. The tarsal canal branch of the posterior tibial artery supplies the neck and the body of the talus. The sinus tarsi artery supplies blood to the head and lateral third of the talus. As a result fractures of the neck and proximal part of the talus carry a high risk of avascular necrosis.

Classification

Fractures of the talus are classified into those of the neck and those of the body, osteochondral fractures, and fractures of the posterior or lateral processes of the talus. In children fractures of the tarsal neck are the most frequent.

Fractures of the talar neck were classified according to Hawkins in 1970 into three types [6]. In this classification blood supply and the risk of avascular necrosis were taken into consideration. A rare type IV was added to the classification in 1978 by Canale and Kelly [7].

Modified Hawkins Classification of Talar Neck Fractures

- Type I: Fractures with no or minimal displacement. Only one source of blood supply entering through the talar neck may be disrupted.
- Type II: Displaced talar neck fracture with subluxation of the subtalar joint but no dislocation of the ankle joint. There may be a medial fracture with multiple fragments. At least two or three sources of blood supply may be damaged.
- Type III: Displaced talar neck fracture with dislocation of the body of the talus from the ankle with a subtalar joints. All three sources of blood supply likely to be damaged and a high risk of avascular necrosis.

F. Fernandez Fernandez (✉)
Department of Pediatric Orthopaedic Surgery, Olgahospital Stuttgart, Stuttgart, Germany

M. Benson et al. (eds.), *Children's Orthopaedics and Fractures*,
DOI 10.1007/978-1-84882-611-3_51, © Springer-Verlag London Limited 2010

- Type IV: Displaced talar neck fracture with dislocation of the talar body from the ankle and subtalar joints associated with dislocation of the talar head and neck fragment from the talonavicular joint. All three sources of blood likely to be damaged and high risk of avascular necrosis.

Diagnosis

Clinically the foot and ankle are swollen and painful. There may be obvious deformity.

Standard anteroposterior (AP) and lateral radiographs of the ankle and foot should be taken. For further evaluation particularly if a fracture of the talus is suspected magnetic resonance imaging (MRI) or computed tomography (CT) can be helpful.

Treatment

Fracture of the Talar Neck

A Hawkins type I fracture without displacement should be immobilized in a below-knee leg cast.

A Hawkins type II fracture with medial comminution, displacement, and subtalar subluxation (Fig. 51.1) should be accurately fixed with a screw or K-wire. Open reduction via an anterolateral or anteromedial approach may be necessary. However, a postero-lateral approach avoids further risk to the blood supply.

Hawkins type III fractures must be treated as an emergency. Open reduction is mandatory. A closed reduction should not be attempted because of the limited chance of success and risk of further damage due to malrotation of the talar body and impingement on the tibialis posterior tendon. Open reduction should be performed with great care to avoid further damage to the blood supply. Stabilization should be obtained by screw fixation through a postero-lateral approach.

Hawkins type IV fractures should be treated as an emergency. Displacement of the neck of the talus, in addition to dislocation of the body, makes treatment of this fracture difficult. There is significant soft tissue injury and an even higher risk of avascular necrosis. The stabilization should be done by the postero-lateral approach. Screw fixation and temporary stabilization of the talonavicular joint for 4 weeks with a K-wire is the treatment of choice.

Fractures of the Body (Dome) of the Talus

Fractures of the body of the talus are unusual in children. The mechanism of injury is axial trauma. If the joint surface is damaged, open or arthroscopic reduction is advised.

Fractures of the Head of Talus

Fractures of the talar head are rare injuries (Fig. 51.2). They are often associated with complex injuries of the foot. In addition to cartilage damage, there are often defects of the

Table 51.1 Modified Hawkins classification of talar neck fractures, treatment, and risk of avascular necrosis (Canale and Kelly, 1978)

Type	Description	Treatment	Risk of osteonecrosis (%)
Type I	Undisplaced vertical fractures of the neck	Closed/open reduction	0–10
Type II	Displaced talar neck fracture with subtalar subluxation	Open/closed reduction	20–50
Type III	Displaced talar neck fracture, dislocation of the ankle and subtalar joints	Open emergency reduction	80–100
Type IV	Displaced talar neck fracture, dislocation of ankle, subtalar, and talonavicular joints	Open emergency reduction	90–100

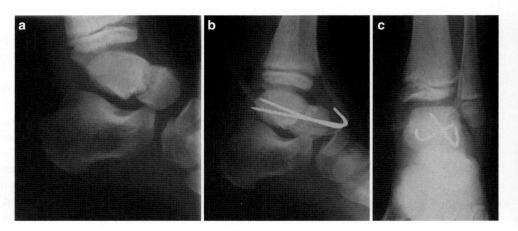

Fig. 51.1 (a) Six-year-old boy with a Hawkins type II fracture of the talar neck. (b) Open reduction and cross-pinning with Kirschner wires

Fig. 51.2 (a) Radiograph of a 10-year-old boy who had fallen from a bicycle and sustained a displaced fracture of the talar head and an infraction of the cuboid. (b) Closed reduction of the talar head and cross-pinning with K-wires

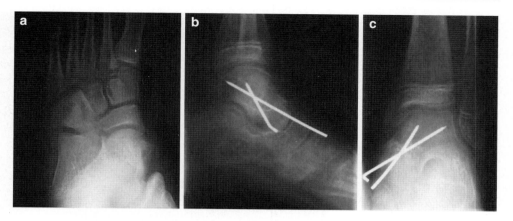

cancellous bone marrow. The aim of surgery is to restore the shape of the talar head and reestablish the medial column.

Fractures of the Lateral Talar Process

Fractures of the lateral talar process are sometimes overlooked or misdiagnosed. With the increase in sports such as snowboarding this injury is becoming more common. The mechanism of injury is dorsiflexion and inversion of the hindfoot. In non-displaced fractures conservative treatment is recommended. Displaced fractures affecting the joint should be reduced and fixed to avoid later joint degeneration [8, 9].

Calcaneus

Epidemiology

The incidence of calcaneus fractures in children varies between 0.05 and 0.15% of all fractures in children [10–12]. The incidence increases with the age and is highest in adolescence [13]. The developing calcaneus is largely cartilaginous, which is one of the reasons for the low incidence. Delayed diagnosis is reported in 43% of children with extraarticular fractures [14]. Some unrecognized calcaneal fractures in infants may be explained by their low morbidity and rapid healing.

Mechanism of Injury

The mechanism of injury depends on the child's age. Wiley and Profitt [14] describe falls from a height in children under the age of 10 years and high velocity injuries in children older

than 10 and in adolescents. Atkins et al. [15] found a correlation between the height of the fall and the grade of injury in adults but this was not observed in children. Twenty to thirty percent of all fractures of the calcaneus in childhood are accompanied by other fractures. In the case of falls from a great height multiple injuries affecting the foot, the lower extremity, or the spine have to be considered. Two associated spinal injuries were found in 34 children with calcaneal fractures [14]. Associated injury to the soft tissues, nerves, and vessels is common [13, 16]. If a compartment syndrome is suspected emergency decompression should be performed (Fig. 51.3).

Classification and Clinical Appearance

Classifications of fractures of the calcaneus in children [13, 14] are shown in Table 51.2 and Fig. 51.4. Foot and ankle are swollen with abrasions or compression marks on the skin.

Imaging

Radiography

Anteroposterior and lateral views of the foot and ankle together with an axial view of the calcaneus should be taken.

It is important to look closely at the posterior facet of the calcaneus. In small children diagnosis can be difficult, in a toddler with a limp the fracture can be overlooked unless an axial view is taken. A follow-up radiograph 10 days after injury may show callus formation. A comparative view of the contralateral side can be helpful in these circumstances.

Fig. 51.3 Classification of fractures of the calcaneus

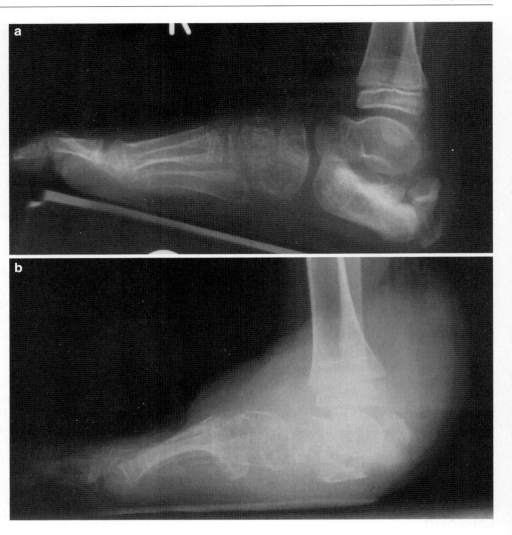

Table 51.2 Fractures of the calcaneus in children

Type I	a. Fracture of the tuberosity or apophysis
	b. Fracture of the sustentaculum
	c. Fracture of the anterior process
	d. Fracture of anterior inferolateral process
	e. Avulsion fracture of the body
Type II	Fracture of posterior and/or superior part of the tuberosity
Type III	Fracture of the body not involving the subtalar joint
Type IV	Fracture through the subtalar joint without displacement
Type V	Displaced fracture through the subtalar joint
Type VI	Fracture with serious soft tissue injury and bone loss

between 2 and 3 mm allow a three-dimensional reconstruction, however, the radiation dose must always be considered (see Chapter 5).

Magnetic Resonance Imaging

If available MRI is helpful to clarify the details of a fracture.

CT Scan

If an intraarticular fracture is suspected a CT scan is indicated to recognize the precise geometry and displacement of the fracture. To facilitate planning of the operation slices

Treatment

The aim of treatment is to restore the bony anatomy and to achieve a pain-free, functional, weight bearing, plantigrade foot.

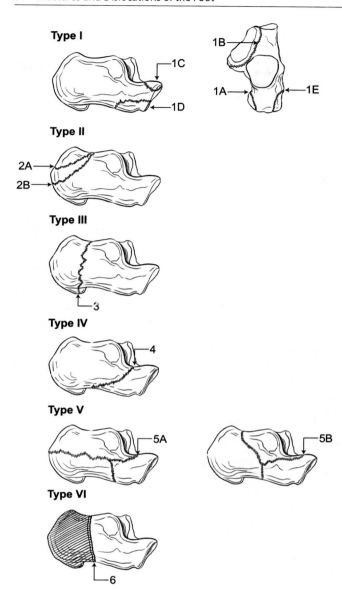

Fig. 51.4 Five-year-old boy who fell from a height sustaining a fracture of the calcaneus in both feet. (**a**) *Right* and (**b**) *left* calcaneus. Following treatment in closed casts in a primary care center he developed bilateral compartment syndrome. After delayed recognition of the compartment syndrome in both feet with major soft tissue necrosis and extensive osteonecrosis of both feet reconstruction with a latissimus dorsi flap was necessary

Undisplaced Fractures of the Calcaneus

In the past conservative treatment was the treatment of choice even for intraarticular fractures. Nowadays this is controversial. There is consensus regarding the management of extraarticular fractures. In non-displaced or minimally displaced extraarticular fractures immobilization in a split below-knee cast or a below-knee splint is indicated. As soon as the swelling subsides a complete below-knee cast

is applied for 4–6 weeks. Weight bearing is allowed after 4 weeks.

Displaced Fractures of the Calcaneus

Treatment of displaced intraarticular fractures is controversial. The published reports have low patient numbers and are retrospective case–control studies (level III for evidence). In two of these long-term studies good outcomes were reported following conservative treatment [17, 18]. In another study, 17 out of 19 fractures of the calcaneus treated conservatively and followed up for 17 years had excellent results [19].

In contrast to this conservative approach, open reduction has been advocated for displaced intraarticular fractures in children [20–22]. Depending on the pattern of fracture a semi-open or open reduction should be performed. When there is a depressed area of the posterior facet with only one fragment, reduction may be performed by a semi-open technique. A Steinmann pin is inserted into the calcaneus carefully avoiding the apophysis. Via an incision 1 cm below the displaced posterior facet a pusher screw is introduced. The pin is used to correct the shortening and varus deformity, the pusher screw straightens the displaced posterior facet and the percutaneous K-wires stabilize the intraarticular surface. The K-wires are left in situ for 4–6 weeks.

When there is a comminuted fracture of the posterior facet open reduction and internal fixation with a titanium plate are recommended (Fig. 51.5).

Fractures of the Midtarsal Bones

Injuries of the midfoot area are rare in children due to the relative shortness of the midtarsal bones and low body weight. The most common mechanism of injury is a crushing injury or direct force during a vehicle accident. Fractures of the midtarsal bones are often associated with injuries to the tarsometatarsal joint (so called Lisfranc joint) or the talonavicular/calcaneocuboid joint(so-called Chopart joint).

Fractures of the Navicular

Fractures of the navicular bone are rare and associated subluxation or dislocation is uncommon (Fig. 51.6). They are sometimes associated with displacement of the talonavicular/calcaneocuboid (Chopart) joint. Forced supination of the forefoot is thought to be the cause of this displacement. The aim of the treatment is to restore the medial and lateral columns using K-wire fixation. The blood supply to the navicular comes from the medial cuneiform and the talus. Variations in the appearance of the ossification center can be mistaken for a fracture particularly when associated with

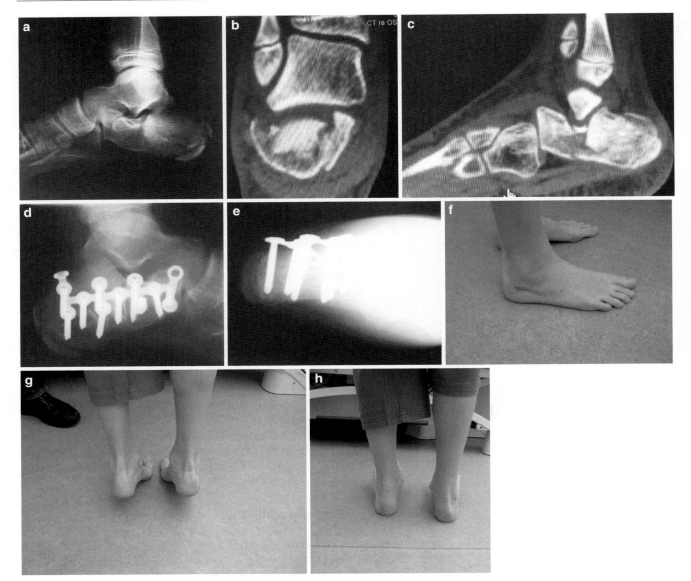

Fig. 51.5 (**a**) Thirteen-year-old boy with a comminuted fracture of the calcaneus. (**b** and **c**) There is considerable shortening and varus deformity on the CT scan. Multiple fragments with a considerable displacement of the posterior joint facet. (**d** and **e**) Open reduction and fixation using a plate. (**f**, **g** and **h**) Clinical picture 11/2 years after fracture. The patient has fully recovered and plays soccer

pain and local swelling as in osteochondritis of the tarsal navicular (Köhler's disease) (see Chapter 30) which is typically seen between the ages of 3 and 7 years.

Fractures of the Cuboid and Cuneiform Bones

The rare fractures of the cuboid are caused by compression. Fractures of the cuboid and cuneiform bones may be associated with dislocation of the Chopart joint. Compression force may cause shortening of the lateral column of the foot. Open or semi-open reduction and K-wire fixation is the treatment of choice.

Tarsometatarsal Injuries

Fracture/Dislocations of the Talonavicular/Calcaneocuboid (Chopart) and Tarsometatarsal (Lisfranc) Joints

Fracture/dislocations of the Chopart and Lisfranc joints are rare in childhood [23, 24]. The incidence in adults is between 0.02 and 0.9% of all fractures [25, 26]. Injuries of the Lisfranc joint are more common than those of the Chopart joint. In children these injuries are even less frequent.

Fig. 51.6 Ten-year-old gril following an injury on a sledge compression fracture of the navicular bone. Treatment in a below-knee cast for 6 weeks

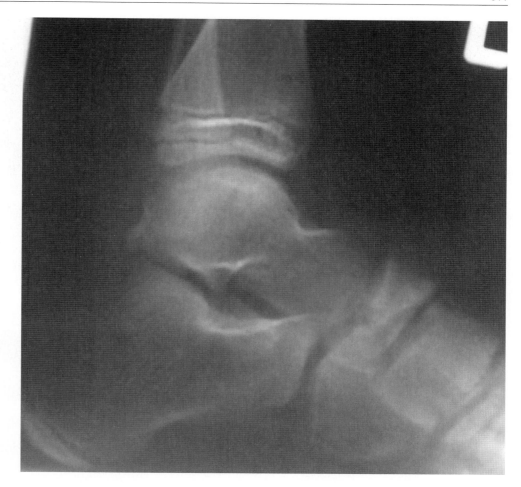

Mechanism of Injury

Fracture/dislocations of the Lisfranc joint are caused by a fall with the foot in a fixed plantarflexed position, a crush injury in a kneeling child, or being run over by a vehicle. The injury is associated with considerable soft tissue damage. The causes of injury to the Chopart joint are falls from a great height, or being run over by motor vehicles (Fig. 51.7)[27].

Classification of Lisfranc Fracture Dislocation

Fracture/dislocations of the Lisfranc joint were classified in 1909 by Quenu and Küss [28]. Zwipp [29] has suggested the following classification for tarsometatarsal fracture/dislocations:

1. Transligamental
2. Transcalcaneal
3. Transcuboidal
4. Transnavicular
5. Transtalar
6. Combination of injuries

Imaging

Three standard radiographic views are suggested for suspected Lisfranc injuries: a true lateral of the foot, a dorsoplantar view of the foot with a caudocranial angle of the X-ray tube of 20°, and a 45° angular view. If there is any doubt concerning a fracture/dislocation of the Lisfranc joint, a CT scan is advised.

For a Chopart joint injury again three views are suggested: a dorsoplantar view with the tube flexed 30°, a 45° angular view, and a true lateral view of the foot. Due to overlap of the tarsal bones interpretation can be difficult and if available, a CT scan is useful.

Treatment

In fracture/dislocation of the Lisfranc joint, the medial and lateral columns and the arch of foot should be reconstructed. The joint has suffered complex bone and ligament injury. If unrecognized and untreated, displacement of the Lisfranc joint produces malalignment of the mid and forefoot, which

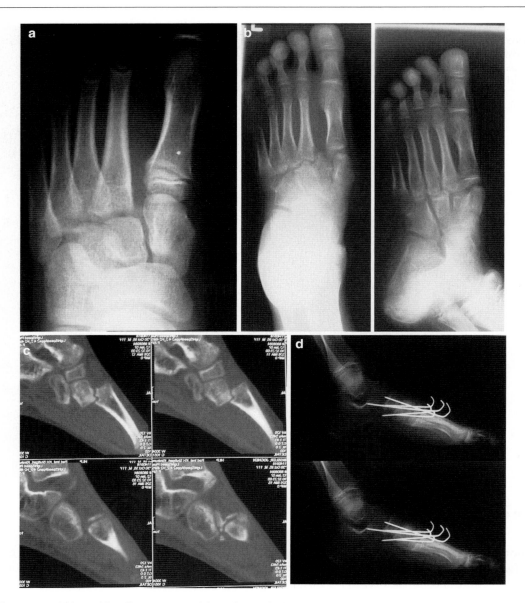

Fig. 51.7 **a**) Eleven-year-old boy with a divergent type Lisfranc fracture. (**b**) The diagnosis of a divergent Lisfranc fracture was not made until 2 months later. (**c**) The CT scans show the extent of the injury including fragmentation of the metatarsal base. (**d**) After open reduction of the fracture and K-wire fixation

causes considerable pain and discomfort. An anatomical reduction should be obtained if possible. If there is instability and a tendency to redisplace, percutaneous K-wire fixation is necessary. The interposition of soft tissue can prevent closed reduction and necessitate open reduction. The key to both closed and open reduction is the second metatarsal bone. The base of the second metatarsal must be correctly aligned with the intermediate (second) cuneiform bone.

Fracture/dislocations of the Chopart joint can be treated conservatively but if closed reduction fails open reduction is necessary followed by transarticular K-wire fixation and cast immobilization for 4 weeks.

Fractures of the Metatarsals

Metatarsal fractures are the second most common injuries to the foot after fractures of the phalanges. Single fractures result from direct or indirect force, while multiple fractures are commonly due to bicycle spoke injuries, participating in sports, or by run over injuries [30].

Single fractures are often minimally displaced and can be treated conservatively. Multiple fractures when displaced up to $\frac{1}{2}$ the diameter of the shaft may also be treated conservatively.

Fig. 51.8 (a) Eleven-year-old girl with displaced metatarsal fractures II–IV after a fall from a bicycle. (b) Closed reduction and percutaneous K-wire fixation

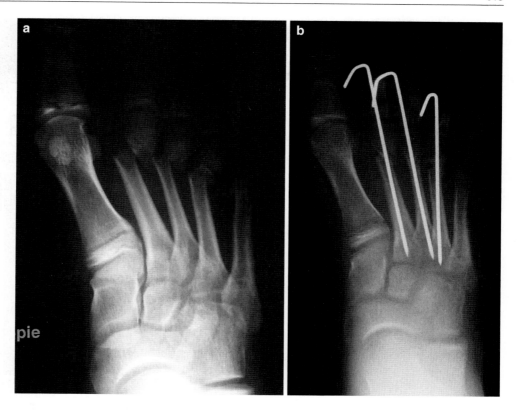

In children older than 10 years K-wire fixation may be indicated to ensure stability (Fig. 51.8).

Fracture of the Base of the Fifth Metatarsal

Mechanism of Injury

Fracture of the base of the fifth metatarsal is commonly caused by an inversion or rotational injury and can be mistaken for a sprained ankle particularly if the ankle and not the foot is radiographed (Fig. 51.9).

Classification

The classification is based on the localization of the fracture. Zone I is the area where the peroneus brevis and abductor digiti minimi tendons insert. Zone II begins distal to the tuberosity and includes the ligamentous attachments to the fourth metatarsal. Zone III is the proximal diaphyseal area.

The apophyseal growth center of the fifth metatarsal is oriented sagittally whereas most fractures of the base of the fifth metatarsal run transversally. This helps to differentiate the apophyseal growth center from a fracture.

Imaging

Two standard views (AP and oblique) are suggested for suspected fractures of the base of the fifth metatarsal. A lateral view is needed rarely.

Treatment

The treatment of a fracture of the base of the fifth metatarsal depends on displacement and zone.

In zone I most of the fractures are minimally displaced (not more than 2–3 mm) and they are avulsion fractures. Conservative treatment with a below-knee cast for 4–6 weeks is the treatment of choice. If the displacement is more than 2–3 mm an operative fixation is recommended.

Fractures in zone II and III are divided into stress fractures and acute injuries.

For stress fractures conservative treatment is usually satisfactory. However, if there is displacement of more than 2 mm operative stabilization with a tension-band technique may be necessary.

Acute injuries without displacement may be treated with a non-weight-bearing below-knee cast for 2–4 weeks followed

Fig. 51.9 (**a** and **b**) Thirteen-year-old girl with fracture of the base of fifth metatarsal after a bicycle accident, She had no treatment initially and presented with non-union 7 month later. (**c** and **d**) After resection of non-union and fixation with two screws

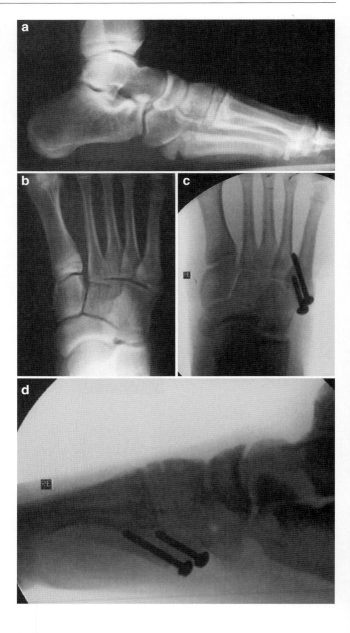

by 2 weeks in a walking cast. Again if there is displacement of more than 2 mm, surgical treatment is indicated.

Fractures of the Phalanges

Fractures of the toes (phalanges) are common. The usual mechanism of injury is crushing or direct injury to the toe. In the uncomplicated fracture taping to the neighboring uninjured toe for 2 weeks is sufficient. However, intraarticular fractures should be reduced and stabilized with one or two K-wires. Malunion should be avoided particularly in the first and fifth toes.

References

1. Anderson M, Blais MM, Green WT. Lengths of the growing foot. J Bone Joint Surg Am 1956; 38:998–1000.
2. De Valentine SJ. Epiphyseal injuries of the foot and ankle. Clin Pediatr Med Surg 1987; 4:279–310.
3. Silas SI, Herzenberg JE, Myerson MS, et al. Compartment syndrome of the foot in children. J Bone Joint Surg Am 1995; 77:356–361.
4. Höllwarth ME , Hausbrand D. Verletzungen der unteren Extremität. Das Verletzte Kind. Sauer (ed.) Stuttgart: Thieme; 1984.
5. Linhart WE, Höllwarth M. Talusfrakturen bei Kindern. Unfallchirurg 1985; 88:168–174.
6. Hawkins LG. Fractures of the neck of the talus. J Bone Joint Surg Am 1970; 52:991–1002.

7. Canale ST, Kelly FB Jr. Fractures of the neck of the Talus: long-term evaluation of seventy-one cases. J Bone Joint Surg Am 1978; 60:143–156.

8. Leibner ED, Symanovsky N, Abu-Sneinah K, et al. Fractures of the lateral process of the talus in children. J. Pediatr Orthop 2001; 10:68–72.

9. Noble J, Royle SG. Fracture of the lateral process of the talus: computed tomographic diagnosis. Br J Sports Med 1993; 26: 245–246.

10. Van Frank E, Ward JC, Engelhardt P. Bilateral calcaneal fracture in children: case report and review of the literature. Arch Orthop Trauma Surg 1998; 118:11–112.

11. Thermann H, Schratt HE, Hüfner T, et al. Frakturen des kindlichen Fußes. Unfallchirurg 1998; 101:2–11.

12. Jarvis JG, Moroz PJ. Fractures and dislocations of the foot. In: Beaty JH, Kasser JR, eds. Rockwood and Wilkins' Fractures in Children, 6th ed. Philadelphia: Lippincott Williams & Wilkins; 2006.

13. Schmidt TL, Weiner DS. Calcaneal fractures in children. An evaluation of the nature of the injury in 56 children. Clin Orthop Relat Res 1982; 171:150–156.

14. Wiley JJ, Profitt A. Fractures of the os calcis in children. Clin Orthop Relat Res 1984; 188:131–138.

15. Atkins RM, Allen PE, Livingstone JA. Demographic features of intra-articular fractures of the calcaneum. Foot Ankle Surg 2001; 7:77–84.

16. Wiley JJ. Tarso-metatarsale joint injuries in children. J Pediatr Orthop 1981; 1:255–260.

17. Schantz K, Rasmussen F. Good prognosis after calcaneal fracture in childhood. Acta Orthop Scand 1988; 59:560–563.

18. Mora S, Thordarson DB, Zionts LE, et al. Pediatric calcaneal fractures. Foot Ankle Int 2001; 22:471–477.

19. Brunet JA. Calcaneal fractures in children. J Bone Joint Surg Br 2000; 82:211–216.

20. Inokuchi S, Usami N, Hiraishi E, et al. Calcaneal fractures in children. J Pediatr Orthop 1998; 18:469–474.

21. Ceccareli F, Faldini C, Piras F. Surgical versus non-surgical treatment of calcaneal fractures in children: a long-term results comparative study. Foot Ankle Int 2000; 21:825–832.

22. Buckinham R, Jackson M, Atkins R. Calcaneal fractures in adolescents. CT classification and results of operative treatment. Injury 2003; 34:454–459.

23. Kay RM, Tang CW. Pediatric foot fractures: evaluation and treatment. J AM Acad Orthop Surg 2003; 9:308–319.

24. Ribbans WJ, Natarajan R, Avala S. Pediatric foot fractures. Clin Orthop Relat Res 2005; 432:107–115.

25. Randt T, Dahlen C, Schikore H, et al. Dislocations fractures in the area of the middle foot-injuries of the Chopart and Lisfranc joint. Zentralbl Chir 1998; 123:1257–1266.

26. Jonson GF. Pediatric Lisfranc injury: "Bunk bed" fracture. AJR Am J Roentgenol 1981; 137:1041–1044.

27. Hosking KV, Hoffman EB. Midtarsal dislocations in children. J Pediatr Orthop 1999; 19:592–595.

28. Quenu E, Kuess G. Etude sur les luxations du metatarse (luxations metatarso-tarsiennes) du diastasis entre le ler et la 2e metatarsien. Rev Chir Orthop 1909; 39:281–336.

29. Zwipp H. Chirurgie des Fußes, Wien, New York: Springer; 1994.

30. Owen RJT, Hickey FG, Finlay DB. A study of metatarsal fractures in children. Injury 1995; 26:537–538.

Chapter 52

Traumatic Disorders of the Cervical Spine

Robert N. Hensinger

Introduction

The child's cervical spine often presents a diagnostic dilemma. The presence of cervical growth plates, lack of complete ossification, unique developmental aspects, and hypermobility are causes of confusion in the interpretation of cervical radiographs in children with neck pain or stiffness [1]. Cervical spine radiographs in children are notoriously difficult to interpret. Lack of familiarity with normal growth and development and poorly positioned films make diagnosis difficult and can lead to problems in management [2].

Normal Development and Variations

Knowledge of normal physeal development is essential when interpreting a child's radiograph. Physeal plates are generally smooth, regular, in predicted locations, and have subchondral sclerotic lines. Fractures are irregular, without sclerosis, and usually in unpredictable locations. The upper two cervical vertebrae are unique in their development (Fig. 52.1); the remaining five develop essentially uniformly.

Upper Cervical Vertebrae (C1 and C2)

At birth the atlas is composed of three ossification centers— one for the body (anterior ring) and one for each of the two neural arches. The anterior ring is occasionally bifid and is not usually present at birth, appearing during the first year of life (Fig. 52.1). On rare occasions it is absent and may

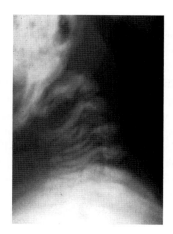

Fig. 52.1 An extension radiograph of a 6-week-old child; the anterior arch of the atlas may slide upward to protrude beyond the ossified part of the dens, giving a mistaken impression of odontoid hypoplasia. Note that the anterior portion of the ring of C1 is not yet ossified

close by fusion of the neural arches anteriorly. The posterior arch of the first cervical vertebra usually closes by the third year. Occasionally its development is incomplete or remains completely absent throughout life. The neurocentral synchondroses link the neural arches to the body of the atlas and are best seen in the open-mouth view. They close by the seventh year of life and should not be mistaken for fractures [2].

The developing axis has four ossification centers at birth; one for each neural arch, one (occasionally two) for the body, and another for the dens. In the anteroposterior (AP) open-mouth view of a young child, the dens (odontoid process) is "sandwiched" between the neural arches. It surmounts the body of the axis and is separated from it by a synchondrosis, or vestigial disc space of the odontoid. Below this are the synchondroses between the body and the neural arches, which together combine to form the letter H.

The epiphysis or synchondrosis of the odontoid runs well below the level of the articular processes of the axis. In the adult, a persistent epiphyseal line is not seen at the base of the odontoid process where fractures often occur, but within the

R.N. Hensinger (✉)
Department of Orthopaedic Surgery, University of Michigan, Ann Arbor, MI, USA

M. Benson et al. (eds.), *Children's Orthopaedics and Fractures*,
DOI 10.1007/978-1-84882-611-3_52, © Springer-Verlag London Limited 2010

body of the axis well below the level of the articular facets. Cattell and Filtzer [1] found that this basilar epiphysis of the odontoid may persist up to 11 years of age as a narrow, sclerotic line and can resemble an undisplaced fracture.

The odontoid fuses with the neural arches and the body of the axis between 3 and 6 years of age, essentially the same time that the remainder of the vertebral body joins the neural arches. Therefore, no epiphysis or synchondrosis should be present in the axis in the open-mouth view of a child over 6 years of age. The normal synchondrosis between the dens and the arch of C2 is not seen on the lateral view of the cervical spine, but is easily visible on the oblique view and should not be mistaken for a fracture [3]. The ossification center of the inferior vertebral ring (ring apophysis) of the second cervical vertebra should cause little confusion. It ossifies during the late years of childhood and fuses with the body at approximately 25 years of age.

The tip of the odontoid is not ossified at birth and it has a V-shaped appearance. A mistaken impression of odontoid hypoplasia may be given by a lateral extension radiograph in a very young child because the anterior arch of the atlas slides upward and protrudes beyond the ossified portion of the dens to lie against the unossified tip [1] (Fig. 52.1). A small ossification center, known as the summit ossification center, appears at its tip at age 3–6 years and fuses with the main portion or the odontoid by age 12 years. Its persistence is referred to as an ossiculum terminale and should not be confused with an os odontoideum [4].

Lower Cervical Vertebrae (C3–C7)

The third to seventh cervical vertebrae ossify from three centers: one from the body and one from each neural arch. The neural arches close at the second or third year, and the neurocentral synchondroses between the neural arches and the vertebral body fuse from the third to sixth years. In the lateral radiograph, the ossified portion of the vertebral body in the young child is wedge-shaped until it becomes squared off at about 7 years of age [1]. The bodies, neural arches, and pedicles enlarge radially by periosteal apposition, similar to the periosteal growth seen in long bones.

At birth, the vertebral bodies possess superior and inferior cartilage plates firmly bonded to the disc [5]. The interface between vertebral body and endplate is similar to the physis of a long hone. The vertebral body is analogous to the metaphysis and the clear space between it and the endplate represents the physeal plate where longitudinal growth occurs [6]. Clinically as well as experimentally, stress applied to the vertebral bodies results in splitting of the cartilage endplate at the growth zone in the area of columnar

and calcified cartilage rather than at the stronger junction between it and the vertebral disc.

The apophyseal rings on the upper and lower surfaces of the vertebral body begin to ossify late in childhood and fuse to the vertebral body by the age of 25 years. Apophyseal fractures in the cervical spine have been reported. The inferior endplates are believed to be more susceptible to fracture than the superior because of the mechanical protection afforded by the developing uncinate processes [7].

Mobility

The cervical region is normally the most flexible area of the spine, especially in children. It may be difficult to determine normal from abnormal mobility in a young child's neck. The most mobile articulation in the cervical spine is between the atlas and axis. Half of all cervical rotation occurs here. Some side-to-side bending is also present, but hyperextension is limited by the dens. In 3- to 10-year-old children, subluxation is present if there is more than 10° of forward flexion at C1–C2 or if the distance between the posterior spines or C1 and C2 is greater than 10 mm in the neutral radiograph. The atlanto-occipital joint allows some flexion and extension but very little rotation. The C2–C3 joint is slightly mobile in flexion and extension, but not in rotation. Thus, the relatively mobile C1–C2 joint is located between two relatively stiff joints. This concentrates forces at the atlanto-axial joint, and partly explains the high percentage of cervical injuries at this level.

The anterior arch of the atlas is firmly held against the odontoid process by the transverse atlantal ligament [8]. This space is called the atlanto-dens interval (ADI) and on the lateral radiograph is measured from the anterior edge of the dens to the posterior edge of the anterior arch of the atlas (Fig. 52.2). Further stability is provided by accessory ligaments such as the alar ligaments that connect the tip of the odontoid process with the medial aspect of the occipital condyles and the capsular ligaments. In the adult, anterior displacement of the ring of C1 up to 3 mm from the odontoid is within the range of normal [8]. When the distance between the odontoid process and the anterior arch of C1 is 4.5 mm or greater, the transverse ligament is ruptured and when the distance is 10–12 mm, all ligaments have failed [8]. Radiographic surveys of children suggest that an ADI of up to 4 mm may be normal [9]. (If the space between the dens and anterior arch of C1 is not symmetrical on the flexion view, the ADI should he measured at the mid-portion of the dens.) The larger normal limit in children is probably due to greater ligamentous laxity and incomplete ossification. A slight increase in the neutral ADI may indicate an injury of

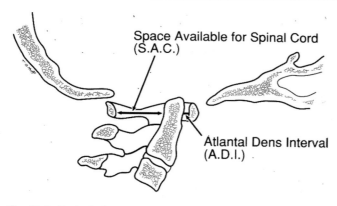

Fig. 52.2 Sagittal views of the atlanto-axial joint demonstrating the atlanto-dens interval (ADI). The space available for the cord (SAC) is the distance between the posterior aspect of the odontoid and the posterior ring of C1. From: Hensinger RN, Fielding JW. The cervical spine. In: Morrisey RT (ed). Lovell and Winter's Pediatric Orthopaedics, 3rd edition, 1990:718

the transverse atlantal ligament. This can be a useful sign of acute injury, where flexion-extension views are potentially hazardous.

The ADI is not helpful in chronic atlanto-axial instability due to congenital anomalies, rheumatoid arthritis, or Down's syndrome. In these conditions, the odontoid is frequently found to be hypermobile with a widened ADI, particularly in flexion [10] (Fig. 52.3). Here attention should be directed to the amount of space available for the spinal cord (SAC) by measuring the distance from the posterior aspect of the odontoid or axis to the nearest posterior structure (foramen magnum or posterior ring of the atlas) (Fig. 52.2).

This measurement is particularly helpful in non-union of the odontoid or os odontoideum because the ADI may be normal in either condition, yet in flexion or extension there is considerable reduction in the space available for the spinal cord (Fig. 52.4). McRae [11] measured the distance from the posterior aspect of the odontoid to either the posterior arch of the atlas or the posterior lip of the foramen magnum, whichever was closer (Fig. 52.2). He found that a neurological deficit was present if this distance was less than 19 mm. It should be measured in flexion because this position most dramatically reduces the SAC.

Patients with a normal odontoid process and an attenuated or ruptured transverse atlantal ligament are particularly at risk; with anterior shift of the atlas over the axis, the spinal cord is easily damaged by direct impingement against the intact odontoid process.

Steel [12] called attention to the check-rein effect of the alar ligaments and how they form the second line of defense after disruption of the transverse atlantal ligament. This secondary stability no doubt plays an important role in patients with chronic atlanto-axial instability. Steel defined the *rule of thirds;* he recognized that the area of the vertebral canal at the first cervical vertebra can be divided into one-third cord, one-third odontoid, and one-third "space" [12]. The one-third spinal space represents a safe zone in which displacement can occur without neurological impingement and is roughly equivalent to the transverse diameter of the odontoid [4]. In chronic atlanto-axial instability it is important to recognize when the patient has exceeded the "safe zone" and enters the area of impending spinal cord compression. At this point the second line of defense, the alar ligaments, has failed and there is no longer a margin of safety.

Fig. 52.3 Atlanto-axial instability with intact odontoid. (**a**) Extension—the ADI and SAC return to normal as the intact odontoid provides a bony block to subluxation in hyperextension. From: Hensinger RN, Fielding JW. The cervical spine. In: Morrisey RT (ed). Lovell and Winter's Pediatric Orthopaedics, 3rd edition, 1990:718. (**b**) Flexion—forward sliding of the atlas with an increased ADI and decreased SAC

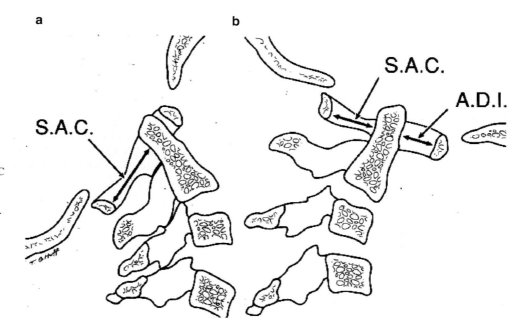

Fig. 52.4 Atlanto-axial instability with os odontoideum, absent odontoid, or traumatic non-union. (**a**) Extension—posterior subluxation with reduction in SAC and no change in the ADI. From: Hensinger RN, Fielding JW. The cervical spine. In: Morrisey RT (ed). Lovell and Winter's Pediatric Orthopaedics, 3rd edition, 1990:719. (**b**) Flexion—forward sliding of the atlas with reduction of the SAC, but no change in ADI

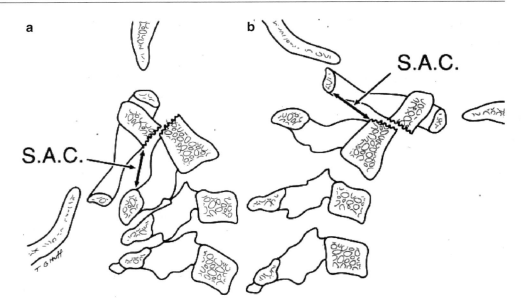

Pseudosubluxation

One of the most frequently misinterpreted findings on paediatric cervical spine films is hypermobility of C2 on C3 in flexion. While this injury pattern can occur in children, the more common explanation is C2–C3 pseudosubluxation (Fig. 52.5). Cattell and Filtzer [1] reported that 9% of children between the ages of 1 and 16 years (19% of children from 1 to 7 years) had marked forward displacement of C2 on C3 in flexion, "clearly resembling" a subluxation. Forty percent of normal children under the age of 8 years demonstrated a definite tendency toward excessive anterior displacement of C2 on C3 in flexion. While pseudosubluxation is a well-recognized phenomenon in small children, it has also been reported in teenagers.

Swischuck [13] described the importance of the posterior cervical (spinolaminar) line (Fig. 52.5) as a helpful guide to differentiate pathological subluxation from normal pseudosubluxation. The posterior cervical line in flexion and extension should have all three of the anterior edges or the spinous processes of C1, C2, and C3 line up within 1 mm of each other [9].

The facet joint angles are shallow in children. This relative flatness adds to the greater mobility and forward translational motion that children demonstrate in their cervical spine (Fig. 52.5).

Lower Cervical Instability

The criteria for lower cervical instability in the adult have been delineated by White et al. [14] in their classic study in 1975, but may not be entirely appropriate for the young child.

In children, the interspinous distance posteriorly can help to diagnose traumatic ligamentous tears. At any given level, the interspinous distance may be 1.5 times greater than the distance one level above or below [9]. Increased interspinous distance, divergence of the articular processes, and widening of the posterior aspect of the disc space are indicative of instability in paediatric cervical spine injuries [9].

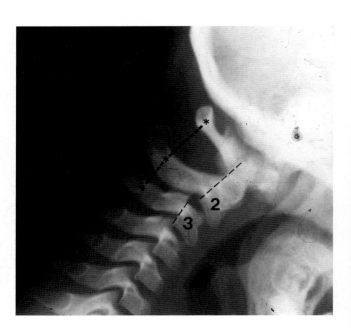

Fig. 52.5 Pseudosubluxation of C2 on C3. Hypermobility is common in children under the age of 8 years. Specific measurement of the movement of the vertebral bodies (*thin dotted line*) is unreliable whereas the relationship with the posterior elements (*thick dotted line*) is more consistent. [13] In flexion the posterior arch of C2 lies in a relatively straight line with C1 and C3. Note the relative horizontal nature of the facet joints which allows greater mobility

Retropharyngeal Soft Tissues

The space between the cervical spine and the pharynx in the region of C3 has been estimated to be a maximum of 5 mm in adults. An increase in width after trauma is presumptive evidence of hemorrhage or edema secondary to fracture or dislocation. Wholey and associates [15] suggest 3.5 mm for the normal retropharyngeal space (opposite the inferior base of C6) as the average value for normal children under 15 years. They suggest further investigation if the retropharyngeal space is wider than 7 mm and the retrotracheal space is over 22 mm.

In inspiration the pharyngeal wall is close to the vertebra while in forced expiration there may be a marked "physiological" increase in the width of the retropharyngeal soft tissue shadow. Crying displaces the hyoid bone and the larynx forward and will increase the width of this shadow.

Cervical Spine Injuries

General Principles

The cervical spine in the adolescent responds to trauma in the same way as in adults. In general, children under the age of 8 years have a higher incidence of injury to the upper cervical spine than the adolescent or adult [16]. The synchondroses tend to be involved. Facet fractures or vertebral dislocations are rare. By the age of 8–10 years the bony

cervical spine has approached adult configuration and most of the cartilage lines have disappeared with the exception of the vertebral ring apophyses. The emphasis, in this section, is on the child's spine from birth to age 10 years.

Incidence and Physical Findings

Injuries to the child's cervical spine are rare and most commonly found in the upper cervical region above C3. Hause et al. [17] reviewed 228 patients with cervical spine or spinal cord injury and found only 10 children under the age of 15 with 70% of children's lesions in the atlas and axis compared with 16% in adults. A more recent review revealed similar findings, with 68% of the injuries in C1–C4 and 25% in C5–C7 [18].

In most series of paediatric cervical fractures, there is a relatively low incidence of neurological deficit, and neurological involvement has a better prognosis in children compared to adults [19]. The younger children tend to sustain more neurological injuries than older teenage patients [20].

In young children, falls and motor vehicle accidents (52%) are the predominant etiology [18, 21]. In older children, sports-related injuries (27%) become more frequent, with football accounting for 29% of all these injuries [18]. Eleraky et al. [19] reported that neck injuries are often associated with trauma to other portions of the body, particularly the head and face (40%) [21, 22]. Evidence of head or facial trauma, especially in the comatose patient, should alert the physician to hidden cervical spine injury (Fig. 52.6). Furnival et al. [23]

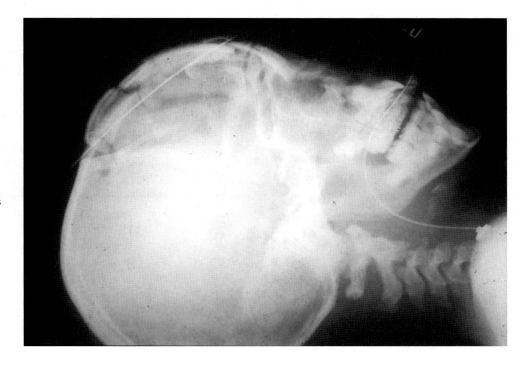

Fig. 52.6 Supine lateral radiograph of a 6-year-old child struck by an automobile. There is an unstable teardrop fracture of the body of C3, with kyphosis at the fracture site (C3). Cervical injuries in children are often associated with head or facial trauma as seen in this case of a massive depressed skull fracture. From: Herzenberg JE, Hensinger RN. Pediatric cervical spine injuries. Trauma Quarterly 1989; 5:73–81. Used with permission

reported a high incidence of neck injuries with the use of trampolines. Gonzalez et al. [24] noted that clinical examination of the neck may help to determine significant cervical spine injury in the awake and alert blunt trauma patient. Somatosensory evoked potentials (SSEPs) can be helpful in detecting a spinal cord injury, especially in children with head injuries and in a comatose patient [16].

Radiological Evaluation

Rachesky et al. [25] attempted to identify which injured children require cervical radiographs by reviewing a large series (2133), in which 25 (1.2%) had a documented cervical spine injury They concluded that cervical spine radiographs were indicated if the child had complained of neck pain or if there was head or facial trauma associated with a motor vehicle accident (Fig. 52.6). Whenever the diagnosis of a localized cervical spine injury is made, a careful examination should be made of the remaining cervical spine, as in children there is a high incidence (24%) of multiple level injury (Fig. 52.7). Avellino et al. [2] reported on the misdiagnosis of synchondroses and cervical spine injuries in children over a 12-year period and found that 19% of these injuries were misdiagnosed; 5% were missed fractures and 14% were normal or developmental variations interpreted to be fractures or dislocations. The error rate for infants and children under 8 years of age was 24%, while for children over 9 years of age the error rate was 15%. The occiput to C2 region was the most common site of diagnostic error, including the hangman's fracture or missed C1 ring fracture of the spine.

Further imaging, particularly flexion-extension lateral radiographs, may be required to assess stability. Tomograms

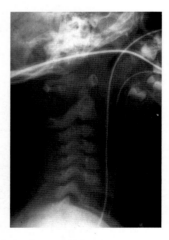

Fig. 52.7 Cervical injury in a 3-year-old. Initial lateral radiograph in traction demonstrating multiple injuries of the cervical spine. Note the distraction at occiput-C1, C1–C2, and C6–C7

have been used to assess the extent of the bony injury, but have been largely replaced by computed tomography (CT). In the past, CT was not recommended as a screening tool [26]. Sanchez et al. [27] recommend using helical CT scans and eliminating plain radiographs. Selective use of CT scanning increased the accuracy of detecting cervical spine injuries from 54 to 100%.

CT may identify occult fractures in the posterior elements that are not clearly seen or appreciated on radiographs. As there is such a high incidence of cervical spine injuries in patients with severe, blunt multiple injury, CT scan can be helpful particularly in the intensive care unit. Woodring noted that, while CT scans were particularly helpful for C1–C2 problems, plain films were better at detecting fractures of the vertebral body, dens, and spinous processes, and subluxation and dislocation [28]. However, plain films may show a vertebral body fracture where CT would show an additional fracture through the posterior elements of the same vertebra. CT is recommended for all fractures of C1 and C7-T1 when plain films are not helpful [29] and for surgical planning. If the patient has a normal CT scan, but a neurological deficit is present, then magnetic resonance imaging (MRI) should be used [27].

CT scans, particularly with flexion and extension views, are very useful to demonstrate atlanto-occipital dislocation, subluxation of the vertebral bodies, and fractures of the lateral masses and processes.

Spinal Cord Injury Without Observable Radiographic Abnormalities

It is well recognized that children may have partial or complete paralysis without radiographic evidence of spine fracture or dislocation. Pang and Wilberger [30] coined the phrase "spinal cord injury without observable radiographic abnormalities" (SCIWORA). Yngve et al.[31] reported SCIWORA in 16 of 17 spinal cord injured children and noted that they tended to be younger than those with osseous fracture. Young children with SCIWORA typically have more severe neurological injury than older children [30–32].

MRI demonstrates parenchymal spinal cord injuries (Fig. 52.8) and disc herniation better than CT. Katzberg et al. [33] noted that MRI is more accurate than radiography in the detection of a wide spectrum of neck injuries [34]. It is superior for hemorrhage, edema, anterior/posterior longitudinal ligament injury, traumatic disc herniation, cord edema, and cord compression. CT remains preferable for the classification of bony injuries. In one study, the predominant neurological presentation of SCIWORA was a mild neurological deficit that resolved within 72 h [35]. MRI revealed

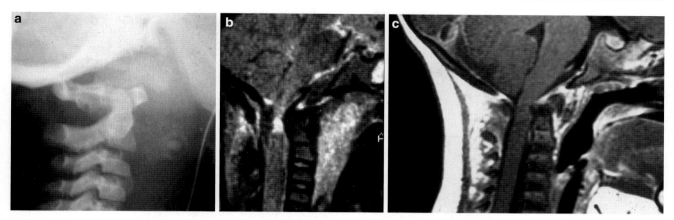

Fig. 52.8 (**a** and **b**) A 9-year-old who sustained an occiput-C1 dislocation in a motor vehicle accident. (**a**) Lateral radiograph demonstrating vertical displacement between the occiput and the ring of C1. (**b**) MRI of the same patient demonstrating a complete spinal cord injury at the level of occiput-C1. (**c**) CT scan of a 2-year-old male who was involved in a motor vehicle accident and sustained a fracture of the odontoid and a C1–C2 dislocation, which resulted in complete quadriplegia

abnormal features only in those patients with complete neurological deficits. These findings suggest that in the acute setting conventional MR images may lack the sensitivity to demonstrate neural and extraneural abnormalities associated with partial or temporary neurological deficits of SCIWORA even when those deficits persist beyond 72 h. MRI helps to exclude lesions that may require emergency decompression, such as hematomas and disc herniations and it serves as a prognosticator for neurological recovery [35]. Some children do not have paralysis immediately after trauma, but only after a latent period of 30 min to 4 days, apparently in the absence of further trauma. In Pang's study [16], the recurrent injury occurred mostly during the first 2 weeks after the initial SCIWORA, but one child had her recurrent injury at 10 weeks. In one large series, most patients' neurological status stabilized, but those who did develop a recurrence recovered back to a baseline [20]. The mean age of the SCIWORA diagnosis was 10.7 ± 4.6 years. Those who had recurrent SCIWORA were older, injured by low energy mechanisms, never had a positive MRI finding and had minor transient neurological deficits on both the initial and recurrent injuries. Twenty of 21 patients with recurrent SCIWORA were over the age of 8 years at the time of recurrence.

Every case of serious permanent SCIWORA had positive findings on CT or MRI [20] and it is very important to rule out spinal instability.

Neonatal Trauma

The normal infant is unable to support the head adequately until about 3 months of age. Infants, therefore, are incapable of protecting the cervical spine and spinal cord against excessive torsional and traction forces that may occur during delivery and the months following birth. Bony injury

usually involves the upper cervical spine, but lower cervical injuries have been reported. These forces may exceed the stretch capability of the neck. According to Stern and Rand [36], the lax ligaments of a child's neck may not be able to protect the less elastic spinal cord, possibly explaining the occurrence of severe cord injuries without skeletal injury. Spinal cords removed from newborns dying from obstetric trauma show changes over long segments, suggesting that longitudinal traction was a major factor.

Skeletal injury due to obstetric trauma is probably underreported because the infantile spine, with its large percentage of cartilage, is difficult to evaluate radiologically, especially if the lesion occurs through cartilage or at the cartilage–bone interface. These injuries commonly occur in the absence of bony injury. They are usually associated (25%) with hyperextension of the fetal head in utero and during delivery [37]. Ultrasound and MRI can be helpful diagnostic tools. Early recognition of hyperextension of the fetal head in utero and a planned cesarean section are important preventive methods. If routine radiographs are normal, then flexion-extension views are necessary. MRI is better than CT in the diagnosis of upper cervical spinal cord compression. A cervical spine lesion should be considered in the differential diagnosis of infants who are found to be floppy at birth, particularly if the delivery was a difficult one. Complete flaccid paralysis with arreflexia is usually followed by the typical pattern of hyper-reflexia once spinal cord shock is over. Brachial plexus birth palsies also warrant a cervical spine radiograph.

Caffey [6] and Swischuck [38] described a form of child abuse called the "whiplash shaken infant syndrome." The weak infantile neck musculature cannot support the head when it is subjected to whiplash stresses. Intracranial and intraocular hemorrhages resulting in death, or latent cerebral injury, retardation, and permanent visual or hearing defects have been reported, together with fractures of the spine and spinal cord injuries.

Fig. 52.9 A 4-year-old who sustained a skull fracture and associated Jefferson fracture in a motor vehicle accident. CT of C1 shows the ring broken at two sites (FX)

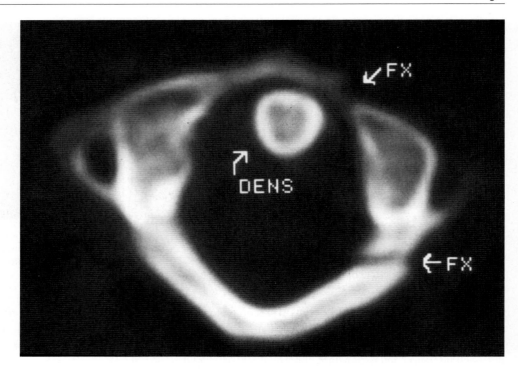

Occiput-C1 Injury

Atlanto-occipital injuries may occur during traumatic deliveries or major blunt trauma and imply an injury to the tectorial membrane and the alar ligaments (Fig. 52.8). Occiput-C1 injury or dislocation is rarely reported in surviving patients as it often results in lethal cervicomedullary cord damage [18]. Many occiput-C1 dislocations may spontaneously reduce and are initially unrecognized. These injuries are probably a result of sudden deceleration. The head is carried forward with a sudden craniovertebral dislocation and immediate spontaneous reduction and, hence, normal radiographic findings. Autopsy findings include disruption of the craniovertebral joints, spinal cord, and vertebral arteries.

For the rare individual who survives this injury, gentle reduction by positioning and minimal traction is recommended. Great care must be taken not to over-distract the injury site (Fig. 52.7). Halo fixation followed by posterior occipital cervical fusion is the definitive treatment. Chronic or late instability of occiput-C1 can be difficult to diagnose. Carefully controlled flexion-extension lateral views or reconstructed CT which allows calculation of the Powers ratio is helpful [39]. Fracture of an occipital condyle is infrequently reported and very difficult to diagnose [40].

Fractures of the Atlas

Fracture of the ring of C1, the so called Jefferson fracture, is not a common paediatric cervical fracture. The etiology is an axial compression load applied to the head, transmitted through the lateral occipital condyles to the lateral masses of C1. The ring of C1 is usually broken at more than one site (Fig. 52.9). In children, isolated single fractures have been described, probably hinging on the synchondroses, which usually heal with immobilization [41]. Fractures have been reported through the synchondroses. As the lateral masses separate, the transverse atlantal ligament may rupture, or be avulsed (Fig. 52.10), and result in C1–C2 instability.

While plain radiography may show the fracture in certain cases, CT is far superior for visualizing the arch of C1 both acutely and in the follow-up period to assess healing (Fig. 52.9). Treatment should consist of a Minerva cast or halo immobilization. Surgery is rarely necessary to stabilize these fractures.

Odontoid Fractures

Odontoid fractures are among the most common cervical injuries in children, occurring at an average age of 4 years and are in reality growth plate injuries of the synchondroses (Fig. 52.11). The injury is frequently associated with head or facial trauma [42]. It may follow trivial head trauma. Children complaining of neck pain should always be radiographed. Clinically, they often resist attempts to extend the neck.

AP radiographs are often of little value since they may show only the normal synchondrotic line. The displacement or angulation may be seen only on the lateral view

Fig. 52.10 A 17-year-old who
sustained a fracture of the ring of
C1 from a direct blow to the
skull. Note the avulsion of the
lateral attachment of the
transverse atlantal ligament
(*arrow*)

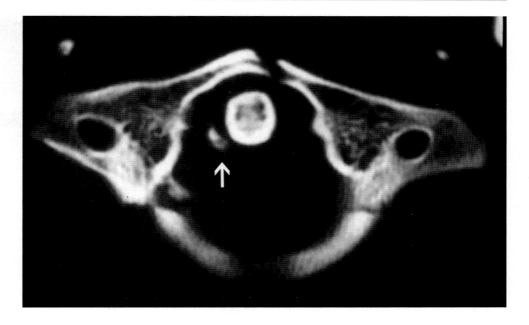

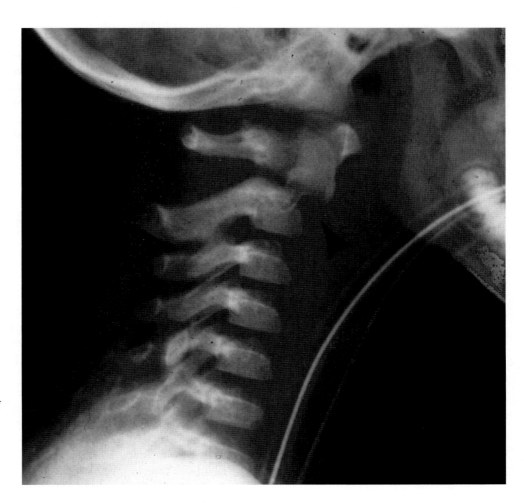

Fig. 52.11 Lateral radiograph of
a young child with a fracture of
the odontoid through the
synchondrosis. This is a
Salter–Harris type I injury and
the periosteum is usually intact
anteriorly

Fig. 52.12 Flexion and extension lateral radiographs of the cervical spine

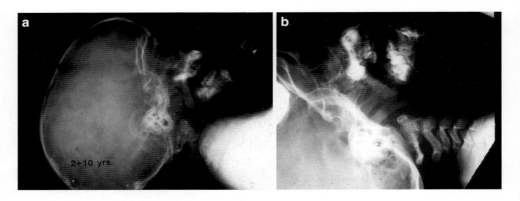

(Fig. 52.11). The displacement is usually anterior with the dens tilted posteriorly. However, posterior angulation of the odontoid process occurs in approximately 4% of normal children and should be interpreted with caution. Dynamic CT or MRI views in flexion and extension with lateral sagittal reconstruction are useful for evaluating instability [27, 35].

The diagnosis of odontoid injuries can be particularly difficult in children with underlying congenital and developmental cervical problems. In Morquio's syndrome, spondyloepiphyseal dysplasia, neurofibromatosis, osteogenesis imperfecta, and Down's syndrome dysplastic appearances of the odontoid make the diagnosis of fracture or instability problematic.

The rarity of complications and the generally good results in young children contrast sharply with complications such as non-union and the occasional late development of neurological sequelae in adults. Griffiths [43] suggested that an intact hinge of anterior periosteum might account for the apparent ease and stability of reduction in extension (Fig. 52.12) and by the early appearance of callus anteriorly.

We recommend reduction of acute odontoid fractures by recumbency in hyperextension as suggested by Sherk et al. [44], followed by a Minerva jacket or halo vest. These injuries should heal in 6 weeks. Following removal of the jacket or vest, healing should be confirmed by flexion-extension stress films. If there is no motion, then a soft collar should be worn for an additional 1–2 weeks. If reduction cannot be obtained by recumbency and hyperextension, then a head halter traction is suggested. Halo traction and, in rare cases, manipulation under general anesthesia should be reserved for those cases that are refractory to more conservative treatment [44]. Excellent long-term results can be expected without growth disturbance, indicating that the cartilage plate at the base of the odontoid contributes little to odontoid growth [5]. Connolly et al. [45] found that the odontoid fracture with anterior angulation does not need to be reduced and can be treated conservatively with excellent long-term follow-up. Many children with odontoid fractures were treated with halo vests for 3 months and did very well.

In the older child, odontoid fractures may cause instability and need stabilization with a screw [46]. Odent et al. [47] recently reported on fractures of the odontoid; 8 of 15 were secured in forward-facing car seats, yet sustained significant injuries in a motor vehicle accident.

Spondylolisthesis of C2 (Hangman's Fracture)

Bilateral spondylolisthesis of C2 has been occasionally reported in children from 6 to 18 months of age. The mechanism of injury is usually hyperextension and few are neurologically compromised [48]. Successful treatment can usually be accomplished through reduction by gentle positioning and immobilization in a halo or Minerva cast (Fig. 52.13). Surgery is only indicated for delayed or non-union union with instability. Traction is unnecessary and can produce a potentially dangerous neural distraction. (Hangman's fracture can occur with abused infants.)

Lower Cervical Injuries (C2–C7)

C2–C3 subluxation is one of the more difficult diagnostic problems in a child's injured neck. The radiographic findings may be similar to those of pseudosubluxation at C2–C3 (Fig. 52.5). The true nature of the lesion may only become apparent with time. It is important to correlate the radiographic picture with the clinical history and examination. A significant subluxation is more likely if the child sustained trauma followed by pain, spasm, limited motion, or tenderness. Persistence of symptoms after adequate conservative therapy is also suggestive of significant injury. Radiographically demonstrable abnormalities may be associated with the subluxation, such as ossification of the posterior longitudinal ligament, avulsion fractures of the tips of the spinous processes, compensatory lordosis, swan neck, or failure to correct the "subluxation" when the spine is placed in

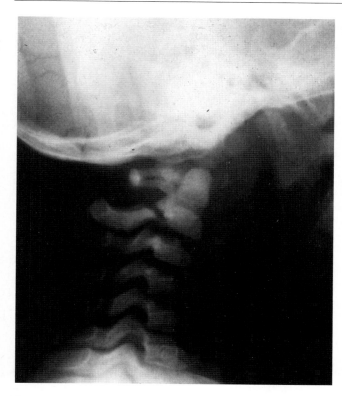

Fig. 52.13 Spondylolisthesis of C2 (hangman's fracture) in a 13-month-old boy. This can be treated with a Minerva cast in extension. From: Herzenberg JE, Hensinger RN. Pediatric cervical spine injuries. Trauma Quarterly 1989; 5:73–81. Used with permission

extension. Absent lordosis or reversal of lordosis may occur in normal subjects and is not always indicative of injury.

Injuries below C2 are less common in children than adults. Most reported injuries occur in teenagers in whom

the cervical spine is near adult in configuration [17]. Many children with vertebral body flexion-compression fractures develop a persistent kyphotic deformity. Kyphosis cannot be prevented or cured by non-operative methods [49].

Hyperextension injuries to the lower cervical spine in children may result in physeal fracture, usually through the inferior vertebral endplate [7].

Many serious injuries below C3 are associated with ligamentous disruption and initially are unrecognized (Fig. 52.14). A ligamentous disruption causes gradual displacement of one segment on the other with secondary adaptive change making reduction difficult. If such lesions are suspected, regular follow-up is recommended with protection in an extension orthosis if necessary (Fig. 52.14). Posterior ligamentous disruption has limited potential for healing and if instability is documented the injury should be stabilized by posterior fusion (Fig. 52.15).

The management of teardrop fractures, facet dislocations, etc. in adolescents is similar to that in adults.

Immobilization

A variety of child-sized cervical stabilization devices are commercially available. They can be divided generally into rigid types made out of plastic and soft types made out of foam [50] (Fig. 52.16). While the rigid types perform better than soft foam in mechanical testing, even the best device allows 17° flexion, 19° extension, 4° rotation, and 6° lateral motion. To gain more control following an acute injury, Huerta et al. [51] recommend that these devices be supplemented with tape, bean bags, and other supports.

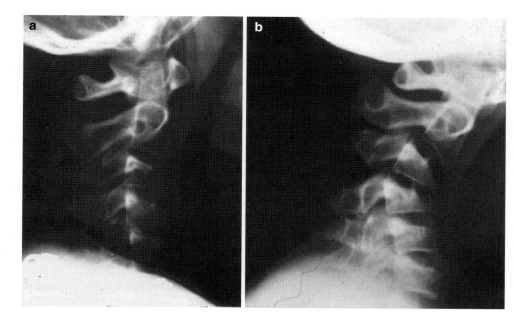

Fig. 52.14 (**a**) Lateral radiograph of a 14-year-old male who sustained a ligamentous injury of the cervical spine while playing football. (**b**) Four weeks later; note the marked cervical kyphosis at C3–C4

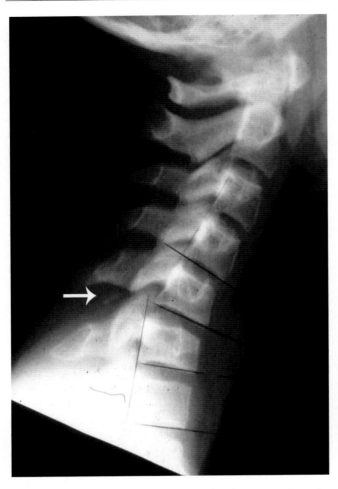

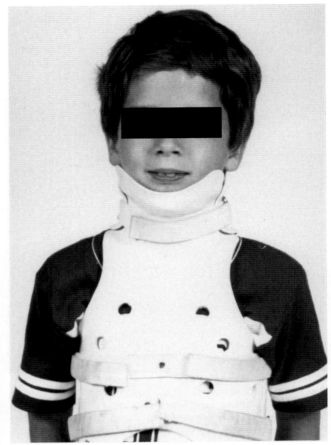

Fig. 52.16 A child immobilized in a SOMI brace

Fig. 52.15 Unstable ligamentous flexion injury in a teenage boy who fell backward while weight-lifting, striking the back of his head on a table. Note the kyphosis at C5–C6 and the small fleck of bone avulsed from the C5–C6 posterior facet joint (*arrow*). This injury would not heal adequately with immobilization alone. From: Herzenberg JE, Hensinger RN. Pediatric cervical spine injuries. Trauma Quarterly 1989; 5:73–81. Used with permission

The child with a cervical injury is at particular risk of further displacement during resuscitation. In a study of four patients with unstable cervical injuries who failed resuscitation in the emergency room, it was found that longitudinal axial traction during emergency intubation actually increased the deformity [52]. The authors recommended that intubation of trauma patients with suspected unstable cervical injuries prior to radiographic evaluation should be attempted first by the nasotracheal route rather than with axial traction and a standard laryngoscope. Cricothyroidotomy is another option.

While adults may be positioned safely supine on a flat backboard to immobilize the cervical spine, small children are different. Young children have disproportionately larger heads and are at risk of developing kyphosis and anterior translation of the upper cervical segment in an unstable fracture pattern (Fig. 52.17a and b). Curran et al. [53] showed

on lateral views of the cervical spine that 60% of the children were immobilized in over 5° of kyphosis and 37% had 10° or more. We must recognize the importance of transferring neck-injured patients safely in a neutral position: Children under 6 years should use a split mattress technique, elevating the thorax 2–4 cm and lowering the occiput (Fig. 52.17c and d). However, this immobilization protocol tends to reduce displaced fractures and makes their recognition more difficult [54]. Bosch et al. [20] do not recommend immobilization of patients with SCIWORA in order to reduce the risk of permanent neurological damage. However, the results of a meta-analysis indicate that external immobilization for 12 weeks seems slightly to reduce recurrence [55].

A plaster Minerva jacket is an excellent means of immobilizing the neck-injured child (Fig. 52.18). Thermoplastic bracing may be of value in the older child [50].

Skull tongs and halo devices can be used in the young child [56]. However, excessive pressure by halo pins or Crutchfield tongs can lead to skull perforation and brain abscess. Biomechanical and anatomical study of halo pin placement in children suggests the pins should be placed

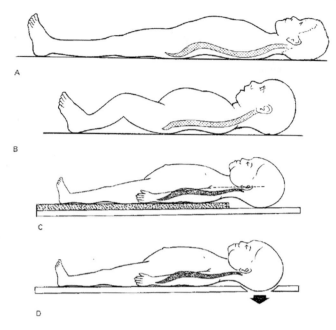

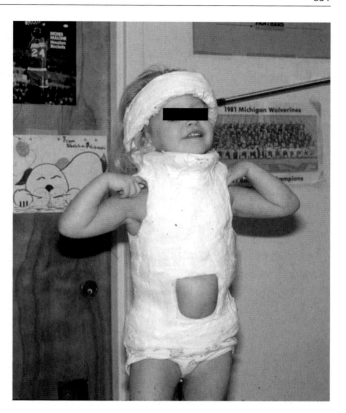

Fig. 52.17 (**a**) Adult immobilized on a standard backboard. (**b**) Young child on a standard backboard. The relatively large head forces the neck into a kyphotic position. (**c**) Young child on a modified backboard that has a double-mattress pad to raise the chest, obtaining safe supine cervical positioning. (**d**) Young child on a modified backboard that has a cut out to recess the occiput, obtaining safe supine cervical positioning. From: Herzenberg et al. [54]. Used with permission

Fig. 52.18 A 3-year-old with a fracture of the odontoid following 6 weeks immobilization in a Minerva cast

anterolaterally, posterolaterally, and perpendicular to the skull (Fig. 52.19). In the small child, a skull CT is needed to ensure there is sufficient bone for pin placement. A modified low-torque multiple pin technique allows the halo to be used in children as young as 7 months.

The halo body cast represents the most rigid form of external immobilization for cervical spine injuries in children. A halo vest does not limit motion sufficiently [56].

Surgical Stabilization

Fusion techniques in children differ little from those in the adult. Their spines fuse easily and it is prudent to expose only the relevant area [57]. Extending the dissection often leads to unwanted creeping fusion to the closely approximated adjacent laminae. Homologous bone grafting is not recommended. Stabler et al. [57] reported pseudarthrosis in six out of seven children aged 6–15 years following posterior wiring and fusion using cadaveric bone graft. Anterior cervical fusion in young children is not recommended for trauma.

Atlanto-axial arthrodesis in children is performed using techniques similar to the adult, but with smaller gauge

wire. In pre-operative planning, CT is essential to determine whether screw placement is feasible: Anderson et al. [58] recommend thin-cut (1 mm) CT scans with 2D sagittal and coronal reconstructions. Some type of stereotactic or other planning workstation helps to determine safe screw trajectories. C1–2 transarticular screws are the first choice whenever possible. They demonstrate resistance to all three planes of movement. This construct has provided excellent outcomes in adults and in a large number of children. The technique is not possible in 7–22% of patients because of variable location of the foramen transversarium and vulnerability of the vertebral artery [58–61]. Alternatives, which combine C1 lateral mass screws and C2 pars screws or C2 translaminar and subaxial lateral mass screws have been well less well studied (Anderson et al. [58]).

The vertebral arteries are locked in a groove on the upper surface of the posterior arch of C1 approximately 2 cm from the midline in the young child which leaves a narrow margin of safety. While halo immobilization may increase the rate of successful fusion, some use neither halo nor brace and report satisfactory results [58]. Many children who undergo posterior spine fusion for cervical fracture experience long-term mild chronic neck pain. McGrory and Klassen [62] reported 76% of children in a large series had excellent results after

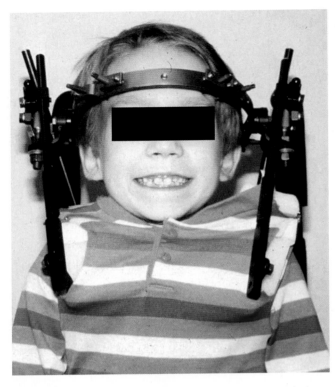

Fig. 52.19 Child immobilized in a halo cast following surgical stabilization of C1–C2 for instability secondary to Morquio's syndrome. Eight halo pins, four anteriorly and four posteriorly, help to distribute the forces on the skull over a larger area

neck fusion for fractures and dislocations. Complications included spontaneous extension of the fusion mass, continued pain at the iliac crest donor site, and superficial infection of the bone graft.

References

1. Cattell HS, Filtzer DL. Pseudosubluxation and other normal variations in the cervical spine in children. A study of one hundred and sixty children. J Bone Joint Surg Am 1965; 47: 1295–1309.
2. Avellino AM, Mann FA, Grady MS, et al. The misdiagnosis of acute cervical spine injuries and fractures in infants and children: the 12-year experience of a level I pediatric and adult trauma center. Childs Nerv Syst 2005; 21: 122–127.
3. Swischuk LE, Hayden CK Jr, Sarwar M. The dens-arch synchondrosis versus the hangman's fracture. Pediatr Radiol 1979; 8: 100–102.
4. Fielding JW, Hensinger RN, Hawkins RJ. Os odontoideum. J Bone Joint Surg Am 1980; 62: 376–383.
5. Sherk HH, Schut L, Lane JM. Fractures and dislocations of the cervical spine in children. Orthop Clin North Am 1976; 7: 593–604.
6. Caffey J. The whiplash shaken infant syndrome: manual shaking by the extremities with whiplash-induced intracranial and intraocular bleedings, linked with residual permanent brain damage and mental retardation. Pediatrics 1974; 54: 396–403.
7. Lawson JP, Ogden JA, Bucholz RW, et al. Physeal injuries of the cervical spine. J Pediatr Orthop 1987; 7: 428–435.
8. Fielding JW, Cochran GB, Lawsing JF 3rd, et al. Tears of the transverse ligament of the atlas. A clinical and biomechanical study. J Bone Joint Surg Am 1974; 56: 1683–1691.
9. Pennecot GF, Gouraud D, Hardy JR, et al. Roentgenographical study of the stability of the cervical spine in children. J Pediatr Orthop 1984; 4: 346–352.
10. Burke SW, French HG, Roberts JM, et al. Chronic atlanto-axial instability in Down syndrome. J Bone Joint Surg Am 1985; 67: 1356–1360.
11. McRae DL. The significance of abnormalities of the cervical spine. Am J Roentgenol 1960; 84: 3–25.
12. Steel HH. Anatomical and mechanical consideration of the atlanto-axial articulation. Proceedings of the American Orthopaedic Association. J Bone Joint Surg 1968; 50A: 1481–1482.
13. Swischuk LE. Anterior displacement of C2 in children: physiologic or pathologic. Radiology 1977; 122: 759–763.
14. White AA 3rd, Johnson RM, Panjabi MM, et al. Biomechanical analysis of clinical stability in the cervical spine. Clin Orthop 1975; 85–96.
15. Wholey MH, Bruwer AJ, Baker HL Jr. The lateral roentgenogram of the neck; with comments on the atlanto-odontoid-basion relationship. Radiology 1958; 71: 350–356.
16. Pang D. Spinal cord injury without radiographic abnormality in children, 2 decades later. Neurosurg 2004; 55: 1325–1342; discussion 1342–1323.
17. Hause M, Hoshino R, Omata S, et al. Cervical spine injuries in children Clin Orthop 1977; 129: 172–176.
18. Brown RL, Brunn MA, Garcia VF. Cervical spine injuries in children: a review of 103 patients treated consecutively at a level 1 pediatric trauma center. J Pediatr Surg 2001; 36: 1107–1114.
19. Eleraky MA, Theodore N, Adams M, et al. Pediatric cervical spine injuries: report of 102 cases and review of the literature. J Neurosurg 2000; 92: 12–17.
20. Bosch PP, Vogt MT, Ward WT. Pediatric spinal cord injury without radiographic abnormality (SCIWORA): the absence of occult instability and lack of indication for bracing. Spine 2002; 27: 2788–2800.
21. Kokoska ER, Keller MS, Rallo MC, et al. Characteristics of pediatric cervical spine injuries. J Pediatr Surg 2001; 36: 100–105.
22. Carreon LY, Glassman SD, Campbell MJ. Pediatric spine fractures: a review of 137 hospital admissions. J Spinal Disord Tech 2004; 17:477–482.
23. Furnival RA, Street KA, Schunk JE. Too many pediatric trampoline injuries. Pediatrics 1999; 103: e57.
24. Gonzalez RP, Fried PO, Bukhalo M, et al. Role of clinical examination in screening for blunt cervical spine injury. J Am Coll Surg 1999; 189: 152–157.
25. Rachesky I, Boyce WT, Duncan B, et al. Clinical prediction of cervical spine injuries in children. Radiographic abnormalities. Am J Dis Child 1987; 141: 199–201.
26. Berne JD, Velmahos GC, El-Tawil Q, et al. Value of complete cervical helical computed tomographic scanning in identifying cervical spine injury in the unevaluable blunt trauma patient with multiple injuries: a prospective study. J Trauma 1999; 47: 896–902; discussion 902–893.
27. Sanchez B, Waxman K, Jones T, et al. Cervical spine clearance in blunt trauma: evaluation of a computed tomography-based protocol. J Trauma 2005; 59: 179–183.
28. Woodring JH, Lee C. The role and limitations of computed tomographic scanning in the evaluation of cervical trauma. J Trauma. 1992; 33: 698–708.
29. Tan E, Schweitzer ME, Vaccaro L, et al. Is computed tomography of nonvisualized C7-T1 cost-effective? J Spinal Disord 1999; 12: 472–476.

30. Pang D, Wilberger JE Jr. Spinal cord injury without radiographic abnormalities in children. J Neurosurg 1982; 57: 114–129.

31. Yngve DA, Harris WP, Herndon WA, et al. Spinal cord injury without osseous spine fracture. J Pediatr Orthop 1988; 8: 153–159.

32. Osenbach RK, Menezes AH. Spinal cord injury without radiographic abnormality in children. Pediatr Neurosci 1989; 15: 168–174; discussion 175.

33. Katzberg RW, Benedetti PF, Drake CM, et al. Acute cervical spine injuries: prospective MR imaging assessment at a level 1 trauma center. Radiology 1999; 213: 203–212.

34. Buldini B, Amigoni A, Faggin R, et al. Spinal cord injury without radiographic abnormalities. Eur J Pediatr 2006; 165: 108–111.

35. Dare AO, Dias MS, Li V. Magnetic resonance imaging correlation in pediatric spinal cord injury without radiographic abnormality. J Neurosurg 2002; 97: 3 3–39.

36. Stern WE, Rand RW. Birth injuries to the spinal cord: a report of 2 cases and review of the literature. Am J Obstet Gynecol 1959; 78: 498–512.

37. Caird MS, Reddy S, Ganley TJ, et al. Cervical spine fracture-dislocation birth injury: prevention, recognition, and implications for the orthopaedic surgeon. J Pediatr Orthop 2005; 25: 484–486.

38. Swischuk LE. Spine and spinal cord trauma in the battered child syndrome. Radiology 1969; 92: 733–738.

39. Powers B, Miller MD, Kramer RS, et al. Traumatic anterior atlanto-occipital dislocation. Neurosurg 1979; 4: 12–17.

40. Cottalorda J, Allard D, Dutour N. Fracture of the occipital condyle. J Pediatr Orthop B 1996; 5: 61–63.

41. Reilly CW, Leung F. Synchondrosis fracture in a pediatric patient. Can J Surg 2005; 48: 158–159.

42. Nachemson A. Fracture of the odontoid process of the axis. A clinical study based on 26 cases. Acta Orthop Scan 1960; 20: 185–217.

43. Griffiths SC. Fracture of odontoid process in children. J Pediatr Surg 1972; 7: 680–683.

44. Sherk HH, Nicholson JT, Chung SM. Fractures of the odontoid process in young children. J Bone Joint Surg Am 1978; 60: 921–924.

45. Connolly B, Emery D, Armstrong D. The odontoid synchondrotic slip: an injury unique to young children. Pediatr Radiol 1995; 25 Suppl 1:S129–133.

46. Morandi X, Hanna A, Hamlat A, et al. Anterior screw fixation of odontoid fractures. Surg Neurol 1999; 51: 236–240.

47. Odent T, Langlais J, Glorion C, et al. Fractures of the odontoid process: a report of 15 cases in children younger than 6 years. J Pediatr Orthop 1999; 19: 51–54.

48. Kleinman PK, Shelton YA. Hangman's fracture in an abused infant: imaging features. Pediatr Radiol 1997; 27: 776–777.

49. Schwarz N, Genelin F, Schwarz AF. Post-traumatic cervical kyphosis in children cannot be prevented by non-operative methods. Injury 1994; 25: 173–175.

50. Millington PJ, Ellingsen JM, Hauswirth BE, et al. Thermoplastic Minerva body jacket—a practical alternative to current methods of cervical spine stabilization. A clinical report. Phys Ther 1987; 67: 223–225.

51. Huerta C, Griffith R, Joyce SM. Cervical spine stabilization in pediatric patients: evaluation of current techniques. Ann Emerg Med 1987; 16: 1121–1126.

52. Bivins HG, Ford S, Bezmalinovic Z, et al. The effect of axial traction during orotracheal intubation of the trauma victim with an unstable cervical spine. Ann Emerg Med 1988; 17: 25–29.

53. Curran C, Dietrich AM, Bowman MJ, et al. Pediatric cervical-spine immobilization: achieving neutral position? J Trauma. 1995; 39: 729–732.

54. Herzenberg JE, Hensinger RN, Dedrick DK, et al. Emergency transport and positioning of young children who have an injury of the cervical spine. The standard backboard may be hazardous. J Bone Joint Surg Am 1989; 71: 15–22.

55. Launay F, Leet AI, Sponseller PD. Pediatric spinal cord injury without radiographic abnormality: a meta-analysis. Clin Orthop 2005: 166–170.

56. Letts M, Kaylor D, Gouw G. A biomechanical analysis of halo fixation in children. J Bone Joint Surg Br 1988; 70: 277–279.

57. Stabler CL, Eismont FJ, Brown MD, et al. Failure of posterior cervical fusions using cadaveric bone graft in children. J Bone Joint Surg Am 1985; 67: 371–375.

58. Anderson RC, Ragel BT, Mocco J, et al. Selection of a rigid internal fixation construct for stabilization at the craniovertebral junction in pediatric patients. J Neurosurg 2007; 107: 36–42.

59. Brockmeyer DL, York JE, Apfelbaum RI. Anatomical suitability of C1–2 transarticular screw placement in pediatric patients. J Neurosurg 2000; 92: 7–11.

60. Igarashi T, Kikuchi S, Sato K, et al. Anatomic study of the axis for surgical planning of transarticular screw fixation. Clin Orthop 2003:162–166.

61. Madawi AA, Casey AT, Solanki GA, et al. Radiological and anatomical evaluation of the atlantoaxial transarticular screw fixation technique. J Neurosurg 1997; 86: 961–968.

62. McGrory BJ, Klassen RA. Arthrodesis of the cervical spine for fractures and dislocations in children and adolescents. A long-term follow-up study. J Bone Joint Surg Am 1994; 76: 1606–1616.

Chapter 53

Fractures of the Thoracic and Lumbar Spine

Robert N. Hensinger and Clifford L. Craig

General and Basic Principles

Injuries of the thoracic and lumbar spine in children are rare. The potential for continued growth, the presence of healthy disc tissue, the elasticity of the soft tissues, and well-mineralized bone distinguish these injuries from those in the adult. The immature spine has the capacity to remodel the vertebral body, but not the posterior elements. Restoration of height of a compressed vertebra is partly due to the hypervascularity of the reparative response and partly due to apophyseal stimulation. This probably accounts for the infrequent occurrence of kyphosis in children with multiple compression fractures.

The development of the thoracolumbar spine in children is more straightforward than that of the cervical spine. One should be aware of the following: (i) an increased cartilage to bone ratio; (ii) the presence of the ring apophysis; and (iii) hyperelasticity. In the newborn and in early childhood, the vertebrae are largely cartilaginous, and radiographically the intervertebral spaces appear widened in relation to the vertebral bodies (Fig. 53.1). With aging, the ossification centers enlarge and the cartilage to bone ratio gradually reverses. The vertebral apophyses are secondary centers of ossification that develop in the cartilaginous endplates located at the superior and inferior surfaces of the vertebral bodies. They are thicker at their periphery than at the center, and thus appear as a ring with early ossification. They are first seen radiologically between the eighth and the twelfth years and normally fuse with the vertebral bodies by the twenty-first year. They may be confused with avulsion fractures. The vertebral apophysis is equivalent to the epiphysis of a long bone and is separated from the vertebral body (the metaphysis) by a narrow cartilaginous physis. Vertical growth of the vertebrae occurs equally at the top and the bottom.

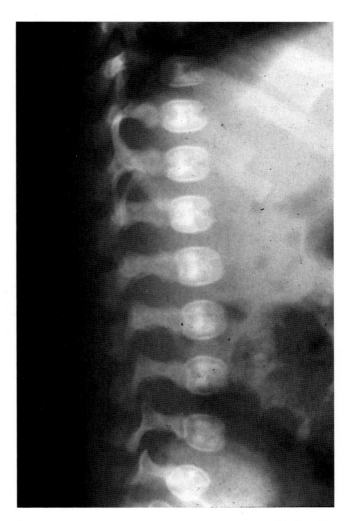

Fig. 53.1 Radiograph of a normal spine in a 10-week-old infant. The superior and inferior vertebral endplates, the vertebral apophyses, are cartilaginous. Thus, the apparent widening of the intervertebral spaces is relative to the ossific portion of the vertebrae. The anterior and posterior notching of the walls of the vertebral body is due to the normal vascular channels and may be confused with fracture

In the infant, on the lateral radiograph, horizontal conical or "notch" shadows of decreased density are seen extending

R.N. Hensinger (✉)
Department of Orthopaedic Surgery, University of Michigan, Ann Arbor, MI, USA

M. Benson et al. (eds.), *Children's Orthopaedics and Fractures*,
DOI 10.1007/978-1-84882-611-3_53, © Springer-Verlag London Limited 2010

835

inward from the anterior and posterior walls of the vertebral bodies, which may be confused with fracture [1] (Fig. 53.1). The posterior notch results from an actual indentation in the posterior vertebra wall at the point of entrance and emergence of the posterior arteries and veins. This indentation is present in all vertebrae and at all ages [1]. In the infant, the anterior conical shadow is usually more obvious than the posterior and represents a large sinusoidal space within the vertebra [1]. It disappears, usually in the first year of life, as the anterior and lateral walls of the vertebral body ossify.

Leventhal [2] demonstrated that in the infant and young child the cervical vertebral bodies function as a series of elastic cartilages which can be stretched up to 5 cm without disruption, while the less elastic cervical spinal cord tolerates only 6 mm. This differential elasticity probably accounts for the frequent occurrence in the young child of spinal cord damage without radiological evidence of bony injury, both in the cervical and in the thoracolumbar spine [3–9]. Magnetic resonance imaging (MRI) has helped to confirm spinal cord lesions in children with traumatic paraplegia from stretching or blunt injury following dislocation and spontaneous reduction or vascular compromise [9, 10].

By 8–10 years, the bony thoracolumbar spine has approached the biomechanical properties of the adult and fracture patterns are very similar, with the exception of late-developing progressive spinal deformity. Paralytic scoliosis occurs in virtually all children who sustain a complete spinal cord injury prior to the adolescent growth spurt age [11]. Possible causes include injury to the vertebral body growth plate as well as muscle imbalance, spasticity, and the influence of gravity [11–13]. As in the neck, thoracic laminectomy increases the likelihood of a progressive kyphosis by 36% [14]. Disc space narrowing and spontaneous interbody fusion after injury are uncommon in children, as the healthy intervertebral discs typically transmit the force to the vertebral bodies [13]. Thus, there is a stronger case for initial conservative management of the spine in children than in adults since up to two-thirds have a stable spine.

Incidence

Childhood spinal fractures are uncommon (2–5% of all spinal injuries [3, 6, 15–17]). While most occur in the cervical spine, significant and disabling injuries take place in the thoracic and lumbar regions. In the series reported by Reddy et al. [18], the thoracic spine was more commonly injured than the lumbar region. The thoracolumbar and cervicothoracic junctions were at risk. There was no relationship to gender or mechanism of injury. The mechanism of injury varies with the age of the patient. Neonates are more prone to cervical than to dorsal or lumbar spine injury [2, 19]. Occasionally, infant spinal injuries are due to

child abuse [20, 21]. The young child in the first decade is more often involved in pedestrian/motor vehicle injuries, as a passenger in a car, or in falls from heights [5, 8, 22–26]. In the second decade, spinal injuries are often (44%) the result of sports and recreational activities, such as tobogganing, cycling, and motorcycling [4, 27–29]. In the United States, American football injuries are the leading cause of sports-related injuries (38%) [24]. Motor vehicle accidents account for 37% of injuries [6]. It is believed that as many as 50% of children who have mild vertebral injuries are never admitted to the hospital and the reported statistics are therefore skewed toward the more severely injured [6, 30]. One should be particularly suspicious of the multiply injured child, as it is easy to overlook significant vertebral fractures. The increased elasticity of children means that the injuring force is transmitted over many segments, with multiple vertebral fractures the rule [13, 17, 25, 31] (Fig. 53.2).

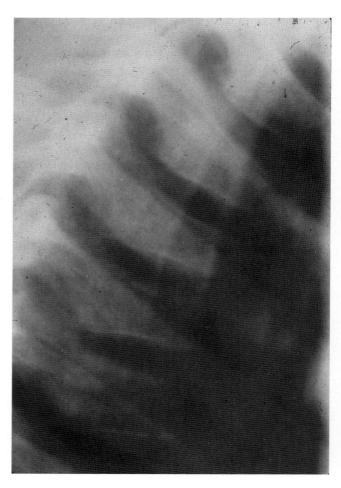

Fig. 53.2 Radiograph of a 5-year-old girl who sustained compression fractures of three vertebrae from a sledging accident. Note reversal of the normally convex endplate, beaking, and wedging of the vertebral bodies. Overlapping of the spongiosum may appear as increased density. The child was asymptomatic within 6 weeks, and complete restitution of the vertebral height can be expected

Similarly, innocuous-appearing fractures of the lumbar or thoracic transverse processes are often associated with serious injury to the abdomen (20%), particularly the spleen and the liver, to the pelvis and urinary tract, or to the chest [24, 32–34].

Mechanisms of Injury

The three-column system described by Denis [35, 36] permits vertebral injuries to be divided into four major types (Fig. 53.3):

1. *Compression fracture*: failure of the anterior column with an intact middle column.
2. *Burst fracture*: failure under compression (usually axial) of both the anterior and the middle columns.

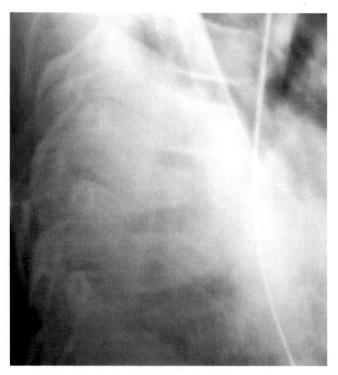

Fig. 53.4 Severe fracture dislocation of the thoracic spine in a 13-year-old male. The patient crashed in a motocross accident at a high rate of speed and was thrown 6 m. Complete paraplegia at the scene. MRI showed complete transection of the spinal cord. The thoracic fracture was reduced and stabilized with internal fixation

3. *Seat-belt fracture*: compression injury of the anterior column with distraction of the middle and posterior columns through either bony or ligamentous elements.
4. *Fracture dislocation*: all three columns fail in compression with rotation and shear of the anterior column, distraction and shear of the middle column, and distraction with rotation and shear of the posterior column (Fig. 53.4).

Compression

Compression injuries due to hyperflexion are more common than distraction, shear, or subluxation/dislocation injuries [26, 37]. In the immature spine, the intact disc is more resistant to vertical compression than is the vertebral body. Roaf [38] experimentally loaded the vertebrae vertically with a slow increase in pressure and demonstrated that the major distortion was a bulge in the vertebral endplate, with only a slight change in the annulus and no alteration in the shape of the nucleus pulposus. He observed that the bulging of the endplate caused the blood to be squeezed out of the cancellous bone. This led him to suggest that the blood in the spongiosa was a major shock-absorbing mechanism.

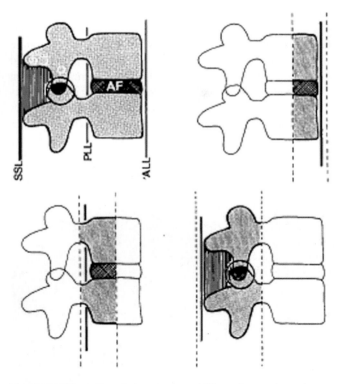

Fig. 53.3 Illustration of the anterior middle and posterior columns after Denis. Supraspinous ligament (SSL), posterior longitudinal ligament (PLL), anterior longitudinal ligament (ALL), and annulus fibrosus (AF). (1) The anterior column includes the anterior longitudinal ligament, the anterior portion of the annulus fibrosis, and the anterior portion of the vertebral body. (2) The middle column is formed by the posterior longitudinal ligament, the posterior annulus fibrosis, and the posterior wall of the vertebral body. (3) The posterior column includes the posterior bony complex, the posterior arch, the posterior ligamentous complex [supraspinous ligament, infraspinous ligament (ISL), capsule (Cl)], and the ligamentum flavum (LF). From: Denis [35]. Used with permission

With greater force, the endplate broke and the nuclear material ruptured into the vertebral body. The two vertebrae moved closer together with a diminution of the disc space (Fig. 53.5). Thus, when a child's spine is hyperflexed, such as during tobogganing or tubing, the blood is squeezed from the vertebra, the shock-absorbing properties are decreased, and less force is required to cause a vertebral injury [27, 28] (Fig. 53.6).

In older patients, Roaf [38] found that the nucleus is no longer fluid, and compression forces are transmitted through the annulus. Applied pressure then led to either tearing of the annulus with general collapse of the vertebrae due to buckling of the sides or a marginal plateau fracture [38]. An even greater or more rapidly applied force caused a bursting injury, similar to that seen in adults [39]. Unstable burst fractures are accompanied by posterior column injuries, such as the seat-belt injuries, resulting from flexion and distraction [40]. Roaf also found that the child's disc has more turgor and is capable of transmitting force through several levels [6, 29, 31, 38, 41]. Clinically, the multiple compression fractures (50–75%) typical of childhood usually occur from the mid-thoracic to the mid-lumbar areas [17, 26, 37, 41]. Roaf [38] noted that, when the immature spine is compressed, the vertebral body always breaks before the normal disc gives way, unless there was pre-injury to the annulus: then it balloons like a tire. This is supported clinically as there are few children reported with posterior herniated discs and these follow significant loading injuries, such as weight lifting and gymnastics [42]. Occasionally, a calcified disc may herniate [43, 44].

Distraction and Shear

Aufdemaur studied children killed by violent injuries (e.g., being hit by a car) and found that their fractures were primarily of the shear type [15]. Typically, the injury did not cause rupture of the intervertebral disc, but rather the vertebrae fractured through the cartilaginous endplate apophysis (Fig. 53.7). Infrequently, children may have a flexion–rotation injury combined with compression, which leads to a shearing injury and spondylolisthesis (Fig. 53.8).

Slipped Vertebral Apophysis

Several authors have described patients, usually adolescent boys, with traumatic displacement of a lumbar vertebral ring apophysis into the spinal canal with associated disc protrusion [45–49] (Fig. 53.9). Most were from the postero-inferior rim of L4 and less commonly from the inferior rim of L3 or L5. The age group and circumstances suggest that the vertebral endplate may be more susceptible during the phase of rapid growth, analogous to the slipped capital femoral epiphysis [50]. Indeed, acute and chronic forms have been described and the problem is often erroneously diagnosed as a herniated disc [51, 52]. Dietemann et al. [51] in their series noted a high association (38%) with lumbar Scheuermann's disease, and a pre-existing marginal Schmorl's node may weaken the edge and lead to the slip [52] (Fig. 53.9a).

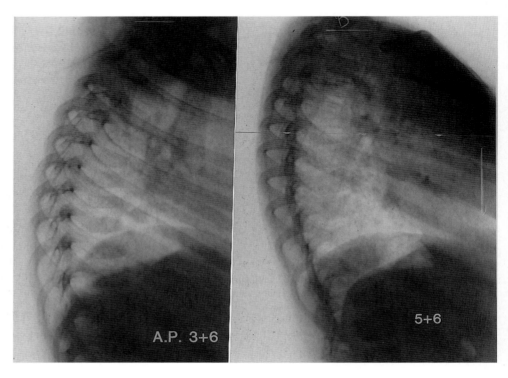

Fig. 53.5 Left: Radiograph of a 3½-year-old girl who was involved in a fall, sustaining multiple compression fractures. Right: The same patient at age 5½. Radiograph demonstrates remodeling of this injury. She was treated conservatively, is asymptomatic, and returned to near-normal vertebral height

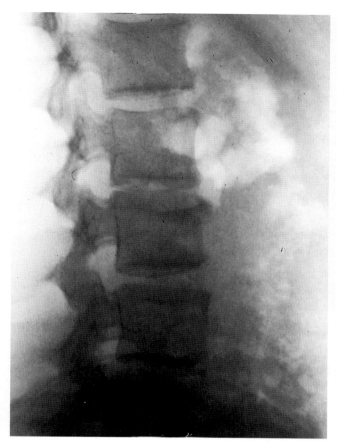

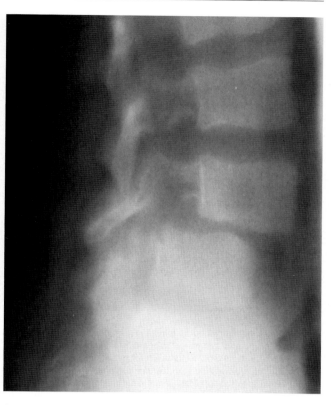

Fig. 53.6 Radiograph of a 15-year-old girl who sustained an injury to the vertebral body from tobogganing, demonstrating a fracture of the apophyseal ring and displacement anteriorly. From: Rockwood CA, Wilkin KE, Beaty JH, eds. Fractures in Children, Volume 3, 4th Edition, Philadelphia: Lippincott-Raven, 1996. Used with permission

Fig. 53.8 Traumatic spondylolysis with severe disruption of the pedicle and the facet. Lateral laminagraphic radiograph of a 13-year-old boy scout who sustained this lumbar fracture when a tree fell directly across his back during a storm. Lateral view demonstrates a shear-type injury with a fracture dislocation of L4–L5. From: Rockwood CA, Wilkin KE, Beaty JH, eds. Fractures in Children, Volume 3, 4th Edition, Philadelphia: Lippincott-Raven, 1996. Used with permission

Fig. 53.7 Distraction injury: Radiograph of the newborn with complete disruption at T3–T4. The patient was a breech delivery with cephalopelvic disproportion, leading to a difficult extraction. (**a**) Anteroposterior view. (**b**) Lateral view, demonstrating that the fracture is through the cartilage endplate. The child is totally paraplegic at that level and also has paralysis of the right hemidiaphragm. From: Rockwood CA, Wilkin KE, Beaty JH, eds. Fractures in Children, Volume 3, 4th Edition, Philadelphia: Lippincott-Raven, 1996. Used with permission

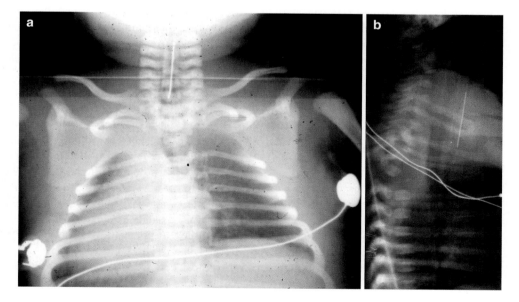

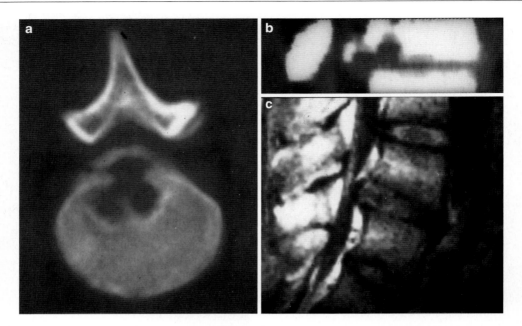

Fig. 53.9 Slipped vertebral apophysis. A 13-year-old with back pain, tight hamstrings, and symptoms suggestive of spinal stenosis. (**a**) CT scan demonstrating a Schmorl's node formation and a fracture of the apophysis with subluxation into the spinal canal. (**b**) CT reconstruction of the same lesion. (**c**) MRI demonstrating slipping of the vertebral apophysis as well as the intervertebral disc with encroachment of the spinal canal. Lateral radiograph of the lumbosacral junction demonstrates Schmorl's node formation and bony changes in the posterior portion of the apophysis of L4. From: Rockwood CA, Wilkin KE, Beaty JH, eds. Fractures in Children, Volume 3, 4th Edition, Philadelphia: Lippincott-Raven, 1996. Used with permission

Radiographically, all cases demonstrate a small bony fragment (edge of the vertebral endplate) within the spinal canal and a large anterior extradural impression or complete block on MRI from the radiolucent protruded disc [50] (Fig. 53.9c). Computed tomography (CT) has proven excellent in confirming the diagnosis [51, 52]. The onset is usually acute after an injury such as during weight lifting or shoveling [50]. The children have the signs and symptoms of a central herniated disc, with muscle weakness, absent reflexes, and limited straight-leg raising [37]. Later findings are similar to spinal stenosis. Laminectomy and decompression by surgical removal of the disc and bony ridge give excellent relief of symptoms [50, 52]. Surgical removal of the disc alone is not sufficient to relieve nerve root impingement [50].

Chance Fractures in Children

The pathomechanics of this injury was first described by Smith and Kaufer [53]. They reviewed lumbar spine injuries associated with seat belts and described the mechanism as forward flexion over a lap belt, producing distraction of the posterior vertebral elements and anterior compression. This injury was previously uncommon in children [54]. As rear seats continue often to have lap belts only, the injury appears to be increasing in children [55]. The fracture levels are primarily the lumbar spine, usually between L1 and L3, but can occur at L4 (Fig. 53.10). In children, the injury is more likely in the mid-lumbar spine, whereas in adults, the injury is at the thoracolumbar junction, which may be due to their having a higher center of gravity [56]. In the rear seats, adult lap belts do not provide protection equivalent to child safety or booster seats. In the absence of this child safety equipment, a shoulder harness should be considered [32]. In adults with this injury, there has been a high association with intra-abdominal pathology (50%), and in children, it would appear even higher [32, 55] (Fig. 53.11). Ecchymosis in a lap-belt distribution should always alert the examiner to look for a chance fracture [32]. In the series by Gumley et al. [57], the abdominal injuries were so severe that they dominated the early clinical picture and the spinal fracture was detected late. The reverse has also been reported. Bilateral facet dislocations are slightly more common than fractures through the lamina. In Betz et al. reported 30–50% of children with lap-belt injuries had associated retroperitoneal injuries [58].

Agran et al. [59] divided the 191 children who were wearing seat belts when they were involved in motor vehicle accidents into the following three groups:

1. Infants and toddlers (0–3 years): these children had proportionally larger heads and higher centers of gravity

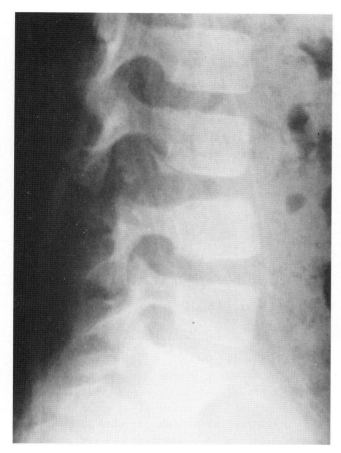

Fig. 53.10 A 3-year-old male sustained a seat-belt fracture at L1–L2 as a restrained backseat passenger. The lateral view demonstrates spreading and angulation of the spinous process and vertebral bodies, suggesting posterior ligamentous disruption similar to the chance fracture in the adult

and sustained injuries to chest and abdominal organs. He noted that children tend to undergo a rotational movement and easily become airborne and move headfirst to the side of the impact.

2. Middle-aged children (4–9 years): the center of gravity is closer to the umbilicus. The iliac crests are not adequately developed and the seat belt tends to slide up and lie over the abdomen.

3. Adolescents (10–14 years): the physique is similar to the adult.

Routine lateral views of the spine are best for making this diagnosis. The CT scan may not reveal the presence of this injury due to limitations in detecting horizontal fractures and dislocations in the axial plane [56]. Distraction and apophyseal injuries are notoriously difficult to exclude with CT scans [60]. Reverse hyperextension injuries of the lumbar spine have been described in children [61]. Similarly, a

fracture through the posterior elements alone without lumbar fracture has been reported in children and adults [22].

Neurological Injury

Between 13 and 20% of all spinal cord injuries occur in children, with higher frequencies in the young child and males predominating (2:1) [6, 26, 62]. In the cervical spine the vertebral column in the young child is more elastic than the spinal cord itself [2]. An infantile spinal canal can be stretched 5 cm, and the cervical cord only 6 mm. Similarly, many children have been reported, particularly those under 10 who have a significant spinal cord injury without observable radiographic injury (SCIWORA) [3–6, 8, 9, 12, 16, 17, 63–65]. MRI has been very helpful to identify the site and extent of the lesion and may show acute hemorrhage or edema of the spinal cord [9, 10, 66, 67].

There are two incidence peaks: (i) those younger than 10 years and (ii) teenagers. In the young child, the lesion is more often at the cervicothoracic junction [9] and the paraplegia is more likely to be permanent. The teenager is more likely to have an incomplete neurological deficit that resolves or improves [17, 62]. Choi et al. [10] reviewed patients with delayed onset of paraplegia (2 h to 4 days) and suggested that this group represents a vascular insult to the spinal cord. The location was typically at the midportion of the thoracic spine (watershed area) and usually associated with a blow to the chest or the abdomen, resulting in shock or profound hypotension from a ruptured spleen or retroperitoneal hematoma. This generally results in complete and permanent paraplegia. The MRI is helpful in delineating the lesion and laminectomy was of no benefit [10, 66].

In the older child, vertebral fracture is the most common cause of neurological injury, and in the majority (83%) a bony injury can be identified radiologically [6]. Fracture dislocations are more commonly the cause of spinal cord injury, usually at the thoracolumbar junction (36%) and the remainder between T4 and L2 [6, 17, 25, 26, 31, 64].

Symptoms and Signs

Several problems peculiar to children may result in diagnostic errors unless a careful clinical and radiographic examination is performed. Failure to recognize paralysis represents the most serious error. An unresponsive or comatose child should be considered to have a spinal injury until proven otherwise. In one study, the most common extraspinal injury was a head injury [62]. Determining paralysis or the extent of paralysis may prove difficult in an uncooperative child.

Fig. 53.11 Seat-belt injury at L1–L2. (**a**) Lateral and (**b**) AP view in a 7-year-old male. Severe disruption of the soft tissue posteriorly with forward translation of L1 on L2. This injury was associated with traumatic paraplegia (complete) and severe abdominal injuries (bowel, pancreas). Many children with seat-belt fractures have serious abdominal injuries, which can be life threatening. From: Rockwood CA, Wilkin KE, Beaty JH, eds. Fractures in Children, Volume 3, 4th Edition, Philadelphia: Lippincott-Raven, 1996. Used with permission

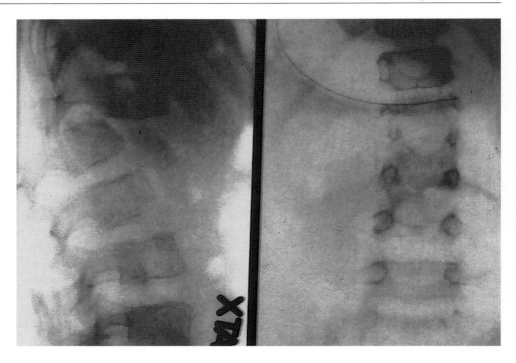

Gross flexion or reflex withdrawal of the limbs may mislead one into thinking that voluntary movement is present.

Stimulation and handling may produce crying and can lead the physician to erroneously assume that sensation is intact. Serial observation over a period of time may be necessary to determine the true neurological status of the patient. The diagnosis of birth injuries of the spinal cord should be suspected in a floppy infant or a child with a nonprogressive neurological lesion following a difficult delivery. The single most important finding is the demonstration of a sensory level. In the older child, pain and tenderness over the spine are usually present, similar to the adult. Inability to walk and muscle spasm are often present with unstable injuries of the spine.

Imaging Features

The radiological appearance depends on the force and mechanism of injury. Compression due to hyperflexion is the most common injury and can range from slight flattening of the normally convex endplates to frank wedging of the vertebrae [16] (Fig. 53.2). Hegenbarth and Ebel [25] suggested a classification of compression fractures in children based on the appearance: (i) wedge shaped or (ii) beak shaped with upper or lower prominent anterior contours. Both types may be asymmetrical on the sagittal view as well as the frontal view. There may be a zone of increased density in the vertebral body due to compression and overlapping of the spongiosa

[25, 26]. In the infant, anterior and posterior notching of the vertebral bodies due to the normal vascular channels may be confused with fracture [1] (Fig. 53.1). Multiply damaged vertebrae are the rule, but clinically observable kyphosis is uncommon unless there is a fracture dislocation [25] (Fig. 53.10). The thoracic spine is often difficult to evaluate with conventional radiographs and careful attention should be paid to this area. CT may be helpful [18]. True fracture lines are seldom seen in the young child prior to puberty (Fig. 53.6). Damage to a vertebral endplate is not likely to be severe enough to cause cessation of growth [40]. Rarely is there an avulsed vertebral corner as might be seen in the adult [26] (Fig. 53.6). With greater force, the endplate ruptures and the disc is extruded into the vertebral body, forming a Schmorl's node, commonly in the lower thoracic and upper lumbar vertebrae [23]. Typical adult fracture patterns are less commonly seen, such as complete fracture of the vertebral body and fracture dislocation and subluxation of the facets. As with the adult, CT and sagittal reconstruction are more accurate in detecting posterior arch fractures and assessing bony fragments and narrowing of the spinal canal [18, 60, 68–70]. Positioning is important, particularly in the injured child. The tomographic cuts must be at right angles to the vertebrae or the lesion will be confused with a pseudo-fracture [68]. MRI is better at detecting injuries to the soft tissue, such as ligaments, intervertebral disc, or spinal cord, and impingement of the spinal cord by the intervertebral disc or epidural hematoma [60, 66, 70, 71]. Sledge et al. [60] conclude that MRI is the imaging modality of choice in patients with thoracolumbar injuries because it can

accurately classify injury to bones and ligaments and because the spinal cord patterns as determined by MRI have predictive value. The younger the patient and the more the vertebral column is composed of cartilage, the harder it is to characterize fully a spinal injury by radiographs and CT scan. Sledge et al. [60] found that posterior fractures were more difficult to rule out by MRI. They missed two that were found on CT. MRI is helpful in predicting whether and how much a patient will improve, but care must be taken in correlating MRI pattern with clinical outcome.

Treatment

Compression fractures heal quickly with little tendency to further progression. Thus, for the mild injury, symptomatic treatment is sufficient with a short period of bed rest or immobilization with a cast or a corset [40]. Many children can be treated at home or require only a short period in hospital. In reports comparing casts to bed rest, the specific treatment did not affect the outcome, and the children were generally asymptomatic in 1–2 weeks [13, 26, 31]. Posterior tenderness in the area of the fracture occasionally persists but does not pose a serious problem [26]. If the endplate is fractured and the disc herniates into the vertebral body, symptoms may persist but can be expected to resolve with symptomatic treatment. However, the kyphotic deformity due to damaged vertebral endplates may not resolve without specific management (see section "Lumbar and Dorsolumbar Scheuermann's Disease"). Thoracic and lumbar vertebral fractures in late adolescence with no or minor neurological deficits have predominantly favorable long-term outcome, even if no remodeling capacity of the fractured vertebral body remains [72]. Sagittal spinal canal width and kyphosis increased in absolute values from baseline to follow-up at all levels, while the disc heights, the degrees of scoliosis, the degree of anterior, posterior, and lateral displacements were unchanged. Prevalence of back pain up to 47 years after vertebral fracture was no higher than expected in a general population [72].

Children who sustain an unstable injury, such as a vertebral subluxation or a fracture dislocation, should undergo reduction in the same manner as an adult with a similar injury [13, 23, 31, 73, 74]. Early surgical treatment, instrumentation, and fusion are mandatory for unstable fractures and injuries associated with spinal cord lesions. In children, a traumatic spinal cord lesion may develop a deformity that is mainly scoliotic, kyphotic, or lordotic in 90% of cases [40]. The child should be nursed on a turning frame or with complete bed rest and logrolling until the acute symptoms subside. The dislocation should be reduced promptly in the neurologically injured child, particularly those with a low

lesion that involves the conus medullaris and nerve roots. Risk of neurological injury increases with canal narrowing, at T1–T12 (35%), L1 (45%), and L2 and below (55%) [71]. The average canal compromise in six adolescents with burst fractures was 55% at the time of injury but only one had an incomplete neurological deficit [75]. Thomas et al. [41] investigated multi-level burst fractures and found neurological deficits in 80% (four of five) patients, which is substantially greater than the 65% reported in single-level burst fractures. Children with burst fractures that result in spinal canal narrowing (greater than 25%) and kyphosis are at increased risk of further canal compromise and should be considered for early correction and decompression [23, 40]. Lalonde et al. [75] found that (a) children who sustain burst fractures tend to develop mild progressive angular deformity at the site of the fracture, (b) operative stabilization prevented further kyphotic deformity as well as decreasing the length of hospitalization without contributing to further cord compromise, and (c) nonoperative treatment of burst fracture was a viable option in neurologically intact children, but progressive angular deformity occurred during the first year after the fracture. In the long term, those who were corrected lost an additional 11% of kyphosis and 12% of anterior vertebral compression. In the nonoperative group, an average of 33% worsened and anterior vertebral compression worsened on average 8%. They concluded that growth proceeded normally in the posterior column and was relatively absent anteriorly. As in the adult, spinal instrumentation is helpful in reducing the deformity and stabilizing the fracture site [11, 12, 76, 77]. Open reduction must be accompanied by a posterior spinal fusion at least one level above and below the fracture site. Spontaneous interbody fusion seldom occurs and should not be depended on to provide long-term stability [13, 31]. Injuries that would be classified as stable in the adult may spontaneously progress in the child. This is common when there has been severe crushing of the vertebral body and endplate (burst fracture) and disruption of the posterior support ligaments or laminectomy [13]. McPhee [13] suggests that this may represent a Salter type IV injury to the vertebral epiphysis, with a growth arrest leading to progressive deformity. Early recognition, reduction, and surgical stabilization will prevent late deformity [13]. In the older child, Lancourt et al. [12] have suggested extending the fusion to include the sacrum as a guard against the late onset of scoliosis. Thomas et al. [41] conclude that multiple burst fractures should be treated individually based on their clinical and radiographic characteristics. Early reduction of the deformity and surgical stabilization will prevent the problems of progressive kyphosis or late neurological injury [73–75].

Laminectomy is seldom helpful, particularly in the child without bony injury [11, 13, 17, 40, 64, 73, 77, 78]. The indications for immediate surgical decompression are the same as those in the adult: (i) an open wound (ii) progressive neurological deficit in an incomplete injury, and (iii) reduction of an unstable fracture dislocation [17, 79]. Removal of the posterior elements frequently accentuates the already unstable condition and may lead to progressive deformity [14]. Laminectomy is not a cause of scoliosis, but many children develop significant kyphosis following the procedure, which is difficult to manage [12, 14, 27, 64, 77]. It would seem advisable that, if a laminectomy is necessary, it should be accompanied by a short segment fusion. Parisini et al. [40] reported on some patients who developed significant kyphoscoliosis at follow-up. The residual deformity involved more segments above and below the level of the lesion. All the patients who progressed had inadequate instrumentation. Distraction-type instrumentation, such as the Harrington rod, was unable to stabilize the lesion.

Neurological Injury

The most devastating problem for the child with a thoracolumbar spine injury is paraplegia, which can be associated with all the problems seen in the adult: increased susceptibility to long bone fractures, hip dislocation, pressure sores, joint contractures, and genitourinary complications [4, 79, 80]. In addition, the child can be expected to develop progressive spinal deformity (scoliosis, kyphosis, and lordosis) that will significantly complicate management [11, 40, 64, 79, 81]. For many, the original injury is often overshadowed by the severity of these late spinal deformities [4]. Scoliosis seriously erodes the child's ability to sit easily, and in the young child, pelvic obliquity leads to subluxation of the hip and ischial pressure sores [12, 82]. Kilfoyle et al.

[82] noted in 1965 that "Surgical intervention is now considered an expression of conservatism." Inexplicably, this recommendation continues to be rediscovered with each subsequent article on the problem of progressive scoliosis in the immature paraplegic and quadriplegic.

In immature children, usually girls under 12 years and boys under 14 years, the incidence of progressive spine deformity following traumatic paraplegia is 86–100% [4, 7, 11, 12, 80] (Fig. 53.12). The onset of curvature has been reported as early as 3 years of age [15]. The fracture seldom determines the direction of the spinal curvature, rather the majority develop a long paralytic thoracolumbar curve believed to be due to the influence of gravity and uneven forces of spasticity [12, 82]. Similarly, on the lateral radiograph the predominant finding (57%) is a reversal of the normal lumbar lordosis with the development of a long thoracolumbar kyphosis, with its apex at the dorsolumbar junction [11, 12]. Progressive lumbar lordosis is less common (18%) and usually associated with hip flexion contractures, particularly in the ambulatory patient [11, 12, 83]. Progression of the spinal curvature is directly related to the age of the child, spasticity, and the level of the lesion [11, 12]. Children with more proximal injuries are more likely to have a progressive deformity than those injured at or below the level of the conus medullaris [4, 79, 83].

In adolescents who are nearly skeletally mature at the time of injury, spinal deformity is more often due to a fracture dislocation [11]. Progressive kyphosis and pain at the fracture site are common (42%), particularly in those who underwent laminectomy [11, 64, 81, 82].

If the kyphotic deformity is progressive, long-term neurological sequelae may develop with further loss of function

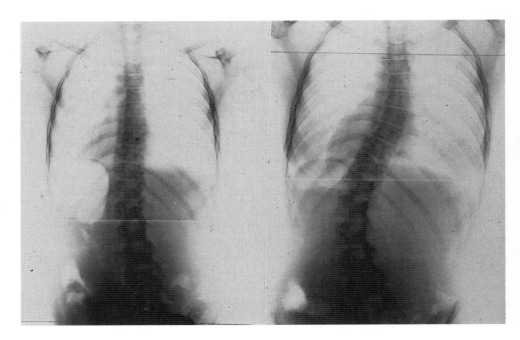

Fig. 53.12 Radiograph of a 9-year-old girl who sustained multiple trauma in a motor vehicle accident. There was no vertebral fracture identified but she had a complete transverse myelitis at T10, believed to be due to vascular injury. (**a**) AP view at 11 years demonstrates a mild collapsing-type curvature. (**b**) At 14 years the curve has increased to 50° despite vigorous management with an underarm orthosis and excellent compliance by the patient. Surgical stabilization and correction of the spine are required to prevent further deformity. From: Rockwood CA, Wilkin KE, Beaty JH, eds. Fractures in Children, Volume 3, 4th Edition, Philadelphia: Lippincott-Raven, 1996. Used with permission

from tenting of the spinal cord over the kyphus. Thus, early surgical stabilization should be considered [11].

Treatment of scoliosis should be initiated soon after the injury, prior to developing a severe curve. The Milwaukee brace has not been effective in controlling a collapsing paralytic curve; however, a total contact underarm plastic orthosis (TLSO) has been helpful [79]. Treatment recommendations are similar to those for idiopathic scoliosis. Curves under 40–45° may be controlled by bracing, or at least surgery can be delayed until the child is of optimum age [12, 19, 81]. Once the curve exceeds 45–50°, surgical stabilization should proceed promptly [11, 79, 81]. In Mayfield's series, 68% required surgical correction [11]. It is helpful if the sacrum is not included in the fusion, as this significantly increases the incidence of pseudoarthrosis.

Post-traumatic Syrinx

With the more frequent use of MRI, the relatively rare problem of post-traumatic syringomyelia is being discovered with greater frequency [66]. Symptoms can develop as late as 17 years after injury (average 4.5 years) [84, 85]. Pain is the initial symptom in over half, followed by progressive neurological deterioration, sweating below the original lesion, and loss of motor function and deep tendon reflexes are indications of a progressive syrinx [85]. MRI is excellent in identifying the lesion and Betz advocates an initial baseline MRI in these children to facilitate later detection [66, 84].

Differential Diagnosis

Child Abuse

Vertebral injuries due to child abuse are less common than those of the extremities [15, 21]. The injuries are usually due to hyperflexion and may be simple compression of the vertebral bodies, avulsion of the secondary center of ossification of the spinous process, less frequently herniation of the nucleus pulposus into the vertebral body, and rarely a fracture dislocation and kyphosis due to severe disruption [21, 86–89] (Fig. 53.13). A striking example is the report of subluxation of T12 on L1 with complete paraplegia from spanking [90]. A thoracolumbar fracture dislocation or listhesis injury resulting from abuse can be misinterpreted as an infectious process or congenital. Levin et al. [20] reported that additional skeletal findings of abuse, while present in some cases, were not universal. There are no radiological vertebral changes specific for battering. Similarly, the classic epiphyseal and metaphyseal fractures of the long bones

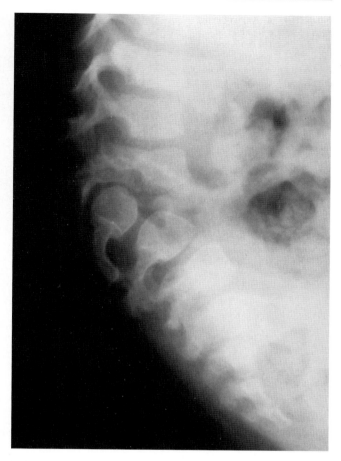

Fig. 53.13 Fracture dislocation of the dorsal lumbar junction (L2–L3), secondary to child abuse. This injury is believed to be secondary to spanking with resultant partial paraplegia

associated with battering are present in only 15% of all abused children [89]. Clinically, a high index of suspicion is more important than a specific radiographic finding (see Chapter 42).

Carrion et al. [91] noted that certain dorsolumbar junction injuries in the young child may be from spanking, representing child abuse, and are analogous to a Salter–Harris type I fracture in a long bone. The fracture is usually through the vertebral body at T12 along the neural central synchondrosis across the inferior endplate and intervertebral disc, exiting anteriorly in the superior (or inferior) endplate of L1 [91] and may slide forward [20].

Systemic Diseases

Spontaneous collapse of a single vertebra should alert one to the possibility of eosinophilic granuloma of the spine. Most of the children are between 2 and 5 years old [43]. Usually there is a complete collapse of the body (vertebra plana), and seldom does one see the lytic appearance that is

Fig. 53.14 (a) An 8-year-old with spontaneous onset of vertebral pain in the thoracic spine. The diagnosis was not confirmed by biopsy, as the clinical presentation was typical of vertebral eosinophilic granuloma. She was treated symptomatically in a TLSO with complete recovery and about 40% reconstitution. No further signs of histocytosis X were found. (b) A 7-year-old child demonstrating a rare herniation of the eosinophilic granuloma into the thoracic spinal column. The child presented with clonus and hyperreflexia. Anterior excision confirmed the eosinophilic granuloma. The lesion was bone grafted and healed without incident

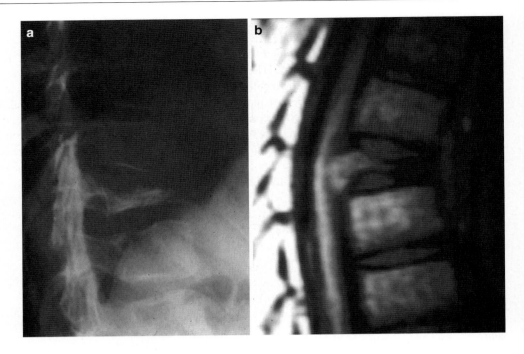

typical of skeletal involvement in other areas (Fig. 53.14). The intervertebral disc is not affected and its thickness is retained. An adjacent soft tissue mass is uncommon, and if present, it suggests an infectious process such as tuberculosis. Several vertebral bodies may be involved, and as many as 11 have been reported [92]. The prognosis is excellent with some growth in height of the vertebral body and little residual deformity. However, complete restitution seldom occurs. We have seen Ewing's sarcoma present as vertebra plana, usually with a soft tissue mass.

Multiple vertebral collapse is commonly seen in Gaucher's disease, mucopolysaccharidoses, lymphoma (Fig. 53.15), and neuroblastoma [93, 94]. The abnormal cells displace normal bone; the vertebra becomes structurally weak and collapses with minor trauma. Usually the children have visceral as well as skeletal involvement at other sites. A bone scan should be obtained to identify other sites. Typical symptoms are persistent back pain localized to the region of the collapse. Neurological complications are rare.

In Gaucher's disease[93], the bone-forming elements are replaced by an infiltrate of carosen-containing reticulum cells. This can usually be confirmed by aspiration of the marrow and finding the atypical cells [93]. One or more vertebrae may collapse, but a gibbus is rare [93] (Fig. 53.16). Schmorl's node formation may occur.

The mucopolysaccharides, chondrodystrophies, and lipidoses are similar to Gaucher's, with cellular storage of an abnormal metabolite and structural weakness. Vertebral changes are typically first noted at the dorsolumbar junction, with anterior herniation of the nucleus pulposus, and

radiologically appear as a "beaking" of the vertebral body (Fig. 53.17). Depending on the severity of the disease, the process may involve the entire spine [23].

Vertebral compression fractures can be seen in a significant number of chronically ill children and are poorly predicted by single bone mineral density (BMD) measurements and clinical history [95]. Seventy-eight percent had a history of treatment with steroids for a median duration of 13 months. Weight and BMD were significantly higher in the group with significant spinal changes. This difference was independent of the cumulative steroid dose, suggesting that increased body weight may predispose these patients to compression fractures [95].

Compression fractures are common in osteogenesis imperfecta (Fig. 53.18) and may develop serially, similar to the storage diseases. However, the children may have typical stigmata such as blue sclerae, fragility of the long bones, and deformity of the extremities (see Chapter 7). Progressive spinal deformity, scoliosis, and kyphosis are common in the severely involved children. Certain conditions are associated with systemic osteoporosis and can lead to compression fractures with kyphosis such as cystic fibrosis or as a consequence of treatment, such as steroid-induced osteoporosis in children with severe juvenile idiopathic arthritis [96, 97] (see Chapter 13).

Assessment of vertebral morphology is recommended as an additional tool in the diagnostic workup of paediatric osteoporosis [95]. Compression fractures occur with idiopathic juvenile osteoporosis, an unusual acquired systemic condition characterized by profound osteoporosis in an

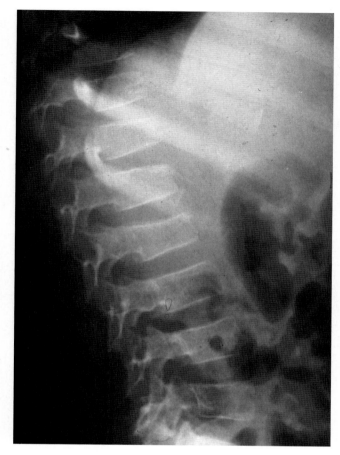

Fig. 53.15 A 6-year-old with acute leukemia who presented with back pain and multiple compression fractures of the lumbar spine. This was a spontaneous onset with no history of trauma initially believed to represent child abuse until leukemia was diagnosed

otherwise normal prepubertal child, typically between age 8 and 15 years [98] (see Chapter 7). Initial complaints are usually related to the spine and the tibia and if the condition is recognized, early treatment with a spine brace will improve appearance and reduce the degree of kyphosis and residual deformity [98].

Lumbar and Dorsolumbar Scheuermann's Disease

Scheuermann's disease is a common cause of thoracic kyphosis. The condition is seldom painful. Typically children present with concerns related to the appearance of the deformity and are found to have the characteristic vertebral changes. Sorenson's radiographic criteria, which include three or more adjacent vertebrae wedged greater than 50%, have been generally accepted to confirm the diagnosis [47,

99, 100]. Endplate irregularity, Schmorl's node formation, and narrowing of the disc space are commonly seen but are not in themselves diagnostic [101]. Lumbar or dorsolumbar osteochondritis is less common but more often accompanied by pain [102, 103]. Several authors, including Scheuermann [104], suggest that the lumbar vertebral changes are the result of trauma [102–104]. By contrast, typical thoracic Scheuermann's disease is limited to the thoracic vertebrae, spontaneous in onset, and due to hereditary influences [100]. Clinically, lumbar or dorsolumbar Scheuermann's disease primarily affects adolescents (13–17 years) and is accompanied by a period of moderately severe pain with activity [100]. Usually the children have a history of previous acute strain or injury [102, 103, 105]. The lumbar vertebral changes are often associated with hard physical labor before the age of 16, suggesting that the maturing endplate and vertebral body are more vulnerable to increased mechanical strain during this period of rapid growth [102, 103]. Hafner [106] coined the term apprentice kyphosis, or kyphosis muscularis, and he found that it occurred more commonly in boys (2:1) between the ages of 15 and 17 during the growth spurt [106]. Micheli found similar lumbar changes to be common in young athletes and suggested that the etiology was a localized stress injury to the vertebral growth plates [107].

The apophyseal bony centers appear first in the lower thoracic region at approximately 9 years of age and fuse with the vertebral body between the age of 17 and 22 years. The ring is thinner in the middle than in the periphery. In the laboratory, Jayson et al. [108] found that mechanically increasing the pressure in the intervertebral disc will force it through the center of the endplate and into the cancellous bone of the vertebral body (Fig. 53.19). The mechanism is analogous to the production of Schmorl's nodes and is accompanied by narrowing of the disc space [108, 109]. Similarly, metabolic and neoplastic diseases that lead to structural weakening of the bone are often associated with Schmorl's node formation [109]. Alexander [110] found that marginal Schmorl's nodes are more often associated with trauma and central nodes are more frequent and consistent with thoracic Scheuermann's disease [74]. Heavy lifting, especially when seated and bending forward, increases the intranuclear pressures to the lower end of the range necessary in experimental models to achieve fracture through the normal vertebral endplate [108] (Fig. 53.20). Micheli [107] noted that the flexion–extension motion of the spine seen in rowers, weight lifters, and gymnasts can achieve these same forces (Fig. 53.21).

In an acute traumatic disc herniation, the disc space is narrowed and the anterior angle of the inferior vertebra slightly flattened, giving an anterior wedged appearance. The Schmorl's node itself may not be visible on plain films and seen only on laminograms or CT reconstruction (Fig. 53.19). After 2–3 months, the radiolucent defect is clearly visible in

Fig. 53.16 Gaucher's disease. The illness is progressive with increased storage of the abnormal metabolite and structural weakening of the vertebral elements. (**a**) Normal appearance of the thoracolumbar spine at age 5 years. (**b**) At age 8 years, a spontaneous compression fracture of L1 has occurred. The patient sustained many similar fractures until her death 3 years later. From: Rockwood CA, Wilkin KE, Beaty JH, eds. Fractures in Children, Volume 3, 4th Edition, Philadelphia: Lippincott-Raven, 1996. Used with permission

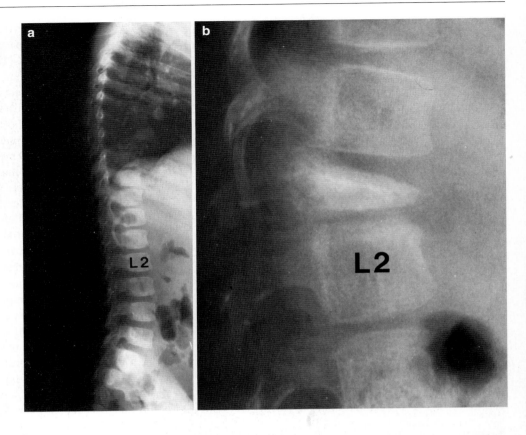

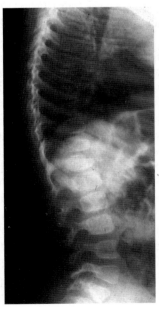

Fig. 53.17 Radiograph of a 13-month-old infant evaluated for delay in motor milestones and subluxation of the hips. Lateral view of the spine demonstrates a beaking of L2 vertebral body. This finding is compatible with a storage disease such as mucopolysaccharidosis, or mucolipidosis, or hypothyroidism. Further clinical and laboratory investigations are indicated. In this child, laboratory studies have confirmed the diagnosis of Hurler's syndrome

the inferior vertebra as the localization has been enhanced by reactive sclerosis in the adjacent bone [105] (Fig. 53.22). There is also buttressing occurring as a thin rim of periosteal new bone under the anterior longitudinal ligament. In some children the disc material may pass peripherally, usually anterior, and submarginally beneath the apophyseal ring [102, 103, 111] (Fig. 53.22). Radiologically, this appears as a separation of the triangular bone fragment from the vertebral body that represents the ring apophysis [111]. Less commonly, posterior separation may occur with narrowing of the spinal canal (see section "Slipped Vertebral Apophysis"). The defect may heal with growth, but typically the apophysis remains separate from the vertebral body, the so-called limbus vertebra [111]. The condition can be encountered at any site, but occurs most often at the dorsolumbar junction, and at more than one level [103, 106, 107].

Clinical symptoms of back pain may extend over 2–6 months, are increased by activity and forward flexion, and are relieved by rest [102, 103].

Conservative treatment such as enforced rest or bracing is usually sufficient. Occasionally, the patient will require bed rest or plaster immobilization. There are no reports of children who have required surgical intervention for the control of symptoms and only a few have required correction for deformity. The vertebral changes improve slowly during

Fig. 53.18 Osteogenesis imperfecta. (**a**) Lateral radiograph of the spine at age 4 years with compression fractures of the lumbar vertebrae. (**b**) At age 7 years, compression fractures of every vertebra, with extreme narrowing of the vertebral body and apparent increase of the intervertebral spaces representing the discs that have retained their normal elasticity. From: Rockwood CA, Wilkin KE, Beaty JH, eds. Fractures in Children, Volume 3, 4th Edition, Philadelphia: Lippincott-Raven, 1996. Used with permission

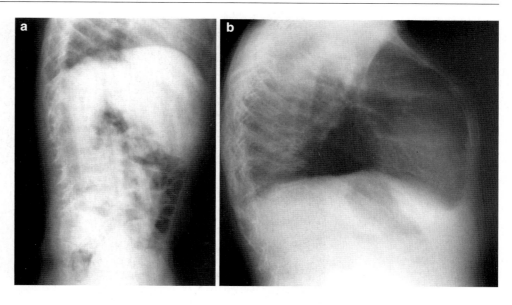

Fig. 53.19 Radiographs of a 15-year-old boy with persistent back pain in the mid-lumbar region following a weight-lifting program. (**a**) Routine lateral view suggests mild endplate changes. (**b**) Laminagraphic view demonstrates Schmorl's node formation and endplate irregularity of T11. Subtle changes in routine films may belie significant endplate changes or disc protrusion into the vertebral body

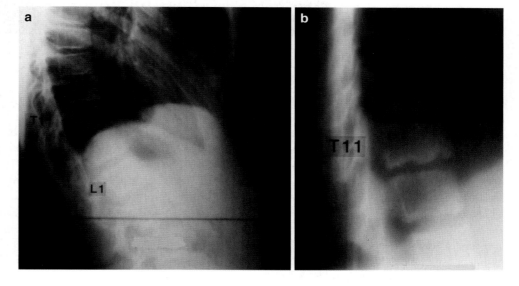

growth. Schmorl's node formation and disc space narrowing generally persist [105]. Similarly, the separate apophyseal fragment at the anterior margin of the vertebral body seldom heals (Fig. 53.17).

Progressive kyphosis may ensue due to two mechanisms: (i) the anterior deformation of the vertebral bodies from the original injury and (ii) the increased pressure on the anterior margin, which may lead to cessation of growth in that region (Fig. 53.23). However, the kyphosis is generally not severe and seldom requires any treatment. If the deformity is significant and the child is skeletally immature, a Milwaukee brace is recommended.

Traumatic Spondylolysis

Spondylolysis at L5 to S1 is often referred to as a congenital anomaly of the spine, yet there is no supporting embryological or anatomical evidence for this assumption. Despite an anatomical incidence of 5% in the general population, only one infant has been discovered to have the pars interarticularis defect [112–114]. Spondylolysis in children occurs after walking age but rarely before 5 years of age and more commonly at 7 or 8 years, suggesting that trauma is an important etiological factor [112, 115]. However, Rowe

Fig. 53.20 A 14-year-old male with back pain following repetitive injury to the lumbar spine by lifting weights. (**a**) Lumbar spine radiograph demonstrates a Schmorl's node on the cephalad portion of the L3 vertebra and on the caudal portion of the L2 vertebra. (**b**) MRI of the same vertebrae demonstrating extensive reaction to the Schmorl's node more acute in the vertebral body of L4 and more chronic in L2

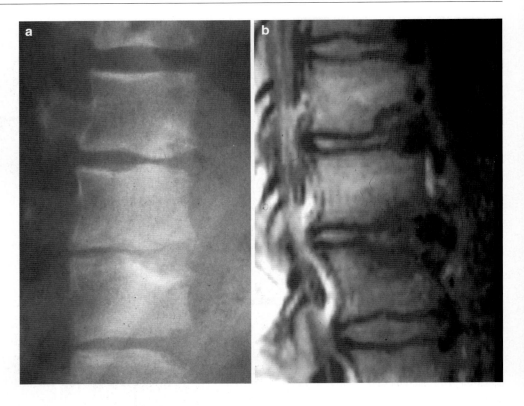

[112] was unable to produce the typical pars interarticularis lesion in infant cadavers despite vigorous flexion and extension. Hitchcock [116] could produce spondylolysis only by forced hyperflexion, and laboratory tests indicate that a high degree of force is required. A history of minor but seldom severe trauma is common (50% of males and 25% of females) and is often related to the onset of symptoms which coincide closely with the adolescent growth spurt [117–120].

There is substantial documentation that spondylolysis represents a "stress" or fatigue fracture of the pars interarticularis [121]. It is postulated that lumbar lordosis is accentuated by the normal hip flexion contractures of childhood. This posture focuses the force of weight bearing on the pars interarticularis, leading to gradual disruptions. Anatomical studies suggest that shear stresses are greater on the pars interarticularis when the spine is extended [121]. In children and adolescents the pars interarticularis is thin, the neural arch has not reached its maximum strength, and the intervertebral disc is less resistant to shear [121]. A fatigue fracture can occur at physiological loads during cyclic flexion–extension of the lumbar spine [121] (Fig. 53.24). Jackson noted spondylolysis to be four times more common (11%) in female gymnasts than expected. Some initially had normal roentgenograms and later developed spondylolysis [122] (Fig. 53.25).

An increased incidence of traumatic spondylolysis (32–50%) has been noted in teenagers with dorsolumbar Scheuermann's disease, a condition believed to be caused by excessive and repetitive mechanical loading of the immature spine [103, 123]. Similarly, dorsolumbar kyphosis is often associated with a compensatory increase in lumbar lordosis [123]. An increased incidence has been noted in those performing heavy physical work such as weight lifters, lumbermen, and football linemen [124].

Several findings favor a congenital origin. A high rate of incidence among family members and certain ethnic groups has been reported by numerous authors: 27–69% in near relatives versus an expected frequency of 4–8% in the general population [125]. There is racial and sex difference, with the lowest incidence in black females and the highest (6.4%) in white males [112]. People with spondylolysis have an increased incidence of sacral spina bifida (28–42%) and a congenital lack of development of the proximal sacrum and superior sacral facets [125].

Thus, there is supporting data in favor of both developmental and congenital origins for spondylolysis. Congenital deficiency of the sacrum and lack of integrity of the posterior structures, on a genetic basis, may predispose a person to spondylolysis. Developmental factors such as trauma, posture, or certain repetitive activities may lead to a stress fracture of the pars interarticularis.

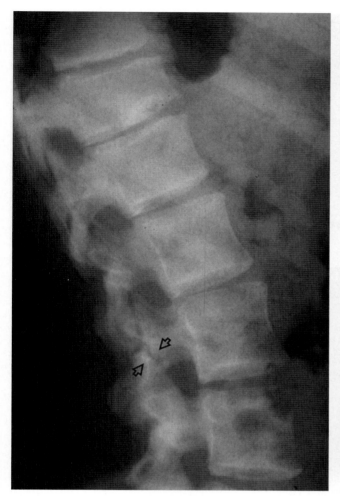

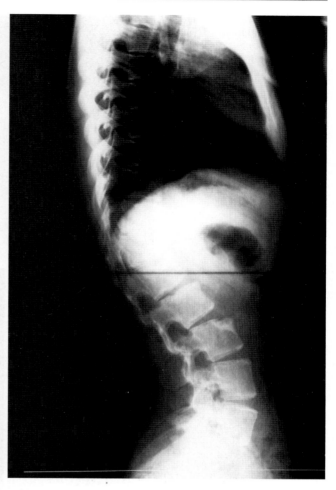

Fig. 53.21 Radiograph of a 13-year-old male who sustained vertebral endplate changes at several levels while playing football. Note the associated spondylolysis (*arrows*). The patient's persistent discomfort responded satisfactorily to bracing

Fig. 53.23 Lumbar Scheuermann's disease in a 16-year-old male who sustained anterior compression and kyphosis at the dorsolumbar junction. He had persistent discomfort over several months that responded to bracing. Note several vertebrae have Schmorl's node formation and the kyphosis is localized at the dorsolumbar junction with increased lumbar lordosis

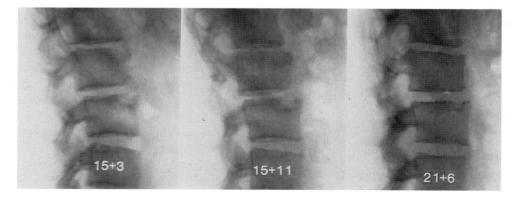

Fig. 53.22 Acute herniated Schmorl's node. (**a**) Radiographs of a 15-year-old weight lifter with back pain and Schmorl's nodes at L2, L3, and L4. (**b**) Eight months later, there has been continued growth of the vertebrae without progressive deformity. (**c**) At 22 years of age the sites of the Schmorl's nodes are still seen, although they appear smaller. The minimal wedging at L2 has not changed in the preceding 6 years. From: Rockwood CA, Wilkin KE, Beaty JH, eds. Fractures in Children, Volume 3, 4th Edition, Philadelphia: Lippincott-Raven, 1996. Used with permission

Fig. 53.24 A 10-year old with spondylolysis. (**a**) Extension and (**b**) flexion views. Note the change in the gap and the flexibility of the disc. The child was asymptomatic. He was not expected to develop symptoms until he is closer to his teenage years, if at all

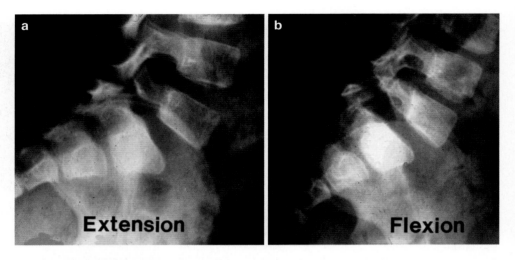

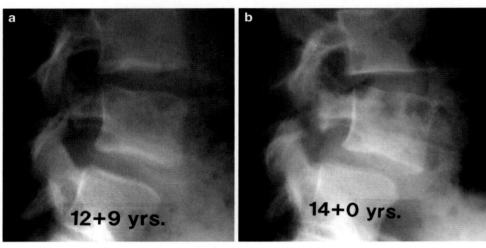

Fig. 53.25 (**a**) Radiograph of a 12-year- and 10-month-old male with normal appearance of the lumbosacral junction. (**b**) The same patient at age 14 years. Spondylolysis and grade I spondylolisthesis have developed in the interim with symptoms referable to the low back.

Spondylolysis in children occurs after walking age, but rarely before 5 years, and more commonly at 7 or 8 years. Onset of symptoms coincides closely with the adolescent growth spurt

Symptoms and Signs

Spondylolysis commonly occurs in late childhood or early adolescence; however, symptoms are relatively uncommon in children and often not sufficiently severe to require medical attention during the teenage years [126, 127]. In a prospective longitudinal study, only 13% of children known to have spondylolysis developed symptoms before 18 years of age [126]. For the occasional child who may develop symptoms, the onset usually coincides with the adolescent growth spurt [117].

Although pain is the predominant complaint in adults, a significant number of children do not have pain and are referred for a postural deformity or abnormality of gait due to hamstring tightness. If the child does complain of pain,

the pain is generally localized to the low back and, to a lesser extent, to the posterior buttocks and thighs [117, 119]. Symptoms are usually related to strenuous exercise, particularly repetitive flexion–extension of the spine common as in rowing, diving, serving in tennis, and gymnastics and are decreased by rest or limitation of activity [107, 117, 121, 122].

Children, unlike adults, seldom have objective signs of nerve root compression, such as motor weakness, reflex change, or sensory deficit [120]. However, examination should include a careful search for sacral anesthesia and bladder dysfunction. Similarly, children with spondylolysis rarely have myelographic evidence of disc protrusion, and in those explored for herniation, none were found [117, 120].

Hamstring tightness (so-called spasm) is commonly found in 80% of symptomatic patients and thought by some to be

Fig. 53.26 (a) Pars interarticularis defect, spondylolysis, as seen on oblique radiograph view (*arrow*), typically found with the isthmic type of spondylolisthesis. (**b**) Similar oblique view of a patient with dysplastic (congenital) spondylolisthesis, demonstrating elongation and attenuation of the pars interarticularis, perhaps a prespondylolytic defect, and possibly representing a "stress" or fatigue fracture of the pars interarticularis. From: Rockwood CA, Wilkin KE, Beaty JH, eds. Fractures in Children, Volume 3, 4th Edition, Philadelphia: Lippincott-Raven, 1996. Used with permission

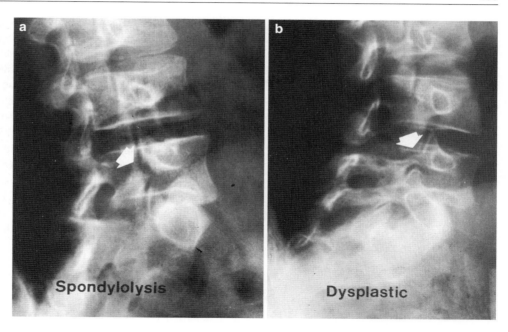

a sign of nerve root irritation but there is no evidence to support this contention [115, 120]. Severe hamstring tightness may be found in patients with spondylolysis or with all grades of spondylolisthesis but is seldom accompanied by neurological signs [115, 117, 119]. Physical examination may demonstrate some tenderness on palpation of the lower back. There may be some splinting, guarding, and restriction of side-to-side motion particularly if the condition is of acute onset. If tightness of the hamstrings is present, there will be marked restriction of forward flexion at the hips.

Imaging Features

Spondylolysis refers to the radiolucent defect in the pars interarticularis (Fig. 53.21). If the defect is large, it can be seen on nearly all radiographs of the lumbar spine. If unilateral, as occurs in 20% of patients, or not accompanied by spondylolisthesis, it can be a very subtle finding requiring special techniques such as oblique views of the lumbar spine [128] (Fig. 53.26). Particularly, in young, symptomatic patients, if oblique views are not obtained, the diagnosis can be missed in up to 20%. The "Scotty dog" of Lachapelle with the defect appearing at the neck is a helpful visual aid to those inexperienced with oblique radiographs (Fig. 53.27). In an acute injury, the gap is narrow with irregular edges, whereas in the long-standing lesion, the edges are smooth and rounded, suggesting a pseudarthrosis (Fig. 53.26). The width of the gap depends on the amount of bone resorption following the fracture and the degree of spondylolisthesis.

Less commonly, children may have poorly developed posterior structures, referred to by Wiltse et al. [114] as the dysplastic (type I), and due to the anomalous development, the posterior facets appear to subluxate on the sacral facets. This is a common finding in children who are symptomatic (26–35%) [124]. In children with the dysplastic type, rather than a gap or a defect in the pars interarticularis, the facets appear to subluxate on the radiograph and the pars interarticularis may become attenuated, the "greyhound" sign of Hensinger [117] (Fig. 53.26), and later a defect may appear in the center. Wiltse et al. [114] suggest that they are different manifestations of the same disease process, as he and Wynne-Davies and Scott [125] have found both lesions present in family members, suggesting that the spondylolytic type represents an acute stress fracture of the pars interarticularis and the dysplastic or elongated type represents a chronic stress reaction with gradual attenuation of the pars.

Deficiency of the posterior elements is a common occurrence in spondylolysis. Easily observable defects, such as dysraphic or malformed laminae, have been found in 32–94% of these patients, and if discovered on routine lumbosacral views, a more detailed radiographic investigation should be performed [125]. CT is rarely indicated in acute fracture of the pars interarticularis, as a combination of bone scan and oblique films will more reliably detect the lesion [129]. Similarly, spondylolysis at other levels, such as L4 or L3, is more difficult to diagnose with CT because the plane of scanning is parallel to the fracture [129]. MRI should be considered if the patient's symptoms or neurological signs do not resolve with bed rest. Similarly, bladder and bowel dysfunction or perineal hypesthesia justify further investigation.

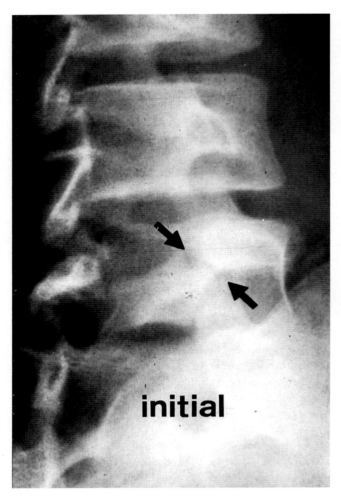

Fig. 53.27 Radiograph of a 13-year-old boy who felt a "snap" in the low back during a swimming racing turn. Radiograph demonstrates spondylolysis of the pars interarticularis (*arrows*). The narrow, irregular appearance suggests recent injury. From: Rockwood CA, Wilkin KE, Beaty JH, eds. Fractures in Children, Volume 3, 4th Edition, Philadelphia: Lippincott-Raven, 1996. Used with permission

Sherman and associates [118] described the unusual appearance of reactive sclerosis and hypertrophy of the pedicle and lamina and contralateral spondylolysis in the same vertebral segment (Fig. 53.28). They suggest that this represents a physiological response to stress, the result of repeated trauma in the presence of an unstable neural arch that will respond to conservative measures and symptomatic treatment [118]. Radiologically, this may be confused with the reactive sclerosis associated with an osteoid osteoma. This is important as excision of a sclerotic pedicle associated with a contralateral spondylolysis may increase instability. The presence of a nidus on the CT scan should confirm the diagnosis of an osteoid osteoma. A bone scan will not be helpful in differentiating between the two, since both will exhibit increased isotope uptake.

Bone Scans

Children who are suspected clinically but cannot be confirmed radiologically, particularly those in the stress reaction (prespondylolytic) stage prior to fracture, may be detected by radioactive bone scan [107, 130]. Those with small, partial, or unilateral fractures can be overlooked on plain radiographs, but bone scan will always demonstrate areas of increased bone turnover, due to the healing fracture. Positive bone scans are associated with a short clinical history and may demonstrate increased uptake in those with only 5–7 days of symptoms [130, 131]. Later the bone scan is helpful to distinguish between those with an established nonunion and those in whom healing is still progressing and may benefit from immobilization [121, 131]. The bone scan is not recommended in those whose symptoms are of more than 1 year duration or for those who do not have symptoms [131]. The bone scan is particularly helpful for those whose activities are particularly associated with spondylolysis, such as gymnasts [122]. Early detection of the stress reaction may lead to appropriate treatment and shorten the recovery period.

Fig. 53.28 Radiographs of a 15-year-old boy with low back pain. Anterior and posterior (**a**) and oblique (**b** and **c**) views demonstrate reactive sclerosis and hypertrophy of one pedicle and lamina (*arrow*), and a contralateral spondylolysis of the same vertebral segment. The oblique view (**b**) demonstrates the reactive sclerosis. Radiologically, this may be confused with an osteoid osteoma

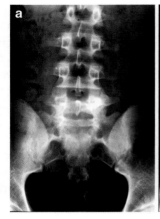
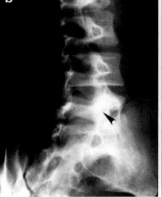
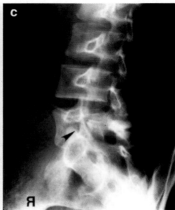

Similarly, the bone scan can be used to assess recovery and prior to the athlete returning to competitions [122]. The bone scan is not indicated once the lesion has become established, unless one suspects bone tumor such as osteoid osteoma, infection, or malignancy.

Treatment

Several authors have reported children and young adults who have been able to heal the spondylolytic defect with a cast or a brace (TLSO) [107, 131]. Typically, the children have an acute onset of symptoms and the episode of injury can be clearly documented. Unfortunately, not all heal with immobilization. However, immobilization should be considered if the injury can be documented to be of recent origin. A bone scan may be helpful to indicate a continuing process versus one of long duration [121].

Although healing is unlikely, in children and teenagers whom the spondylolysis is of long duration, can be expected to respond clinically to simple conservative measures [127]. Restriction of vigorous activities and back and abdominal strengthening exercises are usually successful in controlling those with mild back ache and hamstring tightness [127]. Patients with more severe or persistent complaints may require bed rest, immobilization in a cast or a brace, and non-narcotic analgesics. Hamstring tightness is an excellent clinical guide to the success or the failure of the treatment program. The majority of affected children have excellent relief of symptoms or only minimal discomfort on long-term follow-up [120].

Any child or adolescent with symptoms due to spondylolysis, especially those under 10 years of age, should be followed closely for progression to spondylolisthesis [127]. We do not advise those with asymptomatic spondylolysis or those with minimal symptoms to restrict their activities. About 7.2% of asymptomatic young men aged 18–30 years have a pars defect, and relatively few have persistent symptoms. Thus, limitation of activity in a growing child would not seem justified [107, 127].

It must be emphasized that it is uncommon for spondylolysis to be symptomatic in adolescence, and one should be particularly wary of the child whose symptoms do not respond to bed rest or who has objective neurological findings. In this situation, MRI and electromyographic investigation should be considered.

A small percentage of young people with spondylolysis do not respond to conservative measures or are unwilling to curtail their activities and may require surgical stabilization. If surgery for spondylolysis is found necessary, a lateral column fusion from L5 to S1 employing iliac bone is usually sufficient. In those who also have a spondylolisthesis of grade III or greater, the fusion is usually extended to L4 [127]. Nachemson [132] reported solid healing of the defect using a bone graft coupled with an intertransverse process fusion. In those patients in whom the defect is small (6–7 mm) and the degree of spondylolisthesis is slight, a variety of techniques have been described to reduce the defect directly. These include wiring of the transverse process or screw placement across the pars with bone grafting [133–136]. These procedures are usually recommended for the older teenager and young adult less than 30 years of age with a minimal degree of displacement and degenerative change [135]. The best candidates are those with defects between L1 and L4 [133–136]. This is an attractive alternative to the traditional transverse process fusion because it repairs the defect at one vertebral level rather than involving a second nonaffected vertebrae [134, 136]. In properly selected patients, 80–90% obtain a solid fusion with 80% good–excellent results [134, 136]. The Gill procedure or laminectomy is never indicated without an associated fusion in children [119]. Removal of the posterior elements may in fact be harmful, leading to increased instability and spondylolisthesis in the postoperative period.

References

1. Wagoner G, Pendergrass E P. The anterior and posterior "notch" shadows seen in lateral roentgenograms of the vertebrae of infants: an anatomic explanation. Am J Roentgenol. 1939;42:663–670.
2. Leventhal HR. Birth injuries of the spinal cord. J Pediatr. 1960;56:447–453.
3. Babcock JL. Spinal injuries in children. Pediatr Clin North Am. 1975;22:487–500.
4. Banniza von Bazan UK, Paeslack V. Scoliotic growth in children with acquired paraplegia [proceedings]. Paraplegia. 1977;15:65–73.
5. Glasauer FE, Cares HL. Traumatic paraplegia in infancy. JAMA. 1972;219:38–41.
6. Kewalramani LS, Tori JA. Spinal cord trauma in children. Neurologic patterns, radiologic features, and pathomechanics of injury. Spine. 1980;5:11–18.
7. Melzak J. Paraplegia among children. Lancet. 1969;2:45–48.
8. Scher AT. Trauma of the spinal cord in children. S Afr Med J. 1976;50:2023–2025.
9. Yngve DA, Harris WP, Herndon WA, et al. Spinal cord injury without osseous spine fracture. J Pediatr Orthop. 1988;8:153–159.
10. Choi JU, Hoffman HJ, Hendrick EB, et al. Traumatic infarction of the spinal cord in children. J Neurosurg. 1986;65:608–610.
11. Mayfield JK, Erkkila JC, Winter RB. Spine deformity subsequent to acquired childhood spinal cord injury. J Bone Joint Surg Am. 1981;63:1401–1411.
12. Lancourt JE, Dickson JH, Carter RE. Paralytic spinal deformity following traumatic spinal-cord injury in children and adolescents. J Bone Joint Surg Am. 1981;63:47–53.

13. McPhee IB. Spinal fractures and dislocations in children and adolescents. Spine. 1981;6:533–537.

14. Yasuoka S, Peterson HA, MacCarty CS. Incidence of spinal column deformity after multilevel laminectomy in children and adults. J Neurosurg. 1982;57:441–445.

15. Aufdermaur M. Spinal injuries in juveniles. Necropsy findings in twelve cases. J Bone Joint Surg Br. 1974;56B:513–519.

16. Hachen HJ. Spinal cord injury in children and adolescents: diagnostic pitfalls and therapeutic considerations in the acute stage [proceedings]. Paraplegia. 1977;15:55–64.

17. Hadley MN, Zabramski JM, Browner CM, et al. Pediatric spinal trauma. Review of 122 cases of spinal cord and vertebral column injuries. J Neurosurg. 1988;68:18–24.

18. Reddy SP, Junewick JJ, Backstrom JW. Distribution of spinal fractures in children: does age, mechanism of injury, or gender play a significant role? Pediatr Radiol. 2003;33:776–781.

19. Koch BM, Eng GM. Neonatal spinal cord injury. Arch Phys Med Rehabil. 1979;60:378–381.

20. Levin TL, Berdon WE, Cassell I, et al. Thoracolumbar fracture with listhesis—an uncommon manifestation of child abuse. Pediatr Radiol. 2003;33:305–310.

21. Swischuk LE. Spine and spinal cord trauma in the battered child syndrome. Radiology. 1969;92:733–738.

22. Abel MS. Transverse posterior element fractures associated with torsion. Skeletal Radiol. 1989;17:556–560.

23. Begg AC. Nuclear herniations of the intervertebral disc; their radiological manifestations and significance. J Bone Joint Surg Br. 1954;36-B:180–193.

24. Cirak B, Ziegfeld S, Knight VM, et al. Spinal injuries in children. J Pediatr Surg. 2004;39:607–612.

25. Hegenbarth R, Ebel KD. Roentgen findings in fractures of the vertebral column in childhood examination of 35 patients and its results. Pediatr Radiol. 1976;5:34–39.

26. Horal J, Nachemson A, Scheller S. Clinical and radiological long term follow-up of vertebral fractures in children. Acta Orthop Scand. 1972;43:491–503.

27. Herkowitz HN, Samberg LC. Vertebral column injuries associated with tobogganing. J Trauma. 1978;18:806–810.

28. Odom JA, Brown CW, Messner DG. Tubing injuries. J Bone Joint Surg. 1976;58A:733.

29. Shrosbree RD. Spinal cord injuries as a result of motorcycle accidents. Paraplegia. 1978;16:102–112.

30. Anderson JM, Schutt AH. Spinal injury in children: a review of 156 cases seen from 1950 through 1978. Mayo Clin Proc. 1980;55:499–504.

31. Hubbard DD. Injuries of the spine in children and adolescents. Clin Orthop. 1974:56–65.

32. Santschi M, Echave V, Laflamme S, et al. Seat-belt injuries in children involved in motor vehicle crashes. Can J Surg. 2005;48:373–376.

33. Sclafani SJ, Florence LO, Phillips TF, et al. Lumbar arterial injury: radiologic diagnosis and management. Radiology. 1987;165:709–714.

34. Sturm JT, Perry JF Jr. Injuries associated with fractures of the transverse processes of the thoracic and lumbar vertebrae. J Trauma. 1984;24:597–599.

35. Denis F. The three column spine and its significance in the classification of acute thoracolumbar spinal injuries. Spine. 1983;8:817–831.

36. Denis F. Spinal instability as defined by the three-column spine concept in acute spinal trauma. Clin Orthop. 1984:65–76.

37. Ruckstuhl J, Morscher E, Jani L. [Treatment and prognosis in vertebral fractures in children and adolescents]. Chirurg. 1976;47:458–467.

38. Roaf R. A study of the mechanics of spinal injuries. J Bone Joint Surg. 1960;42B:810–823.

39. Hubbard DD. Fractures of the dorsal and lumbar spine. Orthop Clin North Am. 1976;7:605–614.

40. Parisini P, Di Silvestre M, Greggi T. Treatment of spinal fractures in children and adolescents: long-term results in 44 patients. Spine. 2002;27:1989–1994.

41. Thomas KC, Lalonde F, O'Neil J, et al. Multiple-level thoracolumbar burst fractures in teenaged patients. J Pediatr Orthop. 2003;23:119–123.

42. Bulos S. Herniated intervertebral lumbar disc in the teenager. J Bone Joint Surg Br. 1973;55:273–278.

43. MacCartee CC Jr, Griffin PP, Byrd EB. Ruptured calcified thoracic disc in a child. Report of a case. J Bone Joint Surg Am. 1972;54:1272–1274.

44. Peck FC Jr. A calcified thoracic intervertebral disk with herniation and spinal cord compression in a child; case report. J Neurosurg. 1957;14:105–109.

45. Handel SF, Twiford TW Jr, Reigel DH, et al. Posterior lumbar apophyseal fractures. Radiology. 1979;130:629–633.

46. Keller RH. Traumatic displacement of the cartilagenous vertebral rim: a sign of intervertebral disc prolapse. Radiology. 1974;110:21–24.

47. Lippitt AB. Fracture of a vertebral body end plate and disk protrusion causing subarachnoid block in an adolescent. Clin Orthop. 1976:112–115.

48. Lowrey JJ. Dislocated lumbar vertebral epiphysis in adolescent children. Report of three cases. J Neurosurg. 1973;38:232–234.

49. Techakapuch S. Rupture of the lumbar cartilage plate into the spinal canal in an adolescent. A case report. J Bone Joint Surg Am. 1981;63:481–482.

50. Callahan DJ, Pack LL, Bream RC, et al. Intervertebral disc impingement syndrome in a child. Report of a case and suggested pathology. Spine. 1986;11:402–404.

51. Dietemann JL, Runge M, Badoz A, et al. Radiology of posterior lumbar apophyseal ring fractures: report of 13 cases. Neuroradiology. 1988;30:337–344.

52. Sovio OM, Bell HM, Beauchamp RD, et al. Fracture of the lumbar vertebral apophysis. J Pediatr Orthop. 1985;5:550–552.

53. Smith WS, Kaufer H. Patterns and mechanisms of lumbar injuries associated with lap seat belts. J Bone Joint Surg Am. 1969;51:239–254.

54. Blasier RD, LaMont RL. Chance fracture in a child: a case report with nonoperative treatment. J Pediatr Orthop. 1985;5:92–93.

55. Kolowich P, Phillips, W. Seat belt lumbar fractures in children. Orthop Trans. 1986;10:566.

56. Taylor GA, Eggli KD. Lap-belt injuries of the lumbar spine in children: a pitfall in CT diagnosis. AJR Am J Roentgenol. 1988;150:1355–1358.

57. Gumley G, Taylor TK, Ryan MD. Distraction fractures of the lumbar spine. J Bone Joint Surg Br. 1982;64:520–525.

58. Betz RR, Mulcahey MJ, D'Andrea LP, et al. Acute evaluation and management of pediatric spinal cord injury. J Spinal Cord Med. 2004;27 Suppl 1:S11–15.

59. Agran PF, Dunkle DE, Winn DG. Injuries to a sample of seat-belted children evaluated and treated in a hospital emergency room. J Trauma. 1987;27:58–64.

60. Sledge JB, Allred D, Hyman J. Use of magnetic resonance imaging in evaluating injuries to the pediatric thoracolumbar spine. J Pediatr Orthop. 2001;21:288–293.

61. Ferrandez L, Usabiaga J, Curto JM, et al. Atypical multivertebral fracture due to hyperextension in an adolescent girl. A case report. Spine. 1989;14:645–646.

62. Carreon LY, Glassman SD, Campbell MJ. Pediatric spine fractures: a review of 137 hospital admissions. J Spinal Disord Tech. 2004;17:477–482.

63. Burke DC. Spinal cord trauma in children. Paraplegia. 1971;9:1–14.

64. Burke DC. Traumatic spinal paralysis in children. Paraplegia. 1974;11:268–276.

65. Glasauer FE, Cares HL. Biomechanical features of traumatic paraplegia in infancy. J Trauma. 1973;13:166–170.

66. Betz RR, Gelman AJ, DeFilipp GJ, et al. Magnetic resonance imaging (MRI) in the evaluation of spinal cord injured children and adolescents. Paraplegia. 1987;25:92–99.

67. Akbarnia BA. Pediatric spine fractures. Orthop Clin North Am. 1999;30:521–536.

68. Boechat MI. Spinal deformities and pseudofractures. AJR Am J Roentgenol. 1987;148:97–98.

69. Gellad FE, Levine AM, Joslyn JN, et al. Pure thoracolumbar facet dislocation: clinical features and CT appearance. Radiology. 1986;161:505–508.

70. Tarr RW, Drolshagen LF, Kerner TC, et al. MR imaging of recent spinal trauma. J Comput Assist Tomogr. 1987;11:412–417.

71. McArdle CB, Crofford MJ, Mirfakhraee M, et al. Surface coil MR of spinal trauma: preliminary experience. AJNR Am J Neuroradiol. 1986;7:885–893.

72. Moller A, Hasserius R, Besjakov J, et al. Vertebral fractures in late adolescence: a 27 to 47-year follow-up. Eur Spine J. 2006;15:1247–1254.

73. Jackson RW. Surgical stabilisation of the spine. Paraplegia. 1975;13:71–74.

74. Westerborn A, Olsson, O. Mechanics, treatment and prognosis of fractures of the dorso-lumbar spine. Acta Chirurgica Scandinavica. 1953;102:59–83.

75. Lalonde F, Letts M, Yang JP, et al. An analysis of burst fractures of the spine in adolescents. Am J Orthop. 2001;30:115–120.

76. Bryant CE, Sullivan JA. Management of thoracic and lumbar spine fractures with Harrington distraction rods supplemented with segmental wiring. Spine. 1983;8:532–537.

77. Flesch JR, Leider LL, Erickson DL, et al. Harrington instrumentation and spine fusion for unstable fractures and fracture-dislocations of the thoracic and lumbar spine. J Bone Joint Surg Am. 1977;59:143–153.

78. Bradford DS, McBride GG. Surgical management of thoracolumbar spine fractures with incomplete neurologic deficits. Clin Orthop. 1987:201–216.

79. Campbell J, Bonnett C. Spinal cord injury in children. Clin Orthop. 1975:114–123.

80. Audic B, Maury M. Secondary vertebral deformities in childhood and adolescence. Paraplegia. 1969;7:11–16.

81. Bedbrook GM. Correction of scoliosis due to paraplegia sustained in paediatric age-group [proceedings]. Paraplegia. 1977;15:90–96.

82. Kilfoyle RM, Foley JJ, Norton PL. Spine and pelvic deformity in childhood and adolescent paraplegia: a study of 104 cases. J Bone Joint Surg Am. 1965;47:659–682.

83. McSweeney T. Spinal deformity after spinal cord injury. Paraplegia. 1969;6:212–221.

84. Lyons BM, Brown DJ, Calvert JM, et al. The diagnosis and management of post traumatic syringomyelia. Paraplegia. 1987;25:340–350.

85. Williams B, Terry AF, Jones F, et al. Syringomyelia as a sequel to traumatic paraplegia. Paraplegia. 1981;19:67–80.

86. Cullen JC. Spinal lesions in battered babies. J Bone Joint Surg Br. 1975;57:364–366.

87. Dickson RA, Leatherman KD. Spinal injuries in child abuse: case report. J Trauma. 1978;18:811–812.

88. Kleinman PK, Zito JL. Avulsion of the spinous processes caused by infant abuse. Radiology. 1984;151:389–391.

89. Kogutt MS, Swischuk LE, Fagan CJ. Patterns of injury and significance of uncommon fractures in the battered child syndrome. Am J Roentgenol Radium Ther Nucl Med. 1974;121:143–149.

90. Renard M, Tridon P, Kuhnast M, et al. Three unusual cases of spinal cord injury in childhood. Paraplegia. 1978;16:130–134.

91. Carrion WV, Dormans JP, Drummond DS, et al. Circumferential growth plate fracture of the thoracolumbar spine from child abuse. J Pediatr Orthop. 1996;16:210–214.

92. Nesbit ME, Kieffer S, D'Angio GJ. Reconstitution of vertebral height in histiocytosis X: a long-term follow-up. J Bone Joint Surg Am. 1969;51:1360–1368.

93. Amstutz HC, Carey EJ. Skeletal manifestations and treatment of Gaucher's disease. Review of twenty cases. J Bone Joint Surg Am. 1966;48:670–701.

94. Ribeiro RC, Pui CH, Schell MJ. Vertebral compression fracture as a presenting feature of acute lymphoblastic leukemia in children. Cancer. 1988;61:589–592.

95. Makitie O, Doria AS, Henriques F, et al. Radiographic vertebral morphology: a diagnostic tool in pediatric osteoporosis. J Pediatr. 2005;146:395–401.

96. Ross J, Gamble J, Schultz A, et al. Back pain and spinal deformity in cystic fibrosis. Am J Dis Child. 1987;141:1313–1316.

97. Varonos S, Ansell BM, Reeve J. Vertebral collapse in juvenile chronic arthritis: its relationship with glucocorticoid therapy. Calcif Tissue Int. 1987;41:75–78.

98. Jones ET, Hensinger RN. Spinal deformity in idiopathic juvenile osteoporosis. Spine. 1981;6:1–4.

99. Sørensen HK. Scheuermann's Juvenile Kyphosis. Clinical Appearances, Radiography, Aetiology, and Prognosis. Copenhagen: Munksgaard, 1964.

100. Tribus CB. Scheuermann's kyphosis in adolescents and adults: diagnosis and management. J Am Acad Orthop Surg. 1998;6:36–43.

101. Bradford DS, Moe JH, Montalvo FJ, et al. Scheuermann's kyphosis and roundback deformity. Results of Milwaukee brace treatment. J Bone Joint Surg Am. 1974;56:740–758.

102. Blumenthal SL, Roach J, Herring JA. Lumbar Scheuermann's. A clinical series and classification. Spine. 1987;12:929–932.

103. Greene TL, Hensinger RN, Hunter LY. Back pain and vertebral changes simulating Scheuermann's disease. J Pediatr Orthop. 1985;5:1–7.

104. Scheuermann HW. The classic, kyphosis dorsalis juvenilis. Z Orthop Chir. 1921;41:305–317.

105. McCall IW, Park WM, O'Brien JP, et al. Acute traumatic intraosseous disc herniation. Spine. 1985;10:134–137.

106. Hafner RH. Localised osteochondritis (Scheuermann's disease). J Bone Joint Surg Br. 1952;34-B:38–40.

107. Micheli LJ. Low back pain in the adolescent: differential diagnosis. Am J Sports Med. 1979;7:362–364.

108. Jayson MI, Herbert CM, Barks JS. Intervertebral discs: nuclear morphology and bursting pressures. Ann Rheum Dis. 1973;32:308–315.

109. Resnick D, Niwayama G. Intravertebral disk herniations: cartilaginous (Schmorl's) nodes. Radiology. 1978;126:57–65.

110. Alexander CJ. Scheuermann's disease; a traumatic spondylodystrophy. Skeletal Radiol. 1977;1:209–221.

111. Ghelman B, Freiberger RH. The limbus vertebra: an anterior disc herniation demonstrated by discography. AJR Am J Roentgenol. 1976;127:854–855.

112. Rowe GG, Roche MB. The etiology of separate neural arch. J Bone Joint Surg Am. 1953;35-A:102–110.

113. Wertzberger KL, Peterson HA. Acquired spondylolysis and spondylolisthesis in the young child. Spine. 1980;5:437–442.

114. Wiltse LL, Newman PH, Macnab I. Classification of spondylolysis and spondylolisthesis. Clin Orthop. 1976:23–29.

115. Baker DR, McHollick W. Spondyloschisis and spondylolisthesis in children. J Bone Joint Surg. 1956;38A:933–934.

116. Hitchcock HH. Spondylolisthesis. Observations on its development, progression, and genesis. J Bone Joint Surg. 1940;22:1–16.

117. Hensinger R, Lang, JR, MacEwen, GD. Surgical management of spondylolisthesis in children and adolescents. Spine. 1976;1:207–216.

118. Sherman FC, Wilkinson RH, Hall JE. Reactive sclerosis of a pedicle and spondylolysis in the lumbar spine. J Bone Joint Surg Am. 1977;59:49–54.

119. Sherman FC, Rosenthal RK, Hall JE. Spine fusion for spondylolysis and spondylolisthesis in children. Spine. 1979;4:59–66.

120. Turner RH, Bianco AJ Jr. Spondylolysis and spondylolisthesis in children and teen-agers. J Bone Joint Surg Am. 1971;53:1298–1306.

121. Letts M, Smallman T, Afanasiev R, et al. Fracture of the pars interarticularis in adolescent athletes: a clinical–biomechanical analysis. J Pediatr Orthop. 1986;6:40–46.

122. Jackson DW, Wiltse LL, Cirincoine RJ. Spondylolysis in the female gymnast. Clin Orthop. 1976:68–73.

123. Ogilvie JW, Sherman J. Spondylolysis in Scheuermann's disease. Spine. 1987;12:251–253.

124. Libson E, Bloom RA, Shapiro Y. Scoliosis in young men with spondylolysis or spondylolisthesis. A comparative study in symptomatic and asymptomatic subjects. Spine. 1984;9:445–447.

125. Wynne-Davies R, Scott JH. Inheritance and spondylolisthesis: a radiographic family survey. J Bone Joint Surg Br. 1979;61-B:301–305.

126. Fredrickson BE, Baker D, McHolick WJ, et al. The natural history of spondylolysis and spondylolisthesis. J Bone Joint Surg Am. 1984;66:699–707.

127. Hensinger RN. Spondylolysis and spondylolisthesis in children. Instr Course Lect. 1983;32:132–151.

128. Libson E, Bloom RA, Dinari G, et al. Oblique lumbar spine radiographs: importance in young patients. Radiology. 1984;151:89–90.

129. Rothman SL. Computed tomography of the spine in older children and teenagers. Clin Sports Med. 1986;5: 247–270.

130. Papanicolaou N, Wilkinson RH, Emans JB, et al. Bone scintigraphy and radiography in young athletes with low back pain. AJR Am J Roentgenol. 1985;145:1039–1044.

131. van den Oever M, Merrick MV, Scott JH. Bone scintigraphy in symptomatic spondylolysis. J Bone Joint Surg Br. 1987;69:453–456.

132. Nachemson A. Repair of the spondylolisthetic defect and intertransverse fusion for young patients. Clin Orthop. 1976:101–105.

133. Buck JE. Direct repair of the defect in spondylolisthesis. Preliminary report. J Bone Joint Surg Br. 1970;52: 432–437.

134. Bradford DS, Iza J. Repair of the defect in spondylolysis or minimal degrees of spondylolisthesis by segmental wire fixation and bone grafting. Spine. 1985;10:673–679.

135. Nicol RO, Scott JH. Lytic spondylolysis. Repair by wiring. Spine. 1986;11:1027–1030.

136. Pedersen AK, Hagen R. Spondylolysis and spondylolisthesis. Treatment by internal fixation and bone-grafting of the defect. J Bone Joint Surg Am. 1988;70:15–24.

Index

A

Abbott/Anderson method, 415
Abdominal injury, polytrauma treatment, 680
Abduction contracture of shoulder, 360
Abdul-Kadir, A. H., 179–191
Abnormal visual perception, 307
Abscess on inner side of acetabulum, MRI, 430
Accadbled, F., 687–698
Acetabular osteotomy, 101, 473, 475
    femoral osteotomy, 475
    innominate osteotomy, 475
    limb shortening, 475
    Salter's osteotomy, 475
    Salter–Thompson group B, 475
Acetabular reorientation procedures, 295
Achilles tendonitis, 528
Achondroplasia, 19, 23, 75–78, 82–87, 93, 106, 109, 634
    cause of, 82–83
    C1–C2 fusion, 634
    clinical features
        during adulthood, 84
        at birth, 83
        during childhood, 83–84
    radiographic features of, 84
    spinal stenosis, 634
    thoraco-lumbar kyphosis, 634
    treatment of, 84–85
Achterman and Kalamchi Type II, 396
Acquired brain damage, 233, 236
Acquired dislocation of shoulder, 357
Acquired immunodeficiency syndrome (AIDS), 123–132,
        161–162, 165, 180, 590
    in children
        antiretroviral therapy for, 132
        CD4 lymphocytes, infection of, 131
        classification of HIV disease, 132
        clinical manifestations of, 132
        management of, 132
        by maternal transmission, 131
Acrocephalosyndactyly, see Apert's syndrome

Acromio-clavicular joint disclocation, 381
Acrosyndactyly, 182, 345, 352
Adolescent disc syndrome, 587, 591–592
    ankylosing spondylitis, 592
    dehydration and disc stiffness, 592
    Finnish identical twin cohort, 591
    focal hernia, 592
    nerve root decompression, 592
    radicular pain and paraesthesia, 592
Advanced Pediatric Life Support (APLS), 675
"a la carte" method, 550
Alar ligaments, 574, 820–821, 826
Algodystrophy, see Complex regional pain syndrome
        (CRPS)
Allen, G. M., 49–62
Allodynia, 7, 382, 384
Aluminum osteodystrophy, 122
Amelia, 389
American Orthopaedic Association, 612
Amniocentesis, 53, 270, 541, 542, 544
Amoxicillin, oral antibiotics, 432
Amputation, 147, 182, 187–188, 191, 226, 352, 391, 393,
        395, 397, 399–401, 403, 418, 534, 672, 676, 682
Amputee Medical Rehabilitation Society, 391
Amyoplasia congenita, 327–329
Anatomical leg length discrepancies, 406
Anesthesia and analgesia, in children, 37–48
    and airway management, 38
    central neuraxial blocks
        caudal epidural analgesia, 45
        epidural analgesia, 44–45
        subarachnoid anesthesia, 45
    continuous infusion of opioid, 46
    fluid balance and intravenous fluids, 39–40
        intra-operative fluid administration, 40
        post-operative fluid regimens, 41
        pre-operative fluid resuscitation, 40
    intercurrent disease and, 37–38
    local anesthetic techniques, 42
        Bier's block, 42

M. Benson et al. (eds.), *Children's Orthopaedics and Fractures,*
DOI 10.1007/978-1-84882-611-3, © Springer-Verlag London Limited 2010

drug of choice for, 42
  infiltration analgesia, 42
  topical cutaneous anesthesia, 42
monitoring depth of anesthesia, 39
monitoring protocol, need of, 47
nonsteroidal anti-inflammatory drugs, use of,
    47–48
opioids use, 46–47
patient-controlled analgesia (PCA), 46–47
peripheral nerve blockade
  ankle block, 43–44
  digital nerve block, 42–43
  fascia iliaca compartment block, 43
  femoral nerve block, 43
  sciatic nerve block, 43
pharmacokinetics and, 38
plexus blockade
  brachial plexus blockade, 44
  lumbar plexus blockade, 44
post-operative analgesia, 41–42
pre-operative preparation, 37
tourniquet use, 39
ultrasound-guided nerve blocks, 45–46
venous access, gaining of, 38–39
  internal jugular vein, access via, 38
  intraosseous access, 39
  ultrasound, use of, 38
Aneurysmal bone cysts, 60, 174, 220, 222–223, 433, 517,
    595–597, 636
Angiogenesis, 232
Angulation correction axis (ACA), 409
Ankle
  jerks S1–2, 237
  valgus, 275–276
Ankle and pantalar arthrodesis, 301
Ankle and subtalar valgus, 276–277
Ankle–foot orthosis (AFOs), 255, 273, 312–313, 533
  crouch position of legs in lumbar lesion, 274
Ankle fractures, 654, 682, 793–803
  classification
    of Dias and Tachdjian, 793–794
    of Salter and Harris, 793–794
  incidence and mechanism of injury
  treatment
    displaced/non-displaced fractures, 793
    Salter and Harris Type I and II, 793
    Salter and Harris Types III and IV, 796–797
    transitional and tillaux fracture, 799–800
    triplane fracture, 800–801
Ankylosing spondylitis, 119, 196, 198, 430, 571, 587,
    591–592
Anomalies of ring of C1, 573–574
Anoxia, 383

Antalgic gait, 70, 244, 424, 427, 504
"Anteater's nose," 533
Anterior cruciate ligament (ACL), 394, 397, 507, 511, 778,
    782–784
  rupture, 507
  See also Ruptures of anterior cruciate ligament
Anterior knee pain, 20, 423, 502–513, 515, 780–781
  distinct causes, 501–505
    bipartite patella, 504
    Osgood–Schlatter's condition, 504
    osteochondritis dissecans, 504–506
    Plicae and Bursae, 506–507
    Sinding–Larsen–Johansson, 503
    sleeve and stress fracture of patella, 504–506
  "distinct diagnoses" and "obscure diagnoses," 502
  ligament problems, 509–511
    deformity/growth arrest, 509
    hamstring reconstruction drilling, 509–510
    ligament injuries, 509
    modern bracing techniques, 509
    rehabilitation, 511
    tibial spine avulsion fracture/classification, 510
  meniscal lesions, 507–508
    discoid meniscus, 508–509
    meniscal tears, 507–508
  obscure causes, 512–513
    idiopathic knee pain, 512
    malalignment, 512
    maltracking, 512–513
  other causes, 511–512
Antibiotic therapy, 57, 145, 150–151, 183, 186, 590
Anti-tuberculous drugs, 590
AOCID, see AO Clinical Investigation and Documentation
    (AOCID)
AO Classification Supervisory Committee (CSC), 759
AO Clinical Investigation and Documentation (AOCID),
    759
AO Universal spine system, 616
Apert's syndrome, 345, 357, 534, 536–537, 629
Apical ectodermal ridge (AER), 11–12, 339
Aponeurotomy, 314
Apoptosis, 11–13, 232, 345, 435, 483
Appendicitis, 124, 171, 425
"Apprentice's spine," 603, 625, 640
Arbogast, M. N., 195–211
Arnold–Chiari malformation, 27, 231, 244–245, 265, 571,
    578
Arterial lesion, 383–384
Arthritis
  enthesitis-related arthritis, 591
  psoriatic arthritis, 591
  sacroiliitis, 591
Arthrodesis for foot and ankle deformities, 300–301

Arthrography, 449–450, 454, 457, 471, 473, 505, 704, 725,
        728
    ilio-psoas tendon, 448
    injecting contrast medium into hip joints, 449
    subluxation, progressive degrees, 449
    Y-shaped ligament of Bigelow, 449
    zona orbicularis, 449
Arthrogryposis, 250, 345–346, 354, 438, 454
    Buddha position of child in arthrogryposis, 332
Arthrogryposis multiplex congenita, 268, 277, 327–334,
        354, 765
    differential diagnoses of disorders
        connective tissue, 329
        muscle, 328
        neurological, 328
    etiology, 328
    incidence, 328
    infant with arthrogryposis and fixed extended knees, 330
    investigations, 328
    orthopaedic management
        elbow, 333
        foot, 329–330
        hip, 332
        knee, 330–332
        shoulder, 332–333
        wrist and hand, 333
    See also Hand developmental anomalies
Arthroscopy, 143, 157, 384, 458, 505, 507–509, 510, 516,
        778–779, 782, 784, 785
Articulatory dyspraxia, 235
Ashworth Scale, 240
Association for Spina Bifida and Hydrocephalus (ASBAH),
        30
Atlanto-axial rotary displacement, 580–581
    clinical features, 581
        "cocked robin" position, 581
        "long" sternocleidomastoid, 579
    imaging features, 581–582
        classification of rotary displacement, 581
        flexion–extension stress films, 581
        medial/lateral offset, 581
    ligamentous deficiency, 580
    treatment, 582
        halo traction, 582
        simple soft collar and analgesics, 582
        traction and muscle relaxants, 582
Atlanto-dens interval (ADI), 820–821
Atrophy
        of denervated target organs, 378
        disuse, 242
        and hypertrophy, 252
        spinal muscular atrophy, 23, 241, 249, 252, 255–256,
            328, 523, 561, 630, 632, 707

Autosomal dominant inheritance, 79–80, 259, 262, 349, 533
Avascular necrosis (AVN), 125, 131, 301, 329, 332, 426,
            431–432, 436, 438, 440, 444–446, 448–451,
            454, 457, 462, 476, 481, 490–492, 535, 567,
            759, 762, 771
    decompression/stable internal fixation, prevention
            methods, 762
    Legg–Calvé–Perthes-like appearance, 763
"AVPU" (Alert, response to Voice, response to Pain,
            Unconscious) score, 676
Avulsion fractures of distal fibula, 802–803
Avulsion of pelvic apophysis, 428
Avulsion of tibial tuberosity
    clinical and radiological findings, 785
    mechanism of injury, 785
    treatment, 785–786
    See also Fractures of knee and tibia
Axial dyspraxia, 235
Axial micro motion, 414
Axonal and dendritic development, 232

B
Babinski sign, 237, 252
Back pain in children, 587–597
    adolescent disc syndrome, 591–592
    arthritis, 591
    child assessment, 585
        adolescent disc syndrome, 587
        ankylosing spondylitis, 587
        retroperitoneal sepsis, 587
        roundback deformity, 587
        Scheuermann's disease, 587
        spinal tenderness, 587
    congenital spinal anomalies, 588
    juvenile discitis, 591
    spinal infection, 588–590
        Batson's plexus of veins, 589
        disc resorption, 589
        end plate perforation, 589
        HIV-positive, 589
        pyogenic infection, 590
        spinal cord compression, 589
        tuberculous infection, 590–591
    spinal trauma, 588
        battered baby syndrome, 588
        infancy back trauma, 588
        laminectomy, 588–589
        post-traumatic kyphosis, 588
        Salter type V injury, 588
        SCIWORA, 588
        whiplash flexion injury, 588
    spondylolisthesis, 592–594
        dysplastic spondylolisthesis, 594

isthmic spondylolisthesis, 592–593
   See also Individual
tumors, 594–597
   of bone, 595–597
   intradural, 594–595
   See also Individual
Barlow's test, 440–441
Bartter's syndrome, 658, 660
   stabilization of stress fracture of tibia in, 660
Basal fractures, 747
Basilar impression
   basilar invagination, 571
   clinical features, 571–572
      aqueduct of Silvius, 571
      Arnold–Chiari malformation, 571
      chronic alveolar hypoventilation, 572
      cranial nerves, 571
      foramen magnum, 572
      multiple sclerosis, 572
      occipital nerve, 571
      syringomyelia, 571
      vertebral artery anomalies, 572
   imaging features, 572
      CT reconstruction, 572
      foramen magnum, opening of, 572
   primary, 571
   secondary, 571
Battered baby syndrome, 186, 588
Baumann procedure, 320
Becker muscular dystrophy (BMD), 23, 114, 255, 257–260, 846
Beighton score, 21
Bell's palsy, 432
Below-knee transverse deficiency, 389
Bending fractures, 786–787, 790–791
   See also Fractures of knee and tibia
Bending fractures of proximal tibia
   mechanism of injury and complications
      post-traumatic valgus deformity, theories, 786
   treatment, 786–787
   See also Fractures of knee and tibia
Benign joint hypermobility syndrome (BJHS), 20–21
Benign X-linked (Becker) muscular dystrophy, 258
Benson, M. K. D., 435–463, 481–492, 701–707
Benzodiazepines, 37, 46
Bernard–Horner syndrome, 372
Bier's block, 42, 743
Bilateral congenital pseudarthrosis of olecranon, 361
   See also Elbow, congenital anomalies
Bilateral dislocation, 332, 453
   hip dislocation in 7-year-old girl, 279
   hyperlordotic lumbar spine, 455
Bilateral Perthes disease, 88, 468, 476

Bilhaut–Cloquet procedure, 350–351
Bipartite patella
   sudden flexion injury, 503
   traction apophysitis, 504
   vastus lateralis, 504
Birch, R., 365–384
Birth injuries
   anatomy, 701
   biomechanics, 701
   differential diagnosis of neonatal injury, 707
   etiology, 703–704
   fracture patterns, 702
   healing, 702
   incidence, 703
   specific injuries, 704–707
Birth lesions of brachial plexus (BLBP), peripheral nerve injuries
   clinical assessment, 371–373
      group 1 and 2, 372
      group 3 and 4, 372
   deformity associated with, 378–379
   etiology, 370–371
   lesions of, 381
      arterial lesion, 383–384
      diagnosis, 382–383
   long-term studies, 371
   pain, 384–385
   pathology, 371
   posterior dislocation of shoulder
      operation, 379–380
Bispectral Index™ Monitoring (BIS), 39
Bites, 709
Bleck, E. E., 249–263
Bleeding disorders and musculoskeletal changes
   hemophilia
      acute hemorrhage, treatment of, 126–127
      ankle joint, changes in, 125
      anti-factor VIII antibodies, suppression of, 128
      complications of factor VIII/IX therapy, 127–128
      desmopressin, treatment with, 126–127
      earlier diagnosis of, 124
      elbow, effect on, 124
      genetic basis of, 123
      hemophilia centers, registration at, 125
      hepatic cirrhosis and, 126
      hip joint, acute bleeds into, 124–125
      knee, hemarthrosis of, 124–125
      muscle hematomas, 125–126
      prophylactic factor VIII/IX therapy for, 126
      pseudotumors, and treatment, 126
      and recurrent hemarthrosis, 124
      severity of, 123
      shoulder, acute hemarthrosis of, 125

surgery of patient, 128–129
sickle cell disease (SCD), 129–130
   and avascular necrosis of hip, 131
   and bacterial and joint infection, 130
   osteomyelitis in, 130–131
   and pre-operative procedures, 130
   short stubby fingers in, 130
   use of tourniquets in, 130
thalassemias, 129
Block test, 559
Blount's disease and bow legs, distinction, 19
Bone
   aches, 433
   age, calculation and determination, 410
   bruises, 506
      acute varus angulation, 506
      direct blow/high-velocity fall, 506
   characteristics, child *vs.* adult, 651–652
   cysts, 433
   plug, 412
   scanning with technetium (Tc-99m), 485
   scintigraphy, 52, 426
Bone tumors, 213, 511, 595–597
   aneurysmal bone cyst, 595–596
   benign chondrogenic tumors
      chondroblastomas, 218–219
      chondromas, 218
      chondromyxoid fibroma, 219
      osteochondromas, 217–218
   benign osteogenic tumors
      bone island, 220
      osteoblastomas, 220
      osteoid osteomas, 219–220
      osteomas, 220
   biopsy for, 216–217
      needle or closed biopsy, 217
      open surgical biopsy, 217
   case analysis, information from imaging
      key diagnoses, 216
      number of lesions, 215
      reaction in adjacent bone, 215–216
      site of lesion, 215
      size and shape, 215
   causes of, 213–214
   clinical diagnosis of, 214
   definition of, 213
   eosinophilic granuloma, 597
   Ewing's tumor, or malignancy, 597
   fibrous tumors
      benign metaphyseal cortical lucencies, 220
      eosinophilic granuloma, 222
      monostotic fibrous dysplasia, 221
      non-ossifying fibromas, 220

      osteofibrous dysplasia, 221–222
      periosteal desmoplastic fibromas, 220–221
   Hand–Schüller–Christian disease, 597
   "Histiocytosis X," 597
   imaging for
      angiogram, 215
      CT scan, 214
      MRI, 214
      positron emission tomography (PET), 215
      radiographs, 214
      scintigram, 214
   incidence of, 213
   Letterer–Siwe disease, 597
   malignant tumors, 224
      amputation and rotationplasty, 226
      chemotherapy for, 224–225
      Enneking's resection classification, 225
      Ewing's sarcoma, 224
      Kawaguchi's resection classification, 225
      MRI for, 224
      osteosarcoma, 224
      post-operative treatment, 227
      reconstruction with epiphysis, 226–227
      reconstruction with functional joint, 226
      reconstruction with no functional joint, 226
      tumor resection, 225–226
      tumor staging, 225
   osteoid osteoma/osteoblastoma, 595
   other benign tumors
      aneurysmal bone cyst (ABC), 223
      giant cell tumor, 223–224
      unicameral bone cysts, 222–223
   Pott's disease, 597
   prostaglandin inhibitors, 594
   radiographs and plain films, 596
   soap-bubble trabeculation, 595
   technetium bone scanning, 596
   types of, 213
Bow leg deformity, 19, 498
Brachial plexus injuries, 357, 365–369, 702
   clinical presentation, 365–367
   etiology and pathogenesis, 365
   indications for operation, 367
   spontaneous recovery, 367
   surgical intervention
      anatomical lesions, 368
      complication rate, 369
      late cases, 369
      neurotizations, 367–368
      post-operative care, 368
      results of surgery, 368–369
Brachial plexus lesions, 153, 366, 381, 594
Brachial plexus palsies, 702

Brain development stages, 231–233
Breech presentation, 307, 328, 365, 367, 370, 437, 440, 443, 445, 583, 703
Brittle bone disease, 604, 606, 713
Brooks–Seddon procedure, 291, 292
Brown–Sequard lesion, 575
Bruises, 428, 506, 708–709, 778
Brunner, R., 307–323
Buckle/torus fracture, 743
Burge, P. D., 339–354
Burst fracture, 837, 843

C
Calcaneal apophysis, 428, 528, 529
Calcaneal foot deformity
  calcaneal osteotomy, 300
  Elmslie's procedure, 300
  forefoot equinus, 300
  talectomy, 300
Calcaneo-valgus foot positioning, 437, 565
Calcaneus deformity, 267, 275, 285, 289, 298–299, 554, 556
Calcaneus fractures
  classification and clinical appearance, 807–809
  epidemiology, 807
  imaging techniques
    CT scan, 808
    MRI, 808
    radiography, 807
  mechanism of injury, 807
  treatment of
    cuboid and cuneiform bones, 810
    displaced, 809
    navicular, 809, 811
    the midtarsal bones, 809
    undisplaced, 809
Callus formation, 269, 414, 682, 704, 754, 766–770, 785, 807
Camptodactyly, 340, 344, 347–348
  treatment
    adolescence, 348
    infancy, 348
    long-standing, 348
  See also Hand developmental anomalies
Canale technique, 412
Capitellum osteochondritis, 362
Capsuloplasty, 460–461
  acetabular capsulotomy, 460
  Colonna arthroplasty, 461
  secondary surgery, 461
Capsulorrhaphy, 452–453, 455
Cardio-pulmonary resuscitation (CPR), 711
Care coordination concept, 23
Carpal bone fractures, 745–746

Cartilaginous sulcus, *see* Patello-femoral dysplasia
Cathrin, S. P., 671–685
Catterall, A., 465–478
Catterall classification
  epiphyseal signs, 469
  group 1/2/3/4, 468–469
  "head within a head," appearance, 469
  metaphyseal signs, 469
Caudal regression syndrome, 231
Causalgia, 384–385, 515
Causative bacterium
  Escherichia coli, 140
  Haemophilus influenzae, 139
  Kingella kingae, 140
  methicillin-sensitive S. aureus (MSSA), 139
  Mycobacterium bovis, 140
  Pseudomonas aeruginosa, 140
  Staphylococci, 139
  Streptococci, 139
  See also Infections of bones and joints
Cavendish classification of deformity, 360
Cavovarus deformity as part of myelodysplastic limb, 244
Cavus deformity, 275, 285, 298–300, 381, 546, 552, 559
C5/C6 brachial plexus lesion, 366
Cefuroxime, 145, 147, 150, 154, 432
Center of rotation of angulation (CORA), 408–409
Central core disease, 260
Central neuraxial blocks
  caudal epidural analgesia, 45
  epidural analgesia, 44–45
  subarachnoid anesthesia, 45
Cephalhematoma, 702
Cerebral palsy (CP), children with, 410
  classification, 307
  incidence, 307
  orthotic management, 312–313
  pathology, 307
    deformities in, 308
    Medical Research Council (MRC) scale of, 308
    spastic CP, 308
  physical assessment
    evaluation of gait, 310–311
    static examination, 308–310
  post-operative management and complications, 322–323
  surgery
    for nonwalker, 315–318
    tone management, 313–315
    for walker, 318–321
  upper limb surgery, 321–322
Cervical cord injuries, 703, 707
Cervical spine congenital disorders, 571–584
  anomalies of ring of C1, 573–574
  atlanto-axial rotary displacement, 580–581

basilar impression, 571
congenital muscular torticollis, 582–583
differential diagnosis of torticollis, 579–580
Klippel–Feil syndrome, 576–579
laxity of transverse atlantal ligament, 574
occipito-cervical fusion, 572–573
odontoid anomalies, 574–575
See also Individual
Cervical spine injuries
complications, 832
fusion techniques in children/adults, 831
in infants, 707
SCIWORA
MRI findings, 824–825
Pang's study, 825
Chance fractures in children
bilateral facet dislocations, 840
ecchymosis in lap-belt distribution, 840
motor vehicle accidents, groups, 840–841
reverse hyperextension injuries, 841
routine lateral views of spine for diagnosis, 841
Charcot–Marie–Tooth disease, 247, 249, 559
Cheilectomy, 476
Chemotherapy, 168, 175, 214–215, 224–227, 590, 659
Chevron osteotomy, 535
Chiari malformation and hydrocephalus, 245–246
Chiari medial displacement osteotomy, 459
Chiari osteotomy, 279, 295, 459–460, 475
compression screw, 460
femoral head migration, 460
iliac osteotomy, 457
medial displacement osteotomy, 459
orthopaedic table, 459
pelvic remodeling, 460
skin-crease bikini incision, 459
symptomatic acetabular dysplasia, 459
Child abuse, 428
dorsolumbar junction injuries, 845
fracture dislocation of dorsal lumbar junction secondary
to child abuse, 845
and non-accidental injuries, 708
and polytrauma, 671
risk factors for, 709
suspecting circumstances, 712
thoracolumbar fracture dislocation/listhesis injury, 845
Childhood malignancy, 187, 433
Children, orthopaedic
child centered treatment, in hospital, 3–4
child-friendly clinic rooms, 4
facilties in children's ward, 4
minimum visits and suitable investigations, 4
relaxing atmosphere in hospital, 4
by trained health professionals, 3

differential diagnosis possibilities, in children, 5–6
efficient pre-admission program, 5
history template, for first consultation, 5–6
members of paediatric orthopaedic team, 4
musculoskeletal screening examination, importance of, 5
need and importance of study of, 3
orthotic services, careful planning of, 4–5
pain in children, 6–7
examination of child, 7–8
and proper investigations, 8
physiotherapists, role of, 4
Chondrodiatasis, 414
Chondrodystrophies, 846
Chondroectodermal dysplasia, 537
Chondrolysis, 157, 481–482, 485, 488, 489, 491
Chondromalacia patellae, 502, 514–515
Chopart joint, *see* Talonavicular/calcaneocuboid joint
Chow, W., 287–303
Chronic atlanto-axial instability, 821
Cincinnati approach, 330
Clarke's test, 515
Clark's procedure, 291–292
Clasped thumb, 340, 345–346, 349
Classic metaphyseal lesion (CML), 710–711
Clavicle fractures, 704, 717
congenital pseudarthrosis of, 704
etiology, 717
fracture dislocations of medial and lateral ends, 717
healing and remodeling, 718
obstetrical clavicle fracture, 717
treatment, 717
Cleft hand, 339, 341, 344–345
complex syndactyly with, 344
depth of, 344
See also Hand developmental anomalies
Cleidocranial dyostosis, 358, 392
Clinodactyly, 348–349
angulation, 349
See also Hand developmental anomalies
Clubfoot assessment protocol (CAP), 552
Clubfoot, congenital talipes equinovarus, 541–556
antenatal diagnosis, 541–542
DFAS, 541
functional false positive, 542
Ponseti technique, 542
ultrasonography, 541
in utero diagnosis, 542
assessment of outcome, 551–552
Dimeglio system, 552
grading system, 552
idiopathic foot/complex foot, comparability, 552
Pirani and Dimeglio classification systems, 551
classification systems, 545

Dimeglio and Pirani systems, 545
Flynn systems, 545
Pirani score, 545
Wainwright system, 545
clinical assessment, 544–545
flexibility of foot, 545
"syndromic" foot, 545
decision making in recurrent/relapsed feet, 555–556
etiological theories, 544
imaging, 545
CT and MR scans, 545
"false correction," 545
MMN distance, 545
radiographic measurement, 545
stress radiographs, 545
ultrasound, 545
management of complex case, 551
arthrogrypotic foot deformities, 551
Ponseti program, 551
postoperative splinting program, 551
management of idiopathic foot, 545–551
management of residual or recurrent deformity, 552–555
pathoanatomy, 543–544
dorsalis pedis artery, 543
myofibroblasts, 543
Clubfoot programs, 3
"Cocked robin" position, 581
Cole, W. G., 75–102
Colles fracture, 744
Comminuted fractures, treatment for, 695, 769–770,
781–782, 789, 809–810
Compartment syndrome, 42, 44, 189, 383, 414, 501, 583,
653, 676, 678, 681, 723–724, 744, 747, 775,
788–789, 807–809
Complete syndactyly, 345
Complex clasped thumb, 345–346
Complex regional pain syndrome (CRPS), 384, 515, 654
causalgia, type II, 515
occurrence and treatment, 516
RSD, type I, 515
Compression
due to hyperflexion, 837
immature spine, on, 837
multiple compression fractures, illustration, 838
in older patients, effect of applied pressure, 838
vertebrae loaded vertically, 837
Condylar fractures, 747
Congenital bony deformities, 625–626
failures of
formation, 626
segmentation, 626–627
treatment, 627–628
abdominal ultrasound, 627

antero-convex hemiepiphysiodesis, 628
congenital kyphosis, 628
diastematomyelia, 627
keystone vertebra, 628
MRI/CT myelography, 627
prophylactic fusion, 627
spinal dysraphism, 627
surgical treatment, 628
two-stage wedge resection, 628
Congenital clasped thumb, 345–346
See also Hand developmental anomalies
Congenital constriction band syndrome, 340–341, 345
See also Transverse absence
Congenital Convex Pes Valgus, see Congenital Vertical
Talus
Congenital dislocation of the hip (CDH), 436–437
Congenital dysplasia, 390, 583
Congenital femoral deficiency
congenital fibular deficiency, 396–397
abnormalities associated with, 397
Birch classification of, 397
Taylor spatial frame use in, 398
congenital short femur, 392–394
congenital tibial deficiency/absence of tibia with intact
fibula, 398
abnormalities associated with, 399
classification of, 399–400
idiopathic coxa vara
management, 392
radiological changes, 391–392
management and limb reconstruction, 397–398
management and limb reconstruction, tibial dysplasia
for Type 1a, 399–400
for Type 1b, 400
for Type 3, 401
for Type 4, 401
proximal focal femoral deficiency (PFFD), 392, 394–396
Congenital fiber-type disproportion, 240, 261
Congenital insensitivity to pain, 182–183, 658
Congenital limb deficiencies, 14, 389–391, 394, 411
limb reconstruction for, 394
shortening of lower limb, 390
Congenital muscular dystrophies (CMDs), 252, 260, 328
Congenital myotonic dystrophy, 262
Congenital pseudarthrosis
of clavicle, 357–359, 704
of forearm, 353
See also Hand developmental anomalies
Congenital pseudarthrosis of tibia, 401
clinical and radiological appearances, 402
management, 402
reconstruction techniques with circular fixator,
403–404

Congenital radial head dislocation, 350
    See also Hand developmental anomalies
Congenital radio-ulnar synostosis, 350, 362
Congenital short femur (CSF), 390, 392–395, 657
    bony abnormalities in, 394
    See also Congenital femoral deficiency
Congenital short tibia with absent/hypoplastic fibula, 397
Congenital spinal cord deformities, 628–629
    anterior segmental instrumentation, 628–629
    congenital bony anomaly, 629
    congenital kyphosis of myelomeningocele, 628–630
    congenital spinal deformity syndromes, 629–630
        Apert's syndrome, 629
        congenital intervertebral fusions, 630
        Crouzon's syndrome, 629
        Goldenhar's syndrome, 629
        Klippel–Feil syndrome, 629–630
        Larsen's syndrome, 629
        "sitting Buddha," 630
        Sprengel's shoulder, 629–630
        Treacher–Collins syndrome, 629
    C-shaped paralytic lordoscolioses, 628
    spina bifida syndromes, 628
    spinal surgery, 628
    torso imbalance, 629
Congenital split/cleft foot, 538
    Abraham classification, 538
    cleft lip/cleft palate/deafness, 538
    footwear and cosmesis, 538
Congenital talipes calcaneo-valgus, 526–527
    congenital vertical talus, 527
    "molded baby syndrome," 526
    neuromuscular abnormality, 526–527
Congenital talipes equinovarus, 181, 523, 537, 541–556, 559
Congenital vertical talus, 329, 330, 527, 565–567
    calcaneo-valgus or plano-valgus foot, 565
    Cincinnati incision, 566
    disorders, five, 565
    Eyre–Brook view, 565
    open reduction, deformities, 566
    "rocker bottom" feet, 565
    talonavicular dislocation, 567
    two-stage reduction, 566
Constriction band syndrome, 345, 352
    See also Hand developmental anomalies
Continuous positive airways pressure (CPAP) ventilation, 246
Contralateral epiphysiodesis, 155, 319, 655
Coronal deformity, 502
Cortical dysplasias, 232
Cosmesis, 273, 282, 300, 322, 340–341, 360, 538, 584
"Cot death" syndrome, 523

Cotrel–Dubousset system, 615
Cowboy pattern of ambulation, 233
Craig, C. L., 835–855
Cranio-carpo-tarsal dystrophy, 329
Craniofacial syndromes, 345
C-Reactive protein (CRP), 142, 197, 425, 429, 516
Creepers, 236
Cricothyroidotomy, 830
'Critical ischemia', 383
Crouch gait, 243, 272, 273, 312, 319, 428
Crouzon's syndrome, 361, 629
Cubitus varus and valgus deformity, 362
Curly toes, 534
    clawing of toes, 534
    curly lateral three toes, 534
    over-and understrapping, 534
    persistent deformity, symptoms, 534
    toe deformities, 534
Cutaneous injuries, 708–709
Cyclical steroids, 246

D
Damage-control surgery, 679–680
Dannecker, G. E., 195–211
Danny–Walker malformation, 231
De Bastiani corticotomy method, 414
Deep skin dimples, 328
Deformity analysis, 408–410
    arithmetic method, 410
    bone age, calculation and determination, 410
    error in using growth charts, 411
    Paley's multiplier method, 410–411
    progression, prediction of, 410
    remaining growth, 410
    straight line graph, 410
Deformity in children with motor disorders
    ataxia
        lower limb coordination, 243
        truncal ataxia, 243
        upper limbs, 243
    from cerebral lesions, 241
    contractures, 240–241
    growth failure in cerebral palsy and neurological conditions, 241–242
    muscle fasciculation, 241
    muscle wasting, trophic and growth changes, 241
    observational gait assessment, 243
        fog test, 244
        pes cavus, 244
        spinal curvatures, 244–245
        toe walking, 244
    positional deformities
        "baby buggy spine," 240

"wind sweeping," 240
right hemiplegic gait, 242
sensation
    Charcot joints, 242
Dega pelvic osteotomy, 279, 317, 457
Dejerine–Klumpke (complete paralysis), 366
Dejerine–Sotta type (Type III HMSN), 560
Delta phalanx, 349, 351
Deltoid paralysis, 289, 291
Denckla test, 247
Detailed fetal anomaly scans (DFAS), 541, 542
Development
    brain damage, 233
    gender, 233
    genetic factors, 233
Developmental dysplasia of hip (DDH), 391, 436
Development testing principle, 233
Dextrocardia, 358
Diaphragmatic rupture with peripheral fracture, 681
Diaphyseal fractures of lower leg
    clinical and radiological findings, 788
    See also Fractures of knee and tibia
Diaphyseal fractures of tibia and fibula
    mechanism of injury–remodeling capacity
        stable/unstable fractures, 789
    prognosis, 789–790
    treatment, 789
    See also Fractures of knee and tibia
Diaphyseal (long bone) fractures, 710
    bilateral spiral fractures of tibia, 711
    facial bruising and fractures, 710
    metaphyseal fracture, 711
    periorbital bruising, transverse fracture in, 710
Diastematomyelia, 244
Diastrophic dwarfism, 329, 536
Dick/Jack test, 244
Dickson, R. A., 587–643
Diencephalon division, 232
Dimeglio grade IV foot, 549
Dimeglio system, 545, 552
"Dinner fork deformity," 744
Diplegia, 16, 73, 238, 240–242, 247, 259, 262, 307
Disablility in children, management, 23
    cerebral palsy
        cognitive issues and education, 33
        communication and speech, 31
        control of tone and positioning, 31
        drooling management, 31
        feeding and nutrition, 30–31
        mobility aids, 32–33
        seating, 31–32
    disability registers, creation of, 26
    disabling conditions, 23

nature of, 27
Duchenne muscular dystrophy, 33
    ambulation, maintenance of, 33
    daily living activities, 34
    educational support, 34
    leaving school and adult services, 34–35
    respiratory care, 34
early and continuing intervention
    educational psychologist, 26
    occupational therapist (OT), 26
    paediatric physiotherapist (PPT), 25
    social workers, 26
    specialist children's nurses, 26
    speech and language therapist (SALT), 26
    voluntary organizations, 26
family conditions and, 24
multi-disciplinary assessment, 24–25
    test instruments, to assess development, 25
multi-disciplinary team for, 24
neural tube defects, management of, 27
    from birth, 27–28
    bowel incontinence and constipation, 28
    cognitive issues and education, 29–30
    orthoses, use of, 29
    posture, seating, and mobility, 28–29
    renal tract management, 28
    skin care, 28
    transition to adult services, 30
news to parents, guidelines for giving of, 24
state legislations, 24–25
Discitis, 431–432
Discoid meniscus, 508–509
    congenital malformation, 508
    osteoarthritis, 509
    subtotal meniscectomy, 509
    symptoms and treatment, 509
    Watanabe classification, 508
Distal femoral epiphysis, fracture separation of, 706
Distal femoral osteotomy, 498
Distal femoral physis, 693
    central cancellous bone bridging of, 692
Distal femoral shaft fractures treatment, 769–771
Distal femur, 706
Distal fibula physeal arrest, 655
Distal humerus and elbow, 705
Distal humerus fractures
    supracondylar fractures, 719
        classification, 719
        flexion supracondylar fractures, 725
        neurovascular injury, 723–725
    T-fracture, 728
    treatment, 722–723
Distal physeal fractures, 747

Distal radial fractures, 743–744
 AP and lateral view of metaphyseal, 744
 forearm pronation, 743
 indications for K-wire fixation, 743–744
Distal radio-ulnar subluxation, 745
Distal tibia
 infants, 709
 intra-epiphyseal screws and, 692
 open reduction of type IV triplane fracture of, 694
Distal ulnar epiphysis, 343
Distraction injury, 839
Distraction lengthening of ulna, 343, 353
Distraction osteogenesis, 414, 501
Distraction stress phenomenon, 414
Disuse atrophy, 124, 242
Dorsal root ganglion (DRG), 371
Dorsal wedge carpectomy, 333
Dorsiflexion of ankle, 309–310
Down's syndrome, 242, 438, 574–575, 577, 580, 764, 779,
  821, 828
Doxycycline, oral antibiotics, 432
Doyle, E., 37–48
Duchenne dystrophy, 242, 246, 632
Duchenne gait, 70, 244
Duchenne muscular dystrophy (DMD), 3, 33, 240, 249,
  424–425
 abdomen and lumbar lordosis in, 250
Duncan Ely test, 310
Duncan, R. D., 3–8, 11–21
Dunhill, Z. M., 23–35
Dunn procedure, 488, 490
Dwyer instrumentation system, 617
Dynamic deformities, 240, 308, 321
Dyslexia, 233
Dysmelia, 389
Dysplasia of hip, developmental, 435–463
 avascular necrosis, 444–445
  acetabular dysplasia, 444
  idiopathic necrosis, 444
  Kalamchi/McEwan's classification, 445
  thyroid deficiency/epiphyseal dysplasia, 444
 blood supply, 436
 clinical examination, 440
  Barlow's test, 439
  Ortolani's test, 439
 displacement/dysplasia of hip, 436–437
  CDH/DDH, 436–437
  subluxation/dislocation, 437
 embryology and development, 435–436
  at birth, 435–436
  hip growth after birth, 436
  3, 6, 8, 11, 16, 20-weeks embryo, 435–436
 etiology, 437–438

incidence, 439
 clinical screening, 439–440
 Macnicol's value, 439
 painful dysplasias, 439
 ultrasonographic techniques, 439
investigations, 441–443
  See also Radiological investigations in hip
   dysplasia
outcomes, 462
 avascular necrosis, 462
 closed reduction, 462
 femoral head deformity, 462
 Iowa experience (open reduction), 462
 open reduction and innominate osteotomy, 462
patho-anatomy, 438–439
risk factors for DDH, 440
 Barlow's test, 440
 clinical screening program, 439
 Ortolani's test, 440
salvage procedures, 459–461
 capsuloplasty, 460–461
 chiari osteotomy, 459–460
 shelf arthroplasty, 459
 trochanteric "overgrowth," 461
screening, 439
 neonatal screening programs, 439
 "snap of entry" of dislocated hip, 439
 US screening technique, 439
treatment, 445–461
Dysplasias, 6, 75–78, 81, 88–89, 93, 105, 107, 109,
  111–112, 232, 435, 633–634
 cervical kyphosis, 635
 diastrophic dysplasia, 634–635
 Morquio's syndrome, 634
Dysplastic spondylolisthesis, 593, 640–645
 frank spondylolysis, 641
 hypoplasia or aplasia, 593, 640
 L5 vertebra, 593, 641
 secondary spondylolysis, 641
Dyspraxia, 21, 231, 235, 247
Dystrophia myotonica, 328

E
Early-onset idiopathic scoliosis, 619–623
 clinical features, 619–620
  rib vertebra angle distance, 621
  RVAD/RVAs, 620–621
  severe idiopathic thoracic curve, 620
  "skew" baby, 619
 "malignant" progressive curves, 619
 management, 621–623
  antero-convex hemiepiphysiodesis, 623
  EDF casting, 621–622

epiphysiodesis, 623
   "Luque trolley," 623
   newer generation metalwork systems, 623
   posterior spinal fusion, 622
   "subcutaneous" spinal procedure, 621
Early-onset Werdnig–Hoffmann, 632
Eastwood, D. M., 541–556
Edward's syndrome, 329
Ehlers–Danlos syndrome (EDS), 99, 329, 357, 779
   causes of, 99
   classification of, 100
   clinical features, 99–101
   diagnosis and management, 101
Elastic stable intramedullary nailing (ESIN), 735, 769, 789
   treated children, complications
      mismatched diameters of nail, 771
      obese children, 771
      skin and subcutaneous irritations around the knee, 771
Elbow and forearm fractures
   fractures of radial and ulnar shafts, 733–734
      conservative treatment, 734–735
      surgical treatment, 735–736
   Galeazzi fractures, 736
   Monteggia equivalent (variant) injuries, 738–741
      anatomy, 738
      clinical findings, 738
      congenital dislocation of radial head, 739
      mechanism of injury, 738
      Monteggia lesions, delayed diagnosis of, 739
      persistent dislocation of radial head, treatment, 741
      radiographic findings, 738
      treatment of type I, II and III lesions, 738
      treatment of type IV lesions, 739
   Monteggia fracture dislocation, 737
   olecranon fractures, 733
   radial neck, treatment, 731–733
Elbow, congenital anomalies
   bilateral congenital pseudarthrosis of olecranon, 361
   carrying angle of, 362
   congenital ankylosis, 361
   osteochondritis of capitellum, 362
   supracondylar humeral spur, 361
Elizabethtown classification, 465
Ellis–Van Creveld syndrome, see Chondroectodermal
      dysplasia
Elmslie triple arthrodesis, 562
Elongation-de-rotation-flexion (EDF) casting, 621–622
Emery–Dreifuss muscular dystrophy (EDMD), 258–259
Emery–Dreifuss sex-linked muscular dystrophy, 240
EMLA cream, 42
Enchondromatosis, 96–97
   clinical and radiographic features, 97
   treatment of, 97–98

Endochondral ossification, 12, 687
   diagrammatic view of physis, 688
Endotracheal intubation, indications for, 675
Engelhardt, P. W., 759–764
Enthesopathy, 112, 198, 430
Eosinophil granuloma, 433
Epiphyseal artery, 688
Epiphyseal dysplasias, 88
   multiple epiphyseal dysplasia
      causes of, 88
      clinical features, 88
      diagnosis and treatment of, 88–89
      radiographic features, 88
Epiphyseal fractures, distal radial, 744–745
   neurovascular complications, 744
   Salter–Harris type 2 fracture, 745
Epiphyseal ischemia, 762
Epiphyseal/metaphyseal fractures, polytrauma, 682
Epiphysiodesis, 411–412
   See also Limb equalization
Epiphysiolysis, 95, 379, 656, 702, 704, 760–761, 777, 785
   at proximal tibia
      clinical and radiological findings, 785
      growth disturbances, 786
      mechanism of injury, 785
      treatment, 785–786
   See also Fractures of knee and tibia
   Type I fracture of femoral neck, 760
Epiphysis, blood supply, 690
Equinovarus deformity, 274, 289, 299, 381, 399, 401, 541, 555
Equinus deformity, 126, 239, 244, 285, 297, 298, 300–301, 319, 415, 418, 547, 552, 554, 707
Equinus foot, 497, 559
Erb–Duchenne type paralysis, 365–366
Erythema migrans, 432
Erythrocyte sedimentation rate (ESR), 8, 142, 165, 197, 289, 425, 468, 590–591
Estrogen, 107–108, 482
Etiology, hip dysplasia, 437–438
   environmental and mechanical factors, 437
      breech presentation, 437
      calcaneovalgus foot positioning, 437
      club foot, 437
      eccentric hip movement, 437
      knee dislocation, 437
      plagiocephaly, 437
      postural scoliosis, 437
      torticollis, 437
   genetics and gender, 437
      congenital dislocation, 437
      inherited factors, 437
   hormones, 437–438

maternal hormone concentrations, 437
  syndromic dislocations, 438
    neonatal hip anomalies, 438
    neuromuscular imbalance, 438
    "teratological" dislocations, 438
Etiology, Legg–Calvé–Perthes disease, 362, 466
  growth arrest theory, 466
    decreased birth weight, 466
    delayed bone age, 466
    insulin-like growth factor, 466
    social deprivation, 466
  recurrent infarction, 466
    ischemic necrosis, 466
    tamponade effect theory, 466
  thrombophilia theory, 466
    Factor V Leiden mutation, 466
    partial thromboplastin time, 466
    protein C/S deficiency, 466
    vascular thrombosis, 466
Etiology, slipped upper femoral epiphysis
  biomechanical factors, 481–482
    epiphyseal–metaphyseal junction, 482
    perichondrial fibrocartilaginous ring, 481
    proximal femoral physis, 482
    shear stress, 482
  endocrine factors, 482
    GH treatment, 482
    irradiation therapy, 482
    panhypothyroidism, 482
    Turner's syndrome or chronic renal failure, 482
  immunological factors, 482
    chondrolysis, 482
    generalized inflammatory disorder, 482
    immunoglobulin/complement (C3) production, 482
    synovial fluid assays, 482
    tissue proteoglycan, 482
Euler's laws, 606–607
Ewing's sarcoma, 6, 60, 150, 174, 183, 187, 213, 215–216, 220, 224, 226–227, 428, 846
Exostosis syndromes, 94
  clinical and radiographic features, 96
  diagnosis and management of, 96
  diaphyseal aclasis
    cause of, 94
    clinical features, 94–95
    diagnosis and treatment, 95–96
    radiographic features, 95
  dysplasia epiphysealis hemimelica, 96
Extensive periosteal reaction, 702
Extensor dystonic rigidity, 240
External fixators, 85, 416, 767, 769
External tibial torsion for slipped upper contracted ilial tibial tract, 293

Extra-articular fractures of distal femur
  incidence and mechanism of injury
    hyperextension injuries, 775
    Salter–Harris I and II lesions, 775
    varus–valgus fractures, 775
  prognosis, 775

F

Factor V Leiden mutation, 466
Fairbank's triangle, 391–392
Familial joint laxity and joint dislocation, 357
Fanconi anemia, 341–342
Fasciculation, 241, 246, 249, 252, 256
Fascio-scapulo-humeral (FSH) muscular dystrophy, 259
Femoral deficiency, 390–391, 393, 396, 399
  classification of, 393
Femoral epiphysis
  alternative imaging
    early, 485
    late, 485
  clinical features and classification
    acute-on-chronic slip, 484
    acute slip, 483–484
    chronic slip, 484
    shortening of right leg, 483
  complications
    avascular necrosis, 491
    chondrolysis, 491
    operative, 491
  etiology, *see* Etiology, femoral epiphysis
  measuring slip, 484
    classic lateral projection method, 484
    degree of posterior slip, 484
    Klein's line, 484
    osteopenia, 484
    parallax effect, 484
    Scham's sign, 484
    Shenton's arc, 484
    Southwick angle, 484
    Wilson quantified displacement, 484
  pathophysiology, 482–483
    chronic slip, 483
    impingement, 483
    pre-slip stage, 483
  surgical procedures
    corrective femoral osteotomy, 491
    implant removal, 491–492
  surgical treatment, 485–491
    contralateral prophylactic fixation, 489–491
    later proximal femoral osteotomies, 488
    orthopaedic management, objectives of, 485
    in situ fixation, 485–486
    subcapital osteotomy, 488–489

unstable slip, 486–488
Femoral neck fractures
  assessment, 759
  causes
    high-energy trauma, 759
    pathological conditions, 759
  classification
    proximal epiphyseal/metaphyseal fractures, 759
  complications
    avascular necrosis, 762
    growth arrest/coxa vara, 763
    nonunion, 763
    osteoarthritis, 763
    poorly positioned implants, 763
    screw drilling/removal, 763
  frequency and mechanism of injury
    age-related differences (adult/child ratio), 759
    fractures, cause of, 759
    polytraumatized child, injuries in, 759
  traumatic dislocation of hip, 763–764
  treatment
    diaplaced/undisplaced fractures, 760–761
Femoral osteotomy, 43, 89, 112, 205, 278, 317–318, 414,
    453, 455–457, 473–475, 477–478, 491, 498
  "bone suture," 455
  corrective, 491
    distal segment correction, 491
    intertrochanteric osteotomies, 491
    Southwick, triplane osteotomy, 492
  L-shaped incision, 455
Femoral shaft fractures, 683, 703, 705–706
  classification
    paediatric long bone fractures, 765–766
  clinical findings, 765
  incidence and mechanism of injury
    etiology of femoral fractures (age-dependent), 765
    non-accidental, 765
  radiographic findings, 766
  short oblique humeral fracture after birth, 706
  treatment for fracture during first year of life
    bilateral overhead traction, 766
    Pavlik harness, 766
    spica cast after closed reduction, 766
    vertical traction, 766
  treatment for 1 to 4 years of age
    elastic intramedullary nails/intramedullary Kirschner
      wires, use of, 766
    external fixators, 767
    preferred treatment, 767
    traction, 766
    use of titanium nails, advantage, 766–767
  treatment for 5 to 15 years of age

cast brace/three-point fixation walking spica, use of,
    768–769
  ESIN treated children, complications, 771
  external fixators, 769
  immediate spica cast application, 768
  plate fixation with dynamic compression, 769
  preferred method, 769–771
  submuscular bridge plating, 769
  traction, 767
  use of TENs, 771
Femoral shortening techniques, 413
  See also Shortening osteotomies
Femoral varus osteotomy, 474–475
  flexion deformity, 474
  "head at risk," 474
  initial/fragmentation stage, 474
  limb shortening, 475
  varus derotation osteotomy, 474
Femoral neck fracture, unstable pelvic, 684
Femur fractures, polytrauma, 682
Fernandez, F. F., 793–803, 805–814
Fetal alcohol syndrome, 232
Fetal myopathy and myasthenia, 328
Fetal neuropathy, 328
Fibroblast growth factor (Fgf) signaling in overlying AER,
  339
Fibrodysplasia (myositis) ossificans progressiva, 537
Fibrosis, 115, 124–126, 169, 171, 176, 184, 188–189, 288,
    360, 369, 378, 381, 583, 604, 635, 837, 846
Fibrous dysplasia
  causes of, 101
  clinical and radiographic features, 102
  diagnosis and treatment, 102
Fibrous tumors
  benign metaphyseal cortical lucencies, 220
  eosinophilic granuloma, 222
  monostotic fibrous dysplasia, 221
  non-ossifying fibromas, 220
  osteofibrous dysplasia, 221–222
  periosteal desmoplastic fibromas, 220–221
Fibular bypass grafting, 403
Fibular hemimelia, 389–390, 407
Figure-of-eight bandage, 717
Finger–nose test, 243
Finger-sucking deformities, 353
  See also Hand developmental anomalies
Finnish identical twin cohort, 592
First aid, transport, and hospital facilities, polytrauma,
  674–675
  airway, 675
  breathing, 675
  circulation and hemorrhage control, 675
  disability, 676

exposure, 676
Fish osteotomy, 489
Fixed bony deformity, 313, 318, 321, 323, 561, 577, 580
Fixed extension in knees, 278
Fixed flexion deformity, 277
Fixed lumbar kyphosis, 281
Fixed varus deformity, 274
Fixsen, J. A., 327–334, 357–362, 523–538, 559–562
Flaccid paralysis, 594
Flail undeformed knee, 277
Flat-back deformity, 617
Flat feet, 529–534
    in cerebral palsy, 565
    diagnosis, 530–531
        broad feet, 531
        great toe extension test, 531
        normal testing, 531
        symptoms and treatment, 531
    flexible, 20–21
    management, 531–532
        common flexible flat foot, 531
        Grice type of subtalar arthrodesis, 532
        idiopathic flat foot, 532
        medial displacement osteotomy, 532
        naviculocuneiform fusion, 532
        pathological type of flat foot, 531–532
        reverse Evans operation, 532
    natural history, 530
        calcaneo-valgus, 530
        flattening of medial arch, 530
        flexible flat feet, 530
        tests for joint laxity, 530
    Pes Planus, 529
        joint laxity, 529
    tarsal coalition, 532–533
    See also Tarsal coalition
Flexible steel nails (Ender nails), 771
Flexion–abduction contracture, 277, 292–293
Flexion deformity, 474
    of wrist, 354
Flexion–extension stress films, 581
Flexion supracondylar fractures, 725
Flexor digitorum superficialis (FDS), 349–350
Flexor dystonia, 240
Flexor muscle slide deformity recurrence, 383
Floating thumb, 342, 346–347
Flynn systems, 545
Focused abdominal sonography in trauma (FAST), 676
Foot, 523–538
    congenital split or cleft foot, 538
    congenital talipes calcaneo-valgus, 526–527
    flat feet, 529–534
    foot–thigh angle, 425

in-toe gait, 523–525
    painful heel, 528–529
    progression angle, assessment of, 18
    serpentine/skew/"z-foot," 526
    tip-toe walking, 527–528
    toes, 534–538
    See also Individual
Foot abduction orthosis (FAO), 547
Forceps instrumentation, 583
Forearm shaft fractures, healing, 736
Forefoot varus, 536
"Forward-bending test," 600
Foster, B. K., 687–698
Fracture care, principles, 651
    characteristics of fractures, 651–652
    indications for internal fixation, 655
        age of child, 656
        condition of child, 655–656
        nature of fracture, 656
    internal fixation, 656–657
    management, 652–655
        "R's" of, 653
    pathological fractures, 657
        generalized conditions, 657
        monostotic lesions, 658–659
        single-limb involvement, 657–658
        stress fractures, 659–661
Fracture epidemiology, 665
    etiology
        endogenous factors, 668
        environmental factors, 666
        new trends, 667–668
        secular trends, 668–669
    frequency, 666
    incidence, 665
Fracture of base of fifth metatarsal treatment, 813
Fracture (s)
    age-and sex-specific incidence of, 666
    changes in incidence of fractures in boys and girls, 669
    dislocation, 837
    displacement, delayed treatment, 652
    epidemiology in children by age group, 709
    frequency of various types, 666
    patterns of frequency, 667
Fractures and dislocations of foot
    calcaneus
        classification and clinical appearance, 807
        epidemiology, 807
        imaging techniques, 807–808
        mechanism of injury, 807
        treatment, 807–809
    fracture of base of fifth meta tarsal
        classification based on localization of the fracture, 813

imaging, 813
mechanism of injury, 813
treatment, 813
metatarsals, 812
of phalanges, 814
talus
blood circulation, 805
classification by Hawkin, talar neck fractures,
805–806
diagnosis, 806
epidemiology, 805
mechanism of injury, 805
treatment, 806–807
tarsometatarsal injuries
imaging, 811
Lisfranc fracture dislocation, classification, 811
mechanism of injury, 810
talonavicular/calcaneocuboid (chopart)/
tarsometatarsal (lisfranc) joints, 810
treatment, 811–812
Fracture-separation of distal humeral epiphysis, 705
Fractures of knee and tibia
acute traumatic dislocation of patella
associated injuries, 778–779
clinical findings, 778
epidemiology and mechanism of injury, 778
predisposing factors, 779
prognosis, 780
radiological findings, 778
treatment, 779–780
avulsion of tibial tuberosity
clinical and radiological findings, 785
mechanism of injury, 785
treatment, 785
bending fractures, 790–791
bending fractures of proximal tibia
mechanism of injury and complications, 786
treatment, 786–787
diaphyseal fractures of lower leg
clinical and radiological findings, 788
diaphyseal fractures of tibia and fibula
mechanism of injury–remodeling capacity, 789
prognosis, 789–790
treatment, 789
epiphysiolysis at proximal tibia
clinical and radiological findings, 785
growth disturbances, 786
mechanism of injury, 785
treatment, 785–786
extra-articular fractures of distal femur
incidence and mechanism of injury, 775
prognosis, 775
treatment, 775

intra-articular fractures of distal femur
fracture types, 775–777
treatment, 777–778
intra-articular physeal fractures of proximal tibia,
784–785
isolated tibial fractures
mechanism of injury, fracture pattern and remodeling
capacity, 788–789
treatment, 788–789
osteochondral fractures of knee
clinical and radiological findings, 780
late presentation, 780
mechanism of injury, 780
treatment, 780–781
of patella
fracture types, 781
mechanism of injury, 781
treatment, 781
ruptures of anterior cruciate ligament
prognosis, 783–784
treatment, 783
stress fractures of tibia, 787–788
of tibial spine
clinical and radiological findings, 782
mechanism of injury, 782
prognosis, 782
treatment, 782
toddlers' fractures, 791
torus fractures, 786
Fractures of patella
fracture types
longitudinal/transverse/sleeve, 781
mechanism of injury, 781
treatment, 781
See also Fractures of knee and tibia
Fractures of tibial spine
clinical and radiological findings, 782
mechanism of injury, 782
prognosis, 782
treatment, 782
See also Fractures of knee and tibia
Freeman–Sheldon syndrome, 345–346
Freiberg's disease, 432
Frejka pillow, 446
Friedreich's ataxia, 244, 604, 630–632
Fronto-hypothalamic tract, 232
Functional length discrepancies, 406
Functional Motor Scale (FMS), 272

G
Gadolinium (intra-articular contrast medium), 780
Gait
analysis of, 70

clinical use of, 73
dynamic electromyography, 71
energy consumption, 72
kinematic analysis, 70–72
observational analysis, 70
plantar pressure and foot kinematics, 73
development of
gait maturation, 69
variations of gait, 69–70
diagnostic imaging
bone scintigraphy, 426
computed tomography (CT), 426
magnetic resonance imaging (MRI), 426
radiograph, 425–426
ultrasound imaging, 426
diagnostic investigations
blood tests, 425
joint aspiration, 425
examination of patients, 424
fully mature gait, 424
gait cycle, 67
human gait characteristics, 67
normal gait, 67
description of, 67–69
pathological of
antalgic, 424
cerebral palsy, 424
leg length discrepancy, 424
muscular dystrophy, 424–425
Trendelenburg, 424
physical examination
prone, 425
standing, 425
supine, 425
Gait Arms Legs Spine (GALS) musculoskeletal screening
examination, 5
Galeazzi fractures, 736
Gallie technique, 576
Gastrocnemius–soleus complex, 424–425
Gaucher's disease, 468, 846
Genu recurvatum, 297
secondary, 496–497
equinus foot, 496
flail knee, 496
hyperextended knee, 496
poliomyelitis, hamstring paralysis, 496
Genu varum, 84, 86, 296, 406, 499, 652
Gilbert, A. L., 365–384
Glasgow Coma Scale (GCS), 47, 671, 674
Glenohumeral joint, co-contraction of muscles, 371
Glenoid deformity, 379
Glomus tumor, 515
Gluteal paralysis, 294

Goldenhar's syndrome, 629
Gower's sign, 246, 251
Graf's classification, 441
Graham, H. K., 265–285
Great toe extension test, 531
Green's procedure, 360
Greenstick fractures, 12, 651, 674, 702, 704, 718–719, 739,
743, 786–790
Groove of Ranvier, 654, 701
Gross motor function classification system (GMFCS)
scores, 307
Growth and skeletal development, 11
growth plate, structure of, 12–13
leg length discrepancy, estimation of, 14
limb development, 11–12
antero-posterior axis and, 12
dorso-ventral axis and, 12
factors controlling, 11
in fetus, 11
Hox pathway, role of, 11
proximo-distal development, 11
TBX5, role of, 11
neuromuscular development, 16
normal variants, of growth, 16–17
angular anomalies, 19
flat foot, 19–20
hypermobility syndromes, 20–21
rotational anomalies, 17–18
skeletal growth, control of, 13
role of cytokines, 13
skeletal maturity, assessment of, 15–16
estimation of skeletal age, 15
Greulich and Pyle system, 16
Risser grade, 15–16
Sauvegrain method, 16
Tanner–Whitehouse method, 16
skeleton, structure of, 12
formation of bones, 12
types of bone in, 12
somatic growth, 13–14
spine growth and development, 14–15
Growth hormone (GH) treatment, 482
Growth plate injuries, 653–654
clinical condition
diagnosis and differential diagnosis, 691–692
etiology, 688–691
incidence, 691
pathology, 691
embryology and development, 687
blood supply, 688
fracture through, 654
management of, 687
treatment

complications, 693
 effect of patient's age, 692
 salvage procedures, 694–697
 time of presentation, 692–693
Growth plates (physes), 687
Guillain–Barré syndrome, 242
Gustilo classification, 653

H
Haglund's disease, Sever's disease, 428
Hallux rigidus, 536–537
 chondral/osteochondral injury, 536
 dorsal closing wedge osteotomy, 536
 first metatarsophalangeal joint, 536
 osteochondritis of knee, 537
Hallux valgus, 534–536
 Apert's syndrome, 534
 bilateral hallux valgus, 535
 bunionette/fifth metatarsal bunion, 535
 corrective procedures, 535–536
  Chevron osteotomy, 535
  conservative operation, 535
  hemiepiphysiodesis, 536
  Homann-Thomason, 535
  McBride procedure, 535
  metatarsal osteotomies, 535
  proximal osteotomy, 535
  recurrent deformity, 535
  scarf osteotomy, 535
  splints/insoles/physiotherapy, 535
  Wilson osteotomy, 535
 degree of valgus, 535
 metatarsus primus varus, 535
  congenital talipes equinovarus, 537
  flexor hallucis longus, 537
  peroneus longus, 537
  poliomyelitis and spina bifida, 537
  primary developmental abnormality, 537
Hallux varus, 536
 Apert's syndrome, 536
 bony anomalies, 536
 diastrophic dwarfism, 536
 forefoot varus, 536
 localized fibrous band, 536
 myositis ossificans progressiva, 536
Halo-pelvic/halo-femoral traction, 303
Halo traction, 576, 582, 828
Hamstring reconstruction drilling, 510
Hamstring spasm/contracture, 642
Hand developmental anomalies
 abnormalities and syndromes
  arthrogryposismultiplex congenita, 354
  congenital pseudarthrosis of forearm, 353

  finger-sucking deformities, 353
  Madelung's deformity, 352
  multiple hereditary exostoses, 352–353
 classification, 339–340
 congenitally deficient, 340
 constriction band syndrome, 352
 differentiation failure
  camptodactyly, 347–348
  clinodactyly, 348–349
  congenital clasped thumb, 345–346
  congenital radial head dislocation, 350
  congenital radio-ulnar synostosis, 350
  Kirner deformity, 349
  syndactyly, 345
  thumb hypoplasia, 346–347
  trigger thumb, 349–350
  windblown hand, 346
 duplication, 350
  triphalangeal thumb, 351
 formation failure
  cleft hand, 344–345
  radial dysplasia, 341–343
  transverse absence, 340–341
  ulnar dysplasia, 344
 limb development, 339
 management principles
  aims of treatment, 340
  timing, 340
 overgrowth
  macrodactyly, 351–352
Handicapped child, tetraplegic motor patterns, 248
Hand–Schüller–Christian disease, 597
Hangman's fracture, *see* Spondylolisthesis of C2
Harms construct, 576
Harrington instrumentation, 612–615
Hasler, C. C., 775–791
Hawkins type I, II, III and IV fracture, 806
Head injury, polytrauma treatment, 680
Head lag, 251
Heel, painful
 calcaneal apophysitis, 528–529
  Achilles tendonitis, 528
  Sever's disease, 529
  subacute osteomyelitis, 528
 calcaneal boss, 529
 cause of pain in heel
  bone cysts and osteoid osteoma, 529
  fractures of calcaneus in limb, 529
  sprain/ligamentous injury/Sever's disease, 529
  subacute osteomyelitis of calcaneus, 530
 Köhler's disease, 528
 other cause of pain in heel, 529
Heel–shin test, 243

Hemarthrosis, 124–126, 483, 516, 691, 760, 777–778, 781–782
Hemiepiphysiodesis, 275, 410–413, 536, 623, 628, 787
Hemophilia
    acute hemorrhage, treatment of, 126–127
    ankle joint, changes in, 125
    anti-factor VIII antibodies, suppression of, 128
    centers, registration at, 125
    complications of factor VIII/IX therapy, 127–128
    desmopressin, treatment with, 126–127
    earlier diagnosis of, 124
    elbow, effect on, 124
    genetic basis of, 123
    hepatic cirrhosis and, 126
    hip joint, acute bleeds into, 124–125
    knee, hemarthrosis of, 124–125
    muscle hematomas, 125–126
    prophylactic factor VIII/IX therapy for, 126
    pseudotumors, and treatment, 126
    and recurrent hemarthrosis, 124
    severity of, 123
    shoulder, acute hemarthrosis of, 125
    surgery of patient, 128–129
    See also Bleeding disorders and musculoskeletal changes
Hemophiliacs, 468
Hensinger, R. N., 571–582, 819–832, 835–855
Hereditary motor and sensory neuropathy (HMSN), 527, 559
Hereditary multiple exostosis, 352–353
Herring classification, 469–470
    group A/B/C, 470
    intermediate group, 470
    lateral pillar classification, 470
Heschl's gyrus, 232
Hindfoot surgery, 310
Hip
    abduction of, 316
        posture and internal rotation at, 311
    dislocation, treatment for, 317
    distraction, 476
    hip pointer, 428
    movement, eccentric, 437
    ultrasonography
        bulging joint capsule between, 426
        right antalgic limp with, 426
Hip dysplasia, treatment management in, 450–453
    closed reduction, 450–451
        abduction and avascular necrosis, 450
        hip spica, 450
        safe zone of Ramsey, 450
        subluxation or dislocation, 450
    double half hip spica, 451
    open reduction, 451–453
    anterolateral approach, 452–453
    medial approach, 451–452
    ossification, 451
    posterior approach, 453
    See also Open reduction in hip dysplasia
Hip flexion contractures, 255, 257, 309, 315–316, 424–425, 844, 850
Hip guidance orthosis (HGO), 29, 273
Hip–knee–ankle–foot orthoses (HKAFOs), 255
"Histiocytosis X," 150, 174, 433, 518, 597
Hoffa's fat pad syndrome, 511
Hoi Li, Y., 287–303
Hoke technique, 320
Holt–Oram syndrome, 11, 339, 342
Horner's sign, 366
Hovnanian procedure, 291
Hueter–Volkmann principle, 652
Human immunodeficiency virus (HIV)-positive, 126, 589
Humeral fractures, 703, 719, 723
Humerus shaft fractures, 705–706
    classification, 719
    configuration of elastic nails in, 721
    pathological fracture, 721
    short oblique humeral fracture after birth, 705
    start points for elastic nailing, 721
    treatment, 719–720
Hunt, D. M., 495–518
Hunter, J. B., 717, 731–742
Hybrid mounting for equinus, 416
Hydrocortisone, 533
Hyperkyphosis, 587
Hyperlordosis, 244, 316, 319, 453, 591, 605, 635, 642
Hyperlordotic lumbar spine, 455
Hyperostotic macrodactyly, 351–352
Hypersupination with elbows, 238
Hypertrophic polyneuritis, 632
Hypertrophy, 12, 55, 123–124, 141, 242, 246, 250, 252, 257, 284, 438, 560, 654, 854
Hypophosphatasia, 116
    adult hypophosphatasia, 116
    childhood hypophosphatasia, 116
    infantile hypophosphatasia, 116
    perinatal lethal hypophosphatasia, 116
    treatment of, 117
    See also Metabolic and endocrine bone disease
Hypoplasia of ulna, 344
Hypothyroidism, 89–90, 109–110, 115–116, 233, 252, 468, 482
    See also Metabolic and endocrine bone disease
Hypotonia
    clinical grades of, 239
    See also Posture and movement/mobility
Hypotonic posture, 250–251

Hypoventilation, cause of cardiac arrest, 673

I

Iatrogenic nerve lesions, 383
Ibrahim, S. B., 179–191
Ideomotor/ideational dyspraxia, 235
Idiopathic coxa vara
    management, 392
    radiological changes, 391–392
    See also Congenital femoral deficiency
Idiopathic flat foot, 532
Idiopathic foot, management, 545–551
    Kite's method, 545
    methods of conservative treatment, 550
        Dimeglio scale, 550
        French or functional method, 550
        Kite method, 550
        "manipulating and plastering" techniques, 550
        Ponseti technique, 550
        "stretching and strapping" techniques, 550
    Ponseti method, 545–550
        Achilles tenotomy, 549
        cavus deformity, 546
        Dimeglio grade IV foot, 549
        dorsiflexion, 547
        foot deformities, 545
        percutaneous tenotomy, 547, 549
        post-tenotomy casting, 547
        relative muscle imbalance, 549
        rocker bottom deformity or midfoot breech, 549
        "short, fat foot," 549
        talonavicular alignment, 547
    surgical management, 550–551
        "a la carte" method, 550
        calcaneocuboid relationship, 550
        Cincinnati circumferential incision, 550
        complex foot, 550
        fractional lengthenings, 550
        muscle rebalancing, 551
        surgical approaches and procedures, 550
        talonavicular relationship, 550
        tendo Achilles lengthening, 550
    "traditional" conservative regimes, 545
Idiopathic hyperkyphosis, 623–625
    angular hyperkyphosis, 625
    "apprentice's spine," 625
    lower-limb neurological abnormalities, 625
    pectus carinatum, 625
    postural round back deformity, 624
    pseudarthrosis rate, 625
    Scheuermann's disease, 623–624
        type II, 623
    Schmorl node formation, 625

thoraco-lumbar myelogram, 625
Idiopathic knee pain, 512
    anterior knee pain, 512
    chondromalacia, 512
    conditions, two, 512
Idiopathic necrosis, 444
Idiopathic osteoporosis
    compression fractures of vertebra in, 660
Idiopathic scoliosis, 607–608
    infantile/juvenile/adolescent types, 608
    morbidity and mortality, 608
    reduplication of alveolar tree, 608
Iliac apophysitis, 428
Ilio-psoas transfer, 294
Ilio-tibial tract, 292–293, 295–296
Ilizarov ring fixator, 415
    See also Mechanical devices for leg lengthening
Imaging techniques for children
    angiography, 52
    computed tomography (CT), 51–52
    conventional radiographs, 51
    and CRITOL aide-memoir, 50
    dual X-ray absorptiometry (DEXA), 52
    general principles and challenges, 49–50
    magnetic resonance imaging (MRI), 52
    nuclear medicine studies, 52
    protocols
        antenatal diagnosis, 52–53
        developmental dysplasia of hip (DDH), 53–55
        fractures, 59–61
        irritable hip, 55
        juvenile arthritis, 59
        limb lengthening, 56
        nonaccidental injury, 61–62
        osteomyelitis, 57–58
        scoliosis, 56–57
        slipped upper femoral epiphysis, 55–56
        spinal anomalies, 53–54
        sports injuries, 62
        tumors, 59
    radiation dose and risks of harm, 50
    and recording of deviation from normal, 50
    ultrasound, 51
Immuno-deficiency and sickle cell disease, 516
Incarcerated medial epicondyle
    CT of, 727
Index finger
    deformity
        angular, 349
        rotational, 353
        supination, 353
Index healing period, 414
Indian Hedgehog protein, 12–13, 687

Infants, posture and movement
    practical assessment, 235
Infections
    discitis, 431–2
    Lyme disease, 432
    osteomyelitis, 430–431
    psoas abscess, 432
    septic arthritis, 431
Infections of bones and joints, 135
    acute hematogenous osteomyelitis, 146
        antibiotics, selection of, 146–147
        diagnosis of, 146
        immobilization in, 147
        incidence of, 146
        outcomes of, 147–148
        and re-intervention, 147
        and risk of chronic osteomyelitis, 148–149
        surgery in, 147
    anatomy of bone and joint in child, 136
    causative bacterium
        Escherichia coli, 140
        Haemophilus influenzae, 139
        Kingella kingae, 140
        methicillin-sensitive S. aureus (MSSA), 139
        Mycobacterium bovis, 140
        Pseudomonas aeruginosa, 140
        Staphylococci, 139
        Streptococci, 139
    causative organism, identification of
        aspirates, use of, 138–139
        blood sample, 138
        pus smears, 139
        synovial fluid, 139
        tissue culture, 139
    chronic recurrent multifocal osteomyelitis (CRMO),
            151–152
        diagnosis of, 151
        treatment of, 152
    chronic sclerosing osteomyelitis, 152
    differential diagnoses of, 143
    infants, infection in, 136
    and laboratory tests
        antibody tests, 142
        C-reactive protein (CRP), 142
        DNA-based assays, 142
        erythrocyte sedimentation rate (ESR), 142
        white blood cell count, 142
    management of, 143
        antibiotics, choice of, 143–144
        aspiration and biopsy, 143
        duration of therapy, 145
        routes of administration, 144–145
        surgery, 145–146
    pathology of, 135–136
        septic arthritis, 137
        subacute and chronic osteomyelitis, 136–137
    progress, monitoring of, 142–143
    septic arthritis, in neonates and infants, 152–153
        antibiotic treatment, 154
        diagnosis of, 154
        imaging techniques for, 153–154
        outcome of, 155–156
        recurrence of, 154
        surgical treatment of, 154
        treatment of, 154
    septic arthritis, in older child, 156
        of hip, 156–157
        imaging for, 156
        of knee, 157
        multifocal septic arthritis, 158
        of shoulder, 158
    site of infection, location of, 140
        computed tomography, 141
        conventional radiography, 140–141
        magnetic resonance imaging, 141–142
        radioisotope imaging, 141
        ultrasonography, 140
    subacute osteomyelitis
        classification of, 150
        clinical features, 149
        discitis, 151
        imaging for diagnosis of, 150
        incidence of, 149
        laboratory tests for, 150
        pelvic osteomyelitis, 150–151
        puncture wound osteomyelitis, 151
        treatment of, 150
Inferior scapulo-humeral (ISH) angle, 372
Inflammatory arthritis, 20, 512
Inflammatory synovitis
    transient synovitis of hip
        clinical findings, 429
        differential diagnosis, 429
        infectious etiology, 429
        investigations, 429
        treatment, 429
Inherited disorders of bone, cartilage and fibrous tissue
    biochemical and pathological diagnosis, 77
    clinical diagnosis of, 76
    genetic causes of, 75–76
    and genetic counseling, 77
    management of, 77
    orthopaedic management of, 78
    radiographic diagnosis of, 76–77
    See also specific disorders
Injury mechanisms, thoracic and lumbar spine

anterior middle and posterior columns after Denis,
    illustration, 837
burst fracture, 837
chance fractures in children
    bilateral facet dislocations, 840
    ecchymosis in lap-belt, 840
    ecchymosis in lap-belt distribution, 840
    motor vehicle accidents, groups, 840–841
    reverse hyperextension injuries, 841
    routine lateral views of spine for diagnosis, 841
compression
    due to hyperflexion, 837
    immature spine, on, 837
    multiple compression fractures, illustration, 838
    in older patients, effect of applied pressure, 838
    vertebrae loaded vertically, 837
compression fracture, 837
distraction and shear, 838
distraction injury, 839
fracture dislocation, 837
seat-belt fracture, 837
seat-belt injury, 842
severe fracture dislocation of thoracic spine, 837
slipped vertebral apophysis, 838, 840
    laminectomy and decompression, 840
traumatic spondylolysis with severe disruption of pedicle
    and facet, 839
vertebral body from tobogganing, radigraph, 839
Innominate osteotomy, 456–457
Internal fixation in fracture care, indications, 655
age of child, 656
cannulated screw fixation, 656
condition of child, 655–656
criteria to be considered, 655
elastic nailing of diaphyseal fractures, 656–657
nature of fracture, 656
    clinical characteristics of, 656
primary or delayed, reasons for, 656
smooth wires, usage, 656
International Society for Prosthetics and Orthotics (ISPO),
    389–390
International Society for Study of Lumbar Spine, 639
Interphalangeal joint dislocations, 749
volar plate interposition, 749
Interpositional physeal surgery, 697
In-toe gait, 523–525
metatarsus varus/adductus/adductovarus, 523–524
    congenital talipes equinovarus, 523
    "cot death" syndrome, 523
    forefoot and hindfoot, 523
    neurological conditions, 523
    severe metatarsus varus, 525
treatment, 524–525

knee plastering, 524
long leg plasters, 524
multiple metatarsal osteotomies, 525
persistent deformity, 524
risk factors, surgery, 525
Rushforth's series, 524
serial plasters, 525
tarsometatarsal capsulotomies, 525
In-toeing, in children, 18
Intra-articular fractures of distal femur
fracture types
    Salter–Harris type III, IV, 775–777
treatment, 777–778
    delayed treatment, effects, 778
    See also Fractures of knee and tibia
Intra-articular physeal fractures of proximal tibia, 784–785
    See also Fractures of knee and tibia
Intradural tumors, 594–595
astrocytomas and ependymomas, 594
brachial plexus lesions, 595
cerebrospinal fluid shunting, 595
flaccid paralysis, 595
intramedullary lesion, 595
intrinsic muscle wasting, 595
laminectomy, 595
muscular dystrophy, 595
myelogram, 595
neuroblastoma, 594
pathological reflexes, 595
poliomyelitis, 595
posterior fossa decompression, 595
postural torticollis, 595
spastic paralysis, 595
syringomyelia, 595
tumor or traumatic paraplegia, 595
Intramalleolar triplane fracture, 800
Intramedullary bone lengthening
albizzia nail, 417
fitbone, 417
ISKD nail, 417
    See also Leg lengthening
Intramedullary rodding and grafting, 403
Intramembranous ossification, 12, 414, 687
Intramuscular botulinum toxin A(drug), 314
Intramuscular tendon lengthening, 314
Intra-operative neurophysiological investigation (NPI), 371
Intrathecal baclofen (ITB) therapy, 314
Intravenous antibiotic administration, 590
Intrinsic muscle wasting, 595
Inversion deformity, 532
Irradiation therapy, 482
Irreducible ankle fracture, 800
    See also Triplane fracture

Irreducible hip, 454
    anterolateral approach, 454
    arthrogryposis, 454
    capsular plication, 454
    open reduction, 454
    pelvic osteotomy, 454
    splintage, 454
Ischemic necrosis, 125, 466
Isotope bone scintigraphy, 47, 62
Isthmic spondylolisthesis, 592–594, 639–640
    facet joint orientation, 593
    hypertrophic callus, 640
    local angular kyphosis, 640–640
    lumbosacral orthosis, 593
    "lytic spondylolisthesis," 639
    pars interarticularis, 639
    plain films/CT scan, 592
    plain films of spine, 640
    posterior facet joints, 640
    slippage, 593, 639
    subtypes, 639
    tomogram and CT scan, 640
    type II Scheuermann's disease, 640
    zones of endochondral ossification, 640

J
Jefferson fracture, 826
Jellis, J. E., 123–132
"Jigsaw sign," 575
Joint orientation, 409, 593
Joint pains, 91, 130, 433
Jones' type 2 congenital deficiency, 400–401
Jumper's knee, *see* Patellar tendinitis
Juvenile discitis, 591
    "discitis," 591
    ESR/PV, 591
    rigid lumbar hyperlordosis, 591
    Technetium bone scanning, 591
Juvenile idiopathic arthritis (JIA), 195, 424, 430
    characteristics of, 196
    classification of, 196
    course and prognosis, 201
    drugs for, 199
        abatacept, 201
        anakinra, 200–201
        biological medications, 200
        disease-modifying anti-rheumatic drugs (DMARDs), 200
        glucocorticoids, 200
        intra-articular steroid injections, 200
        leflunomide, 200
        methotrexate (MTX), 200
        NSAIDs, 199–200
        rituximab, 201
        sulfasalazine, 200
    enthesitis-related arthritis, 198
    incidence of, 195
    oligoarthritis, 197–198
    psoriatic arthritis, 198
    rheumatoid factor negative/positive polyarthritis, 198
    surgery in, *see* Surgical treatment, for juvenile arthritis
    systemic arthritis, 195–197
    treatment of, 199
    undifferentiated arthritis, 199
Juvenile osteoporosis, 114–115, 633, 846
Juxta-articular deformities, 409

K
King classification of curve patterns, 614
Kirner deformity, 349
    See also Hand developmental anomalies
Kite's method, 545
Klinefelter's syndrome, 99, 362
Klippel–Feil deformity, 245, 359
Klippel–Feil syndrome, 576–579, 629–630
    associated conditions, 578–579
        cardiovascular abnormalities, 578
        deafness, 578–579
        mirror motions (synkinesia), 579
        renal abnormalities, 578
        scoliosis/kyphosis, 578
        Sprengel's deformity, 578
    clinical features, 577
        abnormalities, 577
        shortening of neck, 577
        Sprengel's deformity, 577
    "hidden" abnormalities, 576
    imaging features, 577–578
        C2–C3 segment, 578
        cervical synostosis, 578
        enlargement of cervical canal, 577–578
        fixed bony deformities, 577
        osteoarthritic spurs, 577
    lesions and defects, 576
    symptoms, 577
        mechanical symptoms, 577
        neurological symptoms, 577
    treatment, 579
Klippel–Trénaunay syndrome, 242
Knee, 495–518
    anterior knee pain, 502–513
    dislocation, infant with, 706
    knee deformity, 495–502
    malfunction, 495
    management, 515
        arthroscopic irrigation, 515

Grade I "closed disease," 515
Grade III/IV, 515
Grade II "open disease," 515
lesion size measurement, 515
Outerbridge classification, 515
patellar mobilizations, 515
physiotherapy, 515
neuropathic pain, 515–516
causes of knee pain, 515
chronic or recurrent pain, 515
"distinct diagnosis," 515
glomus tumor, 515
nerve tumors, 515
"obscure diagnosis," 515
post-surgical peripheral neuropathic pain, 515
patellar dislocation and instability, 513–515
anatomical changes, 514
imaging of knee in older adolescent, 514
ligament laxity, 513
medial patellomeniscal/lateral patellotibial ligaments,
513
microfracturing or drilling, 514
osteoarthritis, 514
patellar subluxation/dislocation, 513
patellofemoral instability syndromes, 514
Roux–Goldthwaite procedure, 514
shortened quadriceps mechanism, 514
skeletal procedures, 514
soft tissue realignment, 514
static soft tissue, 513
tibial tubercle–trochlear groove offset, 514
vastus medialis oblique muscle, 513
plastering, 524
psychogenic pain, 517
swollen knee, 516
acute and transient synovitis, 516
arthroscopy, 516
immuno-deficiency and sickle cell disease, 516
pigmented villo-nodular synovitis, 516
septic arthritis, 516
Staphylococcus aureus, 516
synovial chondromatosis, 516
systemic antibiotics, 516
tumors, 517–518
benign bone tumors, 517
knee neoplasia, 517
leukemia and histiocytosis X, 518
limb angulation, risk of, 518
multiple lesions, 517
osteosarcoma and Ewing's tumor, 518
soft tissue tumors, 518
Knee–ankle–foot orthosis (KAFO), 33, 255, 313
Knee deformity, 495–502

congenital dislocation of knee, 495–496
abnormalities and anomalies, 496
"back to front" joint, 495
congenital short tibia syndrome, 496
degrees of knee hyperextension, 495
dysplastic patella, 496
in infants, 496
Larsen's/Catel–Manzke syndrome, 496
skeletal traction, 496
sloping deformity, 496
splintage, 496
flexion deformity, 497–498
arthrogrypotic deformity, 498
dynamic slings, 497
paediatric deformity, 497
serial plaster splints or slabs, 497
supracondylar extension osteotomy, 497
transverse lazy "S" incision, 497
genu recurvatum, 495
joint laxity, 495
genu varum, 499–502
adolescent Blount's disease, 500
Blount's disease, etiology, 500
bone bar or tether, 500
distal, medial femoral epiphysis, 499
distraction osteogenesis, 500
dome osteotomy, 501
infantile tibia vara, classification, 500
"late correctors," 499
leg length discrepancy, 500
pathological deformity, 499
post-infective genu varum, 502
proximal tibial osteotomy, 502
Scandinavian experience, 500
single tibial osteotomy, 500
Tibia vara or Blount's disease, 499
neurological hyperextension, 496–497
post-traumatic tibial recurvatum, 497
secondary genu recurvatum, 496–497
See also Individual
post-fracture genu valgum, 498–499
asymmetrical physeal growth, 499
post-proximal tibial metaphyseal fracture, 500
proximal, metaphyseal tibial fracture, 498–499
valgus deformity, 498
bow leg deformity, 498
cosmetic problem, 498
distal femoral osteotomy, 498
intermalleolar distance, 498
medial stapling or epiphysiodesis, 498
Knee jerks L3–4, 237
Knee neoplasia, 517
Knee stiffness, 393–394

Köhler's disease, 432, 528, 810
  below-knee walking plaster, 528
  osteochondritis of navicular, 528
  Perthes' disease, 528
Kyphosis, 281, 316, 397, 829

L

Laminograms, 580, 847
Landin, Lennart A., 665–669
Langerhans' cell histiocytosis (LCH), 433
Larsen's syndrome, 495, 526, 629
Laryngeal mask airway, 38
Late-onset idiopathic scoliosis, 608–619
  clinical features, 609–610
    buckling of spinal column, 609
    Cobb angle, 609
    curve patterns, 609–610
    emotional time, 609
    idiopathic lumbar curve, 609
    neoplasm or syrinx, 609
    paraplegia, 610
    spinal dysraphism, 610
    thoracic deformities, rib hump, 609
    three-dimensional surface shape measurements, 610
  conservative treatment, 611–612
    brace trial paper, 612
    "corrective effect," 612
    electro-stimulation, 612
    Milwaukee brace, 611
    two-point fixation, 612
  major spinal surgery, 611
  radiographic assessment, 610–611
  school screening programs, 609
  scoliometer, 609
  screening, 609
  spinal cord monitoring, 611
  surgical treatment, 612–619
    American Orthopaedic Association, 612
    AO Universal spine system, 616
    Cobb angle and buckling, 615
    Cotrel–Dubousset system, 615
    dollar-sign fashion, 614
    double curve patterns, 614
    Dwyer instrumentation system, 617
    flat-back deformity, 617
    Harrington instrumentation, 612–613
    idiopathic thoracic curves, 619
    King classification of curve patterns, 614
    Leeds procedure, 615
    Lenke classification, 614
    Luque twin L-rod system, 614
    massive fusion technique, 614
    modern generation posterior instrumentation, 617

    modern universal spine systems, 618
    Moss–Miami spine system, 616
    multiple anterior discectomies, 619
    plaster treatment, 612
    pre-and postoperative localizer, 612
    pseudarthrosis rate, 612
    scoliosis surgery, 618
    secondary scoliotic deformity, 618
    segmental instrumentation, 619
    sole deformity, 618
    spinal column rotation, 615
    spinal de-rotation, 615
    thoracoscopic techniques, 617
    thoracotomy/mini-thoracotomy, 617
    three dimensional deformity, 615
    transverse plane deformity, 614
    "two-in-one" surgery, 619
    "wake-up test," 618
    Zielke's group, 617
  treatment, 611–619
  "wake-up" test, 611
Lateral ankle sprain, 802
Lateral condyle fractures, 725
  displaced fractures, 725
  K-wire fixation, 726
  posterior screw fixation, 726
  treatment, 725–727
  treatment of late cases, 727
Lateral knee
  radiograph with limp and tenderness, 428
Lauenstein view of hip
  flexion/abduction/external rotation, 468
Laxity of transverse atlantal ligament, 574
  chronic atlanto-axial dislocation, 574
  degree of hypermobility or instability, 574
  Down's syndrome, 574
  neurological injury, 574
  "safe zone of steel,", 574
  surgical stabilization, 574
Leeds procedure, 616
Left congenital short femur, 390, 395
Legg–Calvé–Perthes disease, 362, 423, 429, 465–478
  clinical features, 467–468
  conservative treatment, 473
    bed rest, 473
    pharmacological treatment, 473
    physiotherapy, 473
  containment treatment, 473–476
    acetabular osteotomy, 475
    femoral varus osteotomy, 474–475
    hip distraction, 475
    shelf osteotomy, 475–476
    valgus, extension femoral osteotomy, 475

weight-bearing abduction braces, 473–474
course of disease, 466–467
    Elizabethtown classification, 467
    Waldenström's chronological stages, 467
differential diagnosis, 468
    bilateral Perthes disease, 468
    Gaucher's disease, 468
    hemophiliacs, 468
    hypothyroidism, 468
    mucopolysaccharidoses, 468
    multiple epiphyseal dysplasias, 468
    spondylo-epiphyseal dysplasias, 468
epidemiology, 465–466
etiology, 466
    inherited factors, 466
    See also Etiology, Legg–Calvé–Perthes disease
name description, 465
origin and history, 465
other investigations/value, 471
    Conway tracks, 471
    neovascularization, 471
    radioisotope bone scans, 471
    recanalization, 471
    revascularization, 471
    scintigraphy, 471
    ultrasound scans, 471
pathological findings, 467
    epiphysis, 467
    growth plate cartilage columns, 467
    metaphysis, 467
    synovial tissue, 467
prognosis and "head at risk," 472–473
    Catterall's "head at risk" signs, 473
    "flexion with abduction," 472
    lateral metaphysis, 472
    skeletal maturity, 472
prognosis at maturity, 471–472
    congruency/sphericity, types of, 472
    flat head and steep acetabulum, 471
    Mose rings, 471
    osteoarthritis, 471
    Stulberg classification, 472
published results of treatment regimens, 476–477
    Group A/B/C hips, 477
    Group B and B/C border hips, 477
    Group B/C border hip, 477
radiographic features/classifications, 468–471
    Catterall classification, 468–469
    Herring classification, 469–470
    other systems, 470–471
    Salter and Thompson classification, 469
    See also Individual
signs, 467–468

abduction/internal rotation (extension), 467
no abduction/internal rotation (flexion), 468
Trendelenburg gait, 467
suggested management of child with Perthes disease,
    477–478
    age/clinical findings, 477
    anesthesia and arthrogram, 477–478
    clinical signs, 477
    femoral or innominate osteotomy, 477
    late femoral head deformity, 478
symptoms, 467
treatment procedures, 476
upper femoral epiphysis, infarction of, 465
Legg–Calvé–Perthes Study Group in North America, 477
Leg length discrepancy (LLD), 302, 406
    deformities, 406
    leg length discrepancy gait, 424
    limb-length discrepancy and malalignment, 406
    management of, 411
    orthoradiography for measurement of, 408
    patient assessment
        clinical, 407
        deformity analysis and preoperative planning,
            408–410
        imaging, 407–408
        measurement of, 407
    surgical limb equalization
        epiphysiodesis, 411–412
        leg lengthening, 414–417
        permanent growth plate arrest, 412
        permanent hemiepiphysiodesis, 412
        shortening long leg in children, 411
        shortening osteotomies, 413
        temporary arrest of growth plate, 412–413
Leg lengthening
    distraction, 414
    history, 414
    intramedullary bone lengthening
        albizzia nail, 417
        fitbone, 417
        ISKD nail, 417
    mechanical lengthening device, 414–416
    obstacles in
        pin site infections, 418
        prostheses, 418
        severe stiffness, 418
Leong, J. C. Y., 287–303
Leri–Weill disease, 352
Letterer–Siwe disease, 597
Leukemia, 5, 114, 123, 143, 183, 186, 433, 468, 517, 658
Limb equalization
    epiphysiodesis, 411–412
    permanent growth plate arrest

mini-invasive techniques, 412
 Phemister's open surgery technique, 412
permanent hemiepiphysiodesis, 412
shortening long leg in children, 411
temporary arrest of growth plate
 physeal stapling, 412
 8-plate technique, 412–413
 shortening osteotomies, 413–414
Limb-girdle muscular dystrophy (LGMD), 259–260
Limb hypertrophy, 242
Limb lengthening, 56, 98, 391, 393, 414, 418, 697
Limb-length inequality
 and malalignment
 deformities, 406
 etiologies of, 407
 patient assessment
 clinical, 407
 imaging, 407–408
 measurement of, 407
Limp
 age-specific diagnosis of, 423
 causes of, 426
 child abuse, 428
 leukemia, 433
 osteoid osteoma, 433
 trauma, 427–428
 tumors, 432–433
Lisfranc fracture dislocation, classification, 811–812
Lisfranc joint, see Tarsometatarsal joint
Load–deformation curve, 701
Longitudinal deficiency, 341, 389–390
Lower cervical vertebrae (C3–C7), 820
Ludlam, C. A., 123–132
"Luque trolley," 623
Luque twin L-rod system, 614
Lyme disease, 200, 431–432
"Lytic spondylolisthesis," 639–642, 644

M
Macnicol, M. F., 435–462, 481–492, 495–517, 651–663,
 743–749
Macnicol's value, 439
Macnicol technique, 412s
Macrodactyly, 351–352
 See also Hand developmental anomalies
Madelung's deformity, 95, 340, 352
 See also Hand developmental anomalies
Maffucci's syndrome, see Enchondromatosis
Malalignment, 406–407, 512
 analysis of, 409
 femoral anteversion, 512
 growth and correction of, 651–652
 increased Q angle, 512

successful remodeling in, 651
 tibial tuberosity, 512
Malignant tumors, 224
 amputation and rotation plasty, 226
 chemotherapy for, 224–225
 Enneking's resection classification, 225
 Ewing's sarcoma, 224
 Kawaguchi 's resection classification, 225
 MRI for, 224
 osteosarcoma, 224
 post-operative treatment, 227
 reconstruction with epiphysis, 226–227
 reconstruction with functional/ no functional joint, 226
 tumor resection/ staging, 225–226
 See also Bone tumors
Mallet system of measuring function at shoulder, 368–369
Malmö or von Rosen splint, 446
Malnutrition and fractures, 658
Maltracking, 512–513
 "inverted J" sign, 512
 quadriceps tightness, 513
 "subluxation" and "tilt" of patella, 512
"Manipulating and plastering" techniques, 550
Manual muscle testing, 252
Marfan's and Ehlers–Danlos syndromes, 607
Marfan's syndrome, 329
 cause of, 98
 clinical and radiographic features, 98–99
 management of, 99
McBride procedure, 535
McCune–Albright syndrome, see Fibrous dysplasia
Mechanical axis deviation (MAD), 101–102, 221, 408
Mechanical devices for leg lengthening, 414
 Ilizarov ring fixator, 415
 lengthening over nail, 415
 monolateral devices, 415–416
 Taylor spatial frame, 415
Mechanical lengthening device, 414
Mechano-transduction, 12
Medial epicondyle fractures, 727–728
 complete articular fractures of distal
 humerus–T-fractures, 728
Medial malleolar to navicular (MMN) distance, 545
Medial patellofemoral ligament (MPFL), 778
Medial stapling or epiphysiodesis, 498
Medical Research Council (MRC), 237
 grading, 252
Meniscal tears, 507–508
 ACL rupture, 507
 all-inside techniques, 508
 arthroscopic inside-out technique, 508
 hypermobile medial meniscus, 508
 meniscal repair, 507

prime indications, 507
meniscectomy, 507
minor tears, 507
open repair, 508
preservation, 508
red–red zone and repair, 507
red–white zone, 507
vascularization, 507
white–white zone and repair, 507
Meniscectomy, 507, 509
Menkes' syndrome, 122
Mercedes star, see Three-segmented type TPE
Mesencephalon division, 231–232
Mesenchyme condensations, 687
Metabolic and endocrine bone disease, 105, 110
bone, physiology of, 105
bone cells, 105, 107
bone matrix, 107
calcium homeostasis, 108
mineralization, 107
clinical and biochemical features of, 109–110
ectopic mineralization, 119
fibrodysplasia ossificans progressiva, 119–120
fibrous dysplasia, 119–120
progressive osseous heteroplasia, 119
hormones, action on skeleton, 108
calcitonin, 109
parathyroid hormone (PTH), 108
parathyroid hormone-related peptide, 109
vitamin D, 108–109
hyperphosphatasia, 117
hypophosphatasia, 116
adult hypophosphatasia, 116
childhood hypophosphatasia, 116
infantile hypophosphatasia, 116
perinatal lethal hypophosphatasia, 116
treatment of, 117
hypothyroidism, 115–116
osteopetrosis, 117
marble bone disease, 117–118
mild osteopetrosis, 118
severe infantile osteopetrosis, 118
treatment of, 118
types and features of, 117
osteoporosis, 114
idiopathic juvenile osteoporosis, 114–115
parathyroid disorders
hyperparathyroidism, 115
hypoparathyroidism, 115
rickets, 109
biochemistry and histology, 111
causes of, 110
clinical features, 109–110

diagnosis of, 111
and Fanconi syndrome, 112–113
hypophosphatemic rickets, 112
oncogenic rickets, 114
prevention and treatment, 111
radiographic features, 111
renal glomerular rickets, 113
vitamin D-deficiency rickets, 109, 112–114
vitamins and minerals, excess and deficiency of
aluminum excess, 121–122
copper deficiency, 122
fluorosis, 121
idiopathic hypercalcemia, 121
lead poisoning, 121
vitamin A excess, 121
vitamin C deficiency, 120
vitamin D toxicity, 121
Metacarpal fractures
diaphyseal, 746
reduction, 746
distal phalangeal fractures, 747–749
distal physeal, 747
interphalangeal joint dislocations, 749
proximal (and middle) phalangeal fractures, 747
sites of, 747
Metacarpophalangeal joints deformity, 204, 379
Metaphyseal chondrodysplasias, 93
Schmid type
cause of, 93
clinical and radiographic features of, 93
management of, 93
Metaphyseal–diaphyseal angle (MDA) in bow legs,
measurement of, 19
Metaphyseal lucencies, 97, 433
Metastatic deposit from nephroblastoma/neuroblastoma,
660
Metatarsal osteotomies, 525, 535
Metatarsophalangeal (MTP) joint, 198, 205, 302, 321,
535–537, 554
"Method of Describing Limb Deficiencies Present at Birth",
389
Mid-diaphyseal deformities, 409
Mid-foot break, 320
Midfoot/hindfoot osteotomy, 555
Mikulicz line, 408
Milwaukee brace, 255, 611, 845, 849
Minns, R. A., 231–248
Mitchell posterior displacement osteotomy, 562
Modern universal spine systems, 618
Modified injury severity score (MISS), 671–672
Mok, J. Y.Q., 701–713
"Molded baby syndrome," 247, 526
Molded plastic ankle–foot orthosis, 533

Monolateral devices, 415–416
　See also Mechanical devices for leg lengthening
Monostotic lesions, 660–661
Monozygotic twins, 544
Monteggia equivalent (variant) injuries, 738–739
　anatomy, 738
　clinical findings, 738
　differential diagnosis–congenital dislocation of radial
　　　head, 739
　lesions, delayed diagnosis of, 739–741
　mechanism of injury, 738
　neglected Monteggia fracture, treatment, 741
　radiographic findings, 738
　treatment of persistent dislocation of radial head, 741
　treatment of type I, II and III lesions, 738–739
　treatment of type IV lesions, 739
　variant with displaced fracture of radial neck, 740
Monteggia fracture dislocation, 737–738
Monteggia lesions, 737
　Bado classification of, 737
　delayed diagnosis of, 739–741
　hyperextension theory, 738
　types, 737
Morquio's syndrome, 580, 634, 828
Moseley's straight line method, 14
Moss–Miami spine system, 616
Motor skills pathways, 235
MPS4 (Morquio's syndrome), 580, 634, 828
Mucopolysaccharidoses
　causes of, 91
　clinical and radiographic features, 91–92
　features of, 92
　management of, 92–93
Multi-Axial CorrectionMAC Biomet, 415
Multi-injured child, management
　adjuncts to primary survey, 674
　definitive care, 679–680
　secondary survey, 677–679
Multiminicore disease, 261
Multiple epiphyseal dysplasias, 466, 468
Multiple hereditary exostoses, 350, 352–353
Multiple trauma, 671, 680
Multiplier method, 14, 393, 410–411
Murray, A. W., 651–663
Muscle dystrophies, 250, 254
Muscular dystrophy gait, 424–425
Muscular torticollis, congenital, 582–584
　congenital wry-neck, 582–584
　deformities of face and skull, 583
　etiology, 583
　　breech presentation, 583
　　forceps instrumentation, 583
　　primiparous births, 583

　　uterine crowding or "packing," 583
　　vacuum extraction, 583
　imaging, 583
　　compartment syndrome, 583
　　sternomastoid tumor, 583
　right-sided congenital muscular torticollis, 583
　sternocleidomastoid muscle contracture, 582
　sternocleidomastoid muscle, tumor, 583
　treatment, 584
　　conservative, 584
　　operation, 584
Musculo-aponeurotic release of flexors, 322
Musculoskeletal injury, effective management, 653
Musculotendinous lengthening techniques, 314, 321
Mushroom deformity, 475
Mustard procedure, 294
Myasthenia gravis, 249, 252, 262–263
Myelination, 232–233, 371, 373, 384
Myelodysplasia, 73, 246, 328, 604, 625, 628, 659
Myelomeningocele, 242, 265, 267
Myeloschisis, 266–267
Myotonia congenita, 262, 707
Myotonias, 261
Myotonic dystrophy, 262
Myotubular myopathy, 261

N
Nade, S., 135–158
Nail-patella syndrome, see Onycho-osteodystrophy
Nancy nails, see Elastic stable intramedullary nailing
　　　(ESIN)
Narakas classification, 373
Naviculocuneiform fusion, 532
Neck fractures (femoral), causes
　diaplaced/undisplaced fractures, treatment
　　Watson–Jones' anterolateral approach, 761
　high-energy trauma, 759
　pathological conditions
　　cyst, 759
　　disuse osteopenia, 759
　　neurological disorders, 759
Neck–shaft angle, 84, 317, 392
Neonatal injury, differential diagnosis of, 707
Neovascularization, 471
Nerve action potentials (NAPs), 373
Nerve territory orientated macrodactyly, 351–352
Nerve tumors, 402, 515
Neural crest formation, 231
Neural tube defects
　Chiari 1 malformation, 245–246
　congenital motor disorders
　　hemiplegia, 246–247
　　minimal hemiplegia, 247

transient dystonia following prematurity, 247
Duchenne and muscular dystrophies, 246
hereditary sensory motor neuropathies, 247
"isolated cord"
  type 1/2/3/4 cord, 245
profoundly handicapped child, 247
tethered cord, 246
Neurapraxia, 382
Neuroblastoma, 51, 143, 594, 635, 660
  metastasized to inferior pubic ramus, 661
Neurodevelopment examination
  posture and movement/mobility, 234
Neurofibromatosis, 232
  congenital pseudarthrosis of radius in 3-year-old with, 353
  type NF-1, 632
Neurological injury, thoracic and lumbar spine, 841–842
  incidence peaks, 841
  SCIWORA, 841
  stimulation and handling, 842
  symptoms and signs, 841–842
    uncooperative child, determining paralysis, 841
  vertebral fracture in older child, 841
Neuromuscular deformities, 630–632
  cerebral palsy, 630
  collapsing paralytic scolioses, 631
  C-shaped lordoscoliosis, 630
  idiopathic-type deformity, 630
  muscular dystrophies, 632
    Duchenne dystrophy or congenital myopathies, 632
    spinal deformation, 632
  neuromuscular diseases of childhood, 630
  peripheral neuropathies/Friedreich's ataxia/arthrogryposis, 632
    cardiomyopathy, 632
    Friedreich's ataxia, 632
    segmental instrumentation and fusion, 632
  poliomyelitis, 631–632
    infrapelvic/suprapelvic/transpelvic, 632
    scoliosis and pelvic obliquity, 631
  spinal muscular atrophy, 632
    Becker/limb girdle dystrophies, 632
    chest infection, 632
    early-onset Werdnig–Hoffmann, 632
    later-onset Kugelberg–Welander, 632
    spinal surgery, 632
  two-rod systems, 631
  wheelchair stability, 631
Neuromuscular disorders
  hereditary and developmental
    activity test, 251
    atrophy and hypertrophy, 252
    benign X-linked (Becker) muscular dystrophy, 258
    cardiopulmonary function, 255
    central core disease, 260
    classification and clinical features, 256
    congenital muscular dystrophies (CMDs), 260
    congenital myotonic dystrophy, 262
    differential diagnosis, 254
    Duchenne type, 257–258
    electromyography, 253
    Emery–Dreifuss muscular dystrophy (EDMD), 258–259
    etiology and inheritance, 253
    examination, 249–250
    fasciculations, 252
    gait, 252
    infection and nutrition, prevention of, 255
    limb-girdle muscular dystrophy (LGMD), 259–260
    management, 254
    manual muscle testing, 252
    muscle biopsy, 253
    muscle myopathies, 260
    muscle tone, 252
    muscular dystrophies, 256
    myasthenia gravis, 262–263
    myotonia congenita, 262
    myotonias, 261
    myotonic dystrophy, 262
    nemaline myopathy, 260–261
    orthopaedic management, 256
    orthopaedic surgery, 255–256
    orthotics, 255
    physiotherapy and occupational therapy, 254
    polymyositis–dermatomyositis, 262
    posture, 250–251
    reflexes, 252
    serum enzymes, 252
    spinal muscular atrophy, 256
    symptoms of, 249–250
Neuropathic pain, 377, 382, 515
Neurophysiological investigation (NPI), 371, 375
Neurostenalgia, 384
Neurotizations, 367–368
Neurovascular injury, 723–725
  exploration warranted, 725
Non-accidental fractures, 709
Non-accidental injury (NAI), 708
  diagnosis
    bites, 709
    cutaneous injuries bruises, 708–709
    recognition, 708
    risk factors, 708
  differential diagnosis, 712
  factors suspecting, 708
  skeletal injuries, 709–710

classic metaphyseal lesion (CML), 710–711
   diaphyseal (long bone) fractures, 710
   rib fractures, 711
   skull fractures, 711–712
   subperiosteal newbone formation (SNBF), 710
Nonsteroidal anti-inflammatory drugs (NSAIDs), 41, 47–48,
      199–200
Nonwalker CP surgery
   foot and ankle deformity, 318
   hip, 316–318
   knee, 318
   spinal deformity, 315–316

O

Ober's fasciotomy, 293
Obese baby delivery, vertex presentation, 365
Obscure diagnosis, 515
Obstetrical brachial plexus palsy, 357, 372
Occipital horn syndrome, 100, 122
Occipito-cervical fusion
   clinical features, 572–573
      anomalies, 572
      brain-stem pressure, 573
      kyphosis and scoliosis, 572
      nystagmus, 571
      odontoid migration, 573
      pyramidal tract symptoms and signs, 573
   imaging, 573
      patterns of fusion, 573
   occipitalization, 572
   occipito-cervical synostosis, 572
Occiput-C1 injury
   autopsy findings, 826
   treatment, 826
Oculomotor dyspraxia, 235
Odontoid anomalies, 574–576
   cervical spine syndromes, 575
   clinical features, 575
      neck symptoms, 575
      neurological problems, 575
      transitory paresis, 575
   hypoplasia and os odontoideum, 574
   imaging, 575
      blunt stubby or "cone-shaped" os odontoideum, 575
      Brown-Sequard lesion, 575
      C1–C2 articulation, 575
      hypoplasia, 575
      "jigsaw sign," 575
      myelopathy, 575
      odontoid fracture, 575
   treatment, 576
      C1–2 transarticular screws, 576
      Gallie technique, 576

      Harms construct, 576
      occipito-cervical fusion, 576
      spinal cord pressure, 576
      surgical stabilization, 576
      wiring techniques, 576
Odontoid fractures
   complications in young/older children, 828
   diagnosis in Morquio's/Down's syndrome, 828
   growth plate injuries of synchondroses, 826
Ogden classification, 687
Olecranon fractures, 733–734
   entry point for radial elastic nail/K-wire, 734
Ollier's disease, 96–98, 218, 352, 410, 659
   See also Enchondromatosis
Onycho-osteodystrophy, 537
Open fractures
   classification of, 653
   treatment, quick, 653
Open fractures, polytrauma, 682
Open reduction in hip dysplasia, 451–453
   anterolateral approach, 452–453
      bikini transverse incision, 452
      capsulorrhaphy, 453
      hip dislocation, 452
      plaster immobilization, 453
      pre-osseous cartilage, 452
      radio-opaque dye, 453
      Smith-Petersen approach, 452
      T-shaped incision, 452
   medial approach, 451–452
      avascular necrosis, 452
      capsulorrhaphy, 452
      groin crease, 451
      T incision, 451
   posterior approach, 453
      pelvic procedure, 453
      psoas tenotomy, 453
Opioids use, 46
   continuous infusion of opioid, 46
   monitoring protocol, need of, 47
   patient-controlled analgesia (PCA), 46–47
   See also Anesthesia and analgesia, in children
Oro-facial dyskinesia and normal newborn development,
      235
Orthopaedic injuries, 671
   polytrauma treatment, 681–685
Orthopaedic management of cerebral palsy, 307–323
Orthotic management
   ankle–foot orthosis on crouch gait, 312
Orthotics, 73, 255, 389
Osgood–Schlatter disease, 428, 785
   condition, 503
      acute flexion injury, 503

tibial tuberosity apophysis, 503
warm-up and stretching program, 503
Osseous bar, 655
radiographic projections of, 655
Osteoarthritis, 20, 79, 84, 86–91, 93, 118, 124, 288, 301,
317, 406, 411, 437, 458, 471, 488–491, 498,
506–507, 509, 514–515, 535, 746, 763, 784
Osteochondral fractures of knee, 780
clinical and radiological findings, 780
late presentation, 780
mechanism of injury, 780
treatment, 780–781
See also Fractures of knee and tibia
Osteochondritis dissecans, 504–506
arthroscopy, 505
causes of lesions, 504
drilling or microfracture, 505
four standard radiographic views, 504–505
junevile/adult type, 504
Kirschner wire, 505
lesions and fragments, 505
ligament reconstruction, 505
MRI, 505
osteoarthritis, 506
rehabilitation, 505
separation and fragmentation, 504
technetium bone scan, 504
transarticular drilling, 505
Wilson's sign, 504
Osteochondritis of capitellum, 362
Osteogenesis imperfecta (OI), 78, 357, 657, 779, 846
autosomal dominant mutations in, 78–79
classification and features, 79
type I OI, 79
type II OI, 79
type III OI, 79–80
type IV OI, 80
type V OI, 80–81
type VI OI, 81
type VII OI, 81
type VIII OI, 81
diagnosis of, 81
and mobility, 82
tibial fracture in osteogenesis imperfecta, 658
treatment of, 81–82
upper limb deformity after multiple fracture in, 658
Osteoid osteoma, 52, 214, 216, 219–220, 242, 426,
428–429, 432–433, 517, 533, 588, 595, 611,
636, 854
Osteomyelitis, 57, 430–431
Osteopenia, 33, 55, 81, 93, 137, 141, 211, 269, 483–484,
657, 713, 759, 765
Osteopetrosis, 117

marble bone disease, 117–118
mild osteopetrosis, 118
severe infantile osteopetrosis, 118
treatment of, 118
types and features of, 117
See also Metabolic and endocrine bone disease
Osteotomy
level, 409
triple innominate, 458
varus rotational, 456
Overuse syndromes, 428
See also Trauma
Oxford pelvic bone age score, 481, 489

P
Packaging disorders, 250
Paediatric fracture, quick healing in, 651
trophic changes in physeal growth, 651
Paediatric Trauma Score (PTS), 671–672
Paley's multiplier method, 410–411
for leg length discrepancy, 14
See also Deformity analysis
Panhypopituitarism, 233
Panner's disease, 362
Panton–Valentine leukocidin syndrome, 139
Parallax effect, 484
Paralytic convex pes valgus, 276
Paralytic flat foot, 565
Parathyroid disorders
hyperparathyroidism, 115
hypoparathyroidism, 115
parathyroid hormone-related protein (PTHrP), 108–109, 687
Parsch, K., 135–158, 265–285, 731–741, 743–749,
765–771, 793–803
Parvovirus, 127–128
Patella
sleeve fracture, 503–504
stress fractures, 504
Patellar apicitis, 406
Patellar tendinitis, 511
Patello-femoral dysplasia, 779
Patellofemoral instability syndromes, 514
Patellofemoral pain, 428
Pathological fractures, 657
generalized conditions, 657–659
monostotic lesions, 660–661
single-limb involvement, 659–660
skeletal alterations leading to, 657
stress fractures, 661–663
Patient-controlled analgesia (PCA), 46–47
Pavlik splint, 446
Peak height velocity (PHV), 14, 16
Pectus carinatum, 80, 91, 98, 625

Pediatric Advanced Life Support (PALS), 675
Pelvic fractures
    lesion, CT scan of, 662
    polytrauma, 677, 682–685
    stabilization, 682
Pelvic obliquity, 289, 294, 303, 407
Pelvic osteomyelitis, 431
Pelvic osteotomy, 272, 279, 280, 295, 317, 319, 454–458,
        475, 477
    femoral head deformity, 456
    multiple hip surgery, 456
    Pemberton peri-capsular osteotomy, 455
    redislocation, risk of, 456
    shelf procedure, 456
Pelvic remodeling, 460
Pelvic support osteotomies, 461
Pemberton acetabuloplasty, 457
Penta X syndrome, 362
Periacetabular osteotomies, 458
Pericardial tamponade, 673, 675–676
Perichondrial "bone bark," 701
Peripheral hypotonia, EMG features in, 253
Peripheral nerve blockade
    ankle block, 43–44
    digital nerve block, 42–43
    fascia iliaca compartment block, 43
    femoral nerve block, 43
    sciatic nerve block, 43
Peripheral nerve injuries, 365–385
    clinical presentation, 365–367
    document used for recording progress, 374
    etiology and pathogenesis, 365
    indications for operation, 367
    prognosis, 373–374
    spontaneous recovery, 367
    surgical intervention
        anatomical lesions, 368
        complication rate, 369
        late cases, 369
        neurotizations, 367–368
        post-operative care, 368
        results of surgery, 368–369
Perkins' line, 317
Permanent growth plate arrest
    mini-invasive techniques, 412
    Phemister's open surgery technique, 412
Permanent hemiepiphysiodesis, 412
    See also Limb equalization
Peroneal muscular atrophy, 527, 559
Peroneal spastic flat foot, 532–533
Perthes' disease, 55–56, 410, 528
Pes calcaneocavus, 561–562
    Elmslie triple arthrodesis, 562

Mitchell posterior displacement osteotomy, 562
    neurological conditions, 561
    pistol-grip appearance, 561
Pes cavovarus, 559–561
    angle of Meary, 561
    block test, 559
    fixed bony deformity, 561
    Girdlestone toe flexor to extensor, 561
    HMSN, 559
        Charcot–Marie–Tooth type I and II, 560
        Dejerine–Sotta type, 560
    negative block test, 561
    peripheral neuropathies, 559
    plantar/medial release, 561
    plantigrade forefoot, 561
    Robert Jones tendon, 561
    surgical treatment, 561
    tibialis anterior/posterior, 561
    toe deformities, 561
Pes cavus, 559–562
    pes calcaneocavus, 561–562
    pes cavovarus, 559–560
Pes valgus, 311
Phalangeal fractures, distal, 747–749
    volar splintage, 749
Phasic reflexes, 237
    See also Posture and movement/mobility
Phasic spasticity, 240, 308
Phelp's (gracilis) test, 310
Phemister's open surgery technique, 412
Photon-deficient scan, 426
Physeal displacement, 725
Physeal fractures
    distal ulnar, 745
    flow diagram on clinical management of, 693
Physeal injury
    disproportionate growth of forearm bones after, 655
    incidence according to Salter–Harris classification, 691
Physeal-sparing technique, 783
Physeal stapling, 412
Physiotherapy and occupational therapy, 254
Pin site infections, 418
Pirani and Dimeglio classification systems, 545, 547, 551
Pistol-grip appearance, 561–562
Pistol grip deformity, 299, 491
Plagiocephaly, 247, 437, 445, 449, 542, 619
Plantar flexion–knee extension, 273
Plasma viscosity (PV), 590–591
Plaster of Paris jacket, 377, 380
Plexus blockade, 42–45
    brachial plexus blockade, 44
    lumbar plexus blockade, 44
Plicae and bursae, 502, 506–507

ganglion cysts, 506
Lose capital; plicae, 506–507
popliteal cysts, 506
   asymptomatic fluctuant swelling, 506
   knee surgery, 506
   villonodular synovitis or chondromatosis, 506
Pneumothorax (open), 675
Poland's syndrome, 345
Poliomyelitis, 594
   clinical features
      acute stage, 288
      chronic stage, 288
      convalescent stage, 288
      deformities in, 289
      recovery prognosis, 288
   diagnosis of, 289–290
   differential diagnosis
      acute stage, 290
      chronic stage, 290
   established contractures, management of, 290
   etiology and immunization, 287
   lower limbs
      flail hip, 295
      foot and ankle, 298–300
      hip, 292–294
      knee, 296
      pelvic obliquity, 295
   management, 290
   pathology
      acute stage, 287–288
      chronic stage, 288
   upper limbs
      elbow, 291
      forearm, 292
      shoulder, 291
Pollicization of index finger, 343, 346–347
Polymyositis–dermatomyositis, 262
Polytrauma in children, 671–685
   child abuse, 672
   epidemiology, 671–672
   initial assessment and management, 674
      first aid, transport, and hospital facilities, 674–676
   injuries, 672
   management of multi-injured child
      adjuncts to primary survey, 676–677
      definitive care, 679–680
      SAMPLE history, secondary survey, 678
      secondary survey, 677–679
   outcome, rehabilitation, and long-term course, 685
   physiological and anatomical characteristics, 673–674
      airway and cervical spine, 673
      breathing, 673
      circulation, 673–674

      disability, 674
      exposure/endocrine, 674
      fracture patterns, 674
   principal patterns of injuries, 672–673
   principles of treatment
      abdominal injury, 681
      head injury, 680
      orthopaedic injuries, 681–685
      psychological problems, 685
      spinal cord injuries, 680
      thoracic injury, 680–681
   scoring systems, 671
   systemic response, 674
   victims, statistics, 671
Ponseti method, 181, 274, 329–330, 549–550
Positional deformities, 240, 244, 247
Posterior dislocation (PD), 318, 357, 370, 372–374, 377,
      379, 380, 705, 737, 739, 763–764
Posterior scapulo-humeral (PSH) angle, 372, 375
Post-ganglionic rupture, 371, 377
Post-ischemic fibrosis, 381
Postoperative splinting program, 551
Post-poliomyelitis syndrome, 302
Post-traumatic hemiepiphysiodesis, 410
Post-traumatic neuralgia, 384
Post-traumatic tibial recurvatum, 497
   posterior closing wedge osteotomy, 497
   proximal tibial osteotomy, 497
   Salter–Harris type V fracture, 497
   Taylor spatial frame, 497
Postural torticollis, 594
Posture and movement/mobility
   development of, 234
   deviant locomotor development, 236
   "fly-swatting" movements, 236
   hypertonia, 240
   hypotonia
      clinical grades of, 239
      "floppy baby," 239
   motor skills pathways, 235
   muscle power, 237–238
   muscle tone assessment
      "pithed frog posture," 239
      "popliteal angle," 239
      "scarf sign," 238–239
      "sitting in air," 239
      "straight leg raising" test, 238
      "thumbs up" position, 238
      transient dystonia of prematurity, 239
      "Windsweeping" deformity, 239
      "W sitting," 239
   neuromotor development, 234
   phasic reflexes, 237

primitive reflex, 237
Potts' paraplegia, 591
Prader–Willi syndrome, 242
Premature physeal closure (PPC), 149, 155, 691, 795, 797, 800
Primiparous births, 583
Primitive vesicle formation, 231
Pronation-eversion mechanism, 793
Pronation external rotation injury, 795
Prone/supine discrepancy, 240
Prostaglandin inhibitors, 595
Proximal (and middle) phalangeal fractures, 747
    phalangeal shaft fracture, 748
    sites of, 747
    ulnar collateral ligament avulsion, 747–748
Proximal diplegia, 240
Proximal epiphyseal fractures, 759
Proximal femur, 706
    deformity, 475
    fractures, 701, 761–763
        classification, 765
    ossification, 391
Proximal focal femoral deficiency (PFFD), 390, 392, 394–396, 407
    classification of, 393
    See also Congenital femoral deficiency
Proximal humeral epiphysiolysis, 704
Proximal humeral fractures, 719
    birth fractures of proximal humerus, 719
    classification of, 718
    older child, 718–719
        fully displaced fracture of, 723
Proximal interphalangeal (PIP) joint level, 198, 205–207, 347, 749
Proximal metaphyseal fractures, 759
Proximal pole avascular necrosis, 746
Proximal tibial metaphysis, 219, 416
Proximal tibial osteotomy, 129, 497, 501
Pseudoachondroplasia, 85
    clinical features of, 85–86
    genetic cause of, 85
    mobility in, 88
    radiographic features, 86–87
    treatment of, 87
Pseudohypertrophy, 252, 257
Pseudomonas infection, 432
Pseudoparalysis, 186, 290, 431, 704, 707
Psoas abscess, 168, 172, 184, 432, 587
Psoriatic arthritis, 196, 199, 591
Psychogenesis, 232
Pterygium/popliteal web syndrome, 329
Pulmonary contusion, 672–673, 677, 680–681
Pyogenic infection, 163, 174, 589–590, 635

antibiotic therapy, 590
ESR, 590
intravenous antibiotic administration, 590
pyrexia blood cultures, 590
spinal infection, 590
Pyrexia blood cultures, 590

Q
Quadriceps tendinitis, 511
Quadriplegia, 240, 242, 247, 314, 365
Quasi-athetoid hand movements, 235

R
Radial and ulnar shafts fractures, 733–734
    conservative treatment, 734–735
        forearm shaft fractures, displacement, 734–735
        method of Evans, 735
    surgical treatment, 735–737
        delayed union of forearm fracture caused by high-energy injury, 735
        intramedullary elastic pinning of mid-shaft forearm fracture, 734
        technique for intramedullary nailing of radius and ulna, 735
Radial dysplasia, 341
    anomalies commonly associated with, 342
    bilateral radial absence with floating thumbs, 341
    deformity of, 342
    radiograph of, 342
    surgical treatment, 342–343
    See also Hand developmental anomalies
Radialization
    appearance of forearm of 3 years, 343
    carpus, 343
Radial neck fractures, 731–733
    classification of, 732
    Metaizeau technique for reduction and stabilization of, 732
    semi-closed methods, 731
    sigmoid transverse incision, 733
        vs. scar from anterior open reduction, 732
    treated by Metaizeau technique, 731, 733
Radial physeal stress fractures, 745
Radioisotope bone scans, 471
Radiological investigations in hip dysplasia, 441–444
    radiography, 443–444
        acetabular index, 444
        antero-posterior pelvic radiograph, 443
        center–edge angle of Wiberg, 444
        Severin's radiographic classification, 444
        Shenton's line, 444
    ultrasound, 441–443
        Barlow's test, 441

Graf's classification, 441
    imaging techniques, 443
    mid-sagittal scan, 441
    Morin classification, 441
    Suzuki method scans, 441
    US examination, 443
Radio-ulnar synostosis, 340, 350, 362, 739
Rankin, K. C., 161–168
Reactive arthritis, 6, 8, 430
Realignment surgery, 389, 485
Recanalization, 471
Reciprocating gait orthosis (RGO), 29–30, 273
Recklinghausen's curve, 633
Rectus stretch test, 310
Reducible hip, 279, 445, 454, 462
    double hip spica, 454
    psoas tenotomy, 454
Reflex sympathetic dystrophy (RSD), 7, 515
"Reflex" wasting, 242
Reimer's migration index, 317
Reiter's syndrome, 430
Re-segmentation theory, 625
Residual/recurrent deformity, management, 553–555
    calcaneus, 553
        dorsal soft tissue release, 553
        gastrocsoleus complex, 553
    Coleman block test, 552
    dorsal bunion, 554
        flexor hallucis longus, 554
        Jones tendon, 554
        MTP joint, 554
        split or complete tibialis anterior tendon, 554
        supination deformity, 554
    equinus, 552
        cavus deformity, 552
        flat-topped talus, 552
        Ponseti treatment, 552
    flat-topped talus, 552
    hindfoot valgus, 553
        concomitant forefoot surgery, 553
        forefoot supination deformity, 553
        lengthening calcaneal osteotomy, 553
        triple arthrodesis, 553
    hindfoot varus, 553
    ilizarov method, 555
        law of tension–stress, 555
        midfoot or hindfoot osteotomy, 555
        secondary surgery, 555
        soft tissue distraction techniques, 555
    intoeing gait, 554
    leg length discrepancy, 554
    metatarsus adductus, 554
    parental anxiety, risk factors, 552

recurrent clubfoot deformity, 554
    talectomy, 555
    three-dimensional foot deformities, 552
    triple arthrodesis, 555
        American Orthopaedic Foot/Ankle Society scores, 555
        plantigrade foot, 555
Retroperitoneal sepsis, 587
Retropharyngeal soft tissues
    in inspiration/forced expiration, 823
    optimal retrotracheal space for children (Wholey), 823
Revision arthroplasty, 461
Rhizotomy, 240, 313–314
Rib fractures, 61, 122, 429, 672–673, 680, 711
Rib vertebra angle difference (RVAD), 620–621
Rib vertebra angles (RVAs), 621
Rickets, 109
    biochemistry and histology, 111
    causes of, 110
    clinical features, 109–110
    diagnosis of, 111
    and Fanconi syndrome, 112–113
    hypophosphatemic rickets, 112
    oncogenic rickets, 114
    prevention and treatment, 111
    radiographic features, 111
    renal glomerular rickets, 113
    vitamin D-deficiency rickets, 109, 112–114
    See also Metabolic and endocrine bone disease
Right clavicle pseudarthrosis, 358
Right congenital fibular deficiency, 396
Rim syndrome, 458
Risser–Cotrel table, 644
Robb, J. E., 249–263, 307–323
Robert Jones tendon transfer, 561
Rocker-bottomed foot, 276, 330, 547–549, 565
Roundback deformity, 587
Roux–Goldthwaite procedure, 514
Rubinstein–Taybi syndrome, 779
Rule of thirds (Steel), 821
Ruptures of anterior cruciate ligament
    prognosis, 783–784
    treatment, 783
Rush pin, congenital pseudarthrosis of tibia, 403–404, 418

S
Sacral agenesis, 329
Sacroiliac joint, 142, 151, 172, 196, 198, 430, 459
Sacroiliitis, 196, 432, 591
Salter and Harris Type II, 793–796
    PPC, 795
    preferred method, 795–796
        female athlete after pronation-eversion trauma, 796

pronation-eversion mechanism, 793
supination-inversion mechanism, 793
treatment
non-displaced/displaced SH typeII fractures, 793
Salter and Thompson classification, 469
Group A/B, 469
subchondral fracture, 469
Salter–Harris classification, 654, 687, 691, 719
incidence of physeal injuries according to, 691
I and II lesions, 775
of physeal fracture, 689
type III and IV
fractures, 775–777
treatment, 797
type V fracture, 497
Salter's osteotomy, 456–457, 475
Salter type V injury, 588
Salvage procedures, 694
conservative, 694
epiphysiodesis (contralateral physis), 694
epiphysiodesis (injured physis), 694
limb lengthening, 697
orthoses, 694
physiolysis, 694–696
techniques of surgery, 696–697
Sandifer's syndrome, 240, 580
Sauvegrain method, 16, 410
Sauve–Kapandji procedure, 352
Scaglietti closed cast system, 644
Scaphoid fractures, 746
sites of, 746
waist fracture, 746
Scapula congenital elevation
Sprengel's deformity, 359
treatment, 359–360
Scapula fractures, 718
Scapulo-humeral angle, 375–376
Scapulo-humeral dystrophy, 259
Scarf sign, 238–239, 251
Scham's sign, 484
Scheuermann's disease, lumbar and dorsolumbar, 847–849
acute traumatic disc herniation, 847
apprentice kyphosis, or kyphosis muscularis, 847
back pain in the mid-lumbar region following a
weight-lifting, 849
delay in motor milestones and subluxation of the hips, 13
month old, 848
enforced rest or bracing, conservative treatment, 848–849
Gaucher's disease, 848
limbus vertebra, 848
osteogenesis imperfecta, 849
progressive kyphosis, 849
Schmittenbecher, P. P., 671–685

Schmorl node formation, 604, 625
Scintigraphy, 471
"all right track" scintigraphic pattern, 471
"bad track" scintigraphic pattern, 471
"complications" of healing process, 471
Sclerosis, 433
in diaphysis, 390
Scoliometer, 609
Scoliosis, 260, 281
instrumentation, 644
Scoliosis Research Society, 603
Seat-belt injury, 842
Seat-belt fracture, 837
Secondary lumbar lordosis, 424–425
Segmental instrumentation and fusion, 617, 619, 632
Segmental wiring techniques, 644
Selective dorsal rhizotomy (SDR), 314
Selective posterior rhizotomy, 313–314
Sensory deficits, 307, 551
Septic arthritis, 429, 431, 471, 516
four-parameter assessment, 430
Septic arthritis, in neonates and infants, 152–153
antibiotic treatment, 154
diagnosis of, 154
imaging techniques for, 153–154
outcome of, 155–156
recurrence of, 154
surgical treatment of, 154
treatment of, 154
See also Infections of bones and joints
Septic arthritis, in older child, 156
of hip, 156–157
imaging for, 156
of knee, 157
multifocal septic arthritis, 158
of shoulder, 158
See also Infections of bones and joints
Septicemia, 126, 130, 147, 152, 187, 197, 433, 502, 590,
641
Serpentine/skew/"z-foot," 526
cuneiform opening wedge osteotomy, 526
Larsen's syndrome, 526
"z-or s-shaped" foot, 526
Severe flat foot, 565
Severe knee recurvatum, 297
Severe plano-abducto-valgus, 276
Severe right convex scoliosis with ten-year-old girl, 282
Sever's disease, 428, 528–529
Shelf arthroplasty, 459–460, 475–476
bikini incision, 459
curvilinear slot, 459
rectus femoris, 459
Staheli shelf arthroplasty, 460

Shenton's arc, 484
Shenton's line, 443–444
Shortening osteotomies, 413–414
    femoral shortening techniques, 413
    tibial shortening, 413–414
Shoulder, 101, 153, 188, 218, 289, 360, 357, 379, 380,
            703–704, 717, 720
    abduction contracture of, 360
    congenital and acquired dislocation, 357
    dislocations, 379
    dystocia, 370
    and proximal humerus, 704
Shoulder and humerus, fractures around, 717–728, 759
    clavicle fractures, 704, 717
        etiology, 715
        fracture dislocations of medial and lateral ends of
                clavicle, 715
        obstetrical clavicle fracture, 715
        treatment, 715
    complete physeal displacement, 725
    fractures of distal humerus, 661, 704–705, 709–710,
            719–721, 727, 728
        classification, 720–721
        flexion supracondylar fractures, 725
        neurovascular injury, 723–725
        supracondylar fractures, 720
        treatment, 722–723
    fractures of humerus shaft, 719–720
        classification, 719
        treatment, 719–720
    fractures of medial epicondyle, 727–728
        complete articular fractures of distal
                humerus–T-fractures, 728
    fractures of proximal humerus, 718
        birth fractures of proximal humerus, 718
        classification, 718
        proximal humerus fracture of older child, 718–719
    fractures of scapula, 719
    lateral condyle fractures, 725
        treatment, 725–726
        treatment of late cases, 727
Shufflers, 236
Shuffle trait, 236
Sickle cell disease (SCD), 123, 129–131, 468, 516
    and avascular necrosis of hip, 131
    and bacterial and joint infection, 130
    osteomyelitis in, 130–131
    and pre-operative procedures, 130
    short stubby fingers in, 130
    use of tourniquets in, 130
    See also Bleeding disorders and musculoskeletal changes
Silverskiöld's test, 309–310
Simple syndactyly, 345

Sinding–Larsen–Johansson disease, 428, 781
Single bone mineral density (BMD), 81, 114, 241, 846
Single cannulation screw fixation, 487
Single nucleotide polymorphisms (SNPs), 544
Skeletal dysplasias, 6, 75, 77–78, 88, 105, 107, 111, 407,
            497, 511, 604, 633, 656–657
Skeletal injuries, 709
    classic metaphyseal lesion (CML), 710–711
    diaphyseal (long bone) fractures, 710
    rib fractures, 711
    skull fractures, 711–712
    subperiosteal newbone formation (SNBF), 710
Skeletal shortening of centralization, 343
Skin dimple, 328, 354, 391
Skull fractures, 666, 678, 711–712, 713
Sleeping helmet, 584
Slippage, 55, 481, 482, 485, 592–593, 639–641, 644
Slipped upper femoral epiphysis (SUFE), 55–56, 427, 432,
            482–485, 491–492, 759
Slipped vertebral apophysis, 838–840, 848
    laminectomy and decompression, 840
Slipping of upper (capital) femoral epiphysis (SUFE), 55,
            432, 465, 481–482, 495, 500, 688, 706, 759, 838
    autosomal dominant disorder, 481
    bilaterality, 481
    obesity/radiographic surveillance, 481
    treatment, 479
    zone of hypertrophic cartilage, 479
Smith, R., 80, 105–122, 156, 253, 263, 278, 294, 376, 378,
            452, 508, 762, 840
Smith's fracture, 744
Soap-bubble trabeculation, 595
Soft tissue, 672, 674, 679–680, 682
    contusion, polytrauma, 679
    distraction techniques, 555
    tumors, 517
Sole deformity, 618
Somatosensory evoked potentials (SSEP), 246, 376, 824
Sotos syndrome, 242
Southwick angle, 484
Space available for the spinal cord (SAC), 573, 575, 577,
            821
Spasticity, 68, 73, 236, 240, 242, 244, 245, 247, 252,
            267–269, 271, 273, 307–316, 319–323, 573,
            685, 836, 844
Spastic paralysis, 308, 594
Speech disorders, 307
Spina bifida, 27, 30, 53, 233, 246, 248, 252, 265–285, 328,
            359, 497, 523, 537, 541–542, 544, 559,
            561–562, 604, 625, 628, 641–642, 659, 781, 850
    aims of orthopaedic management, 271–272
    bone fragility, 269–270
    coexistent congenital malformations, 268

arthrogryposis, 268
    traction of nerve roots, 268
coordinated management, 271
deformity
    "diamond posture," 268
    habitually assumed posture after birth, 268
    intrauterine posture, 268
    muscle imbalance due to lowermotor neurone lesions, 267
    muscle imbalance due to uppermotor neurone lesion, 267–268
    "pithed frog position," 268
embryology and pathology, 266–267, 283
    meningocele, 266
    myelomeningocele, 266
    myeloschisis/myelocele, 266
etiology, 75–76
    diet and drugs, 266
    genetic predisposition, 266
gait analysis, 272–273
incidence, 265
management of deformities
    foot and ankle, 274–277
    hip, 278–279
    knee, 277–278
    "pistol grip" heel, 275
    spine, 280–282
    talipes equino varus management in, 275
neonatal management, 271
neurological lesion in, 269
newborn child with, 266
orthoses and mobility aids
    ankle/foot orthosis, 273
    HKAFO, 273
    KAFO, 273
    wheelchairs, 273–274
pathological epiphyseal loosening, 269
pressure sores and chilblains, 269
prevention and counseling, 270–271
types of, 267
Spina bifida and spinal dysraphism, 265–285, 328, 557
Spinal column rotation (CR), 49, 51, 606–607, 615
Spinal cord, 14, 15, 27, 53, 57, 67, 83, 85, 90, 173, 242, 245, 249, 265–267, 283–284, 287, 290, 559, 575, 577, 610, 625, 836, 845
    compression, 634
    injuries, polytrauma treatment, 680
Spinal cord injury without observable radiographic abnormalities (SCIWORA), 588, 680, 824–825, 830, 841
    SCIWORA lesions, 680
Spinal deformities, 78, 82, 93, 302, 315–316, 599–636, 844
    basic principles, 599–604

congenital deformities, 625–630
    congenital bony deformities, 626–628
    congenital spinal cord deformities, 628–630
heritable disorders of connective tissue/mucopolysaccharidoses/skeletal dysplasias, 633–635
    achondroplasia, 634
    other dysplasias, 634–635
    platyspondyly/bullet-shaped vertebra, 634
    severe osteogenesis imperfecta, 634
idiopathic scoliosis, 607–625
    early-onset idiopathic scoliosis, 619–623
    idiopathic hyperkyphosis, 623–625
    late-onset idiopathic scoliosis, 608–619
indications for surgical treatment, 303
infection, deformities, 633
method of treatment, 303
neuromuscular deformities, 630–632
structural spinal deformities, pathogenesis of, 604–607
traumatic spine deformities, 635
tumors, deformities, 635–636
Von Recklinghausen's disease, deformities, 632–633
    See also Individual
Spinal de-rotation, 615
Spinal dysraphism, 604, 627–283, 328
    diagnosis and differential diagnosis, 283–284
    embryology and pathology, 283
    incidence, 283
    management of, 284–285
Spinal infection, deformities, 588–590, 635
    anterior spinal growth, 635
    pyogenic infection, 635
    tuberculous spine, 635
Spinal muscular atrophy, 23, 241, 249, 252, 256, 328, 523, 630, 632, 707
Spine, fractures of, polytrauma, 671–685, 717, 769, 782, 789
Spine–pelvis relationship, 644
Spiral fractures, 428, 702, 711, 719, 767, 769, 771, 788
Splenic rupture, polytrauma, 677
Splintage, 29, 33, 81, 82, 125, 127, 129, 131, 290, 298, 300, 329, 330, 331, 342, 345–346, 348, 440, 445–446, 496, 538, 651, 692, 705, 749
    child after treatment for fixed flexion of knees, 331
Splint types, 446
    Craig splint, 446
    European multicenter trial of 1988, 446
    Frejka pillow, 446
    Malmö or von Rosen splint, 446
    Pavlik splint, 446
    risk of complications, 446
Split hand/split foot malformation (SHSM), 344
Split hook, 340–341

Spondyloarthropathies, 430
Spondyloepiphyseal dysplasia, 75, 77, 85, 88–91, 106, 580,
         634, 828
   spondyloepiphyseal dysplasia congenita, 89
      cause of, 89
      clinical features, 89
      radiographic features, 90
      treatment of, 90
   spondyloepiphyseal dysplasia tarda
      clinical features, 91
      diagnosis and teatment, 91
      genetic cause of, 90
      radiographic features, 91
   stickler syndrome
      clinical and radiographic features, 91
      genetic cause of, 91
      treatment of, 91
Spondylo-epiphyseal dysplasias, 468
Spondylolisthesis, 218, 314, 587, 592–594, 639–645, 661,
         828–829, 838, 853, 855
   clinical features, 642–643
      hamstring spasm or contracture, 642
      lumbosacral kyphosis, 642
      slipping vertebra, 642
      spinal claudication and leg fatigue, 642–643
      spondyloptosis, 642
      thoraco-lumbar hyperlordosis, 642
      z-deformity, 642
   dysplastic spondylolisthesis, 640–641
   isthmic spondylolisthesis, 639–640
   measurement, 641–642
      angle of sagittal rotation, 641–642
      anterior displacement or slip, 641
      lumbo-sacral kyphosis, 642
   treatment, 643–645
      bilateral intertransverse fusion, 644
      bone destructive lesion, 643
      interbody fusion, 644
      intervertebral disc derangements, 643
      isotope bone scanning, 643
      L5 nerve roots, 645
      lumbo-sacral kyphosis, 644
      nerve root decompression, 644
      painkiller and antiinflammatory drugs, 644
      progressive slippage, 644
      Risser–Cotrel table, 644
      Scaglietti closed cast system, 644
      scoliosis instrumentation, 644
      segmental wiring techniques, 644
      solid fusion/body shape, 644
      spinal fusion, 644
      spine–pelvis relationship, 644
      Wiltse-type fusion, 645

Spondylolisthesis of C2, 828, 829
Spondylolysis, 425, 428, 587, 592, 640, 643, 661, 839,
         849–855
Sprengel's deformity, 357, 359, 577, 578, 579
Sprengel's shoulder, 245, 359–360, 629–630
Squint baby syndrome, 239, 240
Stagnara's principle, 602
Staheli hip extension test, 309
      See also Cerebral palsy (CP), children with
Steindler flexorplasty, 333
Steindler's flexorplasty, 291
Steinert disease, 262
Sternomastoid tumor, 583
Straight leg raising test to assess hamstring length, 309
      See also Cerebral palsy (CP), children with
Strayer technique, 320, 435
Streeter's dysplasia, 352, 389
Streptococcal pharyngitis, 430
Stress fractures, 22, 426, 427–428, 502, 504, 535, 592, 639,
         659–661, 745, 759, 766, 787–788, 813, 850, 853
   of proximal tibia, 659, 662
   stabilization of, in Bartter's syndrome, 660
      See also Trauma
      See also Fractures of knee and tibia
Stretching and strapping techniques, 329, 550
Stretch tests for CP, 310
Structural spinal deformities, pathogenesis, 604–607
   biological/mechanical factors, 604
   brittle bone disease, 606
   column buckling, 606
   compensatory lumbar hyperlordosis, 605–606
   epidemiological surveys, 604
   Euler's laws, 606
   lordotic sagittal plane abnormality, 604
   Marfan's and Ehlers–Danlos syndromes, 607
   prismatic-shaped structure, 606
   sagittal plane direction, 605
   Scheuermann's deformity, 605–606
   Schmorl node formation, 604
   schooliosis, 604
   scoliosis screening programs, 604
   spinal column rotation (CR), 606–607
   thoracic kyphosis, 604
   transverse plane geometry of vertebrae, 607–608
   type I Scheuermann's hyperkyphosis, 604
   Von Recklinghausen's disease, 606
Stulberg's classes of deformity, 472
   aspherical congruency, 472
   aspherical incongruency, 472
   spherical congruency, 472
Subacute osteomyelitis, 149–151, 431, 528, 530
   classification of, 150
   clinical features, 149

discitis, 151
imaging for diagnosis of, 150
incidence of, 149
laboratory tests for, 150
pelvic osteomyelitis, 150–151
puncture wound osteomyelitis, 151
treatment of, 150
See also Infections of bones and joints
Subcapital humerus fracture, polytrauma, 677
Subperiosteal newbone formation (SNBF), 710
Subscapularis muscle elongation, 380
Subtalar valgus, 276, 277
Sucking chest wound, *see* pneumothorax (open)
Sugimoto's system, 470
Summit ossification center, 820
Supination-inversion mechanism, 793, 799–800
Supple clasped thumb, 345, 346
Supracondylar fractures, 189, 362, 383–384, 666, 720,
 723–725
 AO and Gartland classification methods for, 722
 classification, 720–722
 configuration of wires to be used, rules, 723
 pinned with lateral wires, 723
 reduction of displaced, 723
 types, 721
 typical AO type 4 (Gartland 3) displaced, 724
Supracondylar humeral spur, 361
 See also Elbow, congenital anomalies
Supracondylar osteotomy for knee flexion contracture, 302
Supramalleolar corrective osteotomy, 797, 799
Surendar, M. T., 161–168
Surgical treatment (femoral epiphysis), 155, 317, 391, 411,
 423, 485–491
 contralateral prophylactic fixation, 489–491
 contralateral fixation, 489
 femoro acetabular impingement, 488
 Oxford pelvic bone age score, 489
 Pistol grip deformity, 491
 later proximal femoral osteotomies, 488
 femoro-acetabular impingement, 488
 intertrochanteric osteotomy, 488
 in situ fixation, 485–486
 cannulated screw, 486
 guide wire or screw, 486
 percutaneous fixation, 485
 pinning or cannulated screw insertion, 486
 posteroinferior quadrant, 486
 subcapital osteotomy, 488–489
 contralateral prophylactic fixation, 488
 distal femoral epiphysiodesis, 488
 Dunn procedure, 488
 fish osteotomy, 489
 plane of dissection, 488

unstable slip, 487–488
double screw fixation, 487
 isotope bone scan, 487–488
 single cannulation screw fixation, 487
 treatment, 488
 trochanteric osteotomy, 488
Surgical treatment, for juvenile arthritis, 59, 202
 joint specific procedures
 ankle and subtalar joints, 209
 elbow, 206–207
 foot, 210–211
 hand and wrist, 206, 208
 hip joint, 206
 knee joint, 206–207, 209–210
 shoulder, 206
 spine, 211
 morphological and pathological changes, in disease, 202
 and postoperative management, 211
 preoperative procedure, 202–203
 surgical procedures
 arthrodesis, 205–206
 corrective osteotomy, 204
 joint replacement, 206
 nerve decompression, 204
 resection arthroplasty, 205
 synovectomy, 203–204
 tendon procedures, 204
Suzuki method scans, 441
Symbrachydactyly, 339, 340, 341, 344
 cleft hand type, 341
 five digital rays, absence of, 341
 frequency of, 345
 monodactylous type, 341
 short finger type, 341
 See also Transverse absence
Syme's amputation, 397
Symphysis pubis, 392, 458, 682, 756
Synaptic pruning, 232
Syndactyly, 11, 37, 182, 340, 345, 534, 536, 577, 629
 See also Hand developmental anomalies
Syndromic foot, 544–545
Synovial chondromatosis, 507, 516
Synovitis, 6, 55, 59, 129, 152, 156, 163, 168, 206, 208, 218,
 424, 427, 506, 516
Syringomyelia, 53, 57, 176, 244, 265, 281, 571, 595, 635,
 845
Systemic diseases, 845–847
 acute leukemia with back pain and multiple compression
 fractures, 847
 assessment of vertebral morphology, 846–847
 BMD, 846
 chondrodystrophies, 846
 compression fractures in osteogenesis imperfecta, 846

Ewing's sarcoma, 846
Gaucher's disease, 846
lipidoses, 846
mucopolysaccharides, 846
multiple vertebral collapse, 846
progressive spinal deformity, scoliosis, and kyphosis, 846
spontaneous onset of vertebral pain in the thoracic spine,
    846
vertebral compression fractures, 846

T
Talar neck fractures
    classification (Hawkin)
        Type I, 805
        Type II, 805
        Type III, 805
        Type IV, 806
    treatment
        and risk of avascular necrosis, 806
Talectomy, 275, 300, 330, 555
Talonavicular/calcaneocuboid joint, 809
Talo-navicular dislocation, 330, 566
Talus fractures
    blood circulation, 805
    classification
        by Hawkin, talar neck fractures, 805–806
        neck/body fractures, 805
    diagnosis
        MRI/CT, 806
    epidemiology, 805
    mechanism of injury, 805
    treatment
        fracture of talar neck, 806
        fractures of the body (dome) of talus, 806
        fractures of the head of talus, 806
        fractures of the lateral talar process, 807
Tamponade effect theory, 466
Tanner and Whitehouse system, 410
Tarsal coalition, 532–533
    anteater's nose, 533
    autosomal dominant inheritance, 533
    bilateral peroneal spastic flat feet, 532
    inversion deformity, 532
    peroneal spastic flat foot, 532
    talocalcaneal coalition, 532
    treatment, 533–534
        beaking of talus, 533
        calcaneal osteotomy, 533
        closing medial wedge osteotomy, 533
        hydrocortisone, 533
        molded plastic ankle–foot orthosis, 533
        osteoid osteoma, 533
        peroneal spastic flat foot, 533

triple arthrodesis, 533
Tarsometatarsal injuries
    imaging, 811
    Lisfranc fracture dislocation, classification, 811
    mechanism of injury
        causes, 810
        talonavicular/calcaneocuboid/tarsometatarsal joints, 810
    treatment, 811–812
Tarsometatarsal joint, 554, 809
Taylor spatial frame, 415–416, 497
    See also Mechanical devices for leg lengthening
T-Box (TBX) transcription factors, role in limb
        development, 11
Technetium bone scan, 151, 504, 591, 596, 787
Technetium bone scanning, 591, 596
Telencephalon division, 232
Temporary arrest of growth plate
    physeal stapling, 412
    8-plate technique, 412–413
    shortening osteotomies, 413–414
    See also Limb equalization
Temporary hemiepiphysiodesis, 410
Temporary paralysis
    of medial rotators by botulinum toxin, 381
Tendo-Achilles
    lengthening, 527
    posteriorly, 330
    shortening, 527
Tendon–bone junctions, 430
Tensioned Kirschner wires, 415
Teratologic dislocation, 565
Tertiary areas maturation, 232
Thalassemias, 129
    See also Bleeding disorders and musculoskeletal changes
Theologis, T. N., 67–73
Thigh–foot angle, 17–18, 310
Thomas's test, 278, 309, 425
Thoracic and lumbar spine, fractures
    differential diagnosis, 845–849
    general and basic principles, 835–836
        development of the thoracolumbar spine, 835
            normal spine in a 10-week-old infant, radiograph,
                835–836
            paralytic scoliosis, 836
            vertebral apophyses, 835
    imaging features, 842–843
        compression due to hyperflexion, 842
        damage to vertebral endplate, 842
        injury to bones and ligaments, classification, 843
        multiply damaged vertebrae, 842
        positioning, 842
    incidence
        American football injuries, 836

compression fractures of three vertebrae, 836
mechanism of injury and age, 836
mechanisms of injury
anterior middle and posterior columns after Denis, illustration, 837
burst fracture, 837
compression fracture, 837
fracture dislocation, 837
seat-belt fracture, 837
severe fracture dislocation of the thoracic spine, 837
neurological injury, *see* Neurological injury, thoracic and lumbar spine
traumatic spondylolysis, *see* Traumatic spondylolysis
treatment, 843–845
See also Treatment for thoracic and lumbar spine fracture
Thoracic injury, polytrauma treatment, 680
Thoraco-lumbar orthoses
spinal alignment in and out, 313
Thoraco-lumbar-sacral orthoses (TLSOs), 255
Thoracoscopic techniques, 617
Three-dimensional gait analysis, 272
Three-ray foot, 397
Three-segmented type TPE, 800
Thrombocytopenia-absent radius (TAR) syndrome, 341, 438
Thumb hypoplasia, 345–347
cigarette grip between adjacent fingers in children, 347
classification of, 346
See also Hand developmental anomalies
Thumb-in-palm deformity, 322
Thumb, Wassel type IV duplication, 351
Tibial tuberosity apophysis, 503
Tibia recurvatum, 404–405
Tillaux fracture
prognosis of, 800
treatment, 799–800
Tinel sign, 382
Tip-toe walking
ankle kinematics and kinetics, 528
degree of hyperextension, 527
idiopathic tip-toe walking, 527–528
muscle biopsies, 527
neuromuscular disorders, 527
perinatal hyperbilirubinemia, 528
persistent tip-toewalking or persistent equinus, 527
heel–toe pattern of gait, 527
toe–heel or toe–toe gait, 527
tip-toe gait, 527
treatment, 527
Titanium elastic nail (TEN), 653, 771
Toddler's fracture, 427, 791
Toe–finger test, 243
Toes, 534–538
accessory navicular, 537–538

Kidner procedure, 538
MR scan, 537–538
symptom-provoking footwear, 538
tibialis posterior tendon, 537
type 1/type 2 ossicle, 537
curly toes, 534
duplication, syndactyly, and accessory toes, 537
chondroectodermal dysplasia, 537
fibrodysplasia (myositis) ossificans progressiva, 537
nail-patella syndrome, 537
polydactyly, surgery, 537
pre/post-axial polydactyly, 537
hallux rigidus, 536–537
hallux valgus, 534–536
hallux varus, 536
interphalangeal valgus of big toe, 537
distal phalanx, 537
proximal phalanx, 537
metatarsus primus elevatus, 537
overriding fifth toe, 534
congenital deformity, 534
congenital elevation of fifth toe, 534
double V-Y plasty, 534
radical bony procedures, 534
V-Y plasty, 534
Y-V plasty, 534
overriding second toe, 536
curly third, fourth, and fifth toes, 536
fixed contracture and tenotomy, 536
fixed flexion deformity, 536
flexor-to-extensor transfer, 536
simple flexor tenotomy, 536
Tomograms, 573, 575, 640, 824
Tonic spasticity, 240, 244, 308, 320–321
Torticollis, differential diagnosis, 579–580
acute pharyngitis, 580
benign paroxysmal torticollis, 580
C1–C2 disc, risk factors, 579
Cl–C2 instability, 580
congenital muscular torticollis, 579
drug intoxication, 580
fracture or dislocation, 580
inflammatory conditions, 580
intermittent torticollis, 580
milder forms, 580
polyarticular juvenile idiopathic arthritis, 580
radiographs, 580
cineradiography, 590
flexion–extension stress films, 580
laminograms, 580
X-ray beam, 580
Sandifer's syndrome, 580
space-occupying lesions, 580

Torus fractures, 786, 790

Traction apophysitis, 504

Transitional fractures
    Tillaux fracture, treatment, 799–800

Transverse absence, 340–341
    digital absence, 341
    proximal forearm, 340–341
    See also Hand developmental anomalies

Transverse atlantal ligament, 574, 820–821, 826

Transverse deficiency, 389–390

Trauma
    fractures, 426
    overuse syndromes, 428
    stress fractures, 427–428

Traumatic dislocation of hip
    anterior/posterior, 763–764
    habitual hip dislocation, cause, 764
    reduction by closed methods, 764

Traumatic dislocation of shoulder, 357

Traumatic disorders of cervical spine
    cervical spine injuries
        fractures of the atlas, 826
        immobilization, 829–831
        incidence and physical findings, 823–824
        lower cervical injuries (C2–C7), 828–829
        neonatal trauma, 825
        occiput-C1 injury, 826
        odontoid fractures, 826–828
        principles, 823
        radiological evaluation, 824
        spinal cord injury without observable radiographic
            abnormalities, 824–825
        spondylolisthesis of C2 (Hangman's fracture), 828
        surgical stabilization, 831–832
    development and variations
        lower cervical instability, 822
        lower cervical vertebrae (C3–C7), 820
        mobility, 820–821
        pseudosubluxation, 822
        retropharyngeal soft tissues, 823
        upper cervical vertebrae (C1 and C2), 819–820

Traumatic spine deformities, 635

Traumatic spondylolisthesis, 639

Traumatic spondylolysis
    acute herniated Schmorl's node, 851
    back pain, repetitive injury to lumbar spine by lifting
        weights, 850
    in children, 849
    congenital anomaly of spine, 849
    in female gymnasts, 850
    high rate
        certain ethnic groups, 850

    teenagers with dorsolumbar Scheuermann's disease,
        850
    increased incidence of sacral spina bifida, 850
    lumbar Scheuermann's disease, 851
    normal appearance of the lumbosacral junction, 852
    spondylolysis (10-year old), 852
    stress or fatigue fracture, pars interarticularis, 853
    symptoms and signs, 852–853
        bone scans, positive, 854–855
        deficiency of the posterior elements, 853
        dysplastic type, chiildren with, 853
        snap in low back during swimming racing turn, 854
        unusual appearance of reactive sclerosis and
            hypertrophy, 854
    teenagers with dorsolumbar Scheuermann's disease, 850
    treatment
        bone graft coupled with intertransverse process
            fusion, 855
        child or adolescent with symptoms, 855
        defects between L1 and L4, 855
        Gill procedure or laminectomy, 855
        hamstring tightness, 855
        restriction of vigorous activities, 855
    vertebral endplate changes at several levels, 851

Treacher-Collins syndrome, 629

Treatment for thoracic and lumbar spine fracture, 843–845
    burst fractures, children with, 843
    compression fractures, 843
    indications for immediate surgical decompression,
        843–844
    in late adolescence, 843
    neurological injury, 844–845
        kyphotic deformity, progressive, 844–845
        multiple trauma in motor vehicle accident, radiograph,
            844
        progressive lumbar lordosis, 844
        treatment of scoliosis, 845
    post-traumatic syrinx, 845
    residual deformity, 844
    spinal instrumentation in adults, 843
    spontaneous interbody fusion, 843
    traumatic spinal cord lesion, 843
    vertebral subluxation or fracture dislocation, 843

Treatment of hip dysplasia, 445–462
    at birth, 445–447
        dislocatable hip, 445
        risk infant, 445
        splintage, 445–446
        teratological hip, 445
        types of splint, 446
    in first few months, 448
    in later childhood, 455–458
        femoral osteotomy, 455

innominate osteotomy, 456–457
  pelvic osteotomy, 455–456
  pemberton acetabuloplasty, 457
before 12 months, 446–453
  arthrography, 449–450
  avascular necrosis, 449
  closed hip reduction, 449
  Galeazzi's sign, 448
  infantile skeletal skew, 448
  ischemic injury, 448
  management, 450–453
  open or closed reduction, 449
  Pavlik harnessing, 448
  porcine model, 448
of toddler, 453–454
  groin lump, 453
  hyperlordosis of lumbar spine, 453
  irreducible hip, 454
  reducible hip, 454
  short leg/Trendelenburg limp, 453
Trendelenburg gait, 70, 391, 424–425, 459, 467, 483
Triceps transfer, 333
Trigger thumb, 349–350
  See also Hand developmental anomalies
Triphalangeal thumb, 351
  See also Hand developmental anomalies
Triplane fracture
  epi/metaphyseal injury identification by MRI, 800
  intraepiphyseal/intraarticular identification by CT, 800
  intramalleolar, 800
  treatment
    arthroscopy-assisted reduction and percutaneous
      fixation, 801
    two/three/four-parts fractures, 800–801
Triplane tibial epiphyseolysis (TPE), 800
  two/three/four-segmented, 800
Triple arthrodesis, 101, 181, 275–276, 298, 300–301, 330,
      533, 553, 555, 561–562
Triple deformity, 566
Trochanteric osteotomy, 90, 102, 280, 461, 488
Trochanteric overgrowth, 445, 461, 467
Trophic limb changes, 241
Tropics, orthopaedic diseases in, 179–180
  acute and chronic osteomyelitis, 183
  amniotic deformity, adhesion, and mutilation complex,
    182
  child abuse, 189
  congenital insensitivity to pain, 182–183
  congenital talipes equinovarus, 181
    Ponseti method for, 181
  countries in tropical belt, 179
    demography of, 179–180
    environment and diseases in, 179

and global health initiatives, 180
developmental dysplasia of hip, 181–182
  and drug therapy, 181
Ewing's sarcoma, 187
hemophilic pseudotumors, 187–188
leprosy, 185–186
musculo-skeletal tumors, 186
necrotizing fasciitis, 184–185
osteosarcoma, 186–187
Perthes' disease, 188
post-injection fibrosis of muscles, 188
road traffic accidents, 190
scoliosis, 188
septic arthritis, 183
snake bites, 188–189
soft tissue sarcomas, 187
supracondylar humeral fractures, 189
syphilis, 186
traditional beliefs and treatment, 180–181
tropical muscle abscess, 183–184
tuberculosis, 185
war injuries, 190–191
workplace accidents, 190
yaws, 186
Tuberculosis of skeletal system, 161
and anti-tubercular drugs, 167–169
  first-line drugs, 169
    multidrug-resistant cases, 169
    second-line drugs, 169
    toxicity and side effects, 169
  areas of predilection, 161
  atypical mycobacteria, diseases by, 164
  causative organism, 164
    sensitivity of, 164
  characteristics and symptoms of, 164–165
  development of, 162
  diagnosis of, 165
    biopsy for, 165
  end result of, 168, 170
  HIV infection and reduced host immunity, 162
    cold abscess, 163
    experimental tuberculosis, 162
    osseous changes and tubercular sequestra, 164
    osteoarticular disease, 162–163
    tubercle, 163
    tuberculous lesion, future of, 164
  investigations for
    biopsy, 166
    blood tests, 165
    clinical trial of treatment, 165
    guinea pig inoculation, 166
    Mantoux Test, 166
    radiography and imaging, 165

management of, 166–167
  abscess, effusion, and sinus, treatment of, 168
  anti-tubercular drugs, 166–167
  rest, mobilization, and bracing, 167–168
  staging and treatment of articular tuberculosis, 168
recurrence of, 170
spinal tuberculosis, 170
  abscesses and sinuses in, 172
  clinical features of, 171
  course of disease, 173–174
  differential diagnosis of, 174
  indications for operations in, 175
  kyphosis in, 177–178
  lateral shift and scoliosis, 173
  myelography and imaging in, 177
  neurological complications and causes, 175–176
  paradiscal type of lesion in, 172
  paraplegia in, 175
  paravertebral shadow in, 172–173
  Potts' paraplegia, treatment of, 177
  prognosis for, recovery of cord function, 177
  radiological healing of, 175
  sites of, 171–172
  symptoms and signs of, 170–171
  treatment for, 175
  vertebral lesions in, 171–172
surgery in, 169–170
  extent and type of, 170
vaccination for, 161–162
  complications of, 162
Tuberculous infection, 590–591
  AIDS, 590
  anti-tuberculous drugs, 590
  chemotherapy, 590
  inflammatory markers, 590
  L1 vertebral body, 590
  Potts' paraplegia, 591
  risk factors, 590
  T10 vertebral body, 590
  vaccination, 590
Tuberous sclerosis, 232–233
Tubesaw method, 412
Tumors, 432–433
  deformities caused by, 635–636
    extradural tumors, 635–636
    gliomas, 635
    idiopathic lordoscoliosis type, 635
    intradural tumors, 635
    MRI scanning, 635
    muscle spasm, 635
    paravertebral tumors, 635
    syringomyelia, 635
    syrinx or excision, 635

    tomography or CT scanning, 636
    Wilms' tumor and neuroblastoma, 636
Turner's syndrome, 329, 362, 482
T10 vertebral body, 590
Type I–acute and chronic infantile disease, *see*
    Werdnig–Hoffmann's disease
Type II and III hypoplasia of thumb, 346
Type III (basocervical) fracture of femoral neck, 762
Type II Scheuermann's disease, 640
Type I (Salter–Harris) fracture, 483–484
Typical z deformity, 561

U
Ulnar dysplasia, 344
  classification of, 344
  See also Hand developmental anomalies
Ulnar osteotomy, 741
Ulnar polydactyly, 350–351
Ulno-carpal fusion, 343
Ultrasonographic (US) screening technique, 439
Undeformed knee with quadriceps weakness, 277
Unicameral bone cysts, 222, 433
Unilateral/asymmetrical abduction contracture, 293
Unilateral dislocation, 455, 462
Unilateral synostosis, 350
Universal screening, 440
Upper cervical vertebrae (C1 and C2)
  ossification centers at birth, 819

V
Vaccination, 140, 161–162, 255, 287, 516, 590
Vacuum extraction, 583
Valgus deformity, 95–96, 101, 148, 178, 189, 204, 274–275,
    278, 293, 296, 298–300, 310, 320, 397, 403,
    407, 412, 416, 496, 498, 511, 533, 555, 727,
    786–790
Valgus, extension femoral osteotomy, 475
  femoral head deformity, 475
  mushroom deformity, 475
  proximal femoral deformity, 475
  rotational and sagittal correction, 475
Valgus feet, 274, 440, 445, 526
  management, 277
Van Nes rotationplasty, 393, 395
Varus–adduction feet, 320
Varus derotation osteotomy (VDRO), 279, 295, 317, 474
Varus–valgus fractures, *see* Extra-articular fractures of distal
    femur
Vascular thrombosis, 466
Vastus lateralis, 188, 252–253, 318, 455, 496, 504
Vertebral artery anomalies, 572
Vertebral compression fractures, 846
Visual observation of gait, 310

Volkmann's ischemic contracture, 126, 189, 383
Von Recklinghausen's disease, deformities, 632–634
    angular Scheuermann's kyphosis, 633
    cervical spine deformities, 633
    deformity kyphoscoliosis, 633
    degree of dystrophic bone change, 632
    neurofibromatosis (type NF-1), 632
    Recklinghausen's curve, 633
Vertical expandable prosthetic titanium rib procedure
    (VEPTR), 623

W
Waddling gait, 85, 89, 93, 116, 239, 246, 250, 252, 424
Wagner device, 415
Wagner technique, 413–415
Wainwright, A. M., 465–478
Wainwright system, 545
Wake-up test, 611, 618
Waldenström's chronological stages, 467
Walker CP surgery
    foot and ankle, 319–321
    hip, 318–319
    knee, 319
Wallerian degeneration, 373, 382
Wassel classification of thumb duplication, 351
Watanabe classification, 508
Watson–Jones' anterolateral approach, 761
Weight-bearing abduction braces, 473–474
    Hinge abduction, 474
    Petrie devise, 473
Werdnig–Hoffmann's disease, 256
Wernicke's and motor association areas, 232
Whiplash flexion injury, 588
Whiplash shaken infant syndrome, 825
Wiberg center–edge angle, 317
Wilson, D. J., 49–62
Wilson osteotomy, 535
Wilson quantified displacement, 484

Wilson's sign, 504
Wiltse-type fusion, 645
Windblown hand, 345–346
    See also Hand developmental anomalies
Windswept deformity, 31, 316
Witherow, Peter J., 701–707
Wnt signaling pathway and dorso-ventral development, 339
Woodward operations, 360
Wrist and hand fractures, 743
    basal fractures, 747
    carpal bone fractures, 745–746
    distal phalangeal fractures, 747–749
    distal physeal, 747
    distal radial epiphyseal fractures, 744–745
    distal radial fractures, 745–746
    distal radio-ulnar subluxation, 745
    distal ulnar physeal fractures, 745
    interphalangeal joint dislocations, 749
    metacarpal fractures
        diaphyseal, 746
    proximal (and middle) phalangeal fractures, 747
    scaphoid fractures, 746
Wrist flexion, 322
Writing dyspraxia, 235

X
X-Ray beam, 580

Y
Yount's procedure, 293

Z
Zellweger syndrome, 232
Z-Lengthening, 314
Zona orbicularis, 449
Zone of hypertrophic cartilage, 481–482
Zones of endochondral ossification, 640
"Z-or s-shaped" foot, 526

Index